Mosby's Canadian Textbook for the Support Worker

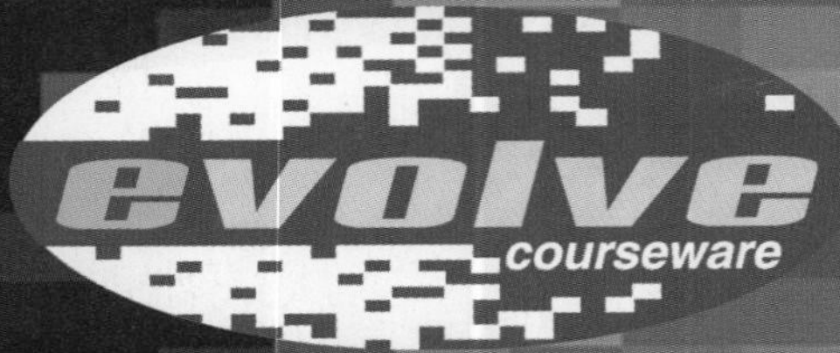

The Latest Evolution in Learning.

Evolve provides online access to free learning resources and activities designed specifically for the textbook you are using in your class. The resources will provide you with information that enhances the material covered in the book and much more.

Visit the Web address listed below to start your learning evolution today!

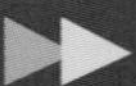 **LOGIN:** ***http://evolve.elsevier.com/Canada/Sorrentino/SupportWorker***

Evolve Online Courseware for Sorrentino: *Mosby's Canadian Textbook for the Support Worker* offers the following features:

- **Content Updates**
  New and updated information related to this textbook.
- **Additional Resources**
  Additional materials to enhance textbook content.
- **Links to Related Websites**
  Links to other sites related to content in this textbook.
- **Links to Related Products**
  See what else Elsevier Science has to offer in a specific field of interest.

Think outside the book . . . evolve.

Mosby's Canadian Textbook for the Support Worker

SHEILA A. SORRENTINO

RN, PhD

Curriculum and Health Care Consultant

Normal, Illinois

Canadian Consultants:

Judith Bowyer, BScN, MEd, The Bowyer Group Inc., Toronto, Ontario

Kathleen Kennedy, RN, BA, MPA (Health Policy Specialization), School of Health Sciences, St. Lawrence College, Kingston, Ontario

First Canadian Edition

With over 740 Illustrations

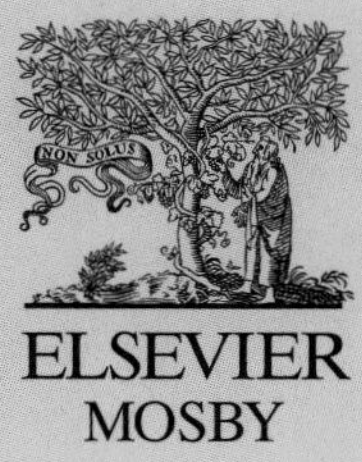

ELSEVIER
MOSBY

National Library of Canada Cataloguing in Publication

Sorrentino, Sheila A.
Mosby's Canadian textbook for the support worker / Sheila A. Sorrentino.

Adaptation of author's Mosby's textbook for nursing assistants, 5th ed.
Includes index.
ISBN-13: 978-0-920513-46-0
ISBN-10: 0-920513-46-8

1. Nurses' aides—Handbooks, manuals, etc. 2. Care of the sick—Textbooks.
I. Title. II. Title: Canadian textbook for the support worker.

RT84.S67 2003 610.73'06'98 C2003-903779-7

Acquisitions Editor: Ann Millar
Developmental Editor: Liz Radojkovic
Production Editor: Shefali Mehta
Production Coordinator: Kimberly Sullivan
Copy Editor: Jim Leahy
Proofreader: Eliza Marciniak
Permissions Editors: Karen Becker and Patricia Buckley
Cover Design: Rivet Art + Design
Typesetting and Assembly: Janette Thompson, Jansom
Beth Crane, Heidy Lawrance Associates
Printing and Binding: Courier

Elsevier Canada
905 King St. W., 4th Floor, Toronto, ON, Canada M6K 3G9
Phone: 1-866-896-3331
Fax: 1-866-359-9534

ISBN-13: 978-0-920513-46-0
ISBN-10: 0-920513-46-8

This book was printed in U.S.A.

4 5 07 06

To my parents

For all that they have done for me
and for so many others

Sheila A. Sorrentino

ABOUT THE AUTHOR

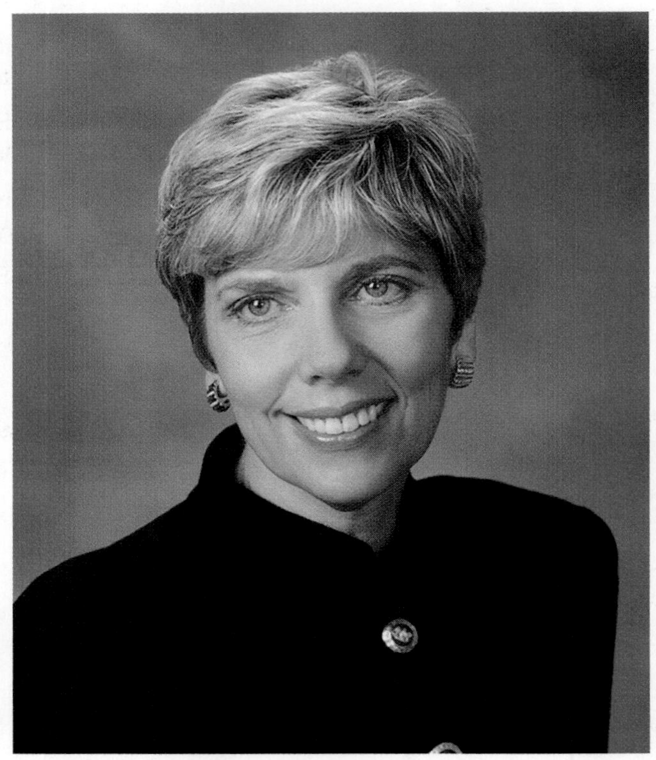

Sheila A. Sorrentino

Sheila A. Sorrentino is currently a curriculum and health care consultant focusing on career ladder nursing programs and effective delegation and partnering with assistive personnel in hospitals, long-term care centres, and home care agencies. She also teaches part-time at Bradley University in Peoria, Illinois.

Dr. Sorrentino was instrumental in the development and approval of CAN-PA-AND programs in the Illinois Community College System and has taught in nursing assistant, practical nursing, associate degree, and baccalaureate and higher degree programs. Her career includes experience as a nursing assistant, staff nurse, charge nurse, head nurse, nursing educator, assistant dean, dean, and consultant.

A Mosby author since 1982, Dr. Sorrentino has written several textbooks for nursing assistants and other assistive personnel. She was also involved in the development of *Mosby's Nursing Assistant Skills Video* and *Mosby's Nursing Skills Videos*. An earlier version of the nursing assistant skills video won the 1992 International Medical Films Award on caregiving.

Dr. Sorrentino has a bachelor of science degree in nursing, a master of arts in education, a master of science degree in community nursing, and a PhD in higher education administration. She is a member of Sigma Theta Tau and a former member and chair of the Central Illinois Higher Education Health Care Task Force. She also served on the Iowa-Illinois Safety Council Board of Directors and the Board of Directors of Our Lady of Victory Nursing Center in Bourbonnais, Illinois. In 1998 she received an alumni achievement award from Lewis University for outstanding leadership and dedication in nursing education. Her presentations at national conferences focus on delegation and other issues relating to assistive personnel.

REVIEWERS

CANADIAN REVIEWERS

The following individuals provided feedback at various stages during the development process:

Mary Boivin, Cambrian College, Sudbury, Ontario

Judith Bowyer, The Bowyer Group, Inc., Toronto, Ontario

Mary Cammaert, Fanshawe College, London, Ontario

Dr. Margaret Crossley, University of Saskatchewan, Saskatoon, Saskatchewan

Marilyn Evans, Brock University, St. Catharines, Ontario

Rosemary Goodacre, Fleming College, Peterborough, Ontario

Nancy Hacking, Conestoga College, Kitchener, Ontario

Sandra Hanna, Mohawk-McMaster Institute for Applied Health Sciences, Hamilton, Ontario

Kelly Kay, Registered Practical Nurses Association of Ontario

Kathleen Kennedy, St. Lawrence College, Kingston, Ontario

Kathy King, Canadore College, North Bay, Ontario

Lori Pollard, Nightingale Academy of Health Services, Edmonton, Alberta

Judy Rantala, Northern College, Timmins, Ontario

Ann Robinson, Academy of Learning, Hamilton, Ontario

Dr. Stephen Sanche, University of Saskatchewan, Saskatoon, Saskatchewan

Maureen Wishart, Durham College, Oshawa, Ontario

Kevin Woo, Mount Sinai Hospital, Toronto, Ontario

OTHER REVIEWERS

Elizabeth Burns, Bonell Good Samaritan Center, Greeley, Colorado

Judy Kramer, San Clemente, California

Susan Lewsen, Utah Health Technology Certification Center, Kaysville, Utah

Rebecca Rastkar, University of Missouri Hospital and Clinics, Columbia, Missouri

Zee Sala, Bonell Good Samaritan Center, Greeley, Colorado

Ginny Scribner, Staff Development Resource, Seattle, Washington

Dorothy Witmer, Healthcare Education and Training, Boise, Idaho

ACKNOWLEDGEMENTS

Textbooks are written and published by the combined efforts of many people. The planning, manuscript development, review, design, and production processes involve the ideas, talents, and contributions of many individuals.

Elsevier Canada is especially grateful to Gail Acton and Jan Chamberlain for suggesting the need for a textbook for the Canadian student. Their vast experience in this field, from developing original material for the Personal Support Worker (PSW) program to promoting and furthering the role of support work as a whole, has been of great benefit in the development of *Mosby's Canadian Textbook for the Support Worker*. Thank you Gail and Jan for your contributions to the project.

Elsevier Canada is also grateful to Judith Bowyer and Kathleen Kennedy for consulting on the project from the idea stage through early sample chapters to final manuscript stage. They spent countless hours poring over the manuscript and providing insight about support work. Their valuable feedback has improved the text immeasurably.

The publisher would also like to thank the staff at the following organizations for their assistance and information.

- Sylvia Acton, Colette Guzik, and Mary Humen, Nightingale Nursing, Saskatoon, Saskatchewan
- Debbie Briere, The Heart and Stroke Foundation of Saskatchewan
- Margo Collver and Magdalen Carter, McCormick Home, London, Ontario
- Sandy McIvor, Winnipeg Deer Creek Lodge
- Melanie Rathgeber, Saskatoon District Health
- Linda Third, Toronto General Hospital
- Sandra Wilson and staff at the HCHSA, Health Care, Health and Safety Association of Ontario

The publisher also wishes to thank Mary Dykes, Heather McWhinney, Ted Patterson, Liz Radojkovic, Joanne Sanche, and Blanche Star for their contributions to the research and development of this textbook.

CREDITS

PHOTO CREDITS

4 (t) Dick Hemingway, 16 Courtesy Victorian Order of Nurses, 19 (l) Tom Stewart/Corbis/Magma, 19 (r) © Tony Freeman/Photo Edit, 24 Keith Brofsky/Photodisc/Getty Images, 27 (b) Dick Hemingway, 28 (t) Al Harvey, 28 (b) Penny Tweedie/Stone/Getty Images, 44 Patricia Barry Levy/Maxx Images, 47 Royalty Free/Corbis/Magma, 52 From Maslow, Abraham H., *Motivation and Personality, 3rd ed.* © 1954, 1987. ©1970 by Abraham H. Maslow. Reprinted by permission of Pearson Education, Inc, Upper Saddle River, NJ., 56 Al Harvey, 57 ©Frank Siteman/Rainbow, 64 From Birchenall, J. & Streight, E. (1997). *Mosby's Textbook for the Home Care Aide.* St. Louis: Mosby. p. 4., 73 Courtesy Credit Valley Hospital, 80 Chris Lowe/Index Stock Imagery/Maxx Images, 84 ©Frank Siteman/Rainbow, 108 (t) Dick Hemingway, Kevin Peterson/Photodisc/Getty Images, Dick Hemingway, Dick Hemingway, Royalty Free/Getty Images, (b) Dick Hemingway, 109 Tom & Dee Ann McCarthy/Corbis/Magma, 110 (t) Dick Hemingway, 110 (b) Leland Bobbé/Magma/Corbis, 174 (t) Courtesy J.T. Posey Co., Arcadia, CA, 174 (b) Courtesy J.T. Posey Co., Arcadia, CA, 187 (t) Courtesy J.T. Posey Co., Arcadia, CA, 187 (b) Courtesy J.T. Posey Co., Arcadia, CA, 189 (t) Courtesy Electromark Company, 189 (b) Adapted from the Canadian Centre for Occupational Health and Safety, http://ccohs.ca/oshanswers/legisl/msds_lab.html. Retrieved January 2003, 196 (t) Courtesy J.T. Posey Co., Arcadia, CA, 196 (c) Courtesy J.T. Posey Co., Arcadia, CA, 196 (b) Courtesy J.T. Posey Co., Arcadia, CA, 200 (tr) Courtesy J.T. Posey Co., Arcadia, CA, 201 (tl) Courtesy J.T. Posey Co., Arcadia, CA, 201 (bl) Courtesy J.T. Posey Co., Arcadia, CA, 201 (br) Courtesy J.T. Posey Co., Arcadia, CA, 202 (t) Courtesy J.T. Posey Co., Arcadia, CA, 202 (b) Courtesy J.T. Posey Co, Arcadia, CA, 203 (b) Courtesy J.T. Posey Co, Arcadia, CA, 205 Courtesy J.T. Posey Co. Arcadia, CA, 214 *practices and additional precautions for preventing the transmission of infection in health care*, Health Canada, (1999) ©. Reproduced with the permission of the Minister of Public Works and Government Services Canada, 2003, 215 Lester V. Bergman/Corbis/Magma, 287 Courtesy J.T. Posey Co., Arcadia, CA, 288 Courtesy J.T. Posey Co., Arcadia, CA, 311 (l) Courtesy J.T. Posey Co., Arcadia, 311 (r) Courtesy J.T. Posey Co., Arcadia, 366 *Canada's Food Guide to Healthy Eating, 1997*, Health Canada ©. Reproduced with the permission of the Minister of Public Works and Government Services Canada, 2003, 368 *Canada's Food Guide to Healthy Eating, 1997*, Health Canada ©. Reproduced with the permission of the Minister of Public Works and Government Services Canada, 2003, 369 The Nutrition Facts Label www.hc-sc.gc.ca/english/media/releases/2003/2003, Health Canada (2003) ©. Reproduced with the permission of the Minister of Public Works and Government Services Canada, 2003, 372 Courtesy Sammons Preston Rolyan, Bolingbrook IL, 440 (l) Courtesy DeRoyal 544, (l) Courtesy Motion Control, Subsidiary of Filauer, Salt Lake City, Utah, 558 Courtesy Northcoast Medical, Ind., Morgan Hill, CA, 558 Courtesy Northcoast Medical, Ind., Morgan Hill, CA, 558 Courtesy Sammons Preston Rolyan, Bolingbrook, IL, 559 Courtesy Northcoast Medical Inc., Mogan Hill, CA, 559 Courtesy Sammons Preston Rolyan, Bolingbrook, IL, 590 Courtesy Mayer-Johnson Inc., Solana Beach, CA, 596 Courtesy Siemen Hearing Instruments Inc., Piscataway, NJ, 613 Joe Wong, 628 © Robin Sachs/Photo Edit, 630 Hattie Young/Science Photo Library/Publiphoto, 660 Dick Hemingway, 687 Source: Courtesy of M. Morison, *A Colour Guide to Nursing Management of Wounds* (London: Wolfe Medical Polishers, 1992), 752 Courtesy Credit Valley Hospital, 777 Courtesy American Heart Association, 786 Courtesy American Heart Association

TEXT CREDITS

17 Helen Heeney (Ed.) (1995). *Life before medicare: Canadian experiences.* Toronto: The Stories Project, ix. Reprinted with permission from Ontario Society (Coalition) of Senior Citizen's Organizations, 48 Based on *Guidelines for Working with Unregulated Care Providers: For Registered Nurses and Registered Practical Nurses in Ontario.* Reprinted with the permission of the College of Nurses of Ontario. 1999, 112 Adapted from The College of Nurses of Ontario, 1999. *Guide to nurses for providing culturally sensitive care.* Ottawa: CNO. p. 11. Reprinted by permission of the College of Nurses of Ontario.

INSTRUCTOR PREFACE

Mosby's Canadian Textbook for the Support Worker is intended to prepare students to function in the role of support worker in community and facility settings across Canada. The text is an adaptation of *Mosby's Textbook for Nursing Assistants*, Fifth Edition, which has been thoroughly revised to reflect the needs of Canadian instructors and students. Although the term *support worker* is used to describe a worker who provides personal care and support, the text addresses programs for nursing attendants, continuing care attendants, home care aides, and other programs across Canada. Like its predecessor, this textbook serves the needs of students and instructors in educational programs taught in community colleges, secondary schools, and other facilities. It is also a resource for support workers already working in facilities or community settings.

Guiding Principles

This textbook is structured around several key ideas and principles:

- *Canadian support workers need to know about Canadian issues.* New chapters address health care in Canada. These include Chapter 2 (The Canadian Health Care System), Chapter 3 (Workplace Settings), and Chapter 10 (Legislation: The Client's Rights and Your Rights). Canadian content appears in other chapters where applicable.
- *Support workers provide services in a variety of community and facility settings.* Because training programs prepare students for a variety of workplaces, multiple workplace settings are discussed throughout the text. Topics are addressed in the context of long-term care, home care, and hospital settings. Focus on Home Care and Focus on Long-Term Care boxes are integrated throughout the text. They highlight information and insights about these settings. The procedures have been written so that they address both facility and community settings.
- *Each client is an individual with dignity and value.* Students are taught that each client is a whole person, with physical, emotional, social, intellectual, and spiritual dimensions. Students are encouraged to appreciate the client as a unique individual with a past, a present, and a future. Students are also taught to recognize a client's basic needs and protected rights. Both the terms *client* and *person* are used when discussing the client. The term *person* is used to remind students that all clients are people first and clients second.
- *An essential part of a support worker's job is to provide compassionate care.* The acronym DIPPS is used to represent the five priorities of support work: recognizing and promoting the client's dignity, independence, preferences, privacy, and safety. These priorities are addressed throughout the text and are highlighted in Providing Compassionate Care boxes. The boxes discuss how to promote the priorities of support work when giving the care described in the chapter.
- *Effective communication skills are necessary to develop good working relationships.* Chapter 12 is devoted to communication skills, and Chapter 35 discusses communication with clients who have speech and language disorders. Case studies and other boxes throughout the text also highlight the importance of communication.
- *Support workers must respect cultural diversity among their clients.* Culture influences people's attitudes and beliefs. Chapter 11 discusses the role of cultural heritage in health and illness practices as well as in other aspects of life, such as communication. Respecting Diversity boxes serve to provide examples of how culture may influence people.
- *Support workers need to understand their scope of practice and the delegation process.* Because agencies and facilities across the country vary in their use of support workers, the responsibilities and limitations of support workers are emphasized throughout the text. The text presents many procedures that support workers across the country need to know. However, some procedures require extra training and supervision. Students are told they must understand and respect their employer's policies as well as provincial or territorial laws governing scope of practice. Chapter 5 addresses scope of practice and delegation issues, Chapter 9 focuses on ethical principles, and Chapter 10 addresses specific legislation that affects support workers in Canada.
- *Providing safe care is at the core of support work.* Providing for the client's safety is a priority of support work and is emphasized throughout the text. Chapter 16 discusses the major types of accidental injuries among clients and how to prevent them. It also discusses how support workers can provide for their own personal safety while on the job. Chapter 17 discusses the safe use of restraints. Chapter 18

discusses how to prevent the spread of infection. Chapter 19 discusses how to recognize and report abuse. Chapter 21 describes the basic principles of body mechanics and how to be safe when moving and transferring clients.

- *Following the client's care plan is critical to providing good care.* Chapter 7 describes the care planning process in both facilities and communities. Students are reminded throughout the text to follow the care plan and their supervisor's directions.
- *Students learn best by reading about real-to-life examples.* Case studies and examples that apply concepts to the real world of support work appear throughout the text. Support Workers Solving Problems boxes discuss how support workers solve problems that may occur in the workplace.

Pedagogical Features and Design

Mosby's Textbook for Nursing Assistants is known for its attractive, four-colour, user-friendly design. Every effort has gone into retaining these features in the Canadian edition. Several features and design elements from previous editions were retained and new ones added to enhance the learning process (see Student Preface, page xiii).

- *Objectives*—explain what is presented in the chapter and what students will learn
- *Illustrations*—the book contains more than 740 full-colour photographs and line art.
- *Key terms with definitions*—appear at the beginning of each chapter. These terms also appear in bold print within the body of the chapter where their definitions are placed in the context of the subject discussed. Terms and definitions appear again in the glossary. Some terms appear in more than one chapter for emphasis. Other important terms appear in italics.
- *Boxes and tables*—are used to list principles, guidelines, signs and symptoms, care measures, and other information.
- *Focus on Children boxes*—provide age-specific information about the needs, considerations, and special circumstances of children.
- *Focus on Older Adults boxes*—provide age-specific information about the needs, considerations, and special circumstances of older adults.
- *Focus on Home Care boxes*—highlight information necessary for safe functioning in the home setting.
- *Focus on Long-Term Care boxes*—highlight information unique to the long-term care setting.
- *Providing Compassionate Care boxes*—remind students of the priorities of support work: respecting and promoting their client's dignity, independence, preferences, privacy, and safety. The acronym DIPPS is used to summarize these five priorities.
- *Support Workers Solving Problems boxes*—present scenarios depicting situations and problems that support workers may face on a typical day. The boxes discuss how these support workers make decisions and solve problems.
- *Respecting Diversity boxes*—help students learn to appreciate the importance of cultural diversity and how culture influences health and illness practices.
- *Case Study boxes*—apply some of the concepts discussed in the text to real-to-life examples of support workers and clients.
- *Icons*—in section headings alert the reader to an associated procedure. Procedure boxes contain the same icon.
- *Procedure boxes*—are divided into pre-procedure, procedure, and post-procedure sections. Colour gradients differentiate the sections. A *Compassionate Care* section in the procedure boxes is a reminder of the priorities of support work. Asterisks are used to delineate steps that are usually not applicable in community settings.
- *Review questions*—are found at the end of each chapter. A page number for the answer section is given.

The editorial staff at Elsevier Canada hopes that this text will serve you and your students well. Our intent is to provide you and your students with the information needed to teach and learn safe and effective care during this time of dynamic change in Canadian health care.

STUDENT PREFACE

This book was designed for you. It was designed to help you learn. The book will be a useful resource as you gain experience and expand your knowledge.

This preface presents some study guidelines and helps you use the book. Your instructor will probably assign chapters or partial chapters from the textbook for you to read before or after class. When given a reading assignment, do you read from the first page to the last page without stopping? How much do you remember? You will learn more if you use a study system. A useful study system has these steps:

- Survey or preview
- Question
- Read and record
- Recite and review

Preview

Before you start a reading assignment, preview or survey the assignment. This gives you an idea of what the assignment covers. It also helps you recall what you already know about the subject. Carefully look over the assignment. Preview the chapter title, headings, subheadings, and terms or ideas in bold print or italics. Also survey the objectives, key terms, introductory paragraph, boxes, and the review questions at the end of the chapter. Previewing takes only a few minutes. Remember, previewing helps you become familiar with the material.

Question

After previewing, you need to form questions to answer while you read. Questions should relate to what might be asked on a test or how the information applies to giving care. Use the title, headings, and subheadings to form questions. Avoid questions that have one-word answers. Questions that begin with what, how, or why are helpful. While reading, you may find that a question does not help you study. If so, just change the question. Remember, questioning sets a purpose for reading. So changing a question only makes this step more useful.

Read and Record

Reading is the next step. Reading is more productive after determining what you already know and what you need to learn. Read to find answers to your questions. The purpose of reading is to:

- Gain new information
- Connect the new information to what you know already

Break the assignment into smaller parts. Then answer your questions as you read each part. Also, mark important information by underlining, highlighting, or making notes. Underlining and highlighting remind you what you need to learn. You need to go back and review the marked parts later. Making notes helps you remember what you learn. When making notes, write down important information in the text margins or in a notebook. Use words and summary statements that will jog your memory about the material.

After reading the assignment, you must remember the information. To accomplish this, you must work with the information. This step involves organizing information into a study guide. Study guides take many forms. Diagrams or charts help show relationships or steps in a process. Much of the information in this text is organized in this manner to help you learn. Note taking in outline format is also very useful. The following is a sample outline:

I. Main heading
   a. Second level
   b. Second level
      1. Third level
      2. Third level
II. Main heading

Recite and Review

Finally, recite and review. Use your notes and the study guides. Answer the questions you formed earlier. Also answer any other questions that came up during the reading and as you answered the review questions at the end of the chapter. Answer all questions out loud (recite). If you are unsure about the answers to any of the questions, ask your instructor.

Reviewing is more about *when* to study than *what* to study. You already decided what to study during the preview, question, and reading steps. Your instructor may have emphasized key points from the reading assignment in class. The best times to review both information in your text and your notes from class are the same day or evening of the class, right after your first study session, one week later, and regularly before a quiz or test, midterm, or final exam. Studying the information many times will help you remember it.

You and support work are important. You and the care you give may be the bright spots in a client's day. This book was designed to help you to learn and study. Special design features are described on the next pages.

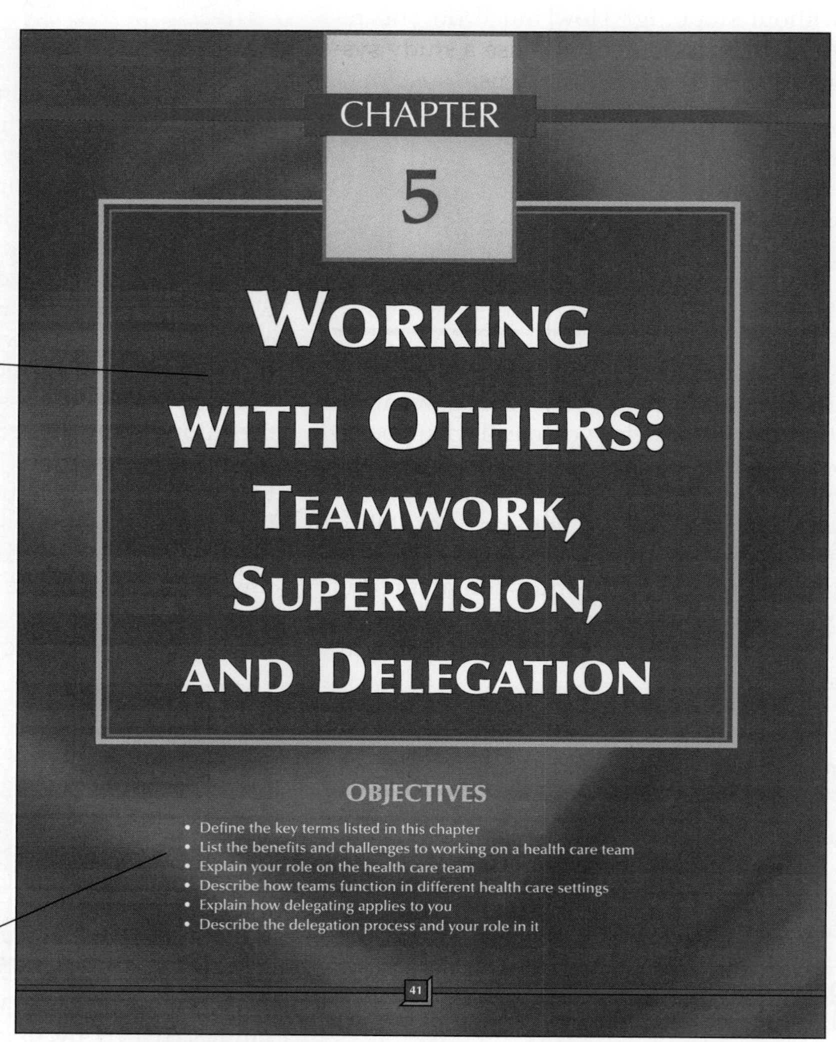

CHAPTER
5
WORKING WITH OTHERS: TEAMWORK, SUPERVISION, AND DELEGATION
OBJECTIVES
• Define the key terms listed in this chapter
• List the benefits and challenges to working on a health care team
• Explain your role on the health care team
• Describe how teams function in different health care settings
• Explain how delegating applies to you
• Describe the delegation process and your role in it
41

Chapter titles and subtitles tell you the subject of the chapter.

Objectives tell you what is presented in the chapter and what you will learn. As a final review of the chapter, see if you have learned the information contained in the objectives.

Key terms are important words and phrases in the chapter. Definitions are given for each term. The key terms introduce you to the chapter content. They are also useful study guides.

KEY TERMS

accountable Being responsible for the outcome; involves answering questions and explaining actions

assigning Giving responsibility for providing care

authority The legal right to do something

case manager A person who assesses, monitors, and evaluates a client's needs in a community care setting; also coordinates team services

delegation A process by which an RN authorizes another health care provider to perform certain tasks; transfer of function

family conference A meeting attended by the health care team and family members to discuss a client's care

multidisciplinary team A team of health care providers from a variety of backgrounds and specialties who work together to meet the client's needs

task A function, procedure, or activity that you assist with or perform for the client

transfer of function Delegation

This chapter discusses the health care team and your role on the team. It also discusses the relationship between you and your supervisor. All health care workers must protect their clients from harm. Understanding the delegation process will help you protect clients and prevent potential legal problems.

The Health Care Team

In most health care settings, you work on a team. A team is a group of people who work together toward a common goal (see Chapter 1). The goal of a health care team is to provide the client with the best possible care and support. When providing care, team members must consider the whole person. You must promote health in all five dimensions of the person's life: physical, emotional, social, intellectual, and spiritual (see Chapter 4). Health care team members depend on each other to perform their roles to the best of their ability. Members of effective teams support one another and communicate effectively.

Members of health care teams vary from setting to setting and from team to team. The client's needs determine who will be on the team. For example, Tom Brown, 15, has mental health problems. Tom, his parents, an RN, psychiatrist, social worker, and support worker work together as a team. Tom's team is different from Mrs. Darby's team. Mrs. Darby, 86, is recovering from hip surgery. She a
team with an RN, social wo
and support workers. The cli
of the team unless he or she i
being involved or chooses no

In some situations, you a
only health care providers on

may be part of a multidisciplinary team. A **multidisciplinary team** includes health care providers from a variety of backgrounds and specialties who work together to meet the client's needs.

Benefits of Working on a Team

There are many benefits to the team approach to health care. A group of people is often better at making decisions and solving problems than one person. The many benefits of a team approach to care include:

- *Opportunities for collaboration.* All team members are encouraged to *collaborate* (to work together toward a common goal). Successful collaboration creates a positive atmosphere that even the client can sense. Staff and clients benefit when team members share information. For example, you find a way to ease a client's discomfort during a bed bath. You share this information with the nurse. The nurse asks other support workers to use your method.
- *Opportunities for communication.* Team meetings provide the opportunity for all team members to share experiences, opinions, and ideas. Without the meetings, valuable ideas might be missed. Box 5-1 contains part of a dialogue from a team meeting. Notice how each team member adds to the complete picture of the client's health.
- *A wide array of abilities, skills, and perspectives.* Team

Terms in bold present the key terms and definitions within the body of the chapter. You again see the key term and its definition. This helps reinforce learning. The key terms are also defined in the glossary starting on page 831. If you come across a term again in a later chapter, you can check the definition in the glossary.

Terms in *italics* present other important terms and information. Pay special attention to these words as you read.

666 Chapter 40 Measuring Height, Weight, and Vital Signs

Taking a Radial Pulse

The radial pulse is used for routine vital signs. Place the first 2 or 3 fingers of one hand against the radial artery. The radial artery is on the thumb side of the wrist (Figure 40-17). Do not use your thumb to take a pulse. The thumb has a pulse. You could mistake the pulse in your thumb for the client's pulse.

You need a good watch or clock with a second hand. Count the pulse for 30 seconds. Then multiply the number by 2. This gives the number of beats per minute. If the pulse is irregular, count it for 1 minute.

Some employers require that all radial pulses be taken for 1 minute. Follow your employer's policy.

Report and record the following after taking a radial pulse:

- The pulse rate
- A pulse rate less than 60 or more than 100 beats per minute (report this at once)
- A pulse rate that is higher or lower than normal for the client (report this at once)
- If the pulse is regular or irregular
- The pulse force—strong, full, bounding, weak, thready, or feeble

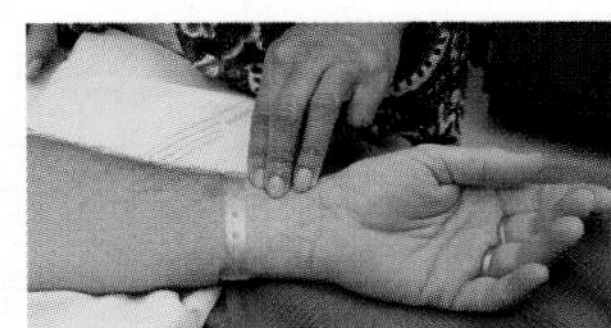

Figure 40-17 Use the middle 2 or 3 fingers to take the radial pulse.

Icons in the headings alert you to an associated procedure. Procedure boxes contain the same icon.

Procedures are written in a step-by-step format. Some procedures are divided into pre-procedure, procedure, and post-procedure sections for easy studying. Those steps that do not apply in community settings are highlighted with an asterisk.

Compassionate Care in the procedure boxes reminds you of the priorities of support work: providing for the client's dignity, independence, preferences, privacy, and safety.

Taking a Radial Pulse

Compassionate Care

Remember to Promote:
- Dignity
- Independence
- Preferences
- Privacy
- Safety

Pre-Procedure

1 Identify the person according to employer policy.
2 Explain the procedure to the person.
3 Wash your hands.
4 Provide for privacy.

Procedure

5 Have the person sit or lie down.
6 Locate the radial pulse. Use your first 2 or 3 middle fingers (see Figure 40-17).
7 Note if the pulse is strong or weak, and regular or irregular.
8 Count the pulse for 30 seconds. Multiply the number of beats by 2. Or count the pulse for 1 minute if required by employer policy.
9 Count the pulse for 1 minute if it is irregular.
10 Record the person's name and pulse on your notepad or assignment sheet. Note the strength of the pulse. Note if it was regular or irregular.

Post-Procedure

11 Provide for safety and comfort.
12 Place the call bell within reach.*
13 Remove privacy measures.
14 Wash your hands.
15 Report and record the pulse rate and your observations according to employer policy.

*Steps marked with an asterisk may not apply in community settings.

- *Attention.* The more a person thinks about the pain, the worse it can seem. Sometimes pain is so severe that it is all a person thinks about. However, even mild pain can seem worse if a person dwells on it. Pain often seems worse at night when there are no distractions.
- *The meaning of pain.* Pain means different things to different people. Some see it as a sign of serious weakness. It also may mean a serious illness. Some people ignore or deny their pain. Sometimes pain is used to avoid certain people or things. Others use pain to get attention.
- *Support from others.* Pain is easier to deal with when family and friends offer comfort and support. The presence of a friend or loved one can be very comforting. People who do not have caring family and friends must deal with pain alone. Being alone can increase fear, anxiety, and suffering. Be especially sensitive to clients who are suffering alone.
- *Culture.* Culture affects how a person responds to pain (see *Respecting Diversity: Pain Reactions* box). In some cultures, people in pain show no reaction. In other cultures, people in pain have strong verbal and nonverbal reactions.
- *Age.* See *Focus on Children: Pain Reactions* and *Focus on Older Adults: Pain Reactions* boxes.

Signs and Symptoms of Pain. Your client may tell you about pain. Or, body language and behaviour may reveal the person is in pain. For example, Ms. Raj grimaces when she moves, but denies having pain. Report any information and observations about pain to your supervisor. Always use the client's exact words when you report and record. Report the following:

- *Location.* Where is the pain? Ask the client to point to the area of pain (Figure 20-9). Remember, pain can radiate. Ask the person if the pain is anywhere else and to point to those areas.
- *Onset and duration.* When did the pain start? How long has the pain lasted?
- *Intensity.* Does the client complain of mild, moderate, or severe pain? Ask the person to rate the pain on a scale of 1 to 10, with 10 being the most severe.
- *Description.* Ask the client to describe the pain. Box 20-1 lists some words used to describe pain. Write down what the person says. Use the person's exact words.
- *Factors causing pain.* Factors causing pain may include moving or turning in bed, coughing or deep breathing, and exercise. Ask what the client was doing before the pain started and when it started.

Respecting Diversity

Pain Reactions

In the Philippines, pain is viewed as the will of God. It is thought that God will give people the strength to bear the pain. In Vietnam, pain relief may not be requested until the pain becomes severe. The people of India accept pain quietly and will accept some relief measures. In China, showing emotion is seen as a weakness of character. Therefore, pain is often suppressed. Pain relief measures must be offered more than once before they are accepted. The people of China find it impolite to accept something the first time it is offered.

Remember, individuals may not follow every belief and practice of their culture and religion. Each person is unique. Do not judge the person by your own standards.

Source: Adapted from E.M. Geissler, *Pocket Guide to Cultural Assessment*, 2nd ed. (St. Louis: Mosby, 1998).

Focus on Children

Pain Reactions

Many children do not understand pain. They have few experiences with pain. They do not know what to expect or how to deal with pain. They must rely on adults for help.

Adults do not always know when children are in pain. Toddlers and preschool children may not know words that express pain. Crying and fussing infants and toddlers can mean many different problems, not just pain. Adults must be alert for behaviours and situations that signal pain.

Focus on Older Adults

Pain Reactions

Older adults may have decreased pain sensations. They may not feel pain, or it may not feel severe. This places them at greater risk for undetected disease or injury. Pain alerts a person to illness or injury. If pain is not felt, the person may not seek health care.

Some older adults have many health problems that cause pain. They may think a new pain is related to an existing health problem. Chronic pain may mask the new pain. They may deny or ignore pain because of what it might mean.

Some older adults have disorders that affect thinking and reasoning. Some cannot communicate verbally. Changes in behaviour may indicate pain. Report changes in clients' behaviour to your supervisor.

Focus on Children boxes provide information about the needs, considerations, and general circumstances of children.

Focus on Older Adults boxes provide information about the needs, considerations, and special circumstances of older adults.

Respecting Diversity boxes contain information to help you learn about the various practices of different cultures.

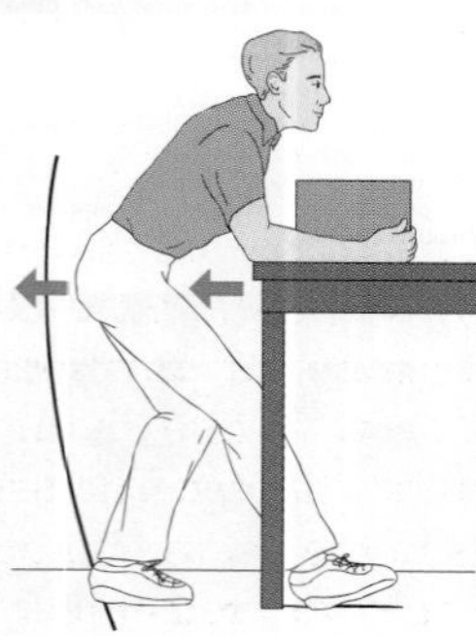

Figure 21-3 Move your rear leg back when pulling an item.

Lifting and Moving Clients in Bed

Many clients can move and turn in bed themselves. Others need help. They cannot move independently, but they can work with you to move. Some clients are unable to move at all. They may be unconscious, paralyzed, or very weak. They cannot help when others move them. Assistive devices may be necessary. For example, a lifting or turning sheet may be used (see page 274). Or a mechanical lift may be required (see page 299). Sometimes two or three people are needed to move the client.

Check with the care plan, your supervisor, and the client to find out if the client can help with moving. Also check if you can safely move the client on your own. Do not attempt a move by yourself if you think you may not be able to do so safely. You must consider the client's safety and your own safety. (See *Focus on Long-Term Care: Lifting and Moving Safety Precautions* and *Focus on Home Care: Getting Help with Lifting and Moving* boxes.)

Focus on Long-Term Care

Lifting and Moving Safety Precautions

In many long-term care facilities, residents have signs in their rooms that say how much assistance is needed to move. The signs state whether the person requires:
- No assistance
- One-person lift
- Two or more people to lift
- Mechanical lift

Comfort and Safety Measures

The client's skin must be protected during lifting and moving. Friction and shearing injure the skin. Both cause infection and pressure ulcers (see Chapter 41). **Friction** is the rubbing of one surface against another. When a person is moved in bed, skin rubs against the sheet. **Shearing** occurs when the skin sticks to a surface and muscles slide in the direction the body is moving (Figure 21-4). Shearing can happen when a person slides down in bed or is moved in bed.

Reduce friction and shearing by rolling or lifting the client. A cotton drawsheet (see Chapter 24) serves as a *lift sheet* (*turning* or *pull sheet*) to move the client in bed and reduce friction (see page 274). Some employ-

Focus on Home Care

Getting Help with Lifting and Moving

You usually will not have a co-worker to help you lift and move home care clients. Plan ahead with your supervisor. Some clients have mechanical lifting devices in their home. Sometimes the primary caregiver or another person in the home helps you lift and move the client.

A nurse or physiotherapist teaches the client's family or primary caregiver about body mechanics and moving, positioning, and transferring the client. You and the family member can then work together. Make sure anyone who helps you has received training.

Focus on Long-Term Care boxes highlight information unique to the long-term care setting.

Focus on Home Care boxes highlight information necessary for safe functioning in the home setting.

Support Workers Solving Problems boxes present scenarios depicting situations and problems that support workers may face on a typical day. The boxes discuss how these support workers make decisions and solve problems. Put yourself in the same situation. What would you do?

Bulleted lists present information in a way that is easy to study and remember.

Boxes and tables contain principles, guidelines, signs and symptoms, care measures, and other information. Many boxes and tables present information in a list format. They are useful study guides for reviewing.

Mosby's Canadian Textbook for the Support Worker Chapter 8 83

Support Workers Solving Problems

DAILY PLANNING

Scenario: Chona is a support worker in a long-term care facility. Before her morning shift begins, she reviews her assignment sheet and the care plans for each of the residents she supports. The care plan notes that Mrs. Paget, a new resident, requires assistance in making decisions for herself. The care plan identifies that all care providers should help Mrs. Paget make decisions by providing choices.

Discussion: Chona considers the choices that she could provide for Mrs. Paget. She decides that she can offer Mrs. Paget two sets of clothes to wear for the day, two different items for breakfast, and she can ask Mrs. Paget whether she would like to participate in the morning or afternoon exercise session. Because she has planned for these choices in advance, Chona is able to concentrate all of her attention on Mrs. Paget during care tasks.

(the night before or just before your shift), you will not have to use valuable time with clients to schedule tasks. This does not mean you should never change a schedule. You must stay flexible and responsive.

Use your planning and scheduling time to think about problems that might arise. Review the tasks on your list. Plan how much time each task will take. To improve scheduling, ask yourself these questions:

- What are the client's needs and priorities?
- How much time will each task or activity require?
- When will I do each task or activity?
- Can I organize my time so that some of the tasks overlap?
- Have I allowed time for the unexpected?
- Is there anyone with whom I should coordinate these activities?

Give each task a time limit. This helps you to stay focused and complete a task in good time. See Box 8-5 for ways to manage your time and stay organized. At the end of your workday, compare what you planned to do with what you actually did. Did you accomplish what you planned? If not, review the reasons. Did problems arise? Were there interruptions? Was scheduling poor?

DECISION MAKING

Support workers make many decisions every day. You make decisions when you organize your time, when you make a schedule, and when you provide care for a client. For example, you decide

- The order in which you are going to carry out tasks
- The equipment and supplies you need for each task
- The amount of time to spend with a client
- When a problem or an observation needs to be reported immediately
- If you need help to complete a task
- If you need to consult with your supervisor
- If you will accept or refuse a delegated task

SKILLS YOU NEED TO MAKE DECISIONS

Do you know people who always seem to make the right decision? They are usually decisive and calm. The following skills will help with decision making:

- *Focus*—Focus requires concentration, involvement, and commitment. Focus on the client and the task to make the right decisions. This involves asking questions and active listening (Figure 8-2 on page 84).
- *Flexibility*—You need to be flexible and responsive. Involve clients in decisions that affect them. Be ready to adapt in response to a client's needs. Remember, each client is an individual with unique needs. Age, culture, and health affect the person's needs. For example, Mr. Johnston, 91, lives in a facility

Box 8-5 Tips to Save Time and Stay Organized

- Follow the assignment sheet and the care plan.
- Remember the client's needs and priorities.
- Know what your supervisor expects you to do and when.
- Know what tasks need to be done at a certain time.
- Set yourself time limits; work within those limits, unless a client's needs are more pressing.
- Develop routines that work for you and the client.
- Allow for more time than you need, when possible.
- Remain flexible at all times.
- Start with the tasks that must get done.
- Remind yourself not to get sidetracked by unessential things.
- Learn to say no—firmly, positively, and tactfully.
- Use a calendar for important dates and reminders.
- Make sure that you have equipment and supplies before you start a task.
- Put equipment and supplies back in their proper place.

462 Chapter 28 Grooming and Dressing

COMPASSIONATE CARE

When helping with grooming and dressing, remember to focus on the whole person rather than only on the task. Promote the person's dignity, independence, preferences, privacy, and safety (see *Providing Compassionate Care Assisting Clients with Grooming and Dressing* box).

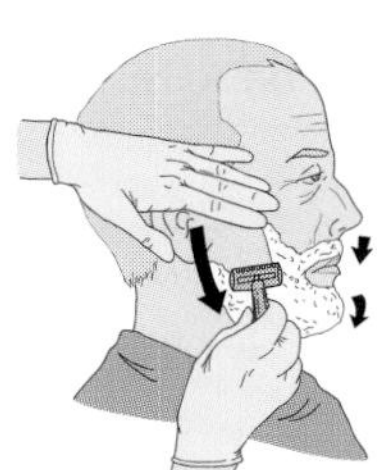

Figure 28-5 Shave in the direction of hair growth. Use longer strokes on the larger areas of the face. Use short strokes around the chin and lips.

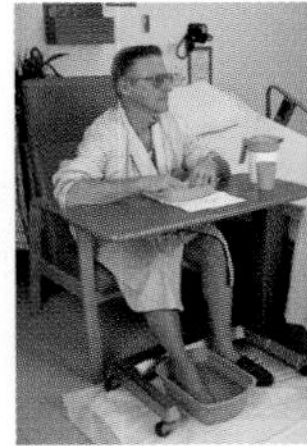

Figure 28-6 Nail and foot care. The feet soak in a foot basin, and the fingers soak in a kidney basin.

Providing Compassionate Care

ASSISTING CLIENTS WITH GROOMING AND DRESSING

Dignity. Being clean and well-groomed helps the person maintain dignity. People often feel good about themselves when they have a neat appearance and clean clothing. When assisting with grooming, carefully handle the person's hygiene products, shaver, hair dryer, brush and comb, perfumes, and other personal care items. Clothing also needs your attention. Do not break zippers, tear clothing, lose buttons, or cause other damage. Treat the person's property with care and respect. If damage occurs, notify your supervisor.

Independence. Encourage the person to be as independent as possible. Only assist when needed. Like other activities of daily living, dressing and undressing stimulate circulation and increase muscle strength and flexibility. They also increase the person's confidence and self-esteem. Sometimes having clients do what they can for themselves requires patience and understanding. Allow the client extra time to dress and undress independently.

If the person has self-care devices, encourage him or her to use them. There are many self-care devices available (see Chapter 32). Devices that promote independence with dressing and undressing include:

- Button hooks (see Figure 32-3, *A* on page 559)
- Sock pullers (see Figure 32-3, *B*)
- Shoe removers (see Figure 32-3, *C*)
- Pantyhose aids
- Trouser pulls
- Pant clips

Preferences. Encourage personal choice whenever possible. Grooming practices vary from person to person. Do not impose your standards on the client. Ask clients how they want their hair styled, what hair or shaving products they use, and what clothing they want to wear.

Privacy. Providing for privacy is important when dressing and undressing the person. Do not expose the person during the procedures in this chapter. Also provide privacy when assisting with grooming.

Safety. Remember to dress the affected side first (DAF) and remove clothing from the unaffected side first (RUF). Also remember to check clients with elastic stockings and bandages often. Check for signs of reduced circulation, swelling, or skin breakdown. Report your observations to your supervisor. This information is needed to meet the person's needs.

Providing Compassionate Care boxes highlight how to promote the client's dignity, independence, preferences, privacy, and safety while giving the care discussed in the chapter. The first letters of the words in the list are bolded and coloured to help you remember DIPPS, the acronym that summarizes the five priorities of support work.

Colour illustrations and photographs visually present key ideas, concepts, and procedure steps. They help you apply and remember the written material. Captions describe the contents of the illustrations.

Chapter 6 Working with Clients and Their Families

Box 6-2 Case Study: Family Conflict

Mei is a support worker. She tells the following story about her experience working with a family in conflict.

"When I look back on the families I've worked with, one in particular stands out. Mr. Skala was an older man with cancer. His wife was his primary caregiver. They had a daughter living nearby who had a family of her own. Just before Mr. Skala became ill, there was a major argument over the family business. The result was that their daughter refused to speak to her parents. The Skalas' son-in-law brought their two young grandchildren to visit, but their daughter never came. She refused all attempts to resolve the conflict.

Mrs. Skala found this situation extremely hard to bear. She asked me to talk to her daughter to try to mend the rift. I felt for Mrs. Skala. I wanted to help, but I had to tell Mrs. Skala that it wasn't my role to get involved with the family's problems. I told my supervisor about Mrs. Skala's family problems. The case manager arranged for a social worker to talk with them. Eventually, the daughter resolved her differences with her parents. In the last three weeks of Mr. Skala's life, the family spent meaningful time together."

Case Study boxes apply some of the concepts found in the text to real-to-life examples of support workers and the people they care for.

REVIEW

Circle T if the answer is true and F if it is false.

1. T F **Ethics apply only to life-and-death situations.**
2. T F **Codes of ethics provide rules and answers to ethical dilemmas.**
3. T F **Ethics are a guide when deciding between right and wrong, good and bad.**
4. T F **Keeping a resident's information confidential is ethical behaviour.**
5. T F **Any decision regarding a client's care is ethical if it does not harm the person.**

Circle the BEST answer.

6. **Providing a safe environment is an example of**
   A. Autonomy
   B. Justice
   C. Beneficence
   D. Nonmaleficence
7. **Showing respect and protecting a person's dignity is an example of**
   A. Autonomy
   B. Justice
   C. Beneficence
   D. Nonmaleficence
8. **Treating all clients with equal care and attention, regardless of their condition or temperament, is an example of**
   A. Autonomy
   B. Justice
   C. Beneficence
   D. Nonmaleficence
9. **Respecting personal preferences is an example of**
   A. Autonomy
   B. Justice
   C. Beneficence
   D. Nonmaleficence
10. **Which question is *not* helpful when deciding an ethical solution to a problem?**
    A. Does the solution respect the client's wishes and stated preferences?
    B. Does the solution treat the client justly and fairly?
    C. Does the solution provide a short-term or long-term benefit to the client?
    D. Does the solution benefit you?

Answers to these questions are on page 822.

Review questions are a useful study guide. They provide a review of the main ideas presented in the chapter. Use them to study for a test or examination. Answers are provided at the back of the book beginning on page 821.

CONTENTS

CHAPTER

1

The Role of the Support Worker

OBJECTIVES

- Define the key terms listed in this chapter
- Explain the goal of support work
- Describe the five main responsibilities of support work
- Explain the goal of the health care team
- List the common members of a health care team
- Explain the difference between regulated and unregulated health care providers
- Explain why scope of practice is important to support work
- Explain what it means to have a professional approach to support work
- Identify the five priorities of compassionate care
- Identify four considerations when solving problems

KEY TERMS

activities of daily living (ADL) Self-care activities people perform daily to remain independent and to function in society

assistive personnel A broad term applied to staff who assist nurses and other health care professionals in giving care

client A person receiving care or support services in a community setting; a general term for all people receiving health care or support services: hospital patients, facility residents, and clients in the community

compassion Caring about another person's misfortune and suffering

confidentiality Respecting and guarding personal and private information about another person

dignity The state of feeling worthy, valued, and respected

discretion Good judgment

licensed practical nurse (LPN) See registered practical nurse

patient A person receiving care in a hospital setting

professionalism An approach to work that demonstrates respect for others, commitment, competence, and appropriate behaviour

registered nurse (RN) A health care professional licensed and regulated by the province or territory to maintain overall responsibility for the planning and provision of client care

registered practical nurse (RPN) A health care professional licensed and regulated by the province or territory to carry out basic nursing techniques and client care; licensed practical nurse

rehabilitation The process of restoring a person to the highest level of functioning possible through the use of therapy, exercise, or other methods

resident A person living in a residential facility

scope of practice The legal limits of your role

support worker A worker who provides personal care and support services

Support workers provide services to people who need help with their daily needs. You provide these services in facilities and in the community. Supervised by a nurse or other professional, you work as part of a health care team. Legislation, employer policies, and the person's condition influence how you function and how much supervision you need. You adapt your work depending on the setting and the needs and wishes of the person receiving care.

The ultimate goal of support work is to improve the person's quality of life. Care is provided in a kind, sensitive, and understanding manner. While tending to the person's physical needs, you also relieve loneliness, provide comfort, encourage independence, and promote the person's self-respect (Figure 1-1). Your services help people in their homes remain independent and with their families. Your services show people in facilities that you care for and about them. You make a difference in people's lives.

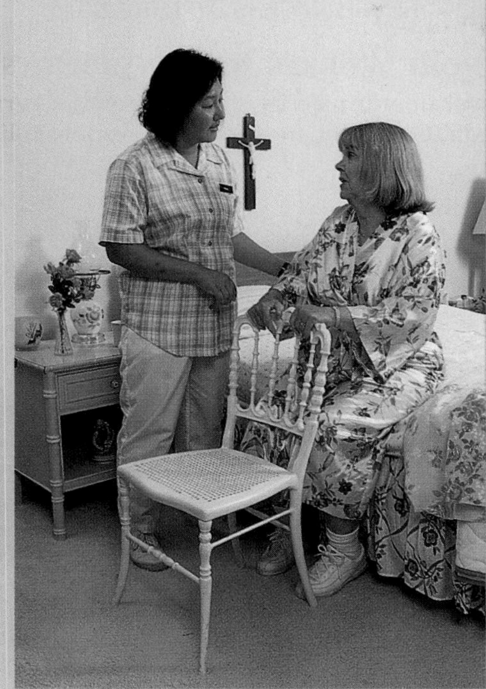

Figure 1-1 A support worker comforting a client.

Support Work across Canada

The nature of support work differs across the country. There are differences in training programs, work settings, job responsibilities, and terms used to describe support workers. Some sections of this text may not apply to support work in your province or territory. If you are unsure about which parts apply, ask your instructor.

Support worker refers to the worker who provides personal care and support services. However, *personal support worker, personal attendant, patient care assistant, resident care aide, health care aide, home care attendant, nursing aide, nursing attendant,* or *continuing care assistant* may be used in your province or territory.

In some parts of Canada, *personal attendant* refers to those workers who are supervised directly by the person for whom they provide services. Generally, personal attendant training is shorter in duration than support worker training. Personal attendants support people who have physical disabilities.

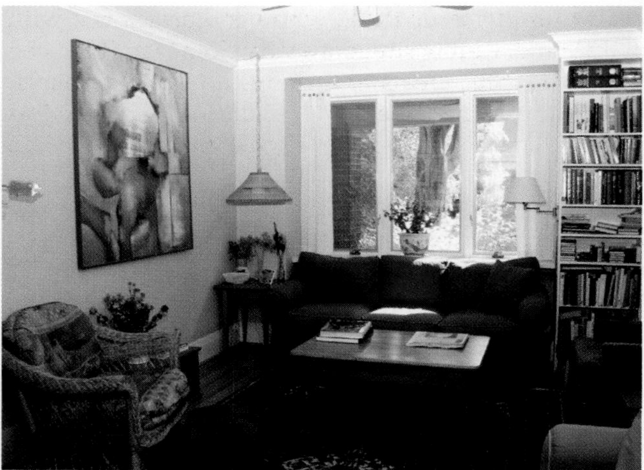

Figure 1-3 Room in a community-based setting; the person's home.

Settings for Support Work

You can work in facility-based and community-based settings (see Chapter 3).

- *Facility-based settings*—workplaces in which accommodations, health care, and support services are provided. Several types of facilities employ support workers. These include hospitals and long-term care facilities (Figure 1-2). A long-term care facility provides services to people who cannot care for themselves at home but who do not need hospital care.
- *Community-based settings*—workplaces within the community, where health care and support services are provided. The most common community setting is the person's home (Figure 1-3).

Support Worker Responsibilities

The tasks performed by support workers vary across Canada. Generally, most of your responsibilities can be grouped into five categories: personal care, support for nurses and other health care professionals, family support, social support, and housekeeping/home management.

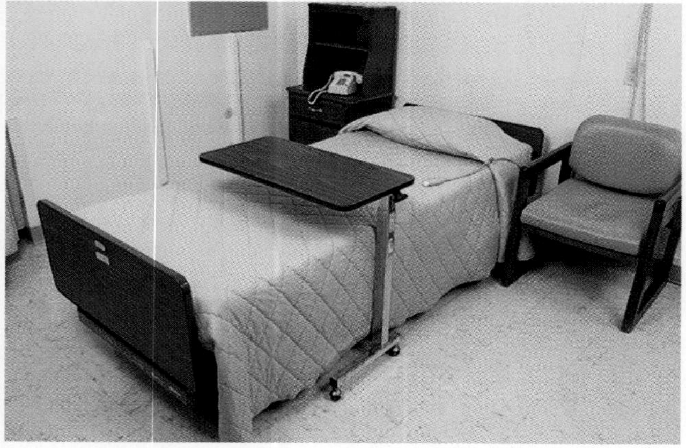

Figure 1-2 Room in a long-term care facility.

Personal Care. Personal care activities include assisting with **activities of daily living (ADL)**. These are the self-care activities that people perform daily to remain independent and to function in society. You help with daily activities such as eating, bathing, grooming, dressing, and toileting (elimination). You assist people with limited mobility to change positions or move from one place to another. You also help promote the person's safety and physical comfort. You are not responsible for deciding what should or should not be done for a person. However, while providing personal care, you observe for and report any changes in the person's behaviour or health. This is important information for the health care team.

Support for Nurses and Other Health Care Professionals. You assist nurses or other health care team members by following the established care plan for each client. For instance, you might clean equipment, measure and report vital signs, or assist with simple wound care. You might also assist with oxygen therapy, heat and cold applications, and range-of-motion exercises.

Family Support. In facilities, you may assist with admissions and discharges. You may introduce the person and family to the facility. You may also show them around and help the person unpack and settle in. In private homes, you help families care for loved ones with health problems or those who need assistance with daily living. Family situations vary. Some families need help preparing meals and doing household chores. Other families need help with childcare. Your services often give family caregivers a break from their duties.

Social Support. You may help people participate in social activities. These activities provide the person with enjoyment, recreation, and a chance to meet with friends. You may organize games and outings. You may be hired privately to be a person's companion.

Housekeeping/Home Management. You may do a variety of housekeeping tasks in a facility setting. These include bed-making, delivering meals, tidying living areas, and maintaining supplies. In a private home, housekeeping is called *home management*. Services depend on the needs of the person and the resources available to provide these services. They may include doing light housekeeping and laundry, and preparing and serving nutritious meals.

The following boxes describe a support worker's typical workday in the community, in a long-term care facility, and in a hospital setting.

(text continues on page 8)

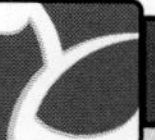

A Day in the Life of a Support Worker

Home Care

Each evening Stephen receives his assignment for the next day from his supervisor. He uses the details in the assignment to plan his day. He consults a city map and plans his route. The people he is assigned to visit have a range of physical, emotional, and social problems and disabilities. Their major problems are briefly described below.

Ms. Lau, 32, has cerebral palsy. She uses a wheelchair. She lives alone. Two days per week she works outside the home. She receives home care to help her prepare for work.

Mr. O'Connor, 59, is recovering at home from a stroke. He is paralyzed on one side of his body and has a speech and language disorder. His wife is his primary caregiver. Mr. O'Connor receives home care three mornings a week. Mrs. O'Connor, 51, is at work during Stephen's visit.

Mr. Horowitz, 71, has dementia. His wife, 67, is caring for him at home. The couple has emotional and social support from family and friends. Mrs. Horowitz looks after her husband's personal care needs. They receive two hours of home care per week to give Mrs. Horowitz a break.

Ms. Adams, 25, is a single mother on social assistance. She is recovering from a Cesarean section. She has very little social and emotional support. She has newborn twins and three young children, ages 1, 3, and 4.

Below are the tasks and activities that Stephen performs on a typical day at work.

0715–0830 (7:15 a.m.–8:30 a.m.)

- Travels to first appointment. Arrives at 0730.
- Assists Ms. Lau with showering, grooming, and dressing.
- Helps Ms. Lau to prepare breakfast, clean up kitchen, and make bed.
- Records care provided, including any relevant observations.

0830–1000 (8:30 a.m.–10:00 a.m.)

- Travels to next appointment. Arrives at 0845.
- Assists Mr. O'Connor with elimination, bathing, shaving, hair care, and mouth care.
- Prepares breakfast for Mr. O'Connor and assists him with eating.
- Cleans up kitchen and makes bed.
- Takes Mr. O'Connor for a brief walk. He is learning to walk with a cane.
- Assists Mr. O'Connor with elimination.
- Records care provided, including any relevant observations.

1000–1215 (10:00 a.m.–12:15 p.m.)

- Travels to next appointment. Arrives at 1015.
- The client's wife, Mrs. Horowitz, is crying and says that she is "worn out."
- Listens to Mrs. Horowitz and suggests she talk to his supervisor. Telephones supervisor who, in turn, calls the Horowitz's case manager. Case manager schedules a visit.
- Assists Mr. Horowitz with elimination, bathing, shaving, hair care, and mouth care.
- Cleans kitchen and does light housework in main living areas.
- Prepares lunch for Mr. Horowitz and assists him with eating.
- Records care provided, including any relevant observations.

1215–1530 (12:15 p.m.–3:30 p.m.)

- Takes break for lunch.
- Travels to next appointment. Arrives at 1300, the same time as the public health nurse.
- Helps children wash face and hands before preparing lunch.
- Prepares lunch for the mother and the three older children while the nurse assists the mother with breastfeeding. Feeds 1-year-old.
- Helps children with oral hygiene after lunch.
- Prepares three dinners. Leaves one in the refrigerator and freezes the others.
- Records care provided, including any relevant observations.
- Drives home.

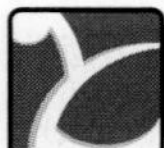

A Day in the Life of a Support Worker

Long-Term Care

Claire works on a unit in which the residents, mostly older adults, require help with activities of daily living. The eight residents assigned to her have a range of physical, emotional, and social problems and disabilities.

Miss McDonald, 94, is partially disabled due to rheumatoid arthritis.

Mr. Schmidt, 82, is recovering from surgery. He is incontinent of urine, which causes him anxiety.

Mrs. Lawson, 88, has a heart condition and osteoarthritis.

Mr. Delgado, 63, is paralyzed on one side due to a stroke. He is unable to speak, but is able to understand written and spoken language.

Mr. Taylor, 71, is in the early stages of Parkinson's disease. He also has diabetes and poor vision.

Mrs. Sanchez, 81, is partially disabled due to multiple leg and hip fractures. She has osteoporosis. She is also depressed.

Mr. Bouchard, 89, is recovering from pneumonia. He has age-related hearing loss.

Mrs. Khan, 44, is severely disabled due to multiple sclerosis. She is incontinent of urine and feces.

Below are the tasks and activities that Claire performs on a typical day at work.

0700–0715 (7:00 a.m.–7:15 a.m.)

- Receives report from RPN on condition of all residents on the unit.
- Receives assignment of care requirements, appointments, and activities scheduled for residents.
- Plans morning's tasks and activities.

0715–0845 (7:15 a.m.–8:45 a.m.)

- Helps seven of the residents to get out of bed.
- Provides partial hygiene care to six residents, a shower for one resident, and a tub bath for another.
- Assists with elimination and changes incontinent briefs.
- Assists residents with dressing, and accompanies them to the dining room.
- Returns to unit. Provides partial hygiene to Mrs. Khan.
- Observes that the cut on Mrs. Khan's arm looks red and swollen and feels warm to the touch. Makes a written record of it. Makes a verbal report to the RPN.
- With help from another support worker, moves Mrs. Khan from her bed to a wheelchair.
- Transports Mrs. Khan to the dining room for breakfast.
- Records care provided, including any relevant observations.

0845–0930 (8:45 a.m.–9:30 a.m.)

- Assists residents with breakfast. Tries to ensure that all residents have a nutritious breakfast and that special diets are followed.
- Prompts Mr. Taylor, Mrs. Lawson, and Miss McDonald to eat.
- Feeds Mrs. Khan.
- Transports Mrs. Khan back to unit.
- Returns to dining room and accompanies other residents back to unit.
- Records each resident's dietary intake in dietary intake record.

0930–1130 (9:30 a.m.–11:30 a.m.)

- Reports to RPN that Mr. Taylor (who has diabetes) did not eat.
- With assistance, lifts Mrs. Khan and settles her in bed.
- Assists residents with elimination and mouth care.
- Changes incontinent briefs.
- Reports on condition of residents to replacement support worker. Takes 15-minute break.
- Completes hygiene and grooming care for residents who received only partial care before breakfast.
- Accompanies residents at 1030 to games room.
- Makes beds and changes linens.
- Repositions Mrs. Khan to prevent pressure ulcers.
- Tidies rooms and living areas.
- Accompanies residents back to unit from games room at 1130.
- Records care provided, including any relevant observations.

1130–1300 (11:30 a.m.–1:00 p.m.)

- Reports on condition of residents to replacement support worker. Takes half an hour break for lunch.
- Checks care requirements for each resident, and plans the afternoon's tasks and activities.
- Accompanies residents to dining room.
- Supervises, assists, and feeds residents as required.
- Accompanies residents back to the unit.
- Assists residents with elimination and changes incontinent briefs.
- Assists with mouth care.
- Makes sure that residents rest after lunch as ordered.
- Records care provided, including any relevant observations.
- Records each resident's dietary intake in dietary intake record.

Continued

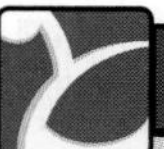

A Day in the Life of a Support Worker — cont'd

1300–1500 (1:00 p.m.–3:00 p.m.)

- Assists residents with elimination and changes incontinent briefs.
- Greets new resident, Mrs. Griffiths, and her family. Introduces them to the facility. Assists Mrs. Griffiths with unpacking.
- Introduces Mrs. Griffiths to the other residents.
- Repositions Mrs. Khan.
- Comforts Mrs. Griffiths, who is upset and lonely.
- Takes Mrs. Sanchez and Mrs. Griffiths for a walk.
- Assists residents with elimination and changes incontinent briefs.
- Records care provided, including any relevant observations.
- Provides a verbal report to the RPN concerning each person's care.

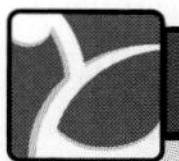

A Day in the Life of a Support Worker

Hospital Care

Gina works on a surgical unit. Most patients on this unit have had surgery for fractures (broken bones). Others have had hip or knee replacement surgery. A few are awaiting surgery. Many patients have additional health problems. Gina assists with the care of ten patients.

Miss Kwan, 66, thigh bone fracture
Mr. McDuff, 76, spine fracture; osteoporosis
Mrs. Sadiq, 46, shoulder and rib fractures; osteoporosis; quadriplegia
Mrs. Clark, 85, hip fracture; osteoporosis; Alzheimer's disease
Mr. Keene, 44, thigh bone and knee fractures
Mr. Cross, 55, knee replacement; arthritis
Mrs. Pocza, 82, hip fracture; osteoporosis
Ms. Hill, 35, multiple fractures: spine, thigh bone, and ankle
Mrs. Leblanc, 74, hip replacement; diabetes
Mr. Paes, 82, hip fracture; hearing loss

Below are the tasks and activities that Gina performs on a typical day at work.

0700–0710 (7:00 a.m.–7:10 a.m.)

- Receives assignment on care requirements.
- Plans morning's tasks and activities.

0710–0800 (7:10 a.m.–8:00 a.m.)

- Provides hygiene care to four patients, including assisting with oral hygiene, hair care, and providing partial bed baths.
- Assists with elimination.
- Records care provided as completed, including any relevant observations.

0800–0845 (8:00 a.m.–8:45 a.m.)

- Accompanies dietary staff as they deliver breakfast trays.
- Positions and arranges trays for patients.
- Assists patients with eating.
- Listens to Mrs. Pocza's concerns about her surgery; calls for the nurse who answers Mrs. Pocza's questions.
- Records food and fluid intake.
- Assists patients with elimination.
- Records care provided, including any relevant observations.

0845–1130 (8:45 a.m.–11:30 a.m.)

- Assists patients with hygiene, elimination, showers, and baths as required.
- Reports on condition of patients and care requirement to replacement support worker. Takes 15-minute break.
- Makes and changes beds.
- Assists with two discharges. Helps patients pack.
- Helps nurse to reposition patients as required.
- Assists patients with leg exercises, coughing, and deep breathing exercises.
- Records care provided, including any relevant observations.

1130–1300 (11:30 a.m.–1:00 p.m.)

- Reports on condition of patients and care requirement to replacement support worker. Takes half an hour break for lunch.
- Checks condition of and care requirements for each patient and plans afternoon tasks.
- Accompanies dietary staff as they deliver lunch trays.
- Positions and arranges trays for patients.
- Assists patients with eating.
- Observes that Mr. McDuff's IV fluid is running low. Notifies the nurse immediately.
- Records food and fluid intake.
- Assists patients with elimination and mouth care.
- Records care provided, including any relevant observations.

Continued

A Day in the Life of a Support Worker — cont'd

1300–1500 (1:00 p.m.–3:00 p.m.)

- Removes Mr. Paes's dentures before his medications are given.
- Assists patients with elimination.
- Observes drainage under Miss Kwan's cast. Notifies nurse immediately.
- Answers call from nurse. Provides comfort to Mrs. Clark (who is upset).
- Assists patients with leg exercises, coughing, and deep breathing exercises.
- Assists with admitting two patients.
- Helps nurse to reposition patients as required.
- Records care provided, including any relevant observations.
- Provides a verbal report to the RN concerning each person's care.

THE PEOPLE YOU SUPPORT

People receiving health care and support services are known by different terms, depending on the workplace setting. A person receiving care in a hospital is called a **patient**. A person living in a residential facility is called a **resident**. A person receiving care or support services in the community is called a **client**. Client is also a general term for all people receiving health care or support services: hospital patients, facility residents, and clients in the community.

Whether the individual receiving care is known as a client, patient, or resident, always remember that he or she is first and foremost a *person*. Every person is unique. The people to whom you provide services have a variety of needs and abilities. They all have unique life experiences and situations. They also have unique wants and opinions. You will work with people from a variety of cultures (see Chapter 11). Part of your job is to accept this diversity among people. Boxes called *Respecting Diversity* appear in this text. These boxes are intended to help you appreciate the importance of diversity and how people's backgrounds influence them.

The people you support can be grouped according to their problems, needs, and ages:

- *Older adults.* Aging is a normal process. It is not an illness or disease. Many older adults enjoy good health. However, body changes normally occur with the aging process. Social and emotional changes may also accur (see Chapter 15). The risks for contracting serious illness and becoming disabled increase with age. Most older adults remain at home as long as possible. Others are unable to manage even with assistance, and move into a residential facility. *Focus on Older Adults* boxes throughout the text discuss issues relevant to older adults
- *People with disabilities.* Some people are disabled due to illness, injury, or conditions present at birth. Disabilities may affect physical or mental functioning, or both. Many adults with disabilities live in their own homes. Many work outside the home. You might help disabled people with activities of daily living.
- *People with medical problems.* Medical problems include illnesses, diseases, and injuries. Medical problems may be short-term (such as a broken bone), long-term (such as diabetes or multiple sclerosis), or progessive and life-threatening (such as some types of cancer).
- *People having surgery.* Surgical patients are those being prepared for or who have recently had surgery. Preoperative care involves preparing the person for what to expect after surgery. The person's fears and anxieties are also addressed. Needs after surgery relate to relieving pain and discomfort, preventing complications, and helping the person adjust to body changes. People recover from surgeries in hospitals and in their homes.
- *People with mental health problems.* Mental health problems vary from mild to severe. Some people function normally but need help making decisions or coping with life stresses. Others are severely affected. They need assistance with activities of daily living.
- *People needing rehabilitation.* **Rehabilitation** is the process of restoring a person to the highest level of functioning possible through the use of therapy, exercise, or other methods. The person may need to regain functions lost from surgery, illness, or accident. Some hospitals have special rehabilitation units. Many people receiving support at home and in long-term care settings require rehabilitation.
- *Children.* When hospital care is needed, children are admitted to the pediatric unit. Some areas of Canada hire support workers to work in pediatric units (Figure 1-4). However, most support work for children occurs in community settings and long-term care facilities. Some children who receive care have physical or intellectual disabilities. Others

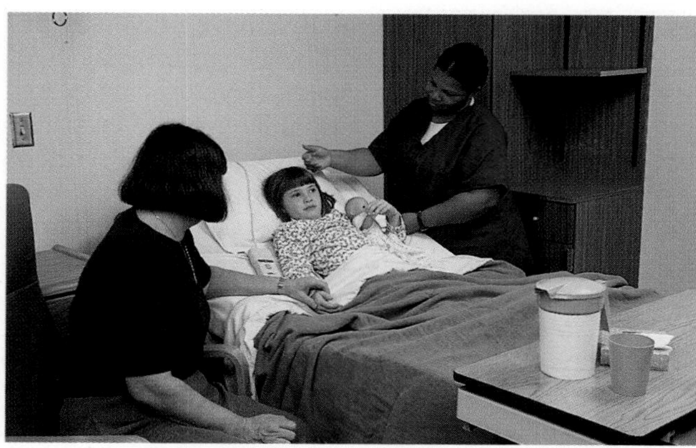

Figure 1-4 The support worker gives care to a sick child.

need care because a parent is ill or disabled or has just had a new baby. *Focus on Children* boxes discuss issues related to caring for children.

- *Mothers and newborns.* Complications and difficulties can occur at any time during pregnancy through the six to eight weeks after childbirth. Some new mothers need assistance with their care or with their newborn's care. Most support work with mothers and newborns takes place in the home.
- *People requiring special care.* Some people who have serious and complex medical conditions need special care and equipment. Hospitals have special care units, including intensive care units, coronary care units, kidney dialysis units, burn units, and emergency rooms. Some areas of Canada hire support workers to work in these units. You might transport people from one unit to another, take specimens to the lab, and assist with special procedures. In some parts of Canada, support workers do not provide personal care to patients in unstable or critical condition.

The Health Care Team

A *team* is a group of people working together toward a common goal. Health care teams include workers with a variety of skills and knowledge who work together to meet the client's needs. Their goal is to provide quality care. Many professionals are involved in the care of one person. Which professionals are involved depends on the needs of the person.

You are an important member of the health care team. The client and family members are also important members of the team. The client is always the focus of the health care team's efforts (Figure 1-5).

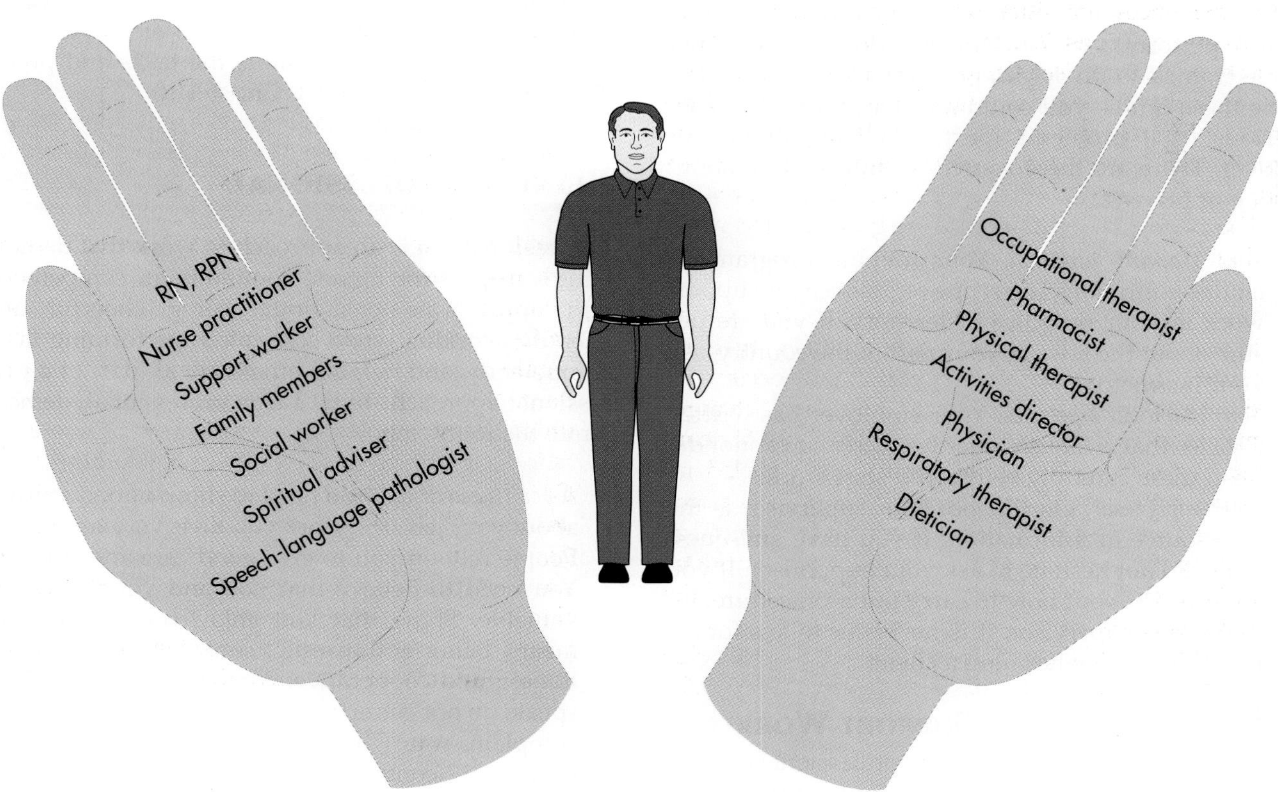

Figure 1-5 Members of the health care team, with the client as the focus of care.

Regulated and Unregulated Workers

Health care professions are either regulated or unregulated. A regulated profession is self-governing. It has a professional organization called a college. The college sets education and licence requirements. It also establishes scope of practice, codes of ethics, and standards of conduct for its members. The college investigates complaints about a member's conduct. If necessary, the college disciplines members guilty of misconduct. Each regulated health profession has legislation that details the roles and responsibilities of its members. Nursing is one of many regulated health care professions.

An unregulated profession does not have a professional college or legislation written specifically for it. There are no official requirements for education and training programs, and there are no codes of ethics. As yet, support workers are unregulated workers. Because you do not have an organization or college that governs your role, you are accountable to your supervisor, your employer, and your clients.

Table 1-1 describes the titles and positions of the common health care team members. It also lists whether they are regulated or unregulated workers.

Scope of Practice

To protect clients from harm, you must understand what you can do, what you cannot do, and the legal limits of your role. This is called **scope of practice**.

Never act beyond the legal limits of your role. Also never perform a function or task that you have not been trained to do. If you perform a task that is outside these limits, you could harm a client and create serious legal problems for yourself and your employer. There are three sources of information about scope of practice:

- *Your training program.* Your training program includes information on scope of practice for support work in your province or territory. If you are unsure about the laws in your part of the country, ask your instructor.
- *Your employer's policies.* Your employer has written policies that establish what you can and cannot do. Read these carefully before you start work.
- *Your supervisor.* On the job, your supervisor is the best source of information. If you have any questions, do not hesitate to ask your supervisor. If you are unsure about how to carry out a procedure, inform your supervisor. It is far better to ask for direction than risk harming a client.

The Supervision of Support Workers

In most settings, nurses or other professionals supervise support workers. A **registered nurse (RN)** is licensed and regulated by the province or territory to maintain overall responsibility for the planning and provision of client care. Some RNs have university degrees. Others have community college diplomas. RNs assess, make nursing diagnoses, develop care plans, and implement and evaluate nursing care. They also carry out physicians' orders. An RN directs the work of registered practical nurses (see below), support workers, and other assistive personnel. **Assistive personnel** is a broad term applied to staff who assist nurses and other health care professionals in giving care.

A **registered practical nurse (RPN)**, also known as a **licensed practical nurse (LPN)**, is licensed and regulated by the province or territory to carry out basic nursing techniques and client care. Some RPNs have a community college certificate. Others have a college diploma. In most parts of Canada, RPNs work under the supervision of RNs. They function with little supervision when caring for stable clients with uncomplicated health problems. RPNs assist RNs in providing care to seriously ill clients and help with complex procedures. Some provinces and territories allow RPNs to supervise support workers in certain situations.

RNs or RPNs are not the only professionals who may supervise you. Depending on the situation, you may be supervised by others. For example, if you work in the recreation department of a long-term care facility, you may report to a recreational therapist. In the community, your supervisor may be a social worker, a physiotherapist, or another health care professional.

Some support workers are hired and supervised directly by clients. You must be aware of provincial or territorial legislation that limits the tasks and procedures you can perform (see Chapter 10).

Being a Professional

Professionalism is an approach to work that demonstrates respect for others, commitment, competence, and appropriate behaviour. Being cheerful and friendly, working when scheduled, performing tasks competently, and helping others are all part of a professional approach. To be a true professional, demonstrate the following:

- *A positive attitude.* You need to show a good attitude about your job. The work you do is very important. People rely on you to give good care and support. You need to believe that you and your work are valuable. Show that you enjoy your work. This means being enthusiastic, considerate, courteous, honest, and cooperative. Always think before you speak, do not gossip about other people, and do not complain. Your words reveal your attitude. Box 1-1 on page 12 contains statements that show a negative attitude and should be avoided.
- *A sense of responsibility.* Never blame others for your problems or mistakes at work. Admit your mistakes,

Table 1-1 Health Care Team Members

Title	Description	Regulated / Unregulated
Activities director	Assesses, plans, and implements recreational needs	Unregulated; provincial/territorial training requirements vary
Dietician	Assesses and plans for nutritional needs; teaches clients about nutrition, food selection, and preparation	Regulated
Nurse practitioner	Registered nurse with advanced education and additional responsibilities for management of client care	Regulated
Occupational therapist	Focuses on rehabilitation; teaches clients skills needed to perform ADL; designs adaptive equipment for ADL	Regulated
Pharmacist	Fills medication orders written by physicians; monitors and evaluates drug interactions; consults with physicians and nurses about drug actions and interactions	Regulated
Physical therapist (Physiotherapist)	Focuses on rehabilitation; assists clients with musculoskeletal problems; focuses on restoring function and preventing disability from illness or injury	Regulated
Physician	Diagnoses and treats clients with illness and injuries	Regulated
Registered nurse (RN)	Assesses; makes nursing diagnoses; plans, implements, and evaluates nursing care; supervises RPNs and support workers	Regulated
Registered practical nurse (RPN)	Provides direct client care, including the administration of medication, under the direction of an RN	Regulated
Respiratory therapist	Focuses on rehabilitation; assists in treatment of lung and heart disorders; gives respiratory treatments and therapies	Regulated
Social worker	Helps clients and families with social and emotional issues related to illness and recovery	Varies according to province/territory
Speech-language pathologist (therapist)	Focuses on rehabilitation; evaluates speech and language and treats people with speech, voice, hearing, communication, and swallowing disorders	Regulated
Spiritual advisor	Assists clients and families with spiritual needs	Determined by religious order
Support worker	Assists clients with personal care, family responsibilities, social and recreational activities, housekeeping/home management; provides support for nurses and other professionals	Unregulated

accept constructive criticism, and learn from others. Always report to work when scheduled and on time. Everyone is affected when one person is late. Have a plan ready for when you are urgently needed at home or your transportation is unavailable. Inform your supervisor immediately if you will be late or unable to work. Also be sure to finish assigned tasks before you leave for the day. The client's care cannot be neglected. Promptly explain to your supervisor if you cannot finish the assignment.

- *A professional appearance.* A professional, appropriate appearance shows respect for the people in your care, your co-workers, and yourself. It signals that you take your job seriously. Your appearance includes your clothes, grooming, and hygiene (Box 1-2 and Figure 1-6 on page 12).

Box 1-1 Statements That Show a Negative Attitude

- "I can't. I'm too busy. Can't somebody else help?"
- "I didn't do it."
- "It's not my fault."
- "Don't blame me."
- "It's not my turn. I did it yesterday."
- "Nobody told me."
- "I work harder than anyone else."
- "No one appreciates what I do."

Box 1-2 Practices for a Professional Appearance

- Follow your employer's dress code policies.
- Wear a clean, well-fitting, modest uniform.
- Wear a name badge or photo ID, as per your employer's policy.
- Wear clean stockings and socks that are in good repair.
- Wear comfortable, well-polished shoes that give you good support.
- Wear underclothing that cannot be seen through your uniform.
- Keep your hair away from your face and up off your collar.
- Use make-up sparingly to avoid a painted, severe look.
- Do not wear perfume, cologne, or aftershave. They may nauseate or cause breathing problems in some clients.
- Keep fingernails clean, short, and neatly shaped. Long nails can scratch the client.
- Do not wear jewellery (even if parts of your body are pierced). Jewellery may scratch or cause injury to your client and yourself. It may offend people.
- Cover tattoos because they may be offensive to others.

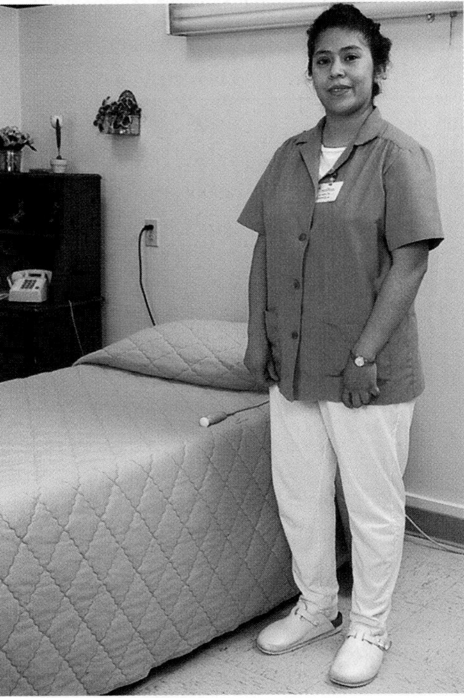

Figure 1-6 This support worker is well-groomed. Her uniform and shoes are clean. Her hair has a simple style and is out of her face and off her collar. No jewellery is worn except for a watch.

- *Discretion about client information.* **Discretion** means good judgment. This means being very careful about what you say, how you say it, when you say it, and where you say it. You need to judge when information should be kept private and when it should be shared. Information about a client is confidential. **Confidentiality** means respecting and guarding personal and private information about another person. Information should be shared only among team members involved in the client's care. Information about your employer, your co-workers, and other clients is also private. Never talk with a client about another client, even if you avoid using names. Avoid talking about clients, co-workers, and your employer where you can be overheard. If you need to discuss a person's care with team members, make sure that other clients, families, and visitors cannot hear you. People overhearing may think you are talking about them or their family members. This can lead to misinformation and confusion, which can be very distressing.
- *Discretion about personal matters.* Discretion in support work includes keeping personal matters out of the workplace. Your role is to focus on your clients and the task at hand. Do not discuss with clients family matters, personal problems, or the problems of others (Box 1-3). No matter how well you think you know a client, remember that your relationship is professional. It is not a friendship (see Chapter 6).
- *Acceptable speech and language.* How you speak at home and in social settings may not be appropriate for a work setting. Your speech and language must be professional. In order not to offend clients or co-workers, never use foul, vulgar, or abusive language. Also avoid using slang. Speak gently and clearly; never yell or shout. Also never fight or argue with a client, family, or co-workers.

The Priorities of Support Work: Compassionate Care

Compassion means caring about another person's misfortune and suffering. Many people who require

Box 1-3 Keeping Personal Matters Out of the Workplace

- Make personal calls only during breaks. Only use a client's phone for urgent matters. Always ask before using the phone.
- Do not discuss personal problems at work.
- Do not let family and friends visit you at work.
- Arrange personal appointments for times when you are not scheduled to work.
- Do not use your employer's supplies or equipment for personal matters.
- Do not raise funds at work, even if the funds are for a good cause.

support are coping with serious illness or disability. They may also have personal problems that make life very difficult. Providing compassionate care means treating people with respect, kindness, and understanding. No matter what kind of care or support you provide, most clients have the following needs:

- *To preserve their dignity.* **Dignity** means the state of feeling worthy, valued, and respected. People need to feel dignified.
- *To live independently.* People need to do what they can for themselves.
- *To express their preferences.* People need to make choices and explain how they want to have things done.
- *To preserve their privacy.* People need to know that their bodies and their affairs are respectfully kept from public view (Figure 1-7).
- *To be safe from harm.* People need to live in an environment as free from hazards as possible. They need to feel secure about the care provided.

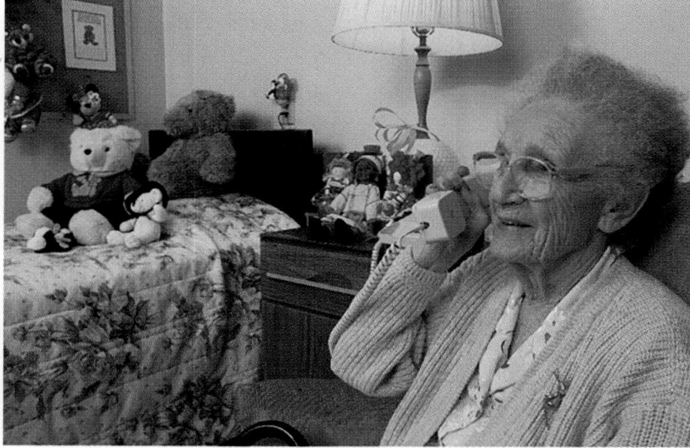

Figure 1-7 A client talking privately on a telephone.

When well and able-bodied, most people take the fulfillment of these five needs for granted. When people become disabled or suffer a serious illness, however, these five needs may be more difficult to fulfill. People who rely on others for personal care may worry about losing their dignity. They may not feel free to express their wishes. For example, people living in long-term care facilities may have to eat what is provided and socialize at prearranged times. When they live in a facility and share a room with another person, they may find that private moments are rare. Safety concerns are serious issues in the lives of people who are ill and disabled. For example, they may worry about reaching the bathroom without falling.

Not all people who are ill and disabled have the same needs. However, most have at least some of the needs just discussed. To help you recognize these needs, *Providing Compassionate Care* boxes discuss the priorities of support work. Most of these boxes discuss how to promote the person's **D**ignity, **I**ndependence, **P**references, **P**rivacy, and **S**afety. The acronym DIPPS reminds you of these five priorities.

Decision Making and Problem Solving

You make many decisions every day. For example, you estimate the time each task will take, and plan the best way to complete your work on time. Many decisions involve solving problems.

When solving problems, consider the following:

- *The priorities of support work.* Solutions to problems should not compromise the five priorities of support work: dignity, independence, preferences, privacy, and safety.
- *The client's viewpoint.* Involve clients in solving problems that concern them. Examine the problem from the person's perspective.
- *Your scope of practice.* Learn and observe the rules of your workplace. Know the limits of your role.
- *Your supervisor's viewpoint.* Decide if the problem is one that you can handle on your own or is one that your supervisor should handle. Your supervisor should provide guidance about the kinds of problems you can deal with on your own.

Decision making and problem solving are crucial to your role, yet are often difficult when you are new to the job. To help you with the problem-solving process, this text includes boxes called *Support Workers Solving Problems.* These boxes present problems faced by support workers and show how they arrive at solutions.

REVIEW

Circle the BEST answer.

1. Activities of daily living are
   A. Physical exercises that people perform daily to keep themselves fit
   B. Activities that support workers perform to prevent injuries
   C. Self-care activities that people perform daily to remain independent and to function in society
   D. Social and recreational activities

2. The following are ways in which support workers assist nurses or other health care team members. Which is *false*?
   A. Measure and report vital signs
   B. Assist with range-of-motion exercises
   C. Assess the client's needs
   D. Report changes in the client's behaviour or health

3. Resident is a term used to describe a person who is receiving care at
   A. Home
   B. A long-term care facility
   C. An outpatient clinic
   D. A hospital

4. The main focus of the health care team is to
   A. Find a cure for the client's illness or condition
   B. See as many clients as possible
   C. Complete assigned tasks as quickly as possible
   D. Provide quality care for the client

5. Support workers are
   A. Unregulated health care workers
   B. Licensed health care workers
   C. Members of a professional college
   D. Members of a regulatory body

6. Scope of practice means
   A. The tasks that are assigned by your supervisor
   B. The tasks that a client asks you to perform
   C. The effort you put into performing a task or procedure
   D. The legal limits of your role

7. Professionalism is
   A. An approach to work used only by members of regulated professions
   B. An approach to work that demonstrates respect for others, commitment, competence, and appropriate behaviour
   C. A commitment made by regulated professionals
   D. Another term for confidentiality

8. Which of the following is *true?*
   A. You can use a client's phone to make personal calls.
   B. Friends can visit you at work.
   C. You must follow your employer's dress code policies.
   D. Sharing your personal problems with a client shows compassion.

9. In a long-term care facility, the client's information should be shared among
   A. Health care team members involved in the client's care
   B. Health care team members and friends who visit the client
   C. Family and friends of the client
   D. All staff members at the facility

10. Compassion means
    A. Caring about another's misfortune and suffering
    B. Keeping one's feelings to oneself
    C. Taking pity on those who are less fortunate
    D. Approaching your work with enthusiasm

11. The acronym DIPPS stands for
    A. Danger, independence, preferences, policies, sympathy
    B. Dignity, independence, preferences, privacy, safety
    C. Difference, individuality, pity, privacy, scope of practice
    D. Disability, individuality, pity, privacy, scope of practice

12. Which is *false?* When solving problems, you should
    A. Not involve the client to prevent causing more problems
    B. Discuss the problem with the client
    C. Consider your scope of practice
    D. Consider the priorities of support work

Answers to these questions are on page 821.

CHAPTER

2

The Canadian Health Care System

OBJECTIVES

- Define the key terms listed in this chapter
- Describe medicare and how it has evolved
- Identify the federal, provincial, and territorial roles in the health care system
- Explain the five principles of medicare described in the *Canada Health Act*
- Identify how the focus of the Canadian health care system is shifting
- Explain why health promotion and disease prevention are important functions of the Canadian health care system
- Recognize the emerging importance of home care and your role in providing some of these services

KEY TERMS

Canada Health Act **(1984)** Federal legislation that clarifies the types of health care services that are insured; it also outlines five principles that must be met for provinces and territories to qualify for federal health money

disease prevention Strategies that prevent the occurrence of disease or injury

health promotion Strategies that improve or maintain health and independence

home care Health care and support services provided to people in their places of residence

medicare Canada's national health care insurance system; publicly funds all the cost of medically necessary health services

Few issues are as important to Canadians as health care. Most Canadians believe that quality health care should be available to all citizens, regardless of their ability to pay. Canada's national health insurance system, known as **medicare**, was developed to achieve this goal. Medicare uses provincial/territorial and federal taxes to pay for all medically necessary health services for all permanent residents. Faced with the ever-increasing costs of providing care, Canadians are re-examining their health care spending and priorities. Support workers have an increasingly important role within Canada's changing health care system.

The Evolution of Canada's Health Care System

When you have a doctor's appointment or are admitted to a hospital, you do not pay for the services out of pocket. Rather, you finance your (and other Canadians') medically necessary health services through your taxes. Rich and poor people have access to the same services.

Health care has not always been this way. In the first part of the last century, individuals paid for their own doctors' bills and hospital fees. Often there were no set fees. Physicians charged whatever they thought the patient could afford to pay. As a result, people often paid different fees for similar services. Those who could not afford to pay had to find charity services through community agencies such as the Victorian Order of Nurses, the Red Cross, and local churches (Figure 2-1).

The spread of the Great Depression across Canada in the 1930s had a dramatic effect on the health care system. Families could not pay their medical bills. A serious illness or stay in a hospital caused financial disaster for many. The cost of care prevented many from seeking medical treatment. Many ill and disabled people depended on family members and neighbours to provide care. Box 2-1 is one woman's memoir of the Depression years. As a child she witnessed the hardships people endured because of their health care system.

These hardships inspired Canadians to create a prepaid medical and hospitalization insurance plan. In 1947, Saskatchewan was the first province to introduce a public insurance plan that covered the costs of hospital services. By 1961, all ten provinces and two territories agreed to provide coverage for in-patient hospital care. The federal government paid about half the cost

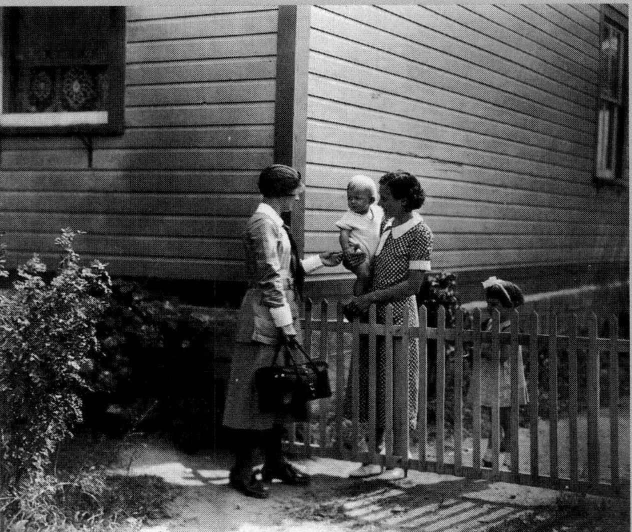

Figure 2-1 In the first part of the last century, charitable services were provided by community agencies such as the Victorian Order of Nurses for Canada.

Box 2-1 Health Care during the Depression

The Depression years were the years of my growing up on an apple farm near a small village in eastern Ontario. Living in the country meant you knew the joys, pains, and sorrows of your neighbours and community. In those years, many were in very difficult circumstances.... The cost of medical care was one of the most painful situations many people faced. Proud and needy people visited the one doctor available only in times of extremity. Recently, I heard that during these years, one-half of Canadians never in all their lives received any medical attention ....

The doctor in our community was caring and very hardworking. Many patients paid him in chickens, eggs, potatoes, or apples. Some were unable to make any payment. It was a situation which was devastating for both patient and doctor. The patient had to beg for medical attention for himself and loved ones. The doctor must have been overstocked with food articles beyond the needs of his family, but without the ready cash for taxes, car upkeep, or clothing for his family.

Source: Helen Heeney, ed., *Life before Medicare: Canadian Experiences* (Toronto: The Stories Project, 1995), p. ix.

of hospital and diagnostic services for each province/territory. The provincial and territorial governments paid for the other half. By 1972, all provinces and territories extended their insurance plans to also cover medical services provided outside hospitals. Again, the provincial/territorial and federal governments shared the health care expenses roughly equally. Modern medicare began that year: all permanent residents now had free access to the same quality of hospital and medical care, regardless of their personal wealth.

THE MODERN HEALTH CARE SYSTEM

The federal government and the ten provincial and three territorial governments share responsibilities within Canada's health care system.

THE FEDERAL ROLE

The federal government is responsible for:

- Delivering health care services to Aboriginal people and people living on reserves, military personnel, veterans, inmates of federal penitentiaries, and members of the RCMP.
- Developing and carrying out government policy and programs that promote health and prevent disease. For example, the federal government approves drugs, assesses health risks posed by environmental hazards, and provides grant money to support public health programs such as prenatal health education.
- Transferring tax money to the provinces and territories to share the cost of medically necessary health care services.
- Ensuring that the provinces and territories provide the same quality and type of care. The ***Canada Health Act* (1984)** is federal legislation that clarifies the types of health care services that are insured. It also outlines five principles that must be met in order for the provinces and territories to qualify for federal money (Box 2-2). The act does not allow service providers (such as physicians) to bill clients for extra charges and user fees.

THE PROVINCIAL/TERRITORIAL ROLE

Each province and territory is responsible for developing and administrating its own health care insurance plan. The provincial or territorial government finances and plans its health care services, following the five basic principles outlined in the *Canada Health Act*. For example, the provincial or territorial governments decide where hospitals or long-term care facilities

Box 2-2 The Principles of Medicare Listed in the *Canada Health Act* (1984)

1. **Public administration.** The insurance plan must be run by a public organization on a nonprofit basis. The public organization must be accountable to the citizens and the government of the province or territory.
2. **Comprehensiveness.** The insurance plan must pay for all medically necessary services. In a hospital, all necessary drugs, supplies, and diagnostic tests are covered. A range of necessary services provided outside a hospital are also covered.
3. **Universality.** Every permanent resident of a province or territory is entitled to receive the insured health care services provided by the plan on similar terms and conditions.
4. **Portability.** People can keep their health care coverage even if they are unemployed, change jobs, relocate between provinces and territories, or travel within Canada or abroad.
5. **Accessibility.** People can receive medically necessary services regardless of their income, age, health status, gender, or geographic location. Additional charges for insured services are not permitted.

will be located and organized; how many physicians, nurses, and other service providers will be needed; and how much money to spend on health care services.

The provincial and territorial health insurance plans pay for hospital and physician costs. They also pay for some of the costs of rehabilitation and long-term care services. Each provincial and territorial plan is unique. Exactly what is covered and by how much varies across the country. For example, coverage for ambulance services, drugs, and home care varies by province. To help pay for services not covered by provincial or territorial insurance, people can buy extra health insurance policies.

Health Care Reform

Many situations challenge the country's ability to provide universal, quality health care. For instance, many rural or remote areas face severe shortages of physicians, nurses, and other health care workers. Long waiting lists are common for surgeries, diagnostics, or medical procedures. The greatest challenge facing the health care system is the steadily rising cost of care. Drugs and technology now exist that treat diseases and disabilities better than ever before. However, these advances come at a high price due to the cost of developing them.

The health care system is changing in response to these challenges. During the 1990s, the government made changes to the health care system to reduce its costs. As part of these reforms, provincial and territorial governments focused on two areas:

- health promotion and disease prevention
- home care

Health Promotion and Disease Prevention

Traditionally, the purpose of a health care system has been to diagnose, treat, and cure illness. A more recent approach to health care, however, involves developing ways to promote health and prevent disease. Preventing illness and injury and keeping people healthy are more effective and cheaper than treating them in hospitals. **Health promotion** refers to strategies that improve or maintain health and independence. **Disease prevention** refers to strategies that prevent the occurrence of disease or injury. Health promotion and disease prevention are now important functions of Canada's health care system.

Research has been done to determine the factors that most affect the health of the population. The following are key factors that determine a person's health:

- Income and social status
- Social support networks (see Chapter 4)
- Education
- Employment and working conditions
- Environment
- Personal health practices and coping skills

Government policy promotes health and prevents illness by improving these areas of people's lives. These policies occur in many sectors of government and industry. Examples of policies that promote health and prevent illness include:

- Immunization programs
- Prenatal and parenting classes
- Information campaigns to reduce drinking during pregnancy, unsafe sex, and tobacco use, and to encourage healthy eating and physical activity
- Efforts to improve housing, decrease poverty, monitor safe drinking water, and protect the environment

Support workers contribute to health promotion and disease prevention. You provide nonmedical care and services that can help prevent major health problems. For example, Mr. Lukovic is on bed rest for a long time. He is at risk for pressure ulcers, pneumonia, and blood clots. To prevent these complications, you help him keep his skin clean and dry, change his position in bed frequently, and perform range-of-motion exercises. You help Mr. Lukovic prevent future illness and disability.

Home Care

The Canadian health care system has seen a shift in focus from hospital care to home care. Traditionally, people entered the health care system through hospitals. However, over the last two decades the role and structure of hospitals have changed dramatically. Hospitals require a tremendous amount of money to operate. Over a third of all health care spending goes into them. Therefore, most provincial and territorial governments have reduced the number of hospitals to cut costs. In the last few years, hundreds of hospitals have closed, merged, or been converted to other types of care facilities.

Partly to save money and partly as a result of technological advances, patients are sent home sooner after hospital procedures. Each year, fewer patients stay in hospital overnight. Those who do stay overnight stay for shorter periods of time than in the past.

To support patients leaving earlier from hospitals, governments have gradually increased spending on home care. **Home care** is health care and support services provided to people in their places of residence. These include private homes, retirement residences, and assisted-living facilities (see Chapter 3). Home care is the most common of the community-based services.

Home care was first created to provide care for people who needed at-home assistance after hospital discharge. Today, home care provides community care and support to a range of people. Clients include older adults; families with children; people who have mental, physical, or developmental disabilities; people with short-term and long-term medical conditions; and people in the recovery, rehabilitative, or final, life-ending stages of a disease. Home care services provide assistance to families who need help with a new baby. They enable people with disabilities to get up in the morning and get ready for school or work. They help people adjust to a disability or recover from an illness. They enable people who are dying to remain at home rather than being admitted to hospital (Figure 2-2).

One major focus of home care is to enable people to remain in their homes, as healthy and as independent for as long as possible. For some people, home care replaces hospital or other facility care. For others, home care enables them to maintain their health and independence, thus delaying or preventing admission to a facility.

Services and funding. Home care includes a range of professional and support services. *Professional services* are therapies and treatments provided by health care professionals. Professional services include:

- Nursing care
- Physiotherapy
- Occupational therapy
- Speech therapy
- Nutrition counselling
- Social work
- Respiratory therapy

Support services offered through home care are non-medical services. Support services include:

- Personal care
- Assistance with activities of daily living
- Assistance with home management

Support workers provide most support services for home care. In most provinces and territories, support services are provided by private or not-for-profit agencies. Public home care agencies hire them to work for eligible clients. Home care agencies may also arrange for volunteer services to be provided for some clients. Examples of volunteer services offered include Meals on Wheels (Figure 2-3) and friendly visiting.

Every province and territory has a publicly funded home care program. Because the *Canada Health Act* does not say what services must be provided, each province and territory has defined and funded its own

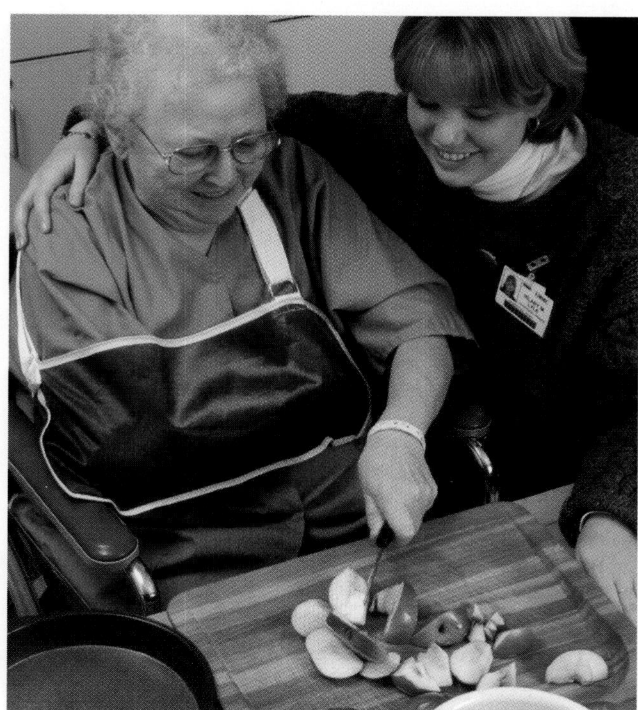

Figure 2-2 This woman receives assistance from home care services so she can live alone at home.

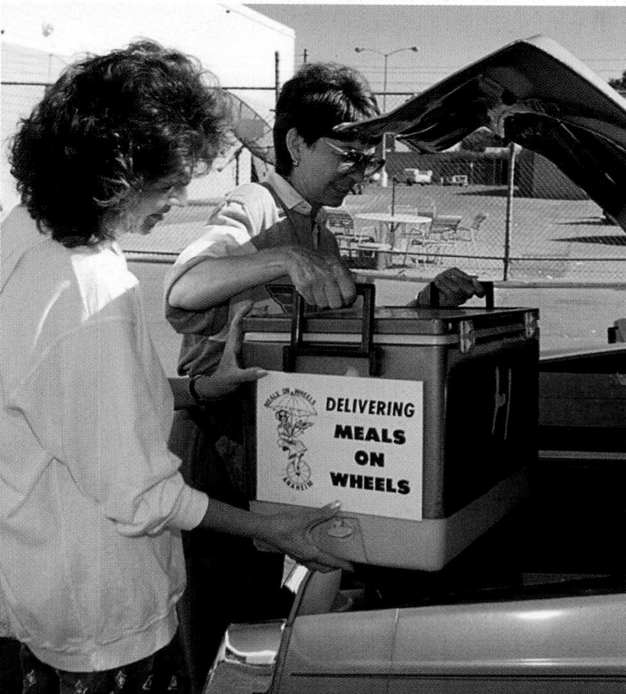

Figure 2-3 A client receives a hot meal delivered to her home.

home care system. The services offered (Table 2-1) and how they are provided (Box 2-3) vary across the country. All provinces and territories, however, offer the following:

- Client assessment—determining if the person is eligible for services
- Case coordination and management (see Chapter 7)
- Nursing services
- Support services for eligible clients

Eligibility and hours of services provided also vary depending on the province or territory. Some people may want home care services that are not funded by their province or for which they do not qualify. They can hire a private agency and pay for these services themselves or with insurance plans.

Table 2-1 Home Care Services Publicly Funded, by Province or Territory

Service	BC	AB	SK	MB	ON	QC	NB	NS	PE	NL	NT	YT
Assessment & case management	*	*	*	*	*	*	*	*	*	*	*	*
Nursing care	*	*	*	*	*	*	*	*	*	*	*	*
Support services/personal care	*	*	*	*	*	*	*	*	*	*	*	*
Occupational/physical therapies	*	*	*	*	*	*	*		*	*		*
Nutrition counselling	*	*	*		*		*					
Speech therapy					*		*					
Respiratory services		*	*	*	*	*	*	*		*		
Social work	*	*	*	*	*	*	*		*	*		*

*Means service is provided.
Information for Nunavut territory not available.
Sources: Adapted from Health Canada, *Provincial and Territorial Home Care Programs. A Synthesis for Canada,* cat. no. H21-147/1999E (June 1999), http://www.hc-sc.gc.ca/homecare/english/syn_7.html; Canadian Institute for Health Information, *Health Care in Canada.* (2001), p. 39.

Box 2-3 How Home Care Is Governed and Delivered

In all provinces and territories, the ministries or departments of health and/or social/community services are responsible for home care services. These departments monitor the services and decide on budgets, policies, and standards of care. In Nova Scotia and the Yukon, they also administer and deliver the services. In the rest of the country, other organizations administer and deliver home care. In British Columbia, Alberta, Saskatchewan, Manitoba, Prince Edward Island, Newfoundland, and the Northwest Territories, local or regional health authorities administer and deliver home care services. Ontario has Community Care Access Centres (CCACs), Quebec has Local Community Services Centres (CLSCs), and New Brunswick has the Extra-Mural Program (EMP) to administer and deliver their services.

Service delivery involves:

- Assessing clients' needs
- Determining clients' eligibility for professional and support services
- Coordinating and monitoring home care services. These services are provided by private or not-for-profit agencies. Eligible clients do not have to pay for these services
- Providing information and referrals to other long-term care services. These include volunteer-based community services such as Meals on Wheels. Some community services charge user fees to the client
- Providing placement services to assisted-living facilities and long-term care facilities (some provinces only)

REVIEW

Circle the BEST answer.

1. Canada's health care system is
   A. Publicly funded through provincial/territorial and federal taxes
   B. Delivered by government employees
   C. Funded by private insurance companies
   D. Strictly a federal responsibility

2. The provincial and territorial governments are responsible for
   A. Delivering health services to Aboriginal people and military personnel
   B. Delivering health services to inmates of federal penitentiaries and the RCMP
   C. Planning, financing, and delivering their own health insurance plans
   D. Paying the full amount of all medical procedures

3. Which law ensures that every citizen has access to health care?
   A. The *Long-Term Care Facilities Act*
   B. The *Canada Health Act*
   C. The *Medical Care Act*
   D. The *Hospital Insurance and Diagnostic Services Act*

4. Canadians who travel to other parts of the country still maintain their provincial/territorial health care coverage. This is an example of which principle of medicare?
   A. Comprehensiveness
   B. Universality
   C. Portability
   D. Public administration

5. The most pressing cause of health care reform has been
   A. Rising costs of providing technology, drugs, and services
   B. The Depression
   C. Lack of available technology
   D. Lack of accessibility

6. A recent trend in health care is to focus on
   A. Cutting back on public health policies
   B. Cutting back on home care services
   C. Opening more hospitals in rural areas
   D. Promoting public policy that promotes health and prevents disease

7. Immunization programs are an example of
   A. Home care services
   B. Disease prevention
   C. Facility-based treatment
   D. Medicare

8. One major focus of home care is to
   A. Enable clients to remain in their own homes
   B. Diagnose and treat disease
   C. Provide accommodation and care for people with disabilities
   D. Provide accommodation for acutely ill people who do not want to go to hospital

9. Support services provided through home care do *not* include
   A. Personal care
   B. Assistance with activities of daily living
   C. Respiratory therapy
   D. Assistance with home management

10. Which of the following is *not* provided by all provincial and territorial home care programs?
    A. Nursing care
    B. Speech therapy
    C. Assessment and case management
    D. Support services

11. In most provinces and territories, support services are delivered by
    A. The provincial or territorial government
    B. The federal government
    C. Private or not-for-profit agencies
    D. Regional health boards

Answers to these questions are on page 821.

CHAPTER

3

Workplace Settings

OBJECTIVES

- Define the key terms listed in this chapter
- Differentiate between community-based care and facility-based care
- List work settings where support workers are employed
- Differentiate between residential facilities and other medical facilities
- Describe the various types of residential facilities
- Identify the issues and challenges support workers encounter in the workplace

KEY TERMS

acute care Health care that is provided for a relatively short time (usually days to weeks) and is intended to diagnose and treat an immediate health issue

acute illness An illness that appears suddenly and lasts a short time, usually less than three months; symptoms can be severe

adult daycare Community day program

assisted-living facility A residential facility where residents live in their own apartments and are provided support services; supportive housing facility

chronic illness An on-going illness, slow or gradual in onset, that usually grows worse over time and cannot be cured

community-based services The health care and support services provided outside of a facility setting and in a community setting

community day program A daytime community-based program for people with physical and/or mental health problems or older adults who need assistance; adult daycare

convalescent care Subacute care

group home A residential facility in which a small number of people with physical and/or mental disabilities live together and are provided with supervision, care, and support services

hospice A facility that provides care for people who are dying

inpatient A patient who is assigned a bed and is admitted to stay in a facility overnight or longer

long-term care Medical, nursing, and/or support services provided over the course of months or years to people who cannot care for themselves

long-term care facility A facility that provides accommodations, 24-hour nursing care, and support services to people who cannot care for themselves at home but do not need hospital care

mental health services Services for people with mental disorders or emotional and behavioural problems

outpatient A patient who does not stay overnight in a facility

palliative care Services for people with progessive, life-threatening illnesses or conditions; these services aim to relieve or reduce uncomfortable symptoms but not produce a cure

rehabilitation services Therapies and educational programs designed to restore or improve the person's independence and functional abilities

residential facility A facility that provides living accommodations and services; includes assisted-living facilities and retirement residences

respite care Temporary care of a person with a serious illness or disability that gives the person's caregivers a break from their duties

retirement residence A facility that provides accommodation and supervision for older adults

supportive housing facility Assisted-living facility

subacute care Care provided to people who are recovering from surgery, injury, or serious illness; convalescent care

Support workers are employed in many settings. Each setting has different goals and services. This chapter describes common community-based and facility-based workplace settings. It also explores issues and challenges you may encounter in these settings. Wherever you work, you provide people with vital services that enable them to be as safe, comfortable, dignified, and independent as possible.

Working in Community-Based Settings

As discussed in Chapter 2, the current trend within the Canadian health care system is to decrease hospital costs and increase resources in **community-based services**. These include the health care and support services provided outside of a facility and in a community setting. For example, community-based services are provided in schools, community health centres, and doctors' offices. Home care agencies and day programs are the community-based services most likely to hire support workers.

HOME CARE

Home care is a vital part of Canada's health care system (see Chapter 2). Support workers have a central role within home care. Health Canada estimates that support workers are responsible for 80% of the total hours worked by all home care workers.[1] You provide a range of home care services, including assisting with personal care (Figure 3-1), activities of daily living, child care, transportation, and home management.

Support workers providing home care services are hired on a full-time, part-time, and casual basis. You must follow agency policies and procedures. Many agencies offer additional training. Box 3-1 describes some of the issues and challenges associated with working in home care.

COMMUNITY DAY PROGRAMS

A **community day program** (also called **adult daycare**) is a daytime program for people with physical and/or mental health problems or older adults who need assistance. Day programs meet the client's needs and provide a break for family caregivers. Programs are held in hospitals, nursing homes, community and recreational centres, church basements, and other settings.

Each day program is unique. Some programs offer rehabilitation for people with disabilities. Others offer counselling for people with mental illness. Many day programs offer recreational activities (Figure 3-2). Arts and crafts, social events, films, and board or card games are examples.

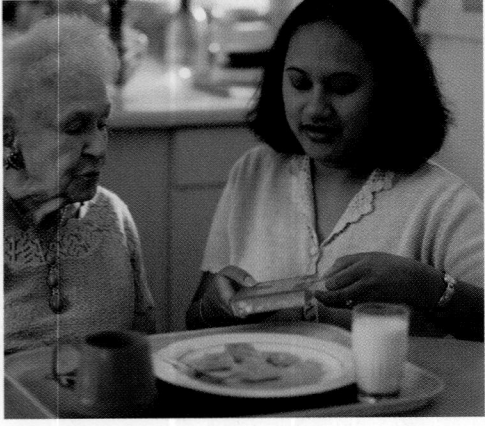

Figure 3-1 With the assistance of support workers, many people are able to remain in their own homes.

Box 3-1 Issues and Challenges Associated with Working in Home Care

- **Working on your own.** Home care work can be lonely and isolating. Many support workers prefer the hustle and bustle of a facility setting. Others like working one-on-one with a client by providing home care services. Not having a supervisor present may also present a challenge. Although your supervisor can be reached by phone, you sometimes need to use your own judgment to solve problems.
- **Taking direction from different health care professionals.** You may be expected to take directions from your supervisor and a number of different health care professionals. For example, the client's physiotherapist visits during your shift. He or she asks you to perform tasks that your supervisor has not asked you to do. These tasks are unfamiliar to you or not allowed by agency policy. Before taking on new tasks, always check with your supervisor.
- **Maintaining professional boundaries.** You often work closely with clients and family members. However, it is never appropriate to become personally involved in the client's life decisions and family relationships. You should always be caring and compassionate, but respect that a boundary does exist in your relationship with clients and their families. Do not mix professionalism with friendship. Clients and their families need your skills, services, and your undivided attention. Do not discuss your personal problems or ask them for advice. Keep these matters private and to yourself.
- **Providing for client safety.** Homes may have many safety hazards. Frayed electric cords and unsafe smoking practices are examples. Discuss any safety concerns with the client and your supervisor.
- **Providing for your personal safety.** In home care, you do not have control over the environment that you will enter. You will travel to unfamiliar areas. You may have to drive in hazardous weather conditions. Abuse or violence may occur in unfamiliar homes. You must look out for your own safety (see Chapter 16).

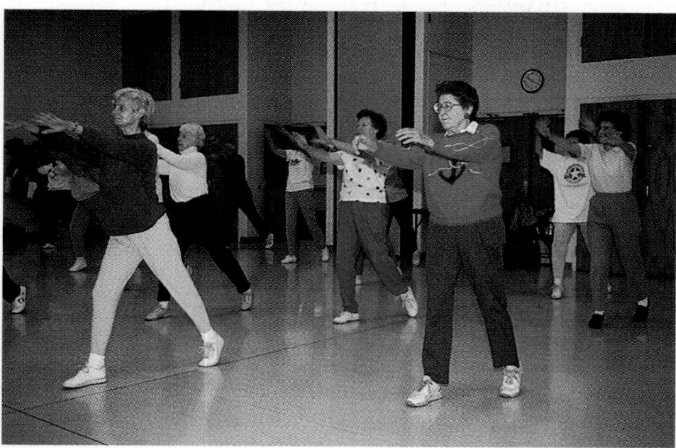

Figure 3-2 Community day programs provide recreational or other activities for clients during the day.

Support workers often work in community day programs. You provide personal care and assistance to people attending the program. You may assist with recreational and social activities. Follow all employer policies and procedures. Box 3-2 lists common issues and challenges associated with working in a community day program.

Working Directly for Clients

You may work directly for a client or the client's family. These people select and supervise their own support workers. People may hire their own support workers if they need a service that is not provided by the local agencies. Or, their province may provide funding assistance directly to them, not an agency. Box 3-3 describes issues and challenges associated with working directly for clients.

Box 3-2 Issues and Challenges Associated with Working in a Community Day Program

- **Working closely with a team and supervisor.** In most community day programs, you work closely with a supervisor and team members. This could be either a challenge or a benefit. Teamwork can be a success if team members have a common goal and work well together. It can be difficult if conflicts occur within the team. Good communication skills are necessary (see Chapter 5).
- **Working in a structured environment**. Many day programs have a highly structured environment, particularly those that provide rehabilitation. People with conditions such as Alzheimer's disease benefit from a predictable routine. To work in a structured environment, you must be very organized and sensitive to the person's needs.
- **Meeting multiple needs**. You may have to attend to the needs of many people. You must be able to focus on each person and quickly decide whose needs to address first. Good judgment and time management are essential.

Working in a Facility

A health care facility is a building designed or established for the delivery of specific care, treatment, and/or support services. Facilities provide a range of services.

Hospitals and Other Medical Facilities

Patients in hospitals usually have serious illnesses or injuries. They require skilled professional care and complex equipment. Some hospitals do not hire support workers, whereas others do. Support workers work in a variety of hospital departments depending on the role they fulfill. In most circumstances, you report to and are supervised by a nurse.

Your role may be to help people with basic care such as feeding. You may also transport people, take specimens to the lab, and measure vital signs. In some hospitals, you may assist before, during, or after surgical or medical procedures. You may perform other tasks, if requested and supervised by the nurse. You usually do not provide care for people in unstable condition.

Box 3-3 Issues and Challenges Associated with Working Directly for Clients

- **Clarifying the terms of employment.** Some employers may want a contract signed. Read the contract carefully before signing it. Hours and pay may change from week to week. Make sure you understand how many hours you are expected to work and what pay you can expect. If you are hired directly, your employer may be required to pay benefits such as unemployment insurance.
- **Establishing work limits.** Before you begin working for the person, ask what exactly is expected of you and how your performance will be evaluated. Ask for this in writing. Find out as much as you can about the person's preferences and standards.

Health care services are offered to **inpatients** (patients who are assigned a bed and admitted to stay in the facility overnight or longer) and to **outpatients** (patients who do not stay overnight in the facility).

Hospitals and other medical facilities provide a variety of services, including acute care, subacute care, long-term care, respite care, rehabilitation services, palliative care, and mental health services. Not all hospitals provide all these services. In some cities and towns, these services are provided in separate, specialized facilities. You may work in these or other medical facilities. The facility may require or provide additional training.

- *Acute care*—health care that is provided for a relatively short time (usually days to weeks) and is intended to diagnose and treat an immediate health issue. It is provided mainly in hospitals. An **acute illness** appears suddenly and lasts a short time, usually less than three months. Symptoms can be severe. Examples of acute illnesses are pneumonia and influenza.
- *Subacute care (convalescent care)*—health care or rehabilitation for people recovering from surgery, injury, or serious illness. The person's condition is stable, but he or she still needs care requiring complex equipment and procedures. Many hospitals and long-term care facilities (see page 28) provide subacute care. Eventually, the person is discharged home or to another level of care.
- *Long-term care*—health and/or support services provided over the course of months or years to people who cannot care for themselves. Many people who require long-term care have chronic illnesses. A **chronic illness** is an on-going illness, slow or gradual in onset, that usually grows worse over time. There is no known cure. The illness can sometimes be controlled and complications prevented. Examples of chronic illnesses are diabetes, multiple sclerosis, and Alzheimer's disease. Sometimes long-term care is provided for the remainder of the person's life. The goal of long-term care is to help the person cope with the challenges of living with a long-term illness or disability. Some hospitals provide long-term care. More often long-term care is provided in long-term care facilities or through home care services.
- *Respite care*—temporary care of a person with a serious illness or disability. Respite care gives the person's caregivers a break from their duties. Respite care is often provided by support workers in the client's home. Many hospitals and other facilities also offer respite care.
- *Rehabilitation services*—therapies and educational programs designed to restore or improve the person's independence and functional abilities. These services are for people who are or have been ill, injured, or disabled. Hospitals, long-term care facilities, and clinics offer rehabilitation services. Services may include life skills training, behaviour management, speech therapy, physiotherapy, job coaching, and family counselling. You may assist the client with personal care or activities of daily living. You may also assist with program delivery.
- *Palliative care*—services for people living with progressive, life-threatening illnesses or conditions that aim to relieve or reduce uncomfortable symptoms but not produce a cure. (*Palliate* means to soothe or relieve.) The goal of palliative care is to meet the physical, emotional, social, and spiritual needs of the client and family. Workers providing palliative care try to make the person's last days as painless, comfortable, and dignified as possible. You assist with personal care and activities of daily living. You also provide emotional support and encouragement to the client and family. Palliative care may be offered in hospitals, long-term care facilities, or in facilities called hospices. A **hospice** is a facility that provides palliative care to people who are dying. Palliative care is also offered in community-based settings. For example, most home care agencies and hospices provide palliative care to the person at home (see Chapter 46).
- *Mental health services*—services for people with mental disorders (such as schizophrenia, bipolar disorder, and addictions). Entire facilities, health care centres, and hospital units are devoted to caring for people with mental disorders. Assessment and treatment programs enable them to function as independently as possible within the community. Inpatient and outpatient services are provided. Rather than staying in a hospital, people are encouraged to return to the community. Here they have access to community-based care and support services.

Residential Facilities

A **residential facility** is a facility that provides living accommodations, care, and support services. These facilities vary in size and levels of care and support.

People using residential facilities are called *residents* because they reside, or live, in the facility. The facility is their temporary or permanent home. Therefore, these facilities provide care in a comfortable, homelike atmosphere (Figure 3-3). The social and emotional needs of the residents are met.

People require residential care when they cannot care for themselves at home but do not need acute medical care or high level nursing care. They include:

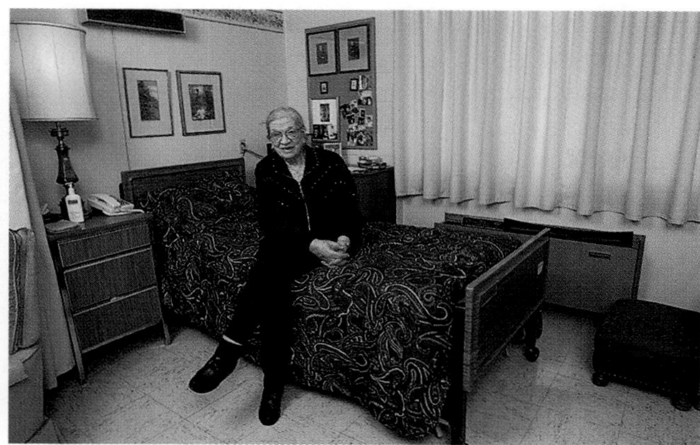

Figure 3-3 The atmosphere of a residential facility is as homelike as possible.

- Frail, older adults
- People of all ages who have physical or mental disabilities or both
- People with mental illness
- People with alcohol or drug problems

The type of facility appropriate for a person depends on the person's needs and level of independence. The types of residential facilities include assisted-living facilities, retirement homes, and long-term care facilities. Facility names vary across Canada.

Assisted-Living Facilities. Also called supportive housing facilities, **assisted-living facilities** are residential facilities where people live in their own apartments and are provided support services. Because they are located in the community, assisted-living facilities are also considered to be community-based services. Residents are usually older adults who require minimal care. Usually the setting is a multi-storeyed apartment building or condominium complex. Because apartments usually have kitchens, residents may cook their own meals. Many assisted-living facilities provide a common living area, activity room, and games room. Residents usually receive the following support services:

- 24-hour monitoring and emergency response services
- Social/recreational programs
- One or two daily meals
- Housekeeping and laundry

Some residents purchase extra support services if required. Not all residents need or want the same services. Some residents in assisted-living facilities may also qualify for home care.

Group homes are another type of assisted-living facility. A **group home** is a residential facility in which a small number of people with physical and/or mental disabilities live together and are provided with supervision, care, and support services. Rather than having their own apartments, residents share a house in a residential neighbourhood (Figure 3-4). Usually residents have private bedrooms and share bathrooms, living, and dining areas. They receive 24-hour supervision, meals, housekeeping and laundry services, and assistance with personal care and activities of daily living.

Residents of group homes are often adolescents or young adults who have disabilities or mental illness. There also are group homes for older adults, women leaving abusive situations, and people with substance abuse problems. The number and type of staff employed by a group home depends on the residents' needs.

All assisted-living facilities must be approved and licensed by the provincial or territorial government. Partial funding is provided by the government. Public or private agencies manage the facility and hire and supervise support workers. Your supervisor may be responsible for one or several assisted-living facilities. Some supervisors work onsite; others visit the facility periodically. Because the level of assistance varies among residents, you often perform a variety of tasks.

Retirement Residences. A **retirement residence** (or retirement home) is a facility that provides accommodation and supervision for older adults. Residents have their own bedrooms and bathrooms and share common living and dining areas (Figure 3-5 on page 28). They do not require nursing care and receive minimal assistance with activities of daily living. The goal of a retirement residence is to allow older people to live as independently as possible, while providing security, support services, and varying degrees of care, as needed.

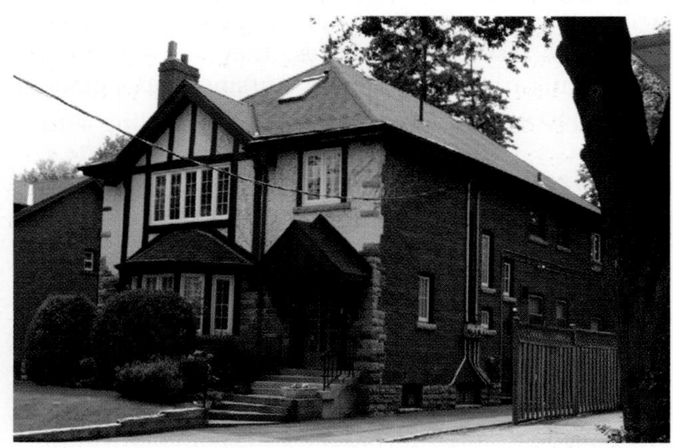

Figure 3-4 Group homes, another type of assisted-living facility, are usually situated in residential neighbourhoods.

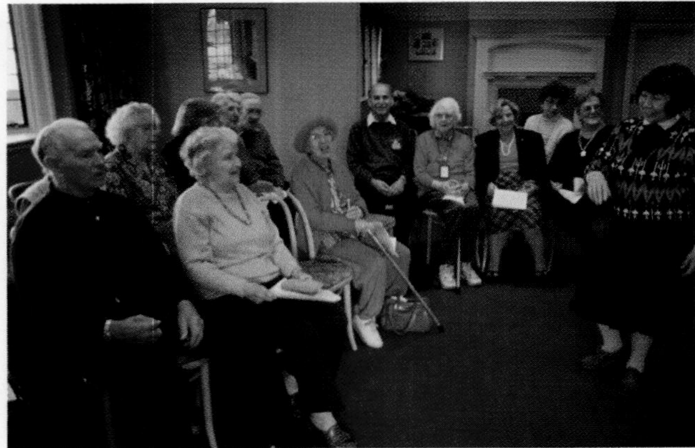

Figure 3-5 Residents living in retirement homes share common living and dining areas in a homelike environment.

Regulations governing retirement residences vary. In some provinces and territories they are privately operated. They are not regulated or financed by the government. Residents must pay the full cost. Standards, prices, and services vary. Some facilities are small, converted houses. Others are high-rise apartment buildings.

Support workers are almost always hired directly by the facility or the resident. If hired by a resident, you provide care only for that person. You perform many functions. You may run errands and provide transportation; assist with activities or social and recreational events; or provide help with various tasks, such as unpacking or organizing bedrooms.

Residents in retirement homes are not ill or disabled. Most can meet their own personal care needs. Usually personal care services are limited. For example, you may help the person get in and out of a bathtub. Once residents need more than minimal daily care, long-term care is needed. Some retirement facilities have a retirement residence and a long-term care facility. When residents need more assistance than the retirement residence provides, they move into the long-term care facility. Here, nursing and personal care services are available 24 hours a day.

Long-Term Care Facilities. These facilities (also called nursing homes, homes for the aged, long-term care homes, and special care homes) provide higher levels of care than retirement residences and assisted-living facilities. **Long-term care facilities** provide accommodations, 24-hour professional nursing care, and support services to people who cannot care for themselves at home but do not need hospital care. Most residents are frail, older adults with many health problems. Some residents are young and middle-aged adults who have severe, chronic health conditions or disabilities. The goals of these facilities are to maintain the residents' health and independence to the greatest extent possible and to meet their physical, emotional, social, intellectual, and spiritual needs.

Residents stay on a ward or in private or semi-private bedrooms. Usually each room has a bathroom with a toilet and sink. Tubs and showers are in common rooms. Besides nursing care, these facilities provide access to medical and rehabilitative care. They also provide assistance with personal care and activities of daily living, meals, laundry service, and recreational and social activities.

Long-term care facilities are licensed, regulated, and funded by the province or territory in which they are located. Medicare pays for some costs. Residents are required to pay a monthly fee. They also must pay for clothing, toiletries, hair dressings, and other incidentals. Government or charitable organizations operate some facilities on a not-for-profit basis. Private companies operate for a profit. Each facility hires its own staff.

Most long-term care facilities serve many residents with various physical or other disabilities. Therefore, the work environment is highly structured. RNs plan and coordinate resident care. You are a member of the health care team and report to a nurse. You provide personal care and assist with activities of daily living (Figure 3-6).

Many long-term care facilities have subacute care units. Some facilities have special care units for residents with specific disabilities. For example, a facility may have a dementia care unit for people with Alzheimer's disease or other dementias. There may also

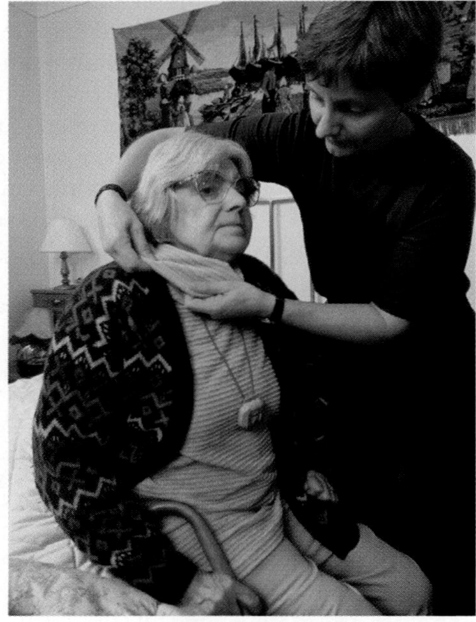

Figure 3-6 Residents in long-term care facilities may need support workers to assist them with activities of daily living.

be respite care and palliative care units. You may work in any of these units. Extra training may be required.

You may also work in the facility's recreation department. You may help organize and carry out recreational outings and activities. Here, you report to the recreation supervisor.

Issues and Challenges Associated with Facility-Based Care

As with working in the community, working in a facility also presents issues and challenges to the support worker (Box 3-4).

Box 3-4 Issues and Challenges Associated with Working in a Facility

- **Working in a structured team environment.** You work on a team with highly skilled professionals. Some people feel intimidated in such an environment. Remember that you are a valuable member of the team and have much to contribute at team meetings. In residential facilities you usually spend more time with residents than do the nurses and physicians. You have valuable insights and observations about the resident's daily needs and possible changes in health.
- **Meeting multiple needs and demands.** You must respond to many needs and demands. It may not be possible to respond immediately to all demands. You must be able to prioritize clients' needs and manage your time. You also must be flexible, diplomatic, and firm. Good organizational and communication skills are essential.
- **Doing many tasks in a short period of time.** You must provide thorough, competent, and respectful care within a short time. This requires self-discipline, dedication, and efficiency.
- **Respecting your scope of practice.** You work closely with nurses and may become familiar with many nursing procedures. Never attempt any procedure that you are not legally allowed to do. Only perform procedures allowed by law and facility policy. Never perform a procedure unless your supervisor has trained you and you are comfortable doing it. The facility has written policies to guide you.
- **Working in shifts.** Most facilities are staffed around the clock. You may have to work evening and night shifts.

Especially in Hospitals or Other Medical Facilities:

- **Dealing with people in distress.** Patients admitted to hospital or other medical facilities may show signs of intense emotional or physical distress. They may be in pain, afraid, upset, angry, or uncooperative. Remain calm and professional no matter how they express themselves. Also be sensitive to their feelings. Try to imagine how they are feeling. Sometimes you can provide emotional support just by holding a person's hand or listening to the person. With palliative care, you need to be strong and supportive in the presence of human suffering and intense emotions. If the person is facing a life-threatening illness, you need to be comfortable with your own feelings and attitudes toward death. Otherwise you may find it very difficult to care for the person.

Especially in Residential Facilities:

- **Making the facility feel like a home.** A residential facility is first and foremost the resident's home. Treat the setting with as much respect as you would your own home. Be careful with personal possessions. Make the facility a cheerful, comfortable place. Every staff member must contribute to a positive, homelike environment.
- **Respecting the person's privacy and dignity.** In any work setting, you must respect your client's privacy and dignity. Lack of privacy can lead to a loss of self-esteem, particularly during personal care. Carefully screen and cover the person. This may seem obvious, but sometimes it is easy to focus more on getting the job done rather than on respecting the need for privacy. As in other care situations, respecting privacy also includes keeping discussions with co-workers confidential and professional, respecting the person's property, and recognizing the person's right to express his or her preferences.
- **Maintaining professional boundaries.** You may care for residents who lack close personal relationships. You work closely with people and form strong attachments with them. This aspect of the job is what attracts many people to support work. However, do not become too personally involved with a resident or family. Always be caring and supportive. But remember that you are responsible for providing care and maintaining a professional outlook.

REVIEW

Circle the BEST answer.

1. A current trend in the Canadian health care system is to
- **A. Increase public spending on hospitals**
- **B. Decrease spending on community-based services**
- **C. Focus on providing more community-based services**
- **D. Promote facility-based services over home care**

2. Home care is an example of
- **A. A community-based service**
- **B. A facility-based service**
- **C. A community day program**
- **D. Palliative care**

3. Which work setting provides acute care?
- **A. Home care**
- **B. Long-term care facilities**
- **C. Assisted-living facilities**
- **D. Hospitals**

4. Which work setting may provide subacute care?
- **A. Retirement homes**
- **B. Long-term care facilities**
- **C. Group homes**
- **D. Hospices**

5. What type of service aims to provide a temporary break to family caregivers?
- **A. Acute-care services**
- **B. Palliative care**
- **C. Respite services**
- **D. Outpatient services**

6. Which of the following is *not* an example of a residential facility?
- **A. Group home**
- **B. Rehabilitation clinic**
- **C. Assisted-living facility**
- **D. Retirement residence**

7. Residents in retirement facilities generally include
- **A. People with mental illness**
- **B. Young adults with physical or other disabilities**
- **C. Frail, older adults with multiple health problems**
- **D. Older adults with limited care needs**

8. Residents in long-term care facilities generally require
- **A. 24-hour nursing care and support services**
- **B. Supervision and limited support services**
- **C. Acute care**
- **D. Housekeeping services, but not meal services**

9. Maintaining a homelike atmosphere is especially important in which setting?
- **A. Hospital**
- **B. Doctor's office**
- **C. Community day program**
- **D. Long-term care facility**

Answers to these questions are on page 821.

CHAPTER

4

HEALTH, WELLNESS, ILLNESS, AND DISABILITY

OBJECTIVES

- Define the key terms listed in this chapter
- Learn how definitions of health have changed
- Understand the concept of holism and explain how it affects your role
- Explain the current concepts of health and wellness
- Understand how health can be achieved in all dimensions of life
- Explain common reactions to illness and disability
- Describe change and loss associated with illness and disability
- Explain the effects of stigma and discrimination on people who are ill and disabled

KEY TERMS

disability The loss of physical or mental function

discrimination Behaviour that treats people unfairly based on their group membership

emotional health Well-being in the emotional dimension achieved when people feel good about themselves

health The state of well-being in all dimensions of one's life

holism A concept that considers the whole person; the whole person has physical, social, emotional, intellectual, and spiritual dimensions

illness The loss of physical or mental health

intellectual health Well-being in the intellectual dimension achieved through an active, creative mind

physical health Well-being in the physical dimension achieved when the body is strong, fit, and free of disease

prognosis The expected course of recovery based on the usual outcome of the illness

social health Well-being in the social dimension achieved when people have stable and satisfying relationships

social support system An informal group of people who help each other or others

spiritual health Well-being in the spiritual dimension achieved through the belief in a purpose greater than the self

stigma A characteristic that marks a person as different or flawed

wellness The achievement of the best health possible in all dimensions of one's life

Your job is to help people achieve or maintain good health. But what exactly is good health? This chapter examines the concepts of health and wellness. It also discusses the experiences of illness and disability. When caring for people who live with illness or disability, it could be easy to focus on the medical condition rather than on the person. Understanding what the person may be experiencing allows you to provide better, more compassionate care.

Health and Wellness

Definitions of health have changed over the years. At the end of the 1800s, health was defined by what it was not: health was the state of *not* being sick. At that time, the leading causes of death were diseases that spread from one person to another. Pneumonia, tuberculosis, and influenza, for example, were frequent killers. Anyone lucky enough to avoid an illness during an outbreak was considered healthy. During the first half of the 20th century, vaccinations, antibiotics, health education, and cleaner living conditions reduced the spread of disease. People were living longer and getting sick less often. But were they healthy? People began to consider that health is more than the absence of disease.

During the latter part of the 20th century, people recognized that health is affected by factors other than disease, such as lifestyle and environment. Discussions of health focused on the person rather than on the disease. There was also a new emphasis on holistic health. **Holism** means *whole*. A whole person has physical, emotional, social, intellectual, and spiritual dimensions. Each dimension relates to and depends on the others. Current views on health are holistic. **Health** is now considered to be a state of well-being in all dimensions of one's life (Figure 4-1). When providing holistic health care, you treat all dimensions of the person, not just the physical.

Health is sometimes referred to as wellness. **Wellness** is achieving the best health possible in all five dimensions of one's life. It is the perfect balance of body, mind, and spirit. Although many people try to achieve wellness, few actually have it. It is difficult to be healthy in all areas of life. At some point, everyone experiences ill health in one or all dimensions.

Seeking wellness is a process that lasts a lifetime. It involves making choices that improve the quality of your life. It also involves becoming the best you can be in all areas of your life, despite limitations. People with diseases or disabilities can still have a high level of wellness. Some individuals with excellent physical health may not achieve wellness. For instance, Soo Hee is an athlete in excellent shape. She eats well and trains daily. However, she does not make time for friends or family. She suffers from loneliness and lacks meaningful relationships. She is not content with her life. She must improve the emotional and social dimensions of her life in order to achieve wellness. Compare her with Michael. He has diabetes. However,

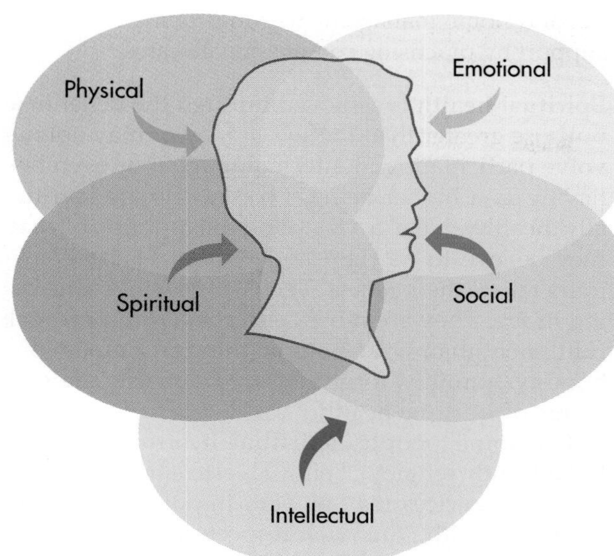

Figure 4-1 A whole person has physical, emotional, social, intellectual, and spiritual dimensions. Health is a state of well-being in all dimensions.

he manages his disease, feels good about himself, and has strong relationships and an active mind. He feels he has a meaningful, productive life. Despite his illness, he has achieved a high level of wellness.

Health is a continuum (Figure 4-2). On one end is optimal (complete) health or wellness. On the other end is extreme ill health. One's place on the continuum shifts, depending on life's circumstances. Remember that health is not constant throughout life. Everyone experiences physical illness and emotional stress during their lives. Most have average health.

However, it is possible to achieve well-being in each dimension of life:

- **Physical health** is achieved when the body is strong, fit, and free of disease. Physical health is influenced by genetics and lifestyle. The following factors contribute to physical health:
  - Following a nutritious diet according to *Canada's Food Guide* (see Chapter 25)
  - Exercising regularly
  - Living in a smoke-free environment
  - Drinking alcohol moderately or not at all
  - Having a good night's sleep
  - Following safety practices, such as using seat belts and bike helmets
  - Seeking medical attention when needed

  You have an important role in maintaining your clients' physical health. For instance, you help maintain a clean, safe, and comfortable environment. You also may prepare nutritious meals and assist with physical activity.

- **Emotional health** results when people feel good about themselves. They have strong self-esteem, self-control, and self-awareness. They are able to

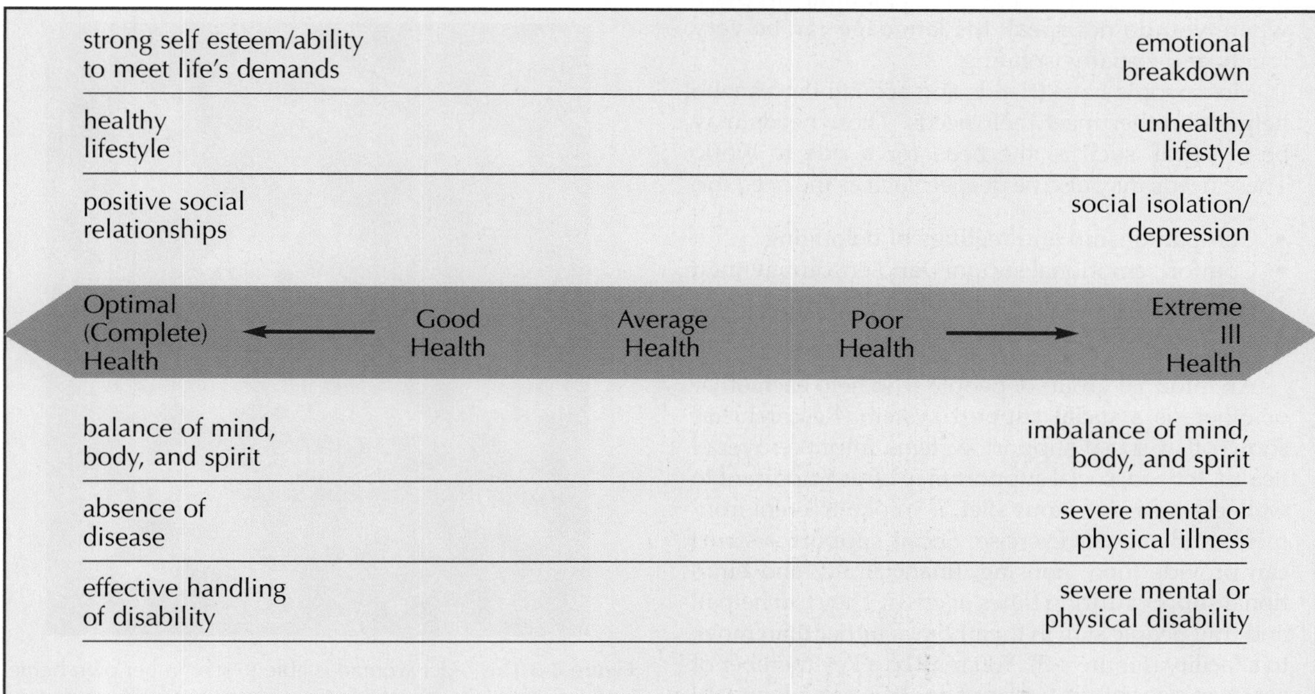

Figure 4-2 Continuum of health

give and receive from others, without worrying about being hurt or rejected. In contrast, emotionally unhealthy people are often insecure. When upset, they may feel overwhelmed and become aggressive.

Emotional health varies throughout one's life. For example, Mr. Szabo was confident, happy, and enjoyed many social relationships. However, at the age of 60, a series of disasters destroyed his emotional health: his daughter died in a car accident, his grandson died from a drug overdose, and he suffered a heart attack. While recovering from the heart attack, he experienced a major depression. This example shows that even emotionally strong individuals cannot always withstand misfortune and suffering.

You will work with emotionally healthy and unhealthy individuals. Some of these individuals will surprise you. For instance, a person who is usually cheerful may sometimes be irritable. Avoid judging people. Instead, learn to read their emotions so that you can respond in a caring manner.

- **Social health** is achieved through stable and satisfying relationships. Socially healthy people approach others with respect, warmth, and openness. They like and trust others. People with poor social health may show little regard for others and may use others for their own gain.

  Few people enjoy strong social health throughout life. Feelings of isolation and loneliness are common among older people and others who have lost their partners, friends, and other social relationships. New immigrants are also vulnerable to poor social health. Being in an unfamiliar place where you do not speak the language can be very lonely and socially isolating.

  Most people have friends and acquaintances who help each other meet their needs. These needs may be practical, such as the need for a ride to work. These needs may also be deeper, such as the need for:

  - Companionship and feelings of belonging
  - Comfort, emotional support, and encouragement
  - Reassurance of one's self-worth
  - Help, guidance, and advice

  An informal group of people who help each other or others is a **social support system.** Research has shown that social support systems improve overall health. Indeed, social support may be as important to wellness as a nutritious diet, a smoke-free environment, and regular exercise. Social support systems can provide food, housing, financial aid, and emotional support during times of crisis. They can help ill and frail people stay in their homes rather than move to a facility (Figure 4-3). You may be a key member of a person's social support system. You provide practical support, such as help with activities of daily living and home management. You provide emotional support by practising compassionate care.

- **Spiritual health** is achieved through the belief in a purpose greater than the self. It may or may not involve participating in a formal religion or even believing in a higher being. People who are spiritually healthy have a clear understanding of what they believe to be right and wrong. Their behaviours reflect their beliefs. They feel they have meaning in life. They are more concerned with personal fulfillment than with material things. Compassion, honesty, humility, forgiveness, and charity are elements of spiritual health.

  For some people, spiritual health is closely linked with religion. Being able to attend regular religious services may be very important for their spiritual health. You must respect people's expressions of their spirituality. In a facility, you may be responsible for transporting people to religious services within the building. Make sure you are not late for this task. In a private home, you may see many signs of the person's faith, such as religious icons. Always treat these items with respect. People in different cultures may express their spirituality in unique ways. (See *Respecting Diversity: Diversity, Health, and Spirituality* box.)

- **Intellectual health** is achieved through an active, creative mind. Recall the last time you talked with a child. You may have marvelled at the curiosity the child showed as he or she asked endless questions.

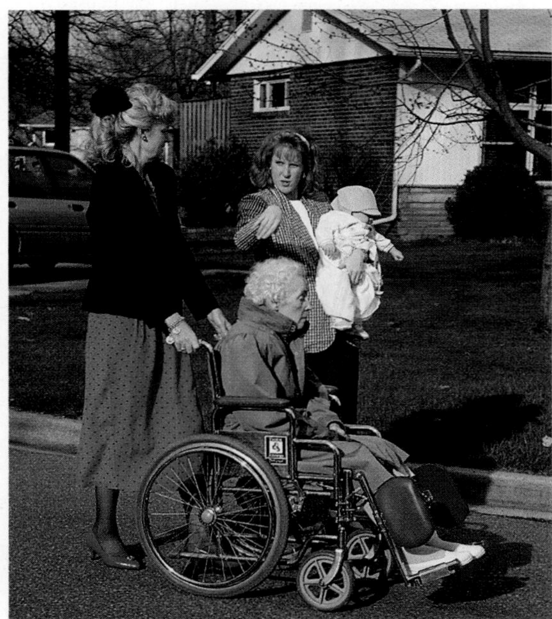

Figure 4-3 This older woman is able to stay in her own home because of her strong social support system. She has help from her daughter, her granddaughter, and support workers.

Respecting Diversity

DIVERSITY, HEALTH, AND SPIRITUALITY

In traditional Aboriginal culture, health and spirituality are closely connected. Illness can be prevented if the mind, body, and spirit are in harmony. Aboriginal healers include herbalists, diagnosticians, and shamans. In the Cree culture, shamans have special powers to bring together the Earth and the spirit world into harmony to aid in the healing process.

Aboriginal peoples recognized the mind/body/spirit connection long before people in Western cultures realized that health was more than the absence of disease. Today, many Aboriginal people combine traditional knowledge with modern health practices.

Source: P.A. Potter, A. Griffin Perry, J.C. Ross-Kerr, and M.J. Wood. *Canadian Fundamentals of Nursing,* 2nd ed. (Toronto: Harcourt Canada, 2001), p. 127.

Intellectually healthy people maintain this curiosity throughout life. They are interested in what is going on around them. They analyze, reason, and solve problems. They are open-minded and eager to learn.

People who lack intellectual health often take a passive approach to life. They do not try to become involved in community and world events. They may not even be involved in the lives of others. They often suffer from poor emotional, social, and physical health as well.

Many residential facilities have recreational programs and activities that promote intellectual and social health. Residents are encouraged to take part in games and outings. They are also encouraged to keep intellectually active when they are in their rooms. Activities such as reading, doing crossword puzzles, caring for indoor plants, doing crafts, and knitting all challenge the mind (Figure 4-4). You can promote your clients' intellectual health by encouraging them to keep their minds active. Talk with them about community and world events. (See *Support Workers Solving Problems: Helping Clients Maintain Intellectual and Social Health* box on page 36.)

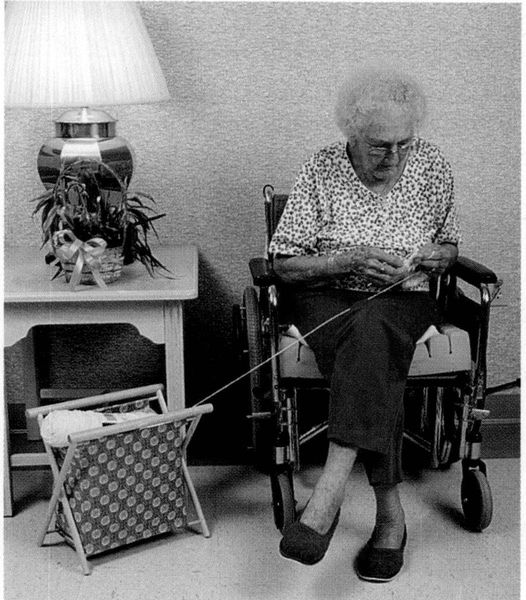

Figure 4-4 Activities such as knitting and reading can help keep the mind active.

Illness and Disability

Illness is the loss of physical or mental health. A **disability** is the loss of physical or mental function. Illness and disability may limit a person's ability to communicate, move, or perform activities of daily living without assistance. Some illnesses (such as influenza) and disabilities (such as a broken arm) last for a relatively short period of time. These are *acute* illnesses and disabilities. Other illnesses or disabilities (such as paraplegia) are *chronic* (permanent) and last for the person's life. Some chronic illnesses and disabilities are progressive: they become worse with time. Others can be managed to prevent further medical problems. Table 4-1 on page 36 lists medical conditions that many of your clients will have. See Chapters 31, 33–36, and 38 for complete descriptions of these and other common illnesses and disabilities.

It is important to remember that people with illness and disability are whole people. They are more than their medical conditions. You help them achieve their best physical health possible, but you also must consider their emotional, social, intellectual, and spiritual health.

The Experience of Illness and Disability

Illness and disability usually affect all aspects of a person's life. For instance, Mr. Spinelli recently suffered severe vision loss. His intellectual health suffers because he no longer reads or pursues his hobbies; his social health is affected because he can no longer travel to meet friends; his emotional health suffers because he is frustrated and depressed; his spiritual life is affected because he is angry at God and no longer wants to attend his church services.

No two people experience illness and disability in the same way. Some severely ill people remain cheerful and calm throughout their illness; others who are not seriously ill complain constantly or grow easily sad or frustrated. Many people who are disabled are

(text continues on page 37)

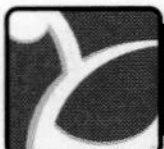

Support Workers Solving Problems

Helping Clients Maintain Intellectual and Social Health

Scenario: Emma is a support worker at a long-term care facility. She works on a floor for residents with physical problems such as arthritis and osteoporosis. Mrs. Davidson is a resident on Emma's floor. She is 92 years old and loves to read. She reads the newspaper every morning. She listens to a book on tape in the afternoon. One day Mrs. Davidson told Emma that she misses talking about books with other people. Emma knows that many other residents like to read and listen to stories. She wonders if there is a way to bring these people together as a group.

Discussion: Emma suggests to her supervisor that the facility start a book club. Emma explains that discussing books will help the residents maintain sharp minds. It will also help them develop friendships. Emma's supervisor likes her idea, and speaks to the recreation director about it. By the end of the month, a weekly book club meeting is up and running, with Mrs. Davidson as leader. The book club becomes so popular that within a year there are two separate clubs—one for fiction, and one for nonfiction.

Table 4-1 Common Illnesses and Disabilities

AIDS	The late stage of infection with the human immunodeficiency virus (HIV). HIV attacks the immune system. People with AIDS are vulnerable to developing infections (such as pneumonias) and cancers. The virus is spread from an infected person to someone else through the exchange of body fluids or through infected needles or blood.
Alzheimer's disease	The most common type of dementia (see below). A disease in which nerve cells in the brain, particularly those responsible for storing memories, are gradually destroyed. Affects a person's ability to understand, think, remember, and communicate.
Anxiety disorders	Disorders in which the person has a high degree of anxiety.
Arthritis	A condition affecting joints and/or connective tissue. Causes inflammation (swelling, redness, heat, and pain) of the joints. The two most common types of arthritis are osteoarthritis and rheumatoid arthritis.
Asthma	A disease in which air passages narrow, causing sudden breathing difficulties.
Bipolar disorder	A mental disorder involving extreme mood swings. Depression is at one extreme (see below); mania (elation) is at the other.
Cancer	An abnormal growth of cells that spread throughout the body.
Cardiovascular disease	Disease affecting the heart and/or blood vessels.
Chronic bronchitis	An inflammation of the bronchi (tubes that bring air into the lungs). Usually caused by smoking and results in chronic cough.
Coronary artery disease	An artery is a vessel that carries oxygen-rich blood. Coronary artery disease occurs when the arteries that supply blood to the heart muscles are narrowed by a build-up of fatty material along their inside walls. This narrowing decreases the amount of blood and oxygen reaching the heart muscle. A heart attack occurs when blood flow is suddenly cut off completely.
Dementia	Progressive impairment of all aspects of brain function. Symptoms include loss of memory, judgment, and reasoning. Dementia also causes changes in mood and behaviour.
Depression	A mood disorder involving feelings of sadness, helplessness, and worthlessness. The person may also experience difficulty concentrating, poor memory, and distorted thinking. Major depression may cause a person to consider or attempt suicide.
Diabetes	A condition in which the body is unable to produce or properly use insulin. Insulin is a hormone that helps cells absorb glucose (sugar) for energy. Without insulin, glucose levels in the body become abnormally high. Left untreated or poorly managed, diabetes damages the small and large blood vessels in the body, resulting in complications like heart disease, blindness, kidney disease, and the need for amputation.
Emphysema	A disease in which air is trapped inside the lungs, resulting in difficulty breathing.
Heart attack	Occurs when part of the heart muscle dies due to lack of oxygen. Usually is caused by a sudden blockage of an artery leading to the heart.

Continued

Table 4-1 Common Illnesses and Disabilities — cont'd

Influenza	An infection of the respiratory tract caused by a virus. It spreads easily through the air when an infected person coughs or sneezes.
Multiple sclerosis (MS)	A disease of the central nervous system in which nerve impulses are disrupted. People with MS can experience a range of symptoms, including balance and coordination problems, fatigue, difficulties with speech and swallowing, and cognitive (thinking) problems.
Osteoporosis	Deterioration of bone tissue caused by lack of calcium in the bones; results in brittle and easily broken bones.
Paraplegia	Paralysis from the waist down; paralysis of the legs.
Parkinson's disease	A chronic disease of the nervous system that gradually impairs body movement. People with Parkinson's disease frequently experience trembling in their hands, arms, and legs; impaired balance and coordination; and difficulty walking, speaking, chewing, and swallowing.
Pneumonia	An infection of the lungs, causing fever and cough. Often the person coughs up sputum (secretions) and has difficulty breathing.
Quadriplegia	Paralysis from the neck down; paralysis of the arms, legs, and trunk.
Schizophrenia	A mental disorder in which thinking and behaviour are disturbed.
Stroke	Occurs when part of the brain is injured due to lack of oxygen. Usually is caused by a blocked or burst artery leading to the brain. People who have had strokes often experience paralysis or weakness on one side of the body, partial vision loss, memory problems, and difficulties learning new information or communicating.

not ill. Nor do they consider themselves ill. People born with disabilities have never known life any other way. Many people disabled later in life adjust to their situation. They need no further medical care. Although people's experiences vary, health care professionals have found common reactions to newly acquired illness and disability (Box 4-1 on page 38).

Factors affecting a person's experience of illness and disability include:

- The nature of the illness or condition
- The person's age
- The person's level of physical fitness
- The amount and degree of pain and discomfort the person experiences
- The **prognosis** (the expected course of recovery based on the usual outcome of the illness)
- The person's emotional, social, intellectual, and spiritual health
- The person's personality and ability to cope with difficulties
- The person's culture; cultural background may influence how the person perceives the illness, seeks treatment, and interacts with caregivers and health care workers (see Chapter 11)
- The presence of emotional, social, and financial support

Change and Loss Associated with Illness and Disability

People with serious illness or recent disability must cope with change and loss. The following are just a few of the many changes these people must face:

- *Change in routine.* Daily routines almost always change. Time previously spent at work or with friends and family is often now filled with doctors' appointments, tests, and treatments. For many people, activities of daily living suddenly become challenges. Concerns such as getting to the bathroom, making meals, eating, and controlling pain are serious issues.
- *Change in work life.* Many people with serious illness or disability quit or limit work. People who feel rewarded and fulfilled by their work may suddenly feel worthless when they can no longer work (Box 4-2 on page 38). The loss of work may also result in financial problems and loss of social interactions.
- *Change in family life.* Serious illness or disability almost always disrupts family life. When one family member is ill, often the lives of everyone at home change greatly. Every family member must adjust and take on new roles. For example, Mrs. Kim has a severe stroke. She can no longer be breadwinner and caregiver for her teenage children. Her role changes to that of patient. While she recovers, her children must now take care of her, with help from professional caregivers. The children may have to give up after-school activities or time with their friends. The changes and new roles often create stress. Sometimes the stress on the family members is so severe that their own health suffers (see Chapter 6).
- *Change in sexual function.* Disability and illness often affect sexual function. A person may feel unfit for closeness and love. The person may be uninterested in sex. He or she may be physically unable to have sex because of the side effects of medications

or illness. Reproductive surgery, heart disease, stroke, spinal cord injuries, and nervous disorders are among the many conditions that can affect sexual function in men and women. Changes in sexual function greatly affect people. Fear, anger, worry, and depression are common. These are normal and

Box 4-1 Common Reaction to Illness and Disability

- **Fear and anxiety.** Even minor illness can cause anxiety. People with serious illnesses have many fears and anxieties: the effects of their illness on their family; how they will manage their daily responsibilities; financial problems; their families' future; death. People with disabilities, disfigurements, or speech or memory problems may worry about embarrassing themselves in front of others. People with mental illnesses often experience severe anxiety. Some client's fears may make sense to you; others may not. To the person experiencing the fear, however, it is real. Some people will communicate their fear and anxiety to you, but many will not. They prefer to keep their concerns to themselves.
- **Sadness and grief.** People facing loss are usually sad. People with serious illness and disabilities often deal with many losses—loss of position, loss of independence, loss of confidence. For some, there is loss of their plans for the future. These losses can cause intense grief. People who are grieving need to mourn. Observe and listen to your clients so you can understand their needs. Some people do not want to talk about their feelings; others find it helpful to talk to an understanding, caring person.
- **Depression.** Fear, anxiety, sadness, and grief can lead to depression. People coping with serious illness, progressive disability, or the challenges of old age are at risk for depression. People who are depressed are often tired, anxious, and uninterested in life. They may avoid contact with other people. People who are severely depressed may be suicidal. Observe closely for any changes in a client's mood, energy levels, and behaviour. Report these changes to your supervisor immediately (see Chapter 33).
- **Denial.** Denial is a refusal to recognize and admit the truth. People who are afraid that they might be seriously ill may downplay or deny symptoms. Even people who know that they are seriously ill may deny their situation. For example, a diabetic teenager may refuse to take her insulin or demand foods that she should avoid. A middle-aged man with heart problems may continue to shovel his driveway even though he is under strict doctor's orders not to do heavy work. This is their way of denying that they have serious health problems. If you think a client is denying his or her condition, be understanding and positive. If the person's denial may cause harm, let your supervisor know.
- **Anger.** People may be angry because they resent their limitations, their illness, and their inability to control their life. They may direct their anger toward their physician, family, friends, or caregivers. Some people direct their anger toward their support worker. You have to be calm, patient, and gentle if this happens. Avoid becoming angry yourself. That will make the situation worse. Try to understand the client's needs and problems. Imagine what life must be like for that person. However, you do not need to accept abuse. Learn how to react when faced with an angry client (see Chapters 12 and 19).

Box 4-2 Case Study: The Effect of Serious Illness on Self-Esteem

On Wednesday, Tony Vitale felt on top of the world. He got up at 6:00 a.m., as usual, and ran for half an hour. Over breakfast, he reviewed the speech he was to give at his company's annual meeting. He was looking forward to announcing that profits were up. At the age of 46, he had achieved his life's goal of becoming chief executive officer (CEO) of a major corporation.

Tony Vitale never gave his speech. As he stepped up to the podium, he let out a short gasp and collapsed to the floor. When he awoke ten hours later, he did not recognize his wife or his two children. He could not speak or understand anything that was said. He had suffered a severe stroke.

Within four months, it became clear that Mr. Vitale would never recover sufficiently to return to his job. Although his memory eventually returned, his speech remained difficult for others to understand. He also had difficulties understanding others. The news that his position had been filled by a new CEO overwhelmed him with sadness. Throughout his adult life, Mr. Vitale's job gave him the recognition, prestige, and status that he craved. Without it, he felt useless and depressed.

During eight months of therapy and rehabilitation, Mr. Vitale made real progress. Although he found long sentences difficult to understand, other people could now understand much of what he said. With the support of his family and a caring health care team, his depression gradually lifted. He began to realize that he still had something to offer the world. He discovered that he enjoyed painting. He also spent time as a volunteer with people suffering from brain injury. His newfound self-esteem came from the knowledge that he was making a useful contribution.

expected reactions. Time, understanding, and a caring partner are helpful. Professional counselling may help a couple adjust.

- *Loss of independence.* Independence is the state of being able to do things for oneself. Losing one's independence can be very hard. It is particularly distressing when the onset of the illness or disability is sudden and there is little or no hope for recovery. You must try at all times to promote your clients' independence to the best of their abilities.
- *Loss of dignity.* Independence and dignity are closely related. For some people, losing their independence can lead to a loss of dignity. This is particularly true when they need help with personal care. It can be extremely difficult to depend on others for private matters, including bodily functions. Always be sensitive to your clients' need for dignity.
- *Change in self-image.* Self-image is the individual's perception of himself or herself. Changes to a person's body caused by illness may affect self-image. People who have lost body parts or have scars due to surgery or accidents may feel unattractive or even repulsive. Others who have conditions that affect the way they look, move, walk, or speak may feel very self-conscious.

You can help clients who are ill and disabled by understanding how their condition affects every aspect of their lives. Do not make assumptions. Do not judge the person's behaviour or compare one person's reaction to illness with another's. Do everything you can to communicate warmth, acceptance, and respect. Always keep the priorities of support work in mind. (See *Providing Compassionate Care: Caring for Clients Who Are Ill or Disabled* box.)

ATTITUDES OF OTHERS TOWARD ILLNESS AND DISABILITY

Some people are uncomfortable or fearful when they are with ill or disabled people. They may stare or avoid eye contact. They may treat ill and disabled people differently than those who are well and able-bodied.

Ms. Leblanc used a wheelchair after injuring her spinal cord. She said that it was very hard getting used to the way some people treated her. "The first time my husband and I went out to dinner after the accident, the waiter asked my husband what I wanted for dinner. To the waiter, I was invisible. Since then I have met many people who ignore me or treat me like a child. I've learned to live with it, but it still hurts."

Some ill and disabled people experience stigma and discrimination. A **stigma** is a characteristic that marks a person as different or flawed. It is often associated with shame or disgrace. **Discrimination** is behaviour that treats people unfairly based on their group membership. People with AIDS, mental illness, and substance abuse disorders are vulnerable to discrimination. Sometimes they are blamed for their misfortunes. They and their families are deprived of much-needed social support. Rejection can lead to isolation, loneliness, and depression. Rejection can also lead to feelings of self-blame and guilt.

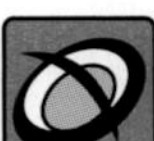

Providing Compassionate Care

CARING FOR CLIENTS WHO ARE ILL OR DISABLED

Dignity. Being helped with bathing, toileting, and other activities of daily living can be extremely embarrassing and harm a person's dignity. Never unnecessarily expose a client's body. Be aware of your facial expressions and gestures. They may reveal that you are disturbed by the person's disfigurement or body odours. This would cause feelings of shame.

Independence. Encourage clients to take part in their care. Tell them what you are about to do and ask how they can help. People may be able to do some of the steps in a procedure themselves. Let clients make decisions for themselves if they are able. For example, people who are paralyzed may not be able to dress themselves, but they can decide what to wear.

Preferences. Ask clients how they want tasks done. You may have to ask for specific information. For example, ask what is important to them, what they enjoy doing, what they are able to do, what they find easy, and what they find difficult.

Privacy. Clients may feel that their privacy is violated. They may need to adjust to all the people around providing care. Never snoop when you are in a client's room or house. The following promote privacy: knocking before entering, drawing curtains and blinds, closing doors and windows, covering people during personal care activities, and keeping client information confidential. People who are ill and disabled still have sexual needs, including the need for touching, caressing, and embracing. Allow privacy for the person's sexual needs.

Safety. All people need to feel safe from harm. People who are ill or disabled have special safety needs. Check with your supervisor and the care plan for specific safety measures for each client. Follow the safety measures described in Chapter 16. Never force people to do more than they are able. Allow time for rest. View the room from their perspective. Ask yourself if there is a safe passage to the bathroom, or if any items could cause falls or injuries. If you are not sure the person's safety needs are being met, talk to the person and to your supervisor.

REVIEW

Circle the BEST answer.

1. **In the 1800s, good health was considered to be**
   A. Well-being in all dimensions of life
   B. Optimal wellness
   C. The absence of disease
   D. Physical, emotional, and social well-being

2. **A holistic approach to health is one that**
   A. Takes a realistic view of a person's health problems
   B. Takes into account the whole person
   C. Focuses on the person's illness or disability
   D. Focuses on the person's physical health

3. **Which of the following is *not* one of the five dimensions of health?**
   A. Emotional health
   B. Spiritual health
   C. Recreational health
   D. Social health

4. **Which factor does *not* contribute to good physical health?**
   A. A good night's sleep
   B. A tobacco-free environment
   C. The regular use of seat belts
   D. A high-fat diet

5. **Which of the following is *false*? People with strong emotional health**
   A. Show their emotions easily
   B. Have strong self-esteem
   C. Exhibit self-control
   D. Are aware of their own strengths and weaknesses

6. **A social support system is**
   A. A group of people who volunteer in the community
   B. A system of social welfare
   C. An informal network of people who help each other or others
   D. Another term for a health care team

7. **An acute illness**
   A. Appears suddenly and lasts a short time
   B. Is a slow, progressive illness
   C. Results in disability
   D. Is another term for influenza

8. **Which of the following is *not true* of chronic illness?**
   A. It is a slow, progressive illness.
   B. The symptoms often appear gradually.
   C. It may result in physical or mental disability.
   D. People usually recover.

9. **Which of the following is a *true* statement?**
   A. People respond to illness and disability in much the same way.
   B. People's response to illness and disability varies.
   C. Almost all ill and disabled people are depressed.
   D. Most ill and disabled people are in denial.

10. **The term stigma means**
    A. Denial
    B. An artificial opening between the colon and the abdominal wall
    C. A characteristic that marks a person as different or flawed
    D. A refusal to admit the truth

Answers to these questions are on page 821.

CHAPTER

5

Working with Others: Teamwork, Supervision, and Delegation

OBJECTIVES

- Define the key terms listed in this chapter
- List the benefits and challenges to working on a health care team
- Explain your role on the health care team
- Describe how teams function in different health care settings
- Explain how delegating applies to you
- Describe the delegation process and your role in it

KEY TERMS

accountable Being responsible for the outcome; involves answering questions and explaining actions

assigning Giving responsibility for providing care

authority The legal right to do something

case manager A health care professional who assesses, monitors, and evaluates a client's needs in a community care setting; also coordinates team services

delegation A process by which an RN authorizes another health care provider to perform certain tasks; transfer of function

family conference A meeting attended by the health care team and family members to discuss a client's care

multidisciplinary team A team of health care providers from a variety of backgrounds and specialties who work together to meet the client's needs

task A function, procedure, or activity that you assist with or perform for the client

transfer of function Delegation

This chapter discusses the health care team and your role on the team. It also discusses the relationship between you and your supervisor. All health care workers must protect their clients from harm. Understanding the delegation process will help you protect clients and prevent potential legal problems.

The Health Care Team

In most health care settings, you work on a team. A team is a group of people who work together toward a common goal (see Chapter 1). The goal of a health care team is to provide the client with the best possible care and support. When providing care, team members must consider the whole person. You must promote health in all five dimensions of the person's life: physical, emotional, social, intellectual, and spiritual (see Chapter 4). Health care team members depend on each other to perform their roles to the best of their ability. Members of effective teams support one another and communicate effectively.

Members of health care teams vary from setting to setting and from team to team. The client's needs determine who will be on the team. For example, Tom Brown, 15, has mental health problems. Tom, his parents, an RN, psychiatrist, social worker, and support worker work together as a team. Tom's team is different from Mrs. Darby's team. Mrs. Darby, 86, is recovering from hip surgery. She and her daughter are on a team with an RN, social worker, physical therapist, and support workers. The client is an active member of the team unless he or she is not mentally capable of being involved or chooses not to participate.

In some situations, you and a nurse may be the only health care providers on the team. In others, you may be part of a multidisciplinary team. A **multidisciplinary team** includes health care providers from a variety of backgrounds and specialties who work together to meet the client's needs.

Benefits of Working on a Team

There are many benefits to the team approach to health care. A group of people is often better at making decisions and solving problems than one person. The many benefits of a team approach to care include:

- *Opportunities for collaboration.* All team members are encouraged to *collaborate* (to work together toward a common goal). Successful collaboration creates a positive atmosphere that even the client can sense. Staff and clients benefit when team members share information. For example, you find a way to ease a client's discomfort during a bed bath. You share this information with the nurse. The nurse asks other support workers to use your method.
- *Opportunities for communication.* Team meetings provide the opportunity for all team members to share experiences, opinions, and ideas. Without the meetings, valuable ideas might be missed. Box 5-1 contains part of a dialogue from a team meeting. Notice how each team member adds to the complete picture of the client's health.
- *A wide array of abilities, skills, and perspectives.* Team members include individuals with a range of abilities, skills, training, and experience. Each team member has ideas and viewpoints that he or she brings to the team. In Box 5-1, notice the support worker's contributions. Because she is the only person who has daily contact with Mrs. Darby, she provides important information. The other team members know more about the health and medical

Box 5-1 Contributions to a Team Meeting

A health care team in a long-term care facility is meeting to discuss a resident's rehabilitation following hip surgery. Mrs. Darby is 86 years old. Her team consists of herself, her daughter, an RN, two support workers, a social worker, and a physical therapist. At the last meeting, the physical therapist suggested exercises to help Mrs. Darby regain mobility. Since then, the physical therapist has shown Mrs. Darby how to do the exercises. A support worker has helped her practise the exercises. Mrs. Darby has chosen not to attend the team meeting. The following team members attended the meeting:

- An RN, who is also the team leader
- A support worker (Meredith)
- A physical therapist
- A social worker
- Mrs. Darby's daughter (Sandra)

RN: I understand that Mrs. Darby is having difficulty with some of her exercises. Meredith, could you please tell the team what you have observed?

Support worker: Well, Mrs. Darby has been having trouble with all the exercises. They give her great pain. She has such a grimace on her face when she attempts them. Let me tell you what she said on Tuesday morning. (Checks notes.) *"I can't do these exercises. They feel like someone is boring holes in my hip."*

Physical therapist: Can you tell me how high she is able to lift her leg?

Support worker: About two inches off the bed.

Physical therapist: Is she taking her pain medication?

RN: Yes, I help her with her medication. She takes it regularly. To me, Mrs. Darby seems much less cheerful than usual. Has anyone else noticed this?

Support worker: Yes, I've noticed that she is much less outgoing than usual. She used to read the newspaper in the mornings. Now, she just sits in her chair. When I ask her how she is feeling, she says she is tired. She told me that she is not attending this meeting because she is so tired.

RN: Perhaps Mrs. Darby is depressed. Sandra, what do you think?

Daughter: I'd say that Mom is definitely feeling down. I just thought it was because of the broken hip and the surgery. Who wouldn't be after what she has been through? She used to be so cheerful and outgoing. Perhaps Mom is depressed. I haven't heard her mention any of her friends lately. Are they keeping in touch?

Social worker: Didn't your mother tell you that her roommate, Mrs. Martino, died suddenly two weeks ago?

Daughter: No, she didn't mention it. That's odd. Gosh, she was close to Mrs. Martino. That must have been a blow.

RN: I think someone needs to talk to Mrs. Darby to find out how she is feeling. Maybe she will have some ideas of ways we might help. She might benefit from some outings and other social activities.

Social worker: I will talk with Mrs. Darby. She may be going through a natural grieving period for her friend. We may also need to discuss this with her family physician.

The discussion continues.

conditions that are discussed. However, only the support worker is in a position to share daily observations about Mrs. Darby.

- *Better decision making and problem solving.* When team members discuss issues, they are more likely to make sound decisions and find appropriate solutions to problems. When information is shared, workable solutions are found.
- *A positive, trusting atmosphere.* Trust develops when team members can be relied upon to do their jobs well, to respect each other, and to share responsibility. The team leader is responsible for fostering a high level of trust. The leader should encourage team members to openly discuss problems. Team members also play a role in creating trust. They must not blame others for their own mistakes. They should take responsibility for their own actions.

Challenges to Working on a Team

Just as there are many benefits to working on a team, there are also challenges:

- *Recognizing role boundaries.* In successful teams, team members understand each other's role. You may become familiar with tasks that support workers are not permitted to perform. Never attempt any task that you are not allowed to perform. You must be aware of your scope of practice and your employer's policies and procedures.
- *Being flexible.* Teams function best when members are willing to meet each other's needs. This requires flexibility. For example, you can help coworkers by exchanging shifts. You might also assist them with certain tasks. Remember, you might need your supervisor's permission first.

- *Handling conflict.* Any group of people is bound to have disagreements. How conflict is handled affects the whole team. The team leader is critical to the resolution of conflict. Team members should feel comfortable addressing problems with their leader. They should also address conflict rather than hope it will go away. This may mean talking to a co-worker with whom you are having problems. If you have hurt someone's feelings, you need to apologize. You also need to admit your mistakes.
- *Expressing your needs and views.* Support workers sometimes feel intimidated on a team that includes physicians and other health care professionals. You are a valuable team member. Often you spend more time with the client than do other team members. You have a great deal to contribute to team meetings.

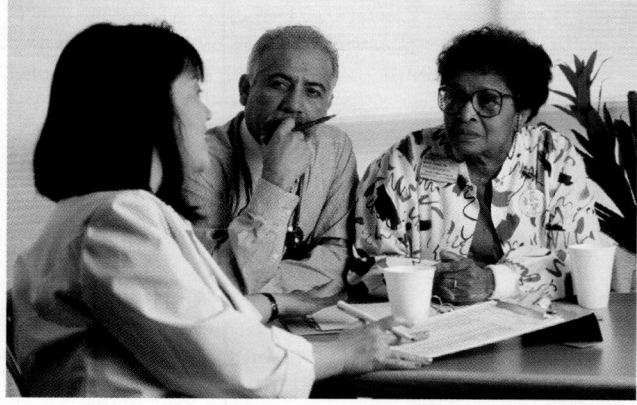

Figure 5-1 A team in a long-term care facility meets to discuss a resident's care.

Teamwork in Facilities

Teams in facilities vary as much as the settings themselves. For example, a team at a retirement home functions differently from a team at a hospital. A hospital team functions differently from a team in a long-term care facility. However, most teams in facilities have one thing in common: team members work in the same location. This makes communication easy. Team members have many opportunities to meet and collaborate.

Long-Term Care Facilities. Most long-term care facilities use a multidisciplinary team approach to care. Teams include physicians, nurses, social workers, support workers, therapists, the resident, and the resident's family. In a large facility, the team may also include the pharmacist, activity director, and other staff members. Usually the team leader is an RN. Often one RN is team leader for all the residents. The same team provides care to all residents. Support workers have many opportunities to work with other team members (Figure 5-1).

Hospitals. Team functions and members vary from hospital to hospital and department to department. Many departments use a multidisciplinary team approach. Specialists and other health care providers are brought together as needed.

Hospices and Palliative Care Units. Most hospices and palliative care units use a multidisciplinary approach. A team usually consists of nurses, support workers, physicians, social workers, volunteers, the client, and family members. Depending on the client's wishes, other individuals may be on the team. A spiritual adviser is an example.

Although hospices and palliative care units are facilities, they are also considered community-based services. Outreach programs provide palliative care to people at home. Team members meet in the facility or in the client's home.

You may be asked to attend a family conference. A **family conference** is a meeting attended by the health care team and family members to discuss the client's care. Family conferences are usually held when difficult situations arise. Family members can ask questions, express feelings, and make difficult decisions. Family conferences are common in hospice and community care settings. They are also held in hospitals and other facilities.

Assisted-Living Facilities. These community-based facilities are usually located in a single building. Being in one building makes communication easier. Staffs in assisted-living facilities (including group homes) are small. They are often multidisciplinary. The make-up of the team depends on the needs of the clients. Teams usually have a supervisor (who may be an RN, an RPN, a social worker, or a qualified youth care worker), and one or two support workers. There may also be other assistive personnel.

Teamwork in Community Settings

Teams in community settings also vary in membership and function.

Home Care. The home care team usually includes the client, family members, the case manager, family physician, nurses, and support workers and their supervisors. Social workers and therapists may also be on the team.

The **case manager** assesses, monitors, and evaluates a client's needs in a community care setting. He or she also coordinates the services of the team. A case manager could be a nurse, but may be a social worker or other professional. Occasionally, the client chooses to be the case manager (see Chapter 7).

Home care teams do not always meet regularly. Team members may communicate with each other by telephone or written reports. The case manager schedules a team meeting when the need arises.

Community Day Programs. Teams in community day programs function differently from home care teams. A rehabilitative program team may include a supervisor (who is often a nurse or other health professional), other professionals, and support workers. A recreational program team may include a supervisor (who is usually a recreational or occupational therapist) and support workers. In a day program, you will probably work with the same team every day. There are regular opportunities to discuss your clients' progress. You may meet before the program starts, after it is over, or weekly.

Working Under Supervision

You are responsible to the client and co-workers. You are also responsible to your supervisor. The supervisor is usually an RN. Some provinces allow RPNs to supervise support workers in long-term care facilities. In some community care settings, you may occasionally be supervised by an RPN, a social worker, or another health care professional.

- *Supervision in a facility.* In many facilities, the team leader is also your supervisor. The team leader (usually an RN) has overall responsibility for the client's care, the work of other RNs, RPNs, support workers, and assistive personnel. The team leader may not be on duty when you are working. You then report to the *charge nurse* (the nurse on duty for that shift).
- *Supervision in a community setting.* In these settings, you report to a supervisor, who is responsible for your work performance. You and your supervisor work for the same agency. Your agency may be hired by a health district, access centre, or community services organization. When this happens, a case manager will arrange with the agency to provide care or support for the client. The case manager is usually, but not always, an RN. The case manager communicates with your supervisor. Your supervisor then gives you information and instructions about specific clients. In some cases, your agency's services may be purchased privately by a client or a client's family. When this happens, your supervisor will be given the overall instructions from the client and/or family. Your supervisor then gives you information and instructions about the client. In some situations, clients directly hire their own support worker. In these circumstances, there is no agency supervisor. The client is your supervisor.

Respecting Your Supervisor and Employer

You must respect your supervisor and your employer. Avoid talking with others about your clients or co-workers. Try not to be negative, even if co-workers complain about a policy or a situation. If you are unhappy with a situation, talk to your supervisor. If you have difficulties communicating with your supervisor, try some of the strategies discussed in Chapters 8 and 12. If you remain unhappy, it might be best for you to find another job with a different facility or agency.

Do not talk about work problems with your clients. You represent your employer. The person trusts that the facility or agency will provide quality care. A negative, disrespectful attitude could destroy this trust and harm your client's health.

Delegation

A **task** is a function, procedure, or activity that you assist with or perform for the client. Your supervisor *assigns* most of your daily tasks. **Assigning** means giving responsibility for providing care or support. The assigned tasks are listed on your assignment sheet. Assigned tasks do not require a nurse's education and professional judgment. For example, you are assigned to assist with or perform the following tasks:

- Activities of daily living—dressing, personal hygiene, mobility, feeding
- Social and recreational activities
- Household management—housecleaning, meal preparation
- Basic nursing care tasks—measuring height, weight, and vital signs, for example

Some care tasks could harm a client if done by unqualified workers. Only nurses have the **authority** (the legal right) to do these tasks. Inserting catheters and giving enemas are examples. However, in certain situations, these tasks may be *delegated* to you. **Delegation (transfer of function)** is a process by which an RN authorizes another health care provider to perform certain tasks. The RN transfers to you the authority to perform a task. This frees the nurse to perform other tasks. It is important to remember that the nurse maintains the authority to delegate to others. The support worker does not.

During the delegation process, you are taught how to perform the task. You are then supervised and monitored to make sure you are performing the task correctly. You are delegated tasks that are routine, require little supervision, and are done for stable clients.

Only some nursing tasks can be delegated. Your employer's policies and guidelines, your job description, and provincial or territorial legislation determine what tasks can be delegated to you. They also determine when and how tasks can be delegated. Although there are many similarities across the country, each province and territory has its own rules for delegation (see the examples described in Box 5-2).

Who Can Delegate?

In most parts of the country, only RNs can delegate to support workers. When making delegating decisions, RNs must protect the client's health and safety. The delegating RN remains accountable for the delegated task. To be **accountable** means to be responsible for the outcome. The RN is accountable for the outcome of the delegated task. If necessary, the RN must answer questions about and explain the actions and decisions involved with the delegated task. However, you are still responsible for your own actions.

Health care professionals other than RNs may *assign* tasks to you. However, only an RN can *delegate* tasks to you. For example, a physician can ask you to help a person with elimination. The physician cannot ask you to give a person an enema. Only an RN can delegate this task to you.

Delegation in a Facility

When an RN delegates a task in a facility, he or she is required to:

- *Teach you the task.* The delegating RN is responsible for providing all necessary teaching. The RN may teach you the delegated task. Or, the RN may have a qualified RPN teach you.
- *Assess your performance.* The RN must determine if you are able to perform the task correctly. If an RPN is teaching, the delegating RN is still responsible for deciding if you are competent.
- *Monitor you over time to ensure you remain able to perform the task correctly and safely.* The monitoring may be achieved in a number of ways, at the discretion of the RN.

Support workers cannot assign or delegate. You cannot authorize someone to perform a task that has been assigned or delegated to you. A co-worker can help you with tasks that have been *assigned* to you. However, only an RN or RPN can help you with tasks that have been *delegated* to you.

Box 5-2 Delegation in British Columbia, Alberta, and Ontario

All provinces and territories have legislation that guides nursing practice, usually called a *Nursing Act.* British Columbia, Alberta, and Ontario also have legislation that applies to all regulated health professions. This legislation prevents unqualified people from performing professional functions.

Regulated health professions legislation and nursing acts list tasks that only nurses are legally able (authorized) to perform. In British Columbia, these authorized tasks are called *reserved acts*; in Alberta they are known as *restricted activities*; and in Ontario they are called *controlled acts.* Only nurses—and *not support workers*—are authorized to do the following:

- Perform a procedure below the skin or mucous membrane. (Cleaning and dressing an open wound is an example.)
- Administer a substance by injection or inhalation. (Giving an insulin injection is an example.)
- Insert an instrument, hand, or finger into a person's body openings, including the person's bladder, esophagus, trachea, nose, ears, bloodstream, or surgically created body openings. (Inserting urinary catheters and rectal tubes are examples.)

Unregulated health care workers (including support workers) are not normally allowed to perform authorized acts. However, unregulated workers may perform an authorized act if an RN properly delegates it. In the delegation process, the RN transfers authority to the unregulated health care worker. However, you are delegated an authorized act only if it is allowed within your job description and employer policy. It remains the responsibility of the RN to determine how and when an unregulated care provider can perform these acts.

Regulated health professions legislation also states that in certain situations, delegation is not necessary. Unregulated workers can be assigned the last two of the above-listed authorized acts if the task is a *routine activity of living.* A routine activity of living is an activity that:

- The client needs done on a regular basis
- Has already been done for the client by a nurse, with consistent and safe results

For example, administering an enema is an authorized act. Mr. Patel is paralyzed. He requires regular enemas to aid with elimination. Because the procedure is a predictable and safe part of his routine, his support worker is assigned to perform the procedure. Ms. Wolfe requires an enema before her surgery. She has never had an enema before. In her situation, the enema is *not* routine. Therefore, a support worker is not legally allowed to administer it. In this case, only a nurse is authorized to give the enema. If necessary, the procedure could be delegated to a support worker by an RN. Support workers are not responsible for deciding when to do a task. You will be assigned or delegated the task as appropriate.

Delegation in the Community

In the community, your supervisor may or may not be an RN. If your supervisor is an RN, he or she follows the same delegation process used in facilities. This involves teaching you the delegated task, assessing your performance, and monitoring your performance over time.

If your supervisor is not an RN and you need to learn a delegated task, the agency may send out an instructor (an RN) to teach you. The instructor teaches the task. He or she assesses and monitors your performance over time or asks your supervisor to do so. The instructor or your supervisor may consult with the client, or the client's family, to determine if you are doing the task correctly.

Some agencies provide educational programs or workshops for support workers. These programs educate workers about specific activities or daily living tasks. For example, you might attend a program given by an RN on how to do catheterizations for clients with paraplegia. You graduate from the program only after the RN is satisfied that you can perform the task safely and competently. The agency is responsible for monitoring your performance over time.

You may be asked to perform tasks by a professional who is not an RN and not your supervisor. Before taking on a task requested by another professional, use your judgment. Usually you can do a simple, noninvasive task that you have done for the client before. Tell the person who made the request that you cannot fulfill the request if:

- You have concerns about your ability to do the task
- It is beyond your scope of practice

Know your employer's policies. If you need clarification, contact your supervisor.

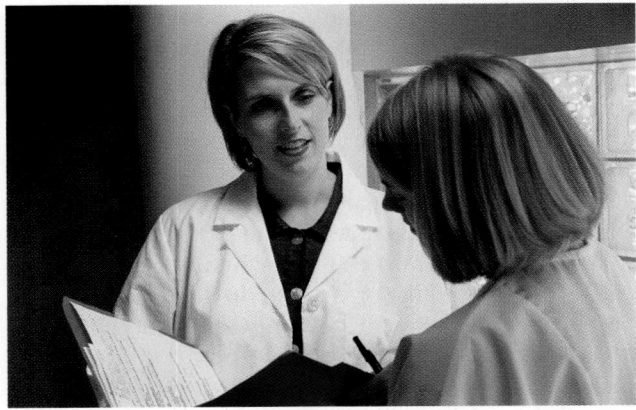

Figure 5-2 This RN is teaching a support worker a delegated task.

The client and caregivers may ask you to do certain tasks. This is common in home settings when no health care professionals are present. You must never perform a task that is beyond your scope of practice. Explain that you are not allowed to perform the task without the authorization of your supervisor. Call your supervisor to discuss the situation.

The Delegation Process

The RN considers factors that are unique to the client's situation when delegating tasks to you. A task that has been delegated is rarely transferable to another client. It must be retaught and redelegated before you can carry it out on another person. For example, you have been taught how to give an enema to Mr. Lau. Mr. Davis is also your client and requires an enema. You cannot give an enema to Mr. Davis without being taught again.

Delegated tasks must be within the legal limits of what you can do. Before delegating tasks to you, the RN must know:

- What tasks your province or territory allows support workers to perform
- The tasks included in your job description
- What you were taught in your training program
- What skills you learned and how they were evaluated
- Your work experiences

Even if a task is in your job description and you have done it before, the RN may or may not decide to assign or delegate it to you. The RN must consider the circumstances when delegating. The RN makes delegation decisions after considering the questions in Box 5-3 on page 48. The circumstances, client's needs, the task, and the person performing the task must all be right. If the person's needs and the task require the knowledge, judgment, and skill of an RN or RPN, a nurse completes the task. You may be asked to assist.

Do not get offended or angry if you are not allowed to perform a task that is part of your job description and that you usually do. The RN makes a decision that is best for the client at that time. This decision is also best for you at that time. You do not want to perform a task that requires a nurse's judgment and critical thinking skills. For example, you often care for Mrs. Mills. You provide personal care and assist with walking. She visits with her son during the weekend. When she returns to the long-term care facility, she has bruises on her face and arms. She reports falling down the stairs. The RN suspects abuse. Instead of assigning you to bathe Mrs. Mills, the RN does so. The RN wants to assess Mrs. Mills for other signs of abuse and to talk with her. Although you are able to give Mrs. Mills a bath, at this time she needs the RN's knowledge and judgment.

Box 5-3 Factors Affecting Delegation Decisions

- What is the client's condition? Is it stable or likely to change?
- What level of knowledge, skill, and judgment is required by the support worker to safely perform the task? Does the support worker have the ability to learn the task?
- What are the risks involved in performing the task? Can the support worker recognize these risks and respond to them appropriately?
- Will the support worker be required to perform the task frequently enough to maintain competency?
- Can the support worker be adequately supervised in the setting?
- Is a nurse available to help or take over if the client's condition changes or problems arise?
- Does the support worker have the time to perform the task safely?
- Does legislation restrict the kinds of acts and procedures support workers are able to perform?
- What tasks are included in the support worker's job description?

Source: Based on College of Nurses of Ontario, *Guidelines for Working with Unregulated Care Providers: For Registered Nurses and Registered Practical Nurses in Ontario* (1999).

The client's circumstances are central factors in making assignment and delegation decisions. These decisions should always result in the best care for the client. Poor decisions could place a client's health and safety at risk and result in serious legal problems.

The Five Rights of Delegation. In the United States, the National Council of State Boards of Nursing identifies five rights of delegation. These rights are relevant in Canada as well.

- *The right task*—Can the task be delegated? Does the provincial nursing act or regulated health professions act allow the RN to delegate the act? Is the task in your job description? Have you been trained to do the task?
- *The right circumstances*—What are the client's physical, emotional, social, intellectual, and spiritual needs at this time? Do you understand the purpose of the task for the person? Do you have the equipment and supplies to perform the task? Do you know how to use the equipment and supplies?
- *The right person*—Do you have the training and experience to safely perform the task for this client? Do you have concerns about performing the task?
- *The right directions and communication*—Does the nurse provide clear directions and instructions? Does the nurse tell you what to do, when to do it, what observations to make, and when to report back? Are the directions legal, ethical, and consistent with employer policies? Can you review the task with the nurse? Do you understand what the nurse expects?
- *The right supervision*—Is a nurse available to answer questions? Is a nurse available if the client's condition changes or if problems occur? After the task is completed, does the nurse assess how the task affected the client? Does the nurse discuss your performance with you, telling you what you did well and how you can improve your work?

Your Role in Delegation

Although the RN is responsible for teaching, supervising, and monitoring your performance, you are responsible for your own actions. You must perform the task safely to protect the client from harm. You are *responsible* for performing the task correctly and safely.

You have two choices when delegated a task. You either *agree* or *refuse* to do the task. Before accepting a delegated task, ask yourself the questions listed in "The Five Rights of Delegation."

Accepting a Task. When you agree to perform a task, you are responsible for your own actions. Remember, what you do or fail to do can harm the client. *You must complete the task safely.* Do not hesitate to ask for help if you are unsure or if you have questions about a task. Always report what you did and your observations.

Refusing a Task. You have the right to say "no." If you have good reasons for not doing a task, refusing to follow the nurse's directions is your right and duty. Use "The Five Rights of Delegation" as a guide, and protect clients and yourself by using common sense. Ask yourself if what you are doing is safe for the client.

You must never ignore an order or request to do something. You must communicate your concerns to the delegating RN. With good communication, you and the nurse should be able to work out the problem. If work problems continue, talk to your supervisor, instructor, or another professional to help you sort out the problems (see Chapters 8 and 12).

You must not refuse a delegated task simply because you do not like or want to do the task. You must have sound reasons for your refusal. Otherwise, you could place the client at risk for harm. You also risk losing your job.

REVIEW

Circle the BEST answer.

1. The membership of a health care team is determined by
   A. The client's needs
   B. The RN's needs
   C. The physician's needs
   D. The needs of the client's family

2. Which of the following is a benefit to the team approach to health care?
   A. Opportunities for confidentiality
   B. Opportunities for delegation
   C. Opportunities for collaboration
   D. Opportunities for assignment of tasks

3. The following statements are about health care teams and facilities. Which is *false*?
   A. Teams are often multidisciplinary.
   B. Family conferences are held when difficult situations arise.
   C. Team members usually work in the same location.
   D. Team members have few opportunities to meet.

4. In a community setting, who usually assesses, monitors, and evaluates a client's needs and coordinates the services of the health care team?
   A. The family physician
   B. The case manager
   C. The occupational therapist
   D. The social worker

5. Delegate means
   A. To give responsibility for providing care
   B. To authorize another worker to perform a task
   C. To transfer responsibility to another worker
   D. To give another worker the power or right to enforce an act, function, or role

6. Which factor does *not* affect delegation decisions made by an RN?
   A. What is the client's condition? Is it stable or likely to change?
   B. Can the support worker be adequately supervised in the setting?
   C. Does the support worker have the time to perform the task safely?
   D. Would the support worker's feelings be hurt if the RN does not delegate the task to him or her?

7. If an RN delegates a task to you, which statement is *true*?
   A. The RN is completely responsible for your actions; you are not responsible.
   B. The RN has overall responsibility for your actions; you are also responsible.
   C. You are completely responsible for your actions; the RN is not responsible.
   D. Neither you nor the RN is responsible.

8. A procedure can be delegated to you
   A. By any regulated health care professional
   B. By a physician
   C. By the client
   D. By an RN

9. An RN delegates a task to you with which you are not comfortable. Which is a *false* statement?
   A. You must perform the task.
   B. You can refuse to perform the task.
   C. You can ask for further training on how to perform the task.
   D. You can ask the nurse to stay while you perform the task.

10. You are assisting Mr. Chiang with personal care in his home. Mrs. Chiang asks you to change her husband's dressing. RNs have delegated dressing changes to you for other clients. What should you do?
    A. Tell Mrs. Chiang that you are not allowed to perform the procedure without the authorization of your supervisor. Call your supervisor.
    B. Tell Mrs. Chiang that you can change the dressing if her husband (your client) asks you to do it.
    C. Tell Mrs. Chiang that you can change the dressing if she stays in the room during the procedure.
    D. Tell Mrs. Chiang she has to obtain permission from your supervisor.

Answers to these questions are on page 821.

CHAPTER

6

Working with Clients and Their Families

OBJECTIVES

- Define the key terms listed in this chapter
- Recognize that each client is an individual and a whole person
- Describe Erikson's developmental stages
- Explain how Maslow's hierarchy of needs applies to support work
- Explain the difference between a professional helping relationship and a friendship
- Explain independence, dependence, and interdependence
- Describe common family patterns
- Explain how the health care team assists the family

KEY TERMS

compassion Caring about another person's misfortune and suffering

competence Performing your job well

dependence The state of relying on others for support; being unable to manage without help

empathy Being open to and trying to understand the experiences and feelings of others

family A biological, legal, or social network of people who provide support for one another

independence The state of not depending on others for control or authority

interdependence The state of depending on one another

need That which is necessary or desirable for maintaining life and psychosocial well-being

primary caregiver A person—usually a family member or close friend—who assumes the responsibilities of caring for an ill or disabled person in the home

psychosocial health Well-being in the social, emotional, intellectual, and spiritual dimensions of one's life

relationship The connection between two or more people, shaped by the roles, feelings, and interactions of those involved

respect Showing acceptance and regard for another person

self-actualization Experiencing one's potential

self-awareness Understanding one's own feelings, moods, attitudes, preferences, biases, and limitations

self-esteem Thinking well of yourself and being well thought of by others

Every person is an individual shaped by a unique blend of genetics and experience. A client's individuality is sometimes overlooked. Too often, health care workers think of the disease or problem rather than the person. For example, Mrs. Porter might be known as "the client with colon cancer" rather than as "Mrs. Porter." Most clients have physical problems. However, to provide good care, you must be aware that clients are more than physical beings. Considering only the physical part ignores the person's ability to think, make decisions, and interact with others. It also ignores the person's experiences, joys, sorrows, and needs.

The client is usually part of a family. Your job often involves helping the person's family. What you do affects the person and the family. It is important to understand your role when working with a family.

Psychosocial Health

A holistic approach to health care takes into account the whole person (see Chapter 4). It considers a person's physical and psychosocial health. **Psychosocial health** is well-being in the social, emotional, intellectual, and spiritual dimensions of one's life. Few people enjoy perfect psychosocial health throughout life. Factors that influence psychosocial health include:

- *Personality.* Personality is the blend of thought patterns, feelings, characteristics, and behaviour that makes a person unique.
- *Family background.* People who grew up in caring, loving families are more likely to have good psychosocial health than those who did not. When there are serious family problems, children may be psychosocially harmed. Problems include abuse, neglect, distrust, anger, and substance abuse. As they grow older, children may have problems with trust and intimacy. They may repeat the patterns learned in childhood. Abused children may abuse their own children. Children of substance abusers may develop their own substance abuse problems in adulthood.
- *Environment.* Experiences outside the family setting strongly influence psychosocial health. For children and adolescents, these nonfamily experiences include school, media influence, and interactions with friends and acquaintances. For adults, they include experiences at work and in the community. Access to social support systems such as health care and social welfare can also influence psychosocial health.
- *Life circumstances.* Some people have experienced devastating loss or tragedy in their lives. The death of a parent during childhood and the death of a child are examples. People who experience such losses may never enjoy strong psychosocial health.

Erikson's Developmental Stages

Erik Erikson was a psychologist who strongly influenced ideas about the development of psychosocial health. In the 1960s, he developed a theory that people move through a series of stages throughout their lives (Table 6-1). Each stage is necessary for the person's identity and psychosocial health. Every stage consists of a task that must be completed before the person can move on to the next stage. For example, a child who never learns to trust others will likely have difficulties forming trusting, intimate relationships later in life.

Maslow's Hierarchy of Needs

Abraham Maslow is another psychologist who has influenced ideas about psychosocial health. Maslow is best known for his theory of needs. A **need** is that which is necessary or desirable for maintaining life and psychosocial well-being. According to Maslow, certain basic needs must be met for a person to survive and function. These needs are arranged in a *hierarchy*, or order of importance (Figure 6-1). Lower-level needs must be met before higher-level needs. These basic needs are, from the lowest level to the highest level:

- Physical needs (low)
- The need for safety
- The need for love and belonging
- The need for self-esteem
- The need for self-actualization (high)

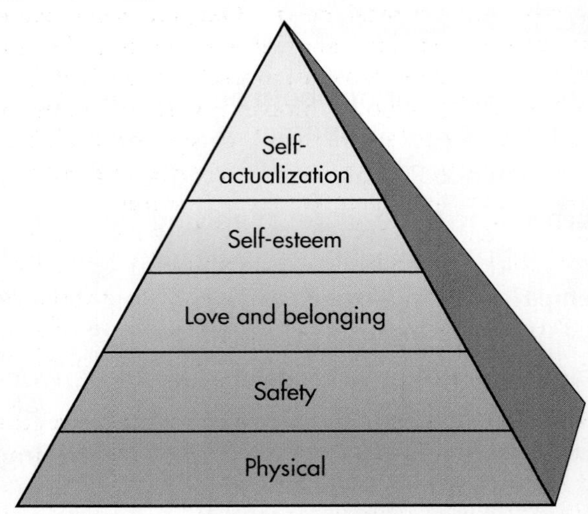

Figure 6-1 Maslow's hierarchy of needs. These needs, from the lowest to the highest level, are physical needs, the need for safety, the need for love and belonging, the need for self-esteem, and the need for self-actualization (the fulfillment of one's potential). Source: A.H. Maslow, *Motivation and Personality,* © 1954, 1987. © 1970 by Abraham H. Maslow.

Table 6-1 Erikson's Theory of Psychosocial Development, from Birth through Old Age

Stage	Age (years)	Psychosocial task	Description of task
1	0–1	Trust versus mistrust	Babies learn to trust that their needs will be met. This shows the infant that the world is a safe place.
2	1–3	Autonomy versus doubt	The toddler learns to become independent and develops self-confidence. Not learning independence creates feelings of shame and doubt.
3	3–6	Initiative versus guilt	The young child learns to initiate his or her activities. Accomplishing this task teaches the child to seek challenges later in life.
4	6–12	Competence versus inferiority	The child develops skill in physical, cognitive, and social areas. This task teaches independence and responsibility.
5	12–19	Identity versus role confusion	The adolescent tries out several roles and forms a single, unique identity.
6	20–40	Intimacy versus isolation	The young adult forms close, permanent relationships, and makes career commitments.
7	40–65	Generativity versus stagnation	The person in middle adulthood helps younger people develop their lives.
8	65 on	Integrity versus despair	The older adult thinks back on life, experiencing satisfaction or disappointment.

Source: Based on M.W. Matlin, *Psychology,* 3rd ed. (Fort Worth, TX: Harcourt Brace, 1999), p. 370.

Physical Needs. The most basic needs in Maslow's hierarchy are physical needs. Oxygen, food, water, elimination, rest, and shelter are required for life. These needs are the most important for survival. They must be met before other needs. For example, people who are starving have no needs except for food. They cannot begin to feel the need for safety, self-esteem, and love until they have satisfied their hunger.

Most adults are able to satisfy their own physical needs. However, children and seriously ill or disabled adults may depend on others to meet these needs. You are often involved in meeting physical needs. For example, you feed people who cannot feed themselves.

Safety Needs. Safety needs relate to protection from harm, danger, fear, and pain. Even minor illness and surgery can make people feel afraid. Most seriously ill people feel extremely fearful. Many people are afraid of health care. Many procedures involve frightening equipment, require invasive techniques, and cause pain and discomfort. Clients feel safer and more secure if they understand the procedure. Even for a simple bed bath, they should know:

- Why a procedure is to be done
- Who will do it
- How it will be performed
- What sensations or feelings to expect

Love and Belonging Needs. Love is a powerful human emotion that includes deep affection, tenderness, and devotion. Romantic love also involves physical desire. The need for belonging includes the need for a rightful place in society, in a peer group, and in a family. A peer group is a group of friends or acquaintances. Humans are social beings who need to be around others. When love and belonging needs are unfulfilled, people often feel lonely and rejected. There are many cases in which people were slow to recover or died because of lack of love and belonging. This is particularly true of children and older adults.

Maslow believed that unfamiliar surroundings create greater love and belonging needs. In long-term care facilities, residents have left their homes, friends, neighbours, pets, belongings, and familiar surroundings. You must be sensitive to the needs of residents who have not settled into their new environment.

Self-Esteem Needs. *Esteem* is the worth, value, or opinion one has of a person. **Self-esteem** is thinking well of yourself and being well thought of by others. When self-esteem needs are fulfilled, a person feels confident, adequate, and useful. Unmet self-esteem needs can result in feelings of inferiority, worthlessness, and helplessness. Depression may occur. People often lack self-esteem when ill or injured. Think about the following:

- How do ill parents feel when they cannot support or care for their children?
- Does a woman feel whole and attractive after having a breast removed?
- Does a person with a leg amputation feel complete, useful, and attractive?

You can help clients meet self-esteem needs by being sensitive to their feelings and encouraging them to be as independent as possible.

Self-Actualization Needs. **Self-actualization** means experiencing one's potential. It involves learning, understanding, and creating to the limit of one's ability. It is the highest need. Rarely, if ever, is it totally met. Most people constantly try to learn and understand more. The need for self-actualization can be postponed and life will continue.

Your Relationship with the Client

A **relationship** is the connection between two or more people. It is shaped by the roles, feelings, and interactions of those involved. Relationships can be either personal or professional. It is rarely a good idea to mix a professional relationship with a personal relationship. You may get to know some of your clients very well. However, even these relationships must remain professional.

A Professional Helping Relationship

Your relationship with your clients is a professional helping relationship. A professional helping relationship is established to benefit the client. It is different from a friendship. A friendship is a personal social relationship that benefits both involved. You relate to a client as a professional helper, not as a friend. Box 6-1 on page 54 compares a professional helping relationship with a friendship.

Although your professional relationship with a client is not a friendship, you should still show your clients that you care about them. Treat them with compassion and consideration. Also recognize that each person is a unique individual. When working with clients, demonstrate the following:

- *Respect*—showing acceptance and regard for another person. Accept your client's values, feelings, lifestyle, and decisions. When people are treated with respect, they feel valued and important. When

Box 6-1 Professional Helping Relationships vs. Friendships

Professional helping relationships	Friendships
One person takes the responsibility for helping the other.	The people involved are not responsible for helping each other. However, they may choose to do so.
There is a specific goal to the relationship.	The relationship is not necessarily goal directed.
Behaviours are based on professional roles, such as support worker and client.	Behaviours are based on personal roles.
The people involved may not choose the relationship.	The people involved choose the relationship.
The helper seeks to fulfill the needs of the person being helped.	Both people in the relationship seek to have their needs fulfilled.
The helper is nonjudgmental.	Both people may be judgmental.

Source: Adapted from E. Arnold and K. Underman Boggs, *Interpersonal Relationships: Professional Communication Skills*, 3rd ed. (Philadelphia: Saunders, 1999), p. 82.

treated with disrespect, they feel ashamed, rejected, or hurt. Showing common courtesy is an important way of being respectful. Remember to always be courteous and polite to your clients. For example, remember to say "please" and "thank you," as appropriate. Being overly familiar with clients can show a lack of respect. Calling clients by their first names without being asked is an example. Failing to recognize a person's need for privacy and independence also shows a lack of respect. Respect your client's preferences for how tasks should be done. As you perform the tasks, check to make sure that the person is comfortable, safe, and satisfied. Encourage people to express preferences, make personal choices, and do as much as they can for themselves.

- *Compassion*—caring about another's misfortune and suffering. Compassion requires an understanding that bad things can happen to people through no fault of their own. Compassion is not the same as pity. To pity someone implies that you are superior to the person. (See *Support Workers Solving Problems: Demonstrating Compassion* box.)
- *Empathy*—being open to and trying to understand the experiences and feelings of others. Empathy involves being receptive to others. It does not involve judging others. Compassion and empathy are similar. Compassion is felt in response to suffering. Empathy may be felt in response to a full range of emotions. For example, a client is told that her son survived a dangerous heart operation. You feel great joy and relief at the news. Your feelings show that you are sensitive to your client's situation. You share her reactions. It is not enough to *feel* empathy for a person. You must also *show* the person that you empathize. Eye contact and physical closeness can show empathy. So can a smile or a kind word. An empathetic response can decrease loneliness and create feelings of well-being and belonging.
- *Competence*—performing your job well. You must safely and skillfully perform tasks. You must be well-organized, punctual, and reliable. You also must know your scope of practice and personal limits. At the same time, be flexible and responsive to the client's needs. You earn the client's trust by being competent.

Support Workers Solving Problems

Demonstrating Compassion

Scenario: Mark Vickers, 16, has Down syndrome. Because his mother recently died of cancer, Mark has moved into a group home. Mark's father long ago abandoned the family. He has no siblings or other family nearby.

Cynthia is a support worker in the group home. She notices that Mark sits all day in his room, staring at the wall. He refuses to join the other residents in the common room.

Discussion: Cynthia has great compassion for Mark. She tries to imagine what it is like to lose the only person you have in the world and to move into a strange, new place. Cynthia recognizes that Mark needs time to deal with his grief and loneliness. She spends as much time as she can with Mark, sometimes simply sitting with him and holding his hand. Her quiet acceptance of his sadness comforts Mark. After a few days, he begins to open up to Cynthia.

- *Self-Awareness*—understanding one's own feelings, moods, attitudes, preferences, biases, and limitations. You must know yourself in order to be genuine and nonjudgmental with others. Self-knowledge requires examining your own feelings and behaviours. (See *Support Workers Solving Problems: Demonstrating Self-Awareness* box.)

Independence, Dependence, and Interdependence

Independence, dependence, and interdependence are fundamental concepts in professional helping relationships.

- **Independence** is the state of not depending on others for control or authority. People who are independent control and direct their lives. They can do things for themselves.
- **Dependence** is the state of relying on others for support; being unable to manage without help.
- **Interdependence** is the state of depending on each other. In most relationships, each person relies upon the other for some things.

These terms must be considered in relation to one another. No one is completely independent, and only infants and very young children and unconscious people are completely dependent. Most people and relationships have elements of all three.

For example, Julie considers herself independent. She feels she is in control of her busy and rewarding life as a support worker, wife, and mother of two young boys. She works full-time and takes her children to daycare. Julie is independent because she is in control of her career and her home life. However, she also depends on others. Without reliable childcare, she could not work full-time. Julie and her husband have an interdependent relationship. They rely on each other for emotional support and companionship. They also rely on each other for help with childrearing, housework, grocery shopping, and cooking.

An important goal of most clients' care is to achieve or maintain as much independence as possible (Figure 6-2). Everyone makes choices about when to do things for themselves and when to rely on others. These choices involve setting goals and priorities. You must respect your client's choices to do some things independently and to accept help with other things. You may not fully understand the reason for these choices.

For example, Elena is hired to help Ms. Godin, 31. Ms. Godin has cerebral palsy. Elena's role is to help Ms. Godin get ready for work in the morning. Elena knows that Ms. Godin is capable of dressing, showering, and preparing breakfast without help. However, each task takes a long time for Ms. Godin. She chooses to put her energies into her work, not into getting ready for work. Elena respectfully accepts Ms. Godin's choices. People make choices according to their wishes and capabilities. They must never feel that you are judging their decisions.

Independence and Self-Esteem

What makes you feel good about yourself? Working hard at your job or at school? Playing a sport? Caring for your family? How would you feel if you could no longer do these things? Good self-esteem often develops when people feel that their life has meaning for themselves and others. It is also closely associated with independence.

For children, attaining power and control over their bodies and environment helps develop self-esteem. Self-esteem can suffer when independence is limited or lost. People's roles and identities can change when they are no longer in control of their lives (see Chapter 4). You must be sensitive to how people feel when they lose their independence through illness or disability.

People who have lost their independence need to find ways to rebuild their self-esteem. Some people who cannot do this become frustrated or depressed.

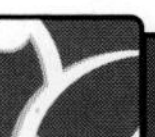

Support Workers Solving Problems

Demonstrating Self-Awareness

Scenario: Mr. Raftis requires assistance with self-care. Maia has been providing care for eight days. One morning Mr. Raftis complains to Maia that she is too rough when shaving him. Maia feels that Mr. Raftis is questioning her competence. She is hurt by his comment. She becomes quiet and withdrawn.

Discussion: Later, Maia thinks about her reaction to Mr. Raftis's comment. She is upset with herself for letting the comment affect how she treated Mr. Raftis. Usually they have a lively conversation while she helps him. After his comment, she barely said a word. She remembers that when she was a child her father criticized her constantly, making her feel incompetent. Once she understands the reason for her hurt feelings, Maia understands that Mr. Raftis's comment was constructive rather than critical. The next day she asks Mr. Raftis to explain how he would like to be shaved. Together they decide how she can increase his comfort.

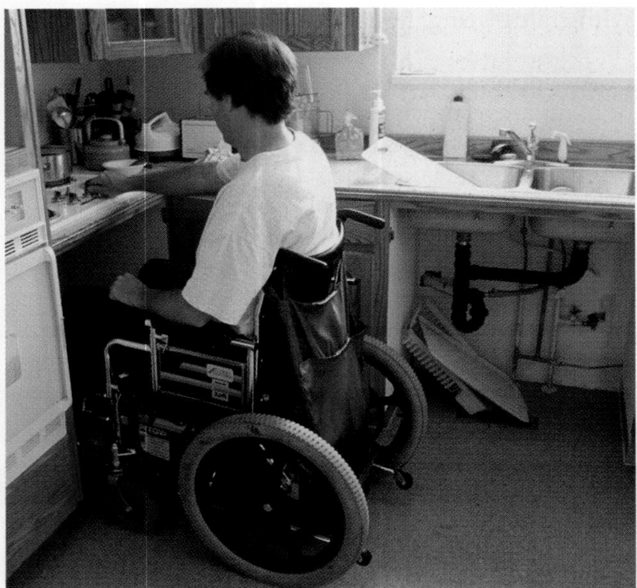

Figure 6-2 This person is able to function independently at home.

Others are able to find a new purpose in life. Ricardo became quadriplegic at the age of 17. He and two friends had been drinking at a party. On the way home, the driver lost control of the car and hit a telephone pole. Ricardo's two friends died at the scene. Ricardo was in hospital for seven months. He was so depressed he wished he had died with his friends in the accident. Then his high school principal asked him to speak to the students about the dangers of drinking and driving. Ricardo agreed. Since then he has spoken to students at every school in his community. This has given his life purpose.

You can reinforce a client's self-esteem by offering encouragement. Praise the person's successes. If the person is not successful yet, you should recognize the person's efforts. You might say, "I can see how hard you are trying." Provide the person with honest, constructive feedback, delivered in a gentle, supportive fashion.

Independence and Balance of Power

In any relationship in which one person is dependent on the other, the balance of power may not be equal. The strong, independent person may control the vulnerable, dependent person. In some situations, this leads to abuse of the dependent person (see Chapter 19).

Be aware of the balance of power in your relationships with clients. Avoid controlling behaviour. It is easy to be controlling without being aware of it. For example, Lynn's client, Mrs. Kerr, insists on wearing a blouse with ten tiny buttons and doing them up herself. Mrs. Kerr takes three minutes to do up the first button. Lynn does not have 30 minutes to help Mrs. Kerr dress. She suggests Mrs. Kerr wear something else. Mrs. Kerr refuses. She is expecting visitors and wants to look good. Lynn undoes the button and removes the blouse. She hands Mrs. Kerr another garment, while saying, "You will look just as nice in this sweater."

Instead of imposing your will on clients, involve them in solving problems that arise. For example, Lynn could have explained to Mrs. Kerr that her time was limited, and together they could have thought of some solutions. Lynn might have suggested that they each do up some of the buttons. Or, she might have suggested doing other tasks (like tidying the room) while Mrs. Kerr dressed herself.

The Client's Family

Close personal relationships are central to the lives of most people. Family and other close relationships involve some forms of dependency. Spouses depend on one another for emotional support, companionship, and financial support. Children depend on their parents to meet their physical, emotional, and financial needs. Older parents may depend on adult children to help them with physical and emotional needs.

The **family** is a biological, legal, or social network of people who provide support for one another. Families can take many forms. They may include people related by blood or marriage. Or, they may include unrelated people who have formed a close personal relationship. Examples of families include:

- A married couple with or without children or stepchildren
- An unmarried couple living together, with or without children
- A widowed grandmother raising two grandchildren
- A divorced parent living with a partner and who has children living elsewhere
- Two women or two men living together in a same-sex relationship
- Older parents, adult children, and grandchildren living together

You may have different ideas about what is a family. You must always respect your client's definition of family. Do not impose your values on the person.

Your Role in Assisting the Family

There are many situations in which you help families. You may care for new mothers and their babies. You may care for toddlers or older children when their parent is ill or unavailable. You may assist or provide needed respite for a **primary caregiver**. A primary caregiver is the person (usually a family member or close friend) who assumes the responsibilities of caring for an ill or disabled person in the home. (See *Focus on Home Care: Assisting the Primary Caregiver* box.) Whatever the situation, when working with a family, you indirectly support their relationships. By providing a family with basic care and support services, you enable family members to invest more time and energy in their relationships.

Chapter 4 discusses how roles change when illness or disability strikes a family. Very often, one family member becomes the primary caregiver of another family member. They form a different relationship, with new patterns of dependency. This is rarely easy. The ill person may feel angry at having to depend on the caregiver. The caregiver may feel burdened by the new responsibility, as well as by other family and work demands.

Professionals on the health care team prepare family members to take on care responsibilities. When helping families cope, they consider the physical, emotional, social, spiritual, and intellectual health of all family members. They also consider relationships within the family, including any conflict and potential for conflict. They may help the family deal with stress by working on communication skills and problem-solving abilities. This sometimes involves bringing family members together in a conference to discuss the ill person's care and its impact on the entire family. You may sometimes be asked to attend family conferences.

Families in Conflict

Some families are coping with conflict. When illness or disability occurs, the stress may be great. Families express conflict by irritation, anger, bickering, and arguments. Conflict may also be hidden. Adult children may care for aging parents with whom they have unresolved conflicts. Siblings who have not spoken in years may be forced to see one another during a parent's illness. Sometimes the health care team can help families resolve their difficulties. Members of palliative care teams are specially trained to help people resolve emotional problems that are causing them distress.

When working with a family, be aware of family relationships and any conflicts, communication difficulties, and stressful situations (Figure 6-3). It is not your role to help families deal with interpersonal problems. However, you can observe and report on family interactions (Box 6-2 on page 58). You must also be alert for signs of abuse (see Chapter 19).

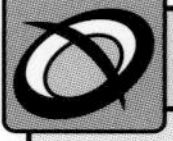

Focus on Home Care

Assisting the Primary Caregiver

Sometimes you work closely with the client's primary caregiver. For example, you assist Mrs. Kalopsis with housekeeping and meal preparation. Now she can spend more time with her ill husband.

Primary caregivers are often relieved to have assistance from the health care team. However, some may have mixed feelings about your presence in their home. Some people may resent the interruption to their routine. Others may feel that you are invading their privacy. Some may also feel like failures for needing help, or regret that someone else is accomplishing tasks that they would like to do if they could.

Try to put the family at ease by showing that you are there to help, not to take over or judge their housekeeping or caregiving skills. Do not do tasks that have not been assigned.

Adapt your work to suit the family's standards and preferences, not your own. Respect the family's routines, schedules, and way of doing things. Consult with your supervisor if you think the family's wishes may affect safety.

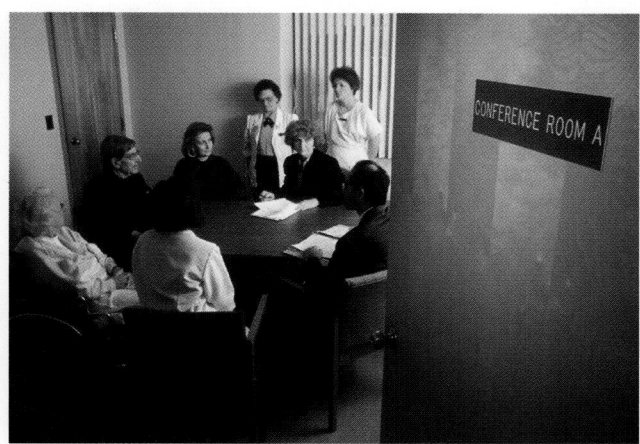

Figure 6-3 A family conference to discuss a loved one's needs and care requirements and their effect on the family.

Box 6-2 Case Study: Family Conflict

Mei is a support worker. She tells the following story about her experience working with a family in conflict.

"When I look back on the families I've worked with, one in particular stands out. Mr. Skala was an older man with cancer. His wife was his primary caregiver. They had a daughter living nearby who had a family of her own. Just before Mr. Skala became ill, there was a major argument over the family business. The result was that their daughter refused to speak to her parents. The Skalas' son-in-law brought their two young grandchildren to visit, but their daughter never came. She refused all attempts to resolve the conflict.

Mrs. Skala found this situation extremely hard to bear. She asked me to talk to her daughter to try to mend the rift. I felt for Mrs. Skala. I wanted to help, but I had to tell Mrs. Skala that it wasn't my role to get involved with the family's problems. I told my supervisor about Mrs. Skala's family problems. The case manager arranged for a social worker to talk with them. Eventually, the daughter resolved her differences with her parents. In the last three weeks of Mr. Skala's life, the family spent meaningful time together."

REVIEW

Circle the BEST answer.

1. Which of the following is *false?*
   A. Every person is a unique individual
   B. People of the same age with the same condition are much the same
   C. Every individual you care for is a whole person
   D. People are influenced by their genetics and their environment

2. Psychosocial health is the achievement of
   A. Well-being in the social, emotional, intellectual, and spiritual dimensions of one's life
   B. Secure, intimate love relationships
   C. Good physical health
   D. Strong social bonds in the community

3. Which is *not* part of Erikson's theory of psychosocial development?
   A. People move through a series of stages throughout their lives
   B. People must successfully complete a task in each stage before moving on to the next
   C. Babies must learn to trust that their needs will be met
   D. Moving to unfamiliar surroundings creates love and belonging needs

4. Maslow's hierarchy of needs can best be described as
   A. Another term for psychosocial health
   B. A system that arranges human needs into categories
   C. Physiological and safety needs
   D. Love and belonging needs

5. Which is *not* part of Maslow's hierarchy of needs?
   A. Financial needs
   B. Self-esteem needs
   C. Safety needs
   D. Physical needs

6. A professional helping relationship is established for the benefit of the
   A. Client and support worker
   B. Client, support worker, and health care team
   C. Client
   D. Client's family

7. Empathy is
   A. Feelings of pity for another person
   B. Being open to and trying to understand the experiences and feelings of others
   C. Showing acceptance and regard for another person
   D. The process of enabling others to set and achieve goals

8. Common courtesy is a sign of
   A. Empathy
   B. Interdependence
   C. Respect
   D. Need

9. Which should *not* be present in a professional helping relationship?
   A. Pity
   B. Respect
   C. Compassion
   D. Self-awareness

10. Independence is
    A. Not depending on others for control or authority
    B. Being unable to manage without help
    C. Relying on others for support
    D. Showing acceptance for another person

11. When supporting clients from families in conflict, your supervisor expects you to
    A. Help family members resolve conflict
    B. Observe and report on family interactions
    C. Ignore any conflict you witness
    D. Take sides in family arguments

Answers to these questions are on page 821.

CHAPTER

7

CLIENT CARE: PLANNING, PROCESSES, REPORTING, AND RECORDING

OBJECTIVES

- Define the key terms listed in this chapter
- Explain the steps in the care planning process in facilities
- Explain the steps in the care planning process in the community
- Explain the function of the care plan
- Describe your role in the care planning process
- Explain why observation is an important part of the support worker's role
- Explain the difference between objective data and subjective data
- Explain what makes an observation effective
- Explain how reporting differs in a facility and a community setting
- List four functions of charts
- Identify the types of documents found in a client's chart
- List the basic rules for recording
- Use the 24-hour clock
- Explain why confidentiality is important to the care planning process
- Explain how computers have affected the care planning process

KEY TERMS

assessment Collecting information about the client; a step in the care planning process

care plan A document that details the care and services the client should receive

care planning process The method used by nurses and case managers to plan and deliver care

chart Document that details a person's condition or illness and responses to care; record

charting Recording

evaluation Assessing and measuring; a step in the care planning process

implementation Carrying out or performing; a step in the care planning process

intervention An action or measure taken by the health care team to help the client meet a goal in the care plan

medical diagnosis The identification of a disease or condition by a physician

nursing diagnosis A statement describing a health problem that is treated by nursing measures

objective data Information that is observed; signs

observation The act of noticing a truth or fact

planning Establishing priorities and goals and developing measures or actions to help the client meet the goals; a step in the care planning process

record Chart

recording The process of documenting care provided and observations made; charting

signs Objective data

subjective data Information reported by a client that cannot be directly observed by others; symptoms

symptoms Subjective data

verbal report A spoken account of care provided and observations made

Safe and effective care requires careful planning and coordination. It does not just happen. Facilities and agencies put systems and processes in place that protect clients from harm and ensure high-quality care. This chapter discusses systems and processes you need to know, including care planning, reporting, and recording.

The Care Planning Process in Facilities

Nurses in facilities use a method called the **care planning process** to plan and deliver care. Its purpose is to meet the client's need for care and support. The care planning process in facilities has the following steps:

1. Assessment
2. Nursing diagnosis
3. Planning
4. Implementation
5. Evaluation

Assessment

Assessment involves collecting information about the client. The nurse meets with the client and takes a health history. This describes the client's past and present health problems. The nurse conducts a physical assessment. This usually includes taking the person's vital signs and making observations about the person's physical health. The nurse also assesses the person's emotional, social, intellectual, and spiritual health. The nurse gathers as much information as possible from various sources. This includes information collected by the physician, social worker, and other health care providers. It also includes information recorded in past medical records and test results.

The nurse usually meets with members of the client's family. The nurse considers the client's needs and the family's needs when preparing the care plan.

Nursing Diagnosis

The nurse uses information from the assessment to make a nursing diagnosis. A **nursing diagnosis** is a statement describing a health problem that is treated by nursing measures. Nursing diagnoses take into account the whole person. Psychosocial health is as important as physical health. For example, a nursing diagnosis may be *low self-esteem, social isolation,* or *spiritual distress*. Most Canadian nurses use nursing diagnoses from the North American Nursing Diagnosis Association or similar lists of diagnoses (Box 7-1 on page 62 contains a partial list).

The client may have a specific health problem or may be at risk for developing a health problem. Some

Box 7-1 Nursing Examples of Diagnoses Approved by the North American Nursing Diagnosis Association (NANDA)

- Anxiety
- Breastfeeding, Ineffective
- Cardiac Output, Decreased
- Caregiver Role Strain
- Communication, Impaired Verbal
- Community Coping, Ineffective
- Constipation
- Diarrhea
- Family Coping, Compromised
- Fatigue
- Grieving, Dysfunctional
- Home Maintenance, Impaired
- Hopelessness
- Incontinence, Urinary, Stress
- Infant Feeding Pattern, Ineffective
- Infection, Risk for
- Injury, Risk for
- Loneliness, Risk for
- Pain, Chronic
- Physical Mobility, Impaired
- Powerlessness
- Social Interaction, Impaired
- Swallowing, Impaired
- Urinary Elimination, Impaired

Adapted from NANDA International (2002), *NANDA Nursing Diagnosis: Definitions and Classification 2003–2004,* Philadelphia: NANDA.

clients have many health problems and nursing diagnoses. A nursing diagnosis and a medical diagnosis are different. A **medical diagnosis** is the identification of a disease or condition by a physician. Medical diagnoses include cancer, pneumonia, bipolar disorder, stroke, heart attack, AIDS, and diabetes. Medications, therapies, and surgery are ordered by physicians to treat diseases or conditions.

PLANNING

Planning involves establishing priorities and goals and developing measures or actions to help the client meet these goals.

Establishing Priorities. The client and the nurse discuss the client's needs. They then decide on the client's priorities. Often family members and the health care team take part in this stage of the planning process. Nurses use Maslow's theory of basic needs to help set priorities (see Chapter 6). The needs necessary for life and survival have priority. They must be met before the other needs can be considered.

Setting Goals. After the nurse and the client agree on priorities, they discuss the goals for the client's care. Goals are practical, achievable, measurable outcomes (results) of the care (Figure 7-1). The goals in Figure 7-1 contain specific actions and dates. If the client does not achieve the goal by the date, the nurse and client will reevaluate the goal. Sometimes the family is involved. Goals focus on promoting health and preventing health problems. Many goals focus on rehabilitation and independence. Goals are aimed at maintaining or improving the client's physical, emotional, social, spiritual, and intellectual health.

Determining Interventions. After the nurse and client have set goals, they discuss interventions. An **intervention** is an action or measure taken by the health care team to help the client meet the goal. An intervention does not need a physician's order. However, some interventions come from a physician's order. For example, a physician orders that Mrs. Jacob walk 100 metres twice a day. The nurse includes this order in the care plan.

Establishing the Care Plan. The **care plan** is a document that details the care and services the client should receive. The plan contains the client's diagnosis, goals, and interventions required to achieve each goal. The care plan has several important functions:

- It lists the care and services the person receives.
- It ensures that the person's care is consistent, no matter who provides the care. For example, Mr. Sayeed's care plan details methods for helping him overcome swallowing difficulties. Each care provider uses the same methods.
- It enables the health care team to communicate details about the person's care. For example, you start a shift in a long-term care facility. The care plan tells you that Mrs. Desormo has achieved the goal of dressing herself.

The care plan is not a finished document. It is continually reviewed and revised. Most care plans change, depending on the client's needs, condition, and progress. For example, Mrs. Atkins's care plan is modified when she does not achieve the goal of bathing herself by May 20.

Usually only the nurse who has the overall responsibility for the client's care makes changes to the care plan.

Nursing diagnosis	Goal	Intervention
Constipation related to lack of privacy.	Resident will have regular bowel movement by 6/30.	Ask resident to use call bell when urge to have bowel movement is felt. Answer call promptly. Assist resident to bathroom. Close bathroom door for privacy. Leave room if resident can be alone; tell resident you are leaving and that you will return if the call bell is turned on.
Sleep pattern disturbance related to noisy environment.	Resident will report a restful sleep by 6/29.	Perform necessary care measures before bedtime. Close door to resident's room. Turn off television or keep volume low if the resident prefers. Ask staff to avoid talking outside the resident's room. Ask staff to speak in low voices. Turn off unneeded equipment.

Figure 7-1 Partial resident care plan in a long-term care facility. Each nursing diagnosis has a goal. There are nursing measures for each goal.

Implementation

At this stage of the process, the actions listed in the care plan are implemented. **Implementation** means carrying out or performing. The nurse in charge of the client's care assigns or delegates tasks to members of the health care team. You are only assigned or delegated tasks that are within the legal limits of your role and job description. To communicate tasks assigned or delegated to you, the nurse uses an assignment sheet. This tells you what tasks need to be done for each client.

There are four main functions of the implementation process:

- Providing the care
- Observing the person during the care
- Reporting and recording that the care has been completed
- Reporting and recording observations made during the care

Observing the client is an important part of the implementation process. Health care providers (including support workers) must report and record their actions and observations after care is completed, according to employer policy.

Evaluation

Evaluation means assessing and measuring. The evaluation step involves determining if the goals in the care plan have been met. The nurse measures the progress made. Goals may be met totally, partly, or not at all. The nurse assesses the reasons why a client may have made no or partial progress towards reaching a goal. Evaluation is an on-going process. As the person's condition or needs change, revisions are made to the diagnoses, goals, and interventions. Changes to the care plan are made in consultation with the client and other members of the health care team.

Team meetings are often part of the evaluation process. The nurse conducts a meeting to share information and ideas about the client's care. The purpose is to develop, evaluate, or revise the person's care plan. You and other members of the health care team are usually included in the meeting. You are encouraged to share your suggestions and observations (see Chapter 5).

The Care Planning Process in Community Settings

Case managers coordinate and manage client care. The care planning process used by case managers usually involves four steps: assessment, planning, implementation, and evaluation.

Assessment

The case manager meets with the client and family members to identify the client's problems and needs. Usually the meeting takes place in the client's home. If the client is coming home from the hospital, the case manager uses information from the hospital record and/or information obtained through a referral sent to the case manager's agency. The referral information may, in some cases, have been completed by a hospital case manager or discharge planner.

The family is very important to the assessment process in community care settings. Serious illness and disability greatly affect family life (see Chapter 4). Family members take on new roles, including the role of caregiver to the ill person. The case manager considers the needs, health, and well-being of the entire family. He or she also considers whether family members need help adjusting to the situation or training to help them care for the ill person. Together, the case manager, client, and family members decide what care and services are needed. For example, they consider nursing and personal care needs and services such as Meals on Wheels, housekeeping, and transportation. The need for special equipment such as oxygen therapy is also considered.

The case manager also considers whether the client's home is a safe environment. For example, the home must be reasonably clean, free of pest infestations, and have hand-washing facilities and adequate heating and cooling systems. The case manager assesses whether the home needs modifications for the person's safety needs. For example, the home may need grab bars installed in the bathroom or a mechanical lifting device in the bedroom. Often, further safety assessments by other specialists are needed. For example, an occupational therapist may assess a home for wheelchair accessibility (see Chapter 32).

Planning

In community care settings, the planning stage can be lengthy and complicated. First, the case manager, client, and family establish priorities, set goals, and determine available resources. Then the case manager develops a master care plan based on the goals and puts together a health care team (Figure 7-2).

The case manager and family members consider resources available for the care. The case manager determines how much publicly funded home care the client and family are eligible for. The family may choose to pay for additional care and services from a private agency.

The care plan includes the care and services that family members, outside professionals, and agencies will perform. These professionals and agencies often develop their own care plans. However, the case manager is in charge of the master plan. For example, the nursing care plan may be one part of the master care plan.

The case manager schedules all outside services and arranges financing for them. If the client needs help from a support worker, the case manager contacts your agency. Your supervisor assigns you to provide care or support for the client. The assignment may be communicated to you by phone or on an assignment sheet.

When clients have multiple needs, several agencies may be involved. For example, Mr. Tremblay is recovering from a stroke. His wife is his primary caregiver. He needs four hours of nursing care a week and visits from respiratory, occupational, speech, and physical therapists. A support worker is also needed to help Mr. Tremblay prepare for bed when his wife is at work. So that Mrs. Tremblay does not have to prepare every meal, arrangements are made for Meals on Wheels.

Some clients choose to coordinate and manage their own care. They may develop their own written care plan. Or they may not write anything down. If there are no written directions, you need detailed instructions from the client.

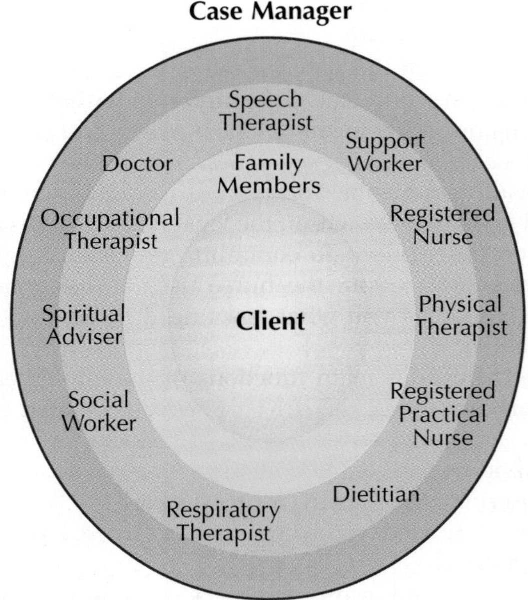

Figure 7-2 The circle of community care. This circle indicates the central role of the case manager, client, and family members on a health care team. Source: J. Birchenall and E. Streight, *Mosby's Textbook for the Home Care Aide* (St. Louis: Mosby, 1997), p. 4.

Implementation

Agency staff provide care and services on the dates and times arranged by the case manager. If any unforeseen needs arise, the client or family member calls the case manager. After assessing the situation, the case manager may ask the agency for an unscheduled visit. For example, Mrs. Tremblay feels too ill to care for her husband one morning. She calls her case manager, who contacts the agency for a support worker to care for Mr. Tremblay.

Evaluation

Evaluation in a home care setting is on-going. The case manager periodically meets with the client and family to assess progress. The case manager also meets with and receives reports from the care and service providers, who continually monitor and evaluate their own care plans.

Your Role in the Care Planning Process

In any health care setting you have an important role in the care planning process. You make observations and provide feedback. Others use this information when reassessing the client's progress, revising goals, and changing the care plan.

Developing Observation Skills

You are often with clients more than are other care providers. Sometimes you are the first to notice a change in a client's condition. You also observe the client's preferences and reactions to interventions. You are expected to make careful and accurate observations for use in the care planning process.

Observation is the act of noticing a truth or fact. Observation requires you to use your sight, hearing, touch, and smell. You see the way the client lies, sits, or walks. You see flushed or pale skin and reddened or swollen body areas. You listen to the person breathe, talk, and cough. You feel changes in the person's skin temperature. With smell, you detect body, wound, and breath odours and unusual odours from urine and bowel movements.

Information observed about a client is called **objective data (signs).** You can feel a pulse and you can see urine. However, you cannot feel or see the person's pain, fear, or nausea. **Subjective data (symptoms)** is information reported by a client that is not directly observed by others. The following comments are examples of subjective data:

- "I hardly slept last night. I lay awake from 1:00 a.m. until the sun came up."
- "With George gone, I just don't feel like living any more. I feel so hopeless."
- "The pain is worse when I move. It is a sharp pain that goes from my ankle to my hip. Thankfully, it comes and goes. I couldn't stand it if I felt it all the time."

When you report or record subjective data, do not interpret the person's comments. Use the person's exact words.

Box 7-2 on page 66 is a guide to follow when making observations. It contains basic observations. However, you may observe other conditions and situations. Be alert to changes in the person's condition or behaviour. Focus your observations on the person's physical, mental, emotional, and social condition. Look for:

- Changes in physical condition—for example, the client's skin is red and blistering
- Changes in mental condition—for example, the client forgets how to use a toothbrush
- Changes in emotional states—for example, the client is crying
- Changes in social condition—for example, a friend does not visit at his or her usual time
- New conditions that you observe—for example, the client develops diarrhea

Describing Your Observations

Your observations are critical to the care planning process. Nurses and case managers use your observations for the assessment and evaluation steps of the care planning process. Remember these points when describing your observations:

- *Be precise and accurate.* Provide details of what you actually see, hear, touch, and smell. Measurements, calculations, and times must be accurate. When describing subjective data, report or record the person's exact words.
- *Do not interpret or make assumptions.* In most cases, your observations are sufficient. You do not need to interpret them. Do not make assumptions. An *assumption* is a guess, usually based on insufficient evidence. When you make assumptions, you jump to conclusions.

Box 7-3 on page 67 contains some examples of ineffective and effective descriptions of observations. After you have studied the box, read the dialogue from the team meeting on page 43. Notice that the contributions the support worker makes to the meeting are observations. She provides precise, accurate details, but she does not make assumptions. The social worker and nurse use the support worker's observations to make a judgment about the client's mental health.

(text continues on page 67)

Box 7-2 Basic Observations

ABILITY TO RESPOND
- Is the person easy or difficult to arouse?
- Can the person give his or her name, the time, and location when asked?
- Does the person identify others accurately?
- Does the person answer questions correctly?
- Does the person speak clearly?
- Are instructions followed correctly?
- Is the person calm, restless, or excited?
- Is the person conversing, quiet, or talking a lot?

MOVEMENT
- Can the person squeeze your fingers with each hand?
- Can the person move arms and legs?
- Are the person's movements shaky or jerky?
- Does the person complain of stiff or painful joints?

PAIN OR DISCOMFORT
- Where is the pain located? (Ask the person to point to the pain.)
- Does the pain go anywhere else?
- When did the pain begin?
- What was the person doing when the pain began?
- How long does the pain last?
- How does the person describe the pain?
  - Sharp
  - Severe
  - Knifelike
  - Dull
  - Burning
  - Aching
  - Comes and goes
  - Depends on position
- Was the medication given?
- Did medication help relieve the pain? Is pain still present?
- Is the person able to sleep and rest?
- What is the position of comfort?

SKIN
- Is the skin pale or flushed?
- Is the skin cool, warm, or hot?
- Is the skin moist or dry?
- What colour are the lips and nails?
- Is the skin intact? Are there broken areas? If so, where?
- Are sores or reddened areas present?
- Are bruises present? Where are they located?
- Does the person complain of itching?

EYES, EARS, NOSE, AND MOUTH
- Is there drainage from the eyes? What colour is the drainage?
- Are the eyelids closed?
- Are the eyes reddened?
- Does the person complain of spots, flashes, or blurring?
- Is the person sensitive to bright lights?
- Is there drainage from the ears? What colour is the drainage?
- Can the person hear? Is repeating necessary? Are questions answered appropriately?
- Is there drainage from the nose? What colour is the drainage?
- Can the person breathe through the nose?
- Is there breath odour?
- Does the person complain of a bad taste in the mouth?
- Does the person complain of painful gums or teeth?

RESPIRATIONS
- Do both sides of the person's chest rise and fall with respirations?
- Is breathing noisy?
- Does the person complain of difficulty breathing?
- What is the amount and colour of sputum?
- What is the frequency of the person's cough? Is it dry or productive?

BOWELS AND BLADDER
- Is the abdomen firm or soft?
- Does the person complain of gas?
- What are the amount, colour, and consistency of bowel movements?
- What is the frequency of bowel movements?
- Can the person control bowel movements?
- Does the person have pain or difficulty urinating?
- What is the amount of urine?
- Does urine have a foul smell?
- Can the person control the passage of urine?
- What is the frequency of urination?

APPETITE
- Does the person like the diet?
- How much of the meal is eaten?
- What are the person's food preferences?
- Can the person chew food?
- How much liquid was taken?
- What are the person's liquid preferences?
- How often does the person drink liquids?
- Can the person swallow food and fluids?
- Does the person complain of nausea?
- What is the amount and colour of material vomited?
- Does the person have hiccups?
- Is the person belching?

ACTIVITIES OF DAILY LIVING
- Can the person perform personal care without help?
  - Bathing?
  - Brushing teeth?
  - Combing and brushing hair?
  - Shaving?
- Does the person use the toilet, commode, bedpan, or urinal?
- Does the person feed himself or herself?
- Can the person walk?
- What amount and kind of assistance are needed?

Box 7-3 Ineffective and Effective Observations Made by Support Workers

Ineffective Observation	Reasons the Observation is Ineffective	Effective Observation	Reasons the Observation is Effective
Mrs. Demarco is having trouble going to the bathroom this morning.	Correct terminology is not used. The statement is vague. No details are provided.	Mrs. Demarco urinated 3 times between 0900 and 0920. She said, "I feel a burning pain when I try to go to the bathroom," and "only a trickle of urine is coming out."	Correct terminology is used. The statement is a direct, precise observation. Both objective and subjective data are used.
Mr. Quennell is having problems remembering things.	The statement is an assumption. There is no supporting evidence.	Mr. Quennell did not remember eating his breakfast. He asked me to make breakfast ½ hour after he had eaten. I told him he had already had breakfast. He said, "I don't remember."	The statement is an observation supported by detailed examples. Both objective and subjective data are used.
Mrs. Witowski seems under the weather today.	Correct terminology is not used. There is no supporting evidence.	Mrs. Witowski did not play bridge today. She took only two bites of her lunch (a turkey sandwich). She said, "I'm not hungry. I feel tired and I don't feel like doing anything."	The statement about Mrs. Witowski's behaviour and condition are observations supported by evidence. Mrs. Witowski's words are quoted exactly.

Verbal Reporting

You report and record your actions and observations. A **verbal report** is the spoken account of care provided and observations made. Employers use different methods for verbal reporting. All have policies about how often to report and what to report. You need to know your employer's policies. There are some circumstances in which you always need to contact your supervisor. These are listed in Box 7-4 on page 68.

Remember that information about a client is confidential. Be careful when communicating client information to members of the health care team. Choose a quiet area where you cannot be overheard by others. Do not discuss a client in his or her room or a common area. Keep all your conversations about clients on a professional level. When making reports by phone in your own home, make sure your family cannot hear you.

Verbal Reporting in a Facility

In a facility, you report your actions and observations to the charge nurse. Reports must be prompt, thorough, and accurate. Always give the client's name, the room and bed number, and the time you made the observation or gave the care. Report only what you observed or did yourself. Prioritize items. Start your report with the most important points. Give reports as often as the client's condition requires or as often as requested by the nurse. Immediately report any changes from normal or changes in the person's condition.

The charge nurse gives a report at the end of shift (called the end-of-shift report). The report includes information about each client's condition, the care given, and the care that must be given on the next shift. Some facilities expect all team members to hear the end-of-shift report as they come on duty.

Verbal Reporting in a Community Setting

Agencies have their own policies for verbal reports. Most agencies do not require support workers to make daily verbal reports. Usually, you call the agency if something out of the ordinary occurs. Call your supervisor immediately if something unexpected happens. Follow agency policy and the guidelines in Boxes 7-4 and 7-5 on page 68.

Charts

A **chart** (also known as a **record)** is a written account of a client's condition or illness and responses to care.

Box 7-4 Guidelines for Contacting Your Supervisor

- There is an emergency
- You observe a change in the client's condition or normal functioning
- The client becomes ill. For example, the person vomits, has diarrhea, or develops a fever
- The client is in distress
- You believe the client's safety is at risk
- A problem arises involving medications
- The client complains about his or her condition or care
- The client asks you a question about his or her diagnosis, condition, or treatment plans
- The client or family member asks you to do something that contradicts the care plan
- You have a conflict with a client or family member
- A question or problem arises with which you need help

Box 7-5 Guidelines for Making Telephone Reports to Your Supervisor

- Keep agency phone numbers and extensions handy.
- Make sure you have a pen and paper handy.
- Identify yourself, the date, and the time of your call.
- Give a concise, accurate, and descriptive report. For example, say what you observed, (client has bruises on buttocks) when you made the observation (when bathing the client) and what the client said ("I fell down the stairs last night").
- Use the client's exact words.
- Speak clearly and slowly. Pause between sentences.
- Write down the instructions from your supervisor.
- Repeat the instructions back to your supervisor.
- Write the instructions on the appropriate document in the client's chart.
- Remember the client's information is confidential. It is shared only with the health care team.

The chart is a permanent, legal record. It provides for the following:

- *Communication.* Health care teams rely on charts to relay information about their clients (Figure 7-3). All team members must be informed about the client's condition and care. Recording is an accurate way to communicate information about the client. The care plan is one part of the chart. Other parts are discussed in Documents Used in Charts.
- *Currency.* Care plans change as the client's needs, preferences, and condition change. Charts enable staff to keep the client's information up-to-date.
- *Accountability.* Charts are signed and dated by members of the health care team. This allows information to be tracked. All team members are accountable for their words and actions.
- *Continuity of care.* Written documentation contains information on the client's past health problems and treatments. This information enables health care providers to detect patterns and changes in the client's health. Team members change over time. Without a written record, care might be fragmented and unreliable.

Documents Used in Charts

Charts vary, depending on the employer. Most employers design their own documents. This section describes some common documents contained in a client's chart.

- *Data forms*—include details about the client's physical, emotional, social, and intellectual health. Long-term care facilities use these forms to record information about residents' health. Activities, interests, medications, treatments, and therapies are examples of information that is recorded.
- *Assessment forms*—used by nurses and case managers to record a client's health problems and needs. Assessments are based on information from the data form and other sources, including observations made by the health care team.
- *Home assessment forms*—documents changes that need to be made to the client's home during rehabilitation (see Box 32-3 on page 562).
- *Care plans*—contain goals and interventions (action plan) based on the assessment. Sometimes the assessment and care plan are on the same form.

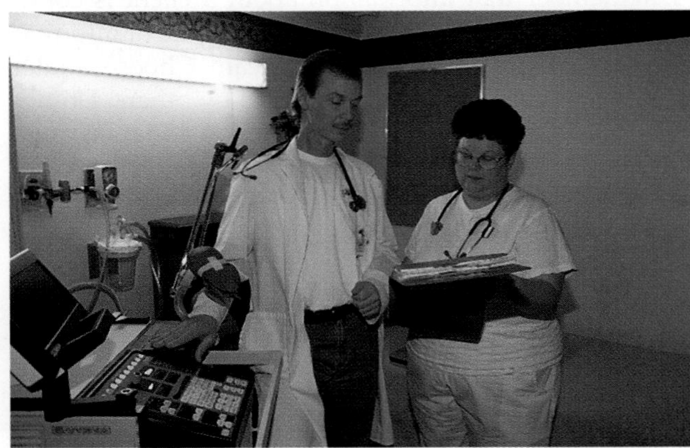

Figure 7-3 The nurse and respiratory therapist review a client's chart.

- *Progress notes*—record information about the care given, the client's response to care, observations, the client's activities, special treatments, and medications. Progress notes also contain areas for the date, time, and initials (Figure 7-4 on page 70). Health care team members from various disciplines may or may not record care and treatment on one set of notes. In some circumstances, progress notes may be separated into disciplines (for example, a section for nursing, a section for physiotherapy, and so on). This enables the disciplines to retain their own progress notes at the end of care. Whether or not you record information on progress notes depends on your employer's policy.
- *Activities-of-daily-living (ADL) checklists and flow sheets*—record actions relating to hygiene, food and fluids, elimination, rest and sleep, mobility, activity, and social interactions. ADL checklists require you to place a check mark in a box. ADL flow sheets use codes for actions, such as "I" for independent and "A" for assist. ADL checklists and flow sheets provide little or no space for writing details. ADL checklists are sometimes called "tick sheets." Some of the items in an ADL flow sheet are shown in Figure 7-5 on page 71.
- *Task sheets*—used by agencies in community settings to record care and services provided. The form has boxes for each day and for care and support activities. You check the box for the day the care or service was given (Figure 7-6 on page 72).
- *Graphic sheets*—record measurements and observations made every shift or three to four times per day. Information may include the client's blood pressure, temperature, pulse, respirations, height, and weight. Some graphic sheets have places to chart the intake and output, routine care, bowel movements, and physician's visits. An example is shown in Figure 7-7 on page 73.
- *Other flow sheets*—record frequent measurements and observations. Some record blood pressure, pulse, and respirations every 15 minutes or more often. Others record intake and output. Flow sheets are used to monitor the condition of seriously ill people.
- *Summary reports*—summarize care and service provided over a period of time. These are used in community settings and by some long-term care facilities to provide summaries of the client's condition monthly, or every second or third month.
- *Incident reports*—written accounts made after an accident, error, or unexpected event. In the community, these reports are commonly called occurrence reports (see Chapter 16).
- *Kardex*—a card file that summarizes information in the chart. It usually includes the person's current diagnosis, medications and treatments, any special equipment needs, and routine care measures. The Kardex system provides a quick source of current information. It can be frequently updated to reflect changes. The Kardex is used in some facilities, but is rarely used in community settings.

Recording

Recording (or **charting**) is documenting care and observations. Employers have their own policies for recording, including when to record, how often to record, what should be recorded, and who should record. Policies address issues like how to abbreviate, what colour of ink to use, and how to make corrections. When recording, focus on:

- What you observed
- What you did
- When you did it
- The client's response

When recording on a document or form, communicate clearly and thoroughly. Make sure that measurements and numbers recorded are absolutely accurate. If there is a space for observations, these should be precise, accurate, and relevant. Use the guidelines in Box 7-6 on page 74, and follow your employer's policies.

Recording Time. The 24-hour clock is used to document care. The 24-hour clock involves using a four-digit number for time (Figure 7-8 on page 74). The first two digits are for the hour: 0100 = 1:00 a.m.; 1300 = 1:00 p.m. The last two digits are for minutes: 0110 = 1:10 a.m. The a.m. and p.m. abbreviations are not used.

As Box 7-7 on page 74 shows, morning hours are the same in the 24-hour clock as they are in the conventional clock, except that a.m. is not used. For p.m. times, add 12 to the first two digits (the hours) of clock time. If it is 2:00 p.m., add 12 to 2 to make 1400. For 8:35 p.m., add 12 to 8 to make 2035.

The 24-hour clock makes communication more accurate. Since health care team members do not have to write a.m. or p.m., there is less chance for confusion.

Terminology and Abbreviations. Medical terminology and abbreviations are used to communicate in health care (see Chapter 48). If a member of the health care team uses a word that you do not understand, be sure to ask the person what the word means. It is a good idea to buy a medical dictionary to use as reference.

Recording in a Facility

In an acute-care setting, you most likely will document care on graphic sheets, flow sheets, and/or progress notes. You may be expected to document, for

(text continues on page 75)

Date	Time	Progress Notes	Name	Signature
4-21	1200	Out for walk and lunch with visitor (niece).	Liz Black (RPN)	Liz Black
	1400	Returned from outing. Said, "I had a good time."	Gerry Krueger (SW)	Gerry Krueger
	1500	Watching TV in lounge. Said, "I don't feel well." Maria Bueno (RN) notified.	Gerry Krueger (SW)	Gerry Krueger
	1505	Took history. Started feeling unwell at 1430. Aches and pains in muscles. No nausea. No cough. Mild headache. T 37.7 orally, radial pulse 85, respirations 16.2. Tylenol given. Dr. Li informed.	Maria Bueno (RN)	Maria Bueno
	1515	Helped resident into bed. Instructed her to use call bell if she feels worse or symptoms occur. Provided drinking water.	Gerry Krueger (SW)	Gerry Krueger
	1540	Resident asleep. Breathing unlaboured.	Liz Black (RPN)	Liz Black
	1600	Resident still asleep. Breathing unlaboured.	Liz Black (RPN)	Liz Black
	1630	Resident awake. Said, "I feel cold." No headache. Still feels aches and pains. Notified RN of resident's condition.	Gerry Krueger (SW)	Gerry Krueger
	1635	Fever has come down. T. 37.2. Headache gone. Aches and pains still felt.	Liz Black (RPN)	Liz Black

Figure 7-4 Progress notes from a long-term care facility.

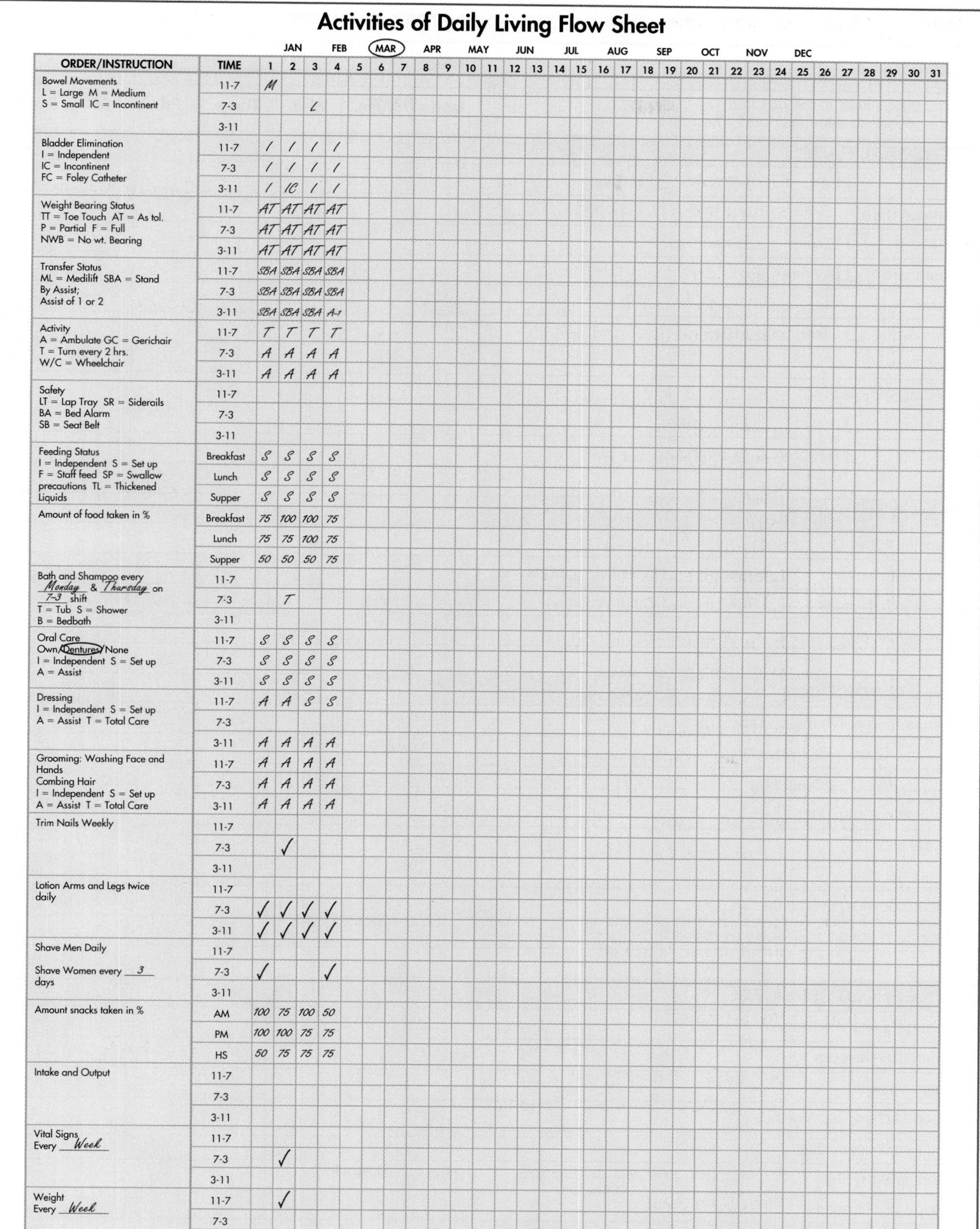

Activities of Daily Living Flow Sheet

JAN FEB (MAR) APR MAY JUN JUL AUG SEP OCT NOV DEC

ORDER/INSTRUCTION	TIME	1	2	3	4	5	6	7	8	9	10	11	12	13	14	15	16	17	18	19	20	21	22	23	24	25	26	27	28	29	30	31
Bowel Movements L = Large M = Medium S = Small IC = Incontinent	11-7	M																														
	7-3			L																												
	3-11																															
Bladder Elimination I = Independent IC = Incontinent FC = Foley Catheter	11-7	I	I	I	I																											
	7-3	I	I	I	I																											
	3-11	I	IC	I	I																											
Weight Bearing Status TT = Toe Touch AT = As tol. P = Partial F = Full NWB = No wt. Bearing	11-7	AT	AT	AT	AT																											
	7-3	AT	AT	AT	AT																											
	3-11	AT	AT	AT	AT																											
Transfer Status ML = Medilift SBA = Stand By Assist; Assist of 1 or 2	11-7	SBA	SBA	SBA	SBA																											
	7-3	SBA	SBA	SBA	SBA																											
	3-11	SBA	SBA	SBA	A-1																											
Activity A = Ambulate GC = Gerichair T = Turn every 2 hrs. W/C = Wheelchair	11-7	T	T	T	T																											
	7-3	A	A	A	A																											
	3-11	A	A	A	A																											
Safety LT = Lap Tray SR = Siderails BA = Bed Alarm SB = Seat Belt	11-7																															
	7-3																															
	3-11																															
Feeding Status I = Independent S = Set up F = Staff feed SP = Swallow precautions TL = Thickened Liquids	Breakfast	S	S	S	S																											
	Lunch	S	S	S	S																											
	Supper	S	S	S	S																											
Amount of food taken in %	Breakfast	75	100	100	75																											
	Lunch	75	75	100	75																											
	Supper	50	50	50	75																											
Bath and Shampoo every Monday & Thursday on 7-3 shift T = Tub S = Shower B = Bedbath	11-7																															
	7-3		T																													
	3-11																															
Oral Care Own/(Dentures)/None I = Independent S = Set up A = Assist	11-7	S	S	S	S																											
	7-3	S	S	S	S																											
	3-11	S	S	S	S																											
Dressing I = Independent S = Set up A = Assist T = Total Care	11-7	A	A	S	S																											
	7-3																															
	3-11	A	A	A	A																											
Grooming: Washing Face and Hands Combing Hair I = Independent S = Set up A = Assist T = Total Care	11-7	A	A	A	A																											
	7-3	A	A	A	A																											
	3-11	A	A	A	A																											
Trim Nails Weekly	11-7																															
	7-3		✓																													
	3-11																															
Lotion Arms and Legs twice daily	11-7																															
	7-3	✓	✓	✓	✓																											
	3-11	✓	✓	✓	✓																											
Shave Men Daily	11-7																															
Shave Women every 3 days	7-3	✓			✓																											
	3-11																															
Amount snacks taken in %	AM	100	75	100	50																											
	PM	100	100	75	75																											
	HS	50	75	75	75																											
Intake and Output	11-7																															
	7-3																															
	3-11																															
Vital Signs Every Week	11-7																															
	7-3		✓																													
	3-11																															
Weight Every Week	11-7		✓																													
	7-3																															

Figure 7-5 Some of the items in an activities-of-daily-living flow sheet

SAMPLE CLIENT CARE TASK SHEET

Client Name: ______________________ **Dates:** ____________ to ____________

Write your initials in the box that corresponds to each task performed.	Mon.	Tues.	Wed.	Thurs.	Fri.	Sat.	Sun.
PERSONAL CARE:							
Bath ☐ Bed ☐ Chair ☐ Shower ☐ Tub							
Perineal Care							
Hair ☐ Groom ☐ Shampoo							
Mouthcare ☐ Denture Care							
Shave							
Nail Care ☐ Clean ☐ File							
Foot Care							
Special Skin Care							
Dressing ☐ Assist ☐ Complete							
Toileting ☐ Bed Pan ☐ Commode ☐ BRP							
Other:							
CLIENT ACTIVITIES:							
Transfer Activity Instructions:							
Assist with walking ☐ Cane ☐ Walker ☐ Crutches							
Assist with exercises ☐ ROM ☐ Other (specify)							
Wheelchair activities							
Other:							
OTHER FUNCTIONS:							
Prepare and serve meal/snack							
Special diet (specify)							
Assist with feeding							
Medications reminder							
Stoma care							
Incontinent care							
Record bowel movements							
Change in condition (office was notified)							
Other:							
HOUSEHOLD SERVICES:							
Change/make client's bed							
Clean client's room							
Clean bathroom							
Clean kitchen; wash dishes							
Vacuum, sweep, dust							
Client laundry							
Shopping/Errands							

Other/Observations: ____

Figure 7-6 Agency task sheet.

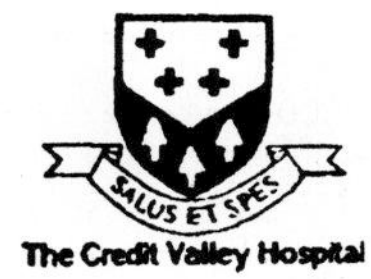

VITAL SIGNS FLOWSHEET

Signature/Status	Initials	Signature/Status	Initials

	Date :												
	Time :												
Temperature (C°)	: 40												
	39												
	38												
	37												
	36												
	35												
Pulse :													
Respirations :													
B.P. :	Lying :												
	Sitting :												
	Standing :												
Weight :													
	Initials												

Figure 7-7 Graphic sheet.

Box 7-6 Guidelines for Recording

- Always use ink. Follow employer policy for the colour of ink to use.
- Include the date and the time whenever a recording is made. Use conventional time (a.m. or p.m.) or 24-hour clock time according to employer policy.
- Make sure writing is legible and neat.
- Use only employer-approved abbreviations.
- Use correct spelling, grammar, and punctuation.
- Never erase or use correction fluid if you make an error. Make a single line through the error. Write "error" or "mistaken entry" over it, and sign your initials. Then rewrite the part. Follow your employer's policies for correcting errors.
- Sign all entries with your name and title as required by your employer's policy.
- Do not skip lines. Draw a line through the blank space of a partially completed line or to the end of a page. This prevents others from recording in a space with your signature.
- Make sure each form is stamped with the client's name and other identifying information.
- Record only what you observed and did yourself.
- Never chart a procedure or treatment until after its completion.
- Be accurate, concise, and factual. Do not record assumptions or opinions.
- Record in a logical manner in the order in which tasks and procedures occurred.
- Be descriptive. Avoid terms with more than one meaning.
- Use the client's exact words. Use quotation marks to show that the statement is a direct quote.
- Chart any changes from normal or changes in the client's condition. Also chart that you informed your supervisor and the time you made the report.
- Do not omit information.
- Record safety measures such as assisting a client when up or reminding someone not to get out of bed. This will help protect you if the person falls.

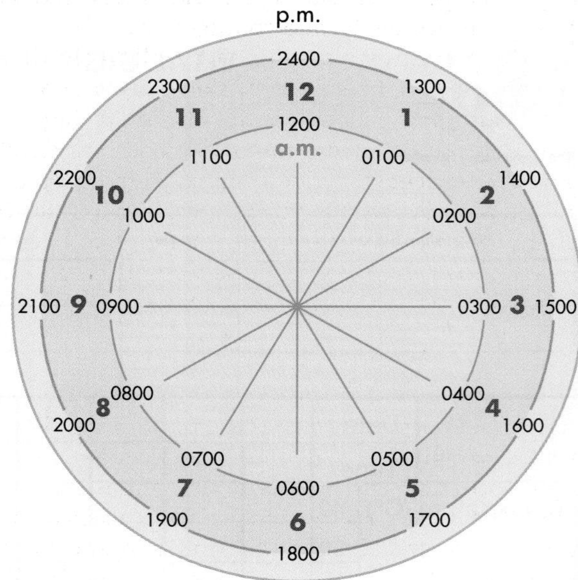

Figure 7-8 The 24-hour clock.

Box 7-7 24-Hour Clock

CONVENTIONAL TIME	24-HOUR CLOCK
1:00 a.m.	0100
2:00 a.m.	0200
3:00 a.m.	0300
4:00 a.m.	0400
5:00 a.m.	0500
6:00 a.m.	0600
7:00 a.m.	0700
8:00 a.m.	0800
9:00 a.m.	0900
10:00 a.m.	1000
11:00 a.m.	1100
12:00 noon	1200
1:00 p.m.	1300
2:00 p.m.	1400
3:00 p.m.	1500
4:00 p.m.	1600
5:00 p.m.	1700
6:00 p.m.	1800
7:00 p.m.	1900
8:00 p.m.	2000
9:00 p.m.	2100
10:00 p.m.	2200
11:00 p.m.	2300
12:00 midnight	2400 or 0000

example, temperature, blood pressure, intake and output, bowel movements, and routine care.

In a long-term care setting, you will likely document care on ADL checklists or flow sheets. If a resident's health status needs frequent monitoring, you may also document on graphic sheets and flow sheets. You may be expected to give summary reports on care provided to residents. Or, your supervisor will ask for your input for the preparation of a summary report from the health care team. These written reports are usually required monthly or every three months.

Recording in the Community

Every agency and case manager keep separate client charts in their organizations. Some parts of the client's chart are usually, but not always, kept in the client's home. Documents in the home are often kept in a binder. The forms in the binder vary according to agency policy and the client's condition and needs. Among other documents, the binder usually contains the care plan, progress notes, ADL checklists, flow sheets, or task sheets. Agency policies differ. Some do not allow support workers to enter anything on the documents that are kept in the binder. Others expect support workers to record tasks and observations on the forms in the binder.

Most agencies have forms called client care task sheets that you carry with you to every assignment (see Figure 7-6 on page 72). You start a new task sheet for each client. As you complete tasks, you check off relevant areas of the form.

Most task sheets contain space for you to record special circumstances or observations. You may be expected to identify whether the client was independent, dependent, or needed some assistance with activities. As mentioned, any changes you observe in a client's normal functioning or condition should be reported by phone to your supervisor. Record on the task sheet any verbal reports that you make, as well as phone instructions received from your supervisor.

You hand in your task sheets monthly or weekly depending on agency policy, along with forms that track mileage and other work expenses. Your supervisor may use your task sheets to help prepare a report on each client. You may be asked for additional information on some of your clients.

Confidentiality

The chart is confidential. You are ethically and legally bound to keep client information confidential. This includes information that you record. All employers have strict guidelines about the confidentiality of charts and client information. You must be particularly careful to observe guidelines about accessing, reporting, and transporting information.

Only health care team members involved in the client's care have access to confidential information. Those not directly involved usually are not allowed access to the client's chart. Housekeeping staff, kitchen staff, and office clerks do not need to see charts or to hear any confidential details about a client. In a home care setting, only certain family members have access to these details. Your supervisor will tell you who can look at the chart.

In a facility, you may transport a document from a central file area to a client's room or other location. In a community setting, you may carry with you confidential information about a client. Be very careful when transporting confidential documents. Concentrate on what you are doing. Remind yourself of the importance of your task. If you become distracted, you could easily leave the documents in an inappropriate place.

Computerized Charts

Charts are on computers in many agencies and facilities. Using a computer is easier, faster, and more efficient than writing on the chart (Figure 7-9). Recordings are more accurate, legible, and reliable. Information can be accessed at the nurse's station, at the agency, and even at the bedside. These computer links reduce clerical work and telephone calls.

In a community setting, you might be expected to send in reports by e-mail. In the future, computer literacy and ownership of a computer may be required for working in these settings.

Computer information is easy to access. Therefore, the client's right to privacy must be protected. Only certain staff members are allowed to use the computer. They have their own codes (passwords) to access computer files. If you are allowed access, you will be trained how to use the computer system. Follow the ethical and legal considerations relating to privacy and confidentiality (see Chapters 9 and 10).

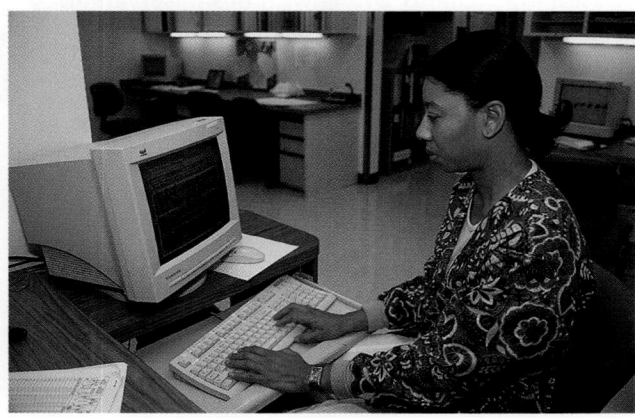

Figure 7-9 The nurse enters information into the computer.

REVIEW

Circle the BEST answer.

1. Assessment involves
   A. Collecting information about the client
   B. Carrying out or performing the elements of the care plan
   C. Implementing the care plan
   D. Evaluating and measuring the effectiveness of the care plan

2. Which is *not* a function of the care plan?
   A. To provide a central reference point on the client's health problems, needs, treatment, and care
   B. To enable the health care team to communicate with each other about the client
   C. To ensure that everyone provides the same care
   D. To provide information about the client that never changes

3. The statement, "Urinary Elimination, Impaired" is on a care plan. This statement is a(n)
   A. nursing diagnosis
   B. assessment
   C. evaluation
   D. medical diagnosis

4. Mrs. Muryama says, "I didn't sleep at all last night because of the pain in my back." This is
   A. A nursing diagnosis
   B. Subjective data
   C. An intervention
   D. Objective data

5. You record the following: "Mr. Munro was better today." What is wrong with this observation?
   A. It does not say better than what.
   B. It is an assumption.
   C. It is an assessment.
   D. Nothing is wrong with this observation.

6. Which statement is *false*?
   A. A chart is discarded after the person is discharged from hospital.
   B. A chart is a permanent, legal document.
   C. A chart is updated as a person's needs and condition change.
   D. A chart provides a record of accountability for health care providers.

7. A graphic sheet
   A. Records a client's activities of daily living (ADLs)
   B. Is used to record measurements and observations made three to four times per day
   C. Contains information about the care given, the client's responses to care, and observations about the client's condition
   D. Summarizes a client's care and services over a period of time

8. A data form
   A. Is used in long-term care settings to detail a person's physical, emotional, social, and intellectual health
   B. Is used in home care settings to assess changes that may be needed to the home
   C. Includes boxes that are checked for the day on which care or services were given
   D. Is another name for Kardex

9. In 24-hour time, 1330 is
   A. 3:30 p.m.
   B. 3:30 a.m.
   C. 1:30 p.m.
   D. 1:30 a.m.

10. If you make an error when recording, you should
    A. Put an X though the error, and write "error" over it.
    B. Erase the error.
    C. Make a single line through the error, and write "error" over it.
    D. Use correction fluid.

11. In a long-term care facility, who has access to the residents' charts?
    A. All staff members
    B. Only the office staff and nursing staff
    C. Nurses, support workers, physiotherapists, occupational therapists, and dieticians
    D. It depends on facility policy and procedures.

Answers to these questions are on page 821.

CHAPTER 8

MANAGING STRESS, TIME, AND PROBLEMS

OBJECTIVES

- Define the key terms listed in this chapter
- Understand how stress can affect all dimensions of life
- List signs of stress
- Discuss defence mechanisms
- Describe common stressors
- Describe how to manage stress
- Define SMART goals
- Describe methods that will improve your decision-making and problem-solving abilities
- Explain how to deal with conflict

KEY TERMS

anxiety A vague, uneasy feeling, including a sense of impending danger or harm

burnout A state of physical, emotional, and mental exhaustion

conflict A clash between opposing interests and ideas

defence mechanism An unconscious reaction that blocks unpleasant or threatening feelings

stress The emotional, behavioural, or physical response to an event or situation

stressor An event or situation that causes stress

Marissa became a support worker because she likes helping people. She feels great compassion for her clients. Most of the time she likes her job. However, she sometimes worries that she is not doing her best. She feels stressed, rushed, and has trouble making decisions. She discusses her feelings with her supervisor, who encourages her to take a time-management course. Her supervisor also offers to help Marissa become a better decision maker and problem solver.

This chapter deals with four key challenges of support work: handling stress, managing time, making decisions, and solving problems. If you can manage time, make wise decisions, and solve problems, you will have less stress.

STRESS

Everyone experiences stress. It is a normal part of life. **Stress** is the emotional, behavioural, or physical response to an event or situation. The event or situation that causes stress is a **stressor**. Events or situations that are perceived to be threatening, new, or exciting are often stressors. Physical conditions like illness, fever, or pregnancy are also stressors.

Although most people do not like stress, it sometimes is helpful. Stress can encourage people to function effectively. For example, the stress caused by a busy schedule can motivate you to work efficiently. However, stress that lasts for a long time or is very intense can cause illness. Headaches, upset stomach, depression, heart disease, and some cancers are examples.

Stress affects the whole person. It can have positive or negative effects in all dimensions—the physical, emotional, social, intellectual, and spiritual (Table 8-1). Severe and prolonged stress can lead to burnout. **Burnout** is a state of physical, emotional, and mental exhaustion. A person with burnout feels discouraged, negative, and powerless.

RESPONSES TO STRESS

People respond differently to the same stressor. Some people have dramatic responses to stress. Others have mild responses. A person's responses to stressors are influenced by several factors, including:

- Health
- Temperament or personality
- Past experiences with the same or similar stressors

Table 8-1 Stress Can Affect All Dimensions

Dimension	Example of stressor	Example of a negative effect	Example of a positive effect
Physical	Pneumonia	Death	Infection resolved
Emotional	Sexual assault	Fear of men; depression	Finds fulfillment as a mentor for others at sexual assault crisis centre
Intellectual	Diagnosis of cancer	Denies presence of cancer and refuses to consider treatment	Learns about the disease to make decisions about care
Social	Alcoholism	Withdraws from family and other social contacts	Participates in Alcoholics Anonymous support group
Spiritual	Injury	Feels abandoned by God	Seeks counselling from spiritual adviser; finds comfort in faith

Source: Adapted from P.A. Potter, A. Perry, J.C. Ross-Kerr, and M.J. Wood, *Canadian Fundamentals of Nursing* (Toronto: Harcourt Canada, 2001), p. 647.

- The number of other stressors the person is experiencing
- The nature, severity, and duration of the stressor

People respond to stress in different ways. There are physical responses to stress (Box 8-1) and emotional and behavioural responses (Box 8-2). Physical responses are the same for most people. However, emotional and behavioural responses vary among individuals. Often the behaviour is the person's way of coping with stress. Some behaviours relieve stress. Crying and talking are examples. Other behaviours are unhealthy. They may eventually increase rather than decrease stress. Smoking and drinking are examples.

It is important to recognize the common responses to stress, both in yourself and in your clients. Tell your supervisor if you notice a client is showing signs of stress. Remember, your role is to observe and report. You do not assess or diagnose. Report only your observations. Do not make assumptions based on your observations. For example, a client complains of headaches and nausea. Do not assume that the client is suffering from stress, as it could be a physical condition. However, it is necessary to note these symptoms. Professionals such as nurses and social workers help clients cope with stress.

Defence Mechanisms

A **defence mechanism** is an unconscious reaction that blocks unpleasant or threatening feelings. Most people use defence mechanisms occasionally, especially when they are under stress. Defence mechanisms help relieve stress. They help the person avoid facing a troubling reality. For example, a resident in a facility is upset that his daughter cannot visit him often. He blames the city bus system. He believes that if the buses were more reliable, his daughter would visit. He focuses his anger on the bus system, but he really is disappointed with his daughter.

When working with clients under stress, it is useful to be able to recognize defence mechanisms. Understanding defence mechanisms gives you insight into what people may really be feeling. You can help by being empathetic to their feelings and providing compassionate care. Report your observations. The following are examples of defence mechanisms:

- *Conversion*—Changing an emotion into a physical symptom. Example: The mother of a seriously ill boy notices she is losing large amounts of hair. Although she appears to be handling the situation very well, her hair loss is in response to the intense stress.
- *Denial*—Refusing to accept an unpleasant or threatening reality. Example: A man in a retirement facility has been told his roommate, John, has died. The man insists that his new roommate *is* John.
- *Displacement*—Directing emotions toward a person or thing that seems safe, instead of toward the person or thing that is the source of the emotions. Example: A client is angry with her husband. Instead of expressing anger at him, she shouts at her support worker.
- *Projection*—Assigning one's feelings to someone or something else. Example: A child says that she needs a night-light because her doll is afraid of the dark.
- *Rationalization*—Making excuses for one's behaviour or a situation while ignoring the real reason. Example: An older man experiences hearing loss. He says he cannot understand what his granddaughter is saying because she is mumbling.

Box 8-1 Physical Signs of Stress

- Rapid pulse
- Rapid respirations
- Increased blood pressure
- Rapid speech, higher-pitched voice
- A "lump" in the throat
- "Butterflies" in the stomach
- Dry mouth
- Sweaty palms
- Sore muscles in neck, arms, and back
- Perspiration
- Nausea
- Diarrhea
- Urinary frequency
- Urinary urgency
- Difficulty sleeping
- Change in appetite
- Change in weight

Box 8-2 Emotional and Behavioural Signs of Stress

- **Anxiety**—a vague, uneasy feeling, including a sense of impending danger or harm
- Depression
- Anger
- Worry
- Fear
- Burnout
- Irritability
- Loss of self-esteem
- Fatigue
- Dissatisfaction
- Forgetfulness
- Poor concentration
- Difficulty focusing or following directions
- Emotional outbursts, including yelling or crying
- Smoking
- Drinking
- Talking about the stressor

- *Reaction formation*—Acting in a way that is opposite to what one feels. Example: A woman ignores a man to whom she is attracted.
- *Regression*—Reverting or moving back to earlier behaviours. Example: A 3-year-old wants a bottle when a new baby comes into the family.
- *Repression*—Keeping unpleasant or painful thoughts or experiences from the conscious mind. Example: A woman who was sexually abused as a child has no memory of the abuse.

Sources of Stress

Many factors cause stress. Common stressors include:

Change. Whether it is positive or negative, change is always a source of stress. For example, getting a promotion, having a baby, and becoming ill create life changes. They all cause stress.

Pressure. Pressure is feeling pushed beyond one's limits or abilities. People feel pressured for many reasons. Being rushed, having too many demands, and feeling unable to fulfill expectations are examples (Figure 8-1). People sometimes put pressure on themselves. They set goals that are very difficult or impossible to meet. For example, Penelope fails to lose 15 pounds in one month. Her goal was too difficult to achieve. She is frustrated with herself. This causes stress.

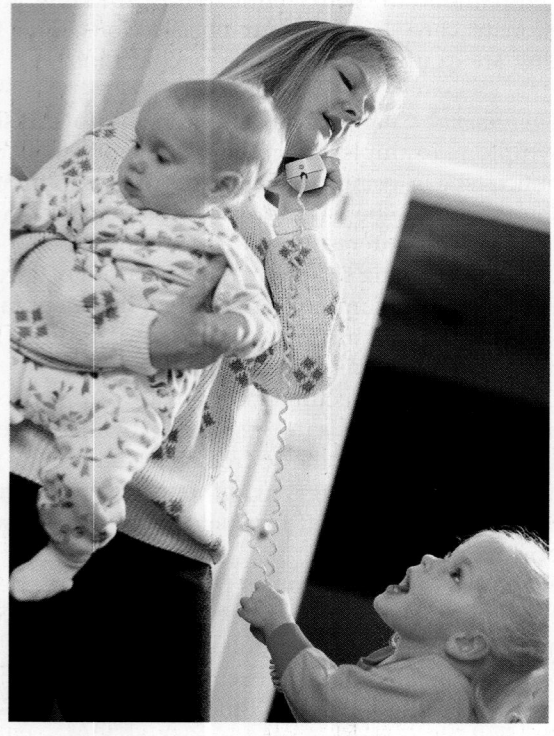

Figure 8-1 This woman is under pressure because she feels unable to fulfill the demands of both her children and her job.

Lack of Control. People feel stress when they cannot control what happens to and around them. Dependency usually causes stress. Stress results from many situations that are out of one's control. For example, loss of work, economic hardships, violence, illness, discrimination, and death of a loved one all cause stress. Not being able to control one's behaviour is also a stressor. For example, Ms. Kumar wants to quit smoking. She tries and fails. She is angry at her apparent lack of self-control. This causes stress, which she responds to by smoking.

Conflict. **Conflict** is a clash between opposing interests and ideas. Conflicts with a partner, friend, child, co-worker, or client are serious sources of stress. People also experience conflict within themselves when working out difficulties or making decisions.

Daily Irritations. The seemingly minor incidents that occur every day sometimes cause stress. For example, you cannot find your car keys. You are stuck in traffic. You oversleep. Depending on your reaction, any frustrating incident can cause stress.

Stressors do not create the same amounts of stress. The more frequent the stressor and the longer it lasts, the more likely the person's health will suffer. Stressors that last for a few minutes to a few hours usually create only mild stress. Daily irritations are examples. Stressors that last for months or years cause severe stress. Chronic illness, disability, and family relationship problems are examples. (See *Focus on Older Adults: Stress* and *Focus on Children: Stress* boxes.)

Managing Stress in Your Life

Burnout is common among health care workers. Support work can be physically and emotionally demanding. You may feel stress from the lifting, moving, and carrying that are required. You may feel stress while trying to do many things at once. For example, a client asks for the bedpan every time you walk by the room, while another needs to be turned and repositioned every 15 minutes. You may feel emotional stress from working with people who are sick, lonely, frail, or dying. You may also work with clients or family members who are angry or distressed. For example, a wife who is the primary caregiver for her ill husband is angry with her boss for insisting she always work late. She may direct her anger toward you. Or, you might feel upset for her. Depending on how you react, situations like this one could cause severe stress.

Managing stress is essential. Do not ignore signs of stress. Letting stress build can result in burnout or illness. Not dealing properly with stress causes some workers to take out their frustrations on their clients or in their personal lives. Abuse or neglect may occur. These situations must not happen.

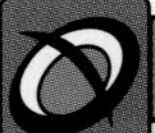

Focus on Older Adults

STRESS

Older adults may face many stressors, including:

- Health problems
- Economic worries, since most older adults are on a fixed income
- Increased dependency if the person becomes frail
- Loneliness and isolation
- Decline in abilities due to the normal aging process

Although they may be faced with many stressors, most older adults can cope with stress as well as other adults. Many older adults rely on their spirituality to cope with illness or severe stress.

Source: Based on P.A. Potter, A. Perry, J.C. Ross-Kerr, and M.J. Wood, *Canadian Fundamentals of Nursing* (Toronto: Harcourt Canada, 2001), p. 655.

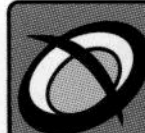

Focus on Children

STRESS

Infants and children also react to stressors. Children may show the same signs of stress as do adults. For example, a child under stress might have stomachaches, irritability, changes in appetite, or changes in sleep patterns.

Children might not be able to communicate their feelings in words. They are more likely to communicate with their actions. Whenever a child behaves out of the ordinary, the behaviour may be a sign of stress. For example, a normally content baby cries for an hour after she was over stimulated. A fully toilet-trained 4-year-old suddenly begins to wet the bed after his mother becomes seriously ill. A usually calm adolescent begins to physically fight with peers after his parents divorce. All these behaviours may be signs of stress.

Good communication with your supervisor will help relieve stress. Talk regularly with your supervisor about stressors at work. Immediately notify your supervisor if you feel overwhelmed by stress or have difficulties coping. Do not expect that you have to manage alone.

The following strategies will help you manage stress in your life:

- *Develop self-awareness.* Know what causes your stress. Think about when you felt under stress. What was the source? Does it occur often? After determining your stressors, you need to decide how to eliminate them, avoid them, or cope with them.
- *Take care of your needs.* A healthy mind and body enable people to cope better with stress. Getting enough sleep is important. Mild irritations may seem like serious problems if you are sleep deprived. Exercising regularly and following a nutritious diet are also important. Do not ignore your social, intellectual, and spiritual needs. For many people, the key to managing stress is finding ways to balance family, work, relaxation, and recreation. Keep track of how you spend your time. What parts of your life get too much time? What parts are neglected? How might you achieve a better balance?
- *Think positively.* A positive attitude can help you manage stress. Focus on what you do well and what you can control. Remember that every person perceives stress differently. Try to change your perspective to see how a stressor can create a positive outcome. Put the stressor into perspective. Try not to let a minor stressor become a major one. Keeping a sense of humour also helps reduce tension.
- *Assert yourself.* Nonassertive people say yes to things when they want to say no. They take on tasks for which they have no time. They also give into the demands of others, without considering their own needs. Never agree to do more than you are able (see Chapter 12).
- *Ask others for help and support.* To avoid stress, you have to accept that you cannot do everything yourself. Assert yourself at work and in your home life. If you need help with an assignment, tell your supervisor. At home, let your family know that you need their help and support. Discuss household duties with your spouse and children. Let them know what you need and expect. Take the time to explain to them how things are done. Be encouraging, and avoid being critical if things are not done to your standard.
- *Practise calming exercises.* As soon as you feel the first sign of stress, find a way to calm yourself (Box 8-3 on page 82). Some people do daily meditation to help cope with stress (Box 8-4 on page 82).

TIME MANAGEMENT

Time management is essential to reducing stress. It is also important in support work. You can use time-management strategies in all aspects of your life. If you reduce your overall stress levels, stress at work will also decline.

To manage your time, you must identify your priorities. They help you stay focused on what is important to you. While at work, providing competent, compassionate care is a priority. To determine your priorities outside of work, ask yourself these questions:

Box 8-3 Calming Yourself When Feeling Stress

- Shut your eyes (if safe to do so) and take deep, slow breaths. Relax your stomach muscles. Breathe in through your nose and out through your mouth. Your stomach should rise about 3 cm (1 inch) as you breathe in. As you inhale, count slowly up to 4. As you exhale, count slowly back down to 1. Pause between breaths. Continue breathing slowly and rhythmically until you can feel yourself relaxing.
- If you feel your muscles tensing, relax them. People tend to clench their jaws and tighten their necks and backs when they are under stress. Relax your muscles, from your face down to your feet.
- If possible, take a few minutes to yourself. Remove yourself from the stressful situation. *However, never leave a client unless it is safe to do so.*

Box 8-4 Meditation

- At home, sit in a comfortable position in a quiet place. Turn the ringer off the phone.
- Pick a word that can be repeated during meditation. Single-syllable words such as *one* are very effective.
- Relax all muscle groups beginning with the head and working progressively down to your feet.
- Breathe in slowly through the nose and exhale slowly through your mouth.
- Silently repeat the chosen word while inhaling and exhaling.
- Focus thoughts on this rhythmic chanting and breathing for ten minutes.
- Allow images and thoughts to flow freely.

Source: Adapted from P.A. Potter, A. Perry, J.C. Ross-Kerr, and M.J. Wood, *Canadian Fundamentals of Nursing* (Toronto: Harcourt Canada, 2001), p. 664.

- What do I value most in life?
- What is my purpose or mission in life?
- What gives me satisfaction?
- What principles do I want to live my life by?

You may identify a large number of priorities. Take some time to decide what are the most important. Assign a number to each, with 1 being the most important and 10 being the least important. Now you are ready to turn your priorities into goals.

Setting SMART Goals

Setting goals for yourself will help you manage time and stress. Your goals should motivate you to take action and give you direction. Start with your number 1 priority and work down the list to number 10. Do not set more than ten goals, or you may lose your focus. Your goals should be SMART: **s**pecific, **m**easurable, **a**chievable, **r**ealistic, and **t**imely.[1]

- ***Specific.*** Goals must be clear. For example, wanting to be assertive is not specific. The goal to "stand up for myself five times by the end of March" is specific. It gives direction and focus.
- ***Measurable.*** Measurable goals tell if you are making progress. The goal stated above is measurable in two ways: "assertive *five* times" and "by the *end of March*."
- ***Achievable.*** Goals should be challenging, yet achievable. When setting goals, consider how much time and effort you can put into them. A goal may need two or more parts to be achievable. For example, you want to learn to play an instrument. You do not expect to be able to play an entire piece right away. First you learn how to read notes. Then you learn how to play a musical scale.
- ***Realistic.*** A realistic goal accounts for time, resources, and skills. For example, your goal is to learn to drive. If you do not have a car to practise with, the goal will be difficult to achieve.
- ***Timely.*** A target date for meeting goals increases commitment. Break goals into parts and set time schedules. As each part is achieved, you will gain confidence and be motivated to reach higher goals.

Planning Your Life and Your Work

Well-organized people include their personal and professional goals in weekly and daily planning. Goals are easier to achieve if you spend some time planning at the start of each week. For example, every Sunday Raj plans his week. He is a busy support worker with a wife and two children. Raj is working the evening shift this week, which means his wife must pick up the children, make dinner, and take them to after-school activities. Raj's wife is out of town on Thursday, so they must arrange for Raj's sister to look after the children that evening. One of Raj's goals is to build a backyard hockey rink, which he has promised his children. He decides to do this during the day before leaving for work. Raj reviews his work schedule for the week. His supervisor has asked him to coach a new support worker this week, which means he will be taking the new support worker on client visits. Since this may cause concern for one of his clients, his supervisor has asked him to call the client to prepare him for the new worker. Raj makes a note for Monday to telephone this client.

Daily planning and scheduling are also important to meeting goals. Review your assignment sheet and the care plan for each client, and decide how you will approach each task. (See *Support Workers Solving Problems: Daily Planning* box.) If you do this ahead of time

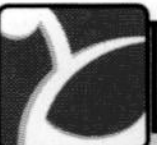

Support Workers Solving Problems

Daily Planning

Scenario: Chona is a support worker in a long-term care facility. Before her morning shift begins, she reviews her assignment sheet and the care plans for each of the residents she supports. The care plan notes that Mrs. Paget, a new resident, requires assistance in making decisions for herself. The care plan identifies that all care providers should help Mrs. Paget make decisions by providing choices.

Discussion: Chona considers the choices that she could provide for Mrs. Paget. She decides that she can offer Mrs. Paget two sets of clothes to wear for the day, two different items for breakfast, and she can ask Mrs. Paget whether she would like to participate in the morning or afternoon exercise session. Because she has planned for these choices in advance, Chona is able to concentrate all of her attention on Mrs. Paget during care tasks.

(the night before or just before your shift), you will not have to use valuable time with clients to schedule tasks. This does not mean you should never change a schedule. You must stay flexible and responsive.

Use your planning and scheduling time to think about problems that might arise. Review the tasks on your list. Plan how much time each task will take. To improve scheduling, ask yourself these questions:

- What are the client's needs and priorities?
- How much time will each task or activity require?
- When will I do each task or activity?
- Can I organize my time so that some of the tasks overlap?
- Have I allowed time for the unexpected?
- Is there anyone with whom I should coordinate these activities?

Give each task a time limit. This helps you to stay focused and complete a task in good time. See Box 8-5 for ways to manage your time and stay organized. At the end of your workday, compare what you planned to do with what you actually did. Did you accomplish what you planned? If not, review the reasons. Did problems arise? Were there interruptions? Was scheduling poor?

Decision Making

Support workers make many decisions every day. You make decisions when you organize your time, when you make a schedule, and when you provide care for a client. For example, you decide:

- The order in which you are going to carry out tasks
- The equipment and supplies you need for each task
- The amount of time to spend with a client
- When a problem or an observation needs to be reported immediately
- If you need help to complete a task
- If you need to consult with your supervisor
- If you will accept or refuse a delegated task

Skills You Need to Make Decisions

Do you know people who always seem to make the right decision? They are usually decisive and calm. The following skills will help with decision making:

- *Focus*—Focus requires concentration, involvement, and commitment. Focus on the client and the task to make the right decisions. This involves asking questions and active listening (Figure 8-2 on page 84).
- *Flexibility*—You need to be flexible and responsive. Involve clients in decisions that affect them. Be ready to adapt in response to a client's needs. Remember, each client is an individual with unique needs. Age, culture, and health affect the person's needs. For example, Mr. Johnston, 91, lives in a facility

Box 8-5 Tips to Save Time and Stay Organized

- Follow the assignment sheet and the care plan.
- Remember the client's needs and priorities.
- Know what your supervisor expects you to do and when.
- Know what tasks need to be done at a certain time.
- Set yourself time limits; work within those limits, unless a client's needs are more pressing.
- Develop routines that work for you and the client.
- Allow for more time than you need, when possible.
- Remain flexible at all times.
- Start with the tasks that must get done.
- Remind yourself not to get sidetracked by unessential things.
- Learn to say no—firmly, positively, and tactfully.
- Use a calendar for important dates and reminders.
- Make sure that you have equipment and supplies before you start a task.
- Put equipment and supplies back in their proper place.

and has no family or friends living nearby. He tells you he feels lonely. You decide to chat with him while helping him bathe. Ms. Chow, 35, is recovering at home after surgery. She tells you she feels exhausted. Since listening and talking can be tiring, you are quiet while helping Ms. Chow with her bath. You ask her if she would like to rest afterwards. She agrees. The same task is done differently because you responded to each client's needs.

- *Decisiveness*—Stick to your decisions unless they are not working. Indecisiveness can upset clients. They want you to be confident and competent.

Decision Making in Different Health Care Settings

You will face similar kinds of decisions in most settings. Some differences exist between facilities and private homes. In a facility, you care for several clients. You also assist nurses as needed. Sometimes you have to decide which person's needs to meet first. For example, a resident is shouting at her roommate. Another resident needs to be shaved. You need to decide whom to help first.

In a home care setting, you must plan your time so you can be on time for the next client. A supervisor is not on site. You have to make many decisions on your own.

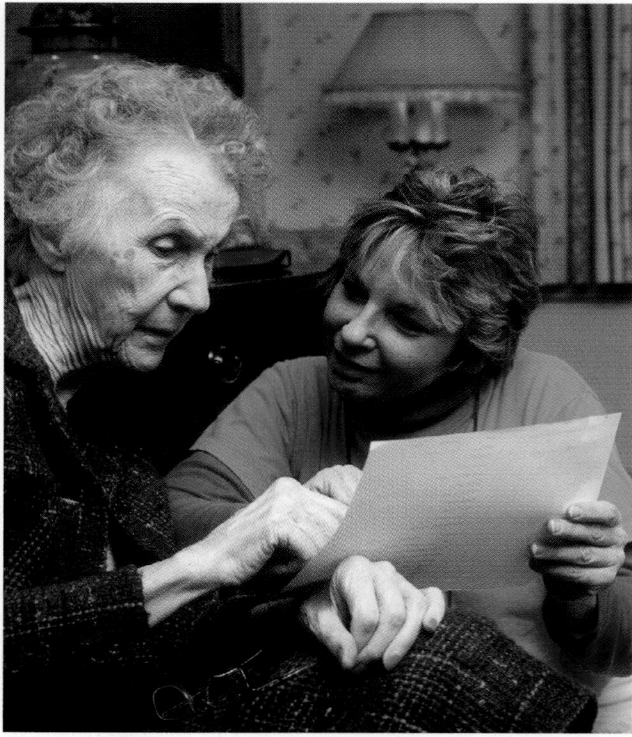

Figure 8-2 This support worker listens carefully to a client in order to make the right decision.

Problem Solving

Problem solving is a process. You identify and analyze a problem. Then you find a solution and devise a plan.

Identify the Problem

You must first determine *if* you have a problem and *what* it is. Ask yourself the following questions:

- Is the situation or issue affecting you, a co-worker, your supervisor, or one of your clients?
- Should you be concerned about the situation?
- Can you influence or contribute to a positive outcome?
- Does the issue require immediate attention?

Consider the following examples. Miles helps Mr. Rossi, 85, get dressed in the mornings. Most days, Mr. Rossi chooses to wear the same tattered sweater. Miles is tired of seeing it on him. He knows that Mr. Rossi has many other sweaters. However, when Miles considers the above questions, he answers "no" to each question. He knows that the sweater is clean. Mr. Rossi enjoys wearing it, and he has the right to choose what he wears. Miles decides that this situation is not a problem.

Cheryl assists Mr. McDonald, 88, with lunch in the dining room of a long-term care facility. He chooses tomato soup for lunch. After one spoonful, he refuses to eat. Cheryl is concerned about the situation. She knows that if Mr. McDonald does not eat, he tends to get dizzy and may fall. She knows this is a problem that requires her attention.

Analyze the Problem

Once you know you have a problem, think about what kind of problem it is. Decide if it is one that you can solve on your own. Consult the assignment sheet and care plan to make sure you know what is expected of you. Remember, consult your supervisor when:

- There is an emergency
- You observe a change in the client's condition or normal functioning
- The client becomes ill. For example, the person vomits, has diarrhea, or develops a fever
- The client is in distress
- You believe the client's safety is at risk
- A problem arises involving medications
- The client complains about his or her condition or care
- The client asks you a question about his or her diagnosis, condition, or treatment plans

- The client or family member asks you to do something that contradicts the care plan
- You have a conflict with a client or family member
- A question or problem arises with which you need help

Your supervisor is always available to provide guidance and solve problems. Even in a community setting, your supervisor is just a phone call away.

Analyzing a problem involves communication. Ask the person questions about the problem. Listen attentively to the answers. Remember to pay attention to verbal and nonverbal messages. (See *Support Workers Solving Problems: Asking, Listening, and Observing* box.) Do not make assumptions about the cause of a problem.

For example, when Cheryl asks Mr. McDonald why he does not want to eat, he says that he has a sore on the inside of his cheek where he bit himself the other day. She can tell by his expression that his mouth is sore. Cheryl knows that Mr. McDonald's care plan does not specify a special diet. He is able to eat anything from the dining room menu. She therefore decides that she can try to solve the problem herself. She does not need to involve her supervisor right now.

Devise a Plan

Think of as many solutions as you can. Decide which is the most practical and helpful. Always be sure that it is safe. Try it and see if it works. For example, Cheryl thinks that the tomato soup is too hot and acidic for Mr. McDonald's sore mouth. She suggests he try a cooler, blander meal. He chooses the macaroni and cheese. He is able to eat this without discomfort. Cheryl later reports to her supervisor that Mr. McDonald has a sore in his mouth.

The planning part of the problem-solving process may involve creativity. Do not be afraid to try a plan, as long as it is safe. Consider Ruth's creative solution to a problem. Ruth's client, Mrs. Klassen, is in the early stages of Alzheimer's disease. Mrs. Klassen is upset because she cannot remember her grandson's name. He will be visiting the next day, and she wants to be able to call him by name. Ruth has the grandson's name listed on the care plan. She then gently suggests a way to help Mrs. Klassen remember it. They find a picture of her grandson and write his name on it. Ruth then tapes the picture to the wall by the phone. Mrs. Klassen will have the picture handy when her grandson visits. Ruth records this on the task sheet. At her next visit with Mrs. Klassen, she asks if their solution worked.

See the *Support Workers Solving Problems: Creative Solutions* box on page 86 for another example of a support worker devising a plan to solve a problem.

Dealing With Conflict

Some problems can be resolved at once. Others take longer. Interpersonal problems may take weeks to solve. They are a common cause of stress.

People bring their own values, attitudes, opinions, experiences, and expectations to the work setting. Differences often lead to conflict. Disagreements, misunderstandings, arguments, and unrest can occur.

Conflicts arise over issues or events. Work schedules, absences, and the amount and quality of work

Support Workers Solving Problems

Asking, Listening, and Observing

Scenario: Salman is a support worker on a surgical ward in a hospital. He is assigned to help Mrs. Kao do range-of-motion exercises following surgery. Mrs. Kao refuses to do the exercises. Salman asks her why she does not want to do the exercises. Mrs. Kao says her legs ache and she does not feel like moving. Salman encourages Mrs. Kao. Salman asks Mrs. Kao if the nurse explained why the exercises are important. Mrs. Kao says she knows why the exercises are important. Salman suggests that Mrs. Kao start by moving her toes. Mrs. Kao moves her toes and grimaces. Salman asks Mrs. Kao if she is in pain. Mrs. Kao says, "No, I'm not in pain."

Discussion: Salman realizes there is nothing more that he can do or say. He has asked Mrs. Kao questions, listened to her responses, and observed her behaviour. It is not his job to assess or diagnose Mrs. Kao's problem. He informs his supervisor of his conversation with Mrs. Kao. He tells his supervisor that Mrs. Kao grimaced when she moved her toes. He is careful to report Mrs. Kao's exact words.

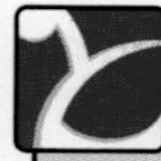

Support Workers Solving Problems

Creative Solutions

Scenario: Josephine's client is Mrs. Samuels, 34, a single mother who is receiving chemotherapy treatments for ovarian cancer. Mrs. Samuels has three boys, ages nine, five, and 20 months. Mrs. Samuels tells Josephine that since becoming ill she does not feel that she is doing enough for her children.

Discussion: Josephine asks Mrs. Samuels what sorts of things she misses doing for her children. Mrs. Samuels says that she wishes she could dress her two little boys in the morning. She also regrets not being able to drive her older boy to after-school activities. Josephine decides to look for opportunities to consult and involve Mrs. Samuels in the care of her children. As the 5-year-old gets ready for school that morning, Josephine suggests that he ask his mother to zip up his coat and help him put on his mittens and hat. Later she asks Mrs. Samuels what she would like the baby to wear that day.

performed are examples. The problems must be worked out. Otherwise, unkind words or actions may occur. The work environment becomes unpleasant, and care is affected.

You may experience conflict with clients or with co-workers. Report all conflicts with clients to your supervisor. Even if you resolved the problem, report what happened. You do not need to report conflicts with co-workers if the problem was resolved. However, if you cannot resolve a conflict, discuss it with your supervisor.

Communication and good work ethics are essential for preventing and resolving conflicts. Identify and solve problems before they become major issues. The guidelines in Box 8-6 can help you deal with conflict.

Box 8-6 Managing Conflict

- Ask your supervisor for some time to talk privately. Explain the situation, and ask for advice in solving the problem. Give facts and specific examples.
- Approach the person with whom you have a conflict. Ask to talk privately. Be polite and professional in your approach.
- Agree on a time and place to talk.
- Talk in a private setting. Others should not see or hear you and your co-worker.
- Explain the problem and what is bothering you. Give facts and specific behaviours. Focus on the problem, not on the person. For example, say "I need to know when you cannot help me so I can make other plans." Avoid criticizing the person—for example, by saying, "You are always late and never call to let me know."
- Listen to the person's response. Do not interrupt the person.
- Identify ways to resolve the problem. Offer your own thoughts and ask for the person's ideas.
- Schedule a date and time to review the situation.
- Thank the person for meeting with you.
- Implement the solutions.
- Review the situation as needed.

REVIEW

Circle the BEST answer.

1. Stress is
   A. The way you cope with and adjust to everyday living
   B. The emotional, behavioural, or physical response to an event or situation
   C. A mental or emotional disorder
   D. A thought or idea

2. A stressor is
   A. An event or situation that causes stress
   B. A coping strategy
   C. A defence mechanism
   D. A reaction to stress

3. Which does *not* influence a person's reaction to a stressor?
   A. Past experiences with the same stressor
   B. The person's sex
   C. The number of stressors present
   D. The person's temperament or personality

4. Which of the following is *not* a physical sign of stress?
   A. Difficulty sleeping
   B. Dry mouth
   C. Diarrhea
   D. Irritability

5. A defence mechanism is used to
   A. Blame others
   B. Block unpleasant or threatening feelings
   C. Solve problems
   D. Make excuses for behaviour

6. You are angry with a co-worker. Instead of responding appropriately, you yell at a friend. Which defence mechanism is this?
   A. Denial
   B. Conversion
   C. Displacement
   D. Compensation

7. Which of the following is *not* an effective way to manage stress?
   A. Balancing family, work, relaxation, and recreation
   B. Improving your decision-making and problem-solving skills
   C. Keeping a positive attitude
   D. Avoiding thinking too much about the stressor

8. Goals should be SMART. What does SMART stand for?
   A. Simple, monthly, allowable, reasonable, timely
   B. Specific, measurable, achievable, realistic, timely
   C. Simple, measurable, achievable, reasonable, topical
   D. Specific, monthly, allowable, realistic, topical

9. When trying to stay organized and save time, it is best *not* to
   A. Save the important tasks until last
   B. Set yourself a time limit for each task
   C. Develop a routine that works for you
   D. Remain flexible

10. The first step in the problem-solving process is to
    A. Call for help
    B. Learn to say no assertively
    C. Identify the problem
    D. Think of as many solutions as you can

11. What is an important part of resolving conflict?
    A. Communication and good work ethics
    B. Focusing on the person, not the problem
    C. Avoiding the person with whom you have a conflict
    D. Confronting the person with your supervisor for support

Answers to these questions are on page 822.

CHAPTER

9

ETHICS

OBJECTIVES

- Define the key terms listed in this chapter
- Explain the purpose of a code of ethics
- Identify the four basic principles of health care ethics
- Describe how each of the four principles applies to support work
- Apply the principles to solve ethical dilemmas

KEY TERMS

autonomy Having free choice involving decisions that affect one's life; self-determination

beneficence Doing or promoting good

ethics The moral principles or values that guide us when deciding what is right and what is wrong, what is good and what is bad

health care ethics The philosophical study of what is morally right and wrong when providing health care services

justice Treating people in a fair and equal manner

nonmaleficence Seeking to do no harm

self-determination Autonomy

The term **ethics** refers to the moral principles or values that guide us when deciding what is right and what is wrong, what is good and what is bad. Your ethics play a part in your everyday life. You apply them when making both big and small decisions. Whether you realize it or not, your ethics have a great impact on your personal and professional relationships. At work, you may have to make difficult choices or decisions. You will rely on your ethics to guide your conduct.

Codes of Ethics

Members of the health care team have special responsibilities. They form professional helping relationships with people who require care and services. To guide health care workers' interactions with people, ethical standards have been established.

Regulated professionals (such as physicians and nurses) have codes of ethics provided by their governing college. These codes describe the ideals of the profession. They also describe standards of conduct that group members must follow.

Support workers do not have a formal code of ethics. However, many employers have an informal code of ethics for their employees. The code describes the values and personal qualities that should guide your work. Codes of ethics vary among employers, but most affirm the priorities of support work identified in this text: promoting the client's dignity, independence, preferences, privacy, and safety. A sample code of ethics for support workers is given in Box 9-1.

Box 9-1 A Sample Code of Ethics for Support Workers

- **Support workers provide high-quality personal care and support services.** They work within their scope of practice. They promptly report to their supervisor any concerns and observations about a client's health and well-being. They perform only those tasks for which they have received the necessary training. They know and follow employer policies and federal, provincial, or territorial laws.
- **Support workers provide compassionate care to all clients.** They promote the person's physical, emotional, intellectual, social, and spiritual well-being. They encourage people to maintain as much independence as possible, during times of normal health and in situations of illness, injury, disability, or while dying. They respect and promote the family's roles and relationships.
- **Support workers value the dignity and value of all clients.** They strive to treat all people in an honest, fair, and just manner. They do not discriminate based on a person's age, colour, religion, sexual orientation, or culture.
- **Support workers respect their clients' choices about how they receive or participate in their care.** They respect and promote the person's wishes.
- **Support workers respect their clients' right to privacy and confidentiality.** Information learned while providing care is not shared outside the health care team.
- **Support workers do not misuse their position of trust.** They do not accept gifts or tips from their clients. They do not buy property from their clients. Nor do they sell products to their clients. They do not try to impose their own religious or other beliefs onto their clients.
- **Support workers are reliable.** They arrive at work on time and complete all assignments. They are patient and courteous with clients. They notify their supervisor if they are going to be late or are unable to work.
- **Support workers promote and maintain their clients' safety.** They report mistakes and unsafe situations immediately. They consider their clients' safety when doing all tasks and activities.

The Principles of Health Care Ethics

Most codes of ethics are based on the principles of health care ethics. **Health care ethics** is the philosophical study of what is morally right and wrong when providing health care services. The four basic principles of health care ethics are:

- Autonomy—respecting the person's right to make choices for himself or herself
- Justice—being fair
- Beneficence—doing good
- Nonmaleficence—doing no harm

Understanding the principles of health care ethics will help you think and behave ethically.

Autonomy

Autonomy (also called **self-determination**) means having free choice involving decisions that affect one's life. It refers to a person's independence. As long as a person is mentally competent, the person has the right to make decisions concerning lifestyle and medical care and services. This concept is critical to health care ethics. There are laws that protect the client's right to autonomy (see Chapter 10). For example, physicians, facilities, and agencies must by law ensure that clients provide informed consent before any procedure is done. Clients decide what kind of treatment they want or do not want.

You must always respect your clients' choices and preferences. The client has autonomy even with routine tasks. For example, a client asks you to use blue sheets to make a bed. It is important that you do so. Using other sheets shows a lack of respect for the person's choices. Or a client wants you to style her hair in a manner that you think is unbecoming. You must respect her choice. It is unethical to ignore her preferences and style her hair according to your own tastes.

Respecting your clients' autonomy is more complicated if you think their decisions are unsafe. The person has the right to make choices and to take risks. For example, an older client refuses to use his cane, knowing that he is at risk for falling. After explaining why he should use the cane, you have to accept his decision. Always consult with your supervisor if you have concerns about the person's safety.

Respecting your clients' autonomy also means that you do not judge their choices or lifestyle. Judgments and opinions are based on your own values and standards. Your clients may have different values and standards than you have. For example:

- A daughter decides that her elderly mother needs nursing home care. In your culture, children take care of aging parents at home. You do not understand why the daughter will not care for her mother at home.
- A client has multiple tattoos and body piercings. You do not approve of tattooing or body piercing.
- A client mentions to you that he has decided not to seek treatment for his cancer. You believe he should try everything possible to save his life.

You must not judge your clients and their decisions by your values or standards. Set aside your biases. Do not give them advice, and never express your disapproval or opinions about their choices, preferences, politics, religion, or lifestyle.

Justice

The principle of **justice** means that all people should be treated in a fair and equal manner. Justice is an ideal that is central to Canada's universal health care system—all Canadians, regardless of ability to pay, receive equal access to the same medical services.

You can uphold the principle of justice by being concerned for all clients, regardless of the their conditions or temperament. Some people are easier to work with than others. You may want to spend less time with a person who is demanding and ungrateful. You may wish to avoid a person whose lifestyle is very different from your own. However, doing so would be unjust and unethical. Each client deserves your attention and care.

Treating people justly also means that you do not betray their trust. Clients trust that you will handle their possessions with care, respect their privacy, perform your services competently and skillfully, and keep all conversations and health information confidential. Do not snoop in the person's home, pry into the person's personal life, or gossip with your friends or co-workers about the person. Share information about the person only with your supervisor and the health care team. Never speak about a client where others may overhear you. This includes dining rooms, lounges, locker rooms, elevators, and other public places. Confidentiality is a basic right. It is so important that laws have been passed to protect the person (see Chapter 10).

Beneficence

Beneficence means doing or promoting good. The principle of beneficence is central to your work. Support work is about promoting wellness, helping people in their daily lives, and supporting them during difficult times.

To apply the principle of beneficence in your work life, always consider meeting the client's needs as your most important function. The client's needs come before even those of his or her family. Consider the following: Mr. Mijovick receives home care services. He lives with his son and daughter-in-law in their home. Marcia is assigned to give Mr. Mijovick a bed bath. His son, however, insists that Marcia does not bathe Mr. Mijovick. The son explains that he wants Marcia to finish early today as he is expecting a visitor. When deciding what to do, Marcia focuses on Mr. Mijovick's needs, not on his son's. She calls her supervisor to report the situation and seek guidance.

The concept of beneficence and professionalism are closely related. To meet your clients' needs, stay within the boundaries of a professional helping relationship (see Chapter 6). Do not ask clients to do something that is in your interests rather than in theirs. For example, your child is selling chocolate bars to raise money for a school trip. Do not ask your client to buy a chocolate bar. Avoid asking clients to do something for you, even if the request appears to benefit others more than yourself or your family. For example, you are canvassing for United Way. Do not ask your client to contribute to the campaign.

When caring for a person, avoid focusing on yourself or burdening the person with your problems and worries. Never take advantage of a client's compassion and generosity. If you tell a client your problems, he or she may try to help you. For example, if you tell a client you are in financial difficulties, the person may offer you money. Never ask for or accept money or loans from clients regardless of how long you have been working with them. To do so is unethical.

Never forget that your relationship with your clients is professional. People can become very attached to their support workers. If family relationships are strained, the client may see the relationship with you as replacing the relationship with a family member. Never take advantage of strained family relationships. Do not take sides with a client against a family member. Never flirt, date, or accept invitations made by a client or the client's partner. When support workers become entangled in their clients' affairs, serious consequences can result. For example, you could be named as a beneficiary in a client's will. This could lead to legal problems for you and your employer.

To do the most good for your clients, always give your best effort at work. Unless the person has unexpected problems or needs to which you must attend, finish all your assigned tasks. Be careful, alert, and exact when following instructions. Also be compassionate and empathetic. Self-discipline is essential, especially when working in home care. Avoid temptations to use your work time for your own interests. This includes watching television, talking on the telephone, and stopping for an extra cup of coffee.

NONMALEFICENCE

Nonmaleficence is seeking to do no harm. Harm can be intentional (abuse) or unintentional (accidental injury or negligence). To avoid harming a client, only perform tasks that you have been trained to do. By recognizing the limits of your role and knowledge, you are protecting your clients from the risk of harm. Clients or family members may ask you to perform functions that are dangerous if not performed correctly. Often such requests are innocently requested. The client may forget that you are not qualified to do certain tasks. This confidence in you as a support worker is commendable. However, it is not safe or wise to take on tasks that you are not trained to do, even if you have the best of intentions.

Clients and their family members may also ask you for information about the client's diagnosis or medical, surgical, or treatment plans. You must never reveal these details, whether you are asked to or not. You could give the wrong information and cause harm or distress. Giving or discussing medical information is outside your scope of practice. It is also unethical. Refer all such questions to your supervisor.

To provide safe and effective care, you must keep your skills and knowledge current. Participate in training programs offered by your employer. Consider enrolling in courses or workshops relevant to your work. Support work is continually changing and so too must your skills and abilities. What you are trained to do this year may be outdated in a few years. The more knowledge and practice you have, the better and safer your skills will be.

You can protect people from harm by practising infection control techniques (see Chapter 18). Recognizing common safety hazards and knowing how to prevent them also protect people (see Chapter 16). You must keep clients as safe as possible.

DEALING WITH ETHICAL DILEMMAS

Codes of ethics only provide guidelines for ethical behaviour. They do not give answers or rules for every situation. When confronted with an ethical dilemma, you need to know how to decide the right thing to do.

When making an ethical decision, carefully consider the four principles of health care ethics. Collect as much information about the situation as possible. Consider all the possible options to the dilemma. Ask yourself these questions about each option:

- Does the option respect the client's wishes and preferences?
- Does the option treat the client justly and fairly?
- Does the option provide the client with a short-term or long-term benefit?
- Could the option cause harm or increase the client's risk of harm?

Answers to these questions may contradict each other. For example, one option may benefit the client but go against his or her wishes. Or an option may reflect the client's preferences but increase the risk of harm. If one option could harm the person, you *must* involve your supervisor in the solution. You must protect the client from harm and avoid serious legal problems for yourself and your employer.

See the *Support Workers Solving Problems: Ethical Dilemmas* box to see how three support workers dealt with ethical dilemmas. Then read the following ethical dilemma. What would you do? Remember to consider the four principles of health care ethics when making your decision.

- You are assigned to work for a family with a 2-year-old boy and newborn twins. You are responsible for helping with the 2-year-old. The mother mentions that since the birth of the twins, the toddler has been having temper tantrums around lunch time. She wants to stop this problem behaviour. She tells you that if the boy has a tantrum or misbehaves, he is to be sent to his room alone for 15 minutes, longer if he has not settled down by the end of that time.

Autonomy: The mother has the right to make parenting decisions.

Justice: Is it fair to the child to leave him in his room for so long?

Beneficence: Will the discipline help the child improve his behaviour? Can other actions improve his behaviour?

Nonmaleficence: Could leaving the child in his room cause harm?

Support Workers Solving Problems

Ethical Dilemmas

Scenario: Miki works at a long-term care facility. Mr. Petrova is a resident on her ward. Miki smells alcohol on Mr. Petrova's breath after he visits his son. She comments on this to Mr. Petrova. He tells her that his son brought him a bottle of liquor. Keeping alcohol in one's room is against facility rules. Mr. Petrova says that alcohol eases his pain. He asks Miki to promise not to tell anyone about the liquor.

Discussion: Telling her supervisor about the liquor would disregard Mr. Petrova's wishes and autonomy. However, not telling her supervisor could harm Mr. Petrova. For example, alcohol may interfere with his medications or cause adverse reactions. Not telling could also harm Miki. She could be fired for not following facility rules.

Miki explains to Mr. Petrova that she is ethically and legally obligated to tell her supervisor about the presence of alcohol in the room. She explains her reasons. Mr. Petrova is upset, but Miki knows she has followed the ethical principle of nonmaleficence. As well, she has not betrayed Mr. Petrova's trust by making a promise she could not keep.

Scenario: John's home care client is Mrs. Jessop. Mrs. Jessop's care plan states that she is not allowed foods with sugars. Today is Mrs. Jessop's birthday, and her neighbour brings a cake. Mrs. Jessop tells John that she goes off her diet every year on her birthday. She asks him to cut her a piece of cake.

Serving Mrs. Jessop a piece of cake would respect her autonomy. However, the cake could harm Mrs. Jessop's physical health.

Discussion: John decides not to serve the cake to Mrs. Jessop. He knows that she can serve herself or her neighbour can serve it to her. John suggests that he call Mrs. Jessop's case manager about the situation. However, Mrs. Jessop does not want John to make the call. She eats the cake. John observes her carefully for any ill effects, but notices no change. He telephones his supervisor to report the incident. His written notes include exactly what happened.

John upholds the principle of autonomy by allowing Mrs. Jessop to eat the cake. He also upholds the principle of nonmaleficence by not serving her the cake and by encouraging her to talk with her case manager before she has a piece. Because he reported what happened, he also followed the principle of beneficence.

Scenario: Tomas is a support worker in a long-term care facility. One afternoon, he observes that Mrs. O'Brian seems upset. He asks if anything is wrong. Mrs. O'Brian starts to cry. She tells Tomas that her 17-year-old grandson has been arrested for drunk driving. She asks Tomas not to tell anyone because the family wants to keep the matter private. She also asks Tomas not to tell the nursing staff that she is upset.

Keeping the information confidential would respect Mrs. O'Brian's privacy. So would not telling about her emotional state. However, Tomas is supposed to report observations about residents' emotional health. Not doing so could cause Mrs. O'Brian harm. She may suffer from the effects of stress.

Discussion: Tomas decides to tell the charge nurse that Mrs. O'Brian is upset about a private family matter. First, Tomas explains to Mrs. O'Brian that he is required to report observations about emotional health. He also assures her that anything he reports is kept confidential by the health care team.

Tomas's solution respects the ethical principles of autonomy and justice. It also upholds the principle of nonmaleficence. By reporting that Mrs. O'Brian is upset, Tomas ensures that someone with authority will take responsibility for Mrs. O'Brian's emotional health.

REVIEW

Circle T if the answer is true and F if it is false.

1. T F Ethics apply only to life-and-death situations.
2. T F Codes of ethics provide rules and answers to ethical dilemmas.
3. T F Ethics are a guide when deciding between right and wrong, good and bad.
4. T F Keeping a resident's information confidential is ethical behaviour.
5. T F Any decision regarding a client's care is ethical if it does not harm the person.

Circle the BEST answer.

6. Providing a safe environment is an example of
   A. Autonomy
   B. Justice
   C. Beneficence
   D. Nonmaleficence
7. Showing respect and protecting a person's dignity is an example of
   A. Autonomy
   B. Justice
   C. Beneficence
   D. Nonmaleficence
8. Treating all clients with equal care and attention, regardless of their condition or temperament, is an example of
   A. Autonomy
   B. Justice
   C. Beneficence
   D. Nonmaleficence
9. Respecting personal preferences is an example of
   A. Autonomy
   B. Justice
   C. Beneficence
   D. Nonmaleficence
10. Which question is *not* helpful when deciding an ethical solution to a problem?
    A. Does the solution respect the client's wishes and stated preferences?
    B. Does the solution treat the client justly and fairly?
    C. Does the solution provide a short-term or long-term benefit to the client?
    D. Does the solution benefit you?

Answers to these questions are on page 822.

CHAPTER

10

Legislation: The Client's Rights and Your Rights

OBJECTIVES

- Define the key terms listed in this chapter
- Explain the basic rights protected by the *Canadian Charter of Rights and Freedoms* and the provincial and territorial human rights codes
- Describe client rights
- Identify ways you can respect your client's rights
- Describe the difference between criminal and civil laws
- Describe how negligence, defamation, assault, battery, false imprisonment, and invasion of privacy apply to your job
- List the types of legislation that address support workers' rights and duties

KEY TERMS

act Another term for a specific law

assault Intentionally attempting or threatening to touch a person's body without the person's consent

autonomy Having free choice involving decisions that affect one's life; self-determination

battery The touching of a person's body without the person's consent

civil law Laws that deal with the relationships between people

consent Agreeing to medical treatment, health care, or personal care services

crime A violation of a criminal law

criminal law Laws concerned with offences against the public and against society in general

defamation Injuring the name and reputation of a person by making false statements to a third person

false imprisonment Unlawful restraint or restrictions of a person's freedom of movement

harassment Troubling, tormenting, offending, or worrying a person by one's behaviour or comments

informed consent Consent based on accurate and complete information

invasion of privacy Violating a person's right not to have his or her name, photograph, private affairs, health information, or any personal information exposed or made public without consent

legislation A body of laws that govern the behaviour of a country's residents

liable Legally responsible

libel Making false statements in print, writing, or through pictures or drawings

negligence Failing to act in a careful or competent manner and thereby harming a person or damaging property

regulation Detailed rules that implement the requirements of a legislative act

right Something to which a person is justly entitled

self-determination Autonomy

slander Making false statements orally

substitute decision maker A person authorized to give or withhold consent on an incapable person's behalf

tort A wrongful act committed by an individual against another person or the person's property

The foundation of a good client–worker relationship is a basic understanding of your client's rights, your rights, and your legal responsibilities. How you conduct yourself at work and how you relate to your clients are determined by:

- Your ethics
- Your employer's policies
- Federal and provincial or territorial laws

Remember, ethics is concerned with what you *should* or *should not do*. Legislation tells you what you *can* and *cannot do*. **Legislation** is a body of laws that govern the behaviour of a country's residents. In Canada, legislation helps to make sure that all clients receive safe and skillful care. Enforced by the courts, legislation also protects clients' rights and your rights.

UNDERSTANDING RIGHTS

A **right** is something to which a person is justly entitled. Some rights are based on a sense of fairness or ethics. These are sometimes called *moral rights*. For example, you and a classmate arrange to study together. You have a right to expect that the classmate will show up and be prepared to work. Or, you discuss a personal matter with a friend. You have the right to expect that your friend will not repeat this information to others. These rights are not based on written laws. They are based on moral principles: commitments should be honoured and secrets should be kept.

Other rights are formally recognized in law. They are *legal rights* based on rules and principles outlined in the law and enforced by society. For example, various laws give you the right to vote, to receive medical care, to own property, and to receive fair treatment if accused of a crime. Laws reflect the values of the society that created them. Canadians enjoy many rights and freedoms that enable a life of equality and dignity.

Basic Human Rights in Canada

The *Canadian Charter of Rights and Freedoms* protects human rights in Canada. The *Charter* is part of the Canadian Constitution and is a constitutional document. It applies at the federal and provincial/territorial levels. All other laws must be consistent with its rules. The *Charter* lists the basic rights and freedoms to which all Canadians are entitled. They include:

- Freedom of conscience and religion
- Freedom of thought, belief, opinion, and expression
- Freedom of peaceful assembly and association (usually these freedoms are associated with the right to form a union or engage in a strike)
- The right to vote
- The right to enter, remain in, and leave Canada
- The right to life, liberty, and security of the person
- The right to equality before and under the law, without discrimination based on race, ethnic origin, colour, religion, sex, age, or mental or physical disability

Every province and territory also has a human rights code. These codes affirm the principle that all people are entitled to equal rights and opportunities without discrimination. Your provincial human rights code protects you and your clients from being treated unfairly because of race, ethnicity, religion, sex, age, or disability. The human rights code affirms that all clients have a right to receive the same type and quality of support services and to be free from discrimination.

Basic Rights of People Receiving Health Services

Your clients are entitled to the same rights and freedoms as all other Canadian residents. However, sometimes they cannot exercise their rights, due to:

- Illness or injury
- Physical or mental disabilities
- Old age, if the person is frail, confused, or isolated

All provinces and territories have legislation that addresses the rights of people using health care services. Legislation governing health care has different names across the country and differs in detail. As well, governments are constantly revising health care legislation and introducing new laws. However, every province and territory protects the rights of people receiving care in facilities and in the community. Examples of this legislation are given in Box 10-1.

Health care legislation consists of acts and regulations. An **act** is another term for a specific law.

Box 10-1 Examples of Long-Term Care and Community Care Legislation

British Columbia
Community Care Facility Act
Continuing Care Act

Alberta
Nursing Homes Act
Social Care Facilities Licensing Act

Saskatchewan
Housing and Special-Care Homes Act
Home Care Act
Personal Care Homes Act
Residential Services Act

Manitoba
Public Health Act
Health Services Insurance Act
The Vulnerable Persons Living with a Mental Disability Act

Ontario
Nursing Homes Act
Charitable Institutions Act
Homes for the Aged and Rest Homes Act
Long-Term Care Act

Quebec
An Act Respecting Health Services and Social Services
An Act Respecting Health Services and Social Services for Cree Native Persons

New Brunswick
Family Services Act
Nursing Homes Act

Nova Scotia
Homes for Special Care Act

Newfoundland/Labrador
Homes for Special Care Act
Private Homes for Special Care Allowances Act
Self-Managed Home Support Services Act
Personal Care Homes Regulations under the *Health and Community Services Act*

Prince Edward Island
Community Care Facilities and Nursing Homes Act

Yukon
Health Act

Northwest Territories/Nunavut
Hospital Insurance and Health and Social Services Administration Act

Regulations consist of detailed rules that implement the requirements of the act. Most health care acts consist of general requirements for maintaining health, safety, and well-being. For example, British Columbia's *Community Care Facility Act* sets out general requirements for the licensing, administration, operation, and inspection of long-term care facilities. It also sets out broad standards of care. *Adult Care Regulations* that accompany the *Community Care Facility Act* set out detailed rules for meeting those broad standards of care. Box 10-2 outlines some of the detailed rules covered in British Columbia's *Adult Care Regulations.*

Some provincial and territorial governments do not have regulations that lay out detailed rules. Instead, they issue standards that expand on their legislation. For example, Alberta's long-term care legislation is accompanied by standards called *Basic Service Standards for Continuing Care Centres*. Regardless of whether detailed rules are contained in regulations or standards, all residential facilities in the province or territory must abide by these rules. Not to do so could result in removal of their licence.

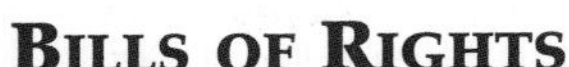

Bills of Rights

There is no single list of rights afforded to all Canadians receiving care in facilities and in the community.

Box 10-2 Some Long-Term Care Facility Issues Controlled by Legislation (British Columbia)

- Bedroom requirements—space, furnishings, privacy, windows, and lighting
- Room and water temperature
- Bathrooms and bathing facilities
- Safety requirements, including fire safety and call systems
- Mobility and access
- Dining area, lounges, recreation, and outside activity area
- Social activities and recreation programs
- Care and supervision; care plans
- Confidentiality and privacy
- Neglect and abuse
- Restrictions on the use of restraints
- Preparation and service of food
- Medication safety; administration of medication; medication records
- Access to health services; oral health

Source: *Adult Care Regulations: Provisions of the Community Care Facility Act,* R.S.B.C. 1996, c.60.

However, some provinces, such as Manitoba and Ontario, have created a bill of rights for clients. These bills of rights take the lengthy rules contained in regulations and standards and condense them into a list of basic rights for people receiving care. For example, consider Ontario's *Resident's Bill of Rights* for long-term care (Box 10-3 on page 98) and *Bill of Rights* for community care clients (Box 10-4 on page 99).

Some facilities and agencies write their own bills of rights based on provincial or territorial laws. Clients must receive a written list of their rights. You must know your provincial or territorial laws and employer policy regarding client rights. Generally, all clients have the following rights, which are a combination of moral and legal rights:

- the right to be treated with dignity and respect
- the right to privacy and confidentiality
- the right to give or withhold informed consent
- the right to autonomy

The Right to Be Treated with Dignity and Respect

All clients have the right to be treated with dignity and respect. This is a guiding principle of caregiving and is emphasized throughout this textbook. It is an ethical principle and a legal obligation. Generally all health care laws protect and promote the client's dignity.

Most health care legislation refers to the client's right to be treated with dignity. For example, British Columbia's *Community Care Facility Act* states that facilities must be operated "in a manner that will maintain the spirit, dignity, and individuality of the person being cared for."[1] Ontario's *Long-Term Care Act* states that the person has the right to be dealt with "in a courteous and respectful manner . . . that respects the person's dignity." The *Act* also states that workers must deal with the person in a manner that "recognizes the person's individuality and that is sensitive to and responds to the person's needs and preferences, including preferences based on ethnic, spiritual, linguistic, familial, and cultural factors."[2]

Many long-term care facilities have policies that promote the dignity of the residents. Because the facility is the residents' home, residents are guaranteed the same freedoms they would have in their own homes. Many long-term care acts, regulations, standards, and facility policies recognize that residents have the following rights:

- To live in a safe and clean environment
- To be properly sheltered, fed, clothed, groomed, and cared for according to their needs

(text continues on page 99)

Box 10-3 Ontario's *Resident's Bill of Rights*

1. Every resident has the right to be treated with courtesy and respect and in a way that fully recognizes the resident's dignity and individuality and to be free from mental and physical abuse.
2. Every resident has the right to be properly sheltered, fed, clothed, groomed, and cared for in a manner consistent with his or her needs.
3. Every resident has the right to be told who is responsible for and who is providing the resident's direct care.
4. Every resident has the right to be afforded privacy in treatment and in caring for his or her personal needs.
5. Every resident has the right to keep in his or her room and display personal possessions, pictures, and furnishings in keeping with safety requirements and rights of other residents of the home.
6. Every resident has the right,
   - To be informed of his or her medical condition, treatment, and proposed course of treatment;
   - To give or refuse consent to treatment, including medication, in accordance with the law and to be informed of the consequences of giving or refusing consent;
   - To have the opportunity to participate fully in making any decision and obtaining an independent medical opinion concerning any aspect of his or her care, including any decision concerning his or her admission, discharge or transfer to or from a home; and
   - To have his or her medical records kept confidential in accordance with the law.
7. Every resident has the right to receive reactivation and assistance toward independence consistent with his or her requirements.
8. Every resident who is being considered for restraints has the right to be fully informed about the procedures and the consequences of receiving or refusing them.
9. Every resident has the right to communicate in confidence, to receive visitors of his or her choice, and to consult in private with any person without interference.
10. Every resident whose death is likely to be imminent has the right to have members of the resident's family present twenty-four hours per day.
11. Every resident has the right to designate a person to receive information concerning any transfer or emergency hospitalization of the resident and, if a person is so designated, to have that person so informed forthwith.
12. Every resident has the right to exercise the rights of a citizen and to raise concerns or recommend changes in policies and services on behalf of himself or herself or others to the resident's council, staff of the home, government officials or any other person inside or outside the home, without fear of restraint, interference, coercion, discrimination, or reprisal.
13. Every resident has the right to form friendships, to enjoy relationships, and to participate in the resident's council.
14. Every resident has the right to meet privately with his or her spouse or same-sex partner in a room that assures privacy and, if both spouses or same-sex partners are residents in the same home, they have a right to share a room according to their wishes, if an appropriate room is available.
15. Every resident has the right to pursue social, cultural, religious and other interests, to develop his or her potential, and to be given reasonable provisions by the home to accommodate these pursuits.
16. Every resident has the right to be informed in writing of any law, rule, or policy affecting the operation of the institution and of the procedures for initiating complaints.
17. Every resident has the right to manage his or her own financial affairs if the resident is able to do so and, if the resident's financial affairs are managed by the institution, to receive a quarterly accounting of any transactions undertaken on his or her behalf and to be assured that the resident's property is managed solely on the resident's behalf.
18. Every resident has the right to live in a safe and clean environment.
19. Every resident has the right to be given access to protected areas outside the home in order to enjoy outdoor activity, unless the physical setting makes this impossible.

Source: *Ontario's Nursing Homes Act,* R.S.O. 1990, c. N. 7, s. 2(2); *Homes for the Aged and Rest Homes Act,* R.S.O. 1990, c. H. 13, s. 1(2); and *Charitable Institutions Act,* R.S.O. 1990, c. C. 9, s. 3.1(2).

Box 10-4 Ontario's *Bill of Rights* for Community Care Clients

Note: The term "service provider" refers to either an agency or a person paid to provide the community service; in other words, a support worker is a service provider.

1. A person receiving a community service has the right to be dealt with by the service provider in a courteous and respectful manner and to be free from mental, physical, and financial abuse by the service provider.
2. A person receiving a community service has the right to be dealt with by the service provider in a manner that respects the person's dignity and privacy and that promotes the person's autonomy.
3. A person receiving a community service has the right to be dealt with by the service provider in a manner that recognizes the person's individuality and that is sensitive to and responds to the person's needs and preferences, including preferences based on ethnic, spiritual, linguistic, familial, and cultural factors.
4. A person receiving a community service has the right to information about the community services provided to him or her and to be told who will be providing the community services.
5. A person applying for a community service has the right to participate in the service provider's assessment of his or her requirements and a person who is determined under this Act to be eligible for a community service has the right to participate in the service provider's development of the person's plan of service, the service provider's review of the person's requirements, and the service provider's evaluation and revision of the person's plan of service.
6. A person receiving a community service has the right to give or refuse consent to the provision of any community service.
7. A person receiving a community service has the right to raise concerns or recommend changes in connection with the community service provided to him or her and in connection with policies and decisions that affect his or her interests, to the service provider, government officials or any other person, without fear of interference, coercion, discrimination, or reprisal.
8. A person receiving a community service has the right to be informed of the laws, rules and policies affecting the operation of the service provider and to be informed in writing of the procedures for initiating complaints about the service provider.
9. A person receiving a community service has the right to have his or her records kept confidential in accordance with the law.

Source: Ontario's *Long-Term Care Act,* 1994, S.O. 1994, c. 26, s. 3(1).

- To keep and display personal possessions, pictures, and furnishings in their rooms
- To have family present 24 hours a day if the person is dying
- To be free from emotional, physical, sexual, and financial abuse
- To discuss problems with or suggest changes to any aspect of the services provided to them

Respecting the person's dignity is a basic and important part of support work. For most people, dignity and independence go together. To respect a person's dignity, encourage the person to be independent. Allow clients to do as much for themselves as possible (Figure 10-1). For example, if a frail, older man can put on his shoes, let him do so. It may be faster for you to put on the shoes for him. However, letting him do so helps him maintain some independence.

Be careful not to make assumptions about people's abilities and limitations. Observe what your client is capable of doing. Check the care plan. A person who is dependent in one area is not necessarily dependent in all areas. For example, Mrs. Mukherjee needs help getting up out of a chair. However, she can cut her food and feed herself. Mr. Simpson needs help shaving. But he can comb his hair and brush his teeth. Do not make assumptions about people's abilities and interests. You may discourage them from doing tasks and activities that they can do.

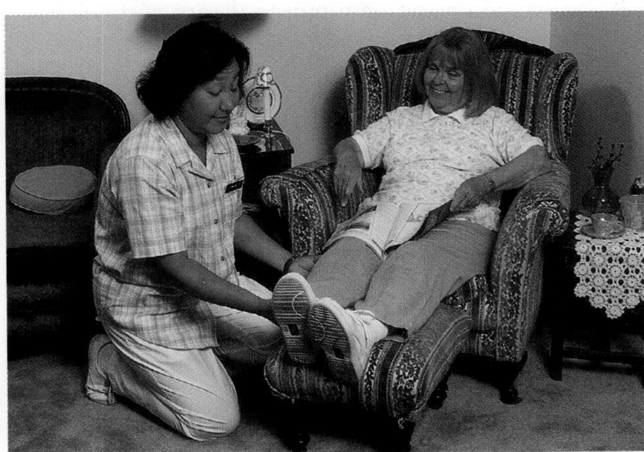

Figure 10-1 Support workers should treat their clients with dignity and respect.

Respecting people's dignity means relating to them the way you would want to be related to if you were in their position. With support work, how you relate to a person is just as important as the care you provide. Treating a person with dignity provides emotional support and greatly contributes to quality of life.

Box 10-5 lists ways to show respect for the client's dignity.

Box 10-5 Respecting the Client's Right to Dignity

- Make eye contact with the person, if culturally appropriate, and listen attentively (Figure 10-2).
- Stand or sit close enough to the person as appropriate. Use touch if you are sure the person would approve. Respect cultural differences regarding touching and personal space preferences (see Chapter 11).
- Be patient. Provide kind and thoughtful care.
- Say "please" and "thank you," and practise other common acts of courtesy.
- Never yell, scold, embarrass, laugh at, or be sarcastic toward the person.
- Respect the person's belongings and property. Do not touch personal possessions unless you have a reason to and have the person's permission. Be sure to put items back where you found them.
- Address an adult by title and last name, unless the person tells you otherwise. Do not call a person honey, sweetie, dear, grandma, grandpa, or other name.
- Tell your supervisor about the person's complaints or concerns about the agency, facility, or services.
- Reinforce the person's independence. Avoid creating dependency. Allow people to do things for themselves.
- Assist the person with personal care and grooming whenever necessary. Make sure the person has:
  - A neat and clean appearance
  - A clean-shaven face or groomed beard
  - Trimmed and clean nails
  - Dentures, hearing aids, glasses, and other prostheses available as appropriate
  - Clean and properly fitted and fastened clothing
  - Shoes and socks or hose properly applied and fastened
  - Extra clothing for warmth as needed, such as sweater or lap blanket

The Right to Privacy and Confidentiality

People using health care services have the right to personal privacy. They have the right to receive care in private and in a way that does not expose their bodies unnecessarily. Only staff members involved in the person's care should see, handle, or examine the person's body.

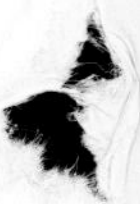

Information about the client's care, treatment, and condition is confidential. Health information must be kept confidential. All provinces and territories have legislation that protects the privacy and confidentiality of clients' health information. This legislation is usually called a *Privacy Act*. Privacy acts provide guidelines to facilities and agencies on how to collect, use, and disclose personal health information. Follow your employer's policies.

Providing for privacy and confidentiality shows respect for the client. It also protects the person's dignity. Box 10-6 lists measures that show respect for privacy and confidentiality.

The Right to Give or Withhold Informed Consent

All people have the right to decide for themselves whether or not they agree to medical treatment, health care, or personal care services. This is called **consent**. All provinces and territories have legislation that describes when and how consent is to be obtained.

For consent to be valid, it must be informed consent. **Informed consent** is consent based on accurate and complete information. This information is provided to the client by the facility, agency, or physician. Consent is informed when the person clearly understands:

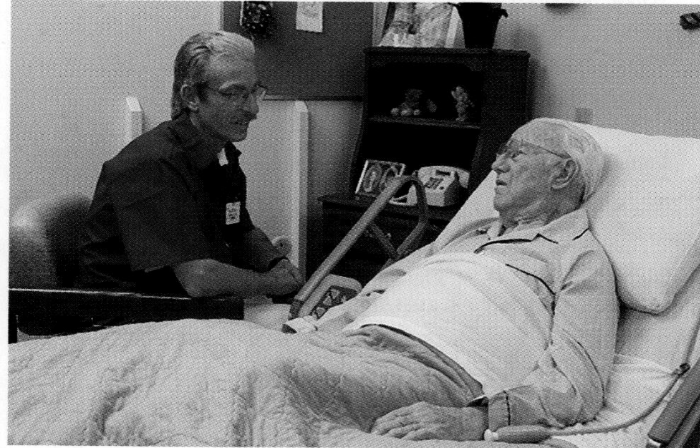

Figure 10-2 Listen by facing the client, having good eye contact, and leaning toward the client.

- The reason for the treatment or service
- What will be done
- How it will be done
- Who will be doing it
- The expected outcomes
- Potential risks and side effects of the treatment
- Other treatment options
- The likely consequences of not having the treatment

Consent is given when the person enters the facility or hires the agency. A form is signed giving general consent to treatment. Special consent forms are required for surgery and other complex and invasive procedures. The physician is responsible for informing the person about all aspects of the surgery or procedure. *The support worker is never responsible for obtaining written consent or giving medical information.* You may or may not be allowed to witness clients' signatures on consent forms. Know your employer's policy.

Box 10-6 Respecting the Client's Right to Privacy

- Knock on the person's door and wait for a reply before entering.
- Ask others to leave the room before giving care. The person must give permission for them to stay.
- Close the door and use curtains or screens when providing care or whenever the person requests. Also close drapes and window shades.
- Drape properly during personal care and procedures. Expose only the body part involved in the treatment or procedure.
- Keep the person covered when moving him or her through a facility's corridors and elevators.
- Close the bathroom door when the person is using the bathroom. If the person needs help, stay in the room with the person and keep the door closed.
- Do not open or read the person's mail or personal documents (Figure 10-3).
- Do not touch or examine the person's belongings without permission.
- Allow the person to visit with others and to use the telephone in private.
- Do not pry into the person's private life or ask for personal information that is not necessary for your work.
- Keep all personal and health care information confidential.
- Do not discuss a client with your family, friends, or the client's family. Only talk about the person with your supervisor and members of the health care team who need to know.

Substitute Decision Makers. Consent is often needed for clients under legal age (usually 18 years of age) and for clients who are unable to make informed decisions for themselves. For example, an unconscious person cannot give consent for a procedure. People with certain mental illnesses, confusion, dementia, or intellectual disabilities may not be able to give informed consent. Such situations require a substitute decision maker. A **substitute decision maker** is a person authorized to give or withhold consent on behalf of the incapable person. Usually the substitute decision maker is a husband, wife, daughter, son, or legal representative. As with consent given by the client, consent given by a substitute decision maker must be informed consent.

Your client may have a substitute decision maker. This person consults with the health care team to make decisions on the person's behalf. All provinces and territories have legislation that addresses substitute decision making.

The Right to Autonomy

Autonomy (also called **self-determination**) means having free choice involving decisions that affect one's life. People using health care services retain their right to autonomy. They have the right to make decisions and choices concerning their care and lifestyle. Clients have the right to be involved with issues concerning their admission, discharge, or transfer to or from a facility (see *Focus on Long-Term Care: Autonomy* box on page 102). All clients have the right to participate fully in assessing and planning their own care and treatment, whether receiving care in a facility or at home.

To have autonomy, people need (and have the right to) complete and accurate information about their health condition, care, and treatment. Make sure your clients know your name and title. Remember to

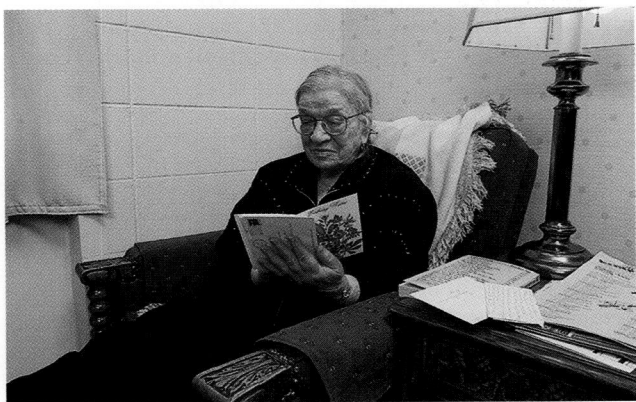

Figure 10-3 A client is reading her mail. Clients have a right to privacy. Never open or read their mail.

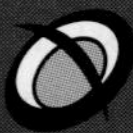

Focus on Long-Term Care

AUTONOMY

Long-term care residents have the right to choose activities, schedules, and care based on personal preferences. They have the right to choose when to get up and go to bed, what to wear, how to spend their time, and what to eat (Figure 10-4). They are also free to form friendships and receive visitors inside and outside the facility. They have the right to share a room with their spouse or partner if they wish and if a room is available. They also have the right to manage their own financial affairs or receive an accounting of transactions done on their behalf.

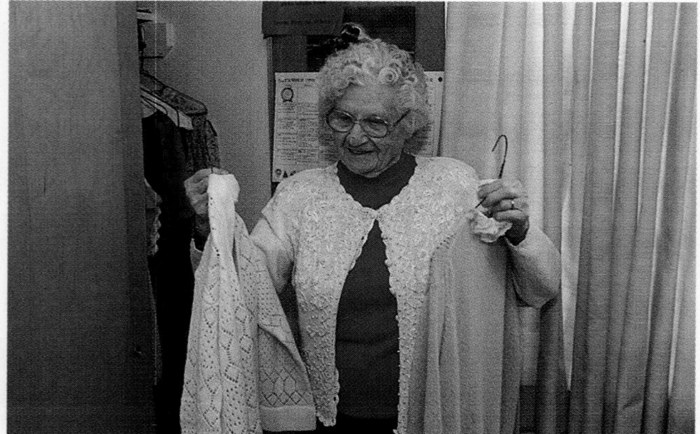

Figure 10-4 Client choosing what clothing to wear.

explain procedures before doing them. Clients may ask you about their condition, care, or your employer's policies. Inform your supervisor. He or she will provide this information. Remember, you must not discuss diagnoses or health conditions with clients.

Personal choice is important for quality of life, dignity, and self-respect. Respect for an individual's personal preference is emphasized throughout this book. You must allow the client to make choices whenever safely possible.

UNDERSTANDING LEGAL ISSUES

Many client rights are based on laws. Like all health care team members, you must act in a legally appropriate manner. If you break the law or violate someone's rights, you are legally responsible (**liable**) for your actions. You could be fined, sued, or imprisoned.

You must obey criminal and civil laws. **Criminal laws** are concerned with offences against the public and against society in general. A violation of criminal law is called a **crime**. A person found guilty of a crime is fined or sent to prison. Theft, murder, rape, and abuse are examples of crimes.

Civil laws deal with the relationships between people. For example, laws relating to business disputes, divorce, or adoption are civil laws. A **tort** is a wrongful act committed by an individual against another person or the person's property. A person who commits such an act can be sued by the injured person. Torts may be intentional or unintentional. An example of an unintentional tort is negligence. Examples of intentional torts are assault, battery, false imprisonment, invasion of privacy, and defamation of character.

NEGLIGENCE

Your clients expect that you will do your job competently and carefully. **Negligence** is when you fail to act in a careful or competent manner and thereby harm the person or damage property. Negligence is an unintentional wrong. The person at fault did not mean or intend to cause harm. The person failed to do what a reasonable and careful person would have done. Or the individual did what a reasonable and careful person would *not* have done. The negligent individual may have to pay damages (a sum of money) to the injured person. Negligence can be caused by:

- *Not performing a task or procedure correctly.* Always perform tasks and procedures exactly as you have been taught. Not following procedures can harm the client. For example, you are taught to keep a urinary drainage bag below the client's bladder level. If you keep it above the bladder, the urine does not drain and the person could develop a urinary tract infection. Such negligence could harm the person. Negligence charges could result.
- *Performing a task or procedure that you are not qualified to do.* You are only legally allowed to do tasks and procedures that you are qualified to do. Do not do more than allowed within your job description, your employer's policies, and legislation within your province or territory. You may be asked to do something beyond your scope of practice. Giving medications is an example. You may be told you are not liable. However, you should remember that *you are responsible for your own actions.* You may, in fact, be liable. In such situations, remember that refusing to follow directions is your right and duty.
- *Making a mistake.* Everyone makes mistakes sometimes. But a mistake that results from carelessness and causes harm is a negligent act. For example, if you do not mop up a spill, the client could slip and fall. Your carelessness could be considered negligent.

Box 10-7 contains examples of negligent acts committed by support workers.

Box 10-7 Example of Negligent Acts Committed by Support Workers

- The support worker leaves the bed in the raised position. The client falls out of bed and breaks a hip.
- A support worker raises the bed rails when the care plan states to leave them down. The client falls while trying to climb over the bed rails.
- A support worker does not raise the bed rails when the care plan states to raise them. The client falls out of bed.
- A support worker does not check the temperature of the bath water. The client is burned.
- A support worker drops a client's dentures. The dentures break.
- A client complains to the support worker of chest pain and difficulty breathing. The complaints are not reported to the support worker's supervisor. The person has a heart attack and dies.
- A client calls for help using the call bell. The support worker ignores the call. The client goes into shock because of sudden, severe bleeding.
- A support worker does not secure a client's garden gate. The client (who has Alzheimer's disease) wanders out on the street and is hit by a car.

A client could be harmed even though you do your job competently and carefully. It is important to accurately record every procedure, following your employer's policy. What you record may protect you from charges of negligence. For example, a client confined to bed develops serious skin injuries. The family thinks she was left lying in the same position for too long. Your charting shows that you repositioned her every hour, as stated in her care plan. This proves you gave the required care and did not cause her injury. If you did not record that you repositioned her every hour, it can be presumed that you did not do it. (Recording is discussed in Chapter 7.)

Assault and Battery

Assault and battery may result in both civil and criminal charges. **Assault** is intentionally attempting or threatening to touch a person's body without the person's consent. The person fears bodily harm. Threatening to "tie down" an uncooperative person is an example of assault. **Battery** is the actual touching of a person's body without the person's consent. Force-feeding a client is an example of battery.

You are not required to obtain written consent. However, you must always be aware of the client's wishes before you perform a task or procedure. A person who has signed a consent form has the right to withdraw his or her consent at any time. Always explain the procedure and what you are going to do. Make sure the client agrees. Consent may be verbal ("yes" or "okay") or a gesture (a nod, turning over for a back rub, or holding out an arm for a blood pressure measurement). If the person objects or declines your services, respect his or her wishes and stop the procedure or task. Immediately tell your supervisor. The person's decision may affect his or her well-being.

False Imprisonment

False imprisonment is the unlawful restraint or restrictions on a person's freedom of movement. Preventing a person from leaving a facility is false imprisonment. So is the unnecessary use of restraints (see Chapter 17).

Invasion of Privacy

Every person has the right not to have his or her name, photograph, private affairs, health information, or any personal information exposed or made public without having given consent. Violating this right is an **invasion of privacy** and is punishable by law. Your employer may require you to sign a document binding you to confidentiality in all dealings with clients and your employer. This document may refer to the provincial or territorial privacy act that protects the privacy of individuals. Signing the document obligates you not to reveal information obtained in the course of your work.

Defamation of Character

Defamation is injuring the name and reputation of a person by making false statements to a third person. **Libel** is making false statements in print, writing, or through pictures or drawings. **Slander** is making false statements orally. Protect yourself from defamation by never making false statements about a client, co-worker, or any other person. Examples of defamation include:

- Implying or suggesting that a person has a sexually transmitted disease
- Saying that a person is insane or mentally ill
- Implying or suggesting that a person is corrupt or dishonest

Your Legal Rights

Federal, provincial, and territorial legislation ensures that Canadian workers receive fair wages and work in a fair and safe environment. There are laws that protect workers' rights and clarify their requirements and duties. These laws have different names across the country and vary in their details. In general, however, all provinces and territories have legislation that addresses human rights, occupational health and safety, employment, labour relations, workers' compensation, long-term care services, and community services legislation.

- *Human rights legislation*. Human rights codes protect workers' basic human rights. This legislation states that employers must treat all workers equally and not discriminate on the basis of the worker's race, colour, sex, sexual orientation, religion, age, or disability. Employers and employment agencies also cannot discriminate at the request of a client. Human rights legislation also declares that workers have the right to be free from harassment in the workplace by the employer, client, or fellow worker. **Harassment** means troubling, tormenting, offending, or worrying a person by one's behaviour or comments.
- *Occupational health and safety legislation*. All provinces and territories have occupational health and safety (OH&S) legislation. This legislation outlines the rights and responsibilities of workers, employers, and supervisors in creating and maintaining a safe work environment. Employers must "take every precaution reasonable in the circumstances for the protection of a worker."[3] Workers have a right to receive (and employers must provide) proper training, instruction, and supervision to ensure their safety. Employers who do not fulfill these duties may be fined. Workers have the right to refuse to work if the work poses a danger to themselves or others. In some provinces, however, health care workers cannot refuse to work if in so doing they endanger a client's health or safety.[4] OH&S legislation also details how hazardous materials used in the workplace are to be identified and managed. WHMIS (Workplace Hazardous Materials Information System) is a national plan developed to provide information on the safe use and potential health risks of hazardous materials (see Chapter 16).
- *Employment standards and legislation*. Employment standards legislation states the minimum employment standards acceptable within the workplace. This legislation covers basic rules about issues such as minimum wage, how wages are paid, how many hours of work per day and per week are acceptable, what is fair overtime pay, how many holidays and vacation days are required, and what situations qualify a worker for a leave of absence.
- *Labour relations legislation*. The provinces and territories have legislation that addresses how employers and employees can resolve workplace issues. According to these laws, all employees have a basic right to form or join a trade union of their choice and to participate in lawful union activities. These unions can negotiate wages and other issues with the employer on all union members' behalf. Labour relations legislation sets out the rules for these negotiations (also called collective bargaining), identifies what obligations must be fulfilled before a legal strike can take place, and identifies unfair labour and employee conduct.
- *Workers' compensation legislation*. The provinces and territories have workers' compensation legislation about how workers are financially compensated for accidental injuries on the job. Generally, an employee is considered on the job from the time of reporting to work until the end of the shift. If travel is work-related, accidents that happen while travelling may also be covered by workers' compensation. This legislation also discusses worker and employer rights when an injury occurs.
- *Long-term care facilities legislation*. All long-term care facilities are regulated by provincial and territorial legislation. These laws address the basic rights of residents and describe requirements for how the facility is operated. Licensing and placement requirements, funding structures, and accountability systems are listed. So are guidelines about creating and maintaining health care records and the level of training required of the staff.
- *Community services legislation*. This legislation sets out the rules and procedures for accessing and providing community services. It defines the different types of community services and details how the services are to be provided. Support work is included.

REVIEW

Circle the BEST answer.

1. Which statement about the *Canadian Charter of Rights and Freedoms* is *false*?
   A. It is part of the Canadian Constitution.
   B. It does not apply at a provincial or territorial level.
   C. It protects Canadians' right to equality before and under the law.
   D. It protects Canadians' right to freedom of expression.

2. Provincial and territorial human rights codes do *not* promote
   A. Freedom from discrimination and harassment
   B. Equal treatment with respect to services and facilities
   C. The right to vote
   D. Equal treatment with respect to age, sex, and ethnicity

3. Which is *not* an example of how to treat a client with respect and dignity?
   A. Assuming that the client needs your help before he or she asks
   B. Listening attentively
   C. Encouraging the client's independence
   D. Being careful with the client's personal possessions

4. Which of the following is *not* required for a person to make informed consent
   A. Information about the nature of the treatment
   B. A discussion of the potential risks and side effects of the treatment
   C. Reassurance that the proposed treatment is the best and only option
   D. Information about the likely consequences of not having the treatment

5. Who decides what kind of recreation activities a long-term care resident will participate in?
   A. The person's family
   B. The person's physician or nurse
   C. The facility
   D. The person

6. If a client complains to you about the home care agency's policy, you should
   A. Inform your supervisor about the complaint
   B. Defend the policy
   C. Ignore the person's complaint
   D. Try to distract the person

7. Which of the following statements about negligence is *false*?
   A. It is an unintentional tort.
   B. The negligent person did not act in a reasonable manner.
   C. Harm was caused to a person or a person's property.
   D. A prison term is likely.

8. The intentional attempt or threat to touch a person's body without the person's consent is
   A. Assault
   B. Battery
   C. Defamation
   D. False imprisonment

9. The illegal restraint of another person's movement is
   A. Assault
   B. Battery
   C. Defamation
   D. False imprisonment

10. Mr. Mohammed's photograph is made public without his consent. This is
    A. Battery
    B. Unintentional tort
    C. Invasion of privacy
    D. Libel

11. Who is responsible for obtaining the person's informed consent?
    A. The physician
    B. The RN
    C. The person's substitute decision maker
    D. The support worker

12. The basic rules about wages, work hours, and vacation days are covered in
    A. Labour relations legislation
    B. Workers' compensation legislation
    C. Employment standards legislation
    D. Regulated health professions legislation

Answers to these questions are on page 822.

CHAPTER

11

Caring about Culture

OBJECTIVES

- Define the key terms listed in this chapter
- Understand the differences between race, ethnicity, and culture
- Recognize the factors that influence a person's culture
- Appreciate that culture influences a person's attitudes and behaviours in many areas
- Describe how culture may affect communication, family organization, religious convictions, and perceptions about illness and health care
- Reflect on how your own cultural biases may affect your relationships with your clients
- Discuss how you can provide culturally sensitive care

KEY TERMS

culture The characteristics of a group of people—the language, values, beliefs, habits, ways of life, rules of behaviour, and traditions—that are passed from one person to the next and from one generation to the next

discrimination Behaviour that treats people unfairly based on their group membership

ethnicity Refers to groups of people who share a common history, language, geography, national origin, religion, and identity

personal space The area immediately around one's body

prejudice An attitude that judges a person based on his or her membership in a group

race Refers to groups of people who share similar features, such as skin colour, hair colour and texture, facial characteristics, and bone structure

stereotype Overly simple or exaggerated impression of a person or a group of people

During your career you will care for people whose lifestyles, beliefs, customs, and rituals are different from your own. Canada has a very diverse population. Whether your client is a third-generation Canadian, an Aboriginal Canadian, or a new immigrant, he or she will have a unique culture and perspective. To provide the best care possible, you should be aware of and respectful toward the person's culture.

Race, Ethnicity, and Culture

Three terms are often confused when discussing diversity: race, ethnicity, and culture. **Race** refers to groups of people who share similar features, such as skin colour, hair colour and texture, facial characteristics, and bone structure. Racial groupings are very general and based mainly on appearances. Examples of racial groups include Caucasians, Aboriginals, Blacks, and Asians.

Ethnicity refers to groups of people who share a common history, language, geography, national origin, religion, and identity. An ethnic group is like a racial subgroup. Examples of ethnic groups include the Irish, Inuit, and Chinese. An ethnic group is not necessarily a nationality. One country may have more than one ethnic group. For example, Canada has many ethnic groups (Table 11-1 on page 108).

Culture is what makes societies distinctive. **Culture** refers to the characteristics of a group of people—the language, values, beliefs, habits, ways of life, rules of behaviour, and traditions—that are passed from one person to the next and from one generation to the next. These characteristics are learned from living within the group and influence a person's attitudes and behaviours.

Everyone has a culture. Some people belong to many cultures at once. Ethnicity is an important influence on a person's culture. However, it is not the only influence. Figure 11-1 shows factors that shape an individual's culture. Every person reacts to the various cultural factors in his or her own way. Therefore, each person is culturally unique. A person's culture can change over time when the person leaves one group and joins another or encounters new life experiences.

Effect of Culture

A person's culture affects how he or she deals with daily situations and problems. It is not possible to understand the beliefs and practices of all cultures. However, it is important to realize that culture affects a person's beliefs and behaviours toward such issues as:

- Communication
- Family and social organization

(text continues on page 109)

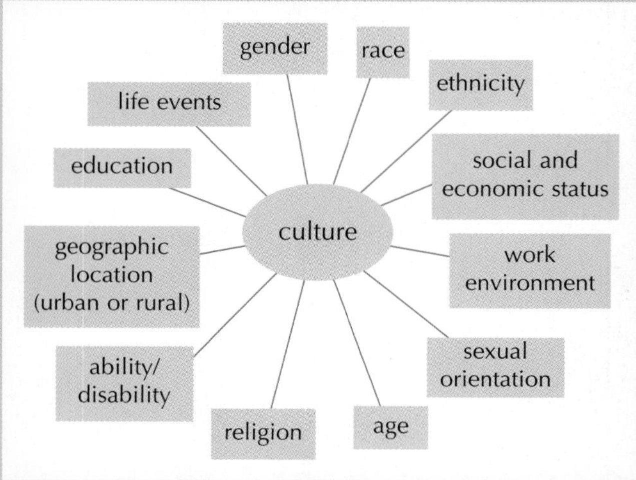

Figure 11-1 Culture is influenced by a number of factors.

Table 11-1 Canada's Most Common Racial and Ethnic Groups

Racial group	Ethnic group
Caucasian	English, French, Scottish, Irish, German, Italian, Ukrainian, Dutch, Polish, Jewish 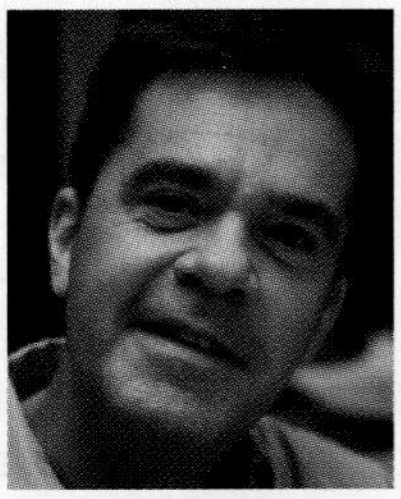
Aboriginal	First Nations, Métis, Inuit 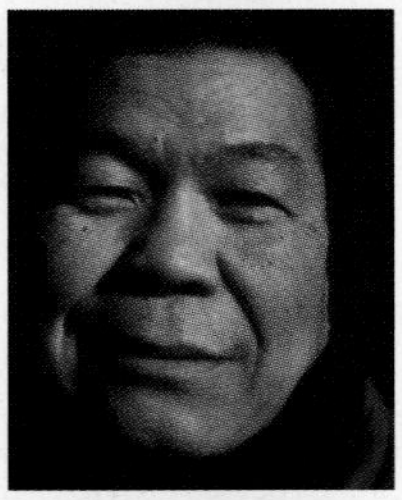
Asian	Chinese, Japanese, Taiwanese, Vietnamese, Thai, Cambodian 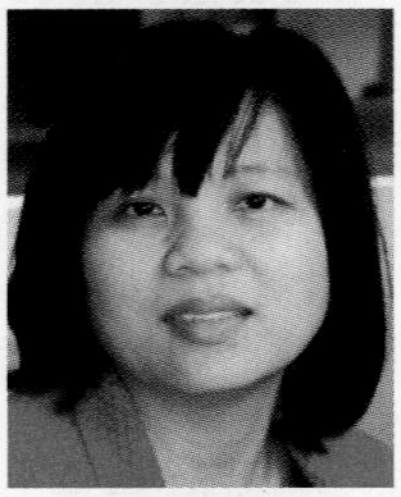
South Asian	Indian, Pakistani, Nepalese 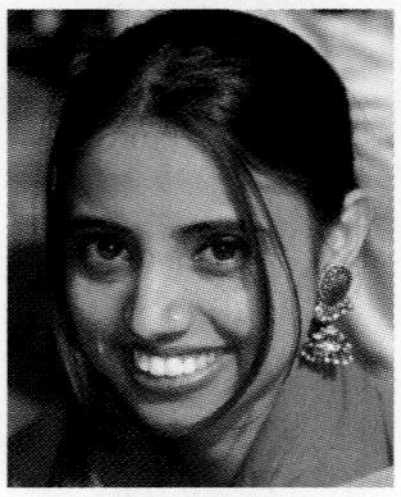
Black	African, Caribbean 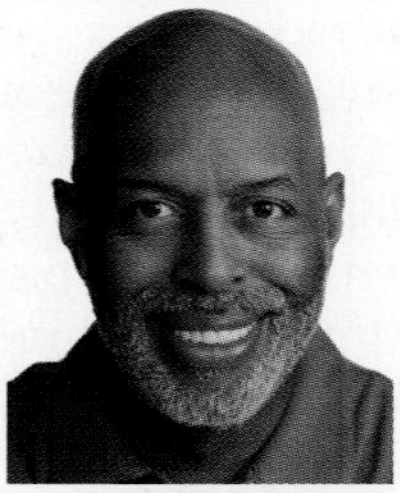
Middle Eastern	Egyptian, Iranian, Palestinian, Saudi Arabian 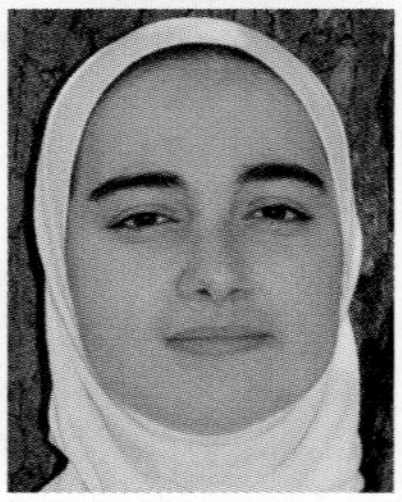

Source: Based on P.A. Potter, A. Perry, J.C. Ross-Kerr, and M.J. Wood, *Canadian Fundamentals of Nursing,* 2nd ed. (Toronto: Harcourt Canada, 2001), pp. 123–33.

- Religion and worship
- Health care practices and reactions to illness

CULTURE AND COMMUNICATION

Many clients may speak a different language or dialect from yours. (See *Respecting Diversity: Communicating with Clients Who Speak a Different Language from Yours* box.) With some clients, you will work with an interpreter. However, information and messages are also sent with many nonverbal cues. For example, touch, the use of space, eye contact, facial expressions, and even silence are used to convey messages. The meanings vary among cultures.

Touch. Touch is a very important form of nonverbal communication. It can convey comfort, caring, love, affection, interest, trust, concern, and reassurance. People are often comforted by being stroked or having their hands held. However, many cultural groups have rules or expectations about who can touch, when touch can occur, and where the body can be touched (Figure 11-2). Some cultures freely use touch. The Spanish, Italian, French, and South American cultures are examples.[1] People in other cultures are embarrassed or uncomfortable with casual touch from strangers and tend to avoid touching. The English, German, and Chinese cultures are examples.[2]

Sometimes the cultural rules of touch depend on the person's gender. For example, in the Indian and Vietnamese cultures, men shake hands with other men, but not with women.[3]

Respecting Diversity

COMMUNICATING WITH CLIENTS WHO SPEAK A DIFFERENT LANGUAGE FROM YOURS

- Convey comfort by your tone of voice and body language.
- Do not speak loudly or shout. It will not help the person understand English.
- Speak slowly and distinctly.
- Keep messages short and simple.
- Be alert for words the client seems to understand.
- Use gestures and pictures.
- Repeat the message in different ways.
- Avoid using medical terms, abbreviations, and slang.
- Be certain the client understands what is going to happen and consents before you begin a procedure. Be alert for signs that the client is pretending to understand. Nodding and answering "yes" to all questions are signs that the client may not understand what you are saying.
- Learn a few useful phrases in the client's language.

You must be aware of what kind and how much touch the person is comfortable with. Ask your supervisor for guidance and watch the person interact with family or other people. Touch should be gentle, not hurried or rough. Touch should not be sexual in nature.

Personal Space. If someone stands too close to you, you probably feel uncomfortable or anxious. Your personal space has been invaded. The same is true for your clients. **Personal space** is the area immediately around one's body. Everyone has personal space preferences.

The exact distance requirements vary among individuals and situations. However, people in the same cultural group tend to have similar personal space requirements.[4] In Western cultures, most people prefer to stand and speak at a distance of about 90 cm (3 feet). People in other cultures may prefer to stand closer or farther away when interacting with others. When providing care, it is important to not invade your client's personal space. If the client steps back from you, does not face you directly, or pulls his or her chair away from you, the client may be sending a message that you are too close.[5]

Eye Contact. Eye contact has different meanings within different cultures. In Western culture, eye contact is a sign of good self-concept, openness, interest in others, attention, and honesty. It also communicates warmth. Lack of eye contact can communicate rudeness, guilt, dishonesty, shyness, or embarrassment. Some cultures are not comfortable with eye contact. For some Asian and Aboriginal cultures, eye contact is considered disrespectful and an invasion of privacy.[6] In certain Indian cultures, eye contact with people of a higher or lower social and economic class is avoided.[7]

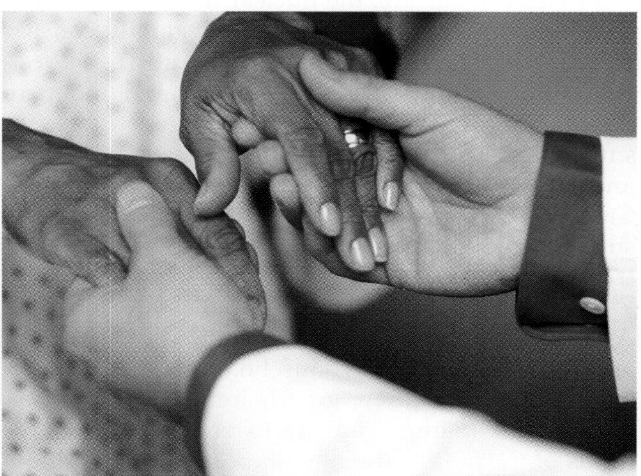

Figure 11-2 Culture may influence how a client responds to touch.

Facial Expressions. Many facial expressions are universal. Expressions of pain, surprise, embarrassment, and happiness are similar around the world. Some cultures are more expressive than others. It therefore may be hard to judge what others are feeling based only on their facial expressions. For example, Italian and Spanish people tend to use many facial expressions and gestures to communicate happiness, pain, or displeasure. In contrast, Irish, English, and northern European people usually use fewer facial expressions, especially with strangers.[8] In some cultures, certain facial expressions may mean the opposite of what the person is feeling. For example, in some Asian cultures people may smile to hide negative emotions.[9]

Silence. Even the use of silence varies among cultural groups. In some cultures, such as the English and Arabic cultures, silence is used for privacy.[10] Among Russian, French, and Spanish cultures, silence means agreement between parties.[11] In some Asian cultures, silence is used as a sign of respect, particularly to an older person.[12] In some Aboriginal cultures, silence is considered a virtue. Speaking is reserved for matters of extreme importance.[13] For some Aboriginal, Chinese, and Japanese people, silence is used as a way to understand a person's needs. For example, if the person is speaking and suddenly stops, the silence may be intended to allow the listener to think about what has just been said before the speaker continues.[14]

Culture and the Family

In your career you will meet many different kinds of families. Culture affects family structure. It also affects roles and responsibilities of various members during times of illness. For example, in some cultures, adult children (especially daughters) are responsible for caring for their older parents.

In Western culture, the nuclear family is the most common family structure. A nuclear family consists of a mother, father, and children (Figure 11-3). Western culture emphasizes self-reliance and independence. Children are usually encouraged to be self-sufficient. Most young adults leave the family home and live independent of their parents and siblings. Care of family members outside the nuclear family—such as grandparents, aunts, or uncles—is often entrusted to others.

In other cultures, extended families are common. Asian, South Asian, and Aboriginal cultures are examples. A family in one household may include parents and their children, grandparents, aunts, uncles, and cousins (Figure 11-4). In extended families, the needs of the family are more important than individual needs. Elders and sick family members are often taken care of by the family. For example, in Vietnam and China, all family members are involved in the ill person's care.[15] Family members bathe, feed, and comfort the person. Canadians of these and other cultures are often surrounded by family during illness.

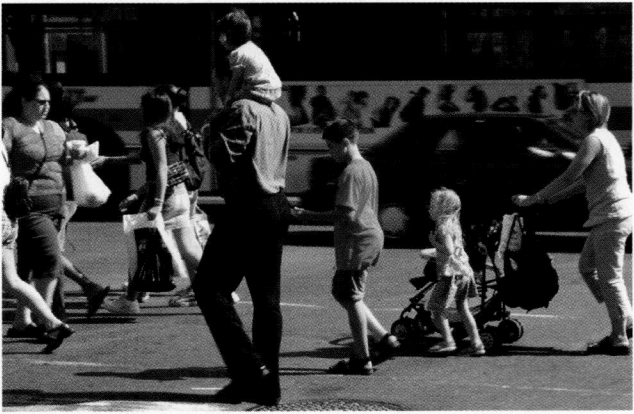

Figure 11-3 A nuclear family.

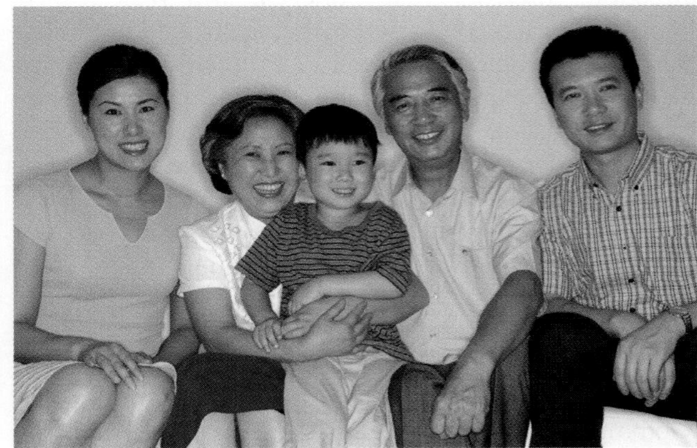

Figure 11-4 An extended family.

Sometimes children rebel against the culture of their parents. Children of first-generation immigrants often reject the roles and behaviours expected of them in favour of the new culture. This can cause great stress for the parents and family. Box 11-1 describes how cultural conflict affected one older person.

Culture and Religion

In most cultures, religion is an extremely important influence. Religion relates to spiritual beliefs, needs, and practices. Religions may promote beliefs and practices related to daily living habits, behaviours, relationships with others, diet, healing, days of worship, birth and birth control, medicine, and death.

Many people rely on religion for support and comfort during illness. They may want to pray and observe certain religious practices. A visit from their spiritual leader or adviser may be helpful. If a client asks to see a religious leader, promptly report the

Box 11-1 Case Study: Cultural Conflict

Mrs. Da Silva is a 75-year-old widow receiving home care. She and her husband moved from Portugal to Canada in the 1960s with their three young children. For the next 30 years, Mr. Da Silva worked on the assembly line of an automobile factory while Mrs. Da Silva worked as a dressmaker. They worked long hours to pay for their children's education. All three children now have successful careers and their own families.

Mrs. Da Silva's health began to decline after her husband died. Severe arthritis in her leg and hip progressed to where she could no longer walk. A family conference was held. The children agreed that their mother no longer could care for herself, even with the aid of a support worker. They thought it was unsafe for her to live alone. None of the children felt that they could manage their mother's care and their own families and careers. They told their mother they thought she should consider moving into a long-term care facility.

This came as a great shock to Mrs. Da Silva. She and her husband took care of her mother years ago. Her mother lived with them until her death. Mrs. Da Silva assumed that one of her children would do the same for her. In Portugal, children take care of their older parents. She felt she was being cast aside. The idea of leaving her home and moving into a facility with strangers made her depressed.

There is a conflict between two cultures. Mr. and Mrs. Da Silva gave their children opportunities to enter and succeed in a new culture. Now a part of the new culture, the children feel that they would have to give up too much in order to care for their mother in their own homes. Many of their friends' parents enjoy living with other people their own age in a retirement facility. They believe their mother will also eventually settle in and feel at home there.

request to your supervisor. Make sure the person's room is neat and orderly for the visit. Ensure privacy during the visit.

Many religions are practised by various groups within Canada. They include Christianity (the Catholic and Protestant faiths), Judaism, Buddhism, Islam, Hinduism, Sikhism, and the Baha'i faith, among others. You will care for clients who have religious beliefs that are different from yours. Some people do not practise a religion. You must always respect the client's beliefs, practices, and religious symbols and items (such as a rosary, prayer rug, or religious medal). Never try to convert your clients to your own belief system.

Culture and Perceptions of Health Care and Illness

Culture greatly affects how people view health care and illness. Some cultures have beliefs about the causes of illness. Culture also affects how people cope with their symptoms and the stresses of being ill.

In Western culture, the general belief is that disease and illness are caused by biological or environmental factors. Illness and disease can often be prevented, and people can be cared for or cured with scientifically proven methods. Some cultures believe that illness is caused by supernatural forces, an imbalance with nature, or disharmony between mind, body, and spirit. People may use charms, rituals, alternative medicines, or traditional or folk medicine. Traditional or folk medicine may include ancient remedies and rituals, passed down through many generations. Many folk remedies involve herbs or a traditional healer or shaman.

Some folk remedies either help the person or do not affect the person's health. If the practice does not harm the client and promotes his or her emotional well-being, the nurse or case manager may include it in the care plan. Other folk remedies may interfere with the client's medical treatment. For example, some herbal medicines may interact with prescription drugs and have harmful results. Many times people try alternative therapies or cultural health care practices without telling their physician, nurse, or case manager.[16] The health care team must be aware of all health care practices to make sure they are not harmful to the client. (See *Support Workers Solving Problems: Culture, Health Care, and Illness* box on page 112.) Tell your supervisor if:

- Your client tells you that he or she is using alternative or folk remedies
- You observe a client using alternative or folk remedies

Providing Culturally Sensitive Care

Providing culturally sensitive care is important. Remember that each client is an individual. People respond to their cultural influences in their own unique way. Do not stereotype a person based on his or her ethnicity, religion, or any other factor. A **stereotype** is an overly simple or exaggerated impression of a person or a group of people. You cannot apply the cultural behaviours of a given culture to all members of the group. That would be stereotyping. *Individuals may not follow every belief and practice of their culture and religion. Each person is unique.*

Support Workers Solving Problems

CULTURE, HEALTH CARE, AND ILLNESS

Scenario: Mrs. Couture has a severe burn on the bottom of her foot. She mentions to her support worker, Nancy, that she has placed a medal of Saint John the Apostle under the top layer of bandage around her foot. Mrs. Couture explains Saint John the Apostle is known for healing burns. She believes that placing the medal in the dressing will help her wound heal quickly and safely.

Discussion: Nancy knows that Mrs. Couture has the right to make her own choices about her care. She also knows that Mrs. Couture's strong spiritual beliefs may help her during her healing process. Nancy is concerned, however, that having the religious medal so close to the wound may be harmful. She calls her supervisor to tell her about the conversation. The supervisor relates the message to the case manager, who was not aware of the situation. The case manager asks Mrs. Couture's nurse to discuss the situation with her.

Source: Adapted from The College of Nurses of Ontario, *Guide to Nurses for Providing Culturally Sensitive Care* (Ottawa: CNO, 1999), p. 11.

Stereotypes are often associated with prejudice. **Prejudice** is an attitude that judges a person based on his or her membership in a group. Making assumptions about a person based on his or her cultural or ethnic group is always wrong and often hurtful. Prejudice frequently leads to discrimination. **Discrimination** is behaviour that treats people unfairly based on their group membership.

Sometimes people do not realize that they are showing prejudice or discrimination. Remember, everyone has a culture. Your attitudes and behaviours are shaped by your culture. Some people react negatively or fearfully to cultural differences. You must resist these reactions and accept a person's differences. You do not have to agree with the client's beliefs and practices. However, you must be tolerant and not make judgments about them.

To be tolerant and understanding of others, you need to understand how your culture influences you. Do you judge people by your own cultural standards? Do you have any prejudices or biases? Consider the following questions:

- Do you assume if something works for you it must work for others?
- Do you think there are "right" and "wrong" ways of doing things?
- Are you ever critical of another person's lifestyle because it is different from your own?
- Do you sometimes consider that other people's lifestyles, religious beliefs, superstitions, and beliefs are silly or odd?
- Do you try to convert others to your religion or way of thinking and doing things?
- Do you believe that people from one race, ethnic group, or religion should not marry people from another?
- Do you avoid trying new things?
- Do you draw conclusions too quickly?
- Do you respect people as individuals or do stereotypes sometimes get in the way?

To accept people of different cultures, you need to learn from them. Communicate with them and listen attentively. Learn as much as possible about their thoughts, beliefs, and values. Respect and show interest in their traditions, foods, dress, and customs. Your clients will feel valued and respected.

REVIEW

Circle T if the answer is true and F if it is false.

1. T F Culture influences people's attitudes and beliefs, but not their behaviours.
2. T F Believing that all members of a group share the same characteristics is an example of stereotyping.
3. T F Everyone has a culture.
4. T F Everyone within an ethnic group shares the same culture.
5. T F Each individual responds differently to cultural influences.
6. T F Everyone responds positively to a hug or pat on the back.
7. T F Although a person's experiences and situation may change over time, his or her culture never changes.

Circle the BEST answer.

8. Which is *false*?
   A. Race refers to a group of people who share similar physical traits.
   B. A country has one ethnic group.
   C. A person's culture influences health and illness practices.
   D. People within an ethnic community often share a common history and identify with one another.
9. Which is *false*?
   A. Culture influences communication.
   B. Culture may affect roles and responsibilities within families.
   C. All people respond to cultural influences in the same way.
   D. Culture affects how people view health care and illness.
10. Mr. Greene asks to see his spiritual adviser. You should
    A. Report his request to your supervisor
    B. Question why he wants the meeting
    C. Offer to introduce him to your spiritual adviser
    D. Call his synagogue to arrange the meeting
11. Which is *false?*
    A. Prejudice is an attitude that judges people based on their group membership.
    B. In some situations, prejudice is acceptable.
    C. Prejudice frequently leads to discrimination.
    D. Stereotypes are often associated with prejudice.

Answers to these questions are on page 822.

CHAPTER

12

INTERPERSONAL COMMUNICATION

OBJECTIVES

- Define the key terms listed in this chapter
- Describe the communication process
- Describe verbal and nonverbal communication
- Explain the methods of and barriers to effective communication
- Explain how to communicate with an angry client
- Explain why assertive communication is important
- Learn to explain procedures and tasks to clients

KEY TERMS

active listening Paying close attention to a person's verbal and nonverbal communication

assertiveness A style of communication in which thoughts and feelings are expressed positively and directly without offending others

body language Posture, appearance, facial expressions, body movements, eye contact, and gestures that send messages to others

closed questions Questions that focus on specific information

empathetic listening Being attentive to a person's feelings

focusing Limiting the conversation to a certain topic

interpersonal communication The exchange of information between two people, usually face to face

nonverbal communication Messages sent without words

open-ended questions Questions that invite a person to share thoughts, feelings, or ideas

paraphrasing Restating someone's message in your own words

verbal communication Messages sent through the spoken word

Good interpersonal communication is needed to provide safe and effective care. Health care team members share information about what was done and what needs to be done for the client. Information about the client's response to care and treatment also is shared. Good communication means better relationships with clients, families, and co-workers. When you communicate with people, you find out about their needs, feelings, likes, and dislikes. You also express your thoughts and ideas. *What* you say and *how* you say it are equally important.

The Communication Process

Interpersonal communication is the exchange of information between two people, usually face to face. A message is sent by one person (the *sender*) and is received and interpreted by another person (the *receiver*). Often the receiver provides information in response to the message (*feedback*). During the exchange of information, each person usually acts as both a sender and a receiver.

Successful interpersonal communication occurs when the receiver understands the meaning of the message. However, sometimes the receiver does not interpret the message in the way the sender intended. Mistakes can happen. Feelings can be hurt. Messages are sometimes misunderstood because many elements influence communication. For example, factors unique to each person affect communication. These include the person's:

- Perceptions (how he or she views events and understands messages)
- Experiences
- Physical and mental health
- Emotions
- Values
- Beliefs
- Culture

The relationship between the sender and the receiver also affects their communication. Communication is easier when the people involved understand and respect each other (Figure 12-1 on page 116).

To effectively communicate with clients, you need to understand and respect them. Be sensitive to each person's unique situation and needs. You must accept and respect the client's culture and religion. You also must appreciate that stresses, problems, and frustrations affect how a message is sent and received. For example, if a client is worried, he or she may not be able to pay close attention to what you are saying.

Remember that clients are whole persons. They are physical, emotional, intellectual, social, and spiritual human beings. You must try to understand their meaning rather than just their words.

Verbal Communication

In **verbal communication**, messages are sent through the spoken word. Sometimes symbols substitute for

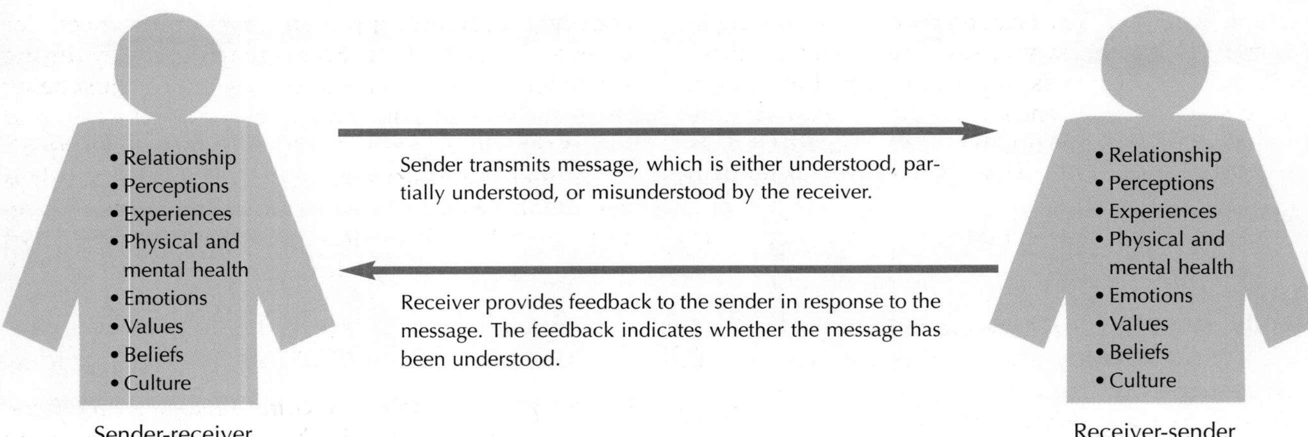

Figure 12-1 Communication is affected by the sender and receiver's relationship, as well as by many other factors.

spoken words. An example is sign language, which is used to speak with a person who cannot hear.

To effectively communicate with words, you need to:

- *Choose your words carefully.* Words must have the same meaning for both you and the other person. Try to avoid words with more than one meaning. For example, the words "small," "moderate," and "large" mean different things to different people. Is small the size of a pea or the size of a walnut? Use words that are specific and descriptive. For example, telling your supervisor that a client's temperature is 37.9° C is clearer than saying, "the temperature is up."
- *Use simple, everyday language.* You will learn medical terminology as you study and gain experience in health care. Do not use medical terms when communicating with clients and their families. Medical terms may be unfamiliar to them. Use correct grammar. Do not use vulgar words or slang.
- *Speak clearly, slowly, and distinctly.* Do not mumble or speak quickly. Move your lips as you speak, slow down your speech, and pause between sentences.
- *Control the volume and tone of your voice.* How your voice sounds sends a message. Do not shout. Shouting can mean irritation or anger. Do not talk in a harsh or abrupt manner. Avoid speaking to adults in high-pitched tones. This may seem like you are treating them like children.
- *Be brief and concise.* Do not add unrelated or unneeded information. Focus on what you are saying, stay on the subject, and do not get wordy. Being brief and concise reduces the possibility of omitting important details. Speak in short sentences to emphasize your words. Short sentences are more clearly understood.
- *Present information in a logical manner.* Organize your thoughts before you speak. Present them in sequence. Think about what will happen or what has happened step by step.
- *Ask one question at a time.* Give the person time to answer. Do not rush the person. Avoid providing the answer for the person.
- *Determine understanding.* Do not assume the person understands what you are saying. Ask the person to repeat the message in his or her own words.
- *Do not pretend to understand.* If you do not understand a term or what the person has said, ask the person to restate or rephrase the message. Repeat the message if needed.

Nonverbal Communication

In **nonverbal communication**, messages are sent without words. Body language, touch, and the use of silence are ways of sending messages without words. The meaning of messages sent through nonverbal communication varies depending on the person's age, gender, and life experiences. It also varies depending on the person's culture (see Chapter 11).

Body Language

Body language includes:

- Posture
- Appearance (dress, hygiene, and adornments such as jewellery, perfume, and cosmetics)
- Facial expressions
- Body movements
- Eye contact
- Gestures

Body language greatly affects communication. It can change the meaning of a verbal message. For example, you say, "Yes, I can do that" while smiling in a friendly manner. Or, you say, "Yes, I can do that" while rolling your eyes and sighing. In both cases, your body language sends a message. If you say one thing with words but another with your body language, you send a *mixed message*. Mixed messages are confusing and unhelpful.

Be sensitive to clients' body language. It can help you understand them better. For example, slumped posture and a slow, shuffling walk may mean the person is not happy or is not feeling well. Or, people may say they feel fine but show that they are in pain with their facial expression.

Nonverbal clues often reflect a person's true feelings. Because they are usually involuntary and unconscious, nonverbal clues may send messages more accurately than words. For example, Mr. Reyes says, "I am looking forward to moving to the nursing home. I am sure I will make some new friends." However, you see tears in his eyes and he looks away from you. His verbal communication suggests that he is happy, but his nonverbal communication shows sadness.

You need to be aware of the messages you send with your body language. You send messages by the way you act and move. Your facial expressions and how you stand, sit, walk, and look at a person all send messages. Your body language should show interest and enthusiasm about your work. It should also show caring and respect for your clients. For example, show respect by physically positioning yourself at the client's level when talking. If the client is in a bed or wheelchair, sit or squat so you are at eye level.

You need to control your body language in many instances. For example, do not react to odours from a client's body. Many odours are beyond people's control. Your client's embarrassment and humiliation increase if you react to odours.

Touch

Touch is a very important form of nonverbal communication. It conveys warmth, comfort, concern, affection, trust, and reassurance. Most people respond well to touch because it helps them feel less alone. Holding a person's hand can provide comfort. Gently stroking a person's shoulder or back can promote rest and relaxation. Touch should be gentle, not hurried or rushed.

Touch means different things to different people. Some people do not want to be touched. Pulling away or tensing the body may mean that the person does not want to be touched. Be sure to find out whether your client wants touch or not.

Silence

The use of silence also conveys messages. Silence can convey acceptance, rejection, fear, or the need for quiet and time to think. Sometimes, especially during sad times, you do not need to say anything. Just being there shows that you care. Silence can give you and others time to organize thoughts or choose words. Silence is useful when making difficult decisions. It is also helpful when a person is upset and is trying to regain control. In these situations, silence on your part shows respect and empathy for the person (Box 12-1).

Communication Methods

Certain methods help you communicate with others. These methods result in better relationships with people.

Active Listening

Active listening means paying close attention to a person's verbal and nonverbal communication. You listen to the content, the intent, and the feelings behind a person's words. You must concentrate on what a person is saying. You also must observe nonverbal clues. Remember, nonverbal clues may show the person's true feelings. For example, Mrs. Gorecki tells you that her knees do not hurt today. However, you

Box 12-1 Case Study: Silence and Touch during Sad Times

How do you show a person that you care? Words may not be enough. You may have to be completely silent and comfort the person with your touch. Holding a person's hand often provides more comfort than words. Jessica, a support worker in a long-term care facility, relates this experience:

"Mrs. Robinson has lived in our facility for 3 years. She is severely disabled with arthritis. She is a friendly, cheerful woman who rarely complains. One morning she didn't reply when I knocked on her door. After knocking three times, I opened the door. I was afraid that she was ill. She was sitting in her wheelchair. She looked very sad. I sensed that something was wrong.

I sat down in a chair beside her and asked if I could help. When there was no reply, I placed my hand on hers. I didn't say anything. After a few minutes, she told me that her son had just called. Her grandson had been killed in a car accident. He was 19, and he had just finished his first year at university. I told Mrs. Robinson that I felt very sad for her. We sat there quietly, my hand on hers, for five minutes. I asked her if anyone else at the facility knew, and if there was anything that I could do. She asked me to tell the nurse. Then she said, 'You are very kind to sit with me. I know how busy you are.' "

observe her rubbing her knees and grimacing. You know that she still has pain.

Active listening requires you to be interested and to show that you care. The following are guidelines for active listening:

- Face the person.
- Make eye contact. (Consider cultural preferences for eye contact.)
- Lean toward the person (Figure 12-2). Do not sit back with your arms crossed.
- Respond to the person. Nod your head. Say "uh huh," "mmm," and "I see." Repeat what the person says, and ask questions.
- Avoid communication barriers (see pages 120–121).

Paraphrasing

Paraphrasing is restating a person's message in your own words. When paraphrasing, use fewer words than the person used to send the message. Paraphrasing serves three purposes:

- It shows that you are listening.
- It lets both you and the person know if you understood the message.
- It promotes further communication.

People usually respond to a paraphrased statement. For example:

Mrs. Cummings: I was a keen reader when I could see. I miss books so much. Those talking books are hard to follow.

You: You love stories, but talking books are not as good as real books.

Mrs. Cummings: Exactly. I wish you had time to read to me.

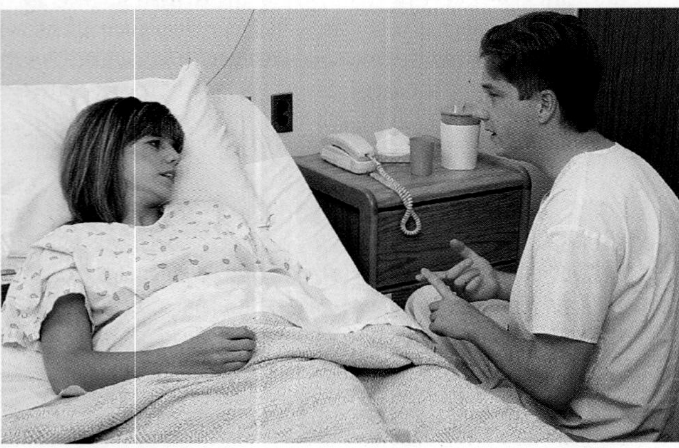

Figure 12-2 Face the person and make eye contact when conversing.

When paraphrasing, try not to interpret. Guide the conversation so that the person feels comfortable expressing thoughts or feelings. If you misinterpret a person's meaning, you could end the conversation or cause offence. See *Support Workers Solving Problems: Using Paraphrasing and Questioning Skills* box for an example of effective paraphrasing.

Empathetic Listening

Empathetic listening means being attentive to a person's feelings. Empathy means being open to and trying to understand the experiences and feelings of others. It involves acknowledging the person's point of view without judging the person. People need to know that they are understood. Empathy can help reduce feelings of loneliness. It can create bonds of trust between you and the people you support.

When paraphrasing, you acknowledge other people's words. When empathizing, you acknowledge their feelings. To show empathy, follow the person's lead. While the person speaks, listen quietly. Do not rush the person or change the subject. Stay focussed on the person and not on your own opinions. For example, if a client mentions a difficult situation, you could say, "I can see you are upset. Do you want to talk about it?" This comment shows that you recognize and care about how the person feels.

Avoid these pat responses:

- "I know how you feel." *(Nobody can ever know how another person feels.)*
- "I feel sorry for you." *(This implies pity.)*
- "I wouldn't want to be in your shoes." *(This suggests superiority and implies pity.)*

Consider these two responses to a complaint:

Mr. Witowski: I can't believe they have made me move to this new room. I was settled in the other room, and I liked the view of the lawn and the pond. Now, all I see when I look out of the window is an asphalt parking lot.

Jane: The move can't be helped, unfortunately. The old wing was falling apart.

Carlos: Being moved is upsetting. Your old room had a lovely view. I can see why you miss it.

Jane's response is not empathetic. She focuses on facts, not on Mr. Witowski's feelings. Carlos's response is empathetic. He paraphrases Mr. Witowski's statement. This lets Mr. Witowski know Carlos has understood his message. Carlos also acknowledges Mr. Witowski's feelings about moving.

Support Workers Solving Problems

Using Paraphrasing and Questioning Skills

Scenario: Sophia provides personal care to Mr. Dupuis, 48. He is severely disabled with multiple sclerosis. This is Sophia's second visit. On her first visit she helped Mr. Dupuis shave and dress. On this visit she is to assist him with bathing and preparing breakfast.

Mr. Dupuis: Oh, it's you. I was still asleep. It's awfully early.
Sophia: A 7:30 start is a little early for you. You're not ready for me. *(paraphrasing)*
Mr. Dupuis: Yes, I've asked the case manager to start the morning care at 8:00 instead.
Sophia: Perhaps she is working on the schedule change. I will check with the agency.
Mr. Dupuis: Thanks.
Sophia: The care plan calls for a bath today. Would you like to have it now or after breakfast? *(closed question)*
Mr. Dupuis: It doesn't matter much. I wish I didn't need a bath. Being bathed by someone else is not much fun.
Sophia: Can you tell me what you dislike about it? *(open-ended question)*
Mr. Dupuis: The lack of privacy really gets to me.
Sophia: We can work together on giving you privacy.
Mr. Dupuis: That would be a good idea. I don't think my last support worker cared much about my privacy.

Discussion: Paraphrasing and questioning skills can help you improve the care you provide your clients. In this case, Sophia listens to Mr. Dupuis. She uses paraphrasing, closed questions, and open-ended questions in her responses. Sophia uses paraphrasing *(A 7:30 start is a little early for you. You're not ready for me.)* to show Mr. Dupuis she has understood his concern and to prompt him to provide more information. She asks a closed question *(Would you like to have your bath now or after breakfast?)* because she needs specific information about Mr. Dupuis's preferences. She asks an open-ended question *(Can you tell me what you dislike about it?)* to encourage Mr. Dupuis to share his feelings about not liking baths. Once Sophia understands Mr. Dupuis's worries about privacy, she can take steps to solve this problem.

Asking Closed Questions

Closed questions focus on specific information. Use these kinds of questions when you need to know something precise. Some closed questions have "yes" or "no" answers. Others require a brief response. For example:

You: Would you like butter on your toast this morning, Mrs. Cummings?
Mrs. Cummings: Yes, please.
You: Would you like strawberry jam or marmalade?
Mrs. Cummings: Marmalade, please.

Asking Open-Ended Questions

Open-ended questions invite a person to share thoughts, feelings, or ideas. The person chooses what to talk about. Answers require more than a "yes" or "no" answer. However, the person controls what is talked about and the information given. Consider these questions: "What was it like to grow up in Scotland, Mrs. Cummings?" (open-ended question) and "Did you like living in Scotland?" (closed question). The first question encourages Mrs. Cummings to talk about herself. It may start a conversation by showing Mrs. Cummings that you are interested in hearing about her life. The second question requires a "yes" or a "no" answer. It does not encourage Mrs. Cummings to talk about herself. Nor does it communicate as much interest in Mrs. Cummings's life.

Use open-ended questions in combination with closed questions to find out about a client's needs and preferences. Use them as well to find out if a client is satisfied with your care. For example, a closed question ("Are you comfortable?") can provide you with necessary information. An open-ended question ("Is there anything I can do to make you more comfortable?") can encourage a client to express thoughts or feelings. The *Support Workers Solving Problems: Using Paraphrasing and Questioning Skills* box shows an example of a support worker using both types of questions to improve a client's care.

Clarifying

Clarifying helps you make sure that you understand a person's message. You can ask the person to repeat the message, say you do not understand, or restate the message as a question. For example:

- "Could you say that again?"
- "I'm sorry, Mr. Hart. I don't understand what you mean."
- "Are you saying that you want to go home?"

FOCUSING

Focusing is limiting the conversation to a certain topic. It is useful when a client rambles or wanders in thought. Take the case of Mr. Reyes, who talks at length about his favourite foods and places to eat. You need to know why he did not feel like eating dinner. You focus the conversation on dinner by saying, "Let's talk about today's dinner. You said you didn't feel like eating." Another example is Mrs. Hooda. The care plan directs you to provide two choices when helping Mrs. Hooda dress. She becomes distracted by the pattern on one of the dresses. You guide the conversation back to the task of dressing by saying, "Would you like to wear the dress with the pretty pattern?" A third example is Mrs. Cummings. She has told you that she does not want to go for a walk. She then reminisces about her early life. Your response encourages her to focus on her reason for not wanting to walk:

Mrs. Cummings: We used to walk for miles in the Lake District. It was usually raining. It rained constantly in Edinburgh too.
You: There is no rain today, and the sun is shining. Is there a reason why you don't feel like walking?

COMMUNICATION BARRIERS

Communication barriers prevent sending and receiving messages so that communication is limited or fails completely. Some barriers cannot be avoided. You must work around these. For example, some people have hearing and vision problems that interfere with communication. Some people have nervous system disorders that limit communication. You must learn special techniques to communicate in these situations (Figure 12-3; see Chapters 35 and 36). Cultural differences can also interfere with communication. The client may attach different meanings to verbal and nonverbal communication (see Chapter 11).

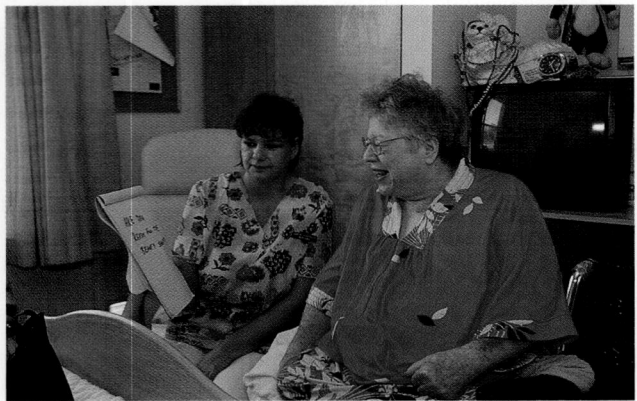

Figure 12-3 The support worker writes a note to a client who is hearing impaired.

Factors in the environment can also limit communication. Loud noises, lack of privacy, and distractions are examples. Try to provide a calm, quiet setting when talking with a client.

Certain behaviours can also create communication barriers. Improve communication by avoiding the following: interrupting, answering your own questions, giving advice, minimizing problems, using patronizing language, and failing to listen.

INTERRUPTING

Interrupting a person stops communication. People interrupt when they:

- Jump to conclusions about what the speaker is trying to say
- Become impatient with the speaker or the way the story is being told
- Become bored and wish to change the subject to something that interests them
- Wish to change the subject because the topic is upsetting
- Feel hurried or stressed
- Focus on a task, not on the person

ANSWERING YOUR OWN QUESTIONS

Avoid answering your own questions. Some people do this routinely in conversation. Others do it only with people who take a long time to respond. Answering questions or completing thoughts for people discourages openness. Notice the following different responses to the same question, phrased slightly differently:

You: How did you sleep last night? Okay? *(answer provided)*
Mrs. Cummings: Yes.
You: How did you sleep last night? *(answer not provided)*
Mrs. Cummings: I was pretty restless. It took me a long time to fall asleep. The last time I looked at the clock it was 3:00 a.m.

GIVING ADVICE

Avoid giving advice to clients and their family members. Let people express their feelings and concerns without adding your opinion. You could create confusion, anxiety, and resentment. Your advice could go against the family's wishes, the physician's orders, or the care plan. Even if a client asks for your advice, do not give it. You could instead suggest that the client speak to your supervisor or his or her case manager. In the following example, the support worker tactfully avoids giving advice to Mrs. Van Doorne:

Mrs. Van Doorne: I don't feel ready to leave my home, but I'm too much of a burden on my daughter. I just don't know what do to. Sometimes I feel that we'd all be better off if I moved into a nursing home. At other times I hate the thought of it. What do you think I should do?

Support worker: I can see what a difficult decision it is, Mrs. Van Doorne. I wish I could help, but it's not my role to give you advice. Is there anyone else you can talk to about it?

Mrs. Van Doorne: I've tried to talk to Anne *(her daughter)*, but she would never admit that I'm a burden.

Support worker: What about talking to Mrs. Stainer *(the case manager)*? I'm sure she could help.

Mrs. Van Doorne: That's a good idea. I'll do that.

Minimizing Problems

Do not minimize a person's problems. Avoid making comments like these: "Everything will be fine," "Don't worry," "It's not really that bad," "Look on the bright side," and "It could be worse." These block communication. They imply that the person is complaining or exaggerating the problem. They also show that you are judging the person or the situation. You have no right to judge others. Minimizing problems makes people feel that you are ridiculing their concerns, feelings, and fears. They think you do not care about what they think or feel. Consider these two responses to a hospital patient's concerns:

Mr. Lam: I'm so nervous about this operation. I've never even been in a hospital before.

Eduardo: Believe me, you have nothing to worry about. The surgeons could do this operation with their eyes closed. You will be just fine. (*Walks away.*)

Helga: Having surgery is frightening, especially when it's your first operation. The doctors and nurses will explain everything to you so that you know what to expect. *(Reports Mr. Lam's concerns immediately to the nurse, who reassures him about the surgery.)*

Eduardo's response minimizes Mr. Lam's worries about his surgery. Helga's response is empathetic. She uses paraphrasing to let Mr. Lam know that she understands his concerns. She also reassures him by expressing confidence in the health care team.

Using Patronizing Language

Sometimes the words you use can make a person feel unimportant and inferior. These words are *patronizing*. They imply that you are better than the other person. To avoid patronizing language:

- Do not address clients as "love," "dear," "honey," or other endearments.
- Do not use a client's first name without his or her permission.
- Do not use terms such as "good girl" or "good boy" or "you guys" with adults.
- Do not use the term "we" when you really mean "you."
- Do not use "baby talk" or terms such as "there, there."
- Do not talk to co-workers or family members as if the client were not present.
- Do not correct a client's speech or language.

Some health care workers mistake patronizing language for warmth and friendliness (Box 12-2).

Failing to Listen

Communication is blocked if you fail to listen with interest and sincerity (Figure 12-4 on page 122). Do not pretend to listen. This conveys a lack of interest and caring. You can miss important complaints of pain, discomfort, or other abnormal sensations that must be reported to your supervisor.

Communicating with Angry People

Anger is a common response to illness and disability (see Chapter 4). It is an emotion often expressed by clients and family members. The many causes of anger include frustration, anxiety, fear, and pain. Loss of body function and losing one's independence can also cause anger. People who are angry often feel helpless.

Anger also is a symptom of diseases that affect thinking and behaviour. People who abuse alcohol

Box 12-2 Avoiding Patronizing Language

Poor Communication Skills

Support worker: Hello, Doris. How are we feeling today, dear?
Mrs. Crossley: I'm feeling much better, thank you.
Support worker: Have you been doing your exercises?
Mrs. Crossley: Yes.
Support worker: Good girl.

Improved Communication Skills

Support worker: Hello, Mrs. Crossley. How are you feeling today?
Mrs. Crossley: I'm feeling much better, thank you.
Support worker: How have your exercises been going?
Mrs. Crossley: Very well, thank you. I'm up to half an hour a day now.
Support worker: That's excellent progress!

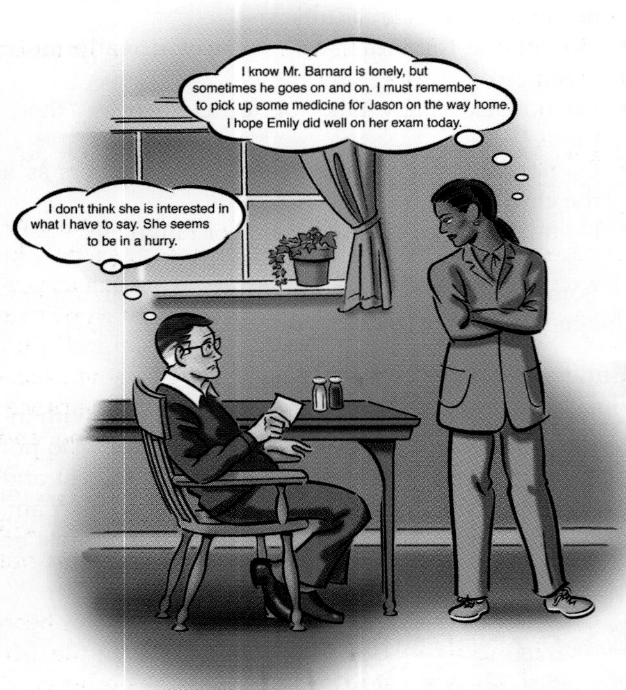
I know Mr. Barnard is lonely, but sometimes he goes on and on. I must remember to pick up some medicine for Jason on the way home. I hope Emily did well on her exam today.
I don't think she is interested in what I have to say. She seems to be in a hurry.

Figure 12-4 This client senses that his support worker is not listening to him.

Box 12-3 Communicating with an Angry Client

- Recognize that the person feels frustrated or frightened. Put yourself in the person's situation. How would you feel? How would you want to be treated?
- Treat the person with respect and dignity.
- Answer the person's questions clearly and thoroughly. Tell the person that your supervisor will answer questions that you cannot answer.
- Keep the person informed. Tell the person what you are going to do and when.
- Do not keep the person waiting for long periods. If you tell the person that you will do something for him or her, do it promptly.
- Stay calm and professional. Speak in a normal tone. Do not respond to a person's anger with your own anger. Try not to take the person's anger personally. Often the anger has more to do with the person's feelings than with you or the care you give.
- Do not argue with the person.
- Listen and use silence. The person may feel better after expressing angry feelings.
- Protect yourself from violent behaviours. Leave the person and call your supervisor if you think you are in danger (see Chapter 16).
- Report the person's behaviour to your supervisor. Discuss how you should deal with the person.

and drugs are likely to show anger. Some people are often angry or unhappy. Few things please them or make them happy. There could be many reasons for their behaviour. Do not judge an angry client. Provide the same high-quality, compassionate care that you provide for all your clients. Report angry behaviour to your supervisor.

Anger is communicated verbally and nonverbally. Verbal outbursts, shouting, raised voices, and rapid speech are common. An angry client may tell you what to do or may threaten you. Some people are silent when angry. Others are uncooperative and may refuse to answer questions. Nonverbal signs of anger include rapid movements, pacing, clenched fists, and a reddened face or neck. The angry person may glare at you or get close to you when speaking. Violent behaviours can occur.

Good communication is important to prevent and deal with anger. Follow the guidelines in Box 12-3 when communicating with an angry client.

Communicating Assertively

Assertiveness is a style of communication in which thoughts and feelings are expressed positively and directly without offence to others. You stand up for your rights while respecting the rights of others.

When you communicate assertively, you appear confident, calm, and composed. You speak gently, firmly, and positively. You do not hesitate or appear anxious. You are respectful.

Being assertive is different from being aggressive and from being passive. When you communicate aggressively, you appear upset, cold, or angry. You may sound threatening. Aggressive communication is usually not respectful.

When you communicate passively, you appear hesitant, apologetic, and timid. A passive person does not want to hurt or offend others. But passive behaviour can make others feel uncomfortable. Assertiveness rarely has this effect. People usually like direct, honest, and sincere communication.

Some people have trouble communicating assertively with people in authority. They feel intimidated. You will have regular contact with physicians, nurses, and other members of the health care team. You need to be confident and assertive when you communicate with them.

Box 12-4 describes three responses to a situation that requires assertiveness.

Box 12-4 Case Study: Communicating Assertively

Kara just graduated as a support worker. Her first job is at a long-term care facility, where she was hired to replace Debbie. Mr. Beruti is a 28-year-old resident. Both his arms were amputated. While Kara is shaving him, he shouts, "Be careful! You almost nicked me. You obviously don't know what you're doing. The nurse told me this is your first job. You're not nearly as good as Debbie. If you don't get better at this I'll report you."

Consider the following responses:

- "Report me if you like, Mr. Beruti. I wouldn't have been assigned to you if I were useless. You're just missing Debbie. I can assure you that I am just as qualified as she is. I won't tolerate your abuse." *(This is an aggressive and hostile response. It makes a judgment by assuming that Mr. Beruti misses Debbie. It shows no empathy or respect. It disregards his safety needs.)*
- "I'm so sorry, Mr. Beruti. I am so clumsy and rough. I'll try to do better." *(This is a passive response. It suggests that Kara lacks confidence. It also implies Kara doubts that she is able to provide safe and competent care.)*
- "I'm sorry, Mr. Beruti. It's hard when caregivers do things in different ways. I can assure you that your safety and comfort are important to me. Can you tell me how you like to be shaved?" *(This is a compassionate yet assertive response. It should reassure Mr. Beruti. It shows that Kara is confident in her ability to adapt her shaving method. It also shows that she is open to Mr. Beruti's preferences for care.)*

Explaining Procedures and Tasks

Part of your role as a support worker is to explain procedures and tasks to clients. Some procedures may be unfamiliar or frightening to them. Some, such as personal care activities, require strangers to touch private body parts. Clients feel safer and more secure if they understand what is going to happen before the procedure is performed. They should know why the procedure is done, who will do it, how it will be done, and what sensations or feelings they can expect. They should also know which parts of the procedure (if any) they will participate in and which parts you will do. For many procedures, you also need to find out your client's preferences before you begin.

You may help clients practise tasks they have been shown by health care professionals. For example, Mr. Krueger, 88, has osteoporosis. His physiotherapist has shown him how to do muscle-strengthening exercises. The physiotherapist has also shown you how to help him with the exercises. As part of Mr. Krueger's care plan, you work with him daily on these exercises.

You may be expected to teach clients simple tasks. For example, Mrs. Ali has hemiplegia (paralysis on one side of her body). She must learn a new method for getting dressed. You have been taught a method for dressing clients with hemiplegia. The care plan calls for you to teach this method to Mrs. Ali. You are to practise it with her until she is able to dress herself.

Whatever the situation, you must give clear, precise explanations and instructions that the client can understand. Organize your thoughts before you speak. Use simple, everyday language. Give your client the chance to discuss the task and to ask questions.

Most people learn tasks best when they are shown how to do them. The following four-step teaching method works for many people:

- Tell the client the steps in the task.
- Show the client how to do each step.
- Have the client try each step.
- Review the client's success with each step.

Follow the guidelines in Box 12-5. Break tasks into steps. Teach one step at a time. Observe your client and listen carefully to make sure he or she understands you. Recognize that people learn in different ways. Recognize as well that illness, disability, and fatigue can affect a person's ability to learn. You may have to explain a task several times and in different ways before the client understands. Even if the client understands, he or she may not be able to do it. You may have to demonstrate a task many times.

Box 12-5 Guidelines for Teaching Clients Tasks

- **Put the client at ease.** Relax and smile. Do not give the impression you are in a hurry. If the person senses you are tense or rushed, learning will be difficult.
- **Start with small steps.** Break the task into small steps. Focus the person's attention on one step at a time.
- **Start with easy steps.** Confidence increases with success. If possible, start with the steps the person is most likely to achieve.
- **Observe and listen.** People do not always tell you when they do not understand. Or they may say they understand when they actually do not. Watch body language and listen actively. Be alert for signs of fatigue.
- **Use positive statements.** Positive statements are easier to follow than negative statements. For example, saying "bend your arm" is more effective than saying "don't use a straight arm."
- **Let the client set the pace.** Be patient. Do not rush the person. Allow time for rest.
- **Provide support and offer encouragement.** Positive comments help the person feel successful. They can also encourage the person to continue trying. It is important to recognize what the person has achieved. Even small achievements deserve recognition and a positive comment.
- **Give time for *practise.*** Allow time for practising a task. Practise helps a person remember.

REVIEW

Circle the BEST answer.

1. During an exchange of information, a message is sent
   A. From a speaker to a receiver
   B. From a receiver to a speaker
   C. From a speaker to a speaker
   D. Without feedback

2. Which is *false?*
   A. Verbal communication involves the spoken word.
   B. Verbal communication is the truest reflection of a person's feelings.
   C. Messages can be sent by facial expressions, gestures, posture, body movements, appearance, and eye contact.
   D. Touch means different things to different people.

3. To communicate with your client, Mr. Long, you should
   A. Use medical words and phrases
   B. Change the subject when he is sharing fears and concerns
   C. Give your opinion when he is sharing fears and concerns
   D. Ask closed questions when you need specific information

4. When talking with Mr. Long, which of the following might mean you are *not* listening?
   A. You sit facing him.
   B. You have good eye contact with him.
   C. You cross your arms and look away.
   D. You paraphrase what he has said.

5. You and Ms. Jones are talking about her surgery. Which of the following is a closed question?
   A. "Do you feel better now?"
   B. "Tell me what your plans are for home."
   C. "What will you do when you fully recover?"
   D. "You said that you will be off work for a while."

6. Your client tells you she is not happy that she has to use a walker. Which of the following responses shows empathy?
   A. You tell her about the time you had to use crutches.
   B. You suggest methods that might help her use her walker more efficiently.
   C. You quickly try to change the subject to something happier.
   D. You listen to her and acknowledge her feelings.

7. Focusing is a useful communication tool when
   A. A person is rambling
   B. You want to make sure you understand the message
   C. You want the person to share thoughts and feelings
   D. You need information

8. Which statement will promote communication?
   A. "Don't worry."
   B. "Everything will be just fine."
   C. "This is a good facility."
   D. "Why are you crying?"

9. Which is *not* a barrier to communication?
   A. Interrupting
   B. Repeating what the person says
   C. Answering for the person
   D. Giving advice

10. A client is angry. Which of the following statements is *true*?
    A. The person probably has a disease that affects thinking and behaviour.
    B. Drug or alcohol abuse is likely.
    C. You should tell the person to calm down and that everything will be fine.
    D. Listening and the use of silence are important.

11. With assertive communication, which is *true*?
    A. You appear upset, cold, or angry.
    B. You appear confident, calm, and composed.
    C. You are usually not respectful.
    D. You appear hesitant, apologetic, and timid.

12. Which is *false?*
    A. It is best not to explain procedures to clients because doing so may upset them.
    B. Most people learn tasks best by being shown how to do them.
    C. Positive statements are easier to follow than negative statements.
    D. People learn in different ways.

Answers to these questions are on page 822.

CHAPTER

13

Body Structure and Function

OBJECTIVES

- Define the key terms listed in this chapter
- Identify the basic structures of the cell, and explain how cells divide
- Describe four types of tissue
- Identify the structures of each body system
- Describe the functions of each body system

KEY TERMS

artery A blood vessel that carries blood away from the heart

capillary A tiny blood vessel; food, oxygen, and other substances pass from the capillaries to the cells

cell The basic functional unit of body structure

digestion The process of physically and chemically breaking down food so that it can be absorbed for use by the cells

hemoglobin The substance in red blood cells that carries oxygen and gives blood its colour

hormone A chemical substance secreted by specialized glands into the bloodstream

immunity Protection against a certain disease or infection; the person will not get or be affected by the disease

menstruation The process in which the lining of the uterus breaks up and is discharged from the body through the vagina

metabolism The burning of food for heat and energy by the cells

organ Groups of tissues that work together to perform special functions

peristalsis Involuntary muscle contractions in the digestive system that move food through the alimentary canal

respiration The process of supplying the cells with oxygen and removing carbon dioxide from them

system Organs that work together to perform special functions

tissue A group of cells with similar functions

vein A blood vessel that carries blood back to the heart

NOTE: Students are responsible for only those terms mentioned in the text. Additional terms used in labelling figures throughout this chapter are for illustrative purposes only.

In your role as support worker, you will help clients meet their basic needs. Their bodies do not work at peak efficiency because of disability, illness, disease, or injury. You provide care to promote comfort, healing, and recovery. You need a basic understanding of the body's normal structure and function. This knowledge should result in safer and more efficient client care. See Chapter 15 for changes in body structure and function that occur with aging.

CELLS, TISSUES, AND ORGANS

The basic functional unit of body structure is the **cell.** Each cell has the same basic structure. However, the function, size, and shape of cells may be different. Cells are so small that a microscope is needed to see them. Cells need food, water, and oxygen to live and perform their functions.

The cell and its basic structures are shown in Figure 13-1 on page 128. The *cell membrane* is the outer covering that encloses the cell and helps it hold its shape. The *nucleus* is the control centre of the cell; it directs the cell's activities. The nucleus is in the centre of the cell. The *cytoplasm* surrounds the nucleus. Cytoplasm contains many smaller structures that perform cell functions. The *protoplasm,* which means "living substance," refers to all of the structures, substances, and water within the cell. Protoplasm is a semiliquid substance much like an egg white.

Chromosomes are threadlike structures within the nucleus. Each cell has 46 chromosomes. Chromosomes contain *genes.* Genes control the physical and chemical traits inherited by children from their parents. Inherited traits include height, eye colour, and skin colour.

Besides controlling cell activities, the nucleus is responsible for cell reproduction. Cells reproduce by dividing in half. Each half becomes a new cell. The process of cell division is called *mitosis.* Cell division is needed for growth and repair of body tissues. During mitosis, the 46 chromosomes arrange themselves in 23 pairs. As the cell divides, the 23 pairs of chromosomes are pulled in half. The two new cells are identical, and each contains 46 chromosomes (Figure 13-2 on page 128).

The cells are the body's building blocks. Groups of cells with similar functions combine to form **tissues.** The body has four basic types of tissue:

- *Epithelial tissue* covers internal and external body surfaces. Tissue that lines the nose, mouth, respiratory

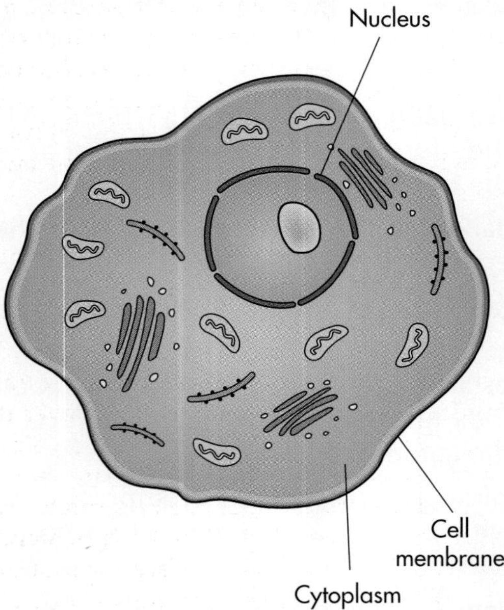

Figure 13-1 Parts of a cell.

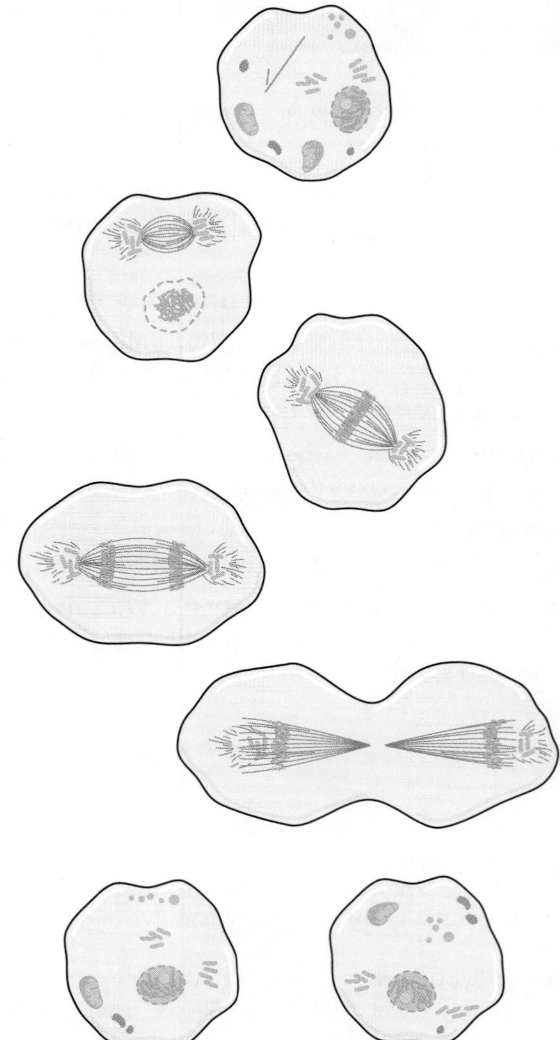

Figure 13-2 Cell division.

tract, stomach, and intestines is epithelial tissue. So are the skin, hair, nails, and glands.

- *Connective tissue* anchors, connects, and supports other body tissues. Connective tissue is found in every part of the body. *Tendons* (tissue that attaches muscles to bones), *ligaments* (tissue that connects bones and supports joints), and *cartilage* (tissue that cushions joints) are examples of connective tissue.
- *Muscle tissue* allows the body to move by stretching and contracting. There are three types of muscle tissue (see page 129).
- *Nerve tissue* relays information to and from the brain and throughout the body.

Organs are groups of tissue that work together to perform special functions. An organ performs one or more functions. Examples of organs are the heart, brain, liver, lungs, and kidneys. **Systems** are formed by organs that work together to perform special functions (Figure 13-3).

THE INTEGUMENTARY SYSTEM

The *integumentary system* is the skin and its appendages—hair, nails, and sweat and oil glands. (A *gland* is a group of cells that produces and secretes a substance. Glands in the skin produce and secrete sweat and oil.)

The integumentary system is the largest system of the body. *Integument* means covering. The skin is the body's natural covering. Skin is made up of epithelial, connective, and nerve tissue. There are two skin layers: the epidermis and the dermis (Figure 13-4). The *epidermis* is the outer layer; it contains living and dead cells. The dead cells were once deeper in the epidermis and were pushed upward as other cells divided. Dead cells constantly flake off and are replaced by living cells. Living cells also die and flake off. Living cells of the epidermis contain *pigment*. Pigment gives skin its colour. The epidermis has no blood vessels and few nerve endings. The *dermis* is the inner layer of the skin and is made up of connective tissue. Blood vessels, nerves, sweat and oil glands, and hair roots are found in the dermis.

The entire body, except the palms of the hands and soles of the feet, is covered with hair. Hair in the nose, eyes, and ears protects these organs from dust, insects, and other foreign objects. Nails protect the tips of fingers and toes. Nails help fingers pick up and handle small objects. Sweat glands help the body regulate

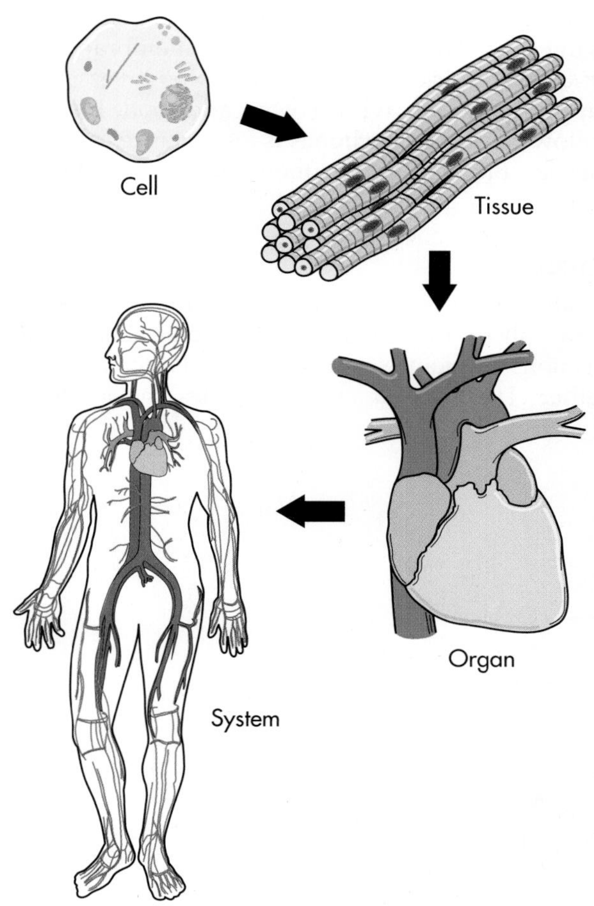

Figure 13-3 Organization of the body.

temperature. Sweat consists of water, salt, and a small amount of wastes. Sweat is secreted through pores in the skin. The body is cooled as sweat evaporates. Oil glands lie near hair shafts. They secrete an oily substance into the space near the hair shaft. Oil travels to the skin's surface, helping to keep the hair and skin soft and shiny.

The skin has many important functions. It is the protective covering of the body. It prevents bacteria and other substances from entering the body. The skin also prevents excessive amounts of water from leaving the body and protects organs from injury. Nerve endings in the skin sense both pleasant and unpleasant stimulation. There are nerve endings over the entire body. The body is protected because cold, pain, touch, and pressure are sensed. The skin helps regulate body temperature. Blood vessels dilate (widen) when the temperature outside the body is high. More blood is brought to the body surface for cooling during evaporation. When blood vessels constrict (narrow), the body retains heat because less blood reaches the skin.

The Musculoskeletal System

The musculoskeletal system provides the framework for the body and allows the body to move. This system also protects and gives the body shape. Besides bones and muscles, the system has ligaments, tendons, and cartilage.

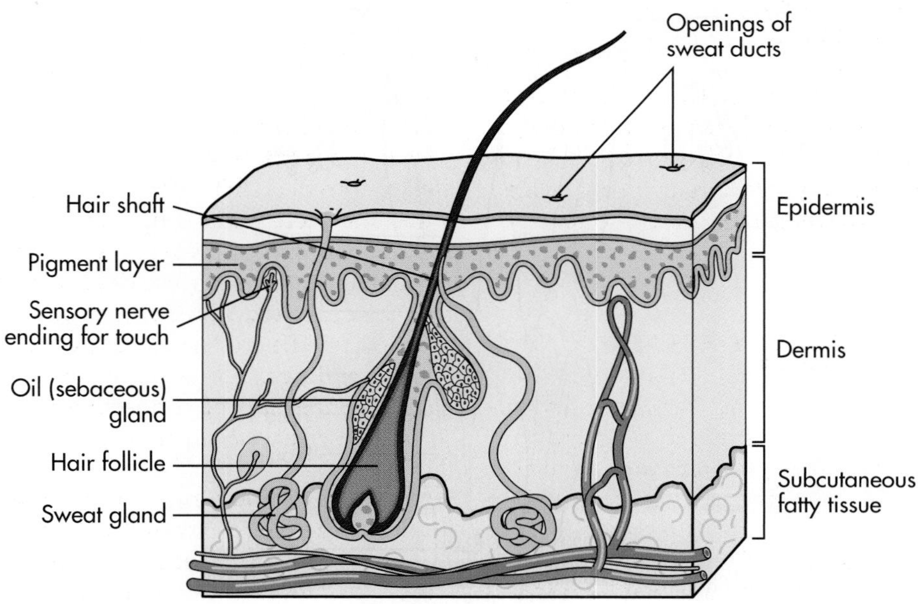

Figure 13-4 Layers of the skin.

Bones

The human body has 206 bones (Figure 13-5). There are four types of bones:

- *Long bones* bear the weight of the body. Leg bones are long bones.
- *Short bones* allow skill and ease in movement. Bones in the wrists, fingers, ankles, and toes are short bones.
- *Flat bones* protect the organs. Such bones include the ribs, skull, pelvic bones, and shoulder blades.
- *Irregular bones* are the vertebrae in the spinal column. They allow various degrees of movement and flexibility.

Bones are hard, rigid structures that are made up of living cells. They are covered by a membrane called *periosteum*. Periosteum contains blood vessels that supply bone cells with oxygen and food. Inside the hollow centres of the bones is a substance called *bone marrow*. Blood cells are manufactured in the bone marrow.

Joints

A *joint* is the point at which two or more bones meet. Joints allow movement (see Chapter 22). *Cartilage* cushions the joint so that bone ends do not rub together. The *synovial membrane* lines the joints. The

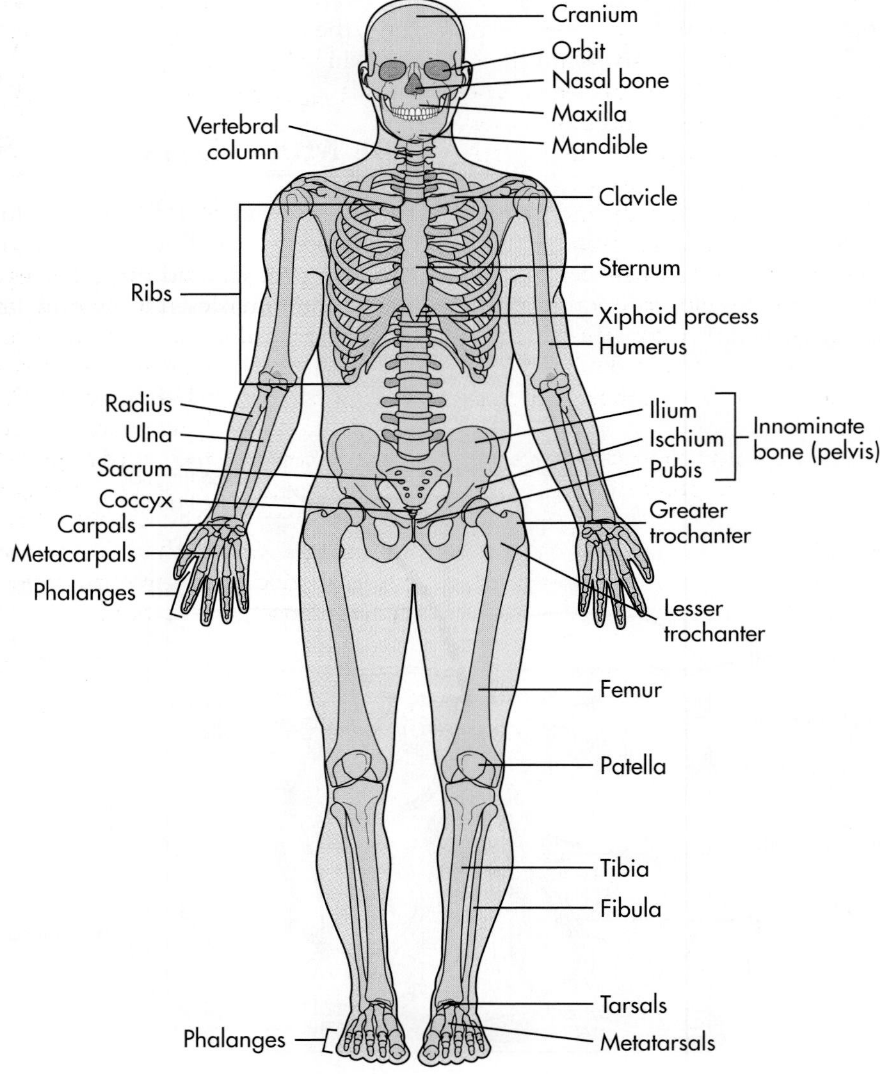

Figure 13-5 Bones of the body.

membrane secretes *synovial fluid.* Synovial fluid acts as a lubricant so the joint can move smoothly. Bones are held together at the joint by strong bands of connective tissue called *ligaments.*

There are three main types of joints (Figure 13-6):

- *Ball-and-socket joint*—allows movement in all directions. It is made up of the rounded end of one bone and the hollow end of another bone. The rounded end of one fits into the hollow end of the other. The joints of the hips and shoulders are ball-and-socket joints.
- *Hinge joint*—allows movement in one direction. The elbow is a hinge joint.
- *Pivot joint*—allows turning from side to side. The skull is connected to the spine by a pivot joint.

Muscles

There are more than 500 muscles in the human body (Figures 13-7 and 13-8 on pages 132 and 133). Some are voluntary, and others are involuntary.

Voluntary muscles can be consciously controlled. Muscles attached to bones *(skeletal muscles)* are voluntary. Arm muscles do not work unless you move your arm; likewise for leg muscles. Skeletal muscles are *striated*; that is, they look striped or streaked.

Involuntary muscles work automatically and cannot be consciously controlled. Involuntary muscles control the action of the stomach, intestines, blood vessels, and other body organs. Involuntary muscles are also called *smooth muscles.* They look smooth—not streaked or striped. *Cardiac muscle* is in the heart. Although it is an involuntary muscle, it appears striated like skeletal muscle.

Muscles can do only one thing: contract. However, muscles perform three important body functions:

- Movement of body parts
- Maintenance of posture
- Production of body heat

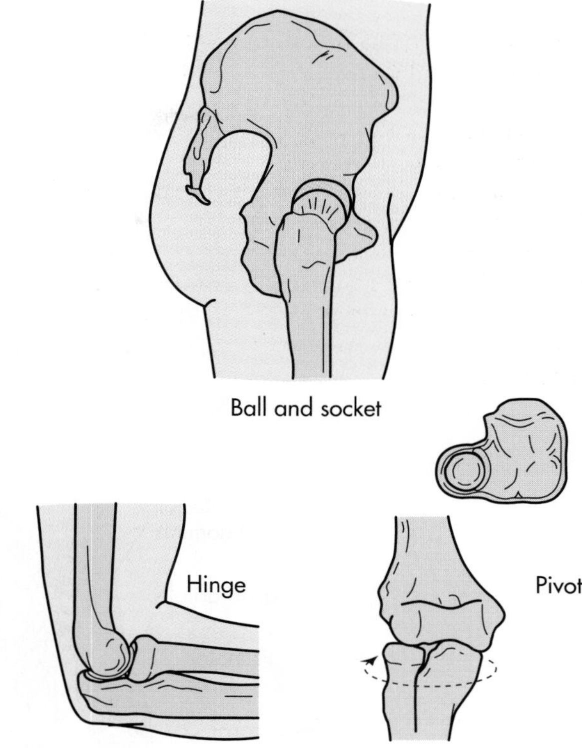

Figure 13-6 Types of joints.

Strong, tough connective tissues called *tendons* connect muscles to bones. When muscles contract (shorten), tendons at each end of the muscle cause the bone to move. The body has many tendons; the Achilles tendon is shown in Figure 13-8 on page 133. Some muscles constantly contract to maintain the body's posture. When muscles contract, they burn food for energy, resulting in the production of heat. The greater the muscular activity, the greater the amount of heat produced in the body. Shivering is a way the body produces heat when exposed to cold. The shivering sensation is from rapid, general muscle contractions.

(text continues on page 134)

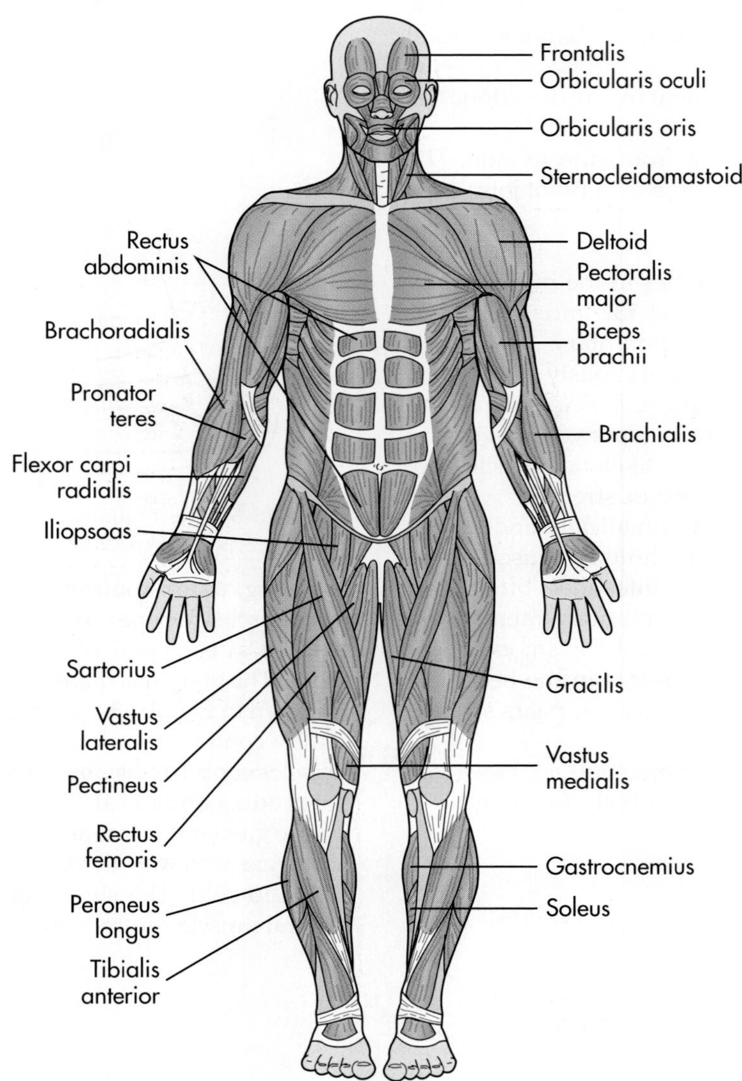

Figure 13-7 Anterior (front) view of the muscles of the body.

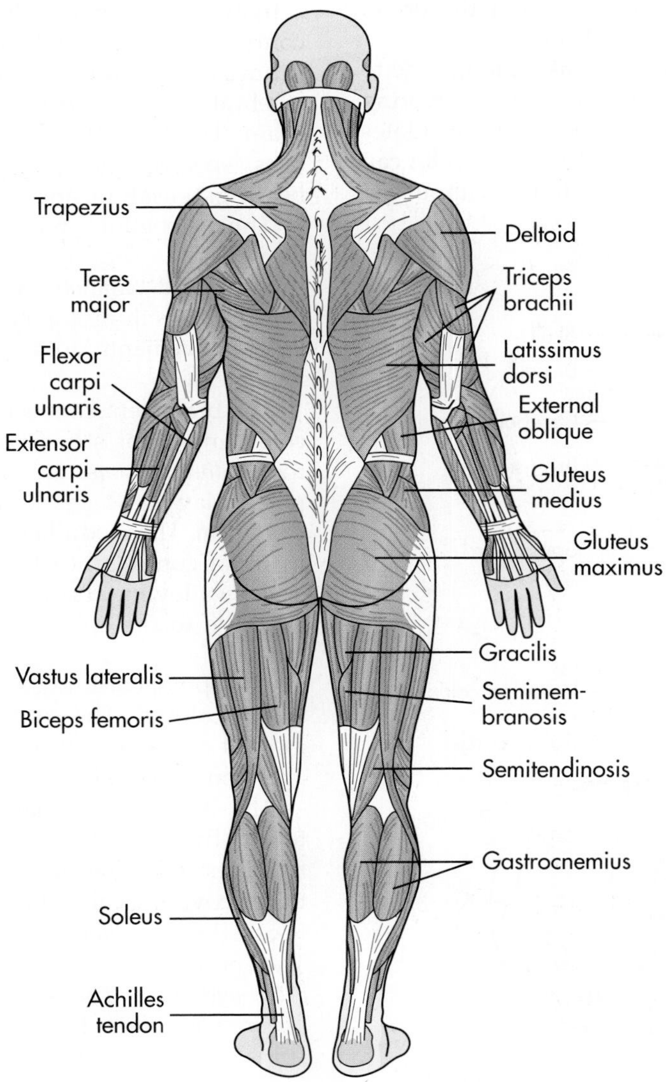

Figure 13-8 Posterior (back) view of the muscles of the body.

THE NERVOUS SYSTEM

The nervous system controls, directs, and coordinates body functions. The two main divisions of the nervous system are the *central nervous system* (CNS) and the *peripheral nervous system* (PNS). The central nervous system consists of the *brain* and *spinal cord* (Figure 13-9). The peripheral nervous system involves the *nerves* throughout the body (Figure 13-10). Nerves carry messages or impulses to and from the brain. Nerves are connected to the spinal cord.

Nerves are easily damaged and take a long time to heal. Some nerve fibres have a protective covering called a *myelin sheath.* The myelin sheath also insulates the nerve fibre. Nerve fibres covered with myelin can conduct impulses faster than those fibres without the protective covering.

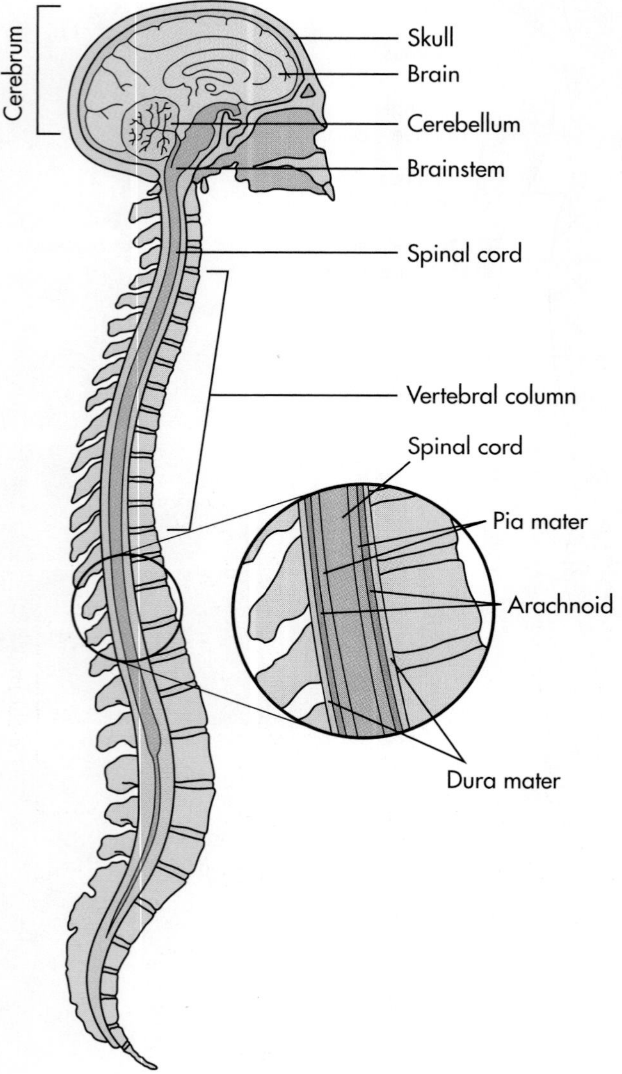

Figure 13-9 Central nervous system.

THE CENTRAL NERVOUS SYSTEM

The central nervous system consists of the brain and spinal cord. The brain is contained in and protected by the skull. The three main parts of the brain are the *cerebrum,* the *cerebellum,* and the *brainstem* (see Figure 13-9).

The cerebrum is the largest part of the brain. It is the centre of thought and intelligence. The cerebrum is divided into two halves called the right and left *hemispheres.* The right hemisphere controls movement and activities on the body's left side. The left hemisphere controls the body's right side. The outside of the cerebrum is called the *cerebral cortex* (Figure 13-11). The cerebral cortex controls the highest functions of the brain. These include reasoning, memory, consciousness, speech, voluntary muscle movement, vision, hearing, sensation, and other activities.

The cerebellum regulates and coordinates body movements. The smooth movements of voluntary muscles and balance are possible because of control by the cerebellum. Injury to the cerebellum results in jerky movements, loss of coordination, and muscle weakness.

The brainstem connects the cerebrum to the spinal cord. Important structures within the brainstem are the *midbrain, pons,* and *medulla.* The midbrain and pons relay messages between the medulla and the cerebrum. The medulla is directly below the pons. The medulla controls heart rate, breathing, blood vessel size, swallowing, coughing, and vomiting. The brain connects to the spinal cord at the lower end of the medulla.

The spinal cord lies within and is protected by the spinal column. The cord is about 45 cm (18 inches) long. It contains pathways that conduct messages to and from the brain.

The brain and spinal cord are covered and protected by three layers of connective tissue called *meninges.* The outer layer lies next to the skull. It is a tough covering called the *dura mater.* The middle layer is called the *arachnoid.* The inner layer is the *pia mater.* The space between the middle and inner layers is the *arachnoid space.* The space is filled with fluid called *cerebrospinal fluid.* It circulates around the brain and spinal cord. Cerebrospinal fluid protects the central nervous system. It cushions shocks that could easily injure structures of the brain and spinal cord.

THE PERIPHERAL NERVOUS SYSTEM

The peripheral nervous system has 12 pairs of *cranial nerves* and 31 pairs of *spinal nerves.* Cranial nerves conduct impulses between the brain and the head, neck, chest, and abdomen. They conduct impulses for smell, vision, hearing, pain, touch, temperature, pressure, and voluntary and involuntary muscle control. Spinal nerves carry impulses from the skin, extremities (a limb of the

(text continues on page 136)

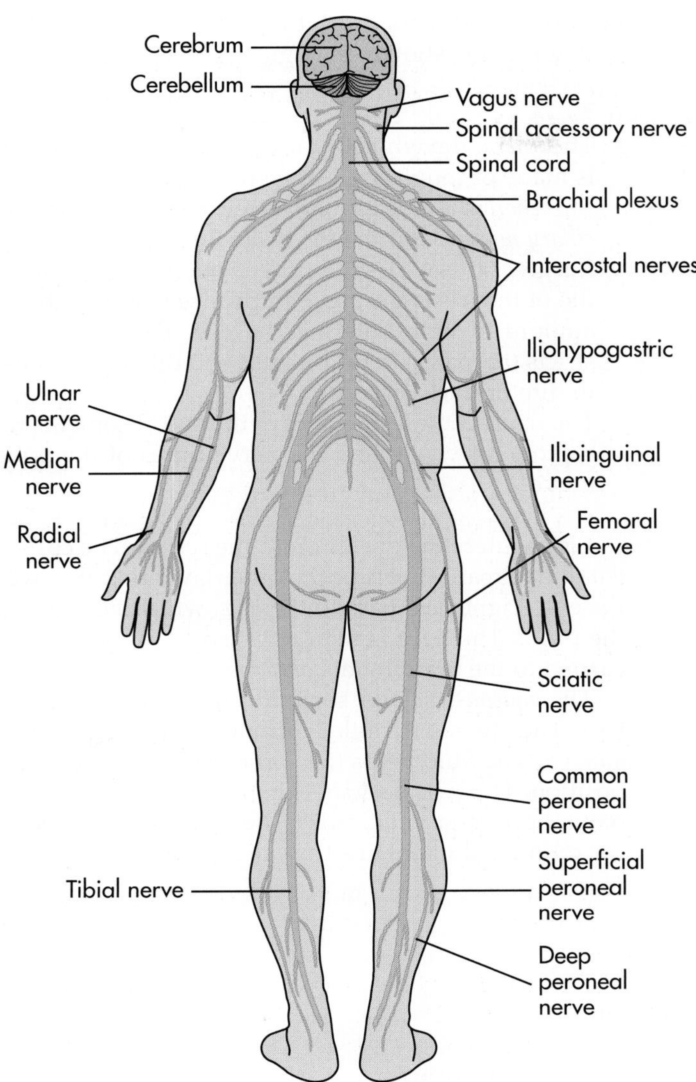

Figure 13-10 Peripheral nervous system.

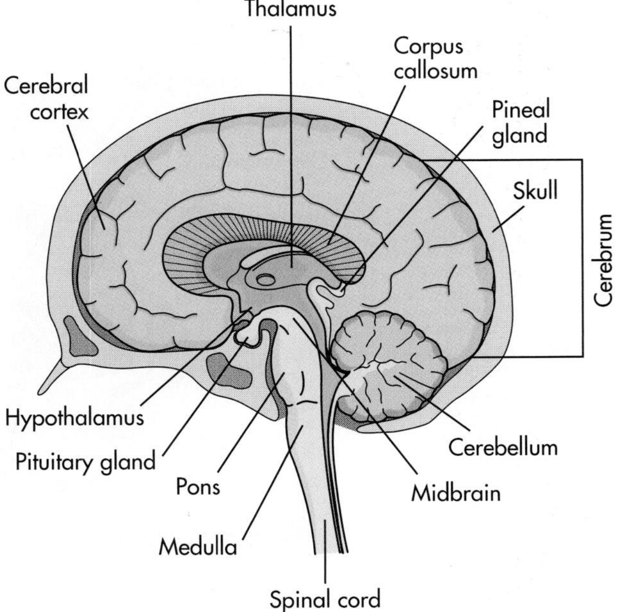

Figure 13-11 The brain.

body, especially a hand or foot), and the internal body structures not supplied by cranial nerves.

Peripheral nerves with special functions form the *autonomic nervous system.* This system controls involuntary muscles and certain body functions. The functions include the heartbeat, blood pressure, intestinal contractions, and glandular secretions. These functions occur automatically.

The autonomic nervous system is divided into the *sympathetic nervous system* and the *parasympathetic nervous system.* These divisions balance each other. The sympathetic nervous system tends to speed up functions. The parasympathetic nervous system slows them down. When you are angry, frightened, excited, or when you are exercising, the sympathetic nervous system is stimulated. The parasympathetic system is activated when you relax or when the sympathetic system is under stimulation for too long.

The Sense Organs

The five senses are sight, hearing, taste, smell, and touch. Receptors for taste are in the tongue and are called *taste buds.* Receptors for smell are in the nose. Touch receptors are found in the dermis, especially in the toes and fingertips.

The Eye. Receptors for vision are in the eyes. The eye is easily injured. Bones of the skull, eyelids and eyelashes, and tears protect the eyes from injury. Eye structures are shown in Figure 13-12. The eye has three layers:

- The *sclera,* the white of the eye, is the outer layer. It is made of tough connective tissue.
- The *choroid* is the second layer. Blood vessels, the *ciliary muscle,* and the *iris* make up the choroid. The iris gives the eye its colour. The opening in the middle of the iris is the *pupil.* Pupil size varies with the amount of light entering the eye. The pupil constricts (narrows) in bright light and dilates (widens) in dim or dark places.
- The *retina* is the inner layer of the eye. It contains receptors for vision and the nerve fibres of the optic nerve.

Light enters the eye through the *cornea.* The cornea is the transparent part of the outer layer that lies over the eye. Light rays pass to the *lens,* which lies behind the pupil. The light is then reflected to the retina and carried to the brain by the *optic nerve.*

The *aqueous chamber* separates the cornea from the lens. The chamber is filled with a fluid called *aqueous humour.* The fluid helps the cornea keep its shape and position. The *vitreous body* is behind the lens. The vitreous body is a gelatin-like substance that supports the retina and maintains the eye's shape.

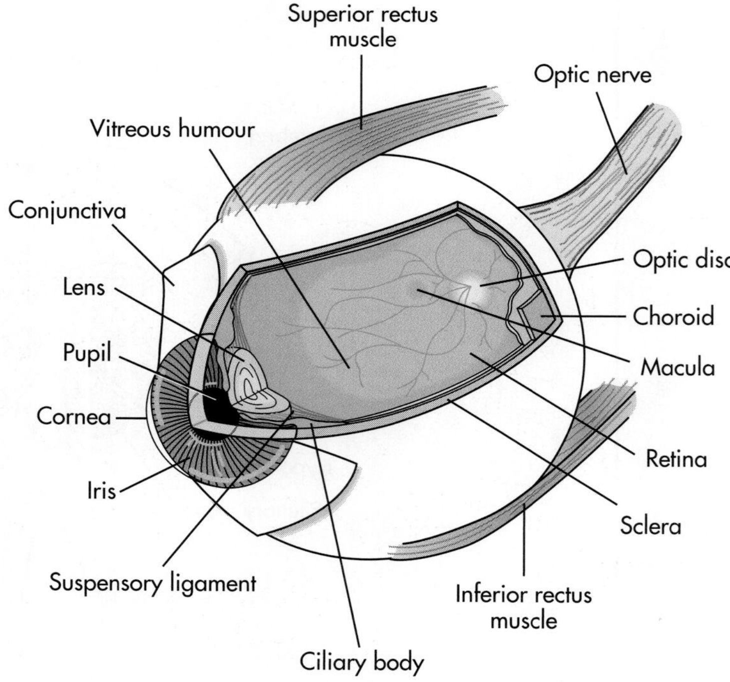

Figure 13-12 The eye.

The Ear. The ear is a sense organ that functions in hearing and balance. It is divided into the *external ear, middle ear,* and *inner ear.* Ear structures are shown in Figure 13-13.

The external ear (outer part) is called the *pinna* or *auricle.* Sound waves are guided through the external ear into the *auditory canal.* Glands in the auditory canal secrete a waxy substance called *cerumen.* The auditory canal extends about 2.5 cm (1 inch) to the *eardrum.* The eardrum *(tympanic membrane)* separates the external ear and middle ear.

The middle ear is a small space that contains the *eustachian tube* and three small bones called *ossicles.* The eustachian tube connects the middle ear and the throat. Air enters the eustachian tube so that there is equal pressure on both sides of the eardrum. The ossicles amplify sound received from the eardrum and transmit the sound to the inner ear. The three ossicles are:

- The *malleus,* which looks like a hammer
- The *incus,* which resembles an anvil
- The *stapes,* which is shaped like a stirrup

The inner ear consists of the *semicircular canals* and the *cochlea.* The cochlea, which looks like a snail shell, contains fluid. The fluid carries sound waves received from the middle ear to the *auditory nerve.* The auditory nerve then carries the message to the brain.

The three semicircular canals are involved with balance. They sense the head's position and changes in position and send messages to the brain.

THE CIRCULATORY SYSTEM

The circulatory system is made up of the blood, heart, and blood vessels. The heart pumps blood through the blood vessels. The circulatory system has many important functions.

- Blood carries food, oxygen, and other substances to the cells.
- Blood removes waste products from the cells.
- Blood and blood vessels help regulate body temperature. Heat from muscle activity is carried by the blood to other body parts. Blood vessels in the skin dilate if the body needs to be cooled. They constrict if heat needs to be kept in the body.
- The circulatory system also produces and carries cells that defend the body from disease-causing microorganisms.

THE BLOOD

The blood consists of blood cells and a liquid called *plasma.* Plasma is mostly water. It carries blood cells to other body cells. Plasma also carries other substances needed by cells for proper functioning. Food (proteins, fats, and carbohydrates), hormones, chemicals, and waste products are among the many substances carried in the plasma.

Red blood cells are called *erythrocytes.* They give the blood its red colour because of a substance in the cell called **hemoglobin**. As red blood cells circulate through the lungs, hemoglobin picks up oxygen. The

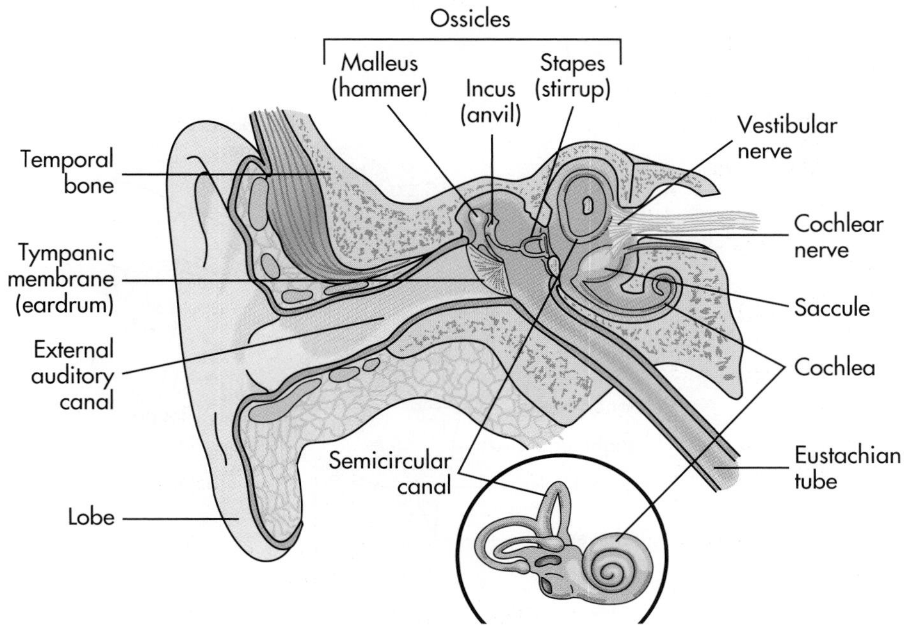

Figure 13-13 The ear.

hemoglobin carries oxygen to the cells. When the blood is bright red, hemoglobin in the red blood cells is saturated (filled) with oxygen. As blood circulates through the body, oxygen is given to the cells. The cells release carbon dioxide (a waste product), which is picked up by the hemoglobin. Red blood cells saturated with carbon dioxide make the blood look dark red.

There are about 25 trillion (25 000 000 000 000) red blood cells in the body. About 4.5 to 5 million cells are in a cubic millimetre of blood (the size of a tiny drop). These cells live for 3 or 4 months. They are destroyed by the liver and spleen as they wear out. Bone marrow produces new red blood cells. About 1 million new red blood cells are produced every second.

White blood cells, called *leukocytes,* are colourless. They protect the body against infection. There are 5000 to 10 000 white blood cells in a cubic millimetre of blood. At the first sign of infection, white blood cells rush to the site of the infection and begin to multiply rapidly. The number of white blood cells increases when there is an infection in the body. White blood cells are also produced by the bone marrow. They live about 9 days.

Platelets (thrombocytes) are necessary for the clotting of blood. They are also produced by the bone marrow. There are about 200 000 to 400 000 platelets in a cubic millimetre of blood. A platelet lives about 4 days.

The Heart

The heart is a muscle. It pumps blood through the blood vessels to the tissues and cells. The heart lies in the middle to lower part of the chest cavity toward the left side (Figure 13-14). The heart is hollow and has three layers (Figure 13-15):

- The *pericardium* is the outer layer. It is a thin sac covering the heart.
- The *myocardium* is the second layer. This layer is the thick, muscular portion of the heart.
- The *endocardium* is the inner layer. The endocardium is the membrane lining the inner surface of the heart.

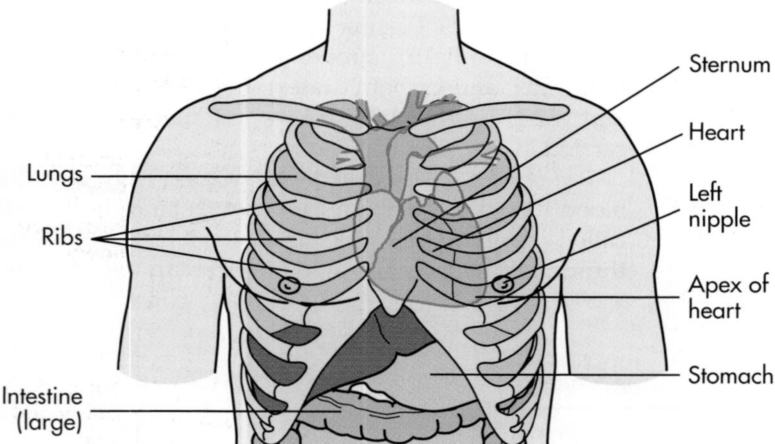

Figure 13-14 Location of the heart in the chest cavity.

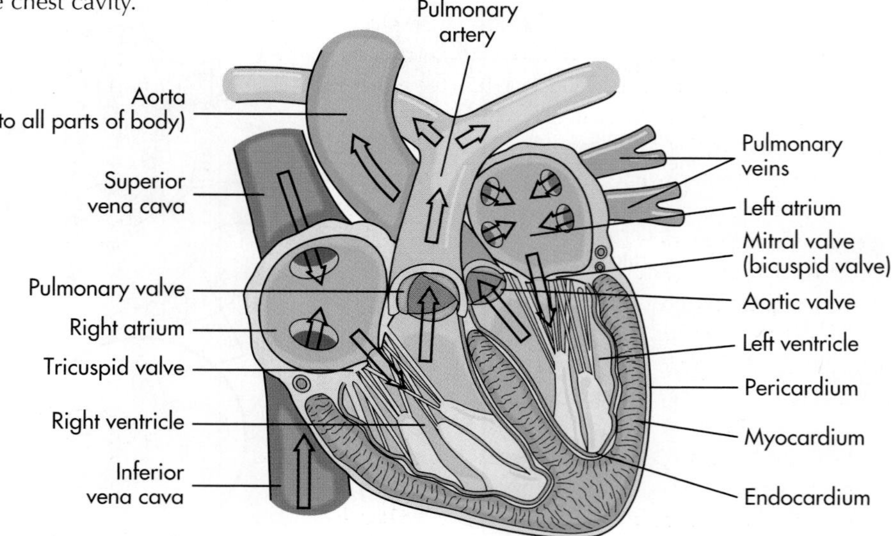

Figure 13-15 Structures of the heart.

The heart has four chambers (see Figure 13-15). Upper chambers receive blood and are called the *atria.* The *right atrium* receives blood from body tissues. The *left atrium* receives blood from the lungs. Lower chambers are called *ventricles.* Ventricles pump blood. The *right ventricle* pumps blood to the lungs for oxygen. The *left ventricle* pumps blood to all parts of the body.

Valves are located between the atria and ventricles. The valves allow blood to flow in one direction. They prevent blood from flowing back into the atria from the ventricles. The *tricuspid valve* is between the right atrium and right ventricle. The *mitral valve (bicuspid valve)* is between the left atrium and left ventricle.

There are two phases of heart action. During *diastole,* the resting phase, heart chambers fill with blood. During *systole,* the working phase, the heart contracts. Blood is pumped through the blood vessels when the heart contracts.

The Blood Vessels

Blood flows to body tissues and cells through the blood vessels. There are three groups of blood vessels: arteries, capillaries, and veins. **Arteries** carry blood away from the heart. Arterial blood is rich in oxygen. The *aorta* is the largest artery. The aorta receives blood directly from the left ventricle. The aorta branches into other arteries that carry blood to all parts of the body (Figure 13-16). These arteries branch into smaller parts within the tissues. The smallest branch of an artery is an *arteriole.*

Arterioles connect with blood vessels called **capillaries.** Capillaries are tiny vessels. Food, oxygen, and other substances pass from capillaries into the cells. Waste products, including carbon dioxide, are picked up from cells by the capillaries. Waste products are carried back to the heart by the veins.

Veins return blood to the heart. They are connected to the capillaries by *venules.* Venules are small veins. Venules begin branching together to form veins. The many branches of veins also branch together as they near the heart to form two main veins (see Figure 13-16). The two main veins are the *inferior vena cava* and the *superior vena cava.* Both empty into the right atrium. The inferior vena cava carries blood from the legs and trunk. The superior vena cava carries blood from the head and arms. Venous blood is dark red because it contains little oxygen and a lot of carbon dioxide.

Blood flow through the circulatory system is diagrammed in Figure 13-15 and can be summarized as follows:

- Venous blood, poor in oxygen, empties into the right atrium.
- Blood flows through the tricuspid valve into the right ventricle.
- The right ventricle pumps blood into the lungs to pick up oxygen.
- Oxygen-rich blood from the lungs enters the left atrium.
- Blood from the left atrium passes through the mitral valve into the left ventricle.
- The left ventricle pumps the blood to the aorta, which branches off to form other arteries.
- The arterial blood is carried to the tissues by arterioles and to the cells by capillaries.
- The cells and capillaries exchange oxygen and nutrients for carbon dioxide and waste products.
- Capillaries connect with venules.
- Venules carry blood that contains carbon dioxide and waste products.
- The venules form veins.
- Veins return blood to the heart, into the right atrium.

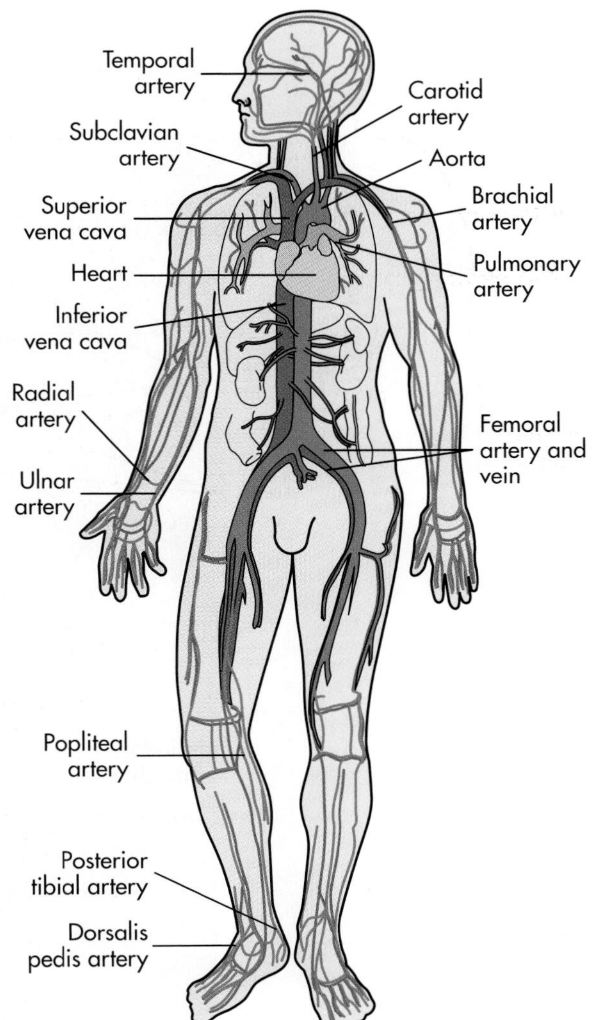

Figure 13-16 Some of the major arteries and veins in the body.

The Respiratory System

Oxygen is needed for survival. Every cell needs oxygen. Air contains about 21% oxygen—enough to meet body needs under normal conditions. The respiratory system brings oxygen into the lungs and eliminates carbon dioxide. The process of supplying the cells with oxygen and removing carbon dioxide from them is called **respiration.** Respiration involves *inhalation* (breathing in) and *exhalation* (breathing out). The terms *inspiration* (breathing in) and *expiration* (breathing out) are also used. The respiratory system is shown in Figure 13-17.

Air enters the body through the *nose.* The air then passes into the *pharynx* (throat), a tube-shaped passageway for both air and food. Air passes from the pharynx into the *larynx* (the voice box). A piece of cartilage called the *epiglottis* acts like a lid over the larynx. The epiglottis prevents food from entering the airway during swallowing. During inhalation the epiglottis lifts up to let air pass over the larynx. Air passes from the larynx into the *trachea* (the windpipe).

The trachea divides at its lower end into the *right bronchus* and *left bronchus.* Each bronchus enters a lung. Upon entering the lungs, the bronchi further divide several times into smaller branches called *bronchioles.* Eventually the bronchioles subdivide and end in tiny one-celled air sacs called *alveoli.*

Alveoli look like small clusters of grapes. They are supplied by capillaries. Oxygen and carbon dioxide are exchanged between the alveoli and capillaries. Blood in the capillaries picks up oxygen from the alveoli. Then the blood is returned to the left side of the heart and pumped to the rest of the body. Alveoli pick up carbon dioxide from the capillaries for exhalation.

The lungs are spongy tissues filled with alveoli, blood vessels, and nerves. Each lung is divided into lobes. The right lung has three lobes; the left lung has

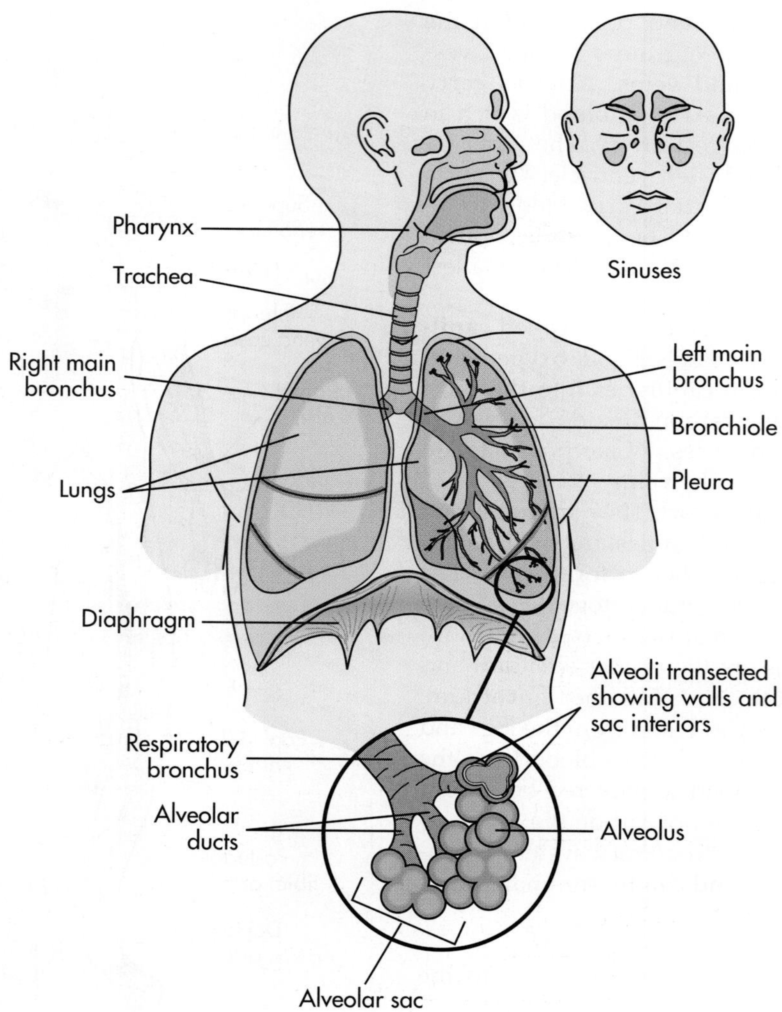

Figure 13-17 Respiratory system.

two. The lungs are separated from the abdominal cavity by a muscle called the *diaphragm.*

Each lung is covered by a two-layered sac called the *pleura.* One layer is attached to the lung and the other to the chest wall. The pleura secretes a very thin fluid that fills the space between the layers. The fluid prevents the layers from rubbing together during inhalation and exhalation. A bony framework consisting of the ribs, sternum, and vertebrae protects the lungs.

The Digestive System

The digestive system breaks down food physically and chemically so it can be absorbed for use by the cells. This process is called **digestion**. The digestive system is also called the *gastrointestinal system (GI system).* The system also eliminates solid wastes from the body.

The digestive system consists of the *alimentary canal (GI tract)* and the accessory organs of digestion (Figure 13-18). The alimentary canal is a long tube extending from the mouth to the anus. Its major parts are the mouth, pharynx, esophagus, stomach, small intestine, and large intestine. The accessory organs of digestion are the teeth, tongue, salivary glands, liver, gallbladder, and pancreas.

Digestion begins in the *mouth.* The mouth is also called the *oral cavity.* The oral cavity receives food and prepares it for digestion. Using chewing motions, the *teeth* cut, chop, and grind food into smaller particles for digestion and swallowing. The *tongue* aids in chewing and swallowing. *Taste buds* on the tongue's surface contain nerve endings. Taste buds allow sweet, sour, bitter, and salty tastes to be sensed. *Salivary glands* in the mouth secrete *saliva.* Saliva moistens food particles for easier swallowing and begins to digest food. During swallowing, the tongue pushes food into the pharynx.

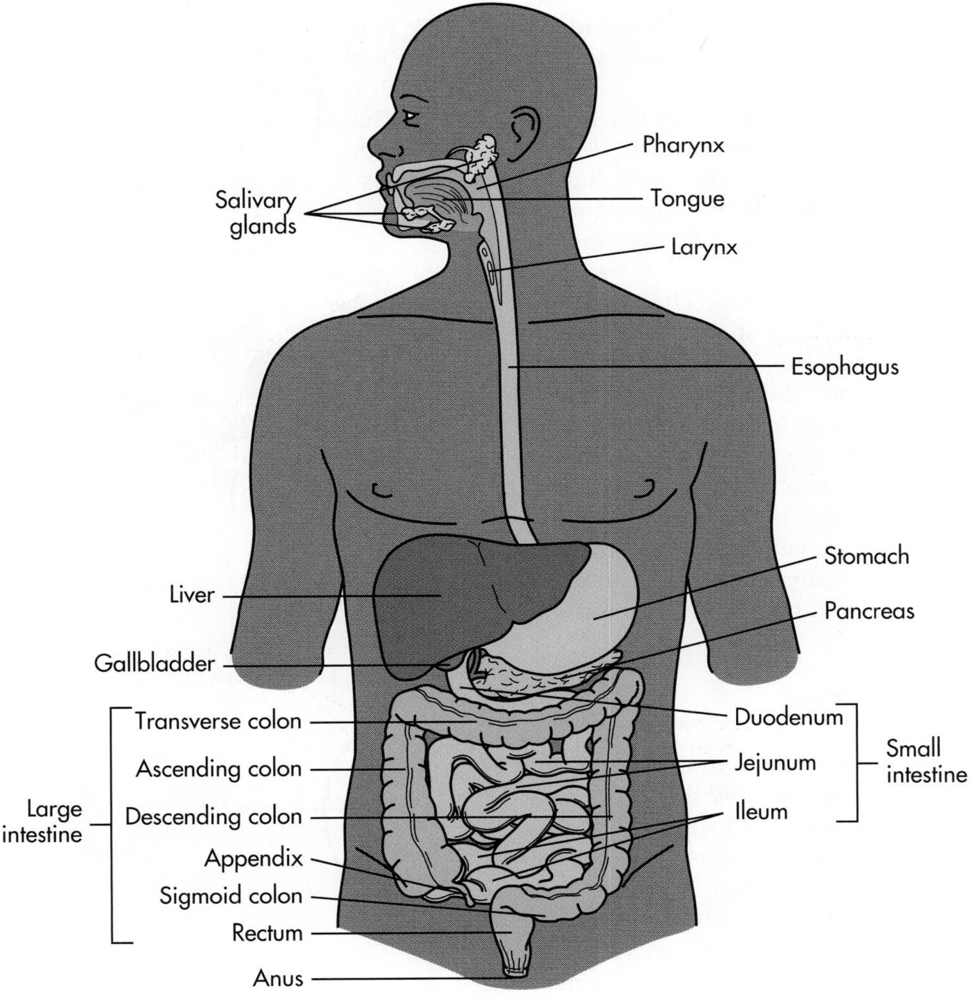

Figure 13-18 Digestive system.

The *pharynx* (throat) is a muscular tube. The act of swallowing is continued as the pharynx contracts. Contraction of the pharynx pushes food into the *esophagus.* The esophagus is a muscular tube about 25 cm (10 inches) long. It extends from the pharynx to the stomach. Involuntary muscle contractions called **peristalsis** move food down the esophagus into the stomach.

The *stomach* is a muscular, pouchlike sac in the upper left portion of the abdominal cavity. Strong stomach muscles stir and churn food to break it up into even smaller particles. The stomach is lined with a mucous membrane containing glands that secrete *gastric juices.* Food is mixed and churned with the gastric juices to form a semiliquid substance called *chyme.* Through peristalsis, the chyme is pushed from the stomach into the small intestine.

The *small intestine* is about 6 metres (20 feet) long and has three parts. The first part is the *duodenum.* In the duodenum, more digestive juices are added to the chyme. One is called *bile.* Bile is a greenish liquid produced by the *liver* and stored in the *gallbladder.* Juices from the *pancreas* and small intestine are also added to the chyme. The digestive juices chemically break down food so that it can be absorbed.

Peristalsis moves the chyme through the two remaining portions of the small intestine: the *jejunum* and the *ileum.* Tiny projections called *villi* line the small intestine. Villi absorb the digested food into the capillaries. Most of the absorption of food takes place in the jejunum and ileum.

Some chyme remains undigested. The undigested chyme passes from the small intestine into the *large intestine (large bowel* or *colon).* The colon absorbs most of the water from the chyme. The remaining semisolid material is called *feces.* Feces consist of a small amount of water, solid wastes, and some mucus and microorganisms. These are the waste products of digestion. Feces pass through the colon into the *rectum* by peristalsis. *Defecation* (bowel movement) is the process of excreting feces from the rectum through the anus. The term *stool* refers to feces that have been excreted.

The Urinary System

Wastes are removed from the body through the respiratory system, the digestive system, and the skin. The digestive system rids the body of solid wastes. The lungs rid the body of carbon dioxide. Water and other substances are contained in sweat. There are other waste products in the blood as a result of body cells burning food for energy. The functions of the urinary system are to remove waste products from the blood and to maintain water balance within the body. The structures of the urinary system are shown in Figure 13-19.

The *kidneys* are two bean-shaped organs in the upper abdomen. They lie against the muscles of the back on each side of the spine. They are protected by the lower edge of the rib cage. The kidneys act as a filtration system for the blood. They cleanse the waste products and toxins (poisons) from the blood.

Each kidney has about a million tiny *nephrons.* The nephron is the basic working unit of the kidney. Nephrons separate nutrients and minerals in the blood (water, sodium, amino acids, glucose) from the toxins and waste products. Most of the water and other neccessary substances are reabsorbed by the blood and recirculated in the body. The toxins and waste products stay in the kidney and form *urine.*

The urine is transported from the kidneys to the *bladder* through the *ureters.* The two ureters are narrow tubes, each about 25 to 30 cm (10 to 12 inches) long. They run from the renal pelvis of the kidneys to the bladder. The bladder is a hollow, muscular sac situated toward the front in the lower part of the abdominal cavity.

Urine is stored in the bladder until the desire to urinate is felt. The need to urinate usually occurs when there is about 250 mL (half a pint) of urine in the bladder. Urine passes from the bladder through the *urethra.* The opening at the end of the urethra is the *meatus.* Urine passes from the body through the meatus. Urine is a clear, yellowish fluid. The amount of urine

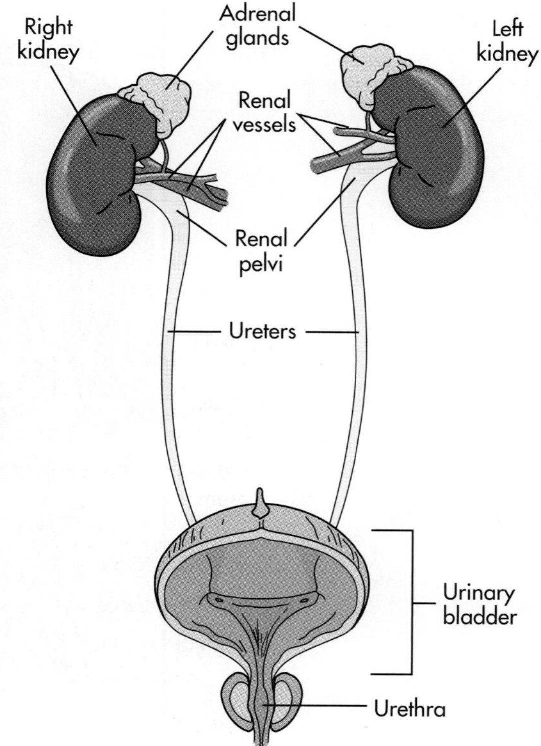

Figure 13-19 Urinary system.

eliminated over a 24-hour period should be close to the amount of fluid consumed.

THE REPRODUCTIVE SYSTEM

Human reproduction results from the union of a female sex cell and a male sex cell. Structures of the male reproductive system and female reproductive system are different. The differences allow for the process of reproduction.

THE MALE REPRODUCTIVE SYSTEM

The structures of the male reproductive system are shown in Figure 13-20. The *testes (testicles)* are the male sex glands. Sex glands are also called *gonads.* The two testes are oval or almond-shaped glands. Male sex cells are produced in the testes. Male sex cells are called *sperm* cells. *Testosterone,* the male hormone, is also produced in the testes. This hormone is needed for the functioning of the reproductive organs and for the development of the male's secondary sex characteristics (see Chapter 14). The testes are suspended between the thighs in a sac called the *scrotum.* The scrotum is made of skin and muscle.

Sperm travel from the testis to the *epididymis.* The epididymis is a coiled tube on top and to the side of the testis. From the epididymis, sperm travel through a tube called the *vas deferens.* Eventually each vas deferens joins a *seminal vesicle.* The two seminal vesicles store sperm and produce *semen.* Semen is a fluid that carries sperm from the male reproductive tract. The ducts of the seminal vesicles unite to form the *ejaculatory duct.* The ejaculatory duct passes through the prostate gland.

The *prostate gland,* shaped like a doughnut, lies just below the bladder. The gland secretes fluid into the semen. As the ejaculatory ducts leave the prostate, they join the *urethra,* which also runs through the prostate. The urethra is the outlet for both urine and semen. The urethra is contained within the penis.

The *penis* is outside of the body and has *erectile* tissue. When a man becomes sexually excited, blood fills the erectile tissue. This causes the penis to become enlarged, hard, and erect. The erect penis can enter the vagina of the female reproductive tract. The semen, which contains sperm, is then released into the female vagina.

THE FEMALE REPRODUCTIVE SYSTEM

The structures of the female reproductive system are shown in Figure 13-21 on page 144. The female gonads are two almond-shaped glands called *ovaries.* There is an ovary on each side of the uterus in the abdominal cavity. The ovaries contain *ova,* or eggs. Ova are the female sex cells. One ovum (egg) is released monthly during the woman's reproductive years. Release of an ovum from an ovary is called *ovulation.* The ovaries also secrete the female hormones *estrogen* and *progesterone.* These hormones are needed for the functioning of the reproductive system and the development of secondary sex characteristics in the female (see Chapter 14).

When an ovum is released from an ovary, it travels through a *fallopian tube.* There are two fallopian tubes, one on each side of the uterus. The tubes are attached at one end to the uterus. The ovum travels through the fallopian tube to the *uterus.* The uterus is a hollow, muscular organ shaped like a pear. The uterus is in the centre of the pelvic cavity behind the

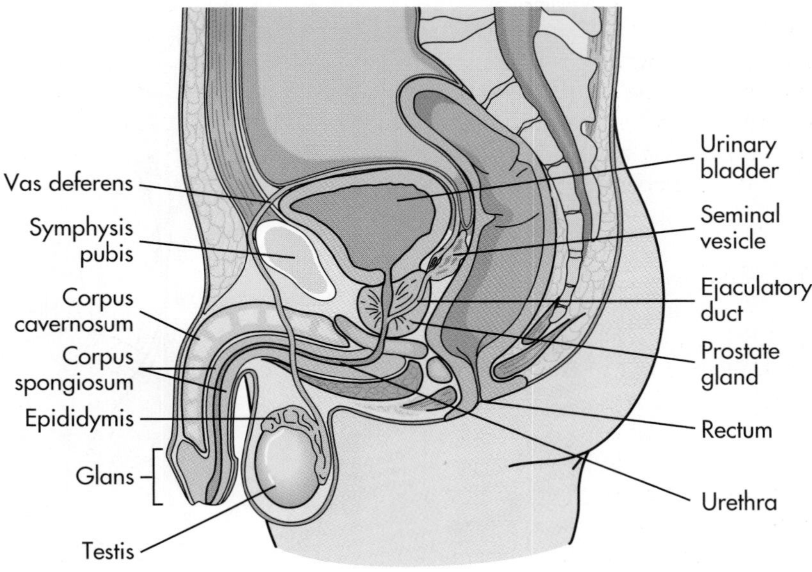

Figure 13-20 Male reproductive system.

bladder and in front of the rectum. The main part of the uterus is the *fundus*. The neck or narrow section of the uterus is the *cervix*. Tissue lining the uterus is called the *endometrium*. There are many blood vessels in the endometrium. If sex cells from the male and female unite into one cell, that cell implants into the endometrium, where it grows into a baby. The uterus serves as a place for the unborn baby to grow and receive nourishment.

The cervix of the uterus projects into a muscular canal called the *vagina*. The vagina opens to the outside of the body and is located just behind the urethra. The vagina receives the penis during sexual intercourse and serves as part of the birth canal. Glands in the vaginal wall keep it moistened with secretions. In young girls, the external vaginal opening is partially closed by a membrane called the *hymen*. The hymen ruptures when the female has intercourse for the first time.

The external genitalia of the female are referred to as the *vulva* (Figure 13-22). The *mons pubis* is a rounded, fatty pad over a bone called the *symphysis pubis*. The mons pubis is covered with hair in the adult female. The *labia majora* and *labia minora* are two folds of tissue on each side of the vaginal opening. The *clitoris* is a small organ composed of erectile tissue. The clitoris becomes hard when sexually stimulated.

The *mammary glands (breasts)* secrete milk after childbirth. They are made up of glandular tissue and

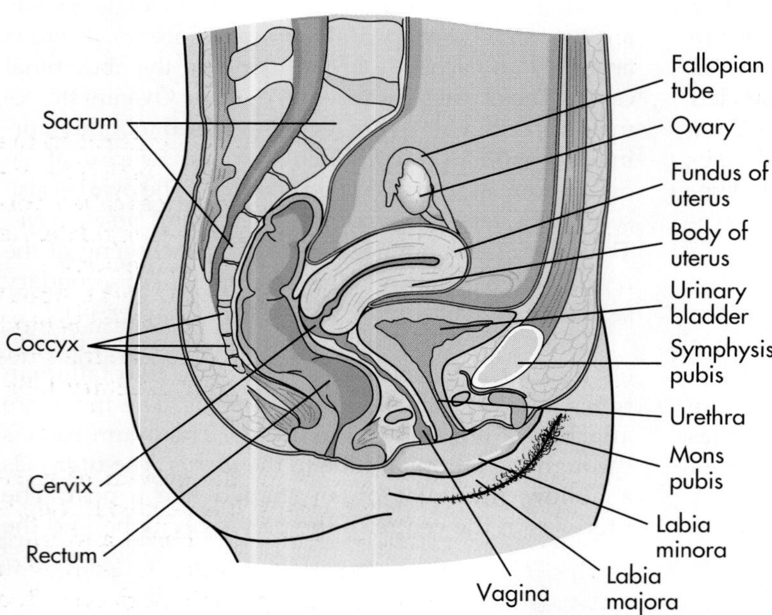

Figure 13-21 Female reproductive system.

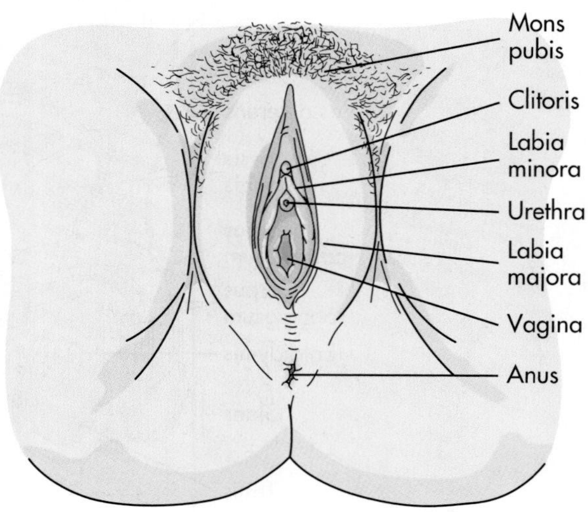

Figure 13-22 External female genitalia.

fat (Figure 13-23). The milk drains into ducts that open onto the nipple.

Menstruation. The endometrium is rich in blood to nourish the cell that grows into an unborn baby *(fetus)*. If pregnancy does not occur, the endometrium breaks up and is discharged through the vagina to the outside of the body. This process is called **menstruation**. Menstruation occurs about every 28 days. Therefore it is also called the *menstrual cycle*.

The first day of the cycle begins with menstruation. Blood flows from the uterus through the vaginal opening. Menstrual flow usually lasts 3 to 7 days. Ovulation occurs during the next phase of the cycle. An ovum matures in an ovary and is released. Ovulation usually occurs on or about day 14 of the cycle.

Meanwhile, estrogen and progesterone (the female hormones) are secreted by the ovaries. These hormones cause the endometrium to thicken for possible pregnancy. If pregnancy does not occur, the hormones decrease in amount. Blood supply to the endometrium decreases because of the decrease in hormones. The endometrium breaks up and is discharged through the vagina. Another menstrual cycle begins.

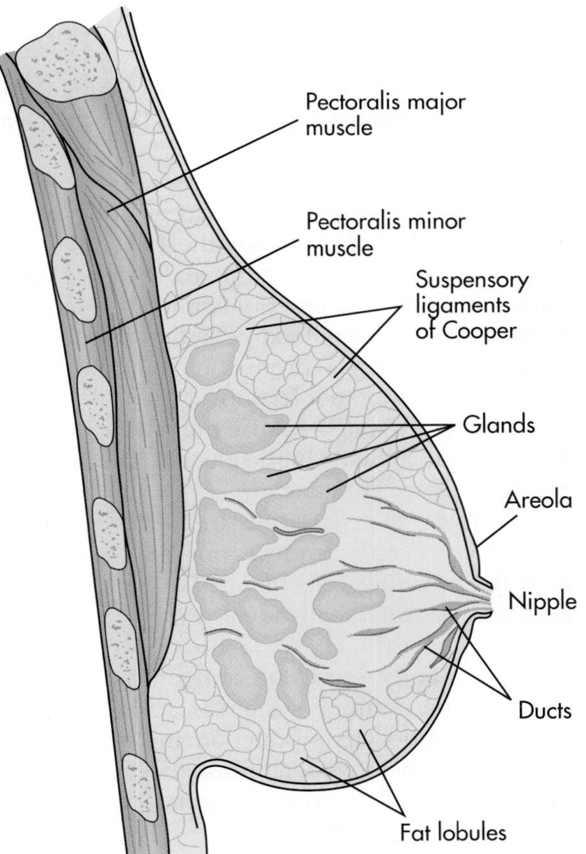

Figure 13-23 The female breast.

FERTILIZATION

For reproduction to occur, a male sex cell (sperm) must unite with a female sex cell (ovum). The uniting of the sperm and ovum into one cell is called *fertilization*. A sperm and an ovum have only 23 chromosomes each, which is exactly half the number that all other cells have. When the two sex cells unite, the fertilized cell has 46 chromosomes.

During intercourse, millions of sperm are deposited in the vagina. Sperm travel up the cervix, through the uterus, and into the fallopian tubes. If a sperm and an ovum unite in a fallopian tube, fertilization occurs and results in pregnancy. The fertilized cell travels down the fallopian tube to the uterus. After a short time, the fertilized cell implants in the thick endometrium and grows during pregnancy.

THE ENDOCRINE SYSTEM

The endocrine system is made up of glands called the *endocrine glands* (Figure 13-24 on page 146). The endocrine glands secrete chemical substances called **hormones** into the bloodstream. Hormones regulate the activities of other organs and glands in the body.

The *pituitary gland* is called the *master gland*. About the size of a cherry, it is at the base of the brain behind the eyes. The pituitary gland is divided into the anterior pituitary lobe and the posterior pituitary lobe. The *anterior pituitary lobe* secretes:

- *Growth hormone*—needed for the growth of muscles, bones, and other organs. It is needed throughout life to maintain normal-size bones and muscles. Growth is stunted if a baby is born with deficient amounts of the growth hormone. Too much of the hormone causes excessive growth.
- *Thyroid-stimulating hormone* (TSH)—needed for thyroid gland function.
- *Adrenocorticotropic hormone* (ACTH)—stimulates the adrenal gland.
- Hormones that regulate growth, development, and function of the male and female reproductive systems.

The *posterior pituitary lobe* secretes *antidiuretic hormone* (ADH) and *oxytocin*. ADH prevents the kidneys from excreting excessive amounts of water. Oxytocin causes the uterine muscles to contract during childbirth.

The *thyroid gland*, shaped like a butterfly, is in the neck in front of the larynx. *Thyroid hormone* (TH) is secreted by the thyroid gland. *Thyroxine* is another term for thyroid hormone. Thyroid hormone regulates **metabolism**. Metabolism is the burning of food for heat and energy by the cells. Too little thyroid hormone

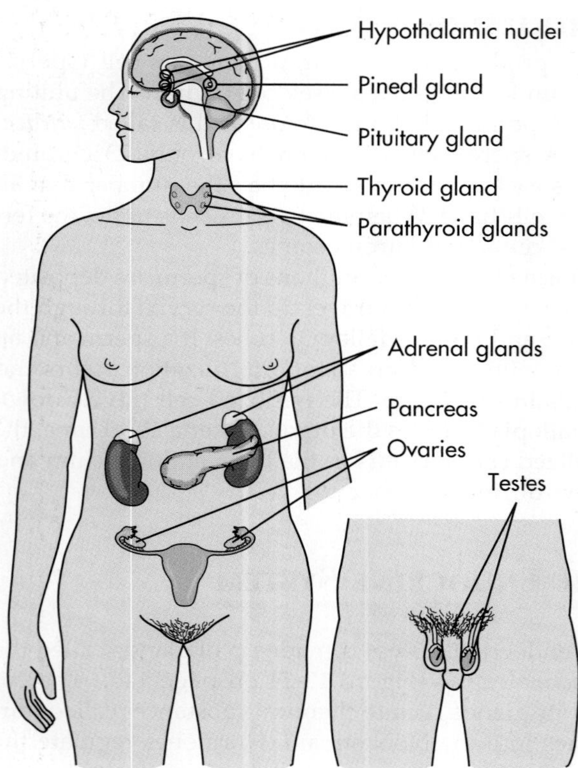

Figure 13-24 Endocrine system.

results in slowed body processes, slowed movements, and weight gain. Too much of the hormone causes increased metabolism, excess energy, and weight loss. If a baby is born with deficient amounts of thyroid hormone, physical and mental growth will be stunted.

The *parathyroid glands* secrete *parathormone.* There are four parathyroid glands. Two are located on each side of the thyroid gland. Parathormone regulates the body's use of calcium. Calcium is needed for the proper functioning of nerves and muscles. Insufficient amounts of calcium cause *tetany.* Tetany is a state of severe muscle contraction and spasm. If untreated, tetany can cause death.

There are two *adrenal glands.* An adrenal gland is on the top of each kidney. The adrenal gland has two parts: the *adrenal medulla* and the *adrenal cortex.* The adrenal medulla secretes *epinephrine* and *norepinephrine.* These hormones stimulate the body to quickly produce energy during emergencies. Heart rate, blood pressure, muscle power, and energy all increase. The adrenal cortex secretes three groups of hormones that are essential for life. The *glucocorticoids* regulate metabolism of carbohydrates. They also control the body's response to stress and inflammation. The *mineralocorticoids* regulate the amount of salt and water that is absorbed and lost by the kidneys. The adrenal cortex also secretes small amounts of male and female sex hormones.

The *pancreas* secretes *insulin.* Insulin regulates the amount of sugar in the blood available for use by the cells. Insulin is needed for sugar to enter the cells. If there is too little insulin, sugar cannot enter the cells. Excess amounts of sugar build up in the blood. This condition is called *diabetes.*

The *gonads* are the glands of human reproduction. Male sex glands (testes) secrete *testosterone.* Female sex glands (ovaries) secrete *estrogen* and *progesterone.*

The Immune System

The immune system protects the body from disease and infection. Abnormal body cells can grow into tumours. Sometimes the body produces substances that cause the body to attack itself. Microorganisms (bacteria, viruses, and other germs) in the environment can lead to an infection. The immune system defends against threats inside and outside the body.

The immune system provides the body with immunity. **Immunity** means that a person has protection against a disease or infection. The person will not get or be affected by the disease or infection. *Specific immunity* is the body's reaction to a specific threat. *Nonspecific immunity* is the body's reaction to anything it does not recognize as a normal body substance.

Special cells and substances provide immunity:

- *Antibodies*—normal body substances that recognize abnormal or unwanted substances. They attack and destroy such substances.
- *Antigens*—abnormal or unwanted substances. An antigen causes the body to produce antibodies. The antibodies attack and destroy the antigens.
- *Phagocytes*—white blood cells that digest and destroy microorganisms and other unwanted substances.
- *Lymphocytes*—white blood cells that produce antibodies. Lymphocyte production increases as the body responds to an infection.
- *B lymphocytes (B cells)*—cause the production of antibodies that circulate in the plasma. The antibodies react to specific antigens.
- *T lymphocytes (T cells)*—cells that destroy invading cells. *Killer T cells* produce poisonous substances near the invading cells. Some T cells attract other cells that destroy the invaders.

When the body senses an antigen (an unwanted substance), the immune system is activated. Phagocyte and lymphocyte production increases. Phagocytes destroy the invaders through digestion. The lymphocytes produce antibodies that attack and destroy the unwanted substances.

REVIEW

Circle the **BEST** answer.

1. The basic unit of body structure is the
   A. Cell
   B. Neuron
   C. Nephron
   D. Ovum

2. The outer layer of the skin is called the
   A. Dermis
   B. Epidermis
   C. Integument
   D. Myelin

3. Which parts allow movement?
   A. Bone marrow and periosteum
   B. Synovial membrane and tendons
   C. Joints
   D. Ligaments

4. Skeletal muscles
   A. Are under involuntary control
   B. Appear smooth
   C. Are under voluntary control
   D. Appear striped and smooth

5. The highest functions of the brain take place in the
   A. Cerebral cortex
   B. Medulla
   C. Brain stem
   D. Spinal nerves

6. Besides hearing, the ear is involved with
   A. Regulating body movements
   B. Balance
   C. Smoothness of body movements
   D. Controlling involuntary muscles

7. The liquid part of the blood is the
   A. Hemoglobin
   B. Red blood cells
   C. Plasma
   D. Alveolus

8. Which part of the heart pumps blood to the body?
   A. Right atrium
   B. Right ventricle
   C. Left atrium
   D. Left ventricle

9. Which carry blood away from the heart?
   A. Capillaries
   B. Veins
   C. Venules
   D. Arteries

10. Oxygen and carbon dioxide are exchanged
    A. In the bronchi
    B. Between the alveoli and capillaries
    C. Between the lungs and the pleura
    D. In the trachea

11. The process of digestion begins in the
    A. Mouth
    B. Stomach
    C. Small intestine
    D. Colon

12. Most food absorption takes place in the
    A. Stomach
    B. Small intestine
    C. Colon
    D. Large intestine

13. Urine is formed by the
    A. Jejunum
    B. Kidneys
    C. Bladder
    D. Liver

14. The male sex gland is called the
    A. Penis
    B. Semen
    C. Testis
    D. Scrotum

15. The endocrine glands secrete substances called
    A. Hormones
    B. Mucus
    C. Semen
    D. Insulin

16. The immune system protects the body from
    A. Low blood sugar
    B. Disease and infection
    C. Falling and loss of balance
    D. Stunted growth and loss of fluid

Answers to these questions are on page 822.

CHAPTER

14

GROWTH AND DEVELOPMENT

OBJECTIVES

- Define the key terms listed in this chapter
- Understand the principles of growth and development
- Identify the stages of growth and development and the normal age ranges for each stage
- Identify the developmental tasks for each age group
- Describe the normal and typical growth and development for each age group

KEY TERMS

adolescence A time of rapid growth and psychological and social maturity

development Changes in a person's psychological and social functioning

developmental task An activity that must be mastered during a stage of development

ejaculation The release of semen

growth The physical changes that can be measured and that occur in a steady, orderly manner

menarche The time when menstruation first begins

menopause The time when menstruation stops

primary caregiver The person who is mainly responsible for providing for the child's basic needs; the person assuming the parental role

puberty The period when the reproductive organs begin to function and secondary sex characteristics appear

reflex An involuntary movement in response to a stimulus

As a support worker, you will care for people in different stages of development. A basic understanding of growth and development helps you give better care. The client's needs also are easier to understand. This chapter presents the basic changes that occur in normal, healthy people from birth through old age.

Human growth and development are presented in nine stages. Age ranges and normal and typical characteristics are given for each stage. Only basic descriptions are given. The stages overlap. This makes it hard to see clear-cut endings and beginnings of the stages. Also, the rate of growth and development varies with each person.

Children grow and develop within the structure of the family. In our society, the family can take many forms (see Chapter 6). Sometimes parents are unable to raise their children. Another person such as a grandparent, aunt, uncle, or court-appointed guardian takes on the parental role.

In this chapter, the term **primary caregiver** is often used when referring to the person who is mainly responsible for providing for the child's basic needs. The primary caregiver may be a parent or other person assuming the parental role.

PRINCIPLES

Growth refers to the physical changes that can be measured and that occur in a steady and orderly manner. Growth is measured in height and weight. Changes in physical appearance and body functions also are measures of growth.

Development refers to changes in psychological and social functioning. A person behaves and thinks in certain ways at different stages of development. A 2-year-old thinks in simple terms and needs a primary caregiver for many basic needs. A 40-year-old thinks in complex ways and meets most basic needs without help from others.

Growth and development affect the entire person. Although each has its own definition, growth and development:

- Overlap
- Depend on each other
- Occur at the same time

For example, an infant cannot say simple syllables (development) until the physical structures needed for speech are strong enough (growth). The basic principles of growth and development are:

- Growth and development occur from the moment of fertilization until death.
- The process proceeds from the simple to the complex. A baby learns to sit before standing, to stand before walking, and to walk before running.
- Growth and development occur in certain directions:
  - From the head to the foot—babies learn to hold up their heads before they learn to sit. After learning to sit, they learn to stand.
  - From the centre of the body outward—babies control shoulder movements before they control hand movements.
- Growth and development occur in a sequence, order, and pattern. Certain **developmental tasks** must be completed during each stage. A stage cannot be skipped. Each stage lays the foundation for the next stage.

- The rate of growth and development is uneven—it does not occur at a set pace. Growth is more rapid during infancy. Also, children have growth spurts. Some children develop rapidly; others develop slowly.
- Each stage of growth and development has its own characteristics and developmental tasks.

Infancy (Birth to 1 Year)

Infancy is the first year of life. Rapid physical, psychological, and social growth and development occur during this time. The developmental tasks of infancy are:

- Learning to walk
- Learning to eat solid foods
- Beginning to talk and communicate with others
- Beginning to have emotional relationships with primary caregivers, brothers, and sisters
- Developing stable sleep and feeding patterns

The *neonatal period* of infancy is the first 28 days after birth. A baby is called a *neonate* or a *newborn* during this time.

The average newborn is 48 to 53 cm (19 to 21 inches) long and weighs 3200 to 3600 grams (7 to 8 pounds) at birth. Birth weight usually doubles by the age of 5 to 6 months and triples by the first birthday. Babies are usually 51 to 76 cm (20 to 30 inches) long at the end of the first year.

The newborn's head is large compared with the rest of the body. The skin is wrinkled, and the baby appears red. Arms and legs seem short compared with the trunk. The abdomen is large and round. Skin and eye colour vary depending on the baby's racial and genetic background and may change during the first year. The newborn has fat, pudgy cheeks, a flat nose, and a receding chin (Figure 14-1).

The central nervous system is not well developed. Movements are uncoordinated and lack purpose. Infants can see at birth, although vision is not clear. They seem attracted to patterns. As they develop, infants prefer colours. Infants hear well. They are startled by loud noises and soothed by soft sounds. They respond better to female than to male voices. Infants react to touch, and the senses of smell and taste are developed.

Newborns have certain **reflexes** (involuntary movements in response to a stimulus). These reflexes decline and then disappear as the central nervous system develops.

- The *Moro reflex (startle reflex)* occurs when an infant is frightened by a loud noise or sudden movement. The arms are thrown apart, the legs extend, and the head is thrown back.
- The *rooting reflex* is stimulated when the infant's cheek is touched at or near the mouth. The infant's head turns toward the touch. The rooting reflex is necessary for feeding; it helps guide the infant's mouth to the nipple.
- The *sucking reflex* is produced by touching the cheeks or side of the lips.
- The *grasping reflex* occurs when the infant's palm is stimulated, causing the fingers to close around the object. This reflex begins to decline around the second month and disappears by the third month.

Infants sleep most of the time during the first few weeks of life. They awaken when hungry and fall asleep right after eating. The time between feedings lengthens as infants grow and develop. They stay awake more and sleep less as growth and development occur.

Body movements are initially uncoordinated and without purpose. They are generally involuntary. As the central nervous system and muscular system develop, infants develop specific, voluntary, and coordinated movements. Newborns cannot hold their heads up. At 1 month, infants can hold their heads up when held and can lift and turn their heads when lying on their stomachs. At 2 months, they can smile and follow objects with their eyes.

Three-month-old infants can raise their heads and shoulders when lying on their stomachs. They can sit for a short while when supported and can hold a rattle. Infants 4 months of age should be able to roll over. They can sit up if supported and may sleep all night. The Moro and rooting reflexes have disappeared. Infants can hold objects with both hands, put objects into their mouths, and babble when spoken to. At 5 months, infants can grasp objects and play with their toes. Teeth start to come through.

Six-month-old infants usually have two lower front teeth and start to chew and bite finger foods. They can

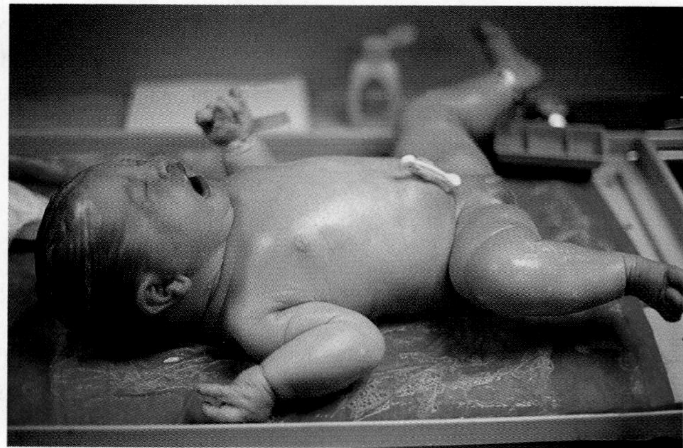

Figure 14-1 A newborn.

hold a bottle for feeding and can sit alone for a short time. At 7 months the upper teeth start to erupt. Infants respond to their names, can say "dada" and "mama," and show a fear of strangers. At age 8 months, infants may be able to stand when holding onto something. They respond to the word "no." Infants at this age often do not like to be dressed or have diapers changed. Nine-month-old infants usually crawl, and more upper teeth appear.

At 10 months, most infants can walk around while holding on to furniture (Figure 14-2). They understand more words than they can say. They communicate what they want by pointing or gesturing. They smile when looking into a mirror. Infants at 11 months of age may begin to take steps. Many infants start to walk at 1 year of age. They can hold a cup for drinking. One-year-olds know more words, can say "no," and shake their heads for "no." They try to imitate words.

During the first 6 months, the infant's diet is mainly breast milk or formula. Solid foods (strained fruits and vegetables) are usually added at 5 to 7 months. Junior foods are added during the ninth and tenth months. A 1-year-old can eat table foods.

TODDLERHOOD (1 TO 3 YEARS)

Physical growth during the second year of life is not as rapid as during infancy. The developmental tasks during this period are:

- Tolerating separation from the primary caregiver
- Gaining control of bowel and bladder function
- Using words to communicate with others
- Becoming less dependent on the primary caregiver

Toddlers have the need to assert independence. The ability to move about and walk increases. So does the child's curiosity. Toddlers get into anything and everything. They touch, smell, and taste everything within reach. As toddlers become more coordinated, they start to climb. These new and increasing skills allow exploration of the environment. The child ventures farther away from the primary caregiver. The toddler also learns that some things can be done without the primary caregiver. By the age of 3 years, the toddler can run, jump, climb, ride a tricycle, and walk up and down stairs.

Increased hand coordination gives toddlers new skills. The need to feel, smell, and taste things is shown in their increasing ability to feed themselves. They progress from eating with fingers to using a spoon (Figure 14-3). Toddlers can drink from cups. They can scribble, build towers with blocks, string beads, and turn book pages. Right- or left-handedness is seen during the second year.

Toilet training is a major developmental task for toddlers. Bowel and bladder control is related to central nervous system development. Children must be psychologically and physically ready for toilet training. The process starts with bowel control. Bowel control is easier because the frequency of bowel movements per day is less than that of urination. Bowel training usually is complete at about 2½ years of age. Bladder control during the day occurs before bladder control at night. Bladder training is complete usually at about 3 years of age.

Speech and language skills increase. Speech is clearer, and vocabulary increases. Words are learned by imitating others. Toddlers understand more words than they use. They are capable of 2- or 3-word sentences. By 3 years of age, children should be able to speak in short sentences.

Play ability increases. The 2-year-old plays alongside other children but does not usually play with them. The toddler is very possessive and does not understand sharing. The word "mine" is often used.

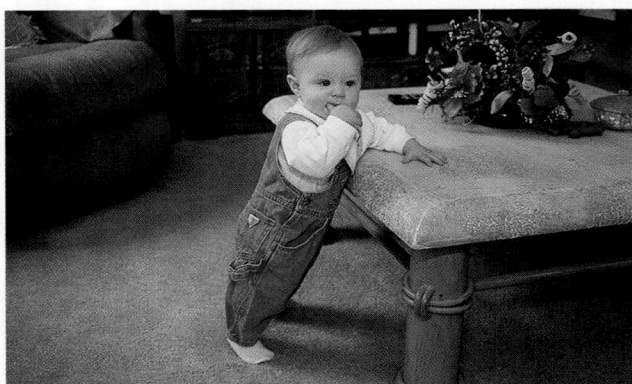

Figure 14-2 A 10-month-old infant can walk while holding on to furniture.

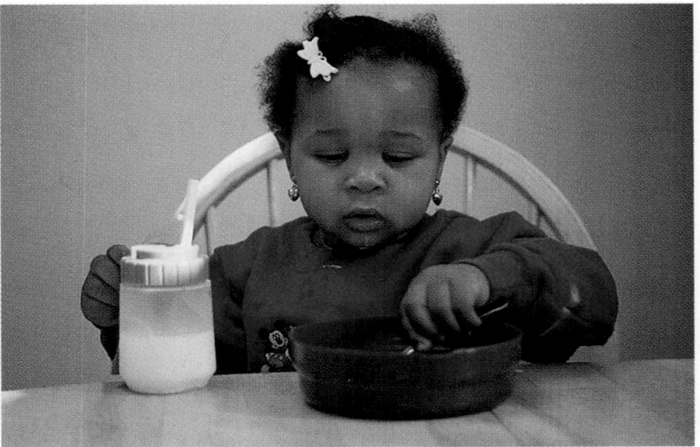

Figure 14-3 A toddler is able to use a spoon.

Temper tantrums and saying "no" are common during this stage. When disciplined, the toddler may kick and scream. The temper tantrum is the child's way of objecting to having independence challenged. The use of "no" and the temper tantrums can frustrate primary caregivers. The toddler years have many such power struggles between caregiver and child. Therefore the toddler years are known as the "terrible twos."

Another developmental task is tolerating separation from the primary caregiver. As toddlers start to explore their environments, they tend to venture away from primary caregivers. When discomfort, frustration, or injury occurs, they quickly return to primary caregivers or cry for their attention. If the primary caregiver is consistently present whenever needed, a child learns to feel secure. Thus toddlers learn to tolerate brief periods of separation.

Preschool (3 to 6 Years)

The preschool years (early childhood) are from the ages of 3 to 6. Children grow taller but gain little weight. Preschoolers are thinner, more coordinated, and more graceful than toddlers. The developmental tasks of the preschool years include:

- Increasing the ability to communicate and understand others
- Performing self-care activities
- Learning the differences between the sexes
- Learning right from wrong and good from bad
- Learning to play with others
- Developing family relationships

The 3-Year-Old

Three-year-olds become more coordinated. They can walk on tiptoe, balance on one foot for a few seconds, and run, jump, and climb with ease. Personal care skills increase. They can put on shoes, dress themselves, manage buttons, wash their hands, and brush their teeth with help. They can feed themselves, pour from a bottle, and help set the table without breaking dishes. Hand skills also include drawing circles and crosses.

Most 3-year-olds know about 1000 words, imitate new words, and talk and ask questions constantly. A favourite question repeated many times a day is "why?" Sentences are brief—usually 3 or 4 words. Three-year-olds can name body parts, family members, friends, and animals.

Play is important. Three-year-olds are able to play with other children instead of just playing beside them. They are developing an understanding that others have feelings. They are more cooperative than toddlers. With an adult's encouragement, they are able to share toys and take turns. They play simple games and can follow simple rules. They enjoy using colouring books and crayons, child-safe scissors and paper, age-appropriate puzzles, and participating in role-playing games such as "house" and "dress-up" (Figure 14-4).

Three-year-olds have vivid imaginations and often play make-believe games. Imaginary friends are common at this age. They may be so involved with their make-believe worlds that they sometimes confuse fantasy and reality. For example, a child may believe that a character in a picture book is real. Their developing imaginations may cause some children at this age to have nightmares or daytime fears and insecurities. They may need a night-light at bedtime.

At 3 years old, children know that there are 2 sexes. They are beginning to identify with their own sex. During role-playing games, girls will often pretend to be women (such as a mom or a princess) and boys will pretend to be men (such as a dad or a cowboy). This is their way of exploring the gender differences seen in their families and in the world around them (such as in books, television, and videos).

The concept of time develops. Three-year-olds may speak of the past, present, and future. "Yesterday" and "tomorrow" are still confusing.

Three-year-olds are less fearful of strangers. They tolerate separation from primary caregivers for short periods. They are less jealous than toddlers of a new baby. They want to please their primary caregivers.

The 4-Year-Old

Four-year-olds can hop, skip, and throw and catch a ball. They can lace shoes, draw faces, copy a square, and try to print letters. They can bathe with some help and usually tend to toileting needs with help.

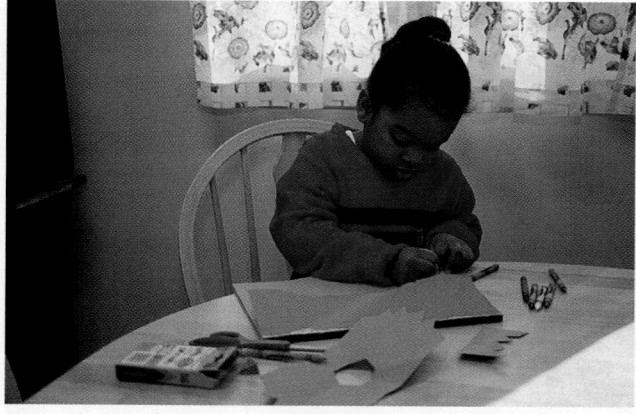

Figure 14-4 Three-year-olds have increased coordination. Many enjoy doing crafts such as cutting paper and using colouring books and crayons.

Vocabulary increases to about 1500 words. The 4-year-old can sing simple songs, repeat 4 numbers, count to 3, and name a few colours. The child continues to ask many questions and tends to exaggerate when telling stories. Many 4-year-olds can tell long and complex stories. Their constant chatter shows that they are learning the power of words. Sometimes they may seem bossy as they use their developing language skills to tease, tattle, or tell others (including caregivers) what to do.

A 4-year-old's hand and finger coordination are well developed. They like to make crafts, build with blocks, and try to "write" with a pencil or pen. Children in this age group still enjoy playing "dress-up" and imitating adults (Figure 14–5). They still have vivid imaginations, but are now better able to know the difference between reality and fantasy. They are more social than they were at 3 years of age and usually enjoy playing in groups of 2 or 3. They also begin to develop close friendships. They may try to be like their friends or show off to impress them.

At this age, many children express curiosity about sexuality. They may ask persistent questions about how babies are made and why boys' and girls' genitals are different. Playing "doctor and nurse" is common as curiosity about sexuality continues.

Four-year-olds may show a strong preference for the parent of the opposite sex. Rivalries with brothers and sisters are seen, especially when siblings take the 4-year-old's possessions. Rivalries also occur when older children have more and different privileges.

The 5-Year-Old

Coordination continues to develop. Five-year-olds can jump rope, skate, tie shoelaces, dress, and bathe. They can use a pencil well and copy diamond and triangle shapes. They can print a few letters and numbers and their first names. Drawings of people include the body, head, arms, legs, and feet.

Communication skills also increase. Vocabulary consists of about 14 000 words. Sentences have 6 to 8 words. Five-year-olds ask fewer questions than before, but questions have more meaning. They want definitions for unknown terms and wish to take part in conversations. They can name 4 or more colours, coins, days of the week, and months. They specify what they draw and give detailed descriptions of drawings.

Five-year-olds are generally responsible and truthful, and they quarrel less than before. There is greater awareness of rules and an eagerness to do things the right way. They want to please others, especially teachers and caregivers. They have manners, are independent, and can be trusted within limits. Five-year-olds have fewer fears but may still have nightmares. They are also proud of their accomplishments.

Many 5-year-olds enjoy simple number and word games. Although they may cheat to win, they like rules and try to follow them. They imitate adults during play and have a greater interest in watching television. They also enjoy activities with the primary caregiver of the same sex (Figure 14-6). Such activities include cooking, housecleaning, shopping, yard work, and sports.

These children tolerate brothers and sisters well. Although younger children are sometimes considered a nuisance, 5-year-olds usually protect them and enjoy playing with them.

Middle Childhood (6 to 8 Years)

Preschoolers often have nursery school and kindergarten experiences. However, middle childhood is the time for school. Children enter the world of peer

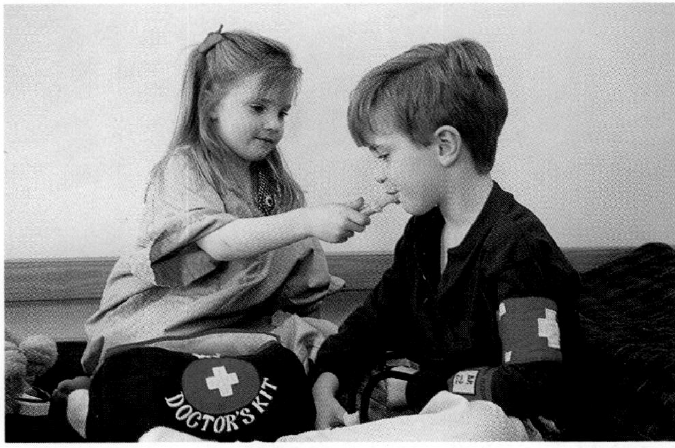

Figure 14-5 Four-year-olds play "dress-up" and imitate adults.

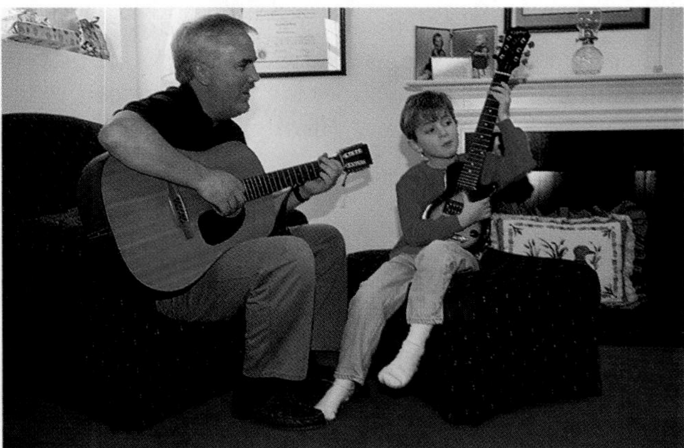

Figure 14-6 Five-year-olds enjoy doing things with the parent of the same sex.

groups, games, and learning. The developmental tasks of middle childhood are:

- Developing the social and physical skills needed for playing games
- Learning to get along with other children of the same age and background (peers)
- Learning behaviours and attitudes appropriate to one's own sex
- Learning basic reading, writing, and arithmetic skills
- Developing a conscience and morals
- Developing a good feeling and attitude about oneself

The 6-Year-Old

Between the sixth and seventh birthdays, a child will grow about 5 cm (2 inches) and gain 1 to 3 kg (3 to 6 pounds). Baby teeth are lost, and permanent teeth begin to erupt. Children are very active and are skilled at running, jumping, skipping, hopping, and riding a bicycle. They seem to be constantly on the go. Sitting is tolerated for only a short time.

Six-year-olds enter the first grade and the world of school, activities, and other children. Children this age are often described as bossy, opinionated, charming, argumentative, and "know-it-alls." They have set ways of doing things and like to have their own way. They may have temper tantrums. Six-year-olds play well with children of both sexes. However, they begin to prefer playing with children of the same sex (Figure 14-7). There is more sharing with others, and the child may have a "best friend." A child may cheat to win or leave a game before it is over to avoid losing. Tattling is common.

Six-year-olds have a vocabulary of about 16 500 words. They know the alphabet and begin to read and spell. They communicate thoughts and feelings better than before.

Play interests range from rough play to quiet activities such as playing with cards, paints, clay, and computer games. Collections are started of odds and ends rather than specific things like stamps, rocks, or butterflies. More active play includes tag, hide-and-seek, playing with balls, skating, and playing in mud or sand.

The 7-Year-Old

Seven-year-olds grow about 5 cm (2 inches) in height during the year. The average 7-year-old weighs about 22 to 25 kg (49 to 56 pounds) and is 119 to 124 cm (47 to 49 inches) tall. Hand coordination increases. Children learn to write rather than print. They are quieter than 6-year-olds and spend more time alone. They are more serious, less stubborn, and more concerned about being well liked. Seven-year-olds are more aware of themselves, their bodies, and the reactions of others. They do not like being teased or criticized and are sensitive about how others treat them. They usually like going to school, learning, and reading. They may worry about grades and what the teacher thinks about them. Reading skills increase, and the child can tell time.

Play includes swimming, biking, collecting and trading objects, playing ball and games with rules, and working puzzles and video games. They play in groups. However, boys prefer to play with boys and girls prefer to play with girls.

The 8-Year-Old

The 8-year-old enters the third grade. Growth in height and weight continues. More permanent teeth appear. Movements are faster and more graceful.

Peer group activities and opinions are important. Being accepted and included in peer groups are important for the fulfillment of love and belonging and self-esteem needs. Children this age get along with adults. However, they prefer peer group fads, opinions, and activities. Boys and girls play separately. Their interests relate to group games, collections, television, and movies.

Eight-year-olds are sometimes described as defensive, opinionated, practical, and outgoing. They give advice freely to others. However, they do not accept criticism well. They are able to help with many household tasks such as vacuuming, cooking, and yard work. They expect more privileges than younger brothers and sisters.

Learning continues. They are curious about science, history, and other places and countries. School also provides social opportunities with peers. Eight-year-olds are daring in the classroom. They may pass notes or talk with others when they think the teacher is not looking. Despite this mischief, they are mannerly, relate well to adults, and take part in adult conversations. They are also friendly and affectionate.

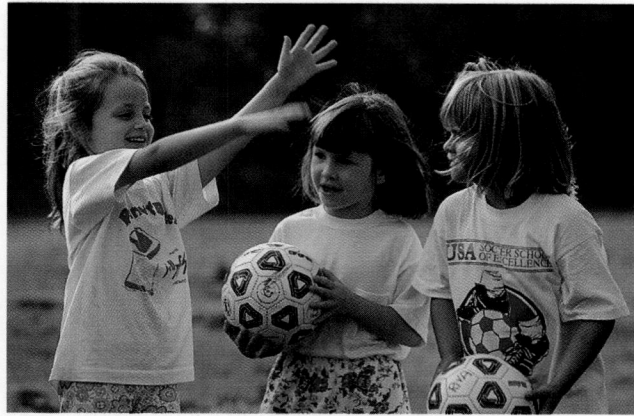

Figure 14-7 In middle childhood, belonging to a peer group is important. Children usually prefer playing with peers of the same sex.

Late Childhood (9 to 12 Years)

Late childhood (preadolescence) is between leaving childhood and dependency on others and entering adolescence. Developmental tasks are similar to those of middle childhood. However, a preadolescent is expected to show more refinement and maturity in achieving the following tasks:

- Becoming independent of adults and learning to depend on oneself
- Developing and keeping friendships with peers
- Understanding the physical, psychological, and social roles of one's sex
- Developing moral and ethical behaviour
- Developing greater muscular strength, coordination, and balance
- Learning how to study

Boys grow about 2.5 cm (1 inch) per year. Girls grow about 5 cm (2 inches) per year. Boys gain about 1.8 kg (4 pounds) each year. Girls gain about 2.3 kg (5 pounds) each year. Girls are usually taller than boys during late preadolescence. Many permanent teeth erupt.

Body movements are more graceful and coordinated (Figure 14-8). Muscular strength and physical skills increase. Skill in team sports is often important to the child.

Body changes occur as the onset of puberty nears. In girls, the pelvis becomes broader, fat appears on the hips and chest, and the budding of breasts occurs. Boys show fewer signs of maturing sexually during this time. Genital organs begin to grow.

Children of this age must have factual sex education. Information about sex that is shared among friends is often incomplete and inaccurate. Parents and children may be uncomfortable discussing sex with each other and may avoid the subject. When children do ask questions, honest and complete answers must be given in terms the children can understand.

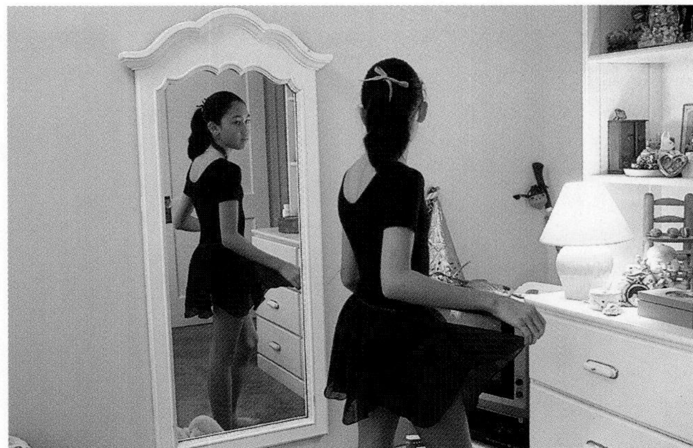

Figure 14-8 Movements are smooth and graceful in late childhood.

Peer groups are the centre of preadolescent activities. The group begins to affect the child's attitudes and behaviour. Preference for companions of the same sex continues. Boys need to show their strength and toughness and may give each other nicknames. Arguments between boys and girls are common, and they often tease each other.

Preadolescents are more aware of the mistakes and weaknesses of adults. They do not accept adult standards and rules without question. Rebellion against adults is common. Disagreements between parents and children increase, although the parents continue to be important for the child's development.

Adolescence (12 to 18 Years)

Adolescence is a time of rapid growth and psychological and social maturity. The stage begins with puberty. **Puberty** is the period during which the reproductive organs begin to function and the secondary sex characteristics appear. Girls experience puberty between the ages of 10 and 14. Most boys reach puberty between the ages of 12 and 16.

Because the age of puberty varies, adolescence ranges from the ages of 12 to 18 years. The developmental tasks of adolescence include:

- Accepting changes in the body and appearance
- Developing appropriate relationships with males and females of the same age
- Accepting the male or female role appropriate for one's age
- Becoming independent from parents and adults
- Developing morals, attitudes, and values needed for functioning in society

Menarche, the beginning of menstruation, marks the onset of puberty in girls. Secondary sex characteristics appear. These include:

- Increase in breast size
- Appearance of pubic and axillary (underarm) hair
- Slight deepening of the voice
- Widening and rounding of the hips

During late childhood, male sex organs begin to increase in size. This growth continues during adolescence. **Ejaculation** (the release of semen) signals the onset of puberty in boys. *Nocturnal emissions* ("wet dreams") occur. During sleep *(nocturnal)*, the penis becomes erect and semen is released *(emission)*. Secondary sex characteristics also appear. These include:

- Appearance of facial hair
- Pubic and axillary (underarm) hair
- Hair on the arms, chest, and legs
- Deepening of the voice
- Increases in neck and shoulder size

A growth spurt occurs. Boys grow about 10 to 41 cm (4 to 16 inches) and gain 7 to 27 kg (15 to 60 pounds). They usually stop growing between the ages of 18 and 21. Some continue to grow until about age 25. Girls grow about 5 to 23 cm (2 to 9 inches) and gain between 7 and 23 kg (15 and 50 pounds). They usually stop growing between the ages of 17 and 18. Some continue to grow until about age 21.

Adolescence is described as the awkward stage. Awkwardness and clumsiness are caused by the uneven growth of muscles and bones. Coordination and graceful body movements develop as muscle and bone growth even out.

Changes in appearance are often hard to accept. Some girls are embarrassed about breast development, especially very large or small breast size. Genital size may be a concern for boys. Height may be a problem for both boys and girls. Boys do not like being much shorter than their peers. Tall girls may feel embarrassed about being taller than other girls and boys. Many adolescents, especially girls, worry about their weight and think they weigh too much. Many try to diet and some develop eating disorders.

Teenagers often feel intense emotions. Emotional reactions vary from high to low. Adolescents can be happy one moment and sad the next. Predicting a reaction to a comment or event is difficult. Teenagers can control their emotions better later in this stage. Older adolescents (15- to 18-year-olds) can still become sad and depressed. However, they can better control the time and place of their emotional reactions.

Adolescents need to become independent of adults, especially their parents. They must learn to function, make decisions, and act in a responsible manner without adult supervision. Many teenagers work toward this independence with part-time jobs, babysitting, going to dances and parties, dating, taking part in school clubs and organizations, shopping without an adult, and staying home alone (Figure 14-9).

Adolescents are increasingly able to use logic and reasoning. They often form passionate opinions on many issues. However, judgment and reasoning are not always sound. Guidance, discipline, and emotional and financial support are still needed from parents. Disagreements with parents are common, especially about behaviour and activity restrictions and limits. Teenagers would rather be with peers than do things with parents and other family members. Adolescents tend to confide in and seek advice from peers or adults other than their parents.

Teenage interests and activities reflect the need to become independent, to develop relationships with the opposite sex, and to act like males or females. Both sexes are often interested in parties, dances, and other social activities. Clothing, make-up, and hairstyles are often important to teenagers because their appearance enables them to define their identity and fit in with a crowd. Parents and teenagers often disagree about clothing and hairstyles. Teenagers may spend a lot of time with friends or conversing with them through e-mail, in chat rooms, or on the phone. They also spend time participating in sports or clubs, listening to music, or playing video games.

Dating begins during adolescence. Although the age when dating begins varies, there is usually a dating pattern. "Crowd" dates are common in the seventh and eighth grades. They are usually related to school activities, such as a dance or basketball game. The same group of girls just happens to be with the same group of boys during these social events. In the ninth grade, pairing off is common during crowd dating. The tenth grade is usually when boy–girl couples go to social events together and then join other couples. Double dating occurs in the eleventh grade. Dates involve one couple during the twelfth grade, although there is some double dating.

Many difficult decisions and conflicts result as the adolescent matures physically, psychologically, and emotionally. Parents and teenagers often disagree about dating. Parents worry that dating will lead to sexual activities, pregnancy, and sexually transmitted diseases. Teenagers usually do not understand or appreciate these concerns. "Going steady" helps meet the teenager's need for security, love and belonging, and self-esteem. Teenagers sometimes have difficulty

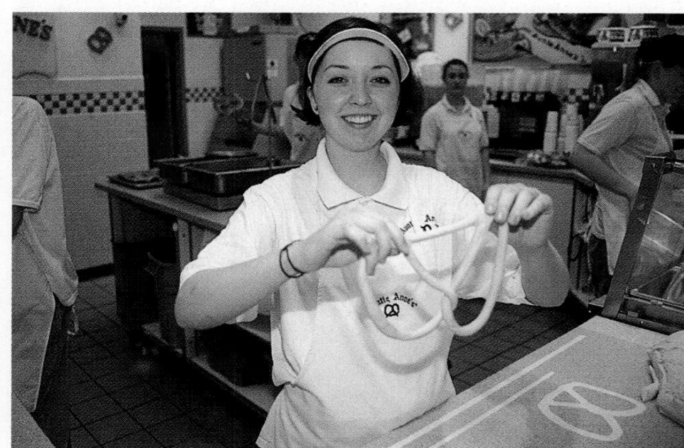

Figure 14-9 This teenager has a part-time job.

controlling sexual urges and considering the consequences of sexual activity.

Adolescents begin to think about careers and what to do after high school graduation. Interests, skills, and talents are some factors that influence the choice of further education and getting a job. Adolescents also need to develop morals, values, and attitudes for living in society. They need to develop a sense about what is good and bad, right and wrong, and important and unimportant. Parents, peers, culture, religion, television, school, and movies are among the many factors influencing teenagers. Drug abuse, unwanted pregnancy, alcoholism, and criminal acts are common problems of troubled adolescents.

Young Adulthood (18 to 40 Years)

Psychological and social development continue during young adulthood. There is little physical growth. Adult height has been reached. Body systems are fully developed. Developmental tasks of young adulthood include:

- Choosing education and an occupation
- Selecting a partner
- Learning to live with a partner
- Becoming a parent and raising children
- Developing a satisfactory sex life

Education and occupation are so closely related that they can rarely be separated. Most jobs require specific knowledge and skills. The amount and kind of education needed depend on the career choice. Most adults find that job choices are greater with adequate educational preparation. Employment is necessary for economic independence and for supporting a family.

Most adults marry at least once. Others choose to remain single. They may live alone, with friends of the same sex, or with a person of the opposite sex. Gay and lesbian people may commit to a partner.

The many reasons for marriage include love, emotional security, wanting a family, sex, wanting to leave an unhappy home life, social status, companionship, and financial security. Some marry to feel wanted, needed, and desirable. Many factors affect the selection of a marriage partner. They include age, religion, interests, education, race, personality, and love. Some marriages are happy and successful, whereas others are not. There are no guarantees that a marriage will work. Therefore, the two people must work together to build a marriage based on trust, respect, caring, and friendship.

Partners (married or unmarried) must learn to live together. Habits, routines, household management, meal preparation, and pastimes are changed or adjusted to "fit" the other person's needs. They must learn how to solve problems and make decisions together. They need to work toward the same goals. Open and honest communication helps create a successful partnership (Figure 14-10).

Adults also need to develop a satisfactory sex life. Sexual frequency, desires, practices, and preferences vary. Understanding and accepting the partner's needs are necessary for a satisfying and intimate relationship.

Most couples decide to have children. Modern birth control methods allow planning about the number of children and when to have them. However, many pregnancies are unplanned. Many couples have a child during the first few years of marriage; some wait several years before starting a family. Other couples decide not to have children. Some have difficulty or cannot have children because of physical problems with one or both partners. Those couples having children need to agree on childrearing practices and discipline methods. They need to adjust to the child and to the child's need for time, energy, and parental attention.

Middle Adulthood (40 to 65 Years)

This stage of development is often stable and comfortable. Children are usually grown and have moved away. Partners now have time to spend alone together. There are fewer worries about children and money. The developmental tasks of middle adulthood include:

- Adjusting to physical changes
- Having grown children
- Developing leisure activities
- Relating to aging parents

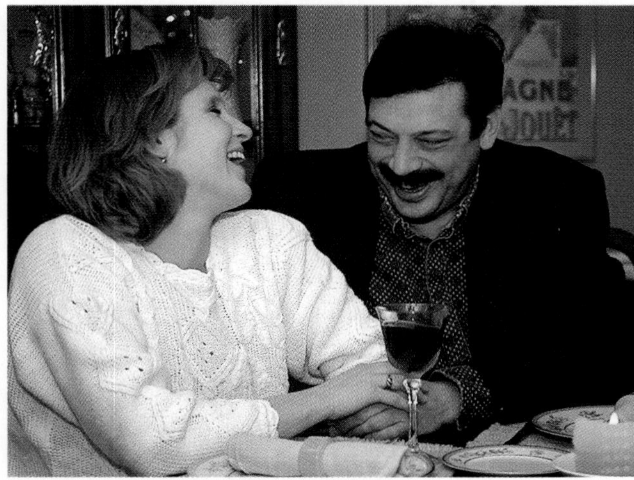

Figure 14-10 Communication is necessary for a successful partnership and a satisfactory sex life.

Several physical changes occur. Many are gradual and go unnoticed; others are seen early. People in their early forties may feel energetic and able to function as they did in their twenties. However, energy and endurance begin to slow down. Weight control becomes a problem as metabolism and physical activities slow down. Facial wrinkles and grey hair appear. The need for eyeglasses is common. Hearing loss may begin. Menstruation stops between the ages of 42 and 55; this is called **menopause**. Ovaries stop secreting hormones, and the woman can no longer have children. Many diseases and illnesses can develop. The disorders can become chronic or life threatening.

Children leave home for school, marry, move to homes of their own, and start their own families. Adults have to cope with letting children go, being in-laws, and becoming grandparents. Parents must let children lead their own lives. However, they need to be available for emotional support in times of need.

Middle-age adults often discover spare time when the demands of parenthood decrease. Hobbies and pastimes such as gardening, fishing, painting, golfing, volunteer work, and membership in clubs and organizations are sources of pleasure (Figure 14-11). Hobbies and pastimes become even more important after retirement and during late adulthood.

Some middle-age adults have parents who are aging and developing poor health. Responsibility for aging parents may begin during this stage. Middle-age adults often have to deal with the death of parents.

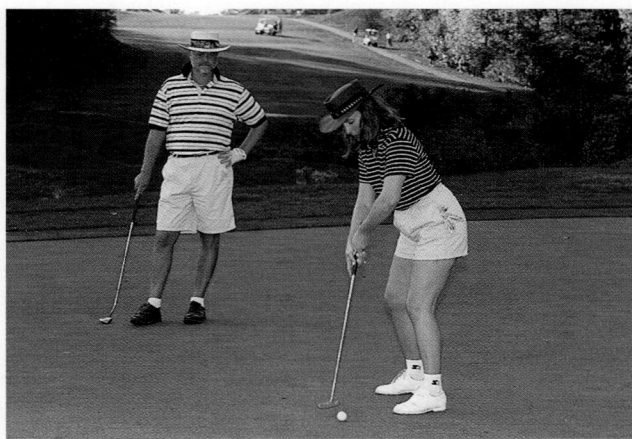

Figure 14-11 Middle-age adults usually have more time for hobbies.

Late Adulthood (65 Years and Older)

Many physical, psychological, and social changes occur during later adulthood. Chapter 15 describes the changes that occur in older adults, as well as the care they may need.

The developmental tasks of this stage are:

- Adjusting to decreased physical strength and loss of health
- Adjusting to retirement and reduced income
- Coping with the death of a partner
- Developing new friends and relationships
- Preparing for one's own death

REVIEW

Circle the BEST answer.

1. Changes in psychological and social functioning are called
   A. Growth
   B. Development
   C. A reflex
   D. A stage

2. Which is *false*?
   A. Growth and development occur from the simple to the complex.
   B. Growth and development occur in an orderly pattern.
   C. Growth and development occur at specific rates.
   D. Each stage has its own characteristics.

3. The stage of infancy is the first
   A. 4 weeks of life
   B. 3 months of life
   C. 6 months of life
   D. Year of life

4. Which reflexes are needed for feeding in the infant?
   A. The Moro and startle reflexes
   B. The rooting and sucking reflexes
   C. The grasping and Moro reflexes
   D. The rooting and grasping reflexes

5. Solid foods are usually given to an infant during the
   A. Fifth to seventh month
   B. Eighth month
   C. Ninth or tenth month
   D. Eleventh or twelfth month

6. The toddler can
   A. Use a spoon and cup
   B. Ride a bike
   C. Help set the table
   D. Name parts of the body

7. Playing with other children begins during
   A. Infancy
   B. The toddler years
   C. The preschool years
   D. Middle childhood

8. Peer group activities become more important at the age of
   A. 6
   B. 7
   C. 8
   D. 9

9. Reproductive organs begin to function and secondary sex characteristics appear during
   A. Late childhood
   B. Preadolescence
   C. Puberty
   D. Early adulthood

10. Which is *false*?
    A. Boys reach puberty earlier than girls.
    B. Most girls reach puberty between the ages of 12 and 13.
    C. Menarche marks the onset of puberty in girls.
    D. A growth spurt occurs during adolescence.

11. Dating usually begins
    A. During late childhood
    B. With "crowd" dating
    C. With "pairing off"
    D. During late adolescence

12. Adolescence is usually a time when parents and children
    A. Talk openly about sex
    B. Express love and affection
    C. Disagree
    D. Do things as a family

13. Which is *not* a developmental task of young adulthood?
    A. Adjusting to changes in the body and in physical appearance
    B. Selecting a partner
    C. Choosing an occupation
    D. Becoming a parent

14. Middle adulthood is from about
    A. 25 to 35 years
    B. 30 to 40 years
    C. 40 to 50 years
    D. 40 to 65 years

15. Middle adulthood is usually a time when
    A. Families are started
    B. Physical energy and free time are gained
    C. Children are grown and leave home
    D. People need to prepare for death

Answers to these questions are on page 822.

CHAPTER

15

Caring for Older Adults

OBJECTIVES

- Define the key terms listed in this chapter
- Describe the effects of retirement
- Identify the social changes common in older adulthood
- Describe how a partner's death affects the survivor
- Describe the changes that occur in the body's systems during aging and the care required
- Explain how aging affects sexuality in older adults
- Describe how the health care team promotes the client's sexuality
- Explain the effect of ageism on older adults

KEY TERMS

ageism Bias and discrimination against older adults

discrimination Behaviour that treats people unfairly based on their group membership

dyspnea Difficult, laboured, or painful breathing

dysphagia Difficulty swallowing

geriatrics The branch of medicine that provides care for older adults

gerontology The study of the aging process

middle-old People between 75 and 84 years of age

old-old People older than 85 years

stereotype An overly simple or exaggerated view of a group of people

young-old People between 60 and 74 years of age

The number of older adults increases every day. People live longer and are healthier and more active than ever before. Most people can expect to live into their seventies. Many live into their eighties and nineties. There also are more 100-year-olds than ever before. Late adulthood is broken down into these age ranges:

- The **young-old**—people between 60 and 74 years of age
- The **middle-old**—people between 75 and 84 years of age
- The **old-old**—people older than 85 years

Gerontology is the study of the aging process. **Geriatrics** is the branch of medicine that provides care for older adults. Aging, or growing old, is a normal process. Normal changes occur in body structure and function. These changes increase the risk for illness, injury, chronic disease, and disability. Usually the changes are gradual. Emotional and social changes also occur. Most older adults adjust to these changes and live healthy and happy lives. Some live in their own homes, alone or with their partners. Others live with their adult children or other family members. Some move into assisted-living facilities. Others require 24-hour care and move into long-term care facilities.

As stated in Chapter 14, the developmental tasks of late adulthood are:

- Adjusting to decreased physical strength and loss of health
- Adjusting to retirement and reduced income
- Coping with the death of a partner
- Developing new friends and relationships
- Preparing for one's own death

EMOTIONAL AND SOCIAL CHANGES

Greying hair, wrinkles, and slow movements are physical reminders of growing old. Retirement and death of a partner, family, and friends are social reminders. Physical and social changes have emotional effects on older adults. They affect the basic needs of love and belonging and self-esteem.

RETIREMENT

Most people look forward to retiring. People usually retire at the age of 65. Some retire earlier. Others work until the age of 70 and beyond. Retirement is a reward for a lifetime of work. The person has earned the right not to work and can now relax and enjoy life. Travel, leisure, and doing what one wants are retirement "benefits." Many people enjoy retirement. Others are not as lucky. Retirement is often a person's first real experience with aging. Some must retire because of chronic disease or disability. Poor health can make retirement very difficult.

Work has social and emotional effects. It helps meet the basic needs of love and belonging and self-esteem. Work brings fulfillment and a feeling of usefulness. There is pride in a day's work or a job well done. Friendships form, and co-workers share daily events. Leisure time, recreation, and companionship often involve co-workers. Some people need work for emotional and social fulfillment. Retirement can be hard for them. Some retired people have part-time jobs or do volunteer work (Figure 15-1 on page 162). Such activities promote usefulness and well-being.

Reduced Income. Retirement income is often less than one-half of the person's working income. The Canada Pension Plan may provide the only

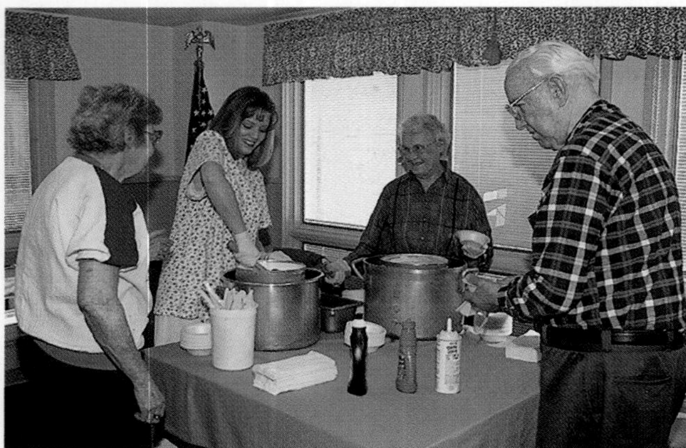

Figure 15-1 These retired people volunteer at a local food bank.

income. Even that has not kept pace with the high cost of living.

Retirement and aging do not mean fewer expenses. Older adults still need to make rent or mortgage payments, buy food and clothing, and pay for transportation, utilities, and taxes. They must also pay for medications that are not covered under government drug plans.

Reduced income may force lifestyle changes. Some people have to limit social and leisure activities. They may have to find cheaper housing or move in with their children or other relatives. Some must rely on family for money or needed items. Others live in poverty.

Some people do not have a reduced income. They were able to plan for their retirement through savings, investments, retirement plans, and insurance. Their retirement years are financially comfortable.

Social Relationships

Social relationships change throughout life. (See *Respecting Diversity: Foreign-Born People* box.) Children grow up, leave home, and have their own families. Many live far away from parents. Older friends and family move away, die, or are disabled. Most older people have regular contact with children, grandchildren, brothers and sisters, nieces and nephews, and other relatives and friends. However, many older adults are lonely. Separation from children and lack of companionship are common causes of loneliness in older adults.

Many older adults adjust to these changes. Hobbies, religious and community activities, and new friends help prevent loneliness. Being a grandparent can bring great love and enjoyment. Taking part in family activities helps prevent loneliness. It also allows the older person to feel useful and wanted. Some home care programs provide a "friendly visitor" program for older adults living alone. Older adults who move to retirement homes and long-term care facilities often make new friends. They can take part in social activities that are offered (Figure 15-2).

> **Respecting Diversity**
>
> **Foreign-Born People**
>
> Older adults who have moved to Canada from another country may not speak English or French. They may have lived and worked in a community with people from their home country. When family and friends move away or die, the person may have no one to talk to. Health care workers may not speak the same language or understand the person's culture. The person feels lonely and isolated. You need to be sensitive to clients in this situation.

Children as Caregivers

Some adult children care for their older parents. Parents and children change roles. The child cares for the parent. This role change and dependency on a child can make the older adult feel more secure. However, others feel unwanted, in the way, and useless. Some lose dignity and self-respect. Tensions may develop among the child, parent, and other household members. Being a caregiver to an elderly parent can be very stressful. Caregivers often have to meet the needs of the parent as well as those of their own children. If the parent has a medical condition, the caregiver has even more responsibilities. Sometimes caregivers must quit work to care for the parent. Loss of income causes financial difficulties. Lack of privacy is also a common problem.

Death of a Partner

As a couple grows older, the chances increase that one partner will die. Women usually live longer than men. Therefore many women will become widows.

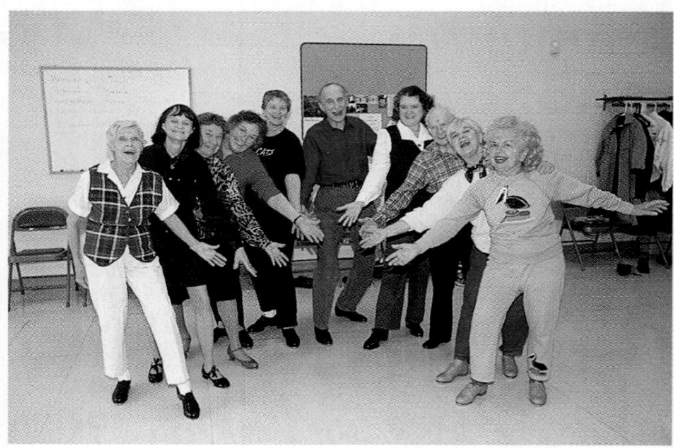

Figure 15-2 Older adults enjoy companionship with people their own age.

A person may try to emotionally prepare for a partner's death. When death occurs, the loss is still devastating. No amount of preparation is ever enough for the emptiness and changes that result. The person loses a friend, lover, companion, and confidant. The survivor's grief may be great. Serious physical and mental health problems can result. The surviving partner may lose the will to live or attempt suicide.

Physical Changes

Certain physical changes are a normal part of aging. The changes occur in everyone (Table 15-1 on page 164). Body processes slow down. Energy level and body efficiency decline. The rate and degree of change vary with each person. Influencing factors include diet, general health, exercise, stress, environment, and heredity. Many changes are gradual and not noticed for a long time. Some older adults also have physical changes caused by disease, illness, or injury.

Normal aging does not mean loss of health. Quality of life does not have to change. The person can adjust to many of the changes. However, many older adults have at least one chronic illness.

The Integumentary System

The skin loses its elasticity, strength, and fatty-tissue layer. This causes the skin to thin and sag. Folds, lines, and wrinkles appear. Dry skin develops because of decreases in oil and sweat glands. The skin is fragile and easily injured. Skin breakdown, skin tears, and pressure ulcers are dangers (see Chapter 41).

Brown spots appear on the skin. These often are called "age spots" or "liver spots." They usually occur on the wrists and hands.

The skin has fewer nerve endings. This affects the person's ability to sense heat, cold, and pain. Bruising and delayed healing result from a decreased number of blood vessels.

Loss of fatty tissues beneath the skin increases sensitivity to cold. Protect the client from drafts and extreme cold. Sweaters, lap blankets, socks, and higher thermostat settings are often needed.

Nails become thick and tough. Feet usually have poor circulation. A nick or cut can lead to a serious infection. Nail and foot care are described in Chapter 28.

Dry skin is easily damaged and causes itching. Older adults with dry skin should avoid daily showers or tub baths. A complete bath twice a week with partial baths on the other days is enough to maintain hygiene. Only mild soaps should be used. Often soap is not used on the arms, legs, back, chest, and abdomen. Lotions, oils, and creams are often recommended to prevent drying and itching. Deodorants usually are not needed because sweat gland secretion decreases (see Chapter 27 for hygiene). Follow the care plan.

An older client may complain of cold feet. Provide socks for warmth. Hot-water bottles and heating pads should not be used because of the risk of burns. Fragile skin, poor circulation, and decreased sensitivity to heat and cold increase the risk of burns.

Most older adults have grey or white hair. Some people colour their hair. Hair loss and thinning occurs in both men and women. Thinning occurs on the head, in the pubic area, and under the arms. Facial hair grows on the lips and chin of some older women. Decreased scalp oils lead to dry hair in older adults. Brushing helps stimulate circulation and oil production. Shampoo frequency depends on personal choice. Shampooing should be done as often as necessary for hygiene and comfort. Follow the care plan.

Signs of age are visible on a person's skin. The older adult and others can see grey hair, bald patches, brown spots, wrinkles, and sagging skin. These reminders of old age can affect an older adult's self-esteem and body image.

The Musculoskeletal System

Muscles atrophy (shrink) and decrease in strength. Bones lose strength, become brittle, and break easily. Sometimes just turning in bed can cause fractures (broken bones). Vertebrae shorten. Joints become stiff and painful. Hip and knee joints flex (bend) only slightly. These changes result in a gradual loss of height, loss of strength, and decreased mobility.

Activity and diet can help slow the rate of these changes. Older adults need to be as active as possible. A regular exercise program is helpful. Bathing, dressing, grooming, and other daily activities are forms of physical activity. Range-of-motion exercises are also helpful (see Chapter 22). An older adult's diet should be high in protein, calcium, and vitamins.

Remember, the bones of older adults can break easily. Protect your older clients from injury and prevent falls (see Chapter 16). Turn and move the person gently and carefully. Some older clients need help and support getting out of bed. Some need help walking.

The Nervous System

Aging affects the senses. Hearing and vision losses occur (see Chapter 36). The senses of taste and smell become dull. Touch and sensitivity to pain and pressure are reduced. So is the ability to feel heat and cold. These changes increase the risk for injury. The older adult may not feel pain when ill or injured. Or pain may be minor. Protect older adults from injury (see Chapter 16). Provide skin care, check for signs of skin breakdown, and prevent pressure ulcers (see Chapters 27 and 41).

(text continues on page 165)

Table 15-1 Physical Changes during the Aging Process

System	Changes
Integumentary	Skin becomes less elastic Skin loses its strength Brown spots ("age spots" or "liver spots") on the wrists and hands Fewer nerve endings Fewer blood vessels Fatty-tissue layer is lost Skin thins and sags Skin is fragile and easily injured Folds, lines, and wrinkles appear Decreased secretion of oil and sweat glands Dry skin Itching Increased sensitivity to heat and cold Decreased sensitivity to pain Nails become thick and tough Whitening or greying hair Loss or thinning of hair Facial hair in some women Drier hair
Musculoskeletal	Muscles atrophy Strength decreases Bones become brittle; can break easily Joints become stiff and painful Gradual loss of height Decreased mobility
Nervous	Vision and hearing decrease Decreased senses of taste, smell, and touch Reduced sensitivity to pain Reduced blood flow to the brain Cell shrinkage Shorter memory; forgetfulness Slower ability to respond Changes in sleep patterns Dizziness
Circulatory	Heart pumps with less force Arteries narrow and are less elastic Less blood flows through narrowed arteries Weakened heart has to work harder to pump blood through narrowed vessels
Respiratory	Respiratory muscles weaken Lung tissue becomes less elastic Difficulty breathing Decreased strength for coughing
Digestive	Decreased saliva production Difficulty in swallowing Decreased appetite Decreased secretion of digestive juices Difficulty digesting fried and fatty foods Indigestion Loss of teeth Decreased peristalsis, causing flatulence and constipation
Urinary	Reduced blood supply to kidneys Kidneys atrophy Kidney function decreases Urine becomes concentrated Urinary frequency, urgency, and incontinence may occur Night-time urination may occur
Reproductive Female	Menstruation stops Decreased estrogen production Ovaries and uterus decrease in size Vaginal walls are thinner, drier, and less elastic Loss of fat and elastic tissue in external genitalia Breasts are less firm
Male	Decreased testosterone production Decreased force of ejaculation Sperm count is reduced Testes are smaller Prostate gland enlarges Erections develop more slowly

Aging affects the cells in the brain. Cells shrink and blood flow to the brain is reduced. These changes affect response time, energy levels, and memory. Reflexes are slower. The person tires more easily. Forgetfulness occurs. The reduction in blood flow may also cause dizziness, which increases the risk for falls. Practise measures to prevent falls (see Chapter 16). Remind your older clients to rise slowly from beds or chairs. This helps prevent dizziness.

Sleep patterns change with age. Many older adults have difficulty falling asleep or wake often during the night. They may rest or nap during the day to prevent fatigue.

THE CIRCULATORY SYSTEM

The heart muscle weakens with age. It pumps blood through the body with less force. A weak heart muscle may not cause problems at rest. Activity, exercise, excitement, and illness increase the body's need for oxygen and nutrients. A weak heart may not be able to meet these needs.

Arteries narrow and become less elastic. Less blood flows through them, causing poor circulation in many body parts. A weak heart must worker harder to pump blood through narrow vessels.

Clients with severe circulatory problems need rest periods during the day. Activities should not cause overexertion. They should not walk long distances, climb many stairs, or carry heavy things. Personal care items, television controls, and other needed items should be kept nearby.

Moderate daily exercise stimulates circulatory, respiratory, digestive, and musculoskeletal functions. Exercise also helps prevent blood clots (thrombi) in leg veins. Many older adults engage in activities such as walking, biking, golf, tennis, swimming, and other forms of exercise. Active or passive range-of-motion exercises are necessary for clients on bed rest (see Chapter 22). Follow the care plan for exercise and activity levels.

THE RESPIRATORY SYSTEM

Respiratory muscles weaken with age and lung tissue becomes less elastic. Lung changes may not be noticed at rest. However, difficult, laboured, or painful breathing (**dyspnea**) may occur with activity. (*Dys* means difficult. *Pnea* means breathing.) Older adults may lack strength to cough and clear the airway of secretions. This puts them at risk for respiratory infections (such as pneumonia) and other diseases, which can be life threatening.

Normal breathing should be promoted. Heavy bed linens should not cover the client's chest because they can prevent normal chest expansion. Turning, repositioning, and deep breathing help prevent respiratory complications from bed rest. Breathing usually is easier in semi-Fowler's position (see Chapter 24). The client should be as active as possible.

THE DIGESTIVE SYSTEM

Changes in the digestive system occur with age. Salivary glands produce less saliva. This can cause difficulty swallowing (**dysphagia**). Secretion of digestive juices decreases. As a result, fried and fatty foods are hard to digest. Peristalsis decreases. Therefore, the stomach and colon empty at a slower rate, leading to flatulence and constipation. Other physical changes also affect appetite and enjoyment of food. Dulled senses of taste and smell decrease appetite and the enjoyment of food. Loss of teeth and ill-fitting dentures make chewing difficult. Chapter 25 discusses diet changes that help older adults address eating and digestive problems.

THE URINARY SYSTEM

Kidney function decreases with age. Blood flow to the kidneys is reduced and the kidneys atrophy. Removal of body wastes is less efficient. Urine is more concentrated. This is caused by decreased kidney function and not drinking enough fluids.

Bladder muscles weaken and the size of the bladder decreases. Therefore the bladder holds less urine. Urinary frequency or urgency may occur. Many older adults have to urinate several times during the night. Urinary incontinence (the inability to control the passage of urine from the bladder) may occur (see Chapter 29).

In men, the prostate gland enlarges, which causes pressure on the urethra. Difficulty urinating and frequent urination are common problems.

Older adults, especially women, are at risk for urinary tract infections. Adequate fluids are necessary. Intake should include water, fruit juices, and milk. Personal choice in beverages is important. Most fluids should be ingested before 1700 (5:00 p.m.). This reduces the need to urinate during the night. Bladder training programs may be necessary for those with urinary incontinence. Indwelling catheters are sometimes needed. Urinary elimination is discussed in Chapter 29.

THE REPRODUCTIVE SYSTEM

In men, the hormone testosterone decreases. This hormone affects strength, sperm production, and reproductive tissues. These changes affect sexual activity. It takes longer for an erection to occur. The phase between erection and orgasm is also longer. Orgasm is less forceful than in younger years. After orgasm, the erection is lost quickly. The time between erections is also longer. Older men may need the penis stimulated for sexual arousal. These changes result in decreased frequency of sexual activity.

Mental and physical fatigue, overeating, and excessive drinking affect erections. Some men fear performance problems. Therefore they may avoid sexual activity.

In women, menopause occurs around 50 years of age. At menopause, a woman stops menstruating. Her reproductive years end. Female hormones (estrogen and progesterone) decrease. Reduced hormone levels affect reproductive tissues. The uterus, vagina, and external genitalia atrophy. Intercourse may be uncomfortable or painful. This is because of thinning vaginal walls and vaginal dryness. Older women also have changes in sexual excitement. Arousal takes longer. The time between excitement and orgasm is longer. Orgasm is less intense. The pre-excitement state returns more quickly.

Frequency of sexual activity decreases for many men and women. Reasons relate to weakness, mental and physical fatigue, pain, chronic illness, and reduced mobility.

The Older Adult and Sexuality

Love, affection, and intimacy are needed throughout life. Sexuality is part of the whole person. The need for love and affection does not disappear in older adults (Figure 15-3). They have the right to be sexual and to form sexual relationships.

Some people cannot have sexual intercourse. This does not mean that sexual needs or desires are lost. They can express their needs in other ways. Handholding, touching, caressing, and embracing bring closeness and intimacy.

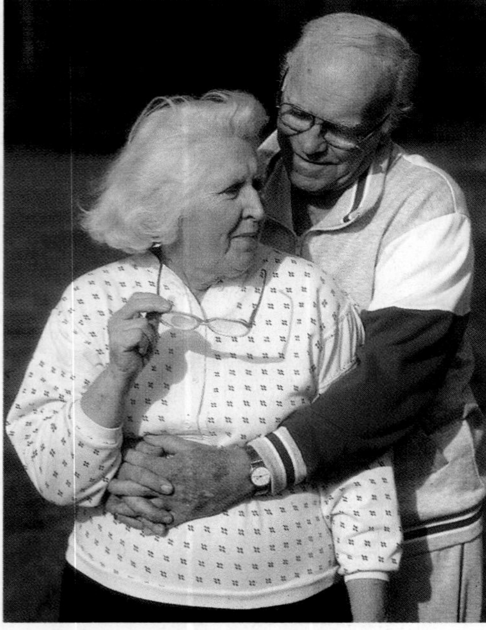

Figure 15-3 Love and affection are important to older adults.

Members of the health care team must respect their clients' sexuality. They allow and promote the meeting of sexual needs (Box 15-1 and *Focus on Long-Term Care: Residents' Sexual Rights* box).

Caring for Older Clients

Mainstream North American culture values youth. This is reflected in media messages that stress the importance of looking and acting young. There are ads for shampoos that cover grey hair and lotions that reduce

Box 15-1 Respecting and Promoting the Client's Sexuality

- Respect your client's clothing and grooming routines. Appearance is often an important part of sexual identity and expression. The client may want to spend extra time on grooming. Assist as needed.
- Accept the client's sexual relationships. He or she may not share your sexual attitudes, values, practices, or standards. The person may have a marital, premarital (before marriage), or extramarital (outside marriage) relationship. Or the person may have a homosexual (same sex) relationship. Do not judge or gossip about relationships.
- Allow privacy. Privacy is key to sexual expression. Knock before entering any room. This shows respect for privacy. It also saves you and the client possible embarrassment. Privacy is sometimes hard to find, especially in a facility. Remember the following if you work in a facility:
  - You can usually tell when two people want to be alone. If the client has a private room, close the door for privacy. Some facilities have *Do Not Disturb* signs for doors. Let the client and partner know how much time they have alone. For example, remind them about meal times or medications. Tell other staff members to avoid disturbing the couple.
  - Consider the client's roommate. Privacy curtains provide little privacy. Arrange for privacy when the roommate is out of the room. Sometimes roommates offer to leave for a while. If the roommate cannot leave, the nurse finds other private areas.
  - Allow privacy for masturbation. It is a normal form of sexual expression and release. Close the privacy curtain and the door. Sometimes people who are confused masturbate in public areas. Lead the person to a private area. Or distract him or her with an activity.

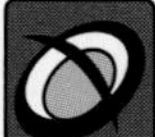

Focus on Long-Term Care

Residents' Sexual Rights

Married couples in long-term care facilities are allowed to share the same room, if one is available. This is required in long-term care legislation (see Chapter 10). The couple has lived together for many years. They have the right to be together in a facility. They can share the same bed if their conditions permit.

Sexual partners are lost through death and divorce. A resident may develop a relationship with another resident. They have the right to spend time together (Figure 15-4).

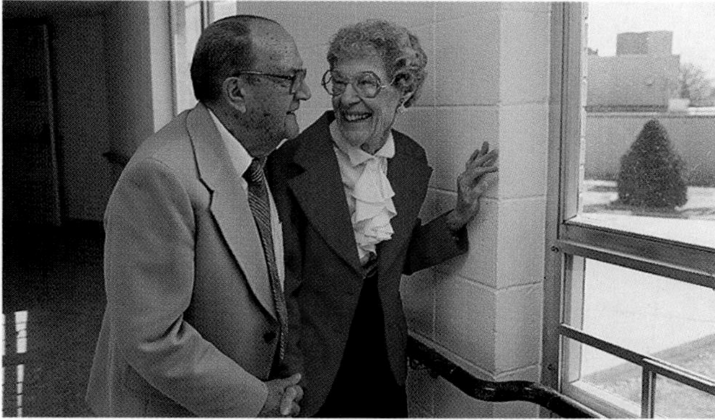

Figure 15-4 Relationships occur in long-term care facilities.

wrinkles. Greeting cards and cartoons often show older adults as grouchy, unproductive, simple, and slow.

Media images like these depict older adults as stereotypes. A **stereotype** is an overly simple or exaggerated view of a group of people. Stereotypes encourage discrimination against older adults. **Discrimination** is behaviour that treats people unfairly based on their group membership. **Ageism** is bias and discrimination against older adults. Treating all older people as boring, useless, or childlike is ageism. Remember, older adults are not all alike. Every person—young, middle-aged, or old—is unique. Every person develops and ages in his or her own way.

Older adults can think and make decisions for themselves. Failure to recognize this can make the person feel like a child. How would you feel if a younger person made decisions for you? Would you feel insulted or angry? Would you feel useless?

When older adults are not treated with respect, their dignity is threatened. The message is that they are no longer useful, productive members of society. Many older people are coping with the loss of loved ones, friends, and health. Loss of dignity and self-esteem can be too much for them to bear. Withdrawal from social contact and depression are risks. By treating older clients with respect, you help them maintain emotional and social health.

You need to understand the emotional, social, and physical changes that occur with aging. You must also be aware of each client's health status and needs. Always follow the care plan (see *Providing Compassionate Care: Supporting Older Clients* box).

Providing Compassionate Care

Supporting Older Clients

D*ignity.* Show respect for your older clients. Avoid using terms, gestures, or a tone of voice that could be considered patronizing (see Chapter 12). For example, never use the term "girl" when addressing an older female client. Some older adults find it rude to be addressed by their first names, especially by younger people. Ask your clients how they would like to be addressed. Never assume you can use a person's first name, even if you have heard your co-workers use it. Do not talk about the client with others. Do not exchange glances with co-workers about something an older client has said or done.

I*ndependence.* Help the client only when necessary. Respect the person's routine. Do things in the way the person is used to doing them. Allow time for rest. Avoid rushing the person.

P*references.* Older adults have the right to make choices. They must consent to all procedures. They make decisions regarding their care. They also choose when to get up and go to bed, what to wear, what activities to participate in, and what to eat. Always ask and accommodate a person's preferences.

P*rivacy.* Provide for privacy and keep information about the client confidential. All clients should be given privacy when visiting with others or when using the telephone. Do not expose the person. Drape and screen the person during procedures. Provide for privacy during elimination.

S*afety.* Be alert to safety hazards in the client's environment. Practise the safety measures in Chapter 16 to prevent falls, burns, poisonings, and suffocation. Only apply restraints if ordered by a physician and properly delegated.

Older adults may not have the usual signs of infection, such as fever, pain, inflammation, and swelling (see Chapter 18). The only signs of infection may be changes in behaviour. Observe for changes in behaviour, including sudden confusion, urinary incontinence, a fall, or a change in mood, energy levels, or eating habits. Be aware that some older adults are lonely and isolated. They are at risk for depression. Immediately report all changes in behaviour and health to your supervisor.

REVIEW

Circle the BEST answer.

1. Which of the following is *not* a usual developmental task of late adulthood?
   A. Adjusting to decreased physical strength
   B. Adjusting to retirement
   C. Seeking employment
   D. Coping with the death of a partner

2. Retirement usually results in
   A. A lower income
   B. Physical changes due to aging
   C. Less free time
   D. Financial security

3. Changes to the skin occur with aging. Care should include the following *except*
   A. Providing for warmth
   B. Applying lotion according to the care plan
   C. Using soap daily
   D. Providing good skin care

4. An older adult has cold feet. You should
   A. Provide socks
   B. Apply a hot-water bottle
   C. Soak the feet in hot water
   D. Apply a heating pad

5. Changes occur in the musculoskeletal system with aging. Which is *false*?
   A. Bones become brittle and can break easily.
   B. Older adults should avoid exercise.
   C. Joints become stiff and painful.
   D. Range-of-motion exercises help to slow the rate of musculoskeletal changes.

6. In older adults, arteries lose their elasticity and become narrow. These changes result in
   A. A slower heart rate
   B. Lower blood pressure
   C. Poor circulation to many body parts
   D. Less blood in the body

7. Mr. Steinberg, 88, has severe circulatory problems. You should do the following *except*
   A. Place personal items nearby
   B. Follow the care plan
   C. Plan activities to avoid exertion
   D. Allow him to carry heavy bags

8. Respiratory changes occur with aging. Which is *false*?
   A. Heavy bed linens prevent normal chest expansion.
   B. The person is turned and repositioned frequently if on bed rest.
   C. The side-lying position is best for breathing.
   D. The person should be as active as possible.

9. Older adults should avoid fried and fatty foods because of
   A. Decreases in saliva
   B. Ill-fitting dentures or loss of teeth
   C. Decreased amount of digestive juices
   D. A decreased sense of taste

10. A physician orders increased fluid intake for an older client. You should
    A. Give most of the fluid before 1700 (5:00 p.m.)
    B. Provide mostly water
    C. Start a bladder training program
    D. Insert an indwelling urinary catheter

11. The health care team in a long-term care facility should
    A. Discourage older residents from sexual expression and activity
    B. Allow and promote sexual expression and activity in older adults
    C. Expect every resident to have the same attitudes toward sex
    D. Not allow residents to masturbate, even in private

12. Which of the following is *false*?
    A. All older adults feel valued when support workers address them as "honey" and "dear."
    B. Patronizing language can harm an older adult's dignity.
    C. Loss of dignity can lead to withdrawal from social contact and depression.
    D. Disrespectful behaviour can make older adults feel undignified and useless.

Answers to these questions are on page 822.

CHAPTER

16

SAFETY

OBJECTIVES

- Define the key terms listed in this chapter
- Describe accident risk factors
- Describe the safety measures to prevent falls, burns, poisoning, and suffocation
- Explain how to prevent equipment accidents
- Identify fire prevention measures
- Explain what to do during a fire
- Describe how identifying the client, providing call bells, and using bed rails correctly promote client safety
- Explain how to protect yourself in the workplace

KEY TERMS

call bell A safety device for hospital patients and long-term care residents that enables them to call for assistance

hazardous material Any substance that presents a physical hazard or a health hazard in the workplace

incident report A report submitted whenever an accident, error, or unexpected problem arises in the workplace; occurrence report

occurrence report Incident report

OH&S (occupational health and safety) legislation Laws designed to protect employees from injuries and accidents in the workplace; these laws outline the rights and responsibilities of employers, supervisors, and workers

suffocation Occurs when breathing stops due to lack of oxygen

Workplace Hazardous Materials Information System (WHMIS) A national system that provides safety information about hazardous materials; includes labelling, material safety data sheets (MSDSs), and employee education

workplace violence Any physical assault or threatening behaviour that occurs in a work setting

Safety is a basic need and right. You, your clients, and your co-workers have the right to a safe setting. Promoting client safety is also one of the priorities of support work. Many clients are at great risk for accidents and injuries. Facilities and community care agencies try to create and maintain a safe environment for their clients. In a safe environment, clients have little risk of accidents or injuries. They feel safe and secure physically and emotionally.

Your employer is also responsible for providing a safe working environment for you. You are responsible for knowing basic safety measures to protect your clients and yourself.

Accident Risk Factors

Anyone can be accidentally injured. The following people, however, are especially vulnerable to accidents: children, older adults, and people living with illnesses or disabilities. Factors that increase these people's risk of accidental injury include:

- *Impaired awareness.* People need to be aware of their surroundings in order to protect themselves from injury. People who are unconscious are unaware of their surroundings and are unable to react or respond to danger. An unconscious person relies on others for protection. Some people who have intellectual disabilities, or who are confused or disoriented, might not be able to recognize and avoid danger. They could harm themselves. For example, a confused client may wander outside in the middle of winter without a coat, gloves, or boots.
- *Impaired vision.* Poor vision can lead to falls. People may not be able to see obstacles in their path (such as toys, furniture, or electrical cords). They may not be able to judge distances or depth. They may also have problems reading labels on medicines, cleaners, and other containers. Poisoning can result.
- *Impaired hearing.* People with impaired hearing have problems hearing explanations and instructions. They may not hear warning signals or fire alarms. If they are not alerted to danger, they do not know that they must move to safety.
- *Impaired taste, smell, and touch.* Diminished taste and smell may cause someone to eat spoiled food or not notice a gas leak. Diminished touch may make someone unable to feel hot and cold, pain and discomfort. For example, Mrs. Gagnon does not feel a blister from her new shoes. She has poor circulation to her legs and feet. The blister can become a serious wound.
- *Impaired mobility. Mobility* means ability to move. Aging, disease, and injury can affect mobility. Some people cannot walk or propel wheelchairs. Being unable to move oneself out of danger is a serious safety risk. Even minor changes in mobility increase accident risks. For example, a person with a sore knee may not be able to recover from a stumble and instead may fall.
- *Medications.* Medications have side effects. They include loss of balance, drowsiness, and lack of coordination. Reduced awareness, confusion, and

disorientation also can occur. The person may be fearful and uncooperative. These side effects increase the risk of accidents. They must be reported to your supervisor.

- *Age.* Children and older adults are at risk for injuries. See *Focus on Children: Accident Risk Factors* and *Focus on Older Adults: Accident Risk Factors* boxes.

Safety Measures

Your employer has safety policies to protect clients. For example, case managers check the client's home for safety hazards during the assessment phase. The case manager and other professionals take measures to correct safety hazards in the home. The care plan lists safety measures needed by the client. It is important to follow all safety policies and care plans.

Despite careful planning and policies, accidents can still happen. To protect clients, co-workers, and yourself, you must recognize common safety hazards. Common sense and simple safety measures can prevent most accidents. The safety measures listed in this chapter apply to facility and community settings.

Preventing Falls

Falls are the most common cause of accidental injuries in all settings. Children and older adults have the greatest risk of falls.

Children. Falls are the leading cause of injuries in children.[1] Infants can easily roll off a change table or bed. Falls out of highchairs and infant seats and falls down stairs are also common accidents among babies and children. Older children often fall when running or playing. Practise the safety measures listed in Box 16-1 on page 172 to prevent falls when caring for infants and children.

Older Adults and Others at Risk. Falls are also very common among older adults. The risk for falls increases with age and illness (Box 16-2 on page 172). Falls may result in death, serious injuries, or changes in the person's quality of life. For example, after a fall an older adult may avoid leaving the house for fear of falling. This may lead to feelings of isolation, anxiety, or depression. It may also lead to increased dependency on others.

Long-term care facility residents are at greater risk for falls than older adults living at home.[3] Residents tend to be older, use more medications, and have greater limits in their activities of daily living. Many have impairments that affect their abilities to think, remember, communicate, or concentrate; people with brain injuries, mental disabilities, dementia, and other conditions that cause confusion and disorientation are examples. All of these increase residents' risk for falls.

Many facilities have fall prevention programs. Patients and residents are assessed to determine their risk for falls. Those who are at high risk need extra supervision and assistance. Methods are used to identify them. The resident or patient may be given a coloured bracelet to wear. Or a sign, sticker, or tag may be placed above the person's bed, at the nurses' station, or on the person's chart.

Most falls occur in bedrooms, bathrooms, and on stairs. Many occur when the client rushes to get to the bathroom or commode without help. Most falls in

Focus on Children

Accident Risk Factors

Accidental injuries are the leading cause of death for Canadian children.[2] Infants are helpless. Young children cannot fully understand danger. They explore their surroundings, put objects in their mouths, and touch new things.

Children are at the greatest risk of being accidentally hurt during times of stress or changes in the family's routine. This is because the caregiver's attention is divided and supervision may not be as careful as usual. For example, when a family member is ill, the caregiver may be focused on the ill person rather than on the child.

Support workers often work with clients and their families during times of stress or change. When you are working with or around children, you must always be aware of possible dangers to them. Practise the safety measures to prevent falls, burns (page 174), poisoning (page 174), and suffocation (page 175). *Always supervise children closely.*

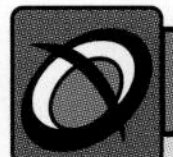

Focus on Older Adults

Accident Risk Factors

In Canada, adults aged 65 and over are killed or hospitalized because of accidental injuries more often than any other age group.[4] Any injury may be serious for older adults because their bodies take longer to heal and recover. An injury that may be minor to a younger person may be life-threatening to an older adult. A broken bone is an example.

Changes that occur with aging increase the risk for falls and other accidents. Joints are stiffer. Muscles are weaker. Movements are slower and less steady. Balance may be affected. Older adults are less sensitive to heat. Poor vision, hearing problems, and dulled senses of smell, taste, and touch are common. Some older adults may have memory problems, which make them more vulnerable to accidents (see Chapter 15).

Box 16-1 Safety Measures to Prevent Falls among Infants and Children

- Do not leave infants and young children unsupervised. Never leave them unattended in highchairs or on a table, couch, bed, or other high surface.
- Secure the child in a highchair or infant seat. Use both the waist and crotch straps. Lock the highchair tray after securing the child in the chair. Keep highchairs away from stoves, tables, and counters. The child could push off against these and fall.
- Do not use baby walkers; they have caused many serious falls and injuries.
- Use safety gates at the top and bottom of stairs. Make sure the child cannot get caught in the slats.
- Keep one hand on a child lying on a scale, bed, change table, or other furniture (Figure 16-1).
- Keep one hand on the baby when changing a diaper. Gather supplies before changing a diaper or bathing an infant. Place supplies within easy reach.
- Keep crib rails up and in the locked position. Check children in cribs often.
- Make sure there is nothing in the crib that the baby can stand on (like large stuffed toys or firm bumper pads). Standing on something in the crib could cause the baby to fall over the top of the railing.
- Do not let children under 6 years of age sleep or play on the top of a bunk bed.
- Keep children away from windows. Do not let them sit on window sills or lean on windows. Window screens are not strong enough to prevent a child from falling out. Do not put furniture underneath or near windows. Children could climb on them to reach the window.
- Do not let children run with objects in their hands or mouths (like baby bottles, soothers, or sticks). The object could cause injury if the child falls.
- Prevent furniture from falling onto children. Injuries and deaths can occur when children climb, pull on, sit on, lean on, or try to move furniture. TVs, bookcases, dressers, and tables are examples. Heavy furniture should be anchored to the wall.

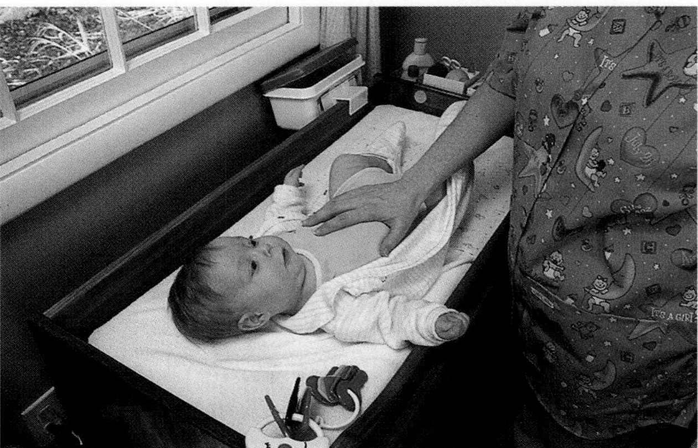

Figure 16-1 Keep one hand on a child lying on furniture.

Box 16-2 Factors Increasing the Risk of Falls

- Accident risk factors listed on pages 170–171
- A history of falls
- Muscle weakness
- Slow reaction time
- Foot problems
- Shoes that fit poorly
- Elimination needs—incontinence or frequent urination
- Dizziness and lightheadedness
- Dizziness on standing
- Joint pain and stiffness
- Low blood pressure
- Balance problems
- Depression
- Poor judgment
- Memory problems
- Strange surroundings
- Treatment equipment (IV poles, drainage tubes and bags, and others)
- Improper use of wheelchairs, walkers, canes, and crutches

facilities occur in the evening, between 1800 (6:00 p.m.) and 2100 (9:00 p.m.). Falls also are more likely during shift changes because confusion can occur about who gives care and answers calls for assistance.

The safety measures listed in Box 16-3 help prevent falls in home and facility settings. Many are included in fall prevention programs and care plans. Always follow the client's care plan for specific safety measures.

Preventing Poisoning

Accidental poisoning occurs most often in children between the ages of 1 and 4.[5] Eating poisonous substances, such as aspirin, cigarette butts, or vitamin pills, is a common cause of childhood poisoning. Poisoning also occurs when certain poisonous substances, such as oven cleaner or pesticide, spill on the skin and are absorbed into the body.

The most common ways adults are poisoned are by eating or drinking contaminated food and water and by overdosing on medications. Carelessness, confusion, and difficulty in reading medication labels can lead to accidental overdose. As a result, the person may take too much of a medication. Sometimes poisoning is a suicide attempt. Confused or disoriented adults may eat poisonous substances.

(text continues on page 174)

Box 16-3 Safety Measures to Prevent Falls among Older Adults and Others at Risk

- Report throw rugs and small mats that are not secure. They can be secured with carpet tape or nonskid backing. Make sure throw rugs and small mats are not in high-traffic areas or at the top of stairways.
- Report loose floor boards and tiles. Report frayed, torn, or bumpy rugs and carpets.
- Keep traffic areas free of telephone and electric cords. Cords and wires can be taped next to the wall so the client will not trip over them.
- Keep the floors and stairways free of clutter. Never leave items on the stairs.
- Use only nonglare and nonslip floor wax.
- Clean up water and other spills immediately.
- Ensure lighting is good, especially near stairways and bathrooms. Offer to replace burned-out light bulbs.
- Turn on night-lights in the halls, especially near the bathroom, in case the client has to get up in the middle of the night.
- Keep a clear path from the bedroom to the bathroom.
- Do not rearrange the client's furniture.
- Use nonslip rubber bathmats or nonslip strips in bathtubs and showers.
- Make sure the client's footwear and clothing fit properly. Shoes and slippers must be nonskid. Long shoelaces should be avoided. Clothing should not be loose or drag on the floor. Belts must be tied or secured in place.
- Ensure crutches, canes, and walkers have nonskid tips. Make sure the client uses these devices correctly.
- Check wheelchair brakes. Make sure you can lock and unlock them. Remind the client to keep the brakes locked when not moving the wheelchair. The brakes prevent the chair from moving if the client wants to transfer to or from the chair. Lock both brakes before you transfer the client to or from the wheelchair. Do not let the client stand on the footrests. Make sure front wheels point forward. This keeps the wheelchair balanced and stable. Remove the armrests and footrests (if removable) when the client transfers to or from the wheelchair (see Chapter 21).
- Encourage the client to wear glasses or hearing aids as needed. Reading glasses should not be worn when the client is up and about.
- Position the client in bed, chair, or wheelchair properly. Use pillows, wedge pads, or seats as the care plan directs.
- Check the client often. Careful and frequent observation is important, especially for those with risk factors.
- Electronic warning devices may be used. Weight-sensitive alarms placed on beds or wheelchairs detect movement or absence of weight and sound an alarm (Figure 16-2 on page 174). Respond to alarms at once.
- Place the call bell within the client's reach (see page 184). Ask the client to call for assistance when getting out of bed or a chair or when walking. Answer calls as soon as possible, before the client tries to get up without help.
- Offer assistance often to clients who need help with elimination. Help them to the bathroom as soon as requested, or offer a bedpan, urinal, or commode at regular times.
- Keep the bedpan or urinal within easy reach of those able to use these devices without help.
- Barriers are used to prevent wandering (Figure 16-3 on page 174).
- Keep beds in the lowest position, except when giving bedside care.
- Never leave the client alone when the bed is raised.
- Use bed rails strictly according to the care plan. If the client tends to get up without calling for assistance, the care plan may state that bed rails be left down. For other clients, the care plan may call for raised bed rails. Know your employer's rules for using bed rails. Bed rails can be unsafe if used incorrectly. Follow the care plan. See pages 185–187 for more safety rules regarding bed rails.
- Encourage clients to use handrails and grab bars. Facilities provide them in hallways, bathrooms, and on both sides of stairways to provide support for those who are unsteady when walking (Figure 16-4 on page 174).
- Lock the wheels on bed legs when giving bedside care and transferring the client.
- Be careful in facilities when turning corners, entering corridor intersections, and going through doors. A person coming from the other direction could be injured.
- In facilities, family and friends are asked to visit during busy times or during the evening and night shifts.
- A warm drink, soft lights, or a back massage is used to calm the client who is agitated.
- Companions are provided to sit with the client.
- In both facilities and homes, safety check the room after visitors leave. They may have lowered a bed rail, removed the call bell, or moved a walker out of reach. Or they may have brought an item that could harm the client.

A

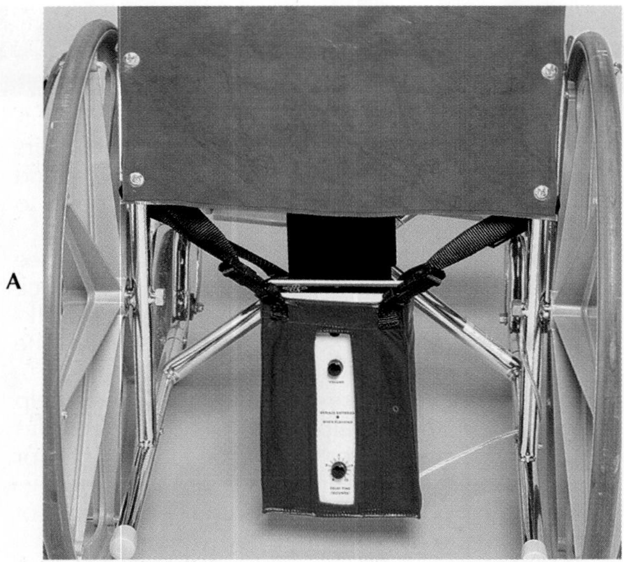

B

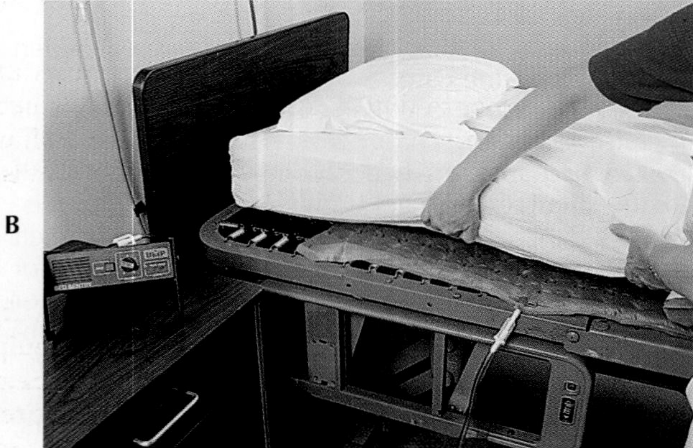

Figure 16-2 Weight-sensitive alarms may be used on wheelchairs or beds.

Common harmful substances include:

- Medications and vitamins
- Household cleaners—such as bleach, drain cleaner, floor wax, furniture polish, soaps, detergents, and toilet, window, and oven cleaners
- Personal care products—such as rubbing alcohol, nail polish and remover, shampoo and conditioner, bath oil, bubble bath, cosmetics, perfumes, deodorant, mouthwash, diaper wipes, and baby oils and powders
- Houseplants
- Insecticides, fertilizers, and insect sprays
- Alcohol and tobacco products, including nicotine gum, patches, and sprays

Follow the safety measures listed in Box 16-4 to prevent poisoning.

Preventing Burns

Burns are the third most common cause of accidental death in Canada.[6] There are varying degrees of burns, depending on the extent of tissue damage they cause (see Chapter 47). Children and older adults are at great risk for burns.

Hot liquids, such as coffee or tap water, are responsible for many childhood burns. For example, an adult carries a hot drink while a child is underfoot. The adult trips over the child and spills the hot liquid onto him or her.

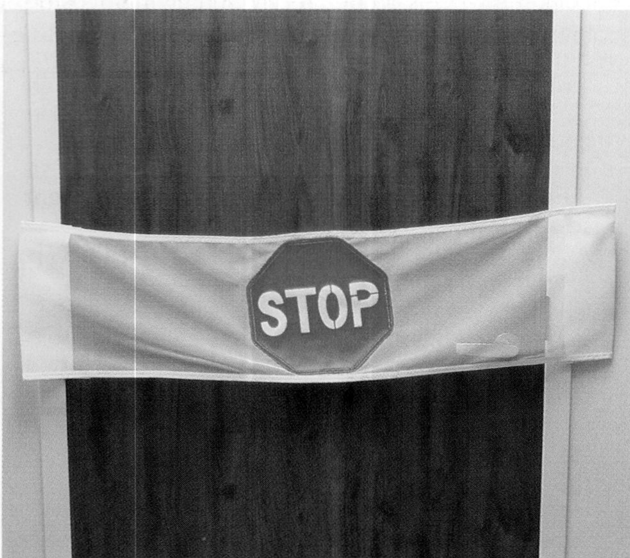

Figure 16-3 Barriers prevent wandering.

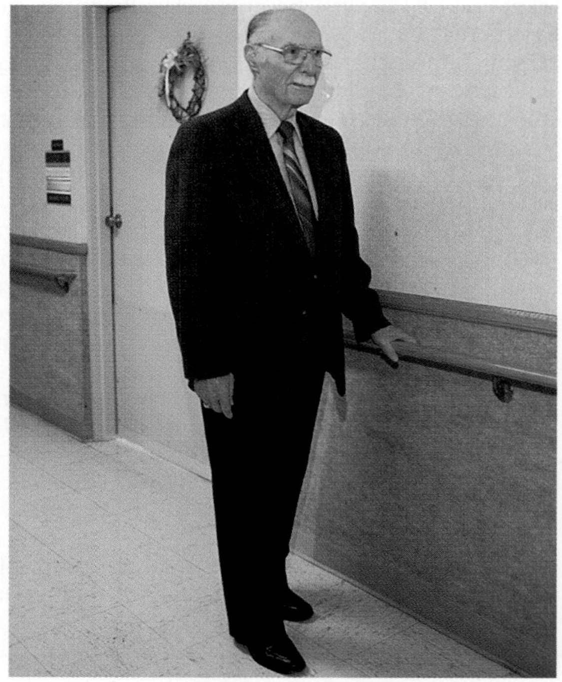

Figure 16-4 Handrails provide support when walking.

Box 16-4 Safety Measures to Prevent Poisoning

- Keep all harmful substances in high, locked areas where children or confused adults cannot see or reach them (Figure 16-5).
- Use and store harmful substances according to the manufacturer's instructions.
- Make sure all harmful substances are labelled and stored in their original containers. Do not store them in food containers or juice bottles. Do not store them near food.
- Keep childproof caps on all harmful substances.
- Put away household cleaners immediately after use.
- Do not mix cleaning products because this could cause harmful fumes.
- Never call medications or vitamins "candy."
- Do not leave your purse or workbag sitting out where children or others at risk can get into it, especially if you are carrying personal care supplies or your own medications.
- Keep plants where clients at risk cannot reach them.
- Do not let children play near walls with chipped paint. The paint may contain lead.
- Discard all food and drinks beyond their expiration dates. (See Chapter 25 for more information about food safety.)
- Keep phone numbers for the local poison control centre, police, and ambulance by the telephone.

Many burns to older adults occur in the kitchen. A common hazard is cooking while wearing loose-fitting sleeves. The sleeves might dangle over the burner and catch on fire. Bathwater and heating pads that are too hot also cause burns. Box 16-5 on page 176 lists safety measures to prevent burns.

Preventing Suffocation

Suffocation occurs when breathing stops due to lack of oxygen. Brain damage or death may occur depending on how long the person is without oxygen. Common causes include choking, drowning, inhaling gas or smoke, strangulation, and electrical shock. Children under 1 year of age and clients with serious mobility or mental impairments are at risk of suffocation. So are clients who have difficulties chewing and swallowing. Box 16-6 on page 177 lists safety measures to prevent suffocation.

Preventing Equipment Accidents

In homes and facilities, you will be required to use equipment such as household appliances, mechanical lifting devices, wheelchairs, and walkers. All equipment is unsafe if broken, not used correctly, or not working properly.

When using any type of equipment, you must know what you are doing. You also must make sure that the equipment is in safe working order. Follow the safety measures in Box 16-7 on page 178 to prevent equipment accidents.

Preventing Fires

Fires are a constant danger in homes and facilities. Unsafe smoking, cooking accidents, faulty electrical equipment and wiring, and heating equipment are major causes. The entire health care team must prevent fires. Box 16-8 on page 179 lists fire prevention measures. (See also *Focus on Home Care: Fire Safety* box on page 179.)

Fires and the Use of Oxygen. Some people have difficulty breathing or do not receive enough oxygen through the air. Physicians order oxygen therapy for them. This means they receive additional

(text continues on page 179)

A 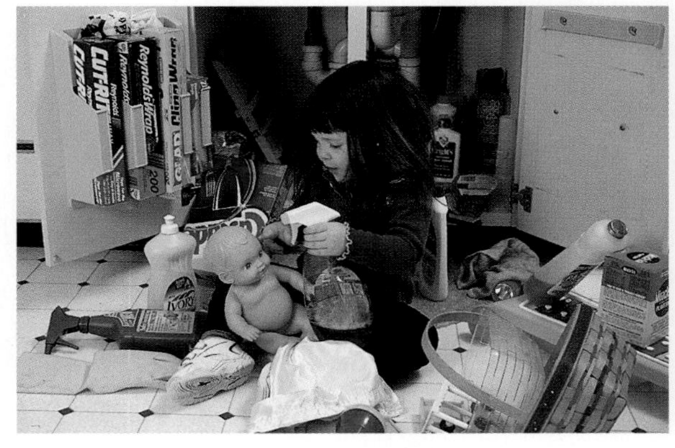

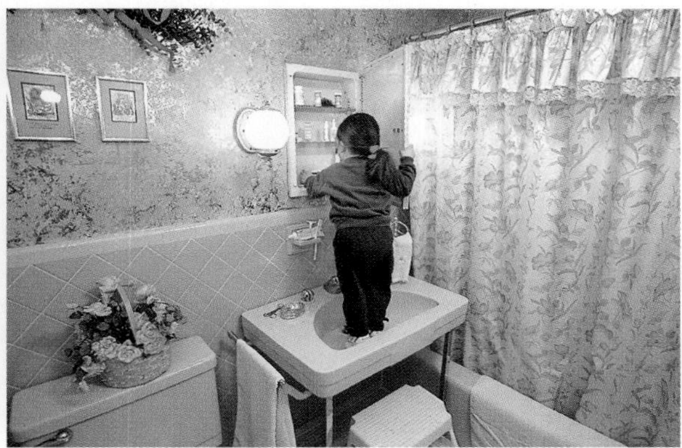 B

Figure 16-5 Harmful substances must be kept in locked areas out of the reach of children and confused adults. **A**, Household cleaners are within reach when in low cabinets. **B**, The bathroom medicine chest holds many hazardous substances.

Box 16-5 Safety Measures to Prevent Burns

PROTECTING CHILDREN

- Do not drink or carry hot liquids near infants and children. Make sure children are not underfoot when you are carrying anything hot, including drinks, clothes irons, or dishes from the oven.
- Do not heat a baby bottle or baby food in a microwave. Always shake the bottle or stir the food before giving it to the baby.
- Keep hot foods and liquids away from counter and table edges where children can reach them.
- Avoid using tablecloths or placemats that can be pulled down by a child.
- Always test bathwater before bathing a child. Position the child facing away from water faucets. Do not let children touch faucet handles.
- Never leave a "live" extension cord lying out (that is, one end is plugged in and the other end is free). A child could pick it up and put it in the mouth, resulting in severe burns to the mouth.
- Put safety plugs in all unused electrical outlets (Figure 16-6).
- Keep pot handles pointed toward the back of the stove. Use the back burners on the stove rather than the front whenever possible. Turn off stove and burners when not in use.
- Do not let children help you cook at the stove.
- Do not let electric cords from irons, coffee pots, toasters, etc., hang down where children could pull on them.
- Do not let children play near hot stoves, space heaters, fireplaces, and other heat sources.

PROTECTING OLDER ADULTS AND OTHERS AT RISK

- Educate clients about the dangers of wearing loose-fitting sleeves while cooking.
- In facilities, be sure clients smoke only in designated smoking areas.
- Supervise clients who smoke and who cannot protect themselves.
- Do not allow smoking in bed. The client could fall asleep and drop the cigarette into the bed sheets or could ignite his or her clothing.
- Follow safety guidelines when applying heat and cold (see Chapter 42).
- Always test the water in the tub, shower, or basin before bathing an adult or helping an adult bathe. Measure water temperature. Check for "hot spots" in water. Move your hand back and forth.
- Assist with eating and drinking as needed. Spilled hot foods and fluids can cause burns.

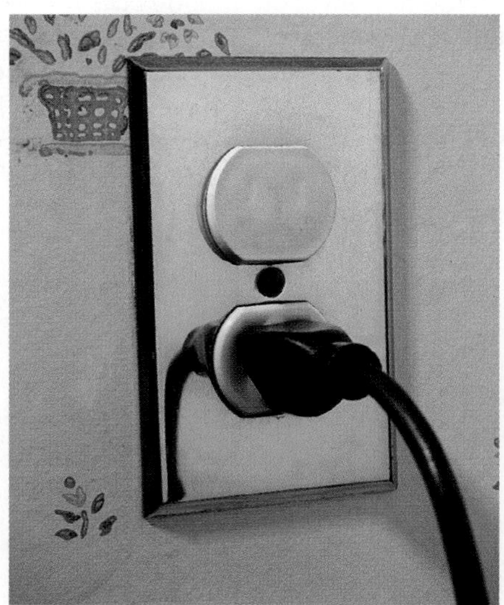

Figure 16-6 Safety plug in an outlet.

Box 16-6 Safety Measures to Prevent Suffocation

Protecting Children

- Always supervise children while they are eating. Grate, mash, blend, or chop food into very small pieces before giving it to a baby. Do not give infants and young children hot dogs, raw carrots, peanuts, popcorn, whole grapes, raisins, hard candy, or gum.
- Do not prop bottles on a rolled towel or blanket. Hold the baby and bottle during feedings.
- Check floors for small objects like coins, buttons, marbles, pins, and paper clips. Children can choke on them.
- Do not allow children to blow up balloons or put one in their mouths. Immediately dispose of any broken balloon pieces.
- Keep all plastic bags and wrappings away from children.
- Do not let children wear necklaces, strings, cords, or other items around their necks. These can become tightly twisted or get caught on furniture. Remove bibs before placing infants in cribs.
- Remove or tie up cords or drawstrings on all articles of children's clothing. This includes drawstrings in the hood, at the neckline, and at the waist.
- Keep cords for blinds, curtains, and drapes out of children's reach. Tie cords up or use a cord shortener. Make sure cribs and playpens are placed far away from blinds, shades, or drapes. Do not hang items with strings, cords, or elastic around cribs or playpens.
- Position infants on their backs for sleep.
- Make sure crib mattresses fit snugly and are very firm. The space between crib rail slats must be no more than 6.3 cm (2⅜ inches). Never let infants sleep on a waterbed. They should sleep only on firm, flat surfaces.
- Do not use pillows to position infants or prevent them from falling off beds or furniture.
- Remove pillows, comforters, quilts, sheepskin, stuffed toys, and other soft items from the crib when the baby is sleeping.
- Always supervise children who are in or near water. This includes tubs, toilets, sinks, buckets and containers, wading pools, and swimming pools.
- Keep bathroom doors closed to prevent drowning in toilets or bathtubs. Keep toilet seats down and use toilet safety locks.
- Keep sinks, tubs, basins, and buckets empty when not in use.
- Keep diaper pails locked.
- Do not leave children unattended in a vehicle. They can suffocate very quickly from high temperatures in the vehicle.

Protecting Others at Risk

- When feeding adults, do not rush them. Cut food into small, bite-sized pieces for clients who cannot do so themselves.
- Make sure the client's dentures fit properly and are in place. Report loose teeth or dentures.
- Check the care plan for swallowing problems before serving food or fluids. The client may ask for something that he or she cannot swallow.
- Tell your supervisor at once if the client has problems swallowing.
- Do not give oral food or fluids to clients with feeding tubes. Follow aspiration precautions (see Chapter 26).
- Open doors and windows if you notice gas odours. Report gas odours to your supervisor.
- Position the client in bed properly (see Chapter 21).
- Use bed rails properly (see pages 185–187).
- Use restraints correctly (see Chapter 17).

Box 16-7 Safety Measures to Prevent Equipment Accidents

- Follow employer policies and procedures.
- Follow the manufacturer's instructions.
- Read all caution and warning labels.
- Do not use unfamiliar equipment. Ask for needed training. Ask for supervision the first time you use the item.
- Use equipment only for its intended purpose.
- Inspect all equipment before use. Check for broken or damaged parts. Check for cracks, chips, rough or sharp edges, or loose bolts or screws. These can cause cuts, stabs, or scratches. Do not use or give damaged items to clients.
- Notify your supervisor immediately about the broken equipment. Follow your employer's policies for reporting equipment in need of repair or equipment-related accidents.
- Do not try to repair broken equipment yourself.
- Make sure electrical cords are not frayed or damaged in any way (Figure 16-7). Make sure there are not too many cords plugged into one electrical outlet (Figure 16-8). Frayed cords and overloaded electrical outlets can cause electrical shocks.
- Make sure all electrical equipment has three-pronged plugs (Figure 16-9). Two prongs carry electrical current. The third prong is the ground. A ground carries leaking electricity to the earth and away from the item, preventing electrical shock.
- Stop using electrical equipment and report it to your supervisor if:
  - It gives you a shock
  - It produces sparks, buzzing sounds, or a burning odour
  - Lights dim or flicker
  - The power shuts down
- Immediately report any shock received while using a piece of equipment.
- Keep electrical equipment away from water (water conducts electricity).
- Hold on to the plug (not the cord) when removing it from an outlet.
- Turn off equipment when you are finished using the item.

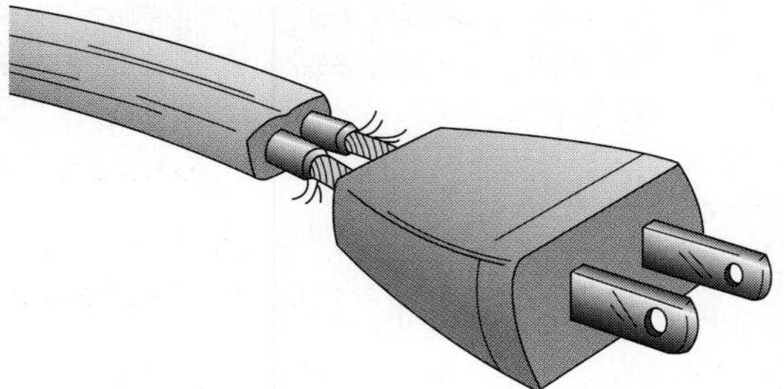

Figure 16-7 A frayed electrical cord.

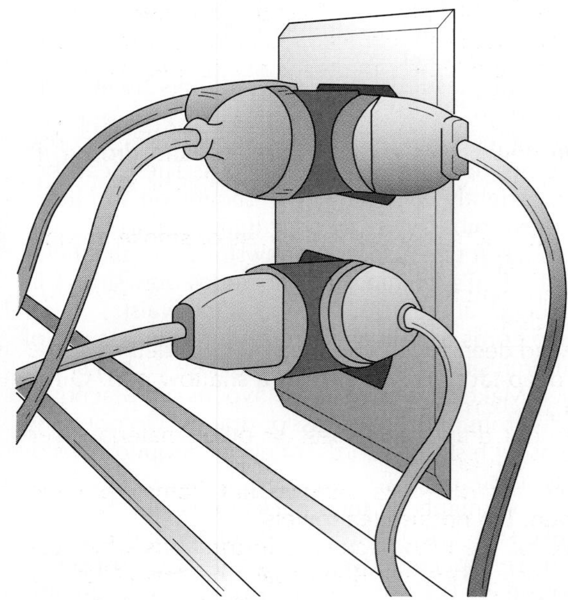

Figure 16-8 An overloaded electrical outlet.

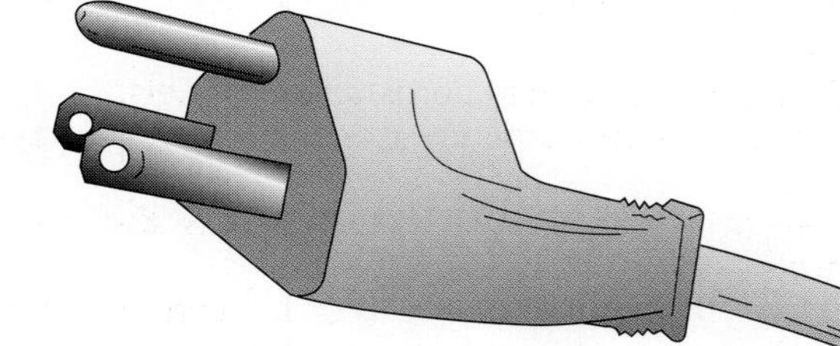

Figure 16-9 A three-pronged plug.

Box 16-8 Safety Measures to Prevent Fires

- Smoke only where allowed to do so. Do not smoke in the client's home.
- Supervise clients who smoke. This is very important for people who are confused, disoriented, or sedated.
- Provide ashtrays for clients who are allowed to smoke.
- Check smoking areas and especially furniture for dropped cigarettes and ashes.
- Be sure all ashes, cigars, and cigarettes are extinguished before emptying ashtrays.
- Empty ashtrays into a metal container partially filled with sand or water. Do not empty them into plastic containers or wastebaskets lined with paper or plastic bags.
- Do not allow clients to smoke in bed or while lying down; they could fall asleep and drop a lit cigarette onto the sheets or cushion, starting a fire.
- Do not light matches or lighters or smoke around flammable liquids or materials.
- Keep matches and lighters out of the reach of children.
- Avoid deep-frying in oil. If you must deep fry, use a deep-fat fryer rather than a shallow pan. Oil is highly flammable.
- Do not drape tea towels or other material over the oven door.
- Use potholders to remove hot items from the oven. Do not use tea towels.
- Follow the manufacturer's instructions when using space heaters. Keep space heaters at least 1 metre (3 feet) away from curtains, drapes, and furniture. Do not leave space heaters unattended.
- Keep flammable liquids and materials away from fireplaces, radiators, registers, and other sources of heat or flame.
- Store flammable liquids in their original containers.
- Do not run electrical cords under carpets.
- Use extension cords only as a temporary measure.
- Prevent equipment accidents. Follow the measures listed in Box 16-7.
- Follow the safety measures for oxygen use (Box 16-9 on page 180 and Chapter 43).

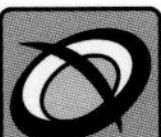

Focus on Home Care

FIRE SAFETY

It is essential to have working smoke detectors on every floor of the home and ideally outside each sleeping area. Always locate smoke detectors in clients' homes. Make sure they are working. Notify your supervisor and the family if a smoke detector does not work.

oxygen through a nasal tube or facemask. The oxygen is supplied through portable oxygen tanks, wall outlets, or oxygen concentrators (see Chapter 43).

Oxygen systems are widely used in facilities and in home care. However, oxygen is a serious fire hazard. It is extremely flammable. It saturates clothing, towels, and sheets, increasing the risk of a fire. Special safety measures are needed where oxygen is used and stored (see Box 16-9 on page 180).

What to Do During a Fire. The health care team must act quickly and responsibly during a fire. The key to surviving a fire is to be prepared before one starts. Know your employer's policies and procedures for fire emergencies. Know where to find fire alarms, fire extinguishers, and emergency exits. Facilities conduct fire drills to practise emergency fire procedures (see *Focus on Home Care: Being Prepared for a Fire* box on page 180).

The acronym RACE will help you remember what to do if you discover a fire in a home or a facility:

- **R**—for *rescue*. Rescue people in immediate danger. Move them to a safe place.
- **A**—for *alarm*. Sound the nearest fire alarm. Notify the switchboard operator. Or call 911 if in a home.
- **C**—for *confine*. Close doors and windows to confine the fire. Turn off oxygen or electrical equipment in use in the general area of the fire.
- **E**—for *extinguish* or *evacuate*. Use a fire extinguisher on a small fire that has not spread to a larger area. If the fire cannot be easily extinguished, evacuation will be necessary.

Always keep equipment away from all exits.

Using a Fire Extinguisher. Facilities require that all employees demonstrate use of a fire extinguisher. Fire extinguishers are readily available in facilities. Home care clients should also have them available. If the client has a fire extinguisher in the home, locate it and make sure it works. Notify your supervisor and the family if the fire extinguisher does not work.

Never attempt to fight a large or spreading fire with an extinguisher. Fire extinguishers are only useful against small fires that have not spread from where they have started. For example, the fire has started and is contained to a wastebasket or cushion. Do not use a fire extinguisher on a fire that is fed by gas or flammable liquid.

Box 16-9 Safety Measures for Using Oxygen

- Never smoke around oxygen equipment. Remove all smoking materials from the room (such as ashtrays and lighters).
- "No Smoking" and "Oxygen in Use" signs are placed on the front door of the client's home, apartment, or room and near where the oxygen is being directly used. Some people ignore such rules. Remind the client, family, and visitors to not smoke around oxygen equipment.
- Keep oxygen tanks away from open flames (such as pilot lights, candles, and incense) and heat sources (such as stoves, heating ducts, radiators, and space heaters).
- Remove materials from the room that easily ignite. Alcohol, nail polish remover, oils, and greases are examples.
- Make sure the client does not use flammable toiletries when receiving oxygen. Perfume, hairspray, and after-shave lotion are examples.
- Turn off electrical items before unplugging them. Sparks occur when electrical items are unplugged while turned on.
- Use electrical equipment only if it has a three-pronged plug and is in good working order. This includes shavers, hair dryers, radios, and stereo equipment.
- Remove all wool and synthetic fabrics from the room because they could create static electricity. Wear cotton uniforms and use cotton blankets and clothing for the client.

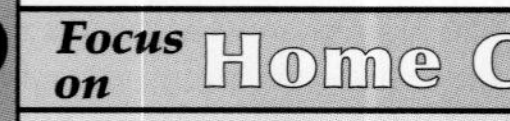

Focus on Home Care

BEING PREPARED FOR A FIRE
Plan what to do in each client's home before an emergency. The first time you enter a client's home, plan two fire escape routes from every room. If the client lives in an apartment building, find the fire alarms in the hallways in case you ever need them.

Different extinguishers are used for different kinds of fires:

- Paper and wood fires
- Oil and grease fires
- Electrical fires

Using the wrong extinguisher on a fire makes the fire worse. Many extinguishers are multipurpose, designed to fight all types of fires. Learn how to use a fire extinguisher *before* an emergency.

Evacuating. When evacuating a facility or home, several safety measures apply (Box 16-10). Facilities have evacuation policies and procedures. If evacuation is necessary, people closest to the danger are taken out first. Those who can walk are given blankets to wrap around themselves. A staff member escorts them to a safe place. Figure 16-11 on page 182 and Figure 16-12 on page 183 show how to rescue people who cannot walk. Once firefighters arrive, they direct rescue efforts.

PROVIDING SAFE CARE DURING PROCEDURES

Safety is a priority when performing procedures. This book describes procedures that you need to know for client care. Certain measures are used to promote the client's safety. These include identifying the client, placing call bells within reach, and using bed rails according to the care plan.

Using a Fire Extinguisher

Procedure

1. Pull the fire alarm. Make sure everyone in danger is moved to safety.
2. Get the nearest fire extinguisher.
3. Carry it upright.
4. Take it to the fire.
5. Make sure you have an escape route behind you.
6. Remove the safety pin (Figure 16-10, A).
7. Direct the hose at the base of the fire (Figure 16-10, B).
8. Push the top handle down to start the spray (Figure 16-10, C).
9. Sweep the nozzle back and forth at the base of the fire.

A

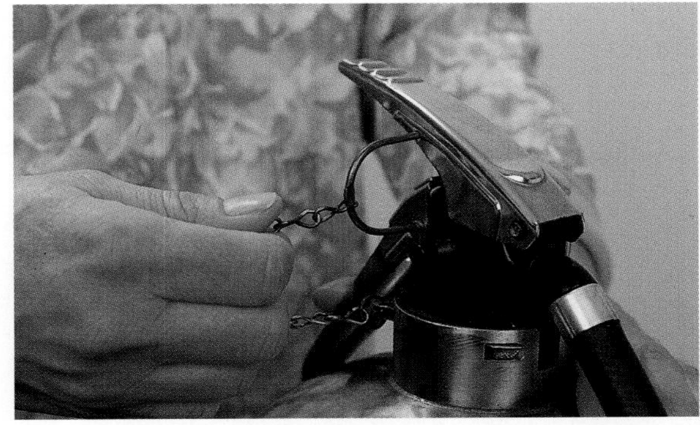

B

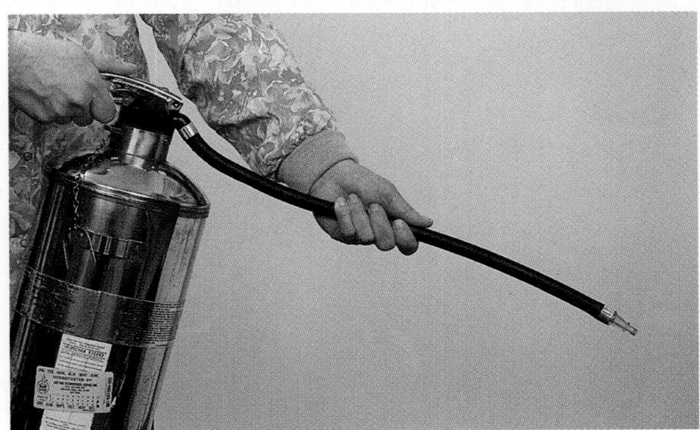

C

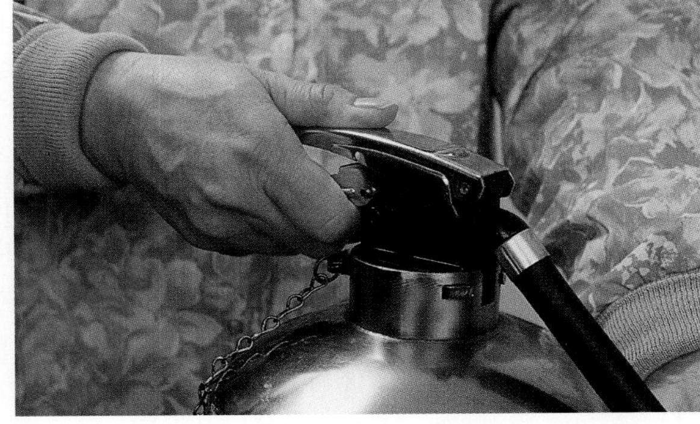

Figure 16-10 Using a fire extinguisher. **A**, Remove the safety pin. **B**, Direct the hose at the base of the fire. **C**, Push the top handle down.

Identifying the Client

You will care for many people. Each has different treatments, therapies, and activity limits. Before doing a procedure, make sure you are giving the right care to the right person. Follow employer policies and procedures for identifying clients. Life and health are threatened if the wrong care is given.

In home care settings, identifying the client is easy. There is usually only one client per home. Make sure you bring the right assignment sheet for the right home. In other community settings like group homes and assisted-living facilities, you might have more than one client in the home. Always make sure you are giving the right care to the right person. Read the name on the care plan carefully.

In long-term care facilities, many residents are receiving care in the same place. You will often care for the same residents over an extended period of time. You will get to know these residents very well and will easily recognize them. Be careful to give the right care to the right person. Check the resident's name and room number on the assignment sheet carefully. Do not confuse one resident's care plan with another's. Some long-term care facilities have a photograph identification system. The resident's picture is taken on admission. The photo is placed in the person's medical record. Other facilities post identifying information in the resident's room. Find out your employer's policies and procedures for identifying residents.

In hospitals, patients usually are admitted and discharged within a short period of time. You may not recognize your clients. Therefore hospitals usually assign identification (ID) bracelets to patients (Figure 16-13 on page 184). Information on the bracelet includes the patient's name, room and bed number, age, gender, and physician.

(text continues on page 184)

Box 16-10 Safety Measures for Evacuating a Building

- Never use elevators in a building on fire.
- Touch doors before opening them. Do not open a hot door. Use another way out. If the door is cool, open it carefully. If heat and smoke rush in, shut the door again.
- If smoke is present, look for another escape route that is smoke-free. If you must exit through smoke, cover your nose and mouth with a damp cloth. Do the same for the client and family. Have everyone crawl to the nearest exit to remain below the smoke.
- If your clothes catch on fire, do not run. Drop to the ground. Cover your face. Roll to smother the flames. If possible, wrap yourself in a rug or blanket. If another person's clothing is on fire, get the person to the floor. Roll the person or cover the person with a blanket or coat.
- Once you and your client get out of the burning building, never go back in.
- If you get trapped in a room by fire or smoke, shut the door and block any cracks with blankets or other thick material that will keep smoke from entering the room. If possible, call 911 or the fire department and tell them exactly where you are in the building. Go to the window and shout for help and hang something from the window, such as a towel, sheet, or clothing. This will attract the firefighters' attention.

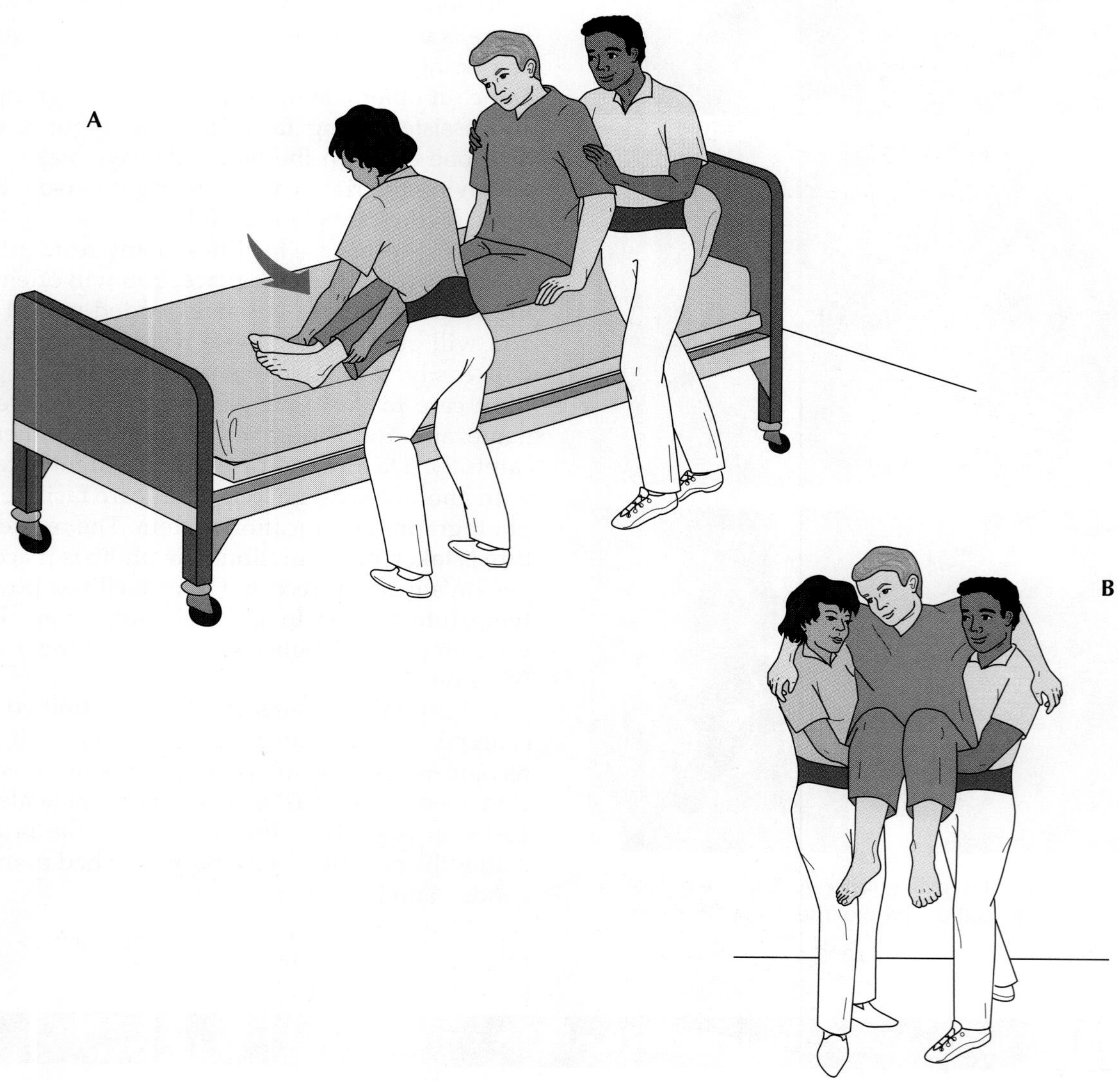

Figure 16-11 Swing carry technique. **A**, Assist the client to a sitting position. A co-worker grasps the client's ankles as you both turn the client so that he sits on the side of the bed. **B**, Pull the client's arm over your shoulder. With one arm, reach across the client's back to your co-worker's shoulder. Reach under the client's knees and grasp your co-worker's arm. Your co-worker does the same.

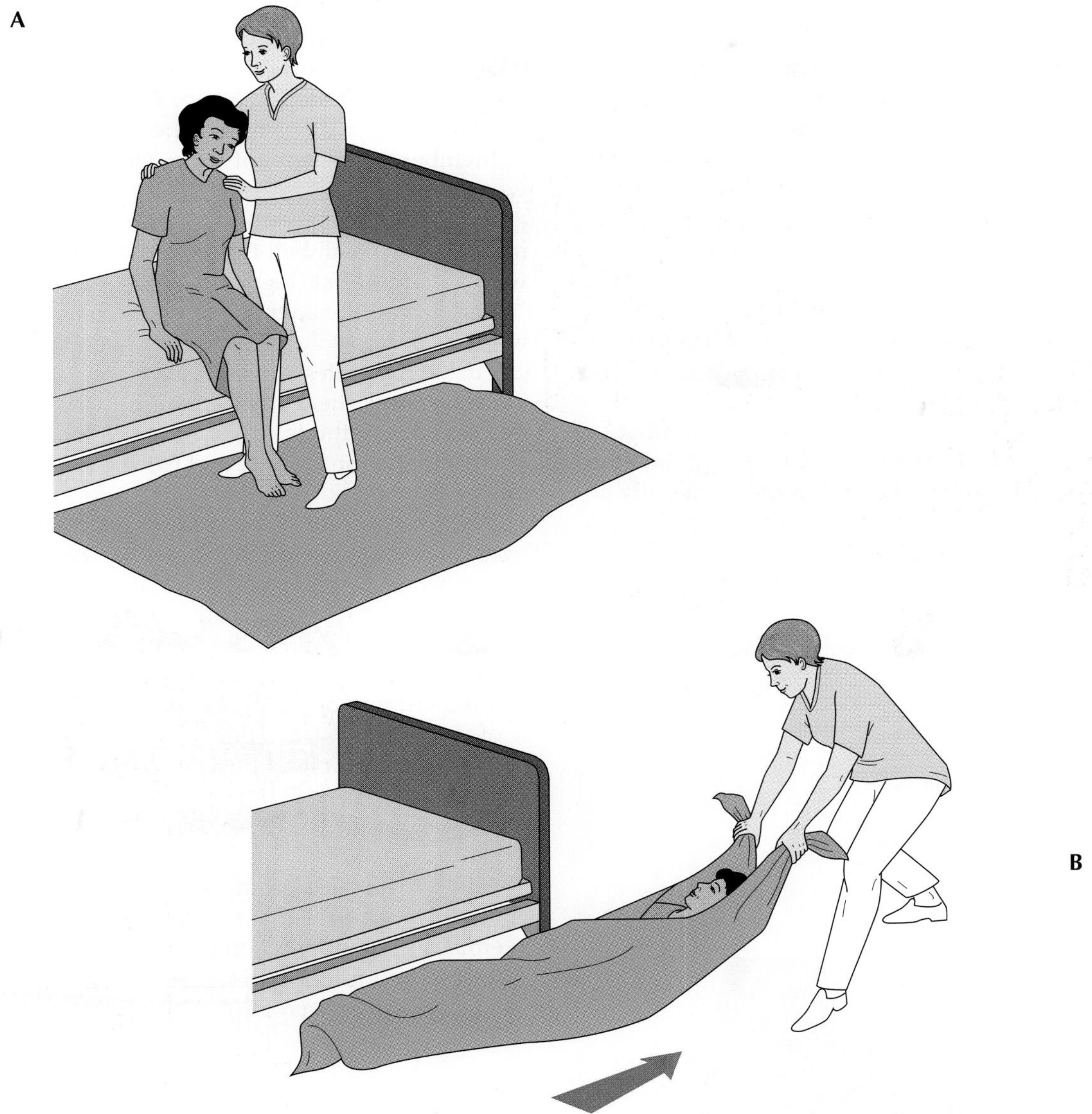

Figure 16-12 One-rescuer carry. **A**, Spread a blanket on the floor. Make sure the blanket will extend beyond the client's head. Help the client sit on the side of the bed. Grasp the client under the arms, and cross your hands over her chest. Lower the client to the floor by sliding her down one of your legs. **B**, Wrap the blanket around the client. Grasp the blanket over the head area. Pull the client to a safe area.

Use the ID bracelet to identify the person before giving care. Treatment cards or assignment sheets state what care to give. To identify a client in a hospital:

- Compare identifying information on the treatment card or assignment sheet with that on the ID bracelet (Figure 16-14). Carefully check the person's full name. Some people have the same first and last names. For example, John Smith is a very common name.
- Call the person by name when checking the ID bracelet. This is a courtesy given as you touch the person and before giving care. However, just calling the person by name is not enough to identify him or her. Confused, disoriented, drowsy, hearing-impaired, or distracted people may answer to any name.

Using the Call Bell

Call bells are important safety devices for hospital patients and long-term care residents. A **call bell** lets a client call for assistance. The term "call bell" is used in this book when referring to any one of a number of call systems that a facility may use. Different facilities use different call systems. However, they generally all consist of a cord that attaches to the bed or chair. A button is at the end of the cord (Figure 16-15). To get help, the client presses the button, which causes a signal to ring at the nurses' station. Or, pressing the button may switch on a light above the client's door and at the nurses' station (Figure 16-16, *A*). These tell the health care team that the client needs assistance.

Some call bells are also connected to an intercom at the nurses' station (Figure 16-16, *B*). Using the intercom, a support worker or a nurse can talk with the client who has called for help. The client can tell you what is needed. Be careful when using an intercom. Remember confidentiality. People nearby can hear what you say.

Some clients have limited hand mobility. They may need a special call bell that is turned on by tapping it with a hand or fist (Figure 16-17).

Patients and residents learn how to use the call bell when admitted to a facility. Some people cannot use call bells. Examples are people who are confused or in a coma. Check the care plan carefully for special communication methods. Check these people often and make sure their needs are met (see *Focus on Home Care: Call Bells* box).

Whenever you finish a procedure and leave the client's room, make sure the call bell is within the client's reach. You must:

- Keep the call bell within the client's reach in the room, bathroom, and shower or tub room. Even if the client cannot use the call bell, keep it within reach of visitors and staff. They may need to call for help.
- Place the call bell on the client's strong (unaffected) side.
- Remind the client to use the call bell when help is needed.
- Answer call bells promptly. The client may have an urgent need to use the bathroom. You can prevent embarrassment by promptly helping the person to the bathroom. A prompt response also helps prevent infection, skin breakdown, pressure ulcers, and falls.

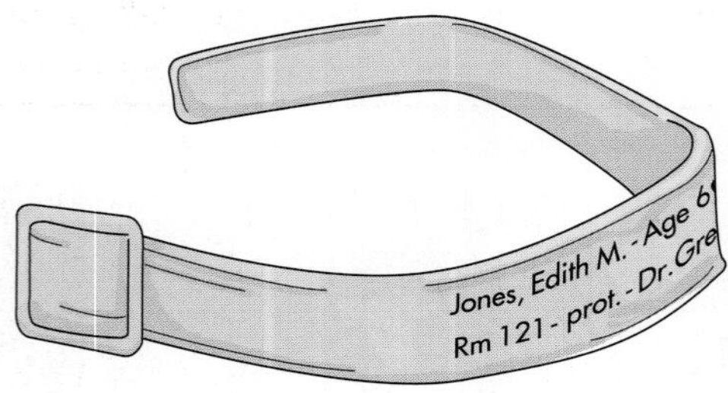

Figure 16-13 ID bracelet.

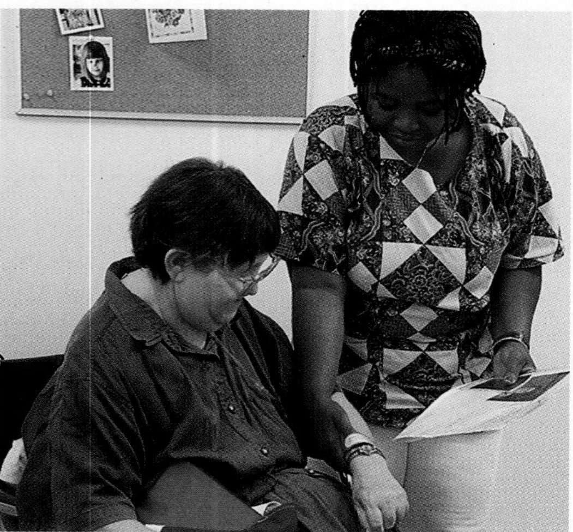

Figure 16-14 In hospitals, compare the ID bracelet against the assignment sheet to accurately identify the client.

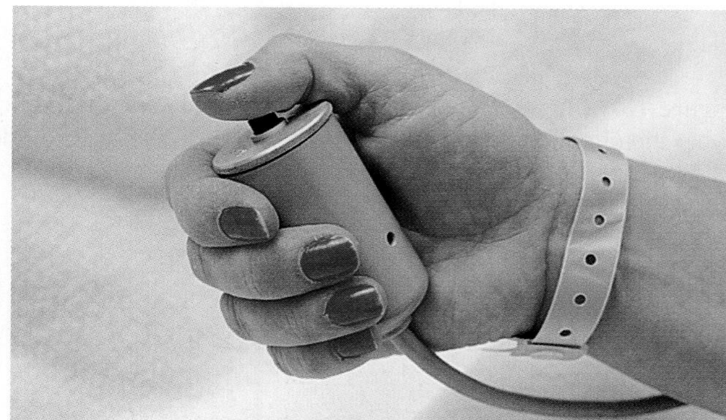

Figure 16-15 A client presses the button when assistance is needed.

A

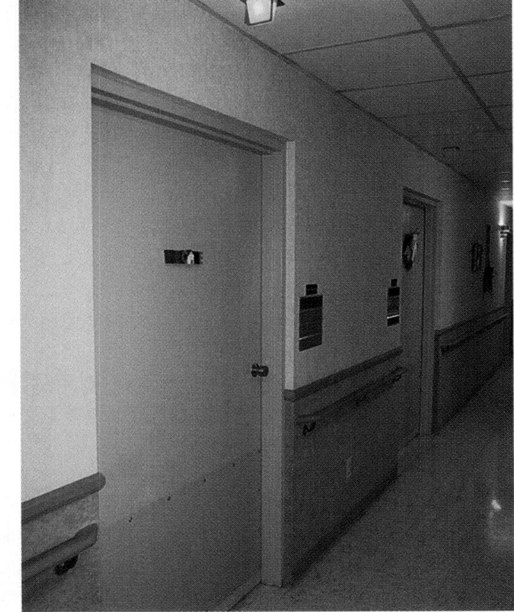

B

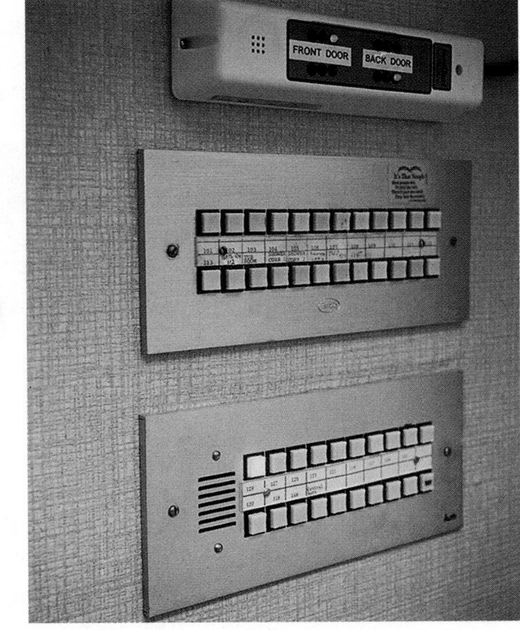

Figure 16-16 **A,** The light above the door of the client's room. **B,** Light panel of intercom system at the nurses' station.

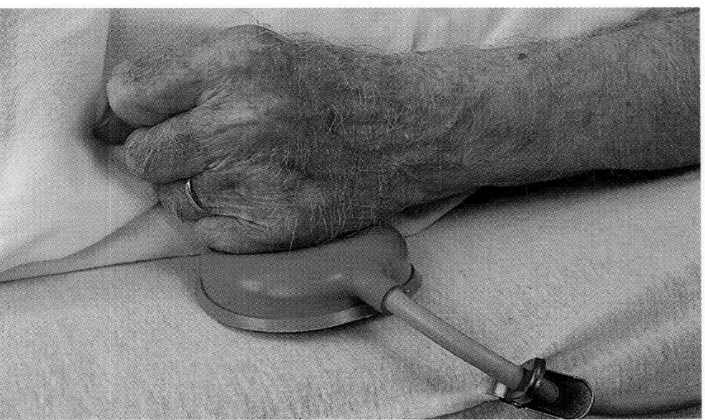

Figure 16-17 Call bell for a client with limited hand mobility.

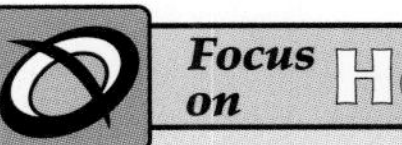

Focus on **Home Care**

Call Bells

Some home care clients stay in bed or in a certain part of the home. They need a way to call for help. Tap bells, dinner bells (Figure 16-18), baby monitors, and other devices are all useful in home care settings. Or, you can give the person a small can with a few coins inside. Children's toys with bells, horns, and whistles may be useful. Whatever the person decides to use, keep the calling device within easy reach.

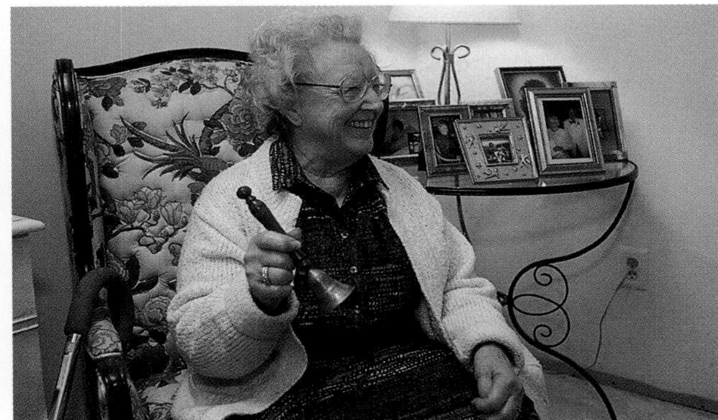

Figure 16-18 This woman rings a dinner bell when she needs assistance.

Using Bed Rails

An important part of safe client care is using bed rails correctly. Bed rails (side rails) are on hospital beds. They are raised and lowered according to the care plan. They lock in place with levers, latches, or buttons. Bed rails are half, three-quarters, or the full length of the bed (Figure 16-19 on page 186). When half-length rails are used, each side may have two rails. One is for the upper part of the bed, the other for the lower part.

Your supervisor and the care plan tell you when to raise bed rails. For example, clients who are unconscious or sedated might need bed rails. Some confused or disoriented clients need them. Some clients feel safer with bed rails up. Others use them to change positions in bed. If the care plan calls for raised bed rails, keep them up at all times except when giving bedside care.

Bed rails present hazards. The client can fall when trying to climb over them. Entrapment is also a risk

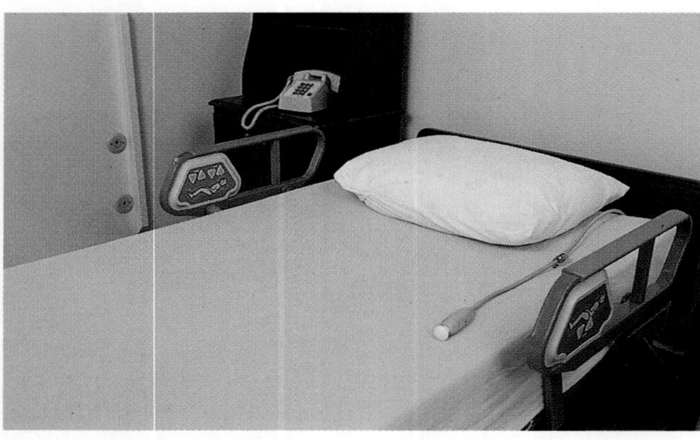

Figure 16-19 Hospital bed with bed rails locked in the raised position.

(Figure 16-20). That is, a person can get caught, trapped, or entangled in the bed rail gaps. Gaps occur between:

- The bars of the bed rail
- The two half-length rails
- The bed rail and the headboard or footboard
- The bed rail and mattress

Injury or death can occur if the person's head, neck, chest, arm, or leg becomes trapped. Clients at greatest risk are those who are:

- Confused or disoriented
- Restrained (see Chapter 17)
- Small in size
- Have poor muscle control or tend to have seizures

For an adult's safety, all bed rail gaps should be no more than 10 cm (4 inches). Sometimes padding is placed over the bed rails to cover gaps in the rails (Figure 16-21). Gap protectors may also be used for split bed rails (Figure 16-22). Follow the manufacturer's instructions and employer policy for the use of gap protectors or padded bed rails.

Because bed rails prevent the client from getting out of bed, they are considered environmental restraints (see Chapter 17). They cannot be used unless they are needed to treat the client's medical symp-

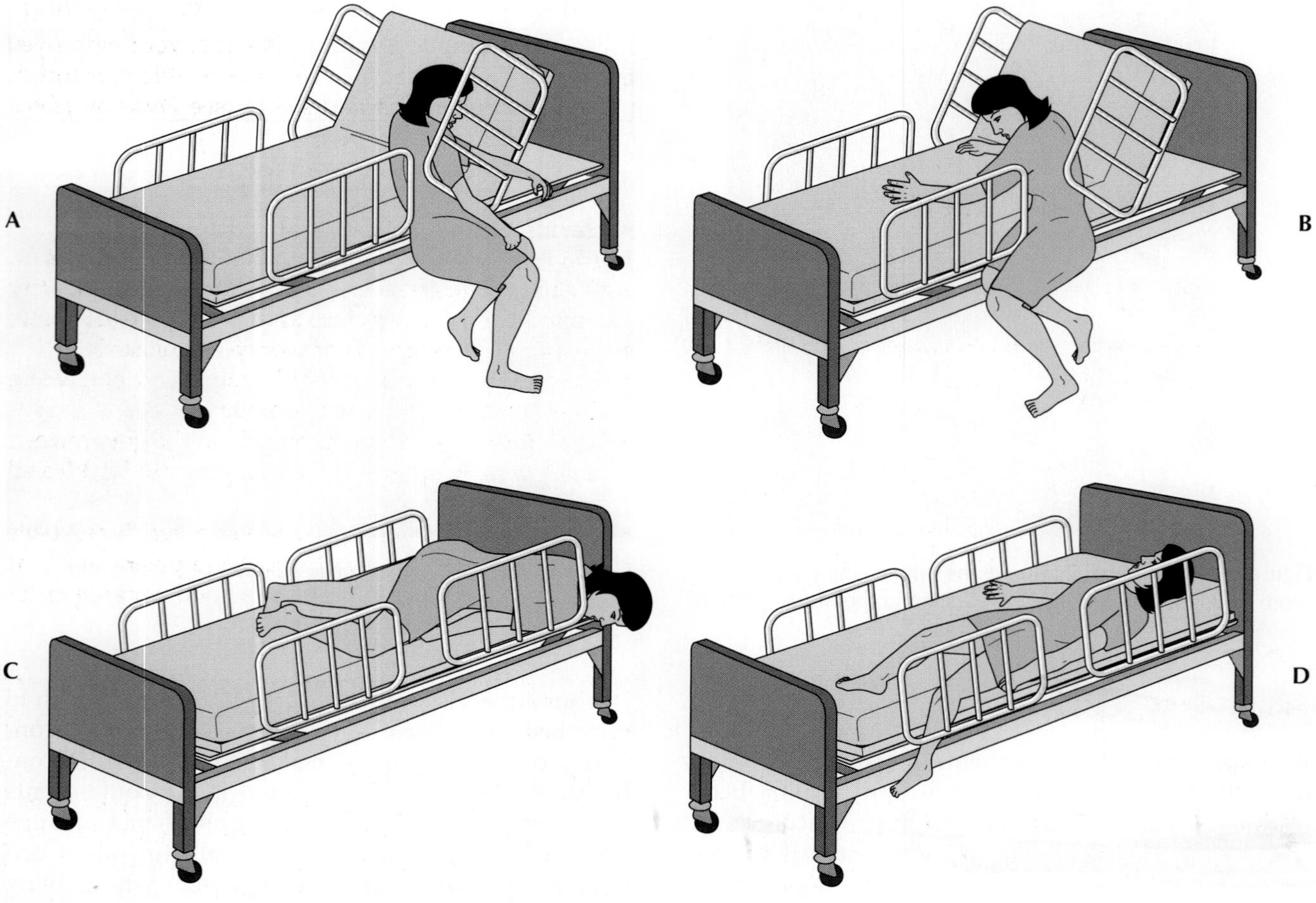

Figure 16-20 Bed rail hazards. **A,** The client is trapped between the bed rail bars. **B,** The client is trapped between two half-length rails. **C,** The client is trapped between the bed rail and the headboard. **D,** The client is trapped between the bed rail and the mattress.

toms. The client or substitute decision maker must give consent for raised bed rails. The need for bed rails must be carefully noted in the client's chart and care plan. Check clients with raised bed rails often.

The procedures in this book include using bed rails. This helps you learn how to use them correctly. Remember, not all beds have bed rails. Not all clients who have beds equipped with bed rails use them. Your supervisor, the care plan, and your assignment sheet tell you which clients use bed rails.

To give care when bed rails are used, lower the rail that is near you. Keep the bed rail raised on the opposite side. Raise both bed rails if you need to leave the bedside for any reason. Remember to raise the rail after completing the procedure.

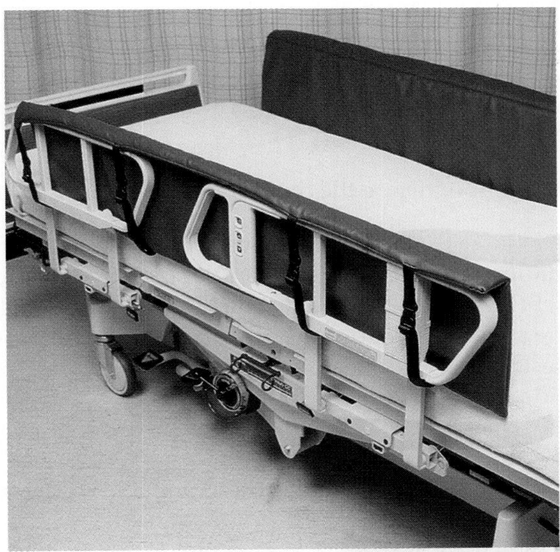

Figure 16-21 Padded bed rails. *(Courtesy J.T. Posey Co, Arcadia, CA.)*

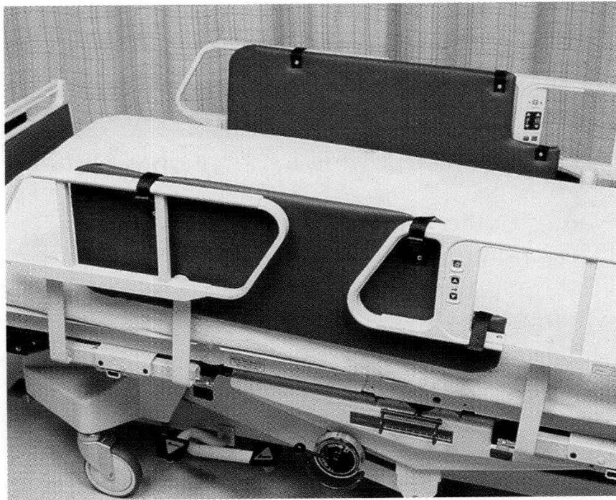

Figure 16-22 Gap protectors. *(Courtesy J.T. Posey Co, Arcadia, CA.)*

Promoting Your Personal Safety

Support workers are sometimes exposed to safety hazards on the job. You could have an accident if your workplace environment is not safe. You could be injured when working with hazardous materials. You might also be at risk for workplace violence.

Creating a Safe Workplace

In Canada, each province and territory has occupational health and safety (OH&S) legislation. **OH&S legislation** is designed to protect employees from injuries and accidents in the workplace. In most places, this legislation is called the *Occupational Health and Safety Act*. However, the name of the act varies across the country.

The details of the legislation also vary from one place to another, but the basic elements are similar. In general, the legislation assumes that all people in the workplace—employers, supervisors, and workers—are responsible for health and safety and have certain rights and duties.

Employers' and Supervisors' Responsibilities. According to OH&S legislation, your employer and supervisor must take every reasonable precaution to protect your health and safety (see *Focus on Home Care: OH&S Legislation* box).

Your employer is responsible for:

- Having written policies that promote safety
- Training and educating you about these policies
- Creating a health and safety committee to identify hazards in the workplace and investigate accidents
- Responding to reports of workplace hazards
- Warning you about safety hazards and correcting these hazards whenever possible
- Reporting all accidents promptly to the government department responsible for occupational health and safety
- Making sure that all necessary equipment is available (including personal protective equipment such as gloves and masks) and is kept in good working order

Focus on Home Care

OH&S Legislation

When you are providing services to a home care client, the client's home is considered a workplace. The home care agency is considered your employer. Therefore, agencies have the same obligations to their employees as do facilities.

ONTARIO HEALTH & SAFETY

Employees' Responsibilities. You are responsible for:

- Following all safety policies and procedures
- Using all recommended protective equipment and clothing
- Reporting all safety hazards and concerns immediately to your supervisor or a representative of your health and safety committee
- Completing an **incident report** (also known as an **occurrence report**). This is a report submitted to your employer whenever an accident, error, or unexpected problem arises in the workplace. Box 16-11 describes the incident report in greater detail.

According to the OH&S legislation, you have the right to refuse to do unsafe work. This applies whether you are working in a facility or a community setting. However, you cannot refuse to work if:

- The danger is a normal part of the job
- Refusing to work would endanger the client

For example, you could not refuse to provide care to a client with a communicable disease because you are afraid of contracting the disease. However, you could refuse to provide care to a client with a communicable disease if protective gloves, masks, and gowns are not available.

Handling Hazardous Materials

A **hazardous material** is any substance that presents a physical hazard or a health hazard in the workplace. Physical hazards can cause fires or explosions. Health hazards are chemicals that can cause acute or chronic health problems. For example, some health hazards can cause kidney or lung damage, cancer, or burns.

OH&S legislation requires that health care employees understand the risk of hazardous materials and know how to safely handle them. In order to provide this information, the Canadian government created the **Workplace Hazardous Materials Information System (WHMIS)**.

WHMIS is a national system that provides safety information about hazardous materials. It includes labelling, material safety data sheets (MSDSs), and employee education. WHMIS applies to hazardous materials that meet certain criteria. These are known as *controlled products*, and include compressed gases and products that are poisonous, corrosive, reactive, or that can catch fire or explode. You may work with or around controlled products. Examples of controlled products include:

- Drugs used in cancer therapy (chemotherapy, anticancer drugs)
- Gases used to sterilize equipment
- Oxygen used in oxygen therapy
- Certain disinfectants and cleaning solutions
- Mercury (found in some thermometers and blood pressure devices)

The following are the three components of WHMIS:

- *Labels*—WHMIS labels provide the essential information needed to safely handle a controlled product (Figure 16-23). The supplier applies the label. If the product is made at the workplace, the employer designs and applies the label. Warning labels provide the following information:
  - Product information—the brand, code, or chemical name of the product
  - Supplier information—the name and address of the supplier
  - Hazard symbols—pictures that show the kind of hazard the product presents (Figure 16-24).
  - Risk phrases—short phrases that describe the physical and health hazards; for example, "Spray may catch fire if used near an open flame."

Box 16-11 The Incident Report

Accidents involving clients, family, visitors, or staff must be reported. You also must report errors in care. These include giving the wrong care to a client, giving care to the wrong client, or forgetting to give care. Broken, lost, or stolen items owned by a client must be reported. (Dentures, eyeglasses, hearing aids, clothing, or money are examples.) Workplace violence and hazardous substance accidents must also be reported.

Notify your supervisor as soon as possible after an incident occurs. Your supervisor will give you an incident form to complete. Or, in community settings, your supervisor might take your account of the incident and complete the report for you. Your employer's policies will guide how you are to complete the form.

Generally, the following information is required:

- Names of those involved
- Date and time of the incident
- Description of the incident (who, what, where, when, how, why)
- Description of follow-up actions taken, such as notifying your supervisor or case manager

The employer and health and safety committees use incident reports to identify recurring problems. For example, they can tell if residents frequently fall in a certain area of a facility. This information is used to revise safety policies as needed.

- Precautionary statements—safety measures to be taken when using or handling the product; for example, "Keep in a cool place." They also list necessary personal protective equipment; for example, "Wear gloves if skin contact may occur."
- First aid measures—measures that are necessary in case of an accident or emergency
- Reference to the MSDS—statement that tells that an MSDS is available

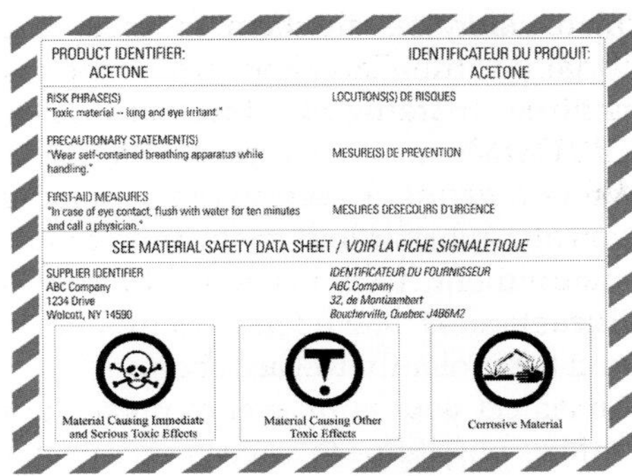

Figure 16-23 Sample WHMIS hazard label.

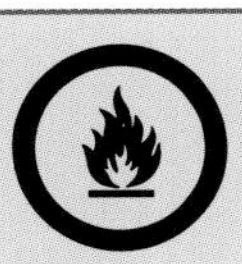	Flammable and Combustible Material	Product may catch fire or burst into flames if exposed to heat, sparks, or flame.
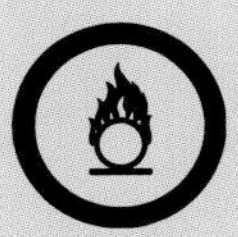	Oxidizing Material	Product may cause a fire or explosion if it is exposed to combustible material.
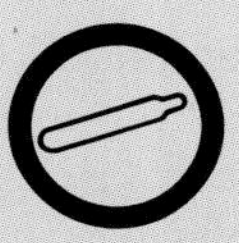	Compressed Gas	Product is under high pressure. May explode or burst when heated, dropped, or damaged.
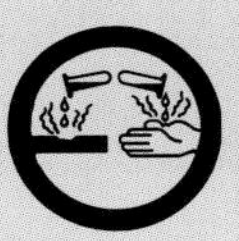	Corrosive Material	Product can cause burns to eyes, skin, or respiratory system.
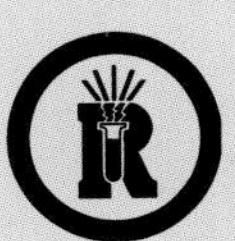	Dangerously Reactive Material	Product may react with light, heat, extreme temperatures, or vibration, causing an explosion, fire, or release of poisonous gases.
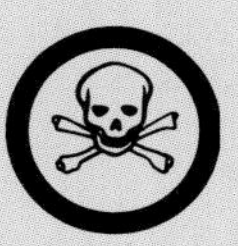	Poisonous and Infectious Material: Immediate and Serious Toxic Effects	Product may be fatal or cause serious or permanent damage to health if exposed to even once.
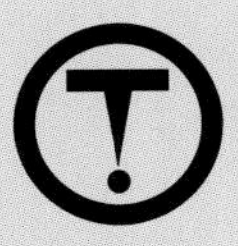	Poisonous and Infectious Material: Other Toxic Effects	Product may cause cancer, birth defects, or other permanent damage if exposed to repeatedly.
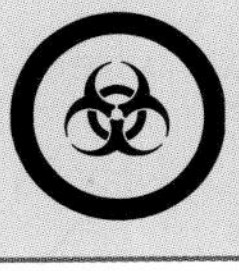	Poisonous and Infectious Material: Biohazardous and Infectious Material	Product may cause disease, serious illness, or death.

Figure 16-24 WHMIS Symbols. Source: Adapted from the Canadian Centre for Occupational Health and Safety, http://www.ccohs.ca/oshanswers/legisl/msds_lab.html (accessed January 2003).

Read and follow all warning labels. A container must have a label. This label must not be removed or damaged in any way. If a warning label is removed or damaged, do not use the product. Take the container to your supervisor, and explain the problem. Do not leave the container unattended.

- *Material Safety Data Sheets (MSDSs)*—These provide detailed information about each hazardous material. They are obtained from suppliers or developed by employers. Each MSDS provides information about the product, says if it can cause a fire or explosion, and describes its health hazards. The MSDS also tells how to safely handle, use, store, and dispose of the product. First aid measures are also listed.
- *Worker education*—Employers must provide WHMIS education to employees who work with controlled products. Information is given about WHMIS labels, MSDSs, and hazard information. The employee also learns how to safely handle, use, store, and dispose of controlled products.

Reducing Personal Security Risks

Workplace violence is any physical assault or threatening behaviour that occurs in a work setting. It includes:

- Murders
- Beatings, stabbings, and shootings
- Rapes
- Kidnapping
- Robbery
- Psychological trauma—threats, obscene phone calls, and harassment of any nature (being followed, sworn at, or shouted at)

Workplace violence can occur in any place where an employee performs a work-related duty. This includes buildings, parking lots, field locations, homes, and travel to and from work assignments.

Home care workers, especially, have personal security risks. They work alone in an unknown, uncontrolled environment. They often work at early or late hours. Clients, family members, or any person in the home could act violently toward them.

You can expect your employer to make your workplace as safe as possible. However, you must also protect yourself from harm. Box 16-12 lists personal safety measures. Follow them all the time. Most of the rules presented apply to support workers working in facilities and in the community.

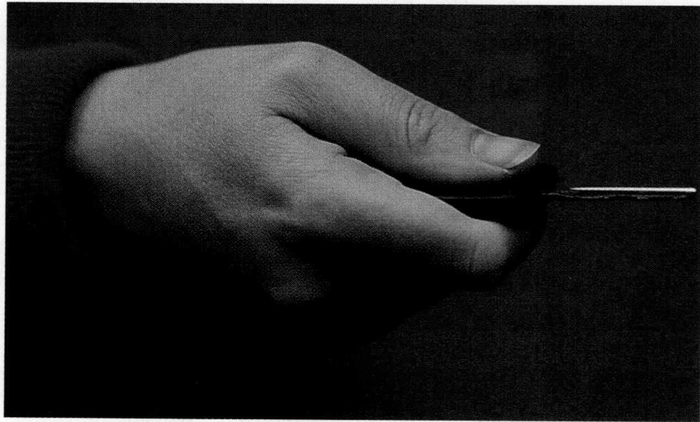

Figure 16-25 Car keys can be used as a weapon.

Box 16-12 Personal Safety Measures

Driving to and from Work

- Know the area where you will be driving. Plan your route in advance, keeping to well-travelled streets and routes that you know. Note the locations of nearby police stations, public telephones, gas stations, and other public buildings that may be of help in an emergency.
- Let your supervisor and a member of your family know the route you will take.
- Carry the number of a reliable tow truck company.
- Keep maps in the car.
- Maintain your car in good working order at all times.
- Always use a seat belt.
- Be prepared for winter driving conditions. Keep a survival kit in the car—booster cables, shovel, extra clothing, sand, and road flares.
- Keep money with you for gas or to make a phone call.
- Have a cellular phone for emergencies on the road. Do not use one while driving. Pull off the road to make an emergency call.
- Pull over to a safe spot away from traffic if you have car trouble. Put on your emergency lights and call for help if you have a cellular phone. Keep your doors locked and windows rolled up until help arrives. Never leave the car and walk off alone for help.
- Check for places to park. Choose a well-lit, busy area. If using a parking garage, park near entrances, exits, and on a lower level. Try to get close to the attendant if possible. Be aware of passengers sitting in parked cars. Avoid parking by these cars if possible. Lock the car doors as you leave.
- Ask for an escort to walk you back to your car after work. Many facilities provide this service. In a home setting, ask a family member to escort you.
- Have your car key ready so you can get into the car quickly. Do not fumble for keys on the way to or at the car. If necessary, you can use your car keys as a weapon. Carry them in your strong hand. Have one key extended (Figure 16-25 on page 190). If you are attacked, slash at the person's face with the key.
- Check for a possible intruder in the front and back seats before getting into your car.
- If you think someone is following you, cross the street or change directions. Head toward a public building or a lighted house. If you are scared, yell for help.
- Lock car doors when you get in the car. Keep windows rolled up.
- Keep purses, backpacks, and other valuables under the seat or near your side. Do not leave them on the seat. They are easy targets for robberies.
- Do not carry valuables. Do not bring your purse or valuables into clients' homes. Leave them at home or in the car trunk. If someone wants what you have, give it. The only thing of value is *you*. Report the crime to the police.
- Carry a whistle or shriek alarm. Carry a travel size can of aerosol hair spray. Go for the attacker's face. If someone tries to force you into a vehicle, do whatever you can to resist being pulled in. Fight back even if you see a weapon (yell, kick, push your thumbs into the attacker's eyes). You are at much greater risk if you are forced into the vehicle.

Visiting Clients

- Call your supervisor when you arrive and leave the client's home.
- Be cautious in hallways, elevators, and stairwells in apartment buildings. Do not get on an elevator with a stranger who makes you anxious.
- Stay in the centre of the hallways and avoid hidden corners in apartment buildings. If someone threatens you, knock on as many doors as possible and yell to get attention. If you are attacked, pull the fire alarm.
- Pause for a few seconds when entering someone's home. Assess the environment. Check any threats to your safety. This includes used syringes, strange odours, clutter, other people, or household items that could be used as weapons. Note the location of the phone. Note any obstacles blocking exits.
- Leave your shoes on. In an emergency, you may need to leave in a hurry. In the winter, bring a pair of shoes for indoor use.
- Leave if a client or anyone else is abusive or makes sexual comments or suggestions.
- If you feel uncomfortable or threatened in any way go to a safe place and immediately call your supervisor.
- Let the client lead the way down corridors, up staircases, etc.
- Leave an exit route or place yourself between the exit and the client. Never allow yourself to be cornered. Decide if you should leave a door opened or unlocked. Tell the client not to shut or lock a door if the action makes you uncomfortable.
- Sit in a hard-backed chair. You can get up faster from a firm chair than from a soft chair or sofa.
- Sit with your strong leg back and your other leg forward. This position lets you get out of your seat quickly without using your hands.
- Ask that pets be restrained or kept out of the room if you are worried about them.
- If a client or family member becomes angry and begins to vent, stay calm. (Follow the measures listed on page 241, Chapter 19.)
- Report any unusual incidents to your supervisor as soon as possible.

Source: Adapted from Health Care Health and Safety Association of Ontario (HCHSA) and Workplace Safety and Insurance Board (WSIB) of Ontario, *Health and Safety in the Home Care Environment* (Toronto: HCHSA, 2000), pp. 13–24, 43–47.

REVIEW

Circle T if the answer is true and F if it is false.

1. T F Older adults are at risk for accidents because of changes in the body.
2. T F The use of medications may increase a client's risk for accidents.
3. T F Children are not at increased risk for accidents during times of stress or change.
4. T F Middle-aged women have the greatest risk for falling.
5. T F Falls in facilities are more likely to occur during the evening.
6. T F Rushing to get to a bathroom or commode is a major cause of falls.
7. T F Socks and bedroom slippers help prevent falls.
8. T F Childproof caps are kept on medications and harmful products.
9. T F Medicines and harmful products can be stored in food containers out of the reach of children.
10. T F Do not carry or drink hot liquids while holding a child.
11. T F You are not responsible for reporting if equipment is broken or damaged.
12. T F To correctly identify a hospital patient, call him or her by name.
13. T F Smoking is allowed where oxygen is used.
14. T F Hazardous materials must have warning labels.

Circle the BEST answer.

15. What is the most common accident in all settings?
    A. Burns
    B. Suffocation
    C. Falls
    D. Poisoning
16. You are caring for Rani, a 6-week-old infant. Which is *unsafe*?
    A. Checking her in her crib often
    B. Laying her on her back for sleep
    C. Propping her baby bottle on a rolled towel when feeding her
    D. Shaking her bottle after warming it
17. Mr. Higgins is 86 years old. Which is *unsafe* for him?
    A. Nonglare, waxed floors
    B. Electrical cords and other items on the floor in high-traffic areas
    C. Safety rails and grab bars in the bathroom
    D. Nonskid shoes
18. To prevent falls, you should do the following *except*
    A. Wipe up spills right away
    B. Turn on night-lights
    C. Encourage the use of hand rails and grab bars
    D. Keep the bed in the highest position
19. Which does *not* prevent falls?
    A. Meeting elimination needs
    B. Answering calls for assistance promptly
    C. Keeping the bed in the highest position
    D. Using bed rails according to the care plan
20. Mrs. Carrera often tries to get up without help. You should do the following *except*
    A. Remind her to call for assistance
    B. Check on her often
    C. Help her to the bathroom at regular intervals
    D. Decide on your own to keep the bed rails up

REVIEW

21. Which is *not* a common cause of burns?
    A. Hot bathwater and heating pads
    B. Spilling of hot liquids
    C. Cooking while wearing long, loose sleeves
    D. Suffocation

22. You are caring for an infant and young children. Which measure is *unsafe*?
    A. Using a safety strap when putting a child in a highchair
    B. Ironing the clothes while the children play at your feet
    C. Removing stuffed animals and toys from the crib at naptime
    D. Using a safety gate at the top and bottom of the stairs

23. To prevent equipment accidents, you should do the following *except*
    A. Use equipment only for its intended purpose
    B. Fix broken items
    C. Stop using electrical equipment if it produces a burning odour
    D. Use three-pronged plugs

24. You are using equipment. Which is *unsafe?*
    A. Following the manufacturer's instructions
    B. Keeping electrical items away from water and spills
    C. Pulling on the cord to remove a plug from an outlet
    D. Turning off electrical items after using them.

25. A fire alarm sounds. Which of the following is *unsafe*?
    A. Turning off oxygen
    B. Moving clients to a safe place
    C. Using elevators for a quick exit
    D. Closing doors and windows

26. Your clothing is on fire. You should do the following *except*
    A. Run to get help
    B. Drop to the floor or ground
    C. Cover your face
    D. Roll to smother the flames

27. Bed rails are raised when
    A. The person tries to get up without assistance
    B. Your supervisor and the care plan tells you to raise them
    C. The person has a seizure
    D. The person is restrained

28. Which of the following is *not* a usual hazard of bed rails?
    A. Entrapment
    B. Suffocation
    C. Infections
    D. Falls

29. According to occupational health and safety legislation, employers are *not* responsible for
    A. Training and educating employees about safety policies
    B. Taking every reasonable precaution to ensure the safety of their workers
    C. Warning employees of any potential and existing safety hazards
    D. Forcing employees to do unsafe work

30. You give Mr. Ford the wrong treatment. What should you do*?*
    A. Report the error at the end of the shift
    B. Take action only if Mr. Ford was injured
    C. Ask Mr. Ford what to do
    D. Complete an incident report

31. You are working with a WHMIS-controlled product. You should *not*
    A. Review instructions on the label
    B. Wear any needed personal protective equipment
    C. Remove the label after using the product
    D. Review instructions on the Material Safety Data Sheet

32. You work the night shift. Which of the following is *unsafe*?
    A. Parking in a well-lit area
    B. Locking your car
    C. Looking for your keys while at the car
    D. Checking the back seat before entering your car

Answers to these questions are on page 823.

CHAPTER

17

RESTRAINT ALTERNATIVES AND SAFE RESTRAINT USE

OBJECTIVES

- Define the key terms listed in this chapter
- Describe the purpose of using restraints
- Describe complications from restraint use
- Identify restraint alternatives
- Explain how to use restraints safely

KEY TERMS

chemical restraints Medications used to control behaviour or movement; they are not otherwise required for a person's medical condition

environmental restraints Barriers, furniture, or devices that prevent free movement

physical restraints Garments or devices used to restrict movement of the whole body or parts of the body

restraint Any device, garment, barrier, furniture, or medication that limits or restricts freedom of movement or access to one's body

A **restraint** is any device, garment, barrier, furniture, or medication that limits or restricts freedom of movement or access to one's body. Restraints are used to protect people from harming themselves or others. Health care professionals decide how best to meet their clients' safety needs. Every effort is made to protect clients without using restraints. However, sometimes restraints are needed.

Restraint use is a sensitive issue. Restraints can cause emotional harm and serious physical injury. They are used *only* as a last resort when other measures have failed.

Support workers never decide if restraints are to be used. Restraints require a physician's order. Nurses apply restraints if ordered by a physician. An RN may delegate this task to you. The RN teaches you how to apply the restraints properly and safely. You are closely supervised and monitored. The RN has full responsibility for applying restraints.

This chapter gives you general information about restraints. Follow your employer's policies and guidelines.

USE OF RESTRAINTS IN CANADA

Current research shows that restraints may cause more harm than good. Studies show that they actually increase incidents of physical injury and psychological harm.[1] Physical injuries such as falls and strangulation may occur. People who are restrained show signs of severe emotional distress. Their quality of life suffers.

Canadian hospitals and long-term care facilities have strict limits on the use of restraints. Each facility writes its own philosophy, policies, and procedures for restraints. These are based on legal guidelines and standards. Generally, facilities have a "least restraint policy." This means that restraints are used only as a last resort when less restrictive measures fail. Restraints are *never* used to discipline a person. Discipline is any action that punishes or penalizes. Restraints are *never* used for staff convenience—they should not be used to make the staff's job easier.

Restraints are not used in community settings. If people are in danger of harming themselves or others, physicians usually advise them to enter a facility, where safe care can be provided.

Restraints are used only when necessary to treat a client's medical symptoms. Symptoms may relate to physical, emotional, or behavioural problems. Some clients may behave in ways that are harmful to themselves or others. The following are examples of harmful behaviour:

- Miss Douris, 88, tries to pull out her IV and feeding tube. The tubes are part of her treatment. If she disconnects the tubes, Ms Douris puts her life in danger.
- Mr. Gorsky, 22, suffers from a severe mental illness. He tries to strangle a staff member. He puts her life in danger.
- Nicole Black, 3, tries to rip out the stitches in her chest. The wound could become infected. This would put her life in danger.

Often there are causes and reasons for harmful behaviours. Knowing and treating the causes can prevent the need for restraints. When determining the causes of harmful behaviour, health care professionals consider some of the following questions:

- Is the client ill, injured, or in pain?
- Is the client afraid?
- Is the client seeing, hearing, or feeling things that are not real?
- Is the client confused or disoriented?
- Are medications causing the behaviour?
- Is the behaviour occurring because the client has not taken medication?
- Does the client need to urinate or have a bowel movement?
- Is clothing or a dressing tight or causing other discomfort?

- Is the client's position uncomfortable?
- Is the client too hot, too cold, hungry, or thirsty?
- Are body fluids, secretions, or excretions causing skin irritation?

The health care professionals caring for the client identify restraint alternatives (Box 17-1). These become part of the care plan. The health care team follows the care plan. Changes to the care plan are made as needed. If restraint alternatives do not protect the client, the physician may, as a last resort, order restraints.

Box 17-1 Alternatives to Restraints

- If the client is living at home, he or she may be admitted to a facility.
- Diversion is provided to calm or distract the client. This includes TV, videos, music, games, books, relaxation tapes, back massages, exercise programs, outdoor time, and simple tasks.
- Lifelong habits and routines are encouraged: for example, showers before breakfast; walks outside before lunch; TV after lunch.
- Attention and companionship are provided. Support workers, family, friends, and volunteers visit with the client. Visits and observations are made every 15 minutes.
- A calm, quiet setting is provided; noise levels are reduced.
- Staff members provide consistent care; they explain procedures and care measures.
- The client spends time in supervised areas: for example, in the lounge and nurses' station.
- The client is allowed to wander in safe areas; the entire staff is kept informed of clients who wander.
- Confused clients are oriented to people, time, and place. Calendars and clocks are provided.
- The call bell is placed within reach.
- Food, fluid, and elimination needs are met; the bedpan, urinal, or commode is within reach.
- Padded hip protectors are worn under clothing (Figure 17-1).
- Rooms and furniture meet safety and comfort needs (e.g., lower bed, reclining chair, padded walls and furniture). Warning devices are used on beds, chairs, and doors; doors have knob guards.
- Pillows, wedge cushions, posture, and positioning aids are used.
- Falls are prevented (see Chapter 16). Floor cushions are placed next to beds (Figure 17-2); roll guards are attached to the bed frame (Figure 17-3).
- Lighting is adjusted to meet the client's needs and preferences.
- Uninterrupted sleep is promoted.

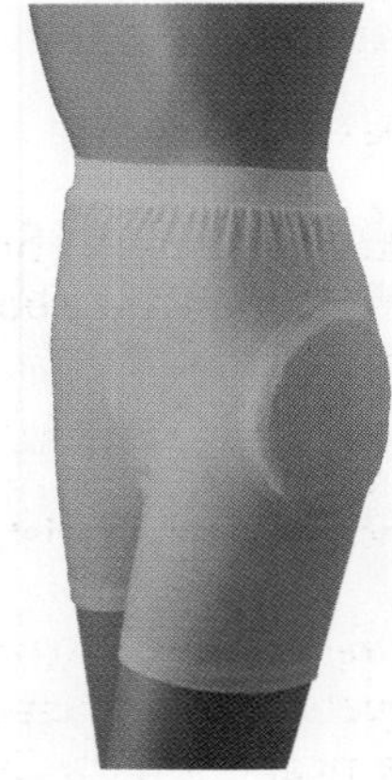

Figure 17-1 Hip protector. *(Courtesy J. T. Posey Company, Arcadia, CA.)*

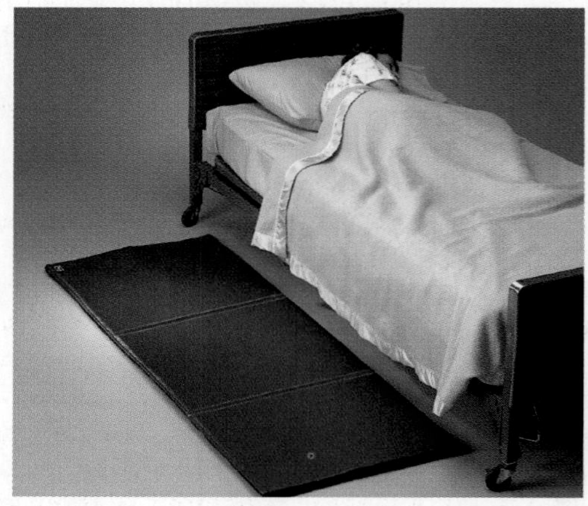

Figure 17-2 Floor cushion. *(Courtesy J. T. Posey Company, Arcadia, CA.)*

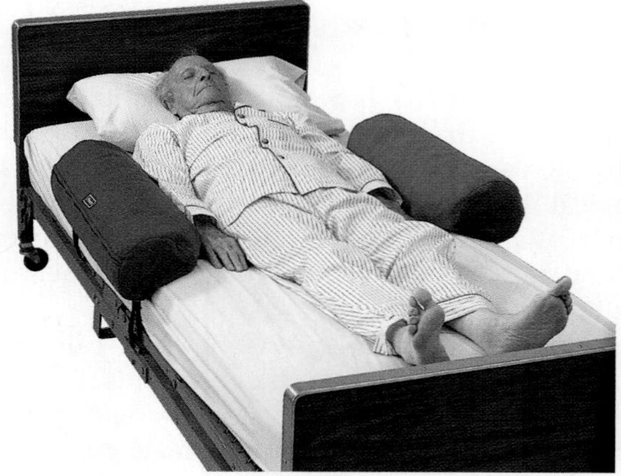

Figure 17-3 Roll guard. *(Courtesy J. T. Posey Company, Arcadia, CA.)*

Types of Restraints

There are three types of restraints:

- **Physical restraints**—garments or devices used to restrict movement of the whole body or parts of the body. They are attached to the body and to a fixed (nonmovable) object. The person wearing the physical device cannot easily remove it. Examples are vests, jackets, and leg, arm, wrist, hand, and some belt restraints.
- **Environmental restraints**—barriers, furniture, or devices that prevent free movement. Environmental restraints are near but not directly attached to the body. They confine the person to a specific place, such as a bed, chair, or room. Examples of environmental restraints include:
  - Geriatric chairs (Geri-Chairs) or chairs with attached trays (Figure 17-4). These are used for people who need support to sit up.
  - Any chair placed close to a wall so that a person cannot move.
  - Bed rails (see Chapter 16).
  - Sheets tucked in tightly in order to restrict movement.
- **Chemical restraints**—medications used to control behaviour or movement; they are not otherwise required for the person's medical condition. Sometimes confused and disoriented clients become anxious, agitated, or aggressive. The physician may order medications to control these behaviours. The goal is to control the behaviour without making the person sleepy or impairing function. Like all restraints, chemical restraints must not be used for discipline or staff convenience. They must not be used if they impair physical or mental function. Giving a chemical restraint is out of your scope of practice. Support workers never administer medications. Only a physician or nurse can administer chemical restraints.

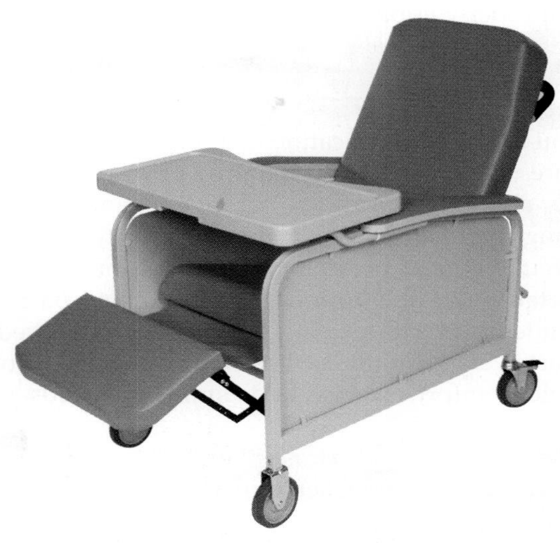

Figure 17-4 A Geri-Chair. *(Courtesy Winco, Ocala, FL.)*

Complications of Restraint Use

Box 17-2 lists complications from restraint use. Injuries occur when people try to free themselves from restraints. Injuries also occur when the wrong restraint is used, when it is applied incorrectly, or when it is kept on too long. The most serious risk is death from strangulation. There are also many emotional effects. Restraints affect a clients's dignity and self-esteem. Often, clients who are restrained feel embarrassed, angry, and depressed. Many begin to mistrust their caregivers. (See *Providing Compassionate Care: Caring for Clients Who Are Restrained* box on page 198.)

Safety Guidelines

If a restraint must be used, the least restrictive method is chosen. While providing protection, it allows the greatest amount of movement or body access possible. When applying restraints or caring for a restrained client, follow the safety measures in Box 17-3 on page 199.

Box 17-2 Complications of Restraint Use

- Bowel and bladder problems (constipation and incontinence)
- Cognitive (intellectual) decline
- Cuts and bruises
- Dehydration
- Emotional harm—agitation, anger, depression, fear, humiliation
- Fractures
- Infections such as pneumonia and urinary tract infections
- Joint problems
- Nerve injuries
- Pressure ulcers
- Strangulation

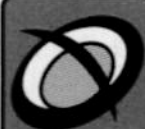

Providing Compassionate Care

Caring for Clients Who Are Restrained

A common misunderstanding is that people do not mind being restrained, especially if they are confused or disoriented. In fact, many people who have been restrained have later reported that they felt angry, afraid, degraded, and uncomfortable. These feelings and memories sometimes last for years afterwards.[2] Another misunderstanding is that restraints will decrease agitated behaviour. In fact, restraints often make people more agitated, confused, or combative. People who are restrained may not understand what is happening to them. They may try to get out of the restraint. They may beg anyone who passes by to free them.

Try to put yourself in the client's situation. Then you can better understand how he or she might feel. Imagine what it would be like to have your hands and arms restrained:

- Your nose itches, but you cannot scratch it.
- You need to use the bathroom, but you cannot get up. You soil yourself.
- You are thirsty, but you cannot reach your water glass.
- You are not wearing your eyeglasses. You cannot identify people coming in and out of your room.
- You are uncomfortable, but you cannot turn or move in bed.
- You hear the fire alarm, but you cannot get up to move to a safe place. You must wait until someone rescues you.

What would you do? Would you calmly lie or sit there? Would you try to get free from the restraint? Would you cry out for help? What would the staff think? Would they think that you are uncomfortable or agitated and uncooperative?

Treat a restrained client like you would want to be treated—with kindness, caring, respect, and dignity. Meet the person's food, fluid, and elimination needs. Make sure the person is as comfortable as possible. Restrained clients need repeated explanations and reassurance. Visit with the person often. Be a good listener. Spending time with the person may have a calming effect.

Also remember the following points about the use of restraints:

- *Restraints are used to protect the client. They are not used for staff convenience or to discipline a person.* Restraining someone is not easier than properly supervising and observing the person. A restrained person requires more staff time for care, supervision, and observation. A restraint is used only when it is the best safety measure for the client. It is not used to punish people for being uncooperative.
- *Restraints require a physician's order.* If restraints are needed, a physician's order is required. The physician explains why the restraint is needed, what to use, and how long to use it. This information is on the care plan and on your assignment sheet.
- *The least restrictive method is used.* For example, most environmental restraints are less restrictive than physical restraints.
- *Restraints are used only after other alternatives have been tried.* Restraints harm a person's dignity. They are used only after other measures fail to protect the person or others (see Box 17-1 on page 196).
- *Unnecessary restraint is false imprisonment* (see Chapter 10). If told to apply a restraint, you must clearly understand the need. If not, politely ask about its use. If you apply a restraint unnecessarily, you could face false-imprisonment charges.
- *Informed consent is required.* Restraints cannot be used without informed consent. The client must understand the reason for the restraint. He or she is told how the restraint will help the planned treatment and what the risks of restraint use are. The client has the choice to give or withhold consent. If the client is not capable of giving informed consent, a family member or substitute decision maker is given the information. This person must decide whether or not to give consent. The physician or nurse provides the necessary information and obtains informed consent.
- *The manufacturer's instructions are followed.* The manufacturer gives instructions about applying and securing the restraint. Failure to follow them could harm the client. You could be found negligent if you improperly apply or secure a restraint.
- *Restraints are applied by knowledgeable workers.* **You must receive proper training and instruction before applying restraints.** Some facilities require you to obtain certification to apply restraints. Make sure you know what is required of you.
- *The client's basic needs are met.* The restraint must be snug and firm but not tight. Tight restraints affect circulation and breathing. The client must be comfortable and able to move the restrained part to a limited and safe extent. The person is checked at least every 15 minutes or as often as required. Food, fluid, comfort, exercise, and elimination needs must be met.
- *More than one staff member may be needed to safely apply the restraint.* Clients in immediate danger of harming themselves or others are restrained quickly. Combative and agitated clients can hurt themselves and the health care worker when restraints are being applied. Two or more workers may be needed to complete the task safely and quickly.

(text continues on page 202)

Box 17-3 Safety Measures for Using Restraints

- Use the restraint noted in the care plan. The least restrictive device is used.
- Follow employer policies and procedures.
- Apply a restraint only after you have been instructed about its proper use.
- Demonstrate proper application of the restraint to the RN before applying it.
- Use the correct size. The RN and care plan tell you what size to use. Small restraints are tight. They cause discomfort and agitation. They also restrict breathing and circulation. Strangulation is a risk from big or loose restraints.
- Use only restraints that have manufacturer instructions and warning labels.
- Read the manufacturer's warning labels. Note the front and back of the restraint.
- Follow the manufacturer's instructions. Some restraints are safe for bed, chair, and wheelchair use. Others are used only with certain equipment.
- Do not use sheets, towels, tape, rope, straps, bandages, or other items to restrain a client.
- Use intact restraints. Look for tears, cuts, or frayed fabric or straps. Look for missing or loose hooks, loops, or straps, or other damage.
- Do not use restraints to position a client on a toilet.
- Do not use restraints to position a client on furniture that does not allow for correct application. Follow the manufacturer's instructions.
- Position the client in good body alignment before applying the restraint (see Chapter 21).
- Pad bony areas and skin. This prevents pressure and injury from the restraint.
- Secure the restraint. It should be snug but allow some movement of the restrained part.
  - If applied to the chest, make sure that the client can breathe easily. A flat hand should slide between the restraint and the client's body (Figure 17-5 on page 200).
  - For wrist and mitt restraints, you should be able to slide one or two fingers under the restraint.
- Follow the manufacturer's instructions to check for snugness.
- Crisscross vest restraints in front (Figure 17-6 on page 200). Do not crisscross restraints in the back unless indicated in the manufacturer's instructions (Figure 17-7 on page 200). Crisscrossing vests in the back can cause death from strangulation.
- Tie restraints according to employer policy. The policy should follow the manufacturer's instructions. Quick-release buckles or airline-type buckles are used (Figure 17-8 on page 201). So are quick-release ties (Figure 17-9 on page 201).
- Secure straps out of the client's reach.
- Secure the restraint to the movable part of the bed frame at waist level (see Figure 17-9). For chairs, secure straps to the wheelchair or the chair frame (Figure 17-10 on page 201).
- Make sure that straps will not slide in any direction. If straps move or are slack, the client can slide off the mattress or chair (Figures 17-11 on page 201 and 17-12 on page 202). Strangulation can result.
- Never secure restraints to the bed rails. The client could reach the bed rails to release knots or buckles. Also, injury to the client could occur when bed rails are raised or lowered.
- Keep full bed rails up when the client is restrained by a vest, jacket, or belt restraint. Also use bed rail covers or gap protectors (see Chapter 16). Otherwise the client could fall off the bed and strangle on the restraint. If half-length bed rails are used without a gap protector, the client could get caught between them.
- Use a belt restraint with chairs or wheelchairs. Position the client in the chair so that his or her hips are well to the back of the chair. Apply the belt restraint at a 45-degree angle over the hips (Figure 17-13 on page 202).
- Do not use back cushions when a client is restrained in a chair. If the cushion moves out of place, the straps could become loose. Strangulation could result if the client slides forward or down from the extra slack (see Figure 17-12 on page 202).
- Bed rails are environmental restraints. Only use them if indicated in the care plan. Check with your supervisor and the care plan for instructions on when to raise or lower bed rails. Use bed rail covers or gap protectors according to your supervisor's instructions. These prevent the client from getting trapped between the rails or the bed rail bars.
- Check the client's circulation every 15 minutes if mitt, wrist, or ankle restraints are applied. You should feel a pulse at a pulse site below the restraint. Fingers or toes should be warm and pink. Tell the nurse at once if:
  - You cannot feel a pulse
  - Fingers or toes are cold, pale, or blue in colour
  - The client complains of pain, numbness, or tingling in the restrained part
  - The skin is red or damaged
- Check the client at least every 15 minutes if a belt, jacket, or vest restraint is used. The client should be able to breathe easily. Also check the position of the restraint, especially in the front and back.
- Check the client at least every 15 minutes for safety and comfort.
- Clients who are in the supine position should be monitored constantly. They are at great risk for aspiration if vomiting occurs. If the client vomits, call for the nurse at once.
- Do not use a restraint near a fire, flame, or smoking materials. Restraint fabrics could ignite easily.

Continued

Box 17-3 Safety Measures for Using Restraints—Cont'd

- Keep scissors in your pocket. In an emergency, cutting the tie may be faster than untying the knot. Never leave scissors at the bedside or where the client can reach them.
- Remove the restraint and reposition the client every 2 hours. Meet the person's basic needs during this time and whenever necessary:
  - Meet elimination needs.
  - Give skin care.
  - Perform range-of-motion exercises or ambulate the client (see Chapter 22). Follow the care plan.
  - Offer food and fluids.
  - Record what was done, the care given, your observations, and the time and details of what you reported to the nurse. Follow employer policy for recording.
- Keep the call bell within the client's reach.
- Report to the nurse every time you checked the client and released the restraint. Report your observations made and the care given. Follow employer policy for reporting.

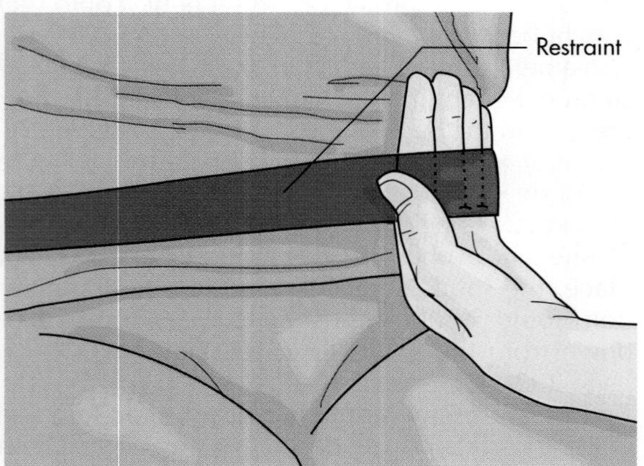

Figure 17-5 A flat hand slides between the restraint and the client.

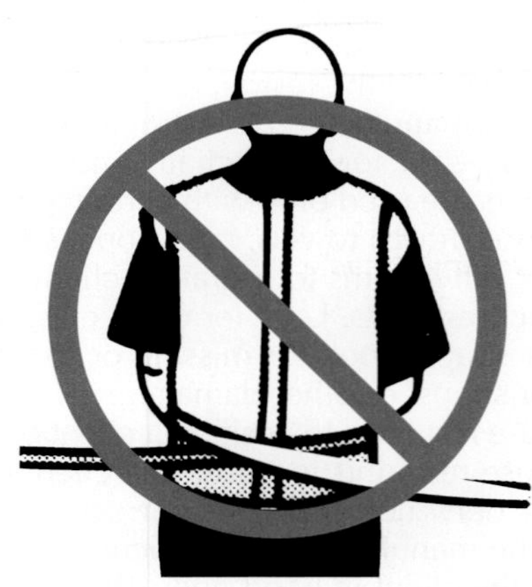

Figure 17-7 Never crisscross vest or jacket straps in back. *(Courtesy J. T. Posey Company, Arcadia, CA.)*

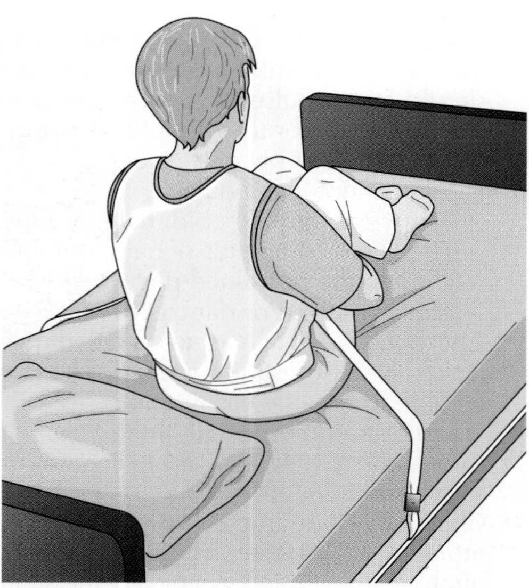

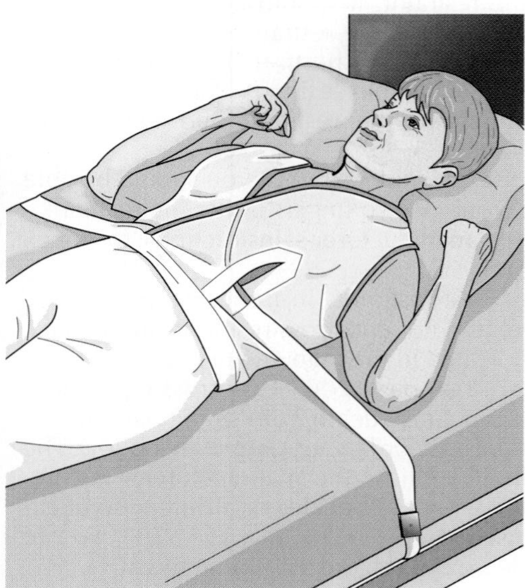

Figure 17-6 Vest restraint crisscrosses in front.

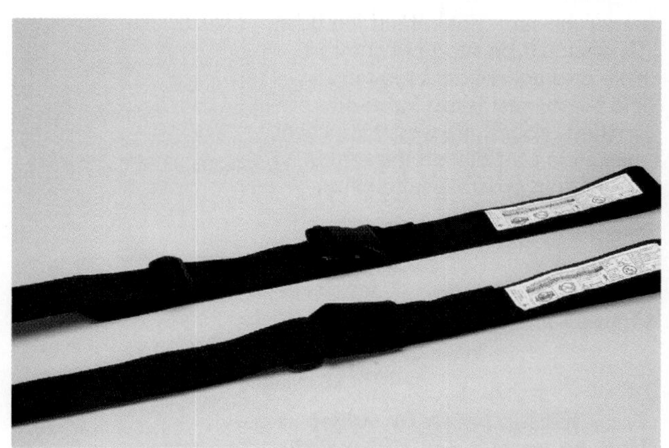

Figure 17-8 Quick-release and airline-type buckles. *(Courtesy J. T. Posey Company, Arcadia, CA.)*

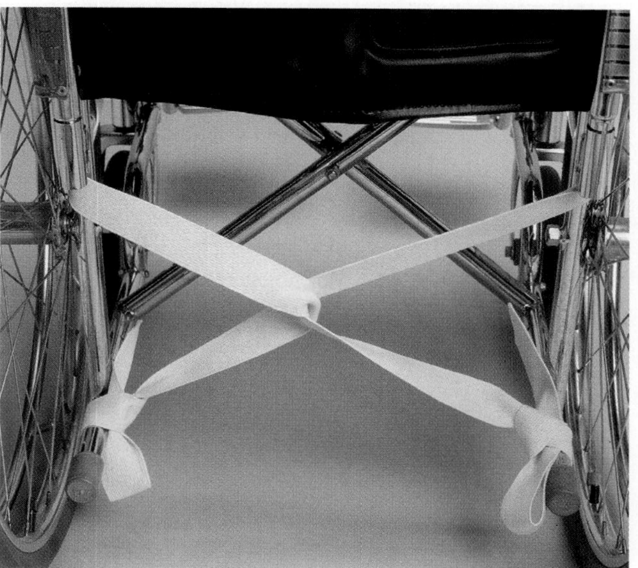

Figure 17-10 The restraint straps are secured to the wheelchair frame with quick-release ties. *(Courtesy J. T. Posey Company, Arcadia, CA.)*

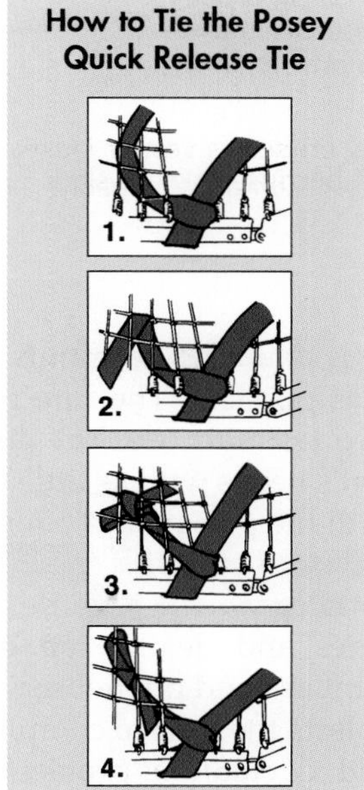

Figure 17-9 The Posey quick-release tie.

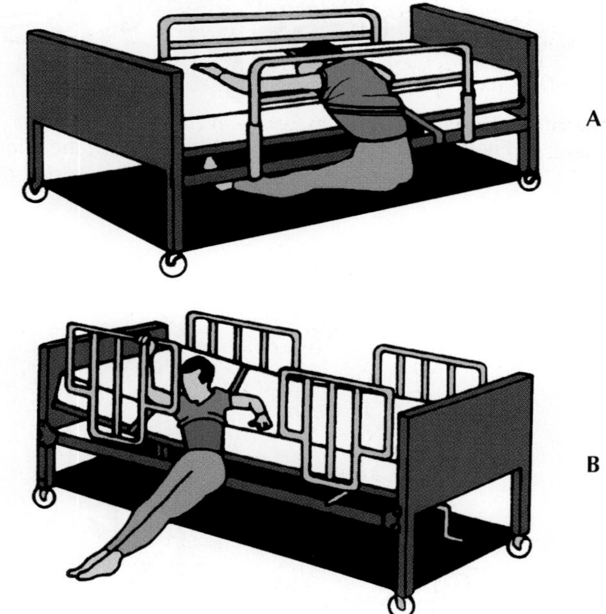

Figure 17-11 Restraint straps must not move in any direction. Strangulation could result. **A**, The client can get suspended and caught between bed rail bars. **B**, The client can get suspended and caught between half-length bed rails. *(Courtesy J. T. Posey Company, Arcadia, CA.)*

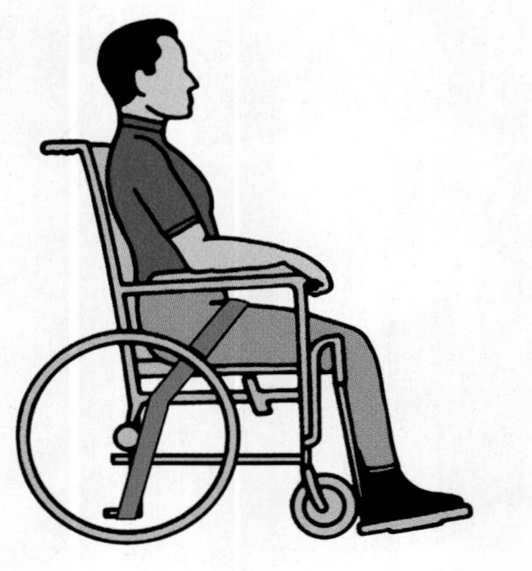

Straps to prevent sliding should always be over the thighs—NOT around the waist or chest. Straps should be at a 45-degree angle and secured to the chair under the seat, not behind the back. They should be snug but comfortable and not restrict breathing. If a belt or vest is too loose or applied around the waist, the client may slide partially off the seat—resulting in possible suffocation and death.

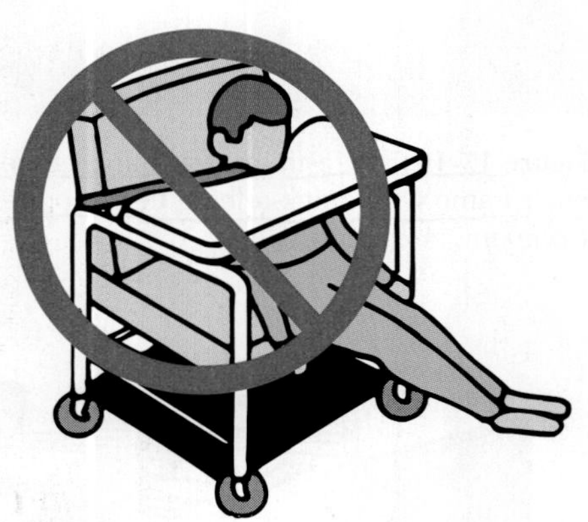

Tray tables (with or without a belt or vest) pose potential danger if the person should slide partly under the table and become caught. This could result in suffocation and death. Make sure the client's hips are positioned at the back of the chair—this may necessitate the use of an anti-slide material (Posey Grip), a pommel cushion, or a restrictive device if the client shows any tendency to slide forward.

Figure 17-12 Strangulation could result if the client slides forward or down because of extra slack in the restraint. *(Courtesy J. T. Posey Company, Arcadia, CA.)*

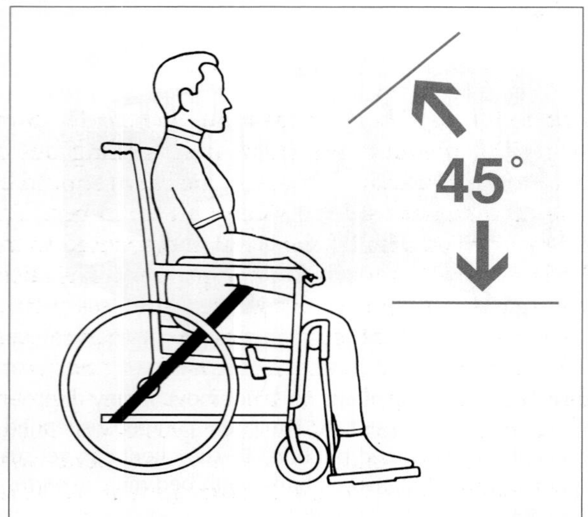

Figure 17-13 The safety belt is at a 45-degree angle over the hips. *(Courtesy J. T. Posey Company, Arcadia, CA.)*

- *Quality of life is protected.* Restraints are used for as short a time as possible. The care plan must show how to reduce restraint use. The goal is always to meet the client's needs with as little restraint as possible. Visit with the person and offer reassurance.
- *The client is observed at least every 15 minutes or more often, as required by the care plan.* Restraints are dangerous. Injuries and deaths can occur from improper restraint use and poor observation. Frequent observation alerts the staff to complications such as breathing and circulation problems. Practise the safety measures in Box 17-3 on page 199.
- *The restraint is removed, the client is repositioned, and basic needs are met at least every 2 hours.* These needs include food, fluid, elimination, skin care, and range-of-motion exercises. The person is ambulated (walked) according to the care plan.
- *Information about restraints is recorded in the client's chart.* When caring for restrained clients, give ver-

bal reports to your supervisor on the following. If you are allowed to chart, include this information:
- The type of restraint applied
- The reason for the application
- Safety measures taken, as listed in the care plan (e.g., bed rails padded and up)
- The time you applied the restraint
- The time you removed the restraint
- The care given when the restraint was removed
- Skin colour and condition
- The pulse felt in the restrained part
- Complaints of a tight restraint, difficulty breathing, and pain, numbness, or tingling in the restrained part (report these complaints to your supervisor at once)

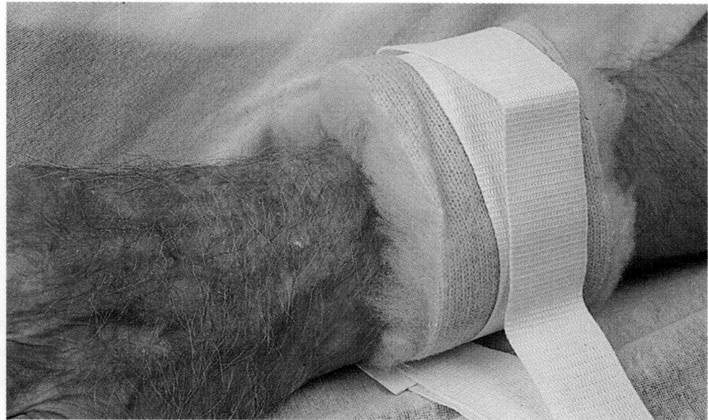

Figure 17-14 Wrist restraint. Note the soft part is toward the skin.

Applying Physical Restraints

Physical restraints are made of cloth or leather. Cloth restraints (soft restraints) are mitts, belts, straps, and vests. They are applied to the wrists, ankles, hands, waist, chest, and elbows. Leather restraints are applied to the wrists and ankles. They are used in cases of extreme agitation and combativeness. (See *Focus on Older Adults: Physical Restraints* box.) The following are the most commonly used physical restraints:

- *Wrist restraints.* Wrist restraints (limb holders) limit arm movement (Figure 17-14). They may be used when a client continually tries to pull out tubes used for treatment (IV, feeding tube, catheter, wound drainage tubes, or monitoring lines). They also prevent the client from trying to scratch, pick at, pull at, or peel the skin, a wound, or a dressing. This can damage the skin or the wound and place the person's life in danger.
- *Mitt restraints.* Hands are placed in mitt restraints. They prevent finger use, but do not prevent hand, wrist, or arm movements. They are used for the same reasons as wrist restraints. Most mitts are padded (Figure 17-15).

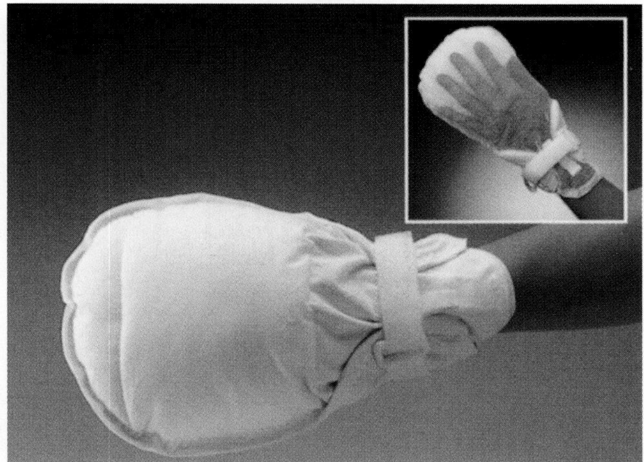

Figure 17-15 Mitt restraint. *(Courtesy J. T. Posey Company, Arcadia, CA.)*

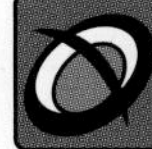

Focus on Older Adults

Physical Restraints

Some older adults have dementia. Restraints may increase their confusion and agitation. They do not understand what is happening to them. They may resist staff efforts to apply a restraint and actively try to get free from it. This can cause serious injury and even death.

Never use force to apply a restraint. Ask your supervisor for help if the client is confused and agitated. Report any problems to your supervisor at once.

- *Belt restraints.* The belt restraint (Figure 17-16 on page 204) prevents the client from getting out of bed or out of a chair. However, the client should be able to turn from side to side or sit up in bed. The belt is applied around the waist and secured to the bed or chair. It is applied over a garment. The client can release the quick-release type. It is less restrictive than those that only staff members can release.
- *Vest restraints and jacket restraints.* Vest and jacket restraints are applied to the chest. They prevent the client from turning in bed or getting out of bed or a chair. They may also be used for clients who need positioning for medical treatment. A jacket restraint is applied with the opening in the back. For a vest restraint, the vest crosses in front (see Figure 17-6). *The straps of vest and jacket restraints always cross in the front.* They must *never* cross in the back. Vest and jacket restraints are never worn backward. Strangulation or other injury could occur

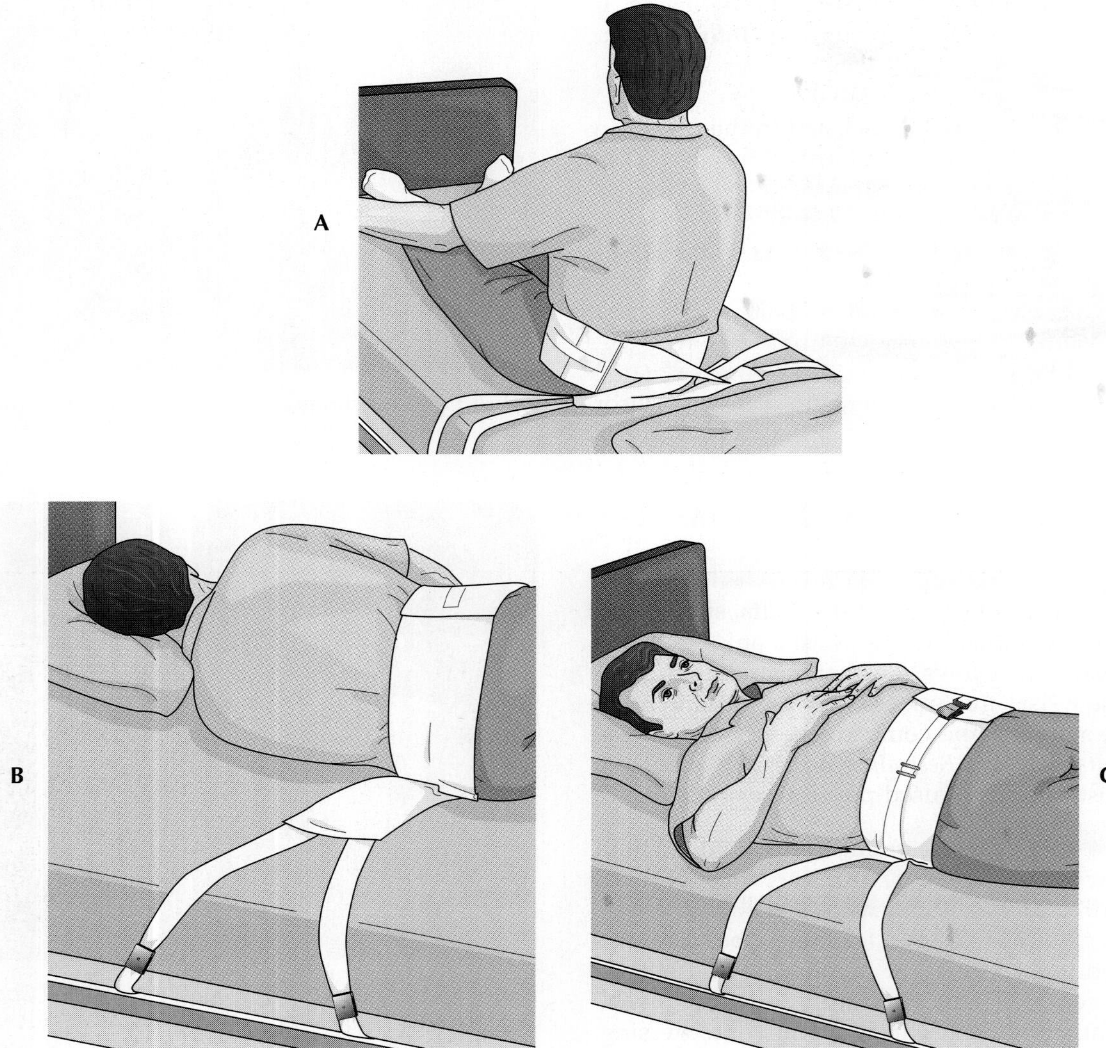

Figure 17-16 Belt restraint. *(Courtesy J. T. Posey Company, Arcadia, CA.)*

if the person slides down in the bed or chair. The restraint is always applied over a garment. *(Note: A vest or jacket restraint may have a positioning slot in the back. Crisscross the straps according to the manufacturer's instructions.)*

Vest and jacket restraints are especially dangerous. Death can occur from strangulation. If the client gets caught in the restraint, it can become so tight that the person's chest cannot expand to inhale air. The person could quickly suffocate and die. Restraints must be applied correctly. For vest and jacket restraints, this is critical.

- *Elbow restraints.* Elbow restraints limit arm movements (Figure 17-17). The person cannot bend the elbows. Elbow restraints are useful in preventing infants and small children from bending their elbows to scratch and touch incisions or pull out tubes. Both arms are restrained to achieve the desired effect. Elbow restraints wrap around the arm. They are secured in place with hook and loop fasteners or ties.

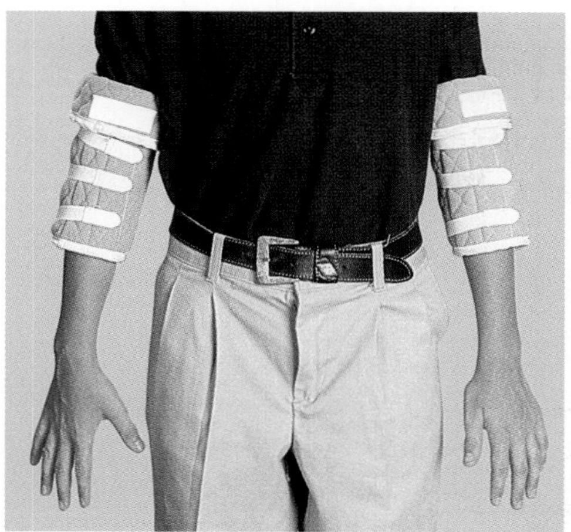

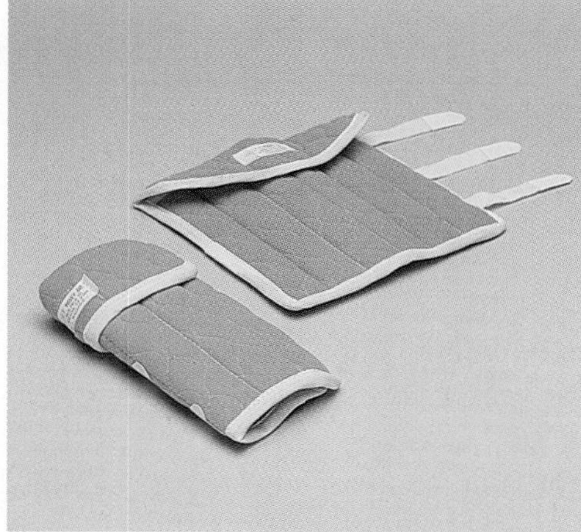

Figure 17-17 Elbow restraints. *(Courtesy J. T. Posey Company, Arcadia, CA.)*

Applying Physical Restraints

Compassionate Care

Remember to Promote:
- Dignity
- Independence
- Preferences
- Privacy
- Safety

Pre-Procedure

1 Identify the person according to employer policy.
2 Explain the procedure to the person.
3 Wash your hands.
4 Collect the following as instructed by the nurse:
- Correct type and size of restraints
- Padding for bony areas
- Bed rail pads or gap protectors

5 Provide for privacy.

Continued

Applying Physical Restraints—cont'd

Procedure

6 Make sure the person is comfortable and in good body alignment (see Chapter 21).

7 Put the bed rail pads or gap protectors on the bed if the person is in bed, if needed. Follow the manufacturer's instructions.

8 Pad bony areas according to the nurse's instructions.

9 Read the manufacturer's instructions. Note the front and back of the restraint.

10 *For wrist restraints:*
- a Apply the restraint following the manufacturer's instructions. Place the soft part toward the skin (see Figure 17-14).
- b Secure the restraint so it is snug but not tight. Make sure you can slide one or two fingers under the restraint (Figure 17-18). Follow the manufacturer's instructions.
- c Tie the straps to the movable part of the bed frame out of the person's reach. Use an employer-approved knot. Leave 2.5 to 5 cm (1 to 2 inches) of slack in the straps.
- d Repeat steps 10 a, b, and c for the other wrist.

11 *For mitt restraints:*
- a Make sure the person's hands are clean and dry.
- b Apply the mitt restraint. Follow the manufacturer's instructions.
- c Tie the straps to the movable part of the bed frame. Use an employer-approved knot. Leave 2.5 to 5 cm (1 to 2 inches) of slack in the straps.
- d Make sure the restraint is snug. Slide a finger between the restraint and the wrist. Adjust the straps if the restraint is too loose or too tight. Check for snugness again.
- e Repeat steps 11 b, c, and d for the other hand.

12 *For a belt restraint:*
- a Help the person to a sitting position.
- b Apply the restraint with your free hand. Follow the manufacturer's instructions.
- c Remove wrinkles or creases from the front and back of the restraint.
- d Bring the ties through the slots in the belt.
- e Help the person lie down if he or she is in bed.
- f Make sure the person is comfortable and in good body alignment (see Chapter 21).
- g Secure the straps to the movable part of the bed frame out of the person's reach or to the chair or wheelchair. Leave 2.5 to 5 cm (1 to 2 inches) of slack in the straps. If secured to the bed frame, the straps are secured at waist level out of the person's reach. Use an employer-approved knot.

13 *For a vest restraint:*
- a Help the person to a sitting position.
- b Apply the restraint with your free hand. Follow the manufacturer's instructions. The "V" part of the vest crosses in front.
- c Make sure the vest is free of wrinkles in the front and back.
- d Help the person lie down if he or she is in bed.
- e Bring the straps through the slots.
- f Make sure the person is comfortable and in good body alignment (see Chapter 21).
- g Secure the straps to the chair or to the movable part of the bed frame. Leave 2.5 to 5 cm (1 to 2 inches) of slack in the straps. If secured to the bed frame, the straps are secured at waist level out of the person's reach. Use an employer-approved knot.
- h Make sure the vest is snug. Slide an open hand between the restraint and the person. Adjust the restraint if it is too loose or too tight. Check for snugness again.

14 *For a jacket restraint:*
- a Help the person to a sitting position.
- b Apply the restraint with your free hand. Follow the manufacturer's instructions. Remember, the jacket opening goes in the back.
- c Close the back with the zipper, ties, or hook and loop closures.

Continued

Applying Physical Restraints—cont'd

Procedure—Cont'd

- **d** Make sure the side seams are under the arms. Remove any wrinkles in the front and back.
- **e** Help the person lie down if he or she is in bed.
- **f** Make sure the person is comfortable and in good body alignment (see Chapter 21).
- **g** Secure the straps to the chair or to the movable part of the bed frame. Leave 2.5 to 5 cm (1 to 2 inches) of slack in the straps. If secured to the bed frame, the straps are secured at waist level out of the person's reach. Use an employer-approved knot.
- **h** Make sure the jacket is snug. Slide an open hand between the restraint and the person. Adjust the restraint if it is too loose or too tight. Check for snugness again.

15 *For an elbow restraint:*

- **a** Wrap the restraint around the person's elbow. Follow the manufacturer's instructions.
- **b** Secure the restraint. Follow the manufacturer's instructions. Leave 2.5 to 5 cm (1 to 2 inches) of slack in the straps.
- **c** Repeat steps 15 a and b for the other arm.

Post-Procedure

16 Place the call bell within the person's reach.

17 Raise or lower the bed rails according to the care plan and the manufacturer's instructions.

18 Remove privacy measures.

19 Wash your hands.

20 Check the person and the restraints at least every 15 minutes.

- **a** For wrist, mitt, and elbow restraints: check the pulse, colour, and temperature of the restrained parts.
- **b** For vest, jacket, and belt restraints: check the person's breathing. *Call for the nurse at once if the person is not breathing or is having difficulty breathing.* Make sure the restraint is properly positioned in the front and back.

21 Do the following at least every 2 hours:

- Remove the restraint.
- Reposition the person.
- Meet food, fluid, hygiene, and elimination needs.
- Give skin care.
- Perform range-of-motion exercises or ambulate the person. Follow the care plan.
- Reapply the restraints.

22 Report and record your actions and observations according to employer policy.

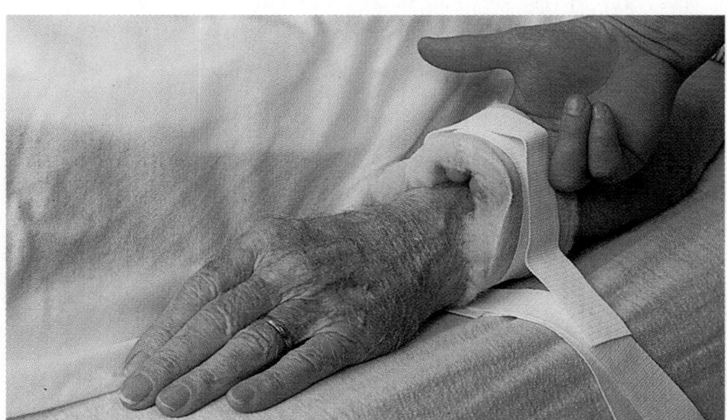

Figure 17-18 Two fingers fit between the restraint and the wrist.

REVIEW

Circle T if the answer is true and F if it is false.

1. T F Restraints can be used for staff convenience.
2. T F A device is a restraint only if it is attached to the person's body.
3. T F Bed rails are restraints.
4. T F Restraints can be used to protect the person from harming others.
5. T F Unnecessary restraint is false imprisonment.
6. T F Informed consent is needed for restraint use.
7. T F You can apply restraints when you think they are needed.
8. T F You should remove restraints every 2 hours to reposition the person and give skin care.
9. T F Some medications are restraints.
10. T F Bed rails are left down when vest restraints are used.

Circle the BEST answer.

11. These statements are about restraints. Which is *false*?
    - A. A restraint can be a barrier, device, garment, or medication.
    - B. A restraint limits or restricts a person's movement.
    - C. Some medications are restraints.
    - D. A restraint is used to make the staff's workload easier.
12. Which is *not* a restraint alternative?
    - A. Positioning the client's chair close to a wall
    - B. Answering calls promptly
    - C. Taking the client outside in nice weather
    - D. Padding walls and corners of furniture
13. Environmental restraints
    - A. Involve medications
    - B. Are attached to the person and fixed to a nonmovable object
    - C. Confine a person to a specific place
    - D. Are used for discipline or staff convenience
14. A belt restraint is applied to a person in bed. Where should you tie the straps?
    - A. To the bed rails
    - B. To the head board
    - C. To the movable part of the bed frame at waist level
    - D. To the foot board
15. Mrs. Kwon has a restraint. You should check her and the position of the restraint at least
    - A. Every 15 minutes
    - B. Every 30 minutes
    - C. Every hour
    - D. Every 2 hours
16. Mrs. Kwon has mitt restraints. Which of these is especially important to report to the nurse?
    - A. Her heart rate
    - B. Her respiratory rate
    - C. Why the restraints were applied
    - D. If you felt a pulse in the restrained extremities
17. Which restraints prevent turning and getting out of bed?
    - A. Wrist restraints
    - B. Jacket restraints
    - C. Belt restraints
    - D. Mitt restraints
18. Mr. Boyd has a vest restraint. It is not too tight or too loose if you can slide
    - A. A fist between the vest and the person
    - B. One finger between the vest and the person
    - C. An open hand between the vest and the person
    - D. Two fingers between the vest and the person

Answers to these questions are on page 823.

CHAPTER

18

Preventing Infection

OBJECTIVES

- Define the key terms listed in this chapter
- Distinguish between pathogens and nonpathogens
- Explain what microbes need to live and grow
- Recognize the signs and symptoms of infection
- Describe the chain of infection
- List ways in which microbes are transmitted
- List risk factors for infection
- Describe common aseptic practices
- Explain why hand washing is so important
- Describe when to wash your hands and general guidelines for hand washing
- Describe cleaning, disinfection, and sterilization methods
- Understand the principles and practices of Standard Precautions and Transmission-Based Precautions
- Explain how to use personal protective equipment (PPE)
- Describe the principles and practices of surgical asepsis
- Learn the procedures described in this chapter

KEY TERMS

asepsis The state of being free of pathogens; clean

aseptic technique Medical asepsis

biohazardous waste Items that may be harmful to others because they are contaminated with blood, body fluids, secretions, or excretions; *bio* means life and *hazardous* means dangerous or harmful

clean technique Medical asepsis

communicable disease A disease caused by microbes that spread easily; a contagious disease

contagious disease Communicable disease

contamination The process of being exposed to pathogens

disinfection The process of destroying pathogens

infection A disease state resulting from the invasion and growth of microbes in the body

infection control Policies and procedures used to prevent the spread of infection within health care settings

isolation precautions Guidelines for preventing the spread of pathogens; includes Standard Precautions and Transmission-Based Precautions

medical asepsis Practices that reduce the number of microbes and prevent their spread; clean technique or aseptic technique

microbe Microorganism

microorganism A form of life (*organism*) that is so small (*micro*) it can be seen only with a microscope; a microbe

multi-resistant organism (MRO) A strain of bacteria that is very difficult to treat with common antibiotics; examples are MRSA and VRE

nonpathogen A microbe that does not usually cause infection

nosocomial infection An infection acquired after admission to a health care facility

pathogen A microbe that can cause an infection

personal protective equipment (PPE) Special clothing and equipment that act as a barrier between microbes and your hands, eyes, nose, mouth, and clothes; includes gloves, gowns, masks, and eye protection

reservoir The environment in which microbes live and grow; host

Routine Practices Standard Precautions

sharp Equipment or item that may pierce the skin; includes needles, razor blades, and broken glass

Standard Precautions Guidelines to prevent the spread of infection from blood, body fluids, secretions, excretions, nonintact skin, and mucous membranes; Routine Practices

sterile Free of all microbes—pathogens and nonpathogens

sterile field A work area free of all microbes—pathogens and nonpathogens

sterile technique Surgical asepsis

sterilization The process of destroying *all* microbes

surgical asepsis Practices that keep equipment and supplies free of *all* microbes; sterile technique

Transmission-Based Precautions Guidelines to contain pathogens within a certain area, usually the client's room

Infection can be a serious safety and health hazard. Some infections cause only minor symptoms. Others are serious. They may delay a person's recovery, create long-term health problems, or cause death. Older adults, people who are ill, and people with disabilities are at great risk. Infections can easily spread from worker to client, from client to client, or from client to worker.

All members of the health care team must protect clients and themselves from infection. To prevent infection, you must understand how infections spread. You also must follow your employer's infection control policies. **Infection control** refers to policies and procedures used to prevent the spread of infection within health care settings.

Microorganisms

A **microorganism** (**microbe**) is a form of life (*organism*) that is so small (*micro*) it can be seen only with a microscope. Microbes live and grow everywhere. They are in water, air, food, soil, plants, and animals. They are on inanimate objects like clothing, furniture, medical equipment, and personal care items. Microbes also live and grow in and on people. They are in the mouth, nose, respiratory tract, stomach, intestines, and on the skin.

Most microbes usually do not cause infection. These are called **nonpathogens**. Some microbes are harmful and can cause infection. These are called **pathogens**. They are also known as "germs" or "bugs."

Types of Microorganisms

Within health care settings, the three types of microbes that cause the greatest risk for infection are bacteria, viruses, and fungi.

- *Bacteria*—single-celled microbes that naturally occur on living, dead, or inanimate objects. They multiply rapidly. They can be nonpathogenic or they can cause serious infections in any body system. Infections caused by bacteria are usually treated with antibiotics.
- *Viruses*—microbes that grow only inside living cells. They take over the cells' machinery to produce new virus particles. AIDS, hepatitis, influenza, and the common cold are examples of infections caused by viruses. Antibiotics are not effective against viruses. Some viral diseases (such as measles, polio, and many types of influenza) can be prevented by vaccination.
- *Fungi*—microbes that live only on organic matter, such as plants and animals. Certain types of yeasts and moulds are common fungi that can be pathogens. In humans, fungi can infect the mouth, vagina, skin, feet, and other body areas. Many fungal infections are mild, such as athlete's foot. However, fungi can also cause life-threatening infections.

Requirements of Microorganisms

Microbes require certain conditions to live and grow. The **reservoir** (host) is the environment where the microbe lives and grows. Microbes grow in reservoirs that are *warm* and *dark*. They need *water* and *nourishment*. Most microbes also need *oxygen*, although some microbes thrive without it. Many microbes grow best at body temperature. They are destroyed by heat and light.

Normal Flora

Normal flora are microbes that naturally live and grow in a certain location. They are nonpathogens when they are in or on this natural location. Certain microbes, for example, are found in the respiratory tract, in the intestines, and on the skin. These are harmless or even beneficial to the body. When a nonpathogen is transmitted from its natural site to another site or host, it becomes a pathogen. For example, *Escherichia coli* is a bacteria normally found in the colon. It helps with food digestion. If *E. coli* enters a different body system (for example, if it is ingested through contaminated food or water), it can cause a serious infection.

Multi-Resistant Organisms

Bacteria reproduce very quickly and in large numbers. Therefore, they can change to protect themselves from antibiotics. Certain strains of bacteria are now very difficult to treat with common antibiotics. These bacteria are known as **multi-resistant organisms (MROs)**.

Multi-resistant organisms are becoming increasingly common. They are a serious threat to patients and residents in health care facilities. Infections caused by MROs are sometimes fatal. They are easily spread among people at risk for infection. The two most common multi-resistant organisms are MRSA (methicillin-resistant *Staphylococcus aureus*) and VRE (vancomycin-resistant *Enterococci*). You will be trained to follow special precautions when in contact with clients infected or suspected of being infected with MROs.

The Spread of Pathogens

An **infection** is a disease state resulting from the invasion and growth of microbes in the body. A *local infection* is infection in one body part. A *systemic infection* involves the whole body. The person has signs and symptoms of infection. Some or all of the signs and symptoms in Box 18-1 on page 212 are present. (See also *Focus on Older Adults: Signs and Symptoms of Infection* box on page 212.)

Many common illnesses are infections. The common cold, influenza, and chicken pox are examples. So are hepatitis, pneumonia, tuberculosis, and AIDS. These are communicable diseases. A **communicable disease (contagious disease)** is a disease caused by microbes that spread easily. For example, pneumonia is an infection in the lungs.

Being exposed to pathogens *does not always* result in an infection. The body can protect itself from infection. There are three possible outcomes when exposed to a pathogen:

- *The immune system destroys the pathogen.* The pathogen does not live and grow within the body.

Box 18-1 Signs and Symptoms of Infection

- Fever and/or chills
- Increased pulse and respiratory rates
- Aches, pain, or tenderness
- Fatigue and loss of energy
- Loss of appetite
- Nausea
- Vomiting
- Diarrhea
- Rash
- Sores on mucous membranes
- Redness and swelling of a body part
- Discharge or drainage from the infected area that may have a foul odour
- New or increased cough, sore throat, or runny or stuffy nose
- Burning pain when urinating or the need to urinate more often or with increased urgency

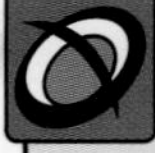

Focus on Older Adults

Signs and Symptoms of Infection

Older adults are especially at risk for infections. The normal changes associated with aging place them at high risk. They are also more likely than other adults to become seriously ill or die from an infection. For example, pneumonia and influenza are often life-threatening illnesses for older adults.

Older adults often do not show the usual signs of infection. For example, fever, pain, and swelling are usually absent in older adults. This is because they tend to have lower body temperatures, decreased pain sensation, and less immune response to infection.

Sometimes the only sign of infection in older adults is a change in behaviour. If an older client displays any of the following, report it to your supervisor:

- New or increased confusion or delirium
- New or increased incontinence
- Loss of appetite
- Decreased ability to do activities of daily living
- Falls
- Changes in mood; for example, a client who is usually talkative, cheerful, and cooperative becomes unusually quiet, moody, and uncooperative

An infection does not occur. (See Chapter 13 to review the immune system.)

- *The immune system does not destroy the pathogen, but an infection does not develop.* Even though the person remains healthy, the pathogen is still present within the body and can be transmitted to others. In this case, the person is colonized with the pathogen. *Colonization* occurs when a pathogen lives on or in the body but does not cause an active infection. The person is now a *carrier*. He or she is able to transfer the pathogen to others.
- *An infection develops sometime after exposure to the pathogen.* The period of time between exposure and the onset of illness is called the *incubation period*. The incubation period may be relatively short or may last for years. During the incubation period, the person can transfer the pathogen to others.

The Chain of Infection

Many factors work together for an infection to develop. The spread of infection involves a process known as the chain of infection (Figure 18-1). The links in the chain are as follows:

- *Pathogen*—a microbe capable of causing disease.
- *Reservoir*—the environment where the pathogen lives before it infects. Remember, a pathogen can live on or in a person or animal (a *host*), food, water, soil, or inanimate objects.
- *Portal of exit*—the path by which the pathogen leaves the reservoir. Exits in the human body are the body openings (mouth; nose; and rectal, vaginal, and urethral openings), breaks in the skin (a scrape, cut, or other wound), and breaks in the mucous membranes (the skin in the mouth, eyes, nose, vagina, and rectum). Pathogens are carried through the portals of exit by blood, body fluids, excretions, or secretions. These include urine, stool, vomitus, saliva, mucus, pus, vaginal discharge, semen, wound drainage, and sputum (respiratory secretions).
- *Mode of transmission*—how the pathogen travels from the portal of exit to the next reservoir or host. Microbes can be transmitted by physical contact (direct and indirect), droplets in the air, air currents, or by an infected vehicle or vector (Table 18-1 on page 214). The mode of transmission depends on the type of microbe. Some microbes are transmitted in more than one way.
- *Portal of entry*—where the pathogen enters the new host's body. Portals of entry are the same as the exits: body openings and breaks in the skin or mucous membranes.
- *Susceptible host*—a person at risk for infection. Whether or not the pathogen grows and multiplies in the new host depends on the state of the person's immune system. Remember, the immune system protects the body from infection. A person whose immune system is weakened is *immunocompromised*. (*Immuno* comes from *immunity*, which means protection against certain disease. *Compromised* means weakened.) He or she is more likely to ac-

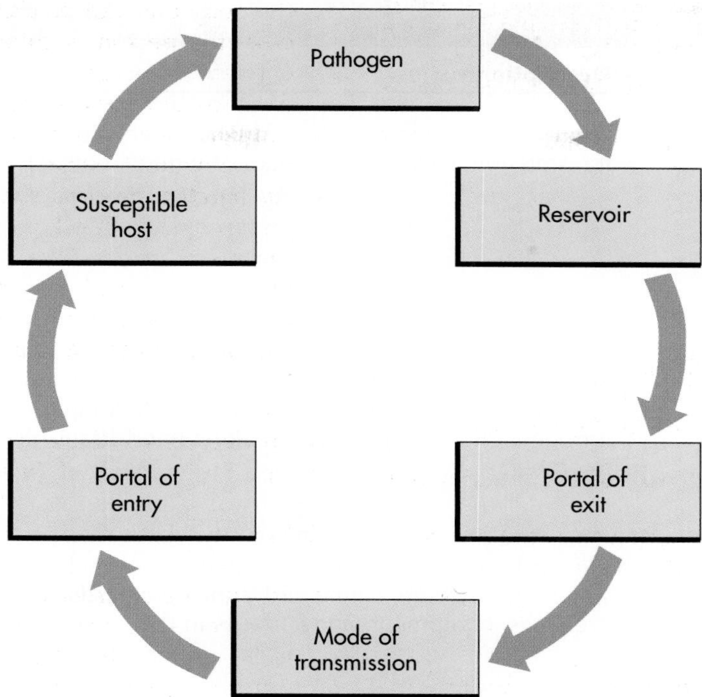

Figure 18-1 The chain of infection.

quire infection. There are many factors that increase the risk of infection (Box 18-2 on page 215).

Infections in Health Care Settings

A **nosocomial infection** is an infection acquired after admission to a health care facility. Infections can also be acquired in home care and other community settings. People in health care settings are usually at high risk for infection. They might have some or all of the risk factors for infection listed in Box 18-2 on page 215.

Microbes can enter the body through equipment used in treatments, therapies, and tests. Therefore equipment must be free of pathogens. Workers can transfer microbes from client to client and from themselves to clients.

The most common infections within health care settings include respiratory tract infections (colds, pneumonia, bronchitis, and influenza), urinary tract infections, gastrointestinal tract infections (resulting in nausea or diarrhea), and skin infections (such as wound or IV site infections).

Sick, frail, and older clients have a hard time fighting infections. Therefore the health care team must prevent the spread of infection. The following help prevent infections in health care settings:

- Medical asepsis
- Isolation precautions
- Surgical asepsis

Medical Asepsis

Asepsis is the state of being free of pathogens. Remember, microbes are everywhere. Therefore measures are needed to achieve asepsis. **Medical asepsis** (**clean technique** or **aseptic technique**) refers to the practices that:

- Reduce the number of microbes
- Prevent the spread of microbes from one person or place to another person or place

Aseptic practices break the chain of infection.

In health care, an aseptic object or area is considered *clean*. There are no pathogens present. The object or area is *contaminated* (unclean) if pathogens are present or if it has been exposed to pathogens. **Contamination** is the process of being exposed to pathogens.

An aseptic (clean) environment is different from a sterile environment. **Sterile** means free of *all* microbes—pathogens and nonpathogens. For example, operating rooms and instruments inserted into the body need to be sterile. Microbes cannot be present during surgery or invasive procedures. Infection is a risk. **Surgical asepsis** (**sterile technique**) refers to the practices that keep equipment and supplies free of *all* microbes (page 232). **Sterilization** is the process of destroying *all* microbes. Both pathogens and nonpathogens are destroyed.

(text continues on page 215)

Table 18-1 Modes of Transmission

Mode of transmission	Description
1. Contact transmission	The transfer of microbes by physical touch. Contact transmission is by direct contact or indirect contact. 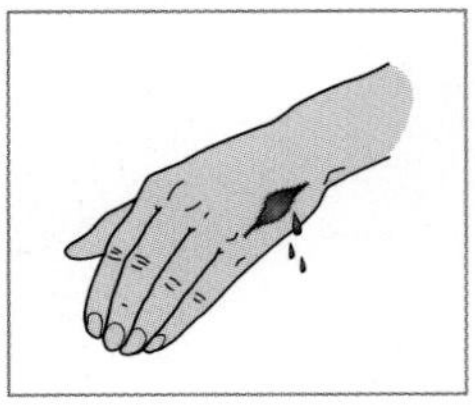
• Direct contact transmission	Occurs by touching an infected or colonized person. Skin-to-skin contact is required. Many personal care activities require direct contact, such as bathing or turning a client in bed. Even shaking hands transmits microbes. 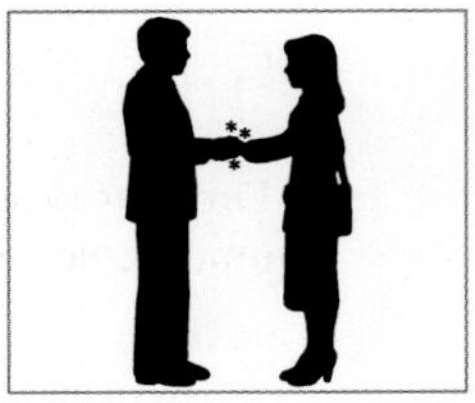
• Indirect contact transmission	Occurs by touching a contaminated object such as soiled linen, tissue, eating and drinking utensils, dressings, equipment, and surfaces in the client's room. 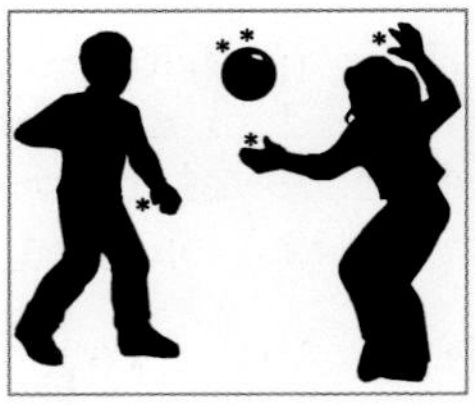
2. Droplet transmission	Occurs when microbes are spread short distances (less than 1 metre) in the air by droplets. Coughing, sneezing, and talking propel droplets from the respiratory system through the air (Figure 18-2). These droplets carry microbes. When the droplets settle on another person or object in the environment, the microbes are deposited on them. 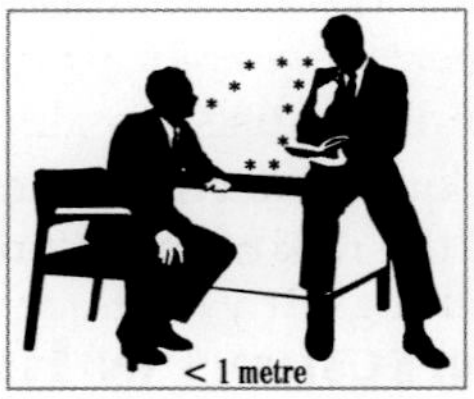
3. Airborne transmission	Occurs when microbes are transmitted long distances (farther than 1 metre) by air currents. These microbes are contained in dust particles or evaporated droplets in the air. Microbes carried in this manner can travel across a room or even farther. People may then inhale the microbes or have contact with them if they are deposited on their skin. 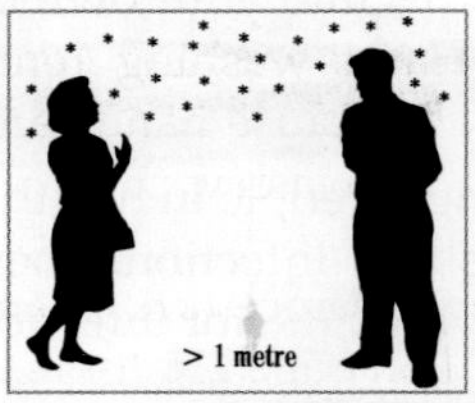
4. Vehicle transmission	Occurs when microbes are transmitted by a contaminated source (vehicle). Common vehicles of transmission include food, water, medication, and invasive medical equipment. One vehicle can transmit microbes to many people, resulting in an outbreak. 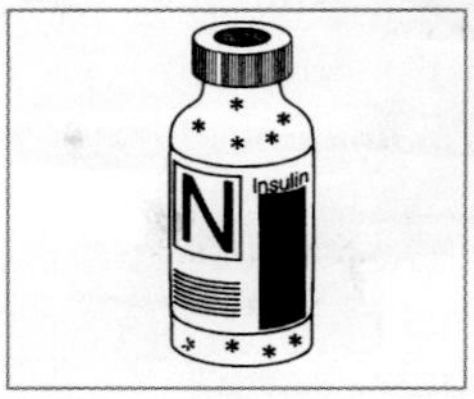
5. Vector-borne transmission	Occurs when insects (fleas, ticks, mites, mosquitoes) or pests (mice) transmit microbes to humans. This type of transmission is rare in health care settings. 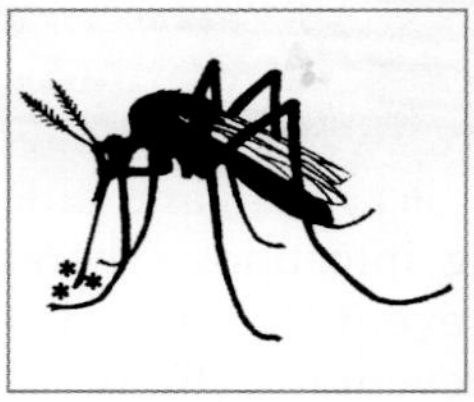

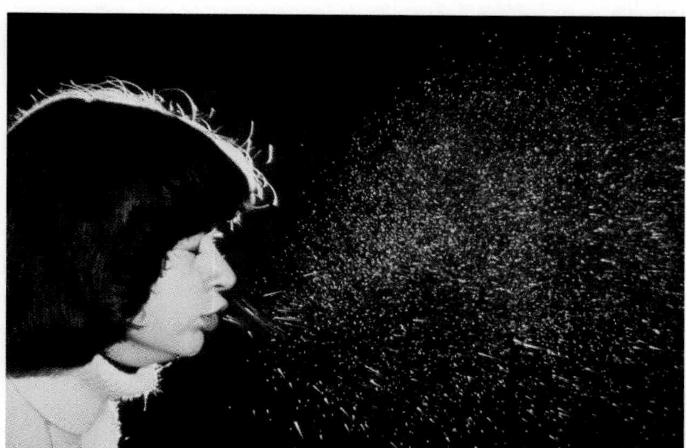

Figure 18-2 Droplets propelled into the air by a sneeze. During a common cold, most of the droplets contain virus particles.

There are many aseptic practices that help prevent the spread of microbes. The following sections describe some of the most important aseptic practices that must be followed.

Hand Washing

Hand washing with soap and water is the easiest and most important way to prevent the spread of infection. Your hands are used in almost every task. They can easily pick up microbes from one person, place, or thing. They can then transmit them to other people, places, or things. If you touch your eyes, nose, or mouth with your contaminated hands, you can also transfer microbes into your own body.

Hand washing removes most microbes from the skin. Because hands are contaminated very easily, you need to wash your hands often (Box 18-3). You also need to wash them properly. Although hand washing is a simple procedure, many people do it incorrectly. Box 18-4 on page 216 lists guidelines for hand washing. (See also *Focus on Home Care: Hand Washing* box on page 217.)

(text continues on page 217)

Box 18-2 Factors That Increase the Risk of Infection

- Extremes of age (young and old are at risk)
- Poor nutrition
- Stress
- Lack of sleep
- The presence of disease or illness. Many diseases or their treatments weaken the immune system, including AIDS, cancer (especially if the person is receiving chemotherapy or radiation therapy), organ transplants, and kidney failure.
- Certain medications
- Invasive procedures—intubations and surgeries are examples
- Invasive devices—intravenous lines (IVs) and urinary catheters are examples
- Open wounds
- Living in close contact with people who have communicable diseases
- Having contact with a number of caregivers

Box 18-3 When to Wash Your Hands

- *Immediately before and after giving care.* This means you wash your hands before caring for a client, after caring for a client, and then again immediately before you care for the next client.
- Whenever your hands are visibly soiled
- After contact with your own or another person's blood, body fluids, secretions, or excretions
- After touching objects that are contaminated, such as soiled linens, tissues, toilet paper, garbage bags, bed pans, or diapers
- Before and after preparing, handling, or eating food
- Before feeding a client
- Before putting on disposable gloves and after removing them
- After personal body functions, such as urinating or having a bowel movement, changing tampons or sanitary pads, sneezing, coughing, or blowing your nose

Box 18-4 Guidelines for Hand Washing

- Wash your hands under warm running water.
- Stand away from the sink. Do not let your hands, body, or uniform touch the sink. The sink is contaminated (Figure 18-3).
- Keep your hands and forearms lower than your elbows. Your hands are dirtier than your elbows and forearms. If you hold your hands and forearms up, dirty water runs from hands to elbows. Those areas become contaminated.
- Rub your palms together to work up a good lather (Figure 18-4). The rubbing action helps remove microbes and dirt.
- Pay attention to areas often missed during hand washing: thumbs, knuckles, sides of the hands, little fingers, and under the nails.
- Clean fingernails by rubbing the fingertips of one hand against the palm of the other hand (Figure 18-5).
- Remember to clean under the fingernails using a nail file, orange stick, or soft nail brush (Figure 18-6). Microbes easily grow under the fingernails.
- Spend enough time lathering and rinsing. The duration of the hand wash is as important as the technique. Check your employer's policy for how long to wash your hands. At least 15 to 20 seconds is needed to remove most microbes on the skin. Wash your hands longer if they are dirty or soiled with blood, body fluids, secretions, or excretions.
- Dry your hands starting at the fingers. Work up to your forearms. You will dry the cleanest area first.
- Use a clean paper towel to turn off each water faucet (Figure 18-7). Faucets are contaminated. Using paper towels prevents clean hands from becoming contaminated again.
- Apply hand lotion or cream after washing your hands. This prevents skin chapping and drying. Skin breaks can occur in chapped and dry skin. Remember, skin breaks are portals of entry for microbes.

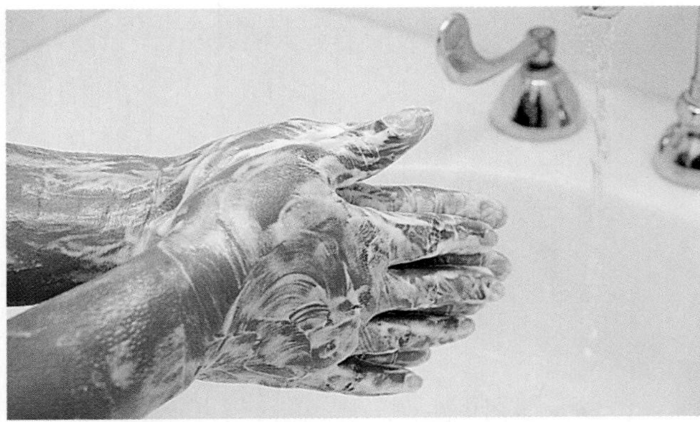

Figure 18-4 Rub your palms together to work up a good lather.

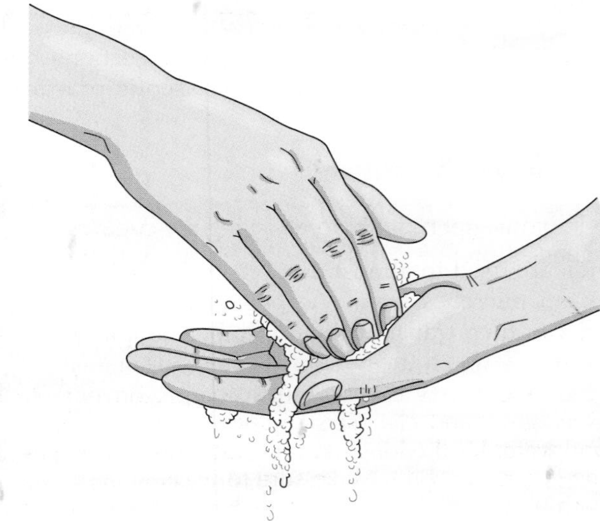

Figure 18-5 Rub your fingertips against your palm to clean underneath the nails.

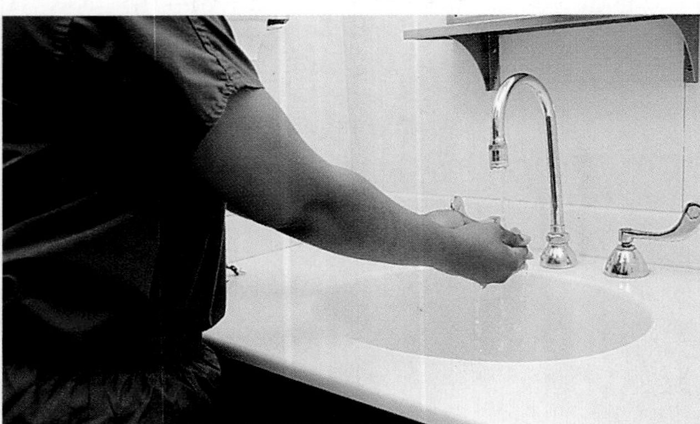

Figure 18-3 Do not touch the sink with your uniform. Keep your hands lower than your elbows.

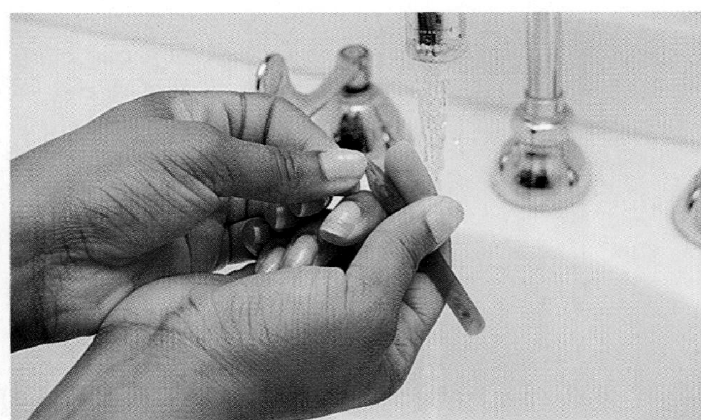

Figure 18-6 Use a nail file to clean under your fingernails.

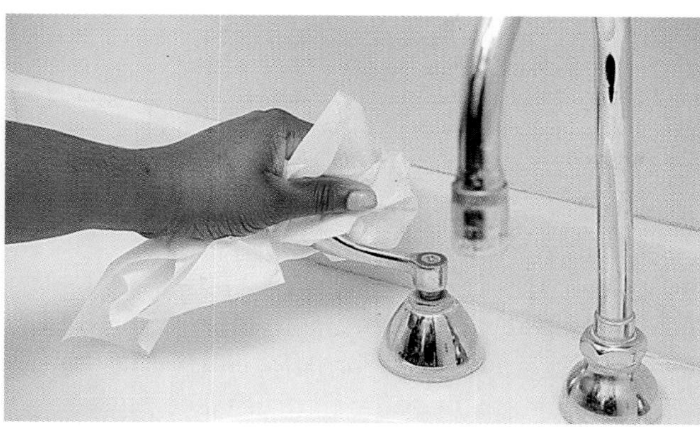

Figure 18-7 Use a clean piece of paper towel to turn off each faucet.

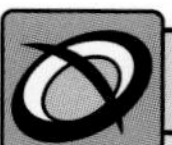

Focus on Home Care

HAND WASHING

A client's home might not have everything you need for proper hand washing. For example, the home might be lacking soap or paper towels. Do not use the client's towels for drying your hands. Bring paper towels with you on home visits. Check with your supervisor before visiting the client. Most agencies provide workers with basic needed supplies to bring with them on visits.

If the home is lacking easy access to warm running water, you should bring along a waterless antiseptic hand cleanser. This product uses alcohol to clean the hands and is effective and convenient. However, hand cleansers should not replace soap and water for the long term because they do not remove dirt build-up. Make sure to wash your hands with soap and water as soon as possible after using the hand cleanser.

Your hands must be dry before you apply a hand cleanser. Moisture dilutes the alcohol and makes it less effective. The hand cleanser is also not effective if your hands are heavily soiled. Apply liquid hand cleansers as follows:

- Pour about 3 to 5 mL ($^1/_2$ to 1 teaspoon) of hand cleanser onto both hands.
- Rub hands together. Make sure that all areas of the hands are covered, including between the fingers.
- Clean under the fingernails by rubbing fingertips on the wet palms.
- Rub hands until they are dry, between 30 seconds and 1 minute.

CARE OF SUPPLIES AND EQUIPMENT

Remember, microbes live on people and on objects. Contaminated equipment and supplies can easily become a source of infection.

Many items used in facilities and home care are disposable. They are used once and then discarded. In these cases, cleaning is not an issue. Some items are reused. These include bedpans, urinals, washbasins, water pitchers, and drinking cups. In facilities, reusable items are labelled with the client's name, room, and bed number. They are never used or "borrowed" for another client.

Reusable items must be decontaminated. There are three levels of decontamination: cleaning, disinfection, and sterilization.

Cleaning. Cleaning reduces the number of microbes present on the item. It also removes organic material such as dirt, blood, body fluids, secretions, and excretions. For some equipment, periodic cleaning is all that is required. For example, items like crutches and blood pressure cuffs need to be cleaned only when visibly soiled and between use on different clients. Follow employer policy about when and how to clean items. The following guidelines apply when cleaning equipment:

- Wear personal protective equipment when cleaning items that may be contaminated with blood, body fluids, secretions, or excretions. **Personal protective equipment (PPE)** is special clothing and equipment that act as a barrier between microbes and your hands, eyes, nose, mouth, and clothes. They include gloves, gowns, masks, and eye protection (goggles or face shields) (see page 224). Follow your employer's policies about the use of PPE when cleaning equipment.
- Rinse the item first in cold water to remove organic material. Warm or hot water makes organic material thick, sticky, and hard to remove.
- Wash the item with soap and hot water.
- Scrub the item thoroughly. Use a brush if necessary.
- Rinse the item in warm water.
- Dry the item.
- Disinfect or sterilize the item.
- Disinfect equipment and the sink used in the cleaning procedure.
- Discard gloves and other PPE.
- Wash your hands.

Hand Washing

Procedure

1. Make sure you have soap, paper towels, wastebasket, and an orange stick, nail file, or soft nail brush.
2. Push your watch and sleeves up well over your wrists. Remove rings.
3. Stand away from the sink so your clothes do not touch it. Stand so the soap and faucet are easy to reach (see Figure 18-3).
4. Turn on and adjust the water until it feels warm.
5. Wet your wrists and hands thoroughly under running water. Keep your hands lower than your elbows (see Figure 18-3).
6. Apply about 5 mL (1 teaspoon) of liquid soap to your hands. If using bar soap, do not touch the soap dish as you pick up the soap. Rinse the bar soap before you use it. Do not touch the soap dish as you put the soap back.
7. Rub your palms together and interlace your fingers to work up a good lather (see Figure 18-4). This step should last at least 15 seconds.
8. Wash each hand and wrist thoroughly. Clean well between the fingers.
9. Clean under the fingernails by rubbing your fingertips against your palm (see Figure 18-5).
10. Clean under the fingernails with a nail file, orange stick, or soft nail brush (see Figure 18-6). This step is necessary for the first hand washing of the day and when your hands are highly soiled.
11. Rinse your wrists and hands well, keeping your hands and forearms down. Water flows from the arms to the hands.
12. Repeat steps 6 through 11, if needed.
13. Dry your hands and wrists with paper towels. Pat dry starting at your fingertips.
14. Discard the paper towels.
15. Turn off faucets with clean paper towels (see Figure 18-7). Use a clean paper towel for each faucet.
16. Discard the paper towels.
17. Apply a small amount of lotion to your hands.

Disinfection. **Disinfection** is the process of destroying all pathogens except spores. *Spores* are bacteria protected by a hard shell. Spores can be destroyed only by the sterilization process. An item must be thoroughly cleaned before it is disinfected.

Reusable items are disinfected with chemicals such as alcohols or chlorines (*chemical disinfectants*). Such items include:

- Metal bedpans
- Glass thermometers
- Commodes
- Countertops
- Tubs
- Room furniture

Follow your employer's policies about when and how to disinfect equipment and supplies. (See *Focus on Home Care: Disinfectants* box.)

Chemical disinfectants can burn and irritate the skin. Wear utility gloves or rubber household gloves to prevent skin irritation. These gloves are waterproof.

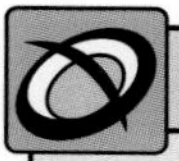

Focus on Home Care

DISINFECTANTS

Detergent and hot water are common disinfectants. They are used for utensils, linens, and clothes. Many commercial products are available for household surfaces. Such surfaces include sinks, countertops, floors, toilets, tubs, and showers. Use the products preferred by the family or as instructed by your supervisor.

Vinegar is also an effective and cheap disinfectant. You can use it to clean bedpans, urinals, commodes, and toilets. To make a vinegar solution, mix 250 mL (1 cup) of white vinegar and 750 mL (3 cups) of water. Make sure you label the container as "vinegar solution." Also put the date on the container and your name.

Do not wear disposable gloves when using disinfectants. Some chemical disinfectants have special measures for use or storage. Check the material safety data sheet before handling a disinfectant (see Chapter 16). Follow your employer's policies.

Sterilization. Sterilizing destroys all nonpathogens and pathogens, including spores. Very high temperatures are used because microbes are destroyed by heat.

Boiling water, radiation, liquid or gas chemicals, dry heat, and steam under pressure are sterilization methods. Items that enter the body or are used during surgery are sterilized. These include IV catheters, urinary catheters, and needles. In facilities, specially trained workers are responsible for the sterilization process. Therefore support workers are not responsible for sterilizing equipment. However, you may be required to clean the item in preparation for sterilization. (See *Focus on Home Care: Sterilization* box.)

OTHER ASEPTIC MEASURES

Hand washing, cleaning, disinfection, and sterilization are important aseptic measures. However, other aseptic measures also prevent the spread of infection and microbes. These measures are listed in Box 18-5 on page 220.

(text continues on page 221)

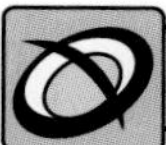

Focus on Home Care

STERILIZATION

In home care, almost all medical items that must be sterile are commercially prepared and disposable. However, you may be required to sterilize noninvasive items such as diapers or glass baby bottles.

Diapers and other colour-fast linens can be sterilized by soaking them in a solution of one part household bleach and 10 parts water. Or one cup of bleach can be added to the wash when laundering items soiled with blood and body fluids. Always check with your client and your supervisor for direction before using bleach. Some linens cannot be bleached. Check labels on clothes before using bleach (see Chapter 23).

Glass baby bottles and other such items can be sterilized in boiling water. Place the items in a large pot filled with cold water. Cover the pot and bring the water to a full boil. Boil the items for at least 15 minutes, then turn off the heat and let the water and items cool. Use tongs to remove the items, and let them air dry on a clean towel. Although boiling water is a convenient and inexpensive method of sterilization in the home, it does not always kill all spores and viruses. Therefore, facilities do not use boiling water for sterilizing items.

Box 18-5 Aseptic Measures

Controlling Reservoirs

- Maintain your personal hygiene. Bathe, shampoo your hair, brush your teeth, and change clothes daily.
- Make sure your vaccinations are up-to-date (Box 18-6).
- Dispose or store soiled tissues, linens, and other materials in leakproof plastic bags.
- Empty garbage at least once a day.
- Keep tables, countertops, wheelchair trays, and other surfaces clean and dry.
- Wash contaminated areas with soap and water. Stool, urine, and blood contain microbes. So do other body fluids, secretions, and excretions.
- Clean work surfaces after completing a task, when they are dirty, and after blood or other potentially infectious material is spilled. Follow employer policies.
- Provide for the client's hygiene (see Chapter 27).
- Keep drainage containers below the drainage site (see Chapter 29).
- Cook meats and poultry adequately. Wash fruits and raw vegetables before eating or serving them. Handle and store all foods safely (see Chapter 25).
- Wash cooking and eating utensils with soap and water after use.

Controlling Portals of Exit

- Cover your nose and mouth when coughing or sneezing. Wash your hands afterward.
- Provide clients with tissues to use when coughing or sneezing.
- Wear personal protective equipment as needed.
- Check your hands frequently for cuts, scrapes, or other breaks in the skin. Report any to your supervisor.

Controlling Transmission

- Wash your hands properly and at appropriate times (see Boxes 18-3 and 18-4).
- Assist clients with hand washing:
  - Before and after handling or eating food
  - After elimination
  - After coughing, sneezing, or blowing the nose
  - After changing tampons, sanitary pads, incontinence products, or other personal hygiene products
  - After contact with blood, body fluids, secretions, or excretions
  - Any time their hands are soiled
- Make sure all clients have their own care equipment, including washbasins, bedpans, urinals, commodes, and glass thermometers. Make sure all clients have their own toothbrush, drinking glass, towels, washcloths, eating and drinking utensils, and other personal care items. Do not share these items among clients or among the client's family members.
- Do not take equipment and supplies from one client's room to use for another client. Even if the item is unused, do not take it from one room to another.
- Hold equipment and linens (clean or contaminated) away from your uniform. This prevents the transfer of microbes from the equipment to your uniform and from your uniform to the equipment (Figure 18-8).
- Prevent dust movement. Dust carries microbes. Do not shake linens. Use a damp cloth for dusting.
- Remove soiled linens by folding them with the dirtiest areas in the centre.
- Clean from the cleanest area to the dirtiest. This prevents soiling a clean area.
- Clean away from your body. Do not dust, brush, or wipe toward yourself. Otherwise you transmit microbes to your skin, hair, and clothing.
- Flush urine and stool down the toilet. Avoid splatters and splashes. Cover bedpans and commodes with a lid when transporting.
- Pour contaminated liquids directly into sinks or toilets. Avoid splashing onto other areas. Clean and disinfect the sink and contaminated areas afterward.
- Avoid sitting on a client's bed. You will pick up microbes and transfer them to the next surface that you sit on, possibly another client's bed.
- Do not use items that have touched the floor. The floor is contaminated. Do not let linens (even soiled linens) touch the floor.
- Disinfect tubs, showers, shower chairs, bedpans, urinals, and commodes after each use. Follow your employer's disinfection procedures.
- Report pests—ants, spiders, mice, and so on.

Controlling Portals of Entry

- Provide good skin care and oral hygiene according to the care plan (see Chapter 27). This promotes intact skin and mucous membranes. Damaged skin and mucous membranes provide portals of entry.
- Do not let the client lie on tubes or other items. This protects the skin from injury.
- Make sure linens are dry and wrinkle-free (see Chapter 24). This protects the skin from injury.
- Turn and reposition the client as directed in the care plan (see Chapter 21). This protects the skin from injury.
- Assist with or clean the client's genital area after elimination as needed (see Chapter 27). This is called perineal care. Wipe and clean from the urethra (the cleanest area) to the rectum (the dirtiest area). This helps prevent urinary tract infections.
- Make sure drainage tubes are properly connected. Otherwise microbes can enter the drainage system.

Protecting the Susceptible Host

- Follow the care plan to meet hygiene needs. This protects the skin and mucous membranes.
- Follow the care plan to meet nutrition and fluid needs. This helps prevent infection.
- Assist with coughing and deep-breathing exercises as directed. This helps prevent respiratory infections.

Box 18-6 Vaccinations

Most health care employers require workers to have their routine vaccinations up-to-date before they start work. In addition, the hepatitis B vaccination (involving three injections over 6 months) is recommended for all people working in health care settings. This vaccination protects you against acquiring hepatitis B from your clients (see Chapter 31). Your antibody levels can be checked periodically after your vaccination to ensure that you are still immune to hepatitis B. A yearly influenza vaccination is also highly recommended (and sometimes required) for anyone working in the health care field. This vaccine is very important to protect both you and your clients from influenza. Influenza can be very dangerous to older adults and people with weakened immune systems.

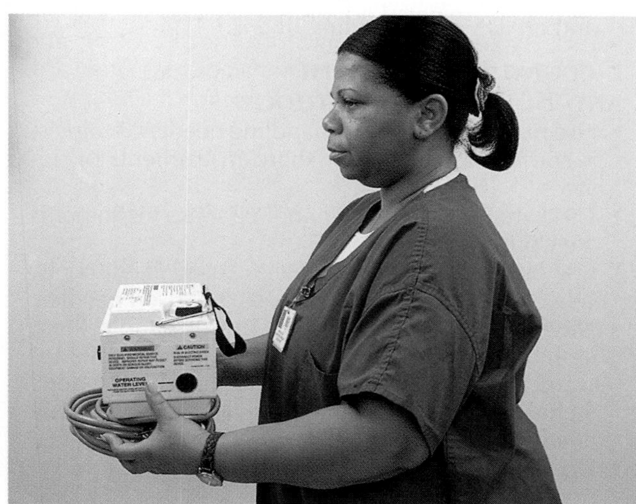

Figure 18-8 Hold equipment away from your uniform.

Isolation Precautions

Along with practising medical asepsis, infection control policies also use isolation precautions to reduce the risk of infection. **Isolation precautions** are guidelines for preventing the spread of pathogens. The most recent isolation precautions were developed in 1996 in the United States by the Centers for Disease Control and Prevention (CDC). These precautions have been accepted by Health Canada and are currently used in most Canadian health care facilities and community care agencies.

There are two types of isolation precautions: Standard Precautions and Transmission-Based Precautions. Both types of precautions provide guidelines on how to contain microbes. Standard Precautions are practised at all times. Transmission-Based Precautions are practised when caring for clients who have certain communicable diseases.

Standard Precautions

Standard Precautions (sometimes also known as **Routine Practices**) are guidelines to prevent the spread of infection from:

- Blood
- All body fluids, secretions, and excretions (except sweat), whether or not blood is visible
- Nonintact skin (skin with open sores, wounds, cuts, scrapes, or other breaks)
- Mucous membranes (including the membranes in the nose, eyes, mouth, vagina, and rectum)

Box 18-7 on page 222 summarizes Standard Precautions. Because you cannot tell by looking at someone whether or not they carry pathogens, everyone must be considered a potential source of infection. Therefore, *Standard Precautions are used when caring for all clients in all settings.*

Standard Precautions stress the following:

- Hand washing
- Appropriate use of PPE (gloves, gowns, masks, and goggles or face shield)
- Proper care and cleaning of equipment, environmental surfaces, and linen
- Safe management of sharps. A **sharp** is a piece of equipment or an item that may pierce the skin. These include needles, scalpels, razors, and broken glass.
- Placing patients or residents who are likely to contaminate the area in private rooms

Transmission-Based Precautions

Some clients have (or are suspected of having) communicable diseases. Remember, these are highly contagious infections. In certain cases, additional isolation precautions are required to protect staff, visitors, and other clients from the infection. **Transmission-Based Precautions** are guidelines to contain pathogens in one area, usually the client's room. Only clients infected or colonized with certain pathogens are placed under Transmission-Based Precautions. These precautions are followed in addition to Standard Precautions. You will be told when Transmission-Based Precautions are ordered for a client.

When a client in a facility is under Transmission-Based Precautions, he or she is usually placed in a private or semi-private room. The isolation room must have hand washing and toilet facilities. It also must have wastebaskets and laundry and garbage containers lined with plastic bags. An isolation sign that states the precautions in place is usually displayed on the outside of the room door.

Sometimes Transmission-Based Precautions are necessary for home care clients to protect other household members and home care workers. For example, if a client is infected with a multi-resistant organism,

(text continues on page 223)

Box 18-7 Standard Precautions

Hand Washing

- Wash your hands after touching blood, body fluids, secretions, excretions, nonintact skin, mucous membranes, and contaminated items. Wash your hands even if you wore gloves.
- Wash hands immediately before putting on gloves and immediately after removing gloves.
- Wash your hands between client contacts.
- Wash your hands whenever necessary to avoid transferring microbes to other people or areas.
- Wash your hands between tasks and procedures on the same client. This prevents cross-contamination of different body sites.
- Use plain soap for routine hand washing. Your supervisor tells you when other types of soap or agents are needed.

Gloves

- Wear gloves when touching blood, body fluids, secretions, excretions, nonintact skin, mucous membranes, and contaminated items. Clean, disposable, nonsterile gloves are adequate.
- Change gloves between tasks and procedures on the same client.
- Change gloves after contact with material that may be highly contaminated.
- Remove gloves promptly after use.
- Remove gloves before touching uncontaminated items and surfaces.
- Remove gloves before going to another client.
- Wash your hands immediately after removing gloves. This prevents the transfer of microbes to other people or areas.

Masks and Eye Protection

- Wear a mask and eye protection (goggles or a face shield) during procedures and tasks that are likely to cause splashes or sprays of blood, body fluids, secretions, or excretions. The mask and eye protection protect your eyes, nose, and mouth from contact with splashes or sprays (Figure 18-9).

Gowns

- Wear a gown during procedures and tasks that are likely to cause splashes or sprays of blood, body fluids, secretions, or excretions. The gown protects the skin. It also prevents contamination of clothing. A clean, nonsterile gown is adequate.
- Remove a used gown as soon as possible.
- Wash your hands after removing the gown. This prevents transferring microbes to other people or areas.

Care of Equipment

- Handle used care equipment carefully. Equipment may be contaminated with blood, body fluids, secretions, or excretions. Do not let the equipment touch your skin, mucous membranes, or clothing. Also prevent the transfer of microbes to other people or areas.
- Do not use reusable items for another client. The item must be cleaned and disinfected or sterilized.
- Discard disposable (single-use) items properly.

Environmental Control

- Follow employer procedures for the routine care, cleaning, and disinfection of surfaces. This includes environmental surfaces, bed rails, bedside equipment, and other frequently touched surfaces.

Linen

- Follow employer policy for linen that is soiled with blood, body fluids, secretions, or excretions. The policy describes how to handle, transport, and process soiled linen.
- Do not touch soiled linen to your skin, mucous membranes, or clothing.
- Prevent the transfer of microbes to other people and areas when handling linens.

Occupational Health and Bloodborne Pathogens

- Use extreme care when handling needles, scalpels, razor blades, and other sharp instruments or devices.
- Use extreme care when handling sharp instruments after procedures.
- Use extreme care when cleaning used instruments.
- Use extreme care when disposing of used needles.
- Never recap used needles. Do not handle them with both hands. Never direct the needle point toward any body part. Use a one-handed "scoop" technique or a mechanical device that holds the needle sheath.
- Do not remove used needles from disposable syringes by hand.
- Do not bend, break, or otherwise handle used needles by hand.
- Place used disposable syringes and needles, scalpel blades, and other sharp items in puncture-resistant containers.
- Place reusable syringes and needles in a puncture-resistant container for transport to the reprocessing area.
- Use barrier devices for rescue breathing (see Chapter 47).

Client Placement

- A private room is used if the client:
  - Contaminates the area
  - Does not or cannot assist in maintaining hygiene or environmental control
- Follow your supervisor's instructions if a private room is not available.

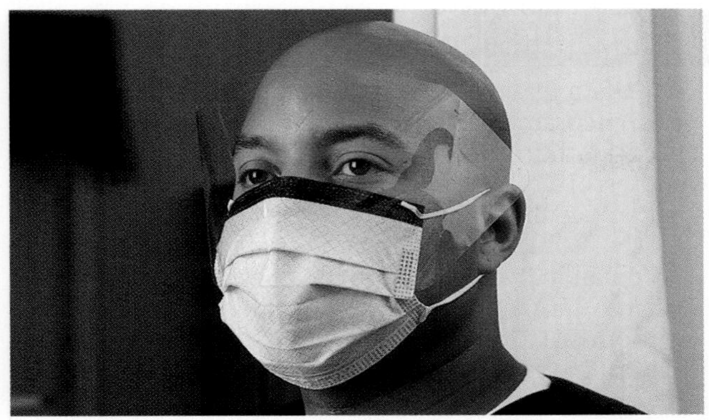

Figure 18-9 A face shield and a mask protect the eyes and mucous membranes of the mouth and nose.

Transmission-Based Precautions might be required. As a member of the home care team, you will be told of the client's need for precautions. An isolation sign is not needed in the home.

There are three types of Transmission-Based Precautions: Airborne Precautions, Droplet Precautions, and Contact Precautions (Box 18-8). The one used depends on how the pathogen is spread. You must understand how certain infections are spread (see Table 18-1). This helps you understand the three types of Transmission-Based Precautions.

The rules in Box 18-9 on page 224 are a guide for giving safe care when Transmission-Based Precautions are used. Your employer may have these or other guidelines. Know your employer's policies about isolation precautions.

Box 18-8 Transmission-Based Precautions

Airborne Precautions

For known or suspected infections caused by microbes transmitted by airborne droplets. Measles, chickenpox, tuberculosis, and SARS (severe acute respiratory syndrome) are examples of infections requiring airborne precautions.

Practices:

- Follow Standard Precautions.
- A private room is required.
- Keep the room door closed and the client in the room.
- Wear respiratory protection (such as an N95 respirator) when entering the room of a client with known or suspected tuberculosis or SARS (see page 227). A disposable surgical mask does not provide enough protection. Follow employer policy for care of clients with tuberculosis.
- Do not enter the room of a client with known or suspected measles or chickenpox if you are susceptible to the disease. If you are susceptible but must enter the room, wear respiratory protection. A disposable surgical mask does not provide enough protection. Respiratory protection is not needed if you are immune to measles or chickenpox.
- Limit moving and transporting the client from the room. The client wears a mask if moving or transporting from the room is necessary.
- For home care clients, revise these precautions as necessary. For example, wear respiratory protection when in the home. Check with your supervisor and the care plan before entering the home.

Droplet Precautions

For known or suspected infections caused by microbes transmitted by droplets produced by coughing, sneezing, or talking. Meningitis, pneumonia, influenza, and mumps are examples of infections requiring droplet precautions.

Practices:

- Follow Standard Precautions.
- A private room is preferred.
- The room door can be open if the bed is more than 1 metre (3 feet) from the door. Otherwise, keep the room door closed.
- Wear a disposable surgical mask when working within 1 metre (3 feet) of the client. (Wear a mask on entering the room if required by employer policy.)
- Limit moving and transporting the client from the room. The client wears a mask if moving or transporting from the room is necessary.
- For home care clients, revise these precautions as necessary. Household members are to avoid sharing common articles or eating utensils. Check with your supervisor and the care plan before entering the home.

Contact Precautions

For known or suspected infections caused by microbes transmitted by:

- Direct contact with the client (skin-to-skin contact that occurs during care)
- Indirect contact (touching surfaces or care items in the client's room)

Multi-resistant organisms and gastrointestinal, respiratory, skin, or wound infections are examples of infections requiring contact precautions.

Practices:

- Follow Standard Precautions.
- A private room is preferred.
- The room door can be open.
- Wear gloves when entering the room.
- Change gloves after touching anything that might have high concentrations of microbes (for example, fecal material or wound discharge).
- Remove gloves before leaving the client's room.

Continued

Box 18-8 Transmission-Based Precautions—Cont'd

- Wash hands immediately after removing gloves. Your supervisor tells you what agent to use (usually an antimicrobial agent or a waterless antiseptic cleanser).
- Do not touch potentially contaminated surfaces or items after removing gloves and washing hands.
- Open the door using a paper towel to touch the doorknob. Discard the paper towel in the garbage pail inside the room as you leave.
- Wear a gown when entering the room if you will have substantial contact with the client, surfaces, or items in the room.
- Wear a gown when entering the room if the client is incontinent or has diarrhea, an ileostomy, a colostomy, or wound drainage not contained by a dressing.
- Remove the gown before leaving the client's room. Make sure your clothing does not touch potentially contaminated surfaces in the client's room.
- Limit moving or transporting the client from the room. Maintain precautions if moving or transporting the client is necessary.
- For home care clients, revise these precautions as necessary. Check with your supervisor and the care plan before entering the home.

Box 18-9 General Rules for Transmission-Based Precautions

- Wear personal protective equipment as required.
- Collect all needed equipment before entering the room. Limit the number of trips in and out of the room.
- Prevent contamination of equipment and supplies. If you drop anything on the floor, consider the item contaminated and do not use it.
- Use mops wetted with a disinfectant solution to clean floors. Floor dust is contaminated.
- Prevent drafts. Pathogens are carried in the air by drafts.
- Use paper towels to handle contaminated items.
- Remove items from the room in sturdy, leakproof plastic bags.
- Double bag items if the outer part of the bag is or can be contaminated (page 231).
- Follow employer policy for removing and transporting disposable and reusable items.
- Return reusable dishes, eating utensils, and trays to the food service department or kitchen. Discard disposable dishes, eating utensils, and trays in the waste container in the client's room.
- Do not touch your hair, nose, mouth, eyes, or other body parts when providing care.
- Do not touch any clean area or object if your hands are contaminated.
- Place clean items or objects that you bring into the room on paper towels.
- Do not shake linen.
- Use paper towels to turn faucets on and off.
- Tell your supervisor if you have fever, cuts, open skins areas, vomiting, diarrhea, a sore throat, or a cough.

PROTECTIVE MEASURES

Standard Precautions and Transmission-Based Precautions involve wearing personal protective equipment (gloves, mask, gown, and/or eye protection). Your supervisor and employer policy will guide you about when to use PPE. Box 18-10 lists the proper order for putting on and taking off a full set of PPE. Standard Precautions also involve careful handling of sharps. Transmission-Based Precautions involve extra measures when removing linens, garbage, and equipment from the room. Special measures are also needed when transporting clients.

Wearing Gloves. Disposable gloves provide a protective barrier between your hands and the client's blood, body fluids, secretions, excretions, nonintact skin, and mucus membranes. They protect you

Box 18-10 Order for Putting on and Taking off a Full Set of PPE

Put on PPE in the following order (wash hands first):
- Mask
- Goggles or face shield
- Gown
- Gloves

Take off PPE in the following order:
- Gloves (wash hands)
- Goggles or face shield
- Mask
- Gown (wash hands)

from acquiring microbes from the client. They also protect the client from acquiring microbes that are on your hands. However, gloves are used as additional protection and not as a substitute for hand washing.

Wear gloves in the following situations:

- When you have nonintact skin on your hands (such as cuts or abrasions)
- When contact with blood, body fluids, secretions, excretions, mucus membranes, or nonintact skin is likely
- When contact with surfaces or items contaminated with blood, body fluids, secretions, or excretions is likely (for example, when handling bedpans, cleaning a bathroom floor, or removing soiled linens)

Gloves are not required for most routine care activities where contact is limited to a person's intact skin. Do not wear gloves when they are not needed. Continuous wear will cause breakdown of the skin on your hands. Your hands will sweat, become dry, and may crack over time if gloves are worn continuously. Remember, cracked skin is a portal of entry for microbes.

Gloves are often made of latex (a rubber product). Some people are allergic to latex. It can cause skin rashes. Asthma and shock are more serious problems. Report skin rashes and difficulty breathing to your supervisor right away. If you have a latex allergy, you need to wear latex-free gloves. Some clients are allergic to latex. You cannot wear latex gloves when caring for them. This information is in the care plan.

No special technique is required to put on disposable gloves. Be careful not to tear them when putting them on. Pathogens can enter the glove through the tear. Carelessness, long fingernails, and rings can tear gloves. Remember the following about wearing gloves:

- Wash and dry your hands before putting on gloves.
- You need a new pair for every client.
- Remove and discard torn, cut, or punctured gloves right away. Wash your hands. Then put on a new pair.
- Wear gloves only once. Discard them after use.
- Put on clean gloves before touching mucous membranes or nonintact skin.
- Put on new gloves whenever gloves become contaminated with blood, body fluids, secretions, or excretions. You may need more than one pair of gloves for a task. This prevents cross-contamination of different body sites.
- Replace gloves if you touch an unclean surface.
- Make sure gloves cover your wrists and the cuff of your sleeve or gown (Figure 18-10).
- Remove gloves so the inside part is on the outside. The inside is *clean*.
- Discard gloves in a container for contaminated waste (see page 231). Follow employer policy.
- Wash your hands after removing gloves.

(text continues on page 227)

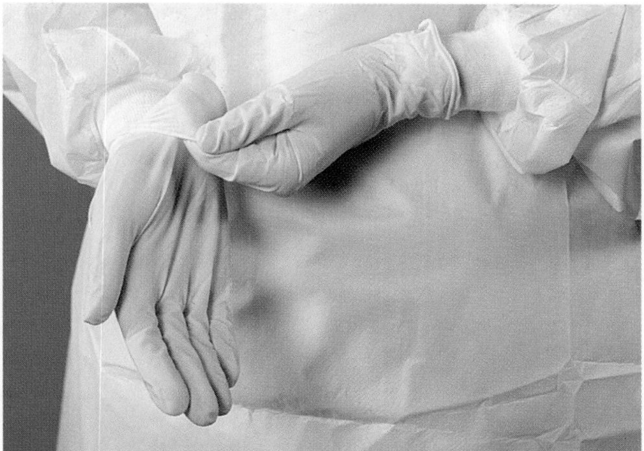

Figure 18-10 The gloves cover the cuffs of the gown.

Removing Gloves

Procedure

1. Make sure that glove only touches glove. Do not let gloves touch skin on your wrists or arms.
2. Grasp a glove just below the cuff with the gloved fingers of your opposite hand. Grasp it on the outside (Figure 18-11, *A*).
3. Pull the glove down over your hand so it is inside out (Figure 18-11, *B*).
4. Hold the removed glove with your other gloved hand.
5. Insert two fingers of your bare hand inside the cuff of the remaining glove (Figure 18-11, *C*).
6. Pull the glove down (inside out) over your hand and the already removed glove (Figure 18-11, *D*).
7. Drop both gloves together into the appropriate container. Follow employer policy.
8. Wash your hands.

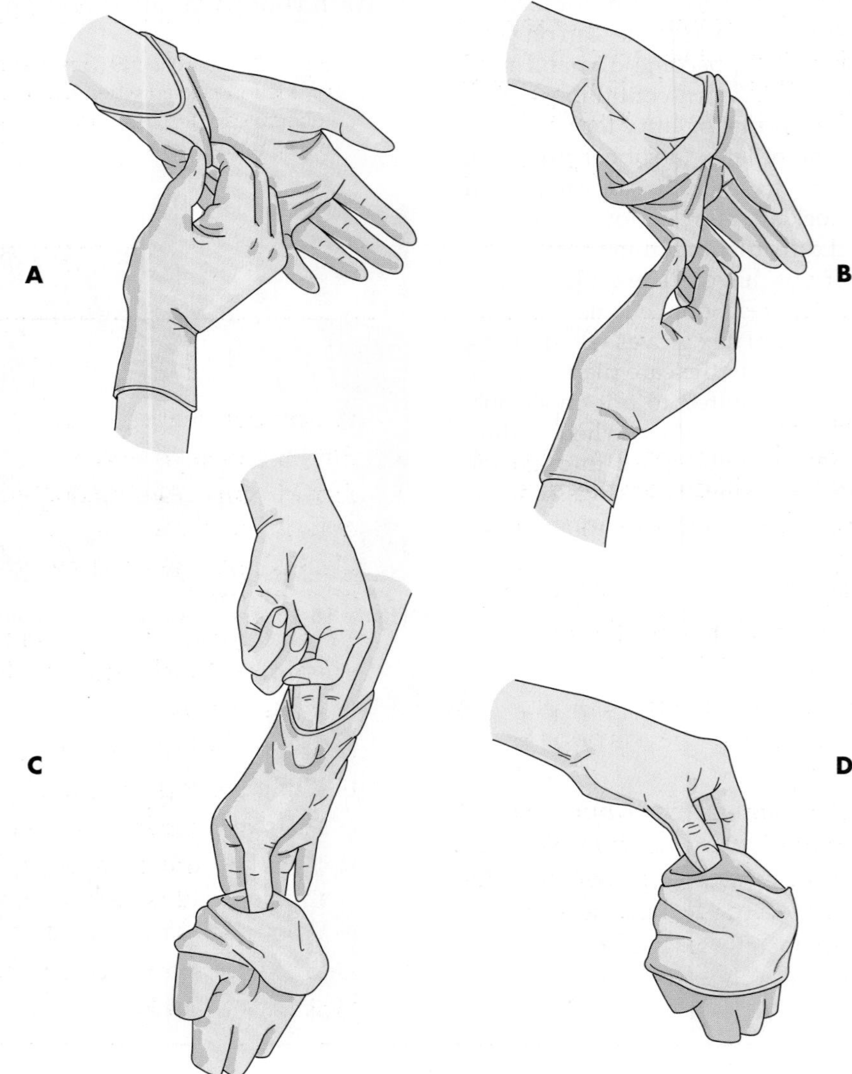

Figure 18-11 Removing gloves. **A,** Grasp the glove below the cuff. **B,** Pull the glove down over the hand. The glove is inside out. **C,** Insert the fingers of your ungloved hand inside the other glove. **D,** Pull the glove down over your hand and the other glove. The glove is inside out.

Wearing Masks and Respiratory Protection. Masks (also called surgical masks) prevent pathogens from entering your mouth and nose. They also prevent the spread of microbes from your respiratory tract. They are used for Airborne and Droplet Precautions. Staff, clients, and visitors wear them. They also protect you from splashes or sprays of blood, body fluids, secretions, or excretions.

Masks are disposable. A wet or moist mask is contaminated. Breathing can cause masks to become wet or moist. Apply a new mask when contamination occurs.

A mask should fit snugly over your nose and mouth. Wash your hands before putting on a mask. To remove the mask, first remove your gloves. Only touch the ties during removal. The front of the mask is contaminated.

Respiratory protection refers to special face masks that filter the air. The N95 respirator is an example (Figure 18-12). Such protection is used for clients under airborne isolation precautions. Follow employer policy regarding the use of respiratory protection.

(text continues on page 229)

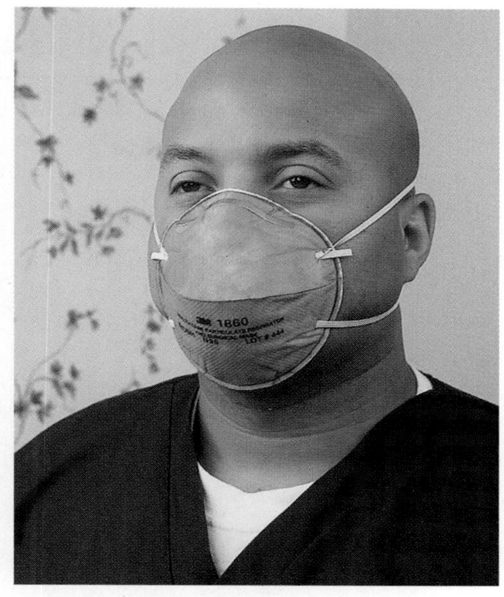

Figure 18-12 The N95 respirator. Respiratory protection is used when caring for clients with tuberculosis and other infections requiring airborne precautions.

Wearing a Mask

Procedure

1. Wash your hands.
2. Pick up the mask by its upper ties. Do not touch the part that will cover your face.
3. Place the mask over your nose and mouth (Figure 18-13, *A*).
4. Place the upper strings over your ears. Tie the strings in the back toward the top of your head (Figure 18-13, *B*).
5. Tie the lower strings at the back of your neck (Figure 18-13, *C*). The lower part is under your chin.
6. Pinch the metal band around your nose. The top of the mask must be snug over your nose. If you wear glasses or protective eyewear, the top of the mask must be snug over your nose and under the bottom edge of the eyewear.
7. Wash your hands.
8. Put on gloves if used.
9. Provide care. Avoid coughing, sneezing, and unnecessary talking.
10. Change the mask if it becomes moist or contaminated.
11. When finished the task, remove and discard the gloves. Wash your hands.
12. Remove the mask:
    - a Untie the lower strings.
    - b Untie the top strings.
    - c Hold the top strings. Remove the mask.
    - d Bring the strings together. The inside of the mask folds together (Figure 18-13, *D*). Do not touch the inside of the mask.
13. Discard the mask. Follow employer policy.
14. Wash your hands.

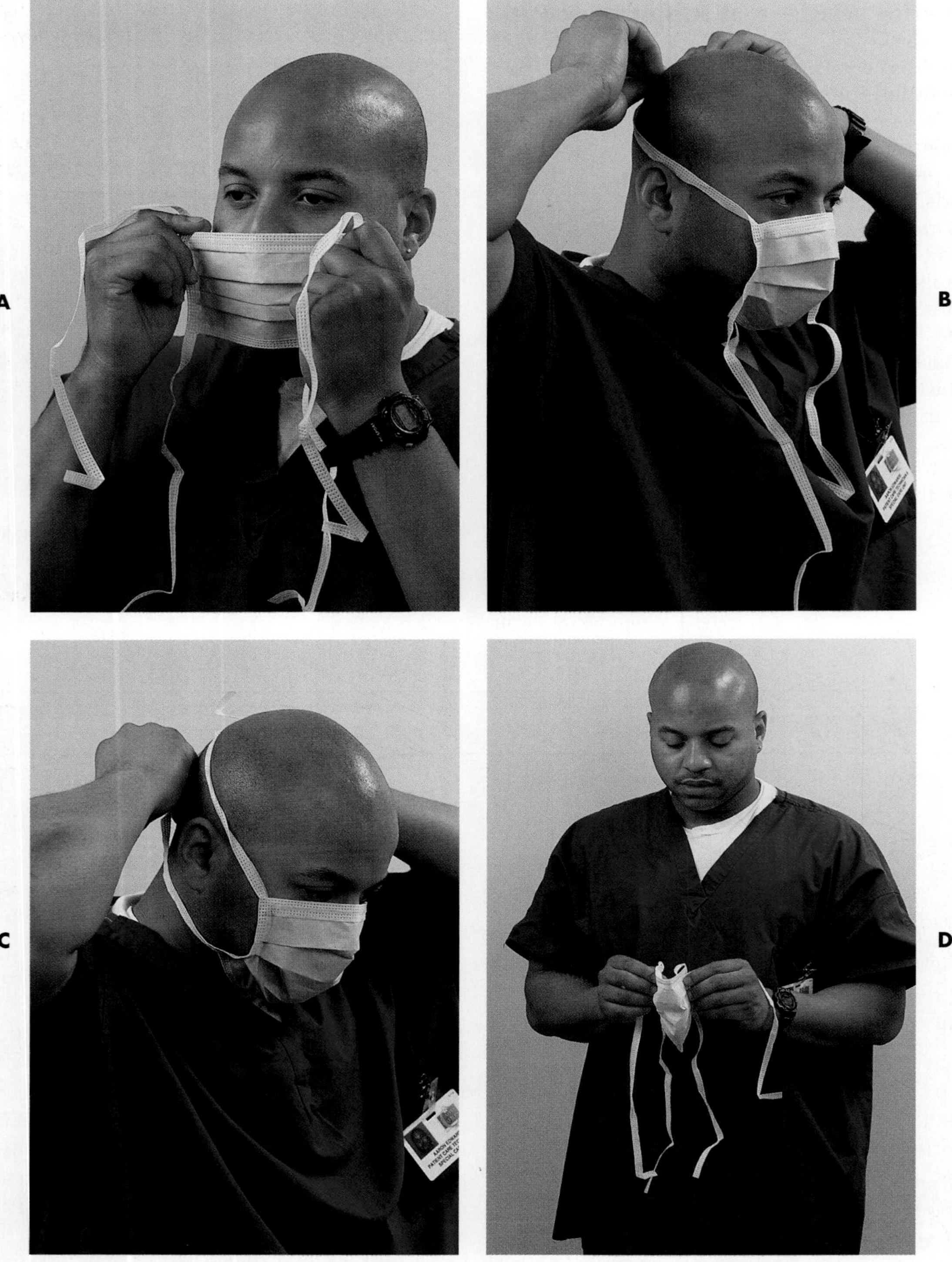

Figure 18-13 Donning a mask. **A,** Cover your nose and mouth with the mask. **B,** Tie upper strings at the back of your head. **C,** Tie lower strings at the back of your neck. **D,** Fold the inside of the mask together after removing it.

Wearing Protective Apparel. Gowns, plastic aprons, shoe covers, boots, and leg coverings prevent the spread of microbes. They protect your clothes, wrists, and arms from contact with blood, body fluid, secretions, and excretions. They also protect against splashes and sprays.

Gowns must completely cover clothing. The sleeves are long with tight cuffs. The gown opens at the back. It is tied at the neck and waist. The inside and neck are *clean*. The outside and waist strings are *contaminated*.

Gowns are used once. A wet gown is contaminated and must be replaced with a dry one. Disposable gowns are made of paper. They are discarded after one use. Reusable gowns are made of cloth and must be laundered before reuse.

Wearing Eye Protection and Face Shields. Goggles and face shields protect your eyes, mouth, and nose from splashing or spraying of blood, body fluids, secretions, or excretions (see Figure 18-9 on page 223). You may need such protection when giving care, cleaning instruments, or disposing of contaminated fluids.

Discard disposable eye protection after use. Reusable eye protection is cleaned before reuse. It is washed with soap and water and then disinfected.

Disposing of Sharps. Although you do not administer needles, you may come across one that is improperly disposed of. This is especially common in home care. For example, while changing sheets for a client who has diabetes, you could find a misplaced needle in the bed. Or while emptying the garbage you could find an IV device that was mistakenly tossed into it. You must always watch out for stray sharps, especially if you know the client frequently uses them.

Standard Precautions say that used needles must not be bent or broken. Place them and other sharps in a container that is:

- Tightly capped
- Puncture-resistant
- Leakproof

This container may be made of steel and provided by your employer. The container should be labelled. Other

(text continues on page 231)

Donning and Removing a Gown

Procedure

1. Remove your watch and all jewellery.
2. Roll up uniform sleeves.
3. Wash your hands.
4. Pick up a clean gown. Hold it out in front of you and let it unfold. Do not shake the gown.
5. Put your hands and arms through the sleeves (Figure 18-14, *A*).
6. Make sure the gown covers the front of your uniform and is snug at the neck.
7. Tie the strings at the back of the neck (Figure 18-14, *B*).
8. Overlap the back of the gown. Make sure the gown covers your uniform. The gown should be snug, not loose (Figure 18-14, *C*).
9. Tie the waist strings at the back.
10. Put on gloves.
11. Provide care.
12. Remove and discard the gloves. Wash your hands.
13. Remove the gown:
    - **a** Untie the waist strings.
    - **b** Wash your hands.
    - **c** Untie the neck strings. Do not touch the outside of the gown.
    - **d** Pull the gown down from the shoulder.
    - **e** Turn the gown inside out as it is removed. Hold it at the inside shoulder seams and bring your hands together (Figure 18-14, *D*).
14. Roll up the gown away from you. Keep it inside out.
15. Discard the gown. Follow employer policy.
16. Wash your hands.

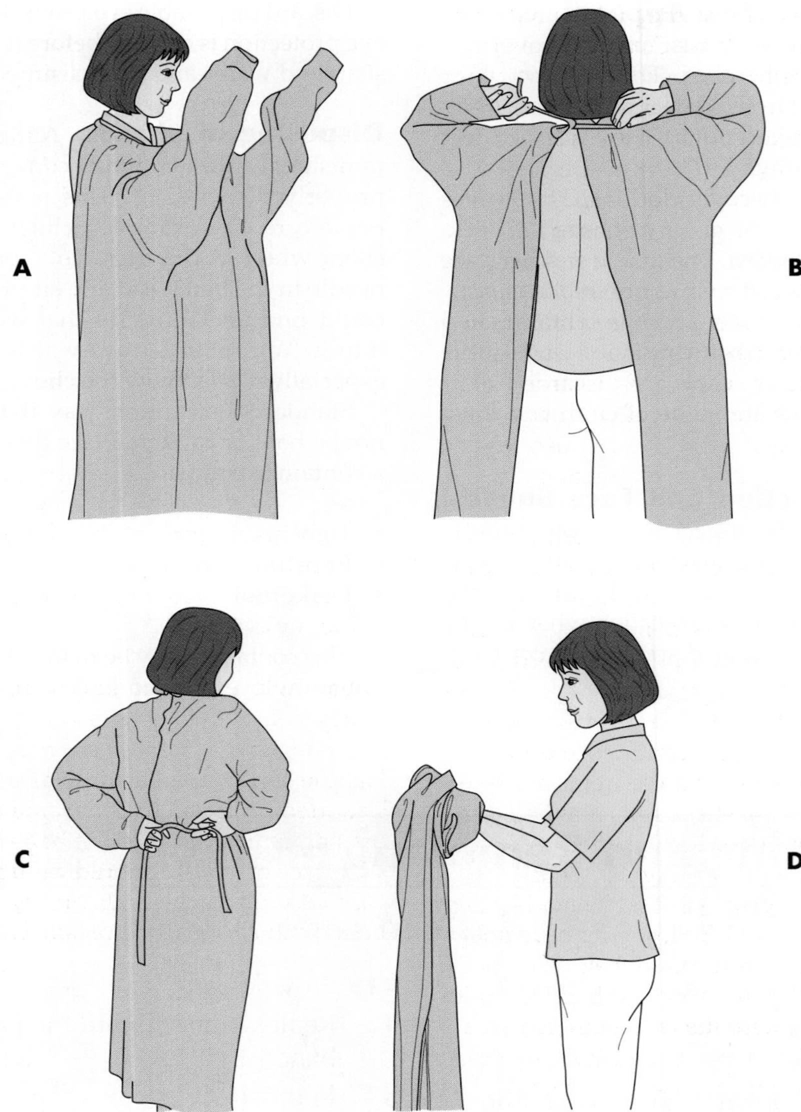

Figure 18-14 Gowning technique. **A,** Put your arms and hands through the sleeves. **B,** Tie the strings at the back of your neck. **C,** Overlap the gown in the back to cover your entire uniform. **D,** Turn the gown inside out as you remove it.

containers can be used as long as they follow the criteria. (See *Focus on Home Care: Sharps Containers* box.)

If your skin is pierced by a needlestick or other sharp, you must report the incident at once. You are at risk for infections, including HIV, hepatitis B, and hepatitis C. Assume that all clients could be potential carriers of these viruses. *Never ignore a sharps injury.*

Immediately after being poked by a sharp, encourage bleeding at the site of your injury and flush it with large amounts of water for about 5 minutes. You should then seek prompt medical attention according to employer policy. Your client may be asked to consent to testing for the above viruses in order to assist with managing your exposure. Confidentiality is important. You are told of evaluation results. You are also told of any medical conditions that may need treatment.

Bagging Items. Items contaminated with blood, body fluids, secretions, or excretions are called **biohazardous waste** and may be harmful to others. (*Bio* means life, and *hazardous* means dangerous or harmful.) These items are considered infectious and must be disposed of in specially marked containers, according to employer policy. Biohazardous waste includes used gloves, dressings, incontinence products, and soiled linen. Containers for these items are lined with sturdy, leakproof plastic bags that may be colour-coded. The containers are labelled with the universal BIOHAZARD symbol (Figure 18-15).

Contaminated waste is placed in a container labelled with the *BIOHAZARD* symbol. Follow employer policy for bagging and transporting. One bag is usually adequate. Double-bagging involves two bags. Double-bagging is not needed unless the contaminated waste touches the outside of the first bag. Two staff members are needed for double-bagging in isolation rooms:

- One worker is inside the room.
- The other worker is at the doorway outside the room.
- The worker in the room places contaminated items into a bag. Then the bag is sealed.

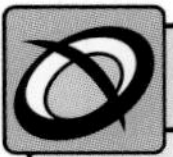

Focus on Home Care

SHARPS CONTAINERS

Home care agencies often use sharps containers that are different from those used in facilities. Safe sharps containers used in home care include empty bleach bottles, coffee cans with the plastic lids taped closed, and plastic milk bottles. Glass or clear plastic containers should not be used. The home care agency is responsible for collecting the containers and disposing of them according to agency policy and local laws.

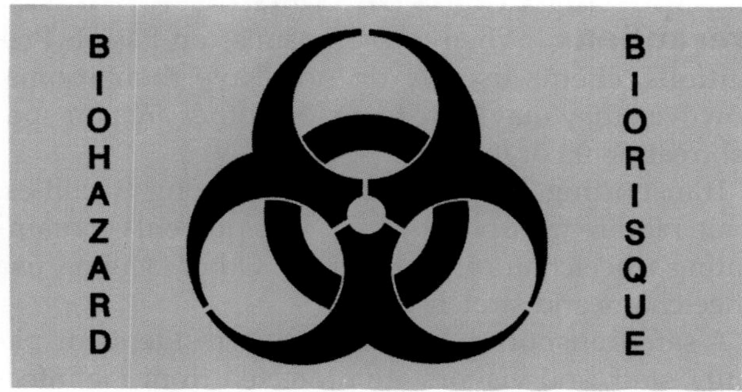

Figure 18-15 BIOHAZARD symbol.

- The worker outside the room holds open another bag. This bag is clean. A wide cuff is made on the clean bag to protect the hands from contamination (Figure 18-16).
- The contaminated bag is placed in the clean bag at the doorway.

Bag and transport linens according to employer policy. All linen bags must have a *BIOHAZARD* symbol. Bag soiled linen in the room where it was used. Handle soiled linen as little as possible. It should not be sorted or rinsed in client care areas. Do not overfill the bag with linen. Tie the bag securely. Linen that is very wet or soiled should be double-bagged to prevent leakage. Place the linen bag in a laundry hamper lined with a biohazard plastic bag.

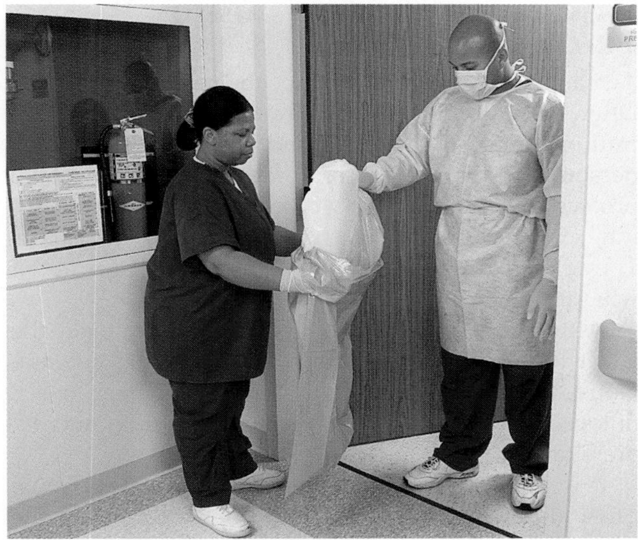

Figure 18-16 Double-bagging. One worker is in the room inside the doorway. The other is outside the room. The contaminated bag is placed inside the clean bag.

Transporting Clients on Transmission-Based Precautions. When on Transmission-Based Precautions, clients usually do not leave their rooms. However, they may have to go to another area for special treatments or tests.

Transporting procedures vary among facilities. Some require transport by bed. This prevents contaminating wheelchairs and stretchers. Other facilities use wheelchairs and stretchers.

A safe transport means that other residents or patients, staff, and visitors are protected from the infection. Follow employer policies and these guidelines to safely transport clients:

- The client wears a clean gown or pyjamas and an isolation gown.
- The client wears a mask if on Airborne or Droplet Precautions.
- Cover any draining wounds.
- Give the client tissues and a leakproof bag. Used tissues are placed in the bag.
- Wear a gown, mask, and gloves as required by the isolation precaution.
- Place an extra layer of sheets and absorbent pads on the stretcher or wheelchair. This protects against draining fluids.
- Do not let anyone else on the elevator. This reduces exposure to the infection.
- Alert staff in the receiving area about the isolation precautions. They wear gowns, masks, protective eyewear, and gloves as needed.
- Disinfect the stretcher or wheelchair after use.

Basic Needs and Transmission-Based Precautions

All clients have love, belonging, and self-esteem needs. Often they are unmet when Transmission-Based Precautions are used. Visitors and staff often avoid the person. The extra effort required to put on personal protective equipment may discourage them from visiting. Some visitors are afraid of getting the disease. They are anxious during the visit and are unsure about what to touch.

Without intending to, visitors and staff can make the client feel ashamed and guilty about having a contagious disease. As a result, he or she can feel lonely, unloved, and rejected. Self-esteem easily suffers and depression is a risk.

It is important to understand the need for Transmission-Based Precautions. Do not be afraid of the client. Remember, the precautions enable you to interact safely with the client. You can help meet the client's need for belonging and self-esteem. The following actions are helpful:

- Remember that the pathogen is undesirable, not the person.
- Treat the person with respect, kindness, and dignity.
- Allow the person to make choices and decisions whenever possible.
- Provide newspapers, magazines, and other reading material.
- Provide hobby materials if possible.
- Place a clock or radio in the room.
- Encourage the person to telephone family and friends.
- Provide a current television schedule.
- Organize your work so you can stay to visit with the person.
- Say hello from the doorway often, if the door can be left open.

Young children and clients with dementia do not understand the need for isolation precautions. Personal protective equipment may frighten children. It also may increase confusion and cause fear and agitation in adults with dementia. These measures can help:

- Let the person see your face before putting on a mask or protective eyewear.
- Tell the person who you are and what you are going to do.
- Use a calm, soothing voice.
- Do not hurry the person.
- Follow the care plan and your supervisor's instructions for individual approaches.
- Report signs of increased confusion or changes in behaviour to your supervisor.

Surgical Asepsis

Surgical asepsis (sterile technique) refers to the practices that keep equipment and supplies free of *all* microbes—pathogens and nonpathogens. Sterile means free of *all* microbes, including spores. Surgical asepsis is required any time the skin or sterile tissues are penetrated.

Some procedures require surgical asepsis. Examples include catheterizations, IVs, suctioning, sterile dressing changes, and blood collection. Support workers are not normally authorized to do these procedures. However, you could be delegated to do them. Or you might assist with these procedures. Therefore, you must understand the principles of surgical asepsis.

Principles of Surgical Asepsis

For sterile procedures, sterile gloves are needed. You also wear personal protective equipment to prevent contact with blood, body fluids, secretions, and excretions.

All items in contact with the client are kept sterile. If an item is contaminated, the client is at risk for infection. A sterile field is needed. A **sterile field** is a work area free of pathogens and non-pathogens (including spores). Box 18-11 lists the principles and practices of surgical asepsis. Follow them to maintain a sterile field when assisting with a sterile procedure.

Box 18-11 Principles and Practices for Surgical Asepsis

- A sterile item can only touch another sterile item.
- If a sterile item touches a clean item, the sterile item is contaminated.
  - A sterile package that is open, torn, punctured, wet, or moist is contaminated.
  - A sterile package is contaminated after the expiration date on the package.
  - Place only sterile items on a sterile field.
  - Use sterile gloves or sterile forceps to handle other sterile items (Figure 18-17).
  - Consider any item to be contaminated if you are unsure of its sterility.
  - Do not use contaminated items. They are discarded or re-sterilized.
- Sterile items or a sterile field are always kept within your vision and above your waist.
  - If you cannot see an item, the item is contaminated.
  - If the item is below your waist, the item is contaminated.
  - Keep sterile gloved hands above your waist and within your sight.
  - Do not leave a sterile field unattended.
  - Do not turn your back on a sterile field.
- Airborne microbes can contaminate sterile items or a sterile field.
  - Prevent drafts. Close the door and avoid extra movements.
  - Ask other staff in the room to avoid extra moving.
  - Avoid coughing, sneezing, talking, or laughing over a sterile field. Turn your head away from the sterile field if you must talk.
  - Wear a mask if you need to talk during the procedure.
  - Do not assist with sterile procedures if you have a respiratory infection.
  - Do not reach over a sterile field.
- Fluids flow downward, in the direction of gravity.
  - Hold wet items down (see Figure 18-17). If held up, fluid flows down into a contaminated area. The contaminated fluid flows back into the sterile field when the item is held up.
- The sterile field is kept dry, unless the area below it is sterile.
  - The sterile field is contaminated if it gets wet and the area below it is not sterile.
  - Avoid spilling and splashing when pouring sterile fluids into sterile containers.
- The edges of a sterile field are contaminated.
  - A 2.5 cm (1 inch) margin around the sterile field is contaminated (Figure 18-18).
  - Place all sterile items inside the 2.5 cm margin of the sterile field.
  - Items outside the 2.5 cm margin are contaminated.
- Honesty is essential to sterile technique.
  - You know when you contaminate an item or sterile field. Be honest with yourself even if no other staff members are present.
  - Remove the contaminated item and correct the situation. If necessary, start over with sterile supplies.
  - Report the contamination to your supervisor.

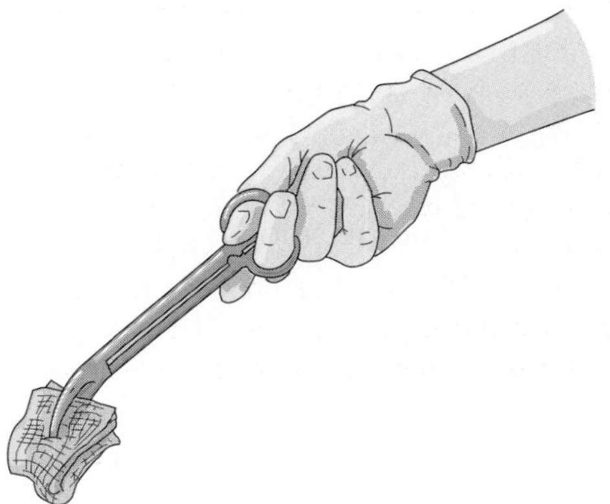

Figure 18-17 Sterile forceps are used to handle sterile items.

Figure 18-18 The 2.5 cm (1 inch) margin around a sterile field is considered contaminated.

Donning and Removing Sterile Gloves

You might need sterile gloves when assisting with a sterile procedure. You put them on after setting up the sterile field. After sterile gloves are on, you can handle sterile items within the sterile field. You cannot touch anything outside the sterile field.

Sterile gloves are disposable. They come in peel-back packaging. They come in many sizes so that they will fit snugly. The insides are powdered for ease in donning the gloves. Also, the right and left gloves are marked on the package.

Always keep sterile gloved hands above your waist and within your vision. Only touch items within the sterile field. If your gloves become contaminated, remove the gloves and put on a new pair. Also replace gloves that are torn, cut, or punctured.

Donning and Removing Sterile Gloves

Procedure

1 Inspect the package for sterility.
   - a Check the expiration date.
   - b See if the package is dry.
   - c Check for tears, holes, punctures, and watermarks.

2 Arrange a work surface.
   - a Make sure you have enough room.
   - b Arrange the work surface at waist level and within your vision.
   - c Clean and dry the work surface.
   - d Do not reach over or turn your back on the work surface.

3 Open the package. Grasp the flaps. Gently peel the flaps back.

4 Remove the inner package. Place it on your work surface.

5 Read the manufacturer's instructions on the inner package. It may be labelled with left, right, up, and down.

6 Arrange the inner package for left, right, up, and down. The left glove is on your left. The right glove is on your right. Have the cuffs near you with the fingers pointing away.

7 Use the thumb and index finger of each hand to grasp the folded edges of the inner package.

8 Fold back the inner package to expose the gloves (Figure 18-19, *A*). Do not touch or otherwise contaminate the inside of the package or the gloves. The inside of the inner package is a sterile field.

9 Note that each glove has a 5 to 7.5 cm (2 to 3 inch) cuff. The cuffs and insides of the gloves are not sterile.

10 Put on the right glove if you are right-handed. Put on the left glove if you are left-handed.
   - a Pick up the glove with your other hand. Use your thumb and index and middle fingers (Figure 18-19, *B*).
   - b Touch only the cuff and inside of the glove.
   - c Turn the hand to be gloved palm side up.
   - d Lift the cuff up. Slide your fingers and hand into the glove (Figure 18-19, *C*).
   - e Pull the glove up over your hand. If some fingers get stuck, leave them that way until the other glove is on. *Do not use your ungloved hand to straighten the glove. Do not let the outside of the glove touch any nonsterile surface.*
   - f Leave the cuff turned down.

11 Put on the other glove with your gloved hand.
   - a Reach under the cuff of the second glove. Use the four fingers of your gloved hand (Figure 18-19, *D*). Keep your gloved thumb close to your gloved palm.
   - b Pull on the second glove (Figure 18-19, *E*). Your gloved hand cannot touch the cuff or any other surface. Hold the thumb of your first gloved hand away from your gloved palm.

12 Adjust each glove with the other hand. The gloves should be smooth and comfortable (Figure 18-19, *F*).

13 Slide your fingers under the cuffs to pull them up (Figure 18-19, *G*).

14 Touch only sterile items.

15 Remove the gloves as in Figure 18-11.

16 Wash your hands.

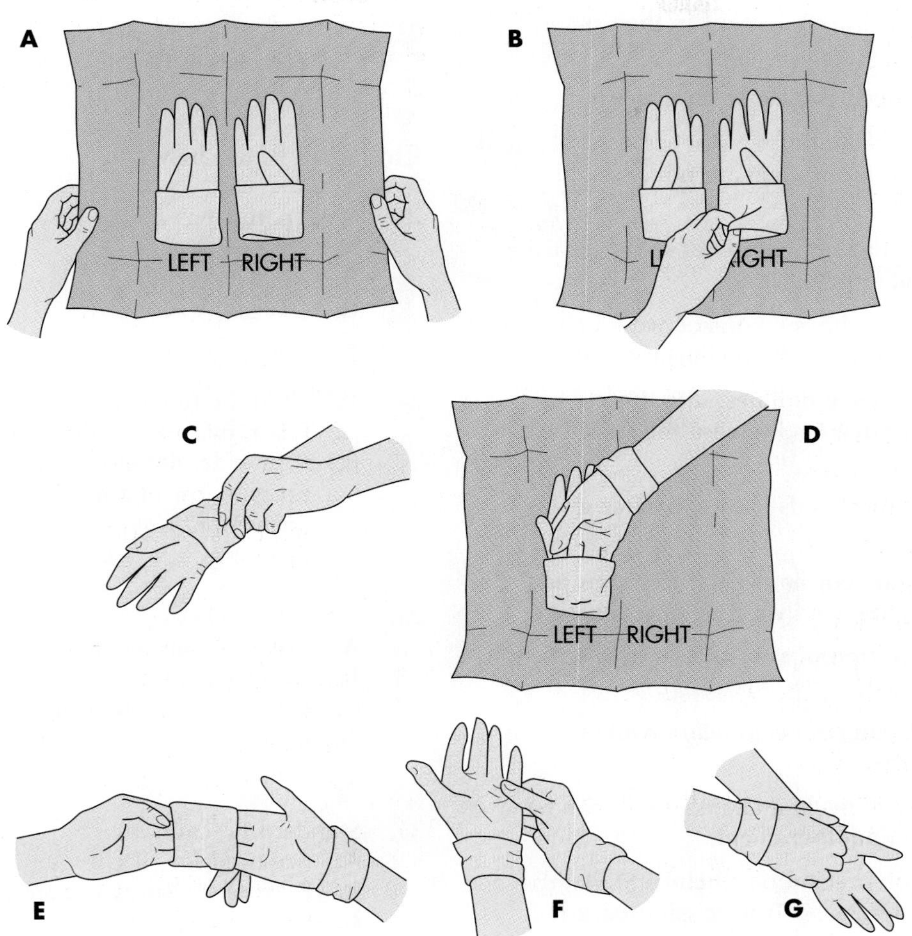

Figure 18-19 Donning sterile gloves. **A,** Open the inner wrapper to expose the gloves. **B,** Pick up the glove at the cuff with your thumb and index finger. **C,** Slide your fingers and hand into the glove. **D,** Reach under the cuff of the other glove with your fingers. **E,** Pull on the glove. **F,** Adjust each glove for comfort. **G,** Slide your fingers under the cuffs to pull them up.

REVIEW

Circle T if the answer is true and F if it is false.

1. T F Pathogens are microbes in their natural sites.
2. T F A pathogen can cause an infection.
3. T F Multi-resistant organisms are easily treated with antibiotics and are not a risk in facilities.
4. T F Older adults often do not show the usual signs of infection.
5. T F A person who is colonized with a pathogen cannot transfer the pathogen to others.
6. T F The presence of illness and the use of invasive devices increase the risk of infection.
7. T F Wash your hands before *or* after giving care.
8. T F You hold your hands and forearms up during the hand washing procedure.
9. T F The duration of the hand wash is not important.
10. T F Disinfecting items usually involves chemicals.
11. T F Unused items in a client's room can be used for another client.
12. T F Isolation precautions include Standard Precautions *and* Transmission-Based Precautions.
13. T F Standard Precautions are used only when the client has a specific contagious disease.
14. T F Transmission-Based Precautions are guidelines that help keep pathogens within one area, usually the client's room.
15. T F Gloves are worn at all times.
16. T F A mask is contaminated when moist.
17. T F Goggles, masks, and gowns are worn when there is a risk of splashing blood or body fluids.
18. T F You do not need to report a sharps injury if the bleeding is not severe.
19. T F Double-bagging of contaminated items is always required.
20. T F An item is sterile if nonpathogens are present.
21. T F A sterile item can touch only another sterile item.
22. T F The 2.5 cm edge around a sterile field is considered contaminated.

Circle the BEST answer.

23. Most pathogens are destroyed by
    A. Water
    B. Heat
    C. Oxygen
    D. Nourishment

24. Which of the following is *not* a sign of infection?
    A. Fever, nausea, vomiting, rash, and/or sores
    B. Pain or tenderness, redness, and/or swelling
    C. Fatigue, loss of appetite, and/or a change in behaviour
    D. Bleeding

25. Aseptic practices
    A. Are a link in the chain of infection
    B. Destroy spores
    C. Reduce the number of microbes
    D. Destroy all microbes—pathogens and nonpathogens

26. Standard Precautions
    A. Are used for all clients
    B. Prevent the spread of airborne pathogens
    C. Involve surgical asepsis
    D. Are not necessary for children or older clients

27. Gloves are worn when in contact with the following *except*
    A. Blood
    B. Body fluids
    C. Secretions and excretions
    D. Sweat

28. Proper use of personal protective equipment involves the following *except*
    A. Washing disposable gloves for reuse
    B. Removing protective equipment before leaving the work area
    C. Discarding cracked or torn gloves
    D. Wearing gloves when touching contaminated items or surfaces

Answers to these questions are on page 823.

CHAPTER

19

ABUSE

OBJECTIVES

- Define the key terms listed in this chapter
- Describe the types of abuse
- Describe the cycle of abuse
- Describe spousal abuse, child abuse, and abuse of older adults
- Describe how clients and health care workers can be abused
- Explain what to do if you have an abusive client
- Identify signs of abuse
- Explain your legal responsibilities when reporting abuse
- Describe what to do if a client tells you that he or she is being abused

KEY TERMS

abuse Physical or mental harm caused by someone in a position of trust—such as a family member, partner, or caregiver

ageism Bias and discrimination against older adults

emotional abuse Words or actions that inflict mental harm; psychological abuse

financial abuse The misuse of a person's money or property

neglect The failure to meet the basic needs (physical or emotional) of a dependent person

physical abuse Force or violence that causes pain, injury, and sometimes death

psychological abuse Emotional abuse

sexual abuse Unwanted sexual activity

sexual harassment Any conduct, comment, gesture, threat, or suggestion that is sexual in nature; a form of sexual abuse

Abuse is physical or mental harm caused by someone in a position of trust—such as a family member, partner, or caregiver. The abuser has power and control over the victim. The victim is usually physically, emotionally, or financially dependent on the abuser. Children, spouses, older adults, and people with disabilities are at risk for abuse.

Abuse occurs in all social levels, in all races, and in all cultures. It can occur in community settings and in health care facilities. You must know how to recognize and report suspected abuse.

TYPES OF ABUSE

There are many ways in which people can be abusive. More than one type of abuse can occur at the same time. The different types of abuse include:

- *Physical abuse*—force or violence that causes pain, injury, and sometimes death. Physical abuse includes pinching, hair pulling, pushing, slapping, hitting, shaking, choking, biting, or kicking. It also includes burning, poisoning, using weapons, or throwing things (like a chair or a hammer).
- *Sexual abuse*—unwanted sexual activity. Rape and attempted rape are sexual abuse. So is unwanted touching, fondling, kissing, and exposure (when the abuser shows his or her genitals to the victim). Sexual harassment is also sexual abuse. **Sexual harassment** is any conduct, comment, gesture, threat, or suggestion that is sexual in nature.
- *Emotional abuse (psychological abuse)*—words or actions that inflict mental harm. Emotional abuse usually involves humiliating or demeaning the victim in public or in private. It diminishes the victim's dignity and self-worth. The victim is called names, yelled at, insulted, mocked, threatened, or sworn at. The victim may be ignored for long periods of time. Or the victim may not be allowed to do activities or visit with family, friends, or others. Threatening to harm someone or something that the victim loves (such as a child or a pet) is another example of emotional abuse.
- *Financial abuse*—the misuse of a person's money or property, usually for the abuser's financial gain. Financial abuse includes stealing; forging signatures; selling property or possessions without permission; and persuading or tricking victims to change their wills or give up control of their finances. Some abusers do not allow their victims access to their own money.
- *Neglect*—failing to meet the basic needs of a dependent person. Victims of neglect are usually children, people with disabilities, and frail older adults. Neglect occurs when a clean, comfortable, and safe environment is not provided. In some cases, the caregiver may withhold or deny food, water, or clothing. Personal care, medical care, education, or attention and love may also be denied or withheld. Sometimes the caregiver knowingly neglects the victim. Other times, the caregiver does not intend to neglect the person, but is unable to provide adequate care.

THE CYCLE OF ABUSE

Abuse usually occurs over and over again. It often follows a pattern known as the cycle of abuse (Figure 19-1). There are three phases in the cycle.

- *The tension-building phase*—Tension starts to build between the abuser and the victim. Everyday

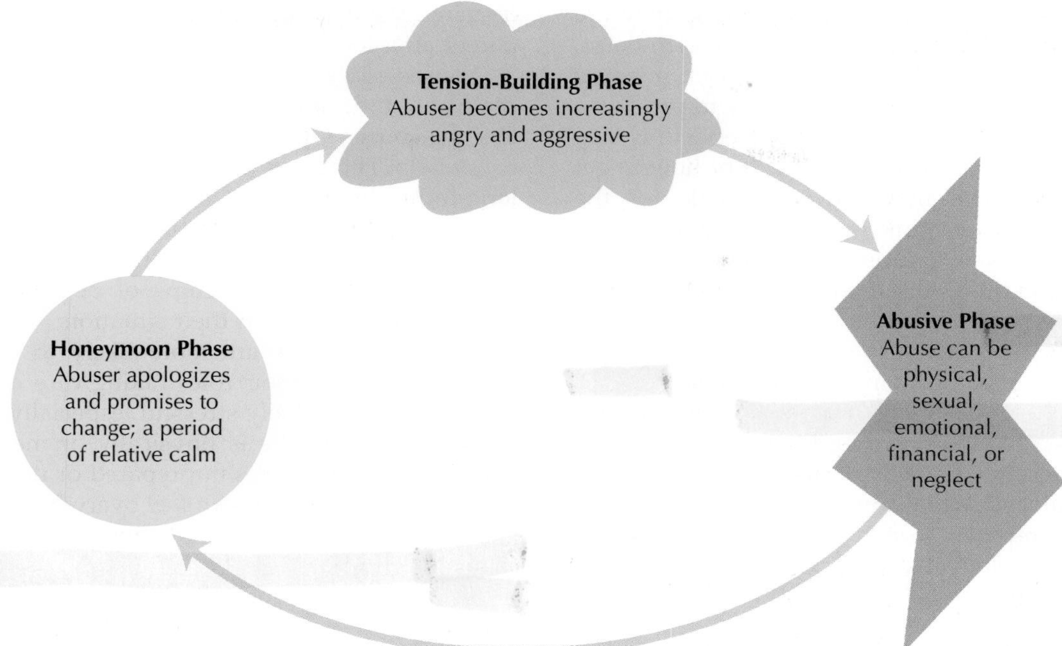

Figure 19-1 The cycle of abuse.

events and comments irritate and anger the abuser. As the abuser becomes more angry and stressed, he or she becomes more aggressive. The victim may try to calm, soothe, and please the abuser. Or, the victim may stay out of the abuser's way. The victim tries not to say or do anything that might anger or upset the abuser.

- *The abusive phase*—Tension explodes into an abusive event. The abuse may involve neglect or physical, sexual, emotional, or financial abuse. Often, the abuse is triggered by an event unrelated to the victim's behaviour.
- *The honeymoon phase*—The abuser feels ashamed or sorry. He or she apologizes and promises never to do it again. The abuser may offer gifts or be very loving and attentive. The abuser and victim may both believe that the abuser can change.

If measures are not taken to stop the abuse, the cycle continues. There may be days, weeks, months, or years between abusive events. Usually, the time between episodes gradually shortens. The abuse becomes more frequent and intense. It is important for the victim and abuser to get help in order to stop the cycle.

Abusive Relationships

Abuse can occur in many different kinds of relationships. Women and men can be abused by their spouses or partners; children can be abused by their parents; older adults can be abused by their adult children; clients can be abused by health care workers; and health care workers can be abused by their clients.

Abusive relationships are complex. There is usually no single cause for the abuse. However, in all relationships, a person is more likely to be abusive if he or she:

- Has problems with alcohol or drugs
- Has a mental illness (for example, major depression) or severe personality flaws (for example, an explosive temper, inability to control impulses, or lack of empathy for others)
- Has been abused as a child
- Is going through a period of high stress, such as divorce, unemployment, poverty, or illness

Spousal Abuse

Spousal abuse is abuse between partners in a marriage or common-law relationship. The types of abuse that occur between spouses or partners may be physical, sexual, emotional, or financial. Usually more than one type of abuse is present in the relationship.

Both women and men can be abused by their partners. A recent Canadian study found that similar numbers of women and men reported being abused by their partners.[1] However, women are usually more severely injured than are men.

People who are abused by their partner often deny the abuse. They also often choose to stay with their partner, even when there is serious physical violence occurring. Some victims may stay because they are afraid of their abuser. The abuser may threaten harm, death, or denial of child custody if the victim leaves the relationship. Or, the victim may stay to provide a two-parent home for the children. Some victims stay because they do not know where to go or how to get help. Others believe they are responsible for the abuse. Or, they may think that no one will believe them. Still others stay because they believe the abuser will change and they want the relationship to work.

Child Abuse

Children are at risk for many types of abuse. Neglect is the most reported form of child abuse. In most child neglect cases, the primary caregiver fails to supervise the child properly. Children are also victims of physical, emotional, and sexual abuse. The abuser is usually a parent, step-parent, or relative. Sometimes the abuser is a nonrelative who is close to the child. Examples are family friends or the parent's partner.

Boys and girls are equally likely to be victims. All age groups from infancy through adolescence are at risk. Child abuse occurs in all types of families: rich and poor, educated and uneducated. However, certain situations increase the risk of child abuse:

- *Family crisis.* Divorce, unemployment, moving, poverty, and crowded living conditions all cause stress. Stress can lead to abuse.
- *Single-parenting.* A recent study found that almost half of all cases of child abuse involved children living in a single-parent family.[2] Possibly this is because some single parents are under great stress.
- *Isolation.* Many abusive parents do not have close relationships with extended family, friends, or community.[3] As a result, they do not understand normal child development and behaviour. They may have unrealistic expectations of the child. For example, they may think a crying baby is being bad. They may believe hitting or slapping are appropriate forms of discipline. They also do not have help during times of stress.
- *Caring for children with special needs.* Children with physical or mental disabilities or chronic illness are especially at risk for being abused. Children with personalities or behaviours that the abuser considers "different" or unacceptable are also at greater risk.

Abuse of Older Adults

Older adults are at risk for all types of abuse: physical, sexual, emotional, and financial abuse, as well as neglect. Financial and emotional abuse are the most common types of abuse reported by older adults. Abusers are usually family members, such as an adult child or grandchild. Often, the abuser is the older adult's primary caregiver. Most abusers of older adults depend on their victims for financial help or housing.[4] For example, an adult son moves in with his parent after losing his job.

Abused older adults sometimes choose not to complain about the abuse. Like abused spouses, they may fear the abuser. Or, they may not know where or how to get help. They may fear being forced to move into a long-term care facility if they report their caregiver. Some older adults are not able to report abuse. They may have physical or mental disabilities that prevent them from reporting. Victims of neglect especially may be unable to report their situation.

Family caregivers are more likely to be abusive when they resent their role. Taking care of an older adult can be extremely stressful, especially when the person receiving care is physically or mentally disabled. If the caregiver is unprepared or unable to fulfill the duties, he or she can feel overwhelmed.

Ageism is another cause of abuse (see Chapter 15). **Ageism** is bias and discrimination against older adults. Caregivers who do not respect the dignity or abilities of older adults are more likely to be abusive. For example, a caregiver who thinks that older adults cannot manage money may take control of the person's finances without permission (financial abuse).

Abuse of Clients

Abuse of clients can happen in a facility or a home care setting. Clients can be abused by any member of the health care team. In facilities, they can also be abused by visitors or a member of the staff.

Clients are at risk for all types of abuse: physical, sexual, emotional, and financial abuse, as well as neglect. Abusive situations include: using restraints inappropriately, handling the client roughly, isolating the client in his or her room, stealing from the client, not reviewing the care plan regularly, not responding to a call for help, not checking on the client for long periods of time, and leaving the client in soiled linen or clothes. *Violating a client's rights* is another form of abuse. Providing care against the person's wishes is an example. So are failing to provide privacy, failing to keep personal or medical information confidential, and not letting residents visit or use the phone in private.

As with all abusive relationships, stress sometimes causes abuse of clients. Some workers may not have received enough training or education. Too much work and too few workers may contribute to a high level of stress. Some clients are uncooperative or abusive toward the staff. For example, they may hit or yell at the worker. Some workers respond to abusive clients by being abusive in return.

However, there is no excuse for abusive behaviour. Sometimes you will work with difficult clients in stressful situations. You must recognize when you are feeling stress. Take time out if you begin to lose your temper. Always treat your clients gently and with respect, even when they resist your care.

To prevent your behaviour from becoming abusive, immediately discuss difficult or aggressive clients with your supervisor. Your supervisor will help you decide how to handle them. If necessary, you can ask for an assignment change. Chapter 8 discusses how to manage stress.

ABUSE OF HEALTH CARE WORKERS

Sometimes health care workers, including support workers, are abused while on the job. You are at risk for physical or verbal abuse from your clients, your clients' family members, or other members of the health care team.

Health care workers are especially at risk for abuse when they work with clients who have a mental illness or condition that affects behaviour. Schizophrenia and dementia are examples. Clients who have problems with drugs or alcohol, who have a history of abusive behaviour, or who are being placed in restraints are also more likely to be abusive toward you.

Abuse should never be ignored or accepted as "part of the job." Examples of abusive behaviours by the client or someone else include:

- Swearing, name calling, and using racial or cultural slurs
- Threatening to harm you or trying to scare you
- Denying meal breaks, drinking water, bathroom use, or hand-washing facilities
- Hitting, pushing, kicking, spitting, biting, pinching, or other physical attacks
- Inappropriate touching
- Sexually assaulting or harassing
- Following you home or finding out your phone number and calling you at home

Your employer will have policies describing what to do if you have an abusive client. Box 19-1 lists general safety measures to follow when dealing with abusive clients.

Box 19-1 What to Do When a Client Is Abusive

- Stay calm.
- Stand up so as not to be dominated by the client. Stand far enough away from the person so he or she cannot hit or kick you, about 2 metres (6 feet).
- Position yourself close to a door in case you have to escape quickly.
- Note the location of call bells, alarms, closed-circuit monitors, and other security devices.
- Keep your hands free. Do not touch the client.
- Listen to the client. Restate what he or she says in your own words.
- Talk to the client calmly. Do not raise your voice or argue, scold, or interrupt the person. Be polite and positive. Avoid such comments as "Calm down" or "You have no reason to be mad at me." Instead, acknowledge the person's frustrations and tell the person you will get your supervisor to speak to him or her.
- Watch the client's body language, including shaking or clenching fists or a change in posture. This may be a sign the person is ready to hit or push.
- If you are in a facility, tell the client that you will get a nurse to speak to him or her. Make sure the client is safe, then quickly leave the room. Tell the nurse or security officer about the situation. If you cannot leave and you suspect the person is going to lose control, sound a call bell, alarm, or other security device.
- If you are in a client's home, leave the house if you think you are in danger. Go to a safe place, and immediately call your supervisor. If you cannot leave the house and you feel threatened, call the police.
- Complete an incident report after an abusive encounter.

The Sexually Aggressive Client. Some clients want the health care team to meet sexual needs. They flirt or make sexual advances or comments. Some expose themselves, masturbate, or touch health care workers. This can anger or embarrass the worker. These reactions are normal. Often there are reasons for the client's behaviour. Understanding this helps you deal with the matter.

Sexually aggressive behaviours have many causes. They include:

- Confusion or disorientation
- Nervous system disorders
- Side effects from medications
- Fever
- Dementia
- Acquired brain injury

Some clients may think someone else is their partner. Others cannot control their behaviour. Changes in mental function cause the behaviour. A healthy person can usually control sexual urges. Changes in the brain make control difficult. Sexual behaviour in these cases is usually not intended to be abusive. However, it still must be dealt with. Notify your supervisor if a client makes sexual advances.

Some people touch and fondle their genitals for pleasure. Masturbation in public is viewed as a sexually aggressive behaviour. However, some clients may not understand that they are offending others. Other clients may touch their genitals because of an underlying health problem. Urinary or reproductive system problems can cause soreness and itching. So can poor hygiene and being wet or soiled from urine or stool. Try to determine the cause of the client's behaviour. Provide for privacy and safety. Tell your supervisor about the situation.

Sometimes clients do not have mental or physical problems that cause sexual aggression, but behave aggressively for other reasons. They may touch workers because they have unmet needs for love and belonging or self-esteem. The person may feel lonely or unloved. For example, a divorced man behaves sexually because he wants to prove that he is attractive and can perform sexually. You must be professional in these situations:

- Ask the person not to touch you. State the places where you were touched.
- Tell the person you will not do what he or she wants.
- Tell the person that the behaviours make you uncomfortable. Politely ask the person not to act in that way.
- If you feel your safety is at risk, leave the room or home. Call your supervisor.
- Tell your supervisor about what happened. She or he can help you decide if further action is necessary. If you are uncomfortable being with the client, you have the right to ask to be reassigned.

Remember, sexual harassment is a form of sexual abuse. Sexual harassment at work is when clients, their families, or co-workers make sexual comments, gestures, threats, or suggestions. If the behaviour offends you or makes you uncomfortable, it is harassment. Explain to the person that his or her conduct is unwelcome and unacceptable. Be firm and assertive. Most people will stop the harassing behaviour if they realize it is unacceptable. If the harassment persists, tell your supervisor. In Canada, employers are legally required to prevent sexual harassment at work. All employers have policies about how to deal with sexual aggression and harassment.

Recognizing Signs of Abuse

You are responsible for recognizing signs of abuse. Box 19-2 lists signs of the various kinds of abuse. These signs generally apply to all abusive relationships in all settings. However, you are not qualified to judge whether or not your client is being abused. If you notice one or some of the signs listed in Box 19-2, it does not mean that abuse has occurred. Rather, these signs suggest that abuse could be a possibility.

Watch for signs of abuse or neglect in your daily work. Immediately report any suspicions or observations to your supervisor. Your supervisor will ensure that the situation is investigated. Know your employer's procedures on reporting observations or suspicions.

Your Legal Responsibilities

You are legally required to report child abuse. You must report if you witness child abuse. You also must report if you suspect child abuse. Each province and territory has rules about what must be reported and to whom. However, *all* require that witnessed and suspected child abuse be reported directly to child protection authorities. (Look up your local child welfare agency or social service agency in the phone book.) Do not rely on your supervisor to report for you. However, consult with your supervisor before making your report. Your supervisor will advise you.

As long as you have reasonable grounds for reporting, no legal action can be taken against you if your suspicions are eventually proved wrong. Your name will be kept confidential. In some provinces, failing to report child abuse can result in fines or imprisonment.

Several provinces and territories also have laws that require health care workers to report witnessed or suspected abuse within facilities. In these provinces, workers must report abuse directly to a public authority. Even if your province or territory does not require public reporting, inform your supervisor about any cases or suspicions of abuse. Know your employer's policy and provincial or territorial law concerning the reporting of abuse within a facility.

With the exception of Nova Scotia and Newfoundland, no provinces or territories have laws requiring the public reporting of abuse of an adult living in the community. It is understood that mentally capable adults can make their own choices and decisions about seeking help. Therefore, in home care settings, you do not need to report abuse of older adults or spouses to a public authority. However, immediately report your suspicions to your supervisor, according to your employer's policies.

How to Report Abuse

Your employer will have specific rules for how to report your observations. It is very important to record all your observations and make your reports in writing. Keep all notes in case you will be asked to remember details later on. In general, when you report abuse—whether to your supervisor or a public authority—you should record the following:

- The alleged victim's name, address, phone number, age, and sex
- The alleged abuser's name, address, phone number, and relationship to the victim
- Description of abuse and neglect, suspicions, and evidence obtained to date; record the date, time, and place; only state the facts that you know or were told by the victim; do not make assumptions

(text continues on page 244)

Box 19-2 Signs and Symptoms of Abuse

Physical Abuse

- Physical injuries (such as burns, bumps, bruises, scratches, cuts, or fractures) that occur frequently, are left untreated, and either are unexplained or have unlikely explanations
- New injuries that appear while older injuries are still healing
- Frequent injuries (such as burns, bruises, welts, or cuts) on the face, neck, inner arms, back, upper arms and inner thighs; people who are abused often try to hide their injuries under clothing or make-up
- Welts, bruises, or burns that appear in the shape of the object that caused the injury; for example, the shape may be of a handprint, belt, or wooden spoon
- Unexplained missing or loose teeth

Sexual Abuse

- Irritation, injury (such as cuts and bruises or scarring) of the thighs, perineum, or breasts
- Intense fear of bathing or perineal care
- Torn, stained, or bloody underwear
- Vaginal discharge, genital odour, and painful urination
- Difficulty walking or sitting
- Avoidance of touching

Emotional Abuse

- A change in behaviour, especially if the person seems depressed or unusually quiet or withdrawn
- The person seems fearful, especially in the presence of the suspected abuser; for example, the person cowers, avoids eye contact, or trembles
- The person does not want to talk or answer questions
- The person's behaviour changes when the suspected abuser enters and leaves the room
- The person is not permitted to socialize with family or friends or has withdrawn from these contacts
- Private conversations are not allowed; the suspected abuser insists on being present or within hearing distance of all conversations
- The caregiver's behaviour changes: on one occasion he or she is pleasant and cooperative; on another occasion he or she is defensive or hostile
- The caregiver does not show any affection toward the person in his or her care, or the affection that is shown seems strained or "put on for show"
- The caregiver often states that the person in his or her care is difficult or demanding

Financial Abuse

- The caregiver refuses to spend money on caring for the person
- The person has many unpaid bills (such as utilities, telephone, or rent) or bounced cheques, even though the person has money
- There is a lack of adequate food, clothing, personal care items, or furnishings, even though the person can afford them
- The suspected abuser seems more concerned about the cost rather than the quality of the person's care
- Personal belongings are missing without explanation
- The suspected abuser does not have a job and is secretive about his or her source of income
- The person must ask for permission to write cheques or spend money

Neglect

- Living conditions are unsafe, unclean, or inadequate
- Personal hygiene is lacking; for example, a neglected client may have ingrown nails, decayed teeth, untreated sores, matted hair, body odour, or dirty clothing
- There are signs of poor nutrition and fluid intake such as weight loss, extreme thirst, a thin, bony appearance, and sunken eyes or cheeks; dehydration may make the skin feel dry and papery
- Pressure sores are present
- Medications are not purchased
- The person is left unsupervised or unattended for prolonged periods of time

Infants and Children

All of the above and the following are signs of abuse or neglect in children and infants:

- Sudden behaviour changes, such as bedwetting, loss of bladder or bowel control during the day, or loss of appetite
- Prolonged vomiting or diarrhea
- Developmental delays, such as not gaining weight or reaching developmental milestones (for example, sitting or standing)
- Lack of energy in infants, shown by lack of interest in the surroundings, infrequent crying, and generally an undemanding disposition

Sources: Virginia Boyack, *Golden Years—Hidden Fears: Elder Abuse. A Handbook for Front-Line Helpers Working with Seniors* (Calgary: Kerby Centre, 1997), p. 7; Mary Joy Quinn and Susan K. Tomita, *Elder Abuse and Neglect: Causes, Diagnosis, and Intervention Strategies*, 2nd ed. (New York: Springer, 1997), pp. 55, 76.

Whenever you report your suspicions, it is essential that you respect and protect your client's right to privacy. Only tell people who need to know. Do not gossip or tell anyone who is not directly involved.

When Clients Speak of Abuse

You should be prepared for the possibility that a client or child may tell you that he or she is being abused. In such situations, it is important that you support the person and know how to offer help immediately. Follow your employer's guidelines and policies. The following are some general guidelines for how to be supportive:

- Listen attentively. Let the person tell you what happened in his or her own words. Recognize the person's feelings.
- Reassure the person that you believe what he or she has said. Stay calm and do not show anger or disgust. Do not deny or ignore the problem. Do not ask what the person did to make the abuser angry. This will only make the victim think the abuse was his or her fault.
- Assure the person that you will do what you can to help. Notify your supervisor at once. Your employer's guidelines and policies will say what should be provided to people who are living with abuse. Helpful community resources include the police, women's shelters, counselling services, telephone help lines, and legal clinics.
- Provide emotional support for the person whatever he or she decides to do. Remember, you cannot force an adult to make a certain decision or take a particular action. People who are capable of making their own informed decisions have the right to decide for themselves whether to live with the abuse or to accept help. Some people choose not to accept help. This is their right. You must accept their decision. People who are not capable of making informed decisions must have a professional help them.

REVIEW

Circle the BEST answer.

1. Which is *not* physical abuse?
   A. Kicking
   B. Pinching
   C. Throwing something at someone
   D. Withholding affection

2. Which is *not* part of the cycle of abuse?
   A. Honeymoon phase
   B. Resolution phase
   C. Tension-building phase
   D. Abusive incident

3. Who are more likely to be abusive?
   A. Women
   B. Men
   C. People who have a problem with alcohol or drugs
   D. Parents with close family and social relationships

4. These statements are about spousal abuse. Which is *true*?
   A. Suspected abuse must be reported to the police.
   B. Abuse only involves violence.
   C. Women and men can be abused.
   D. Only one type of abuse is usually present.

5. These statements are about child abuse. Which is *true*?
   A. You must have proof that abuse has occurred before you report it.
   B. All victims of child abuse are girls.
   C. You must report any suspicions of child abuse directly to the child protection authorities.
   D. Infants are not at risk for child abuse.

6. Which of the following is *not* an example of abuse of a client?
   A. Inappropriate use of restraints
   B. Reviewing the care plan regularly
   C. Taking a coffee break before responding to a call bell
   D. Leaving the client in soiled linen or clothes

7. When confronted by an abusive client, you should *not*
   A. Touch the person
   B. Stand about 2 metres (6 feet) away from the person
   C. Talk to the person calmly
   D. Quickly leave the room or house if you think you are in danger

8. Which is *not* a sign of physical abuse?
   A. Stiff and sore joints
   B. Old bruises and new bruises
   C. Unbelievable explanations for injuries
   D. Frequent or untreated injuries

9. Intense fear of bathing or perineal care may be a sign of
   A. Physical abuse
   B. Emotional abuse
   C. Sexual abuse
   D. Neglect

10. Which is *not* a sign of emotional abuse?
    A. Isolation from family and friends
    B. Low self-esteem
    C. Depression
    D. Pressure sores

11. Mr. Deol states, "My daughter won't give me food until I give her my pension cheque." This is a sign of
    A. Financial abuse
    B. Emotional abuse
    C. Neglect
    D. Physical abuse

12. You suspect an adult client is being abused. What should you do?
    A. Tell the family
    B. Tell your supervisor
    C. Call the police
    D. Ask the person if he or she was abused

Answers to these questions are on page 823.

CHAPTER

20

The Client's Environment: Promoting Well-Being, Comfort, and Rest

OBJECTIVES

- Define the key terms listed in this chapter
- Explain how to promote well-being during the admission, transfer, and discharge procedures
- Explain why comfort is important
- Describe four types of pain
- List the signs and symptoms of pain
- List the care plan measures that relieve pain
- Explain why rest and sleep are important
- Describe the factors that affect sleep
- Describe common sleep disorders
- List care plan measures that promote sleep
- Learn the procedures described in this chapter

KEY TERMS

acute pain Sudden pain due to injury, disease, trauma, or surgery; it generally lasts less than six months

admission Official entry of a person into a hospital or other health care facility

chronic pain Pain that lasts longer than 6 months; it may be constant or occur off and on

discharge Official departure of a client from a hospital or other health care facility

insomnia A chronic condition in which the person cannot go to sleep or stay asleep throughout the night

phantom pain Pain felt in a body part that is no longer there

radiating pain Pain felt at the site of tissue damage and in nearby areas

transfer Moving a client from one room or unit to another

Clients should feel safe, comfortable, and relaxed in their environment. The environment may be any of the settings described in Chapter 3. These include private homes, assisted-living dwellings, apartments, units in long-term care facilities, and hospital rooms. Consider these examples:

- Mr. Kremer, 88, moves from his home to a long-term care facility. He feels like a stranger. You make his room feel more like home and introduce him to other staff and residents. He begins to feel more secure and comfortable.
- Jose Cruz, 17, is admitted to hospital following a car accident. He has some pain and is also anxious and fearful. A nurse gives him medication to control his pain. She explains what to expect during surgery and afterwards. He feels better knowing what will happen next.
- Ms. Lalonde, 35, has a disorder that causes paralysis. You help her to bathe and dress. You change her bed, do her laundry, and clean her house. She feels more relaxed and comfortable in fresh clothes and a clean environment.

Feeling safe, comfortable, and relaxed contributes to well-being. Support workers play a key role in promoting the well-being of their clients.

WELL-BEING DURING TRANSITIONS

Clients often move from one environment to another. For example, they move:

- Into and out of facilities (admissions and discharges)
- From one room or unit in a facility to another (transfers)

Transitions are difficult for most people. Do you remember how you felt the last time you moved? You probably felt sad if you had to leave friends and family behind. You might have felt strange and disoriented in your new environment.

For people who are elderly or unwell, moving from one environment to another can be very difficult. Many people feel anxious, unsettled, and alone. Moving can even cause or increase signs of confusion in some people. You can promote clients' emotional well-being during transitions as you help them with the admitting, transfer, and discharge processes.

ADMITTING A PERSON TO A FACILITY

Admission is the official entry of a person into a health care facility. The process can cause uncertainty, anxiety, and fear. People often worry about medical tests, treatment, and surgery. They may fear pain and serious health problems. People moving to a long-term care facility often feel sad about leaving home. The facility is strange and unfamiliar. They do not know what to expect and where to go. They worry about getting meals, finding the bathroom, and getting help.

The admitting processes in long-term facilities and hospitals are similar. However, there are also differences.

Long-Term Care Facilities. The admitting process in long-term care facilities usually starts several days before the new resident enters the facility. Many facilities have admissions coordinators who make the process as simple as possible. Details are handled before the person arrives. Therefore, the person is not bothered on arrival with forms and procedures.

The staff is told of the admission and room assignment. The room is prepared according to facility policy and the wishes of the new resident and family. Most facilities provide a bed, a bedside stand, and a chair, although residents can use their own if desired.

Residents are encouraged to make their rooms as homelike as possible. Long-term care legislation states that residents have the right to choose their furnishings and display personal items in their rooms (see Chapter 10). Families are often involved in preparing the room. Furniture is delivered in advance. Family members arrange the room and hang pictures. Some install curtains or blinds from the person's home. Some even put up wallpaper.

When the new resident arrives, you might help with the admitting process. The process may become routine for you. Remember that the process is *not* routine for the person. It is a major life event. How would you feel if you had to leave your home and enter a facility? Long-term care residents have left behind their homes. They have also left behind family, friends, neighbours, and pets. Now they must live in a strange place, where they probably have to share a room with a stranger. Their health is probably declining, and they may have little hope for the future. The new resident probably feels anxious and out of place.

First impressions of the facility are important. An uncaring reception could make the new resident feel unwanted. A warm welcome will help reassure and comfort the person. (See *Providing Compassionate Care: Welcoming a New Resident to a Long-Term Care Facility* box.) The procedure on page 249 can be used in long-term care facilities or hospitals.

Hospitals. Except in emergencies, the hospital admission process starts in the admissions office. A member of the admitting staff gives the new patient an ID number and bracelet. The patient signs a consent-for-treatment form. Admitting staff notifies the nursing unit that a patient is being admitted. You may be asked to prepare the room for the person. A porter, support worker, or admitting office staff member brings the patient to the nursing unit. Many people require transport by wheelchair or stretcher.

At the nursing unit, a nurse usually greets and admits the patient. If the patient is not in pain or distress, you may be asked to greet the person and assist with admission procedures. Introduce yourself by name and title. Call the patient by name. Remember that the patient and family may be anxious. Accompany them to the room. Be friendly and gentle. Do not rush. Admission procedures involve:

- Weighing and measuring the person (see Chapter 40)
- Obtaining a urine specimen if ordered (see Chapter 29)
- Orienting the patient to the room, nursing unit, and hospital

(text continues on page 250)

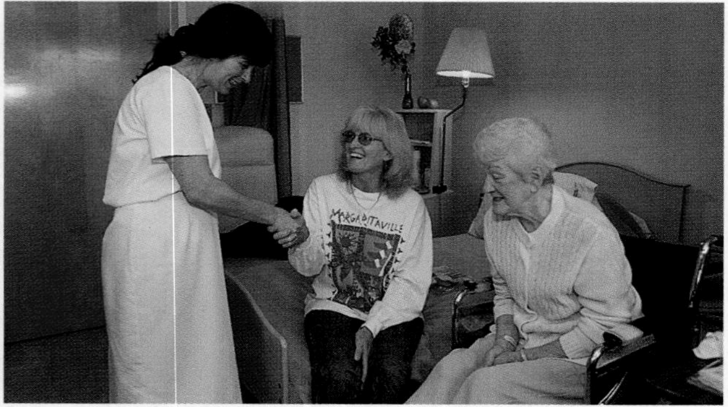

Figure 20-1 A support worker introduces herself to a new resident and family member.

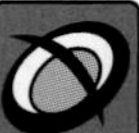

Providing **Compassionate Care**

WELCOMING A NEW RESIDENT TO A LONG-TERM CARE FACILITY

D*ignity.* Treat the new resident and his or her belongings with respect. Greet the person by name. Do not call adults by their first names unless you are asked to do so. Introduce yourself by name and title to the resident and family (Figure 20-1). Do not rush into admission procedures. Treat the resident and family as if they are guests in your home. Offer them refreshments. Tell them the many good things about the facility. Listen to their concerns or questions. Do not overload people with information. Explain details about routines, recreation facilities, and other matters only if the new resident seems eager to listen. Reassure people that they do not need to remember everything. Remind them that they can ask questions and talk to the staff at any time.

I*ndependence.* A homelike setting is important to a person's independence and control. Help new residents feel at home. Show them their room. Explain how to use equipment in the room. Offer to help unpack and arrange their belongings (unless this has been done by the family). Make sure the person can reach the phone, TV, and light controls.

P*references.* Some new residents want to arrange their own rooms. Choice is always allowed in arranging personal items. The health care team makes sure that the resident's choices are safe, will not cause falls or other accidents, and do not interfere with the rights of others.

P*rivacy.* Show the new resident how to draw the privacy curtains. Explain that the health care team respects all residents' right to privacy. Explain how you maintain privacy during personal care and other procedures.

S*afety.* Explain how to use the call bell (see Chapter 16). Ensure it is in easy reach. Show the bathroom and safety features such as grab bars. Review safety and emergency procedures according to facility policy.

Admitting the Person to a Facility

Compassionate Care

Remember to Promote:
- **Dignity**
- **Independence**
- **Preferences**
- **Privacy**
- **Safety**

Pre-Procedure

1 Wash your hands.

Procedure

2 Greet the person by name. Ask if he or she prefers a certain name.

3 Introduce yourself to the person and family or friends who may be present. Give your title, and explain that you assist the nurses in giving care.

4 Introduce the roommate.

5 Call for the nurse immediately if the person complains of any severe pain or appears to be in distress.

6 Proceed if the person's condition does not present an immediate or serious problem.

7 Provide for privacy. Ask relatives or friends to leave the room. Tell them how much time you need and where they can wait comfortably. (Allow family members or friends to stay if the person prefers.)

8 Have a hospital patient put on a gown or pyjamas. Assist as needed. A long-term care resident can stay dressed if his or her condition permits.

9 Provide for comfort. Follow the directions in the care plan. The person should be in bed or in a chair if directed by the nurse.

10 If instructed to do so by the nurse, measure the person's height and weight and vital signs.

11 Complete a clothing and valuables list.

12 Help the person to unpack, hang clothes in the closet, and put personal items in the drawers and bedside stand.

13 Explain any ordered activity limits.

14 Obtain a urine specimen if ordered (see Chapter 29).

15 Take the specimen to the assigned area. Clean equipment and wash your hands.

16 Orient the person to the area:

- a Give names of nursing staff.
- b For long-term care residents, give the names of other residents.
- c Identify items in bedside stand. Explain the purpose of each item.
- d Show how to use the call bell.
- e Show how to operate the bed, television controls, and telephone.
- f Explain policies, including visiting hours.
- g Describe the location of the nurses' station, lounge, dining room, activity area, gift shop, chapel, and other areas.
- h Explain other services (for example, newspaper, library, activities and programs, and religious services).
- i Identify other staff (for example, dietary, housekeeping, physical therapy, and social work).
- j Explain when and where meals and snacks are served.

17 Provide a denture container if needed. Label it with the person's name and room number.

Continued

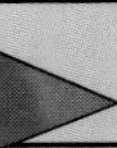

Admitting the Person to a Facility—cont'd

Procedure—cont'd

18 For the long-term care resident, label personal property and personal care equipment with the person's name.

19 Introduce the resident to other residents in the unit (if the person is mobile and the care plan permits).

Post-Procedure

20 Provide for safety and comfort.

21 Place the call bell within reach.

22 Remove privacy measures.

23 Follow the care plan for bed position and bed rails.

24 Fill the water pitcher if oral fluids are allowed.

25 Clean any used equipment. Discard used disposable items.

26 Wash your hands.

27 Report and record your actions and observations according to employer policy.

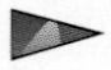

TRANSFERS

A **transfer** occurs when a client is moved from one room or nursing unit to another. Transfers usually occur when a client's condition changes. Some people are transferred for rehabilitation. Some people request a room change. Sometimes roommates do not get along. A client may or may not welcome a transfer. The person's physician, nurse, or social worker usually explains the reason for the transfer. You may assist with the transfer or carry out the entire procedure. Clients are usually transported by wheelchair or stretcher. Sometimes the bed is used. Be sensitive and compassionate as you carry out this procedure. Support and reassurance are needed. The new person does not know the staff on the new unit. Introduce the person to the staff and roommate. Wish the person well as you leave.

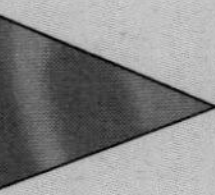

Transferring the Person to Another Nursing Unit

COMPASSIONATE CARE

Remember to Promote:

- **Dignity**
- **Independence**
- **Preferences**
- **Privacy**
- **Safety**

Pre-Procedure

1 Find out where the person is going. Ask if the bed, a wheelchair, or a stretcher will be used.

2 Identify the person according to employer policy.

3 Explain the procedure to the person.

4 Get a stretcher or wheelchair, blanket, and a utility cart if needed.

5 Wash your hands.

Continued

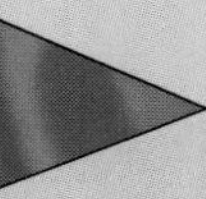

Transferring the Person to Another Nursing Unit—cont'd

Procedure

6 Collect the person's belongings and bedside equipment. Place them on the utility cart.
7 Assist the person to the wheelchair or stretcher. Cover the person with a blanket.
8 Transport the person to the assigned place.
9 Introduce the person to the receiving nurse.
10 Help transfer the person from the wheelchair or stretcher into bed or a chair. Help position the person.
11 Bring the person's belongings and equipment to the new room. Help put them away.
12 Report the following to the receiving nurse:
- a How the person tolerated the transfer
- b Whether a nurse will bring the person's chart and medications

Post-Procedure

13 Return the wheelchair or stretcher and utility cart to the storage area.
14 Wash your hands.
15 Report and record your actions and observations according to employer policy. Include the following:
- The time of the transfer
- Where the person was taken
- How the person was transferred (bed, wheelchair, or stretcher)
- Who received the person
- Any other observations

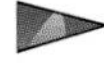

DISCHARGES

Discharge is the official departure of a client from a hospital or other health care facility. Some clients have recovered enough to go home. Some need home care. Others are discharged to another hospital, to a long-term care facility, or to a hospice. The physician, nurse, dietician, social worker, and other health care team members plan the client's discharge. They teach the client and family about diet, exercise, medications, treatments, and dressing changes. The case manager arranges for home care, rehabilitation, special therapy, and equipment, if required.

You may help clients pack their belongings and get ready to leave. You may transport clients out of the facility. In a hospital, the physician must write a discharge order before a patient is allowed to leave. In a long-term care facility, permission must be obtained from the nurse. In some facilities, the chart contains instructions as to when the resident may leave and with whom.

Always use good communication skills when assisting with a client's discharge. Wish the person and family well as they leave the facility.

A client may want to leave without permission. If a person tells you that he or she wants or intends to leave, notify the nurse immediately.

(text continues on page 253)

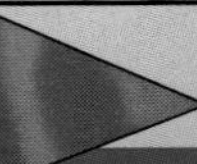

Discharging the Person

Compassionate Care

Remember to Promote:
- **Dignity**
- **Independence**
- **Preferences**
- **Privacy**
- **Safety**

Pre-Procedure

1. Make sure the person is to be discharged. Find out if transportation arrangements have been made.
2. Identify the person according to employer policy.
3. Explain the procedure to the person.
4. Wash your hands.
5. Provide for privacy.

Procedure

6. Help the person dress as needed.
7. Help the person pack. Check all drawers and closets to make sure all items are collected.
8. Check off the clothing and personal belongings list. Ask the person to sign the form indicating that all clothing and personal belongings have been returned.
9. Tell the nurse that the person is ready for the final visit. The nurse:
   a. Gives prescriptions written by the physician
   b. Provides discharge instructions
   c. Gets valuables from the safe
10. Get a wheelchair and a utility cart for the person's belongings. Ask a co-worker to help you.
11. Bring the wheelchair to the bedside and lock the wheels. Lock the bed wheels. Lower the bed to its lowest position.
12. Help the person into the wheelchair.
13. Unlock the wheels.
14. Take the person to the exit area. Lock the wheels of the wheelchair.
15. Help the person out of the wheelchair and into the car.
16. Help put the person's belongings into the car.

Post-Procedure

17. Return the wheelchair and cart to the storage area.
18. Wash your hands.
19. Report and record your actions and observations according to employer policy. Include the following:
    - The time of discharge
    - How the person was transported
    - Who accompanied the person
    - The person's destination
    - Any other observations

Comfort

Comfort is a feeling of contentment. There is no physical or emotional pain. The person is calm and at peace. Age, illness, pain, and inactivity affect comfort. So do factors like temperature, ventilation, odours, noise, and lighting.

- *Temperature.* Most people are comfortable when the room temperature is between 20 and 23° C (68–74° F). Infants, older adults, and ill people generally need higher room temperatures for comfort. Government legislation dictates minimum temperatures in long-term care facilities. In home care settings, clients set the temperature they want. Some people may be concerned with the cost of heat. Help these clients keep warm with extra clothing or blankets.
- *Ventilation.* Stale room air affects comfort. Facilities have ventilation systems that provide fresh air. In home care settings, you can open windows and doors and turn on fans, as the client desires. Protect clients from drafts by making sure they are dressed warmly, covered with blankets, and moved away from drafty areas.
- *Odours.* Many bodily substances and fluids have unpleasant odours that can embarrass people. Body, breath, and smoking odours may also offend people. If you smoke, wash your hands and brush your teeth afterwards. Change your clothes frequently. Good hygiene, housekeeping practices, and ventilation help eliminate odours. To reduce odours:
  - Empty and clean bedpans, urinals, commodes, and kidney basins promptly
  - Change and dispose of soiled linens and clothing promptly
  - Clean clients who are wet or soiled from urine, feces, vomitus, or wound drainage
  - Dispose of incontinence and ostomy products promptly
  - Keep laundry containers closed
  - Provide clients with good personal hygiene
- *Noise.* Ill people are sensitive to noise. Health care facilities can be noisy places. The clanging of bedpans, the clatter of dishes, phones ringing, loud talking, and television sounds can disturb people. Households, too, can be noisy, particularly when young children and teenagers live at home. Help to control noise. Talk quietly. Handle equipment carefully. Answer phones promptly. Noises in facilities can be frightening, especially for new patients and residents. Explain the source of the noise to help the person feel secure.
- *Lighting.* Glares, shadows, and dull lighting can cause falls, headaches, and eyestrain. Dim light often helps people rest better. Bright light is helpful when giving care. It also helps people to feel cheerful and stimulated. Before adjusting the lights, ask clients about their preferences. Make sure light switches are in reach.

Room Furniture and Equipment

Rooms are furnished and equipped for comfort and safety:

- *Bathrooms.* Most facility bathrooms have a sink, call bell, mirror, and toilet with handrails (Figure 20-2). Some bathrooms have showers. Toilets in some facilities are higher than regular toilets. This makes moving to and from wheelchairs easier. They are also helpful for people with joint problems. Some bathrooms are private; others are shared. Most bathrooms in private homes do not have elevated toilets and handrails. You must make sure the client's bathroom is clean and safe.
- *Beds.* For those who are confined to bed, comfort is especially important. Hospital beds have electrical or manual controls that allow people to sit up and lie down without effort. Many home care clients have regular beds. Use pillows to help people sit comfortably in a regular bed (see Chapter 24).
- *Overbed tables.* Hospitals and many long-term care facilities have overbed tables. These tables can be positioned over the bed. The height can be adjusted for a person in bed or in a chair. The overbed table is used for placing meal trays, eating, reading, writing, and other activities. It is also used as a work area for bedside procedures. Never place bedpans, urinals, or soiled linens on an overbed table. Always clean the table carefully after each use.
- *Bedside furniture.* Most hospitals and long-term care facilities have bedside stands for personal items (Figure 20-3). In private homes, bedside furniture

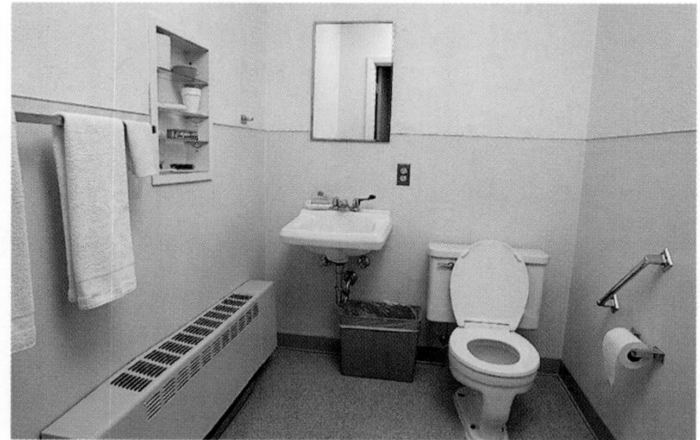

Figure 20-2 A facility bathroom.

varies. Some people have a bedside stand. Others have a small table. Still others have nothing at the bedside.

- *Chairs.* A hospital room usually has one or two chairs. Long-term care residents may bring their own chairs from home (Figure 20-4). Home care clients often have a favourite chair. Make sure that the chair is kept clean and free of food particles. Plump cushions regularly.

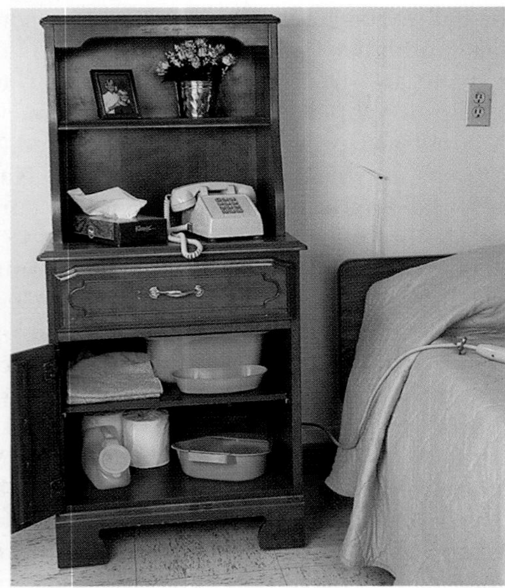

Figure 20-3 A bedside stand in a long-term care facility is used to store personal care items.

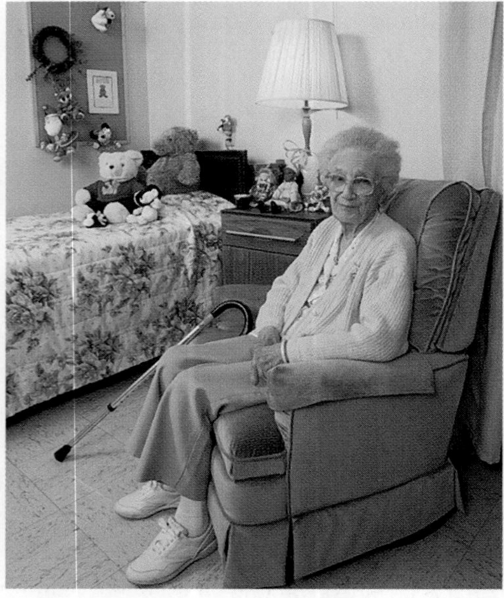

Figure 20-4 A resident's chair from home.

- *Privacy curtains and screens.* Privacy curtains are standard in hospitals and long-term care facilities (Figure 20-5). Suspended from the ceiling, the curtain is pulled around the bed. Pull the curtain around the bed before giving care. Privacy curtains prevent others from seeing the client. However, they do not block sound or prevent conversations from being heard. In home care settings, portable screens can be used for privacy (Figure 20-6).
- *Closet and drawer space.* Hospitals and long-term care facilities provide closet and drawer space for the client's clothing. Government legislation states that long-term care residents must have easy access to the closet and its contents.
- *Medical equipment.* Most hospital rooms have blood pressure equipment mounted on the wall. An IV pole (IV standard) is used to hang an intravenous infusion bag or a feeding bag. Some hospital beds have an IV pole stored in the bed frame. The IV pole may be a separate piece of equipment that is brought to the bedside when needed. Hospital rooms also have wall outlets for oxygen and suction

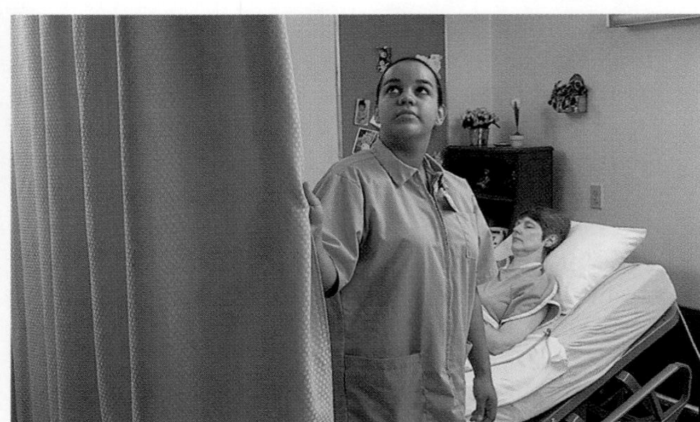

Figure 20-5 Curtains around the bed provide privacy in hospitals and long-term care facilities.

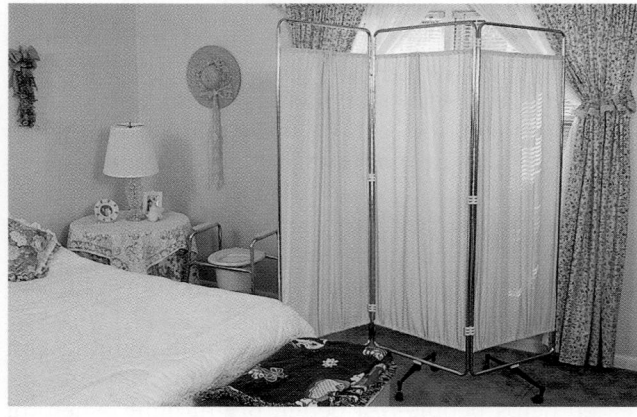

Figure 20-6 Portable screens provide privacy in the home.

(Figure 20-7). Oxygen tanks and portable suction equipment are common in long-term care and home care settings. Only medically necessary equipment is kept in the client's room.

PAIN

To have discomfort or pain means to ache, hurt, or be sore. Discomfort and pain are subjective. You cannot see, hear, touch, or smell a client's discomfort or pain. You must rely on what the person and the person's body language tell you. Report complaints and observations to your supervisor.

Pain is personal. It differs for each person. What *hurts* to one person may *ache* to another. What one person calls *sore*, another may call *burning*. If a client complains of pain or discomfort, the client *has* pain or discomfort. You must believe the person. Remember, you cannot see, hear, feel, or smell the pain. Pain may signal tissue damage.

Pain is not only physical. People also feel emotional, social, and spiritual pain. When suffering, the whole self feels pain. Clients in pain may be sad, impatient, irritable, or angry. You must be especially kind and empathetic.

Types of Pain. There are different types of pain.

- **Acute pain** is felt suddenly from injury, disease, trauma, or surgery. Tissue is damaged. Acute pain usually lasts less than 6 months. It decreases with healing.
- **Chronic pain** lasts longer than 6 months. Pain is constant or occurs off and on. Arthritis and cancer are common causes of chronic pain.
- **Radiating pain** is felt at the site of tissue damage and in nearby areas. Pain from a heart attack is often felt in the left side of the chest, left jaw, left shoulder, and left arm. A diseased gallbladder can cause pain in the right upper abdomen, the back, and the right shoulder (Figure 20-8).
- **Phantom pain** is felt in a body part that is no longer there. A person who has had a leg amputated may still feel leg pain.

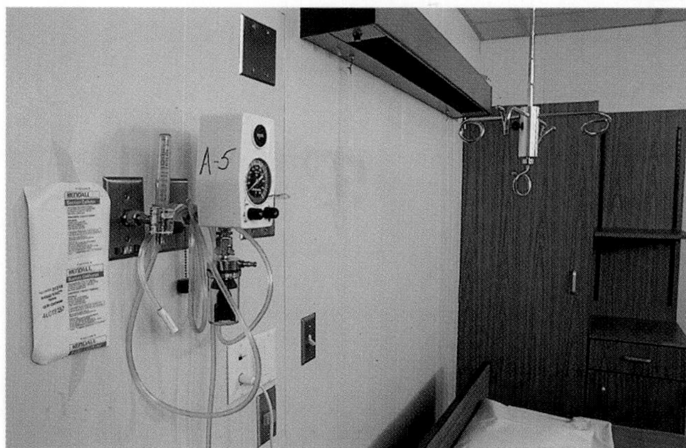

Figure 20-7 This hospital room has blood pressure equipment, an IV pole, and oxygen and suction outlets.

Factors Affecting Pain. Pain does not always affect people the same way. Many factors affect reactions to pain.

- *Past experience.* A person may have had pain before. The severity of pain, its cause, how long it lasted, and whether relief occurred all affect the person's current response to pain. Knowing what to expect can help or hinder a person in handling pain. People who have never experienced pain may be fearful because they do not know what to expect.
- *Anxiety.* An anxious person feels troubled or threatened. Pain and anxiety are related. Pain can cause anxiety. Anxiety can make pain feel worse. Lessening anxiety helps reduce pain. For example, the nurse explains to Mr. Schett that he will have pain after surgery and that he will receive medication for pain relief. When Mr. Schett feels pain after surgery, he knows what to expect. This helps reduce his anxiety and therefore the amount of pain he feels.
- *Rest and sleep.* Rest and sleep restore energy and help the body to repair itself. Ill and injured people need more sleep than usual. Lack of rest and sleep affects how a person copes with pain. Pain seems worse when a person is tired or restless.

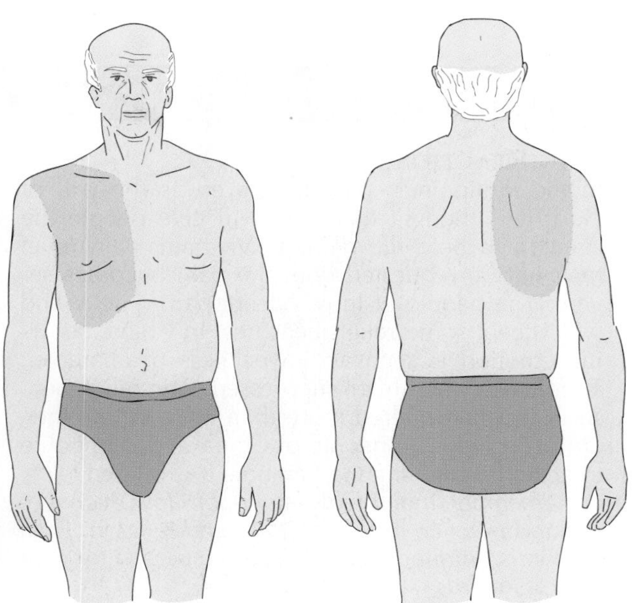

Figure 20-8 Gallbladder pain radiates to the right upper abdomen, the back, and the right shoulder.

- *Attention.* The more a person thinks about the pain, the worse it can seem. Sometimes pain is so severe that it is all a person thinks about. However, even mild pain can seem worse if a person dwells on it. Pain often seems worse at night when there are no distractions.
- *The meaning of pain.* Pain means different things to different people. Some see it as a sign of serious weakness. It also may mean a serious illness. Some people ignore or deny their pain. Sometimes pain is used to avoid certain people or things. Others use pain to get attention.
- *Support from others.* Pain is easier to deal with when family and friends offer comfort and support. The presence of a friend or loved one can be very comforting. People who do not have caring family and friends must deal with pain alone. Being alone can increase fear, anxiety, and suffering. Be especially sensitive to clients who are suffering alone.
- *Culture.* Culture affects how a person responds to pain (see *Respecting Diversity: Pain Reactions* box). In some cultures, people in pain show no reaction. In other cultures, people in pain have strong verbal and nonverbal reactions.
- *Age.* See *Focus on Children: Pain Reactions* and *Focus on Older Adults: Pain Reactions* boxes.

Signs and Symptoms of Pain. Your client may tell you about pain. Or, body language and behaviour may reveal the person is in pain. For example, Ms. Raj grimaces when she moves, but denies having pain. Report any information and observations about pain to your supervisor. Always use the client's exact words when you report and record. Report the following:

- *Location.* Where is the pain? Ask the client to point to the area of pain (Figure 20-9). Remember, pain can radiate. Ask the person if the pain is anywhere else and to point to those areas.
- *Onset and duration.* When did the pain start? How long has the pain lasted?
- *Intensity.* Does the client complain of mild, moderate, or severe pain? Ask the person to rate the pain on a scale of 1 to 10, with 10 being the most severe.
- *Description.* Ask the client to describe the pain. Box 20-1 lists some words used to describe pain. Write down what the person says. Use the person's exact words.
- *Factors causing pain.* Factors causing pain may include moving or turning in bed, coughing or deep breathing, and exercise. Ask what the client was doing before the pain started and when it started.

Respecting Diversity

Pain Reactions

In the Philippines, pain is viewed as the will of God. It is thought that God will give people the strength to bear the pain. In Vietnam, pain relief may not be requested until the pain becomes severe. The people of India accept pain quietly and will accept some relief measures. In China, showing emotion is seen as a weakness of character. Therefore, pain is often suppressed. Pain relief measures must be offered more than once before they are accepted. The people of China find it impolite to accept something the first time it is offered.

Remember, individuals may not follow every belief and practice of their culture and religion. Each person is unique. Do not judge the person by your own standards.

Source: Adapted from E.M. Geissler, *Pocket Guide to Cultural Assessment*, 2nd ed. (St. Louis: Mosby, 1998).

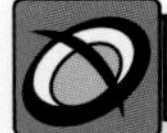

Focus on Children

Pain Reactions

Many children do not understand pain. They have few experiences with pain. They do not know what to expect or how to deal with pain. They must rely on adults for help.

Adults do not always know when children are in pain. Toddlers and preschool children may not know words that express pain. Crying and fussing infants and toddlers can mean many different problems, not just pain. Adults must be alert for behaviours and situations that signal pain.

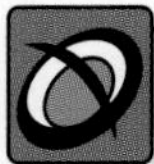

Focus on Older Adults

Pain Reactions

Older adults may have decreased pain sensations. They may not feel pain, or it may not feel severe. This places them at greater risk for undetected disease or injury. Pain alerts a person to illness or injury. If pain is not felt, the person may not seek health care.

Some older adults have many health problems that cause pain. They may think a new pain is related to an existing health problem. Chronic pain may mask the new pain. They may deny or ignore pain because of what it might mean.

Some older adults have disorders that affect thinking and reasoning. Some cannot communicate verbally. Changes in behaviour may indicate pain. Report changes in clients' behaviour to your supervisor.

- *Vital signs.* What are the client's pulse, respirations, and blood pressure? Increases in these vital signs often occur with pain.
- *Other signs and symptoms.* Does the client have other symptoms: dizziness, nausea, vomiting, weakness, numbness, tingling, or others? Box 20-2 lists the signs and symptoms that often occur with pain.

Measures to Relieve Pain. Nurses and case managers use the care planning process to promote comfort and relieve pain. Box 20-3 lists measures that are often part of the care plan. Medications ordered by the physician provide pain relief. However, medications can cause drowsiness, dizziness, and coordination problems. People on pain relief medications must be protected from injury. The care plan alerts you to safety practices.

Measures other than medications also control pain. These include distraction, relaxation, and guided imagery. Nurses and therapists teach clients these measures. You may be trained to assist with some of them.

- *Distraction* means a change in a person's focus of attention. Attention is directed away from the pain. Conversation, music, television, games, and needlepoint are examples of distractions.

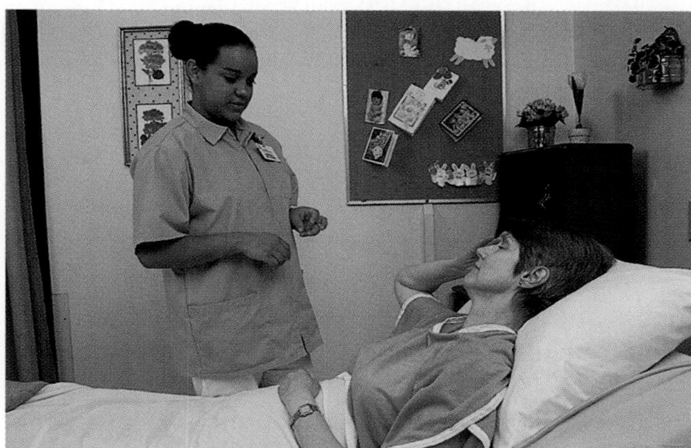

Figure 20-9 A client points to the area of pain.

Box 20-1 Words Used to Describe Pain

- Aching
- Burning
- Cramping
- Crushing
- Dull
- Gnawing
- Knifelike
- Piercing
- Pressure
- Sharp
- Sore
- Squeezing
- Stabbing
- Throbbing
- Viselike

Box 20-2 Signs and Symptoms of Pain

Body Responses
- Increased pulse, respirations, and blood pressure
- Nausea
- Pale skin (pallor)
- Sweating (diaphoresis)
- Vomiting

Behaviours
- Changes in speech; slow or rapid, loud or quiet
- Crying
- Gasping
- Grimacing
- Groaning
- Grunting
- Holding the affected body part (splinting)
- Being irritable
- Maintaining one position; refusing to move
- Moaning
- Being quiet
- Being restless
- Rubbing
- Screaming

Box 20-3 Measures to Promote Comfort and Relieve Pain

- Position the client in good body alignment. Use pillows for support.
- Keep bed linens tight and wrinkle-free.
- Make sure the client is not lying on drainage tubes.
- Assist with elimination needs.
- Provide blankets for warmth and to prevent chilling.
- Use correct lifting, moving, and turning procedures.
- Wait one half-hour after pain medication was given before giving care.
- Give a back massage.
- Provide soft music to distract the client.
- Use touch to provide comfort.
- Allow family and friends to visit as requested by the client.
- Avoid sudden or jarring movements.
- Handle the client gently.
- Practise safety measures if the client is receiving strong pain medication or sedatives:
  - If the client is in a hospital bed, keep the bed in the lowest position.
  - Follow the care plan for bed rail use.
  - Check on the client every 10 to 15 minutes.
  - Provide assistance when the client is up.
  - Provide heat or cold applications as directed.
  - Provide a calm, quiet, darkened environment.

- *Relaxation* means absence of mental or physical stress. A relaxed state reduces pain and anxiety. The nurse or therapist teaches the client to breathe deeply and slowly and to contract and relax muscle groups. A comfortable position and a quiet room are important.
- *Guided imagery* involves creating an image in the mind and focusing on it. The client is asked to think of a pleasant scene such as a warm beach. The nurse uses a calm, soft voice when helping the person focus on the scene. Soft music, a blanket for warmth, and a darkened room may help. The nurse coaches the person to focus on the image and then to do relaxation exercises.

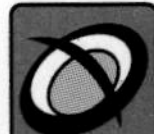

Providing Compassionate Care

Helping Clients to Rest

Dignity. Protecting a person's dignity can promote rest. Some people find hospital gowns embarrassing. Many rest better wearing their own gowns or pyjamas. Many people feel better about themselves when they are clean and groomed. Help clients with personal hygiene and grooming before rest.

Independence. Many people follow rituals or routines before resting. These may include going to the bathroom, brushing teeth, having a snack or beverage, praying, locking doors, or making sure loved ones are safe at home. Some people have a favourite blanket. Ask clients about their preferences. Follow rituals and routines when possible.

Preferences. Allow people to do as much as possible without assistance. The person decides when he or she wants to rest.

Privacy. Lack of privacy can make rest impossible. Close doors and privacy curtains if the person desires.

Safety. Safety needs must be met (see Chapter 16). People trying to rest must feel safe from falls or other injuries. In facilities, the call bell must be within reach. Understanding the reason for treatments can also help a person to feel safe. So can knowing how procedures are done. That is why you explain procedures before they are performed.

Rest and Sleep

To be rested means to be calm, at ease, relaxed, and free from anxiety and stress. Rest involves physical inactivity. However, some people do calming or relaxing activities while resting. Examples include reading, listening to music, and watching television.

A comfortable position and good body alignment are important for rest. A quiet setting promotes rest. So does a clean, dry, and wrinkle-free bed. Some people rest easier in a clean, neat, and uncluttered room.

Basic needs must be met for people to rest. Thirst, hunger, elimination needs, pain, discomfort, anxiety, and fear can affect rest. Unmet love and belonging needs can also affect rest. For people in a facility or living alone, visits or telephone calls from family and friends may promote relaxation. You can promote rest by meeting clients' needs. (See *Providing Compassionate Care: Helping Clients to Rest* box.)

You must plan and organize care so that clients can rest without interruptions. Some people feel refreshed after resting for 15 or 20 minutes. Others need more time. Health care routines usually allow time for an afternoon rest.

Ill or injured people need to rest often. Some need to rest during or after care. For example, a bath tires Mr. Rajan. To gather the energy to dress, he must rest in a chair. Some people need a few hours to complete oral hygiene, bathing, grooming, and dressing. Others need to rest after meals. Do not rush clients or push them beyond their limits. Allow rest periods as needed.

The physician may order bed rest for a client. Bed rest, its complications, and advice on preventing complications are presented in Chapter 22.

Sleep is a basic physical need. It saves the body energy, lets the mind and body rest, and allows body functions to slow. During sleep, vital signs fall, and tissue heals and repairs itself. Sleep lowers stress, tension, and anxiety. After sleep, a person usually feels refreshed, more energetic, and mentally alert.

The amount of sleep required varies for each age group and declines with age (Table 20-1). People may require more sleep when they are sick or recovering from illness or injury. (See *Focus on Older Adults: Sleep* box.)

Several factors affect the amount and quality of sleep. Quality relates to how well the person slept. Did the person sleep soundly and feel refreshed in the morning? Or was the person restless and wakeful?

- *Illness.* Discomfort, pain, nausea, and coughing can affect sleep. Often clients are awakened for treatment or medication.
- *Nutrition.* Some foods and drinks affect sleep. Those with caffeine (coffee, chocolate, tea, and colas) prevent sleep. A protein found in milk, cheese, and beef can help sleep.
- *Exercise.* Exercise makes people tired and helps them sleep. However, it is also a stimulant. Exercising

Table 20-1 Average Sleep Requirements

Age group	Hours per day
Newborns (birth to 4 weeks)	14 to 18
Infants (4 weeks to 1 year)	12 to 14
Toddlers/preschoolers (1 to 6 years)	11 to 12
Middle/late childhood (6 to 12 years)	10 to 11
Adolescents (12 to 18 years)	8 to 9
Young adults (18 to 40 years)	7 to 8
Middle-aged adults (40 to 65 years)	7
Late adulthood (65 years and older)	5 to 7

before bed may disrupt sleep. Allow at least 2 hours between exercise and bedtime.

- *Environment.* Most people sleep better in their own beds and in familiar surroundings. Any change in the environment can affect sleep. So can noise and light.
- *Medications.* Sleeping pills promote sleep. Medications for anxiety, depression, and pain can cause drowsiness. These substances also interfere with sleep. The person may not feel mentally alert or refreshed the next day.
- *Alcohol.* Alcohol disrupts normal sleep patterns. The person may wake up and have difficulties falling back to sleep.
- *Change and stress.* Change disrupts sleep. This can range from small changes in routine, such as staying up late, to stressful life events, such as a new job or a divorce.
- *Emotional problems.* Fear, worry, anxiety, and depression affect sleep. People may have difficulty falling asleep, or they may wake up often and have problems falling back to sleep.

Focus on Older Adults

Sleep

Older adults have less energy than younger people. They may nap during the day. They may nap at a certain time, or nap on and off during the day. Organize care so that naps are not disturbed. Avoid waking an older person from a nap.

Long-term care residents are allowed to choose when they nap and sleep. They also have the right to choose what measures help promote comfort, rest, and sleep. Follow the care plan and the person's wishes.

Residents are sometimes prepared for bed as early as 6:00 p.m. They may not be ready to sleep at this time. They may want to watch television, listen to the radio, or read.

Sleep Disorders

Sleep disorders are chronic problems that affect the amount and quality of sleep. Sleep disorders can cause fatigue, irritability, poor judgment, and other problems. Signs and symptoms of sleep disorders are listed in Box 20-4.

Insomnia. **Insomnia** is a chronic condition in which the person cannot go to sleep or stay asleep throughout the night. The person is unable to fall asleep or to stay asleep, or wakes early and is unable to fall back to sleep. Ill or injured people often have insomnia. They may be depressed or anxious. Pain or discomfort may keep them awake. Or they may be afraid of dying during sleep.

Sleep Deprivation. When people are sleep deprived, the amount and quality of their sleep declines. Illness and hospital care are common causes of sleep deprivation. The light and sound of nighttime care can interfere with sleep.

Box 20-4 Signs and Symptoms of Sleep Disorders

- Hand tremors
- Slowed response to questions, conversations, or situations
- Difficulty finding the right word
- Decreased attention
- Decreased reasoning and judgment
- Irregular pulse
- Red, puffy eyes with dark circles
- Moodiness; mood swings
- Disorientation
- Fatigue and/or sleepiness
- Restlessness and/or agitation
- Irritability
- Hallucinations (see Chapter 33)
- Coordination problems
- Slurred speech

Sleepwalking. Sleepwalkers walk about while they are sleeping, often for several minutes. The person is not aware of sleepwalking and has no memory of doing so on awakening. Children sleepwalk more than adults. Stress, fatigue, and some medications can cause sleepwalking. The risk of falling is great. Ill people may trip or pull out tubes and catheters. Guide sleepwalkers back to bed. Awaken them gently, as they startle easily.

Your Role in Promoting Rest and Sleep

If required, measures to promote sleep are included in the care plan. These are outlined in Box 20-5. Check the care plan to make sure you are giving correct care. Observe the client closely. Report any of the signs and symptoms listed in Box 20-4.

Many people have rituals and routines before bedtime. Some people always have a bedtime snack. Some always watch a television program before bed. Others read a book. Long-term care residents may like to check on friends before going to bed. Whatever the routine, it is important to the person.

Sleep disturbances are common in some types of dementia. Confusion and restlessness often increase at night. Night wandering is common. Night wandering in a safe and supervised setting is helpful for some people (see Chapter 34). The measures listed in Box 20-5 may help.

Box 20-5 Measures to Promote Sleep

- Organize care to allow for uninterrupted rest.
- Encourage the client to avoid physical activity before bedtime.
- Discourage the client from tending to business or family matters before bedtime.
- Allow a flexible bedtime. Bedtime is when the client is ready to sleep.
- Provide a comfortable room temperature.
- Let the client take a warm bath or shower.
- Provide a bedtime snack.
- Have the client avoid caffeine and alcohol.
- Have the client void before going to bed. Make sure incontinent clients are clean and dry.
- Follow bedtime rituals.
- Make sure the client wears loose-fitting nightwear.
- Provide for warmth (blankets, socks).
- Make sure linens are clean, dry, and wrinkle-free.
- Allow the client to read, listen to music, or watch television.
- Sit and talk with the client.
- Reduce noise.
- Darken room: close shades, blinds, and curtains. Shut off or dim lights in the room and hallway.
- Position the client in good body alignment. Support body parts as ordered.
- Implement measures to relieve pain.
- Give a back massage if ordered.
- Assist with relaxation exercises as ordered.

REVIEW

Circle T if the answer is true and F if it is false.

1. T F A person is greeted by name when being admitted to a nursing unit in a hospital or long-term care facility.

2. T F Transfers are usually related to changes in a person's condition.

3. T F A physician must write a discharge order before a patient can leave a hospital.

4. T F Pain affects all people in the same way.

5. T F Moderate exercise, such as walking, is considered rest.

Circle the BEST answer.

6. Most long-term care facilities
   A. Discourage residents from bringing personal items from home
   B. Have strict rules about the appearance of residents' rooms
   C. Encourage residents to make their rooms homelike
   D. Allow residents to bring only one piece of furniture from home

7. A person complains of pain in the left side of the chest, up into the left jaw, and down to the left shoulder and left arm. This is
   A. Acute pain
   B. Chronic pain
   C. Radiating pain
   D. Phantom pain

8. The nurse gives Mr. Smith a medication for pain. A procedure is scheduled for this time. You should
   A. Perform the procedure before the medication is given
   B. Perform the procedure right after the medication is given
   C. Wait one half-hour to let the medication take effect
   D. Omit the procedure for the day

9. You must protect Mr. Smith from injury after he is given medication. You should do the following *except*
   A. Keep the bed in the high position
   B. Follow the care plan for bed rail use
   C. Check on him every 10 to 15 minutes
   D. Provide assistance if he needs to get up

10. Which measure is *not* an example of a distraction?
    A. Talking with the client
    B. Keeping the room well lit
    C. Providing soft music
    D. Giving a back massage

11. Which of the following measures will *not* help Mr. Smith to rest or sleep?
    A. Having him void before rest or sleep
    B. Helping him to assume a comfortable position
    C. Helping him to ambulate (walk) before rest or sleep
    D. Letting him choose sleep attire

12. Mr. Smith tires very easily. His morning care includes a bath, hair care, and getting dressed. His bed is made after he is dressed. When should he rest?
    A. After morning care is completed
    B. After his bath and before hair care
    C. After you make the bed
    D. Whenever he needs to

Answers to these questions are on page 824.

CHAPTER

21

Body Mechanics: Moving, Positioning, and Transferring the Client

OBJECTIVES

- Define the key terms listed in this chapter
- Explain the purpose and rules of using good body mechanics
- Identify comfort and safety measures for lifting, turning, and moving clients in bed
- Explain how to lift and move clients in bed
- Explain why good body alignment and position changes are important for the client
- Identify the comfort and safety measures for positioning clients in bed
- Explain how to position a client in the basic bed positions and in a chair
- Explain the purpose of a transfer belt
- Describe the safety measures for transferring clients
- Learn the procedures described in this chapter

KEY TERMS

base of support The area on which an object rests

body alignment The way in which body parts (head, trunk, arms, and legs) are positioned in relation to one another; posture

body mechanics The movement of the body in an efficient and careful way

dorsal recumbent position Supine position

Fowler's position A semi-sitting position in bed; the head of the bed is elevated 45 to 60 degrees or the person is propped up with a backrest or pillows

friction The rubbing of one surface against another

gait belt A transfer belt used when helping a client to walk

lateral position A side-lying position

logrolling Turning the person as a unit, in alignment, with one motion

posture Body alignment

prone position A front-lying position on the abdomen, with the head turned to one side

shearing The process in which skin sticks to a surface and muscles slide in the direction the body is moving

Sims' position A left side-lying position; the right leg is sharply flexed so it is not on the left leg, and the left arm is positioned along the person's back.

supine position A back-lying position; dorsal recumbent position

transfer To move or help a person move from one place to another

transfer belt A belt used to hold onto a person during a transfer or when walking with the person

A support worker's daily activities include many instances of lifting, moving, and carrying items. For example, you lift grocery bags, push wheelchairs, move the client's bed, or carry garbage or laundry bags. You also lift and move clients. You turn and reposition clients in their beds. You move clients from one place to another. For example, you help clients move from their beds to chairs or wheelchairs.

You must protect yourself and the client during moving, positioning, and transferring activities. Back injuries and muscle and joint strains are serious and common injuries among health care workers and support workers. Use your body correctly. Knowing the proper techniques will help protect you and the client from injury.

Body Mechanics

Body mechanics refers to the movement of the body in an efficient and careful way. It involves good posture and balance. It also involves using the strongest and largest muscles for work. (Review the structure and function of the musculoskeletal system in Chapter 13.) Fatigue, muscle strain, and injury can result from the improper use and positioning of the body during activity or rest. Good body mechanics reduces the risk of injury. You must focus on your client's and your own body mechanics during all activities.

Body alignment (posture) is the way the body parts (head, trunk, arms, and legs) are positioned in relation to one another. Good body alignment lets the body move and function with strength and efficiency. It reduces strain on the muscles and joints and prevents injury. For people with limited mobility, correct body alignment helps prevent disabling complications such as muscle atrophy and contractures (see Chapter 22).

Figure 21-1 on page 264 shows a person standing with good body alignment. Notice that both sides of the body are in line with each other. When a person is standing with good posture:

- Head and neck are erect and straight
- Shoulders and hips are parallel to each other
- Shoulders are back
- Chest is out
- Spine is straight
- Abdomen is tucked in
- Knees are slightly flexed
- Arms are hanging comfortably at the side
- Feet are about shoulder-width apart
- Toes are pointing forward; one foot is slightly forward

Lying down and sitting also require good alignment (see pages 284–287).

The position of the feet is especially important for good body mechanics. Your feet provide your base of support. A **base of support** is the area on which an object rests. A wide base of support provides more stability and balance than a narrow base of support. Therefore—especially when moving, lifting, or transferring weight—stand with your feet and legs apart for a wide base of support.

The strongest and largest muscles are in the shoulders, upper arms, hips, and thighs. Use these muscles for lifting and moving. Otherwise, you place strain and exertion on smaller and weaker muscles, such as those in the lower back. This causes fatigue and injury. Follow the guidelines in Box 21-1 to safely and efficiently move clients and objects.

(text continues on page 266)

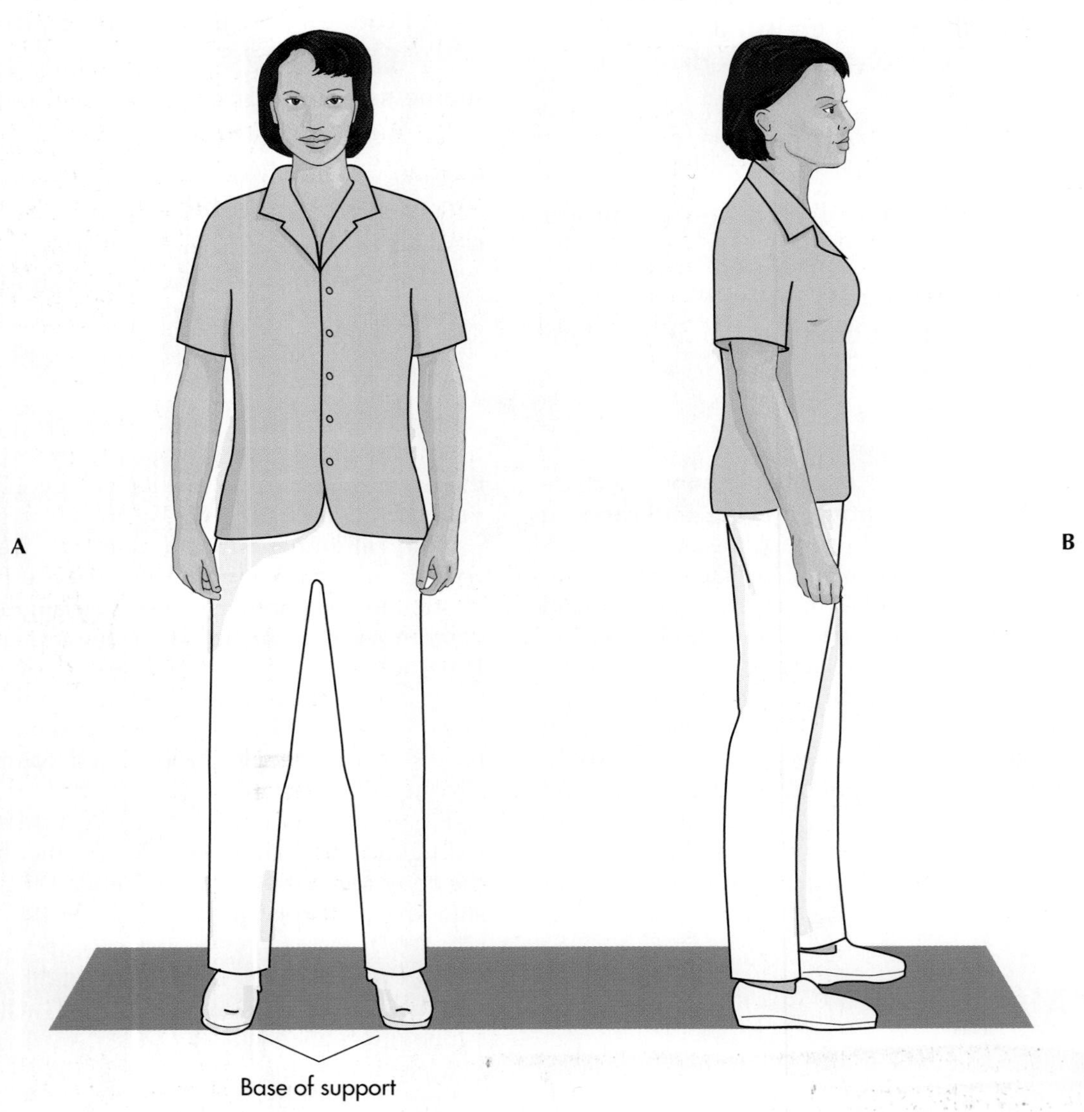

Figure 21-1 A, Anterior (front) view of an adult in good body alignment with feet apart for wide base of support. **B,** Lateral (side) view of an adult with good alignment.

Box 21-1 Guidelines for Good Body Mechanics

- *Assess the situation before you begin lifting.* Get help if you think the weight is more than you can safely lift. Avoid lifting or moving a person alone. Many employers have a "no lift" policy. Workers are not allowed to lift or move clients without help or mechanical aid. Always check the care plan and know employer policy before moving a client.
- *Face your work area.* This prevents unnecessary twisting. Remember to stand with a wide base of support.
- *Bend at your knees and hips and squat when lifting or setting down objects below your waist.* Do not bend forward from your waist or you will strain your small back muscles (Figure 21-2).
- *Tighten your stomach muscles and tuck in your pelvis as you lift.* Keep your back straight. Use your leg and thigh muscles as you lift the item to waist level. You legs should be bearing the weight, not your back.
- *Hold objects close to your body when lifting, moving, or carrying them.* This involves upper arm and shoulder muscles (see Figure 21-2). Holding objects away from your body places strain on small muscles in your lower arms. Do not lift objects higher than chest level. Use both hands and arms to lift, move, or carry heavy objects.
- *Avoid unnecessary bending and reaching.* If your client has a hospital bed, raise the bed so it is close to your waist. Adjust the overbed table so it is at your waist level. Arrange all equipment and supplies in a convenient, easy-to-reach location before you begin a task. If necessary, move a chair next to the bedside and arrange your supplies on it. If an object is higher than chest level, use a step stool to reach it.
- *Turn your whole body as one unit when changing the direction of your movement.* Do not twist your body. Move your feet in the direction of the turn. Work with smooth and even movements. Avoid sudden or jerky motions. Take your time.
- *Push, slide, or pull heavy objects whenever you can, rather than lifting them.* Pushing with your body weight is easier than pulling. Widen your base of support when pushing or pulling. Move your front leg forward when pushing. Move your rear leg back when pulling (Figure 21-3 on page 266).

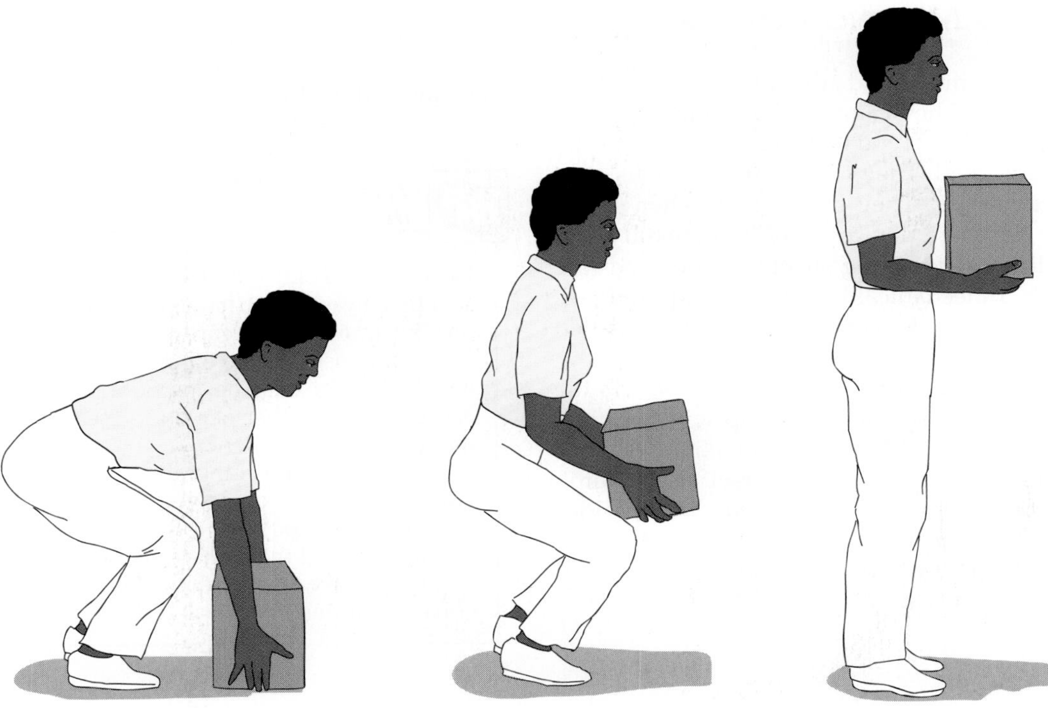

Figure 21-2 Picking up a box using good body mechanics.

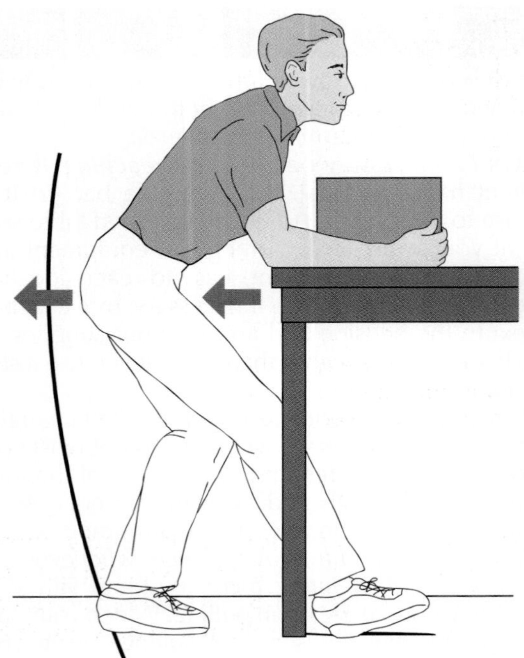

Figure 21-3 Move your rear leg back when pulling an item.

Lifting and Moving Clients in Bed

Many clients can move and turn in bed themselves. Others need help. They cannot move independently, but they can work with you to move. Some clients are unable to move at all. They may be unconscious, paralyzed, or very weak. They cannot help when others move them. Assistive devices may be necessary. For example, a lifting or turning sheet may be used (see page 274). Or a mechanical lift may be required (see page 299). Sometimes two or three people are needed to move the client.

Check with the care plan, your supervisor, and the client to find out if the client can help with moving. Also check if you can safely move the client on your own. Do not attempt a move by yourself if you think you may not be able to do so safely. You must consider the client's safety and your own safety. (See *Focus on Long-Term Care: Lifting and Moving Safety Precautions* and *Focus on Home Care: Getting Help with Lifting and Moving* boxes.)

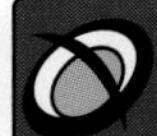

Focus on Long-Term Care

Lifting and Moving Safety Precautions

In many long-term care facilities, residents have signs in their rooms that say how much assistance is needed to move. The signs state whether the person requires:

- No assistance
- One-person lift
- Two or more people to lift
- Mechanical lift

Comfort and Safety Measures

The client's skin must be protected during lifting and moving. Friction and shearing injure the skin. Both cause infection and pressure ulcers (see Chapter 41). **Friction** is the rubbing of one surface against another. When a person is moved in bed, skin rubs against the sheet. **Shearing** occurs when the skin sticks to a surface and muscles slide in the direction the body is moving (Figure 21-4). Shearing can happen when a person slides down in bed or is moved in bed.

Reduce friction and shearing by rolling or lifting the client. A cotton drawsheet (see Chapter 24) serves as a *lift sheet* (*turning* or *pull sheet*) to move the client in bed and reduce friction (see page 274). Some employ-

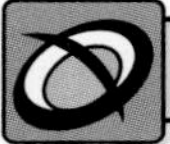

Focus on Home Care

Getting Help with Lifting and Moving

You usually will not have a co-worker to help you lift and move home care clients. Plan ahead with your supervisor. Some clients have mechanical lifting devices in their home. Sometimes the primary caregiver or another person in the home helps you lift and move the client.

A nurse or physiotherapist teaches the client's family or primary caregiver about body mechanics and moving, positioning, and transferring the client. You and the family member can then work together. Make sure anyone who helps you has received training.

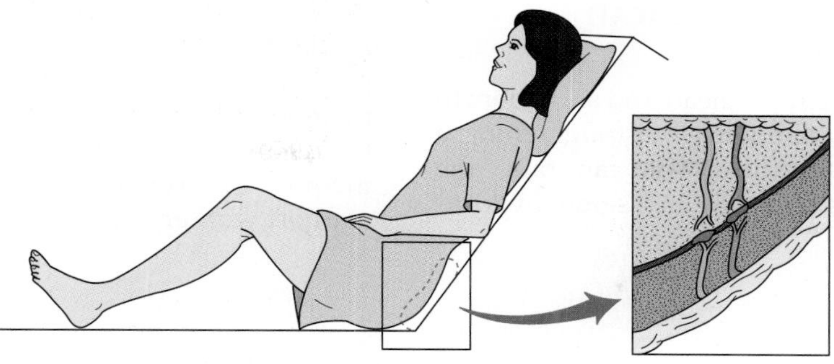

Figure 21-4 Shearing. When the head of the bed is raised to a sitting position, skin on the buttocks stays in place. However, internal structures move forward as the client slides down in bed. Skin is pinched between the mattress and the hip bones.

ers use turning pads for this purpose. (See *Focus on Older Adults: Shearing* box.)

Follow these comfort and safety measures when moving clients in bed:

- Check with your supervisor and the care plan about limits or restrictions in positioning or moving the client. For example, people with severe arthritis and osteoporosis (see Chapter 31) may experience pain or injury when being moved. Your supervisor will tell you what measures to take when moving clients with these conditions.
- Decide how to move the client and how much help you need *before* attempting the move.
- Ask for help *before* starting the move.
- Communicate directions with your helper. Count 1-2-3 and then move together.
- Move the client in small increments. Several small movements may be easier than one large movement.
- Cover and screen the client to protect privacy rights.
- Protect tubes or drainage containers connected to the client. Make sure tubing is not pulled, tangled, or pinched during the move.
- Position clients in good body alignment after lifting or moving them.
- Make sure linens are wrinkle-free after moving. Straighten them as needed.

Focus on **Older Adults**

SHEARING

Older adults are at great risk for shearing. Their skin is fragile and easily torn. Use a lift or turning sheet or turning pad when lifting and moving older adults.

Raising the Client's Head and Shoulders

You may have to raise a client's head and shoulders to give care. For example, removing or straightening a pillow requires this procedure. You can raise the client's head and shoulders easily and safely by locking arms with the client (Figure 21-5). For clients with fragile bones and joints, it is best to have help when performing this procedure. Follow the care plan. Remember, a helper in a facility is a co-worker. A helper in a home care setting is usually a trained family member or primary caregiver. Figure 21-6 shows a support worker and a helper doing the procedure.

(text continues on page 271)

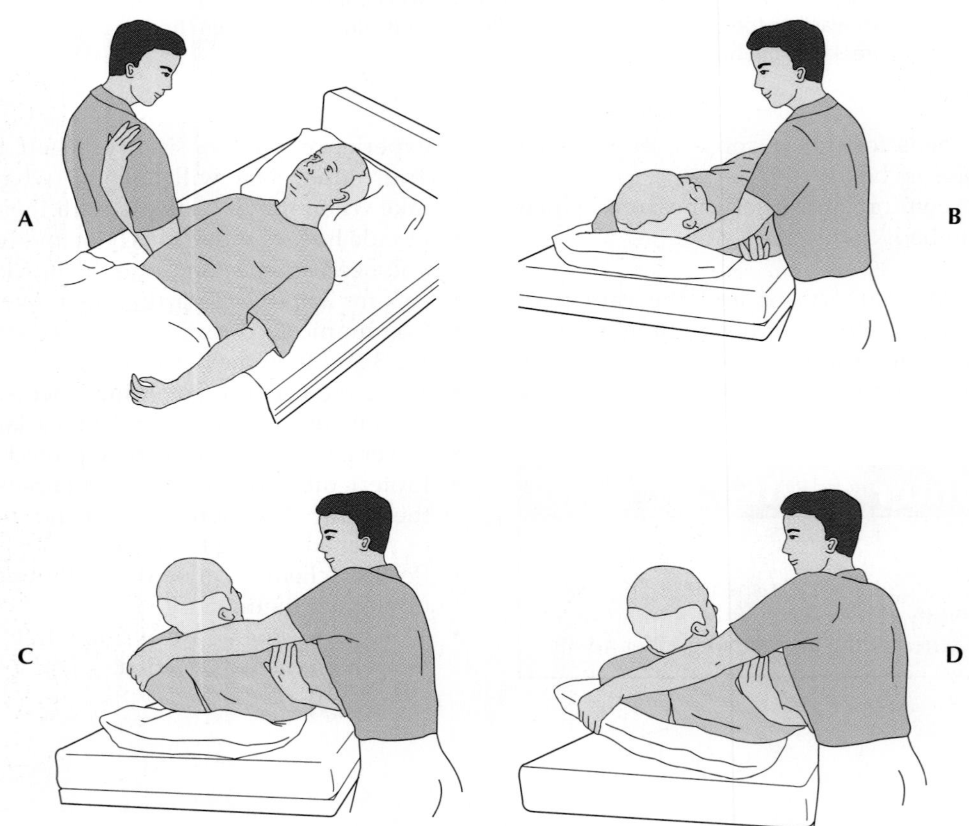

Figure 21-5 Raising the client's head and shoulders by locking arms with the client. **A,** Place your near arm under the client's near arm; have the client rest his or her hand on your shoulder. **B,** Place your far arm under the client's neck and shoulders, with your near arm still under the client's nearest arm. **C,** Raise the client to a semi-sitting position. **D,** Continue supporting the client with your arm locked under the client's shoulder. Use your other arm to lift the pillow.

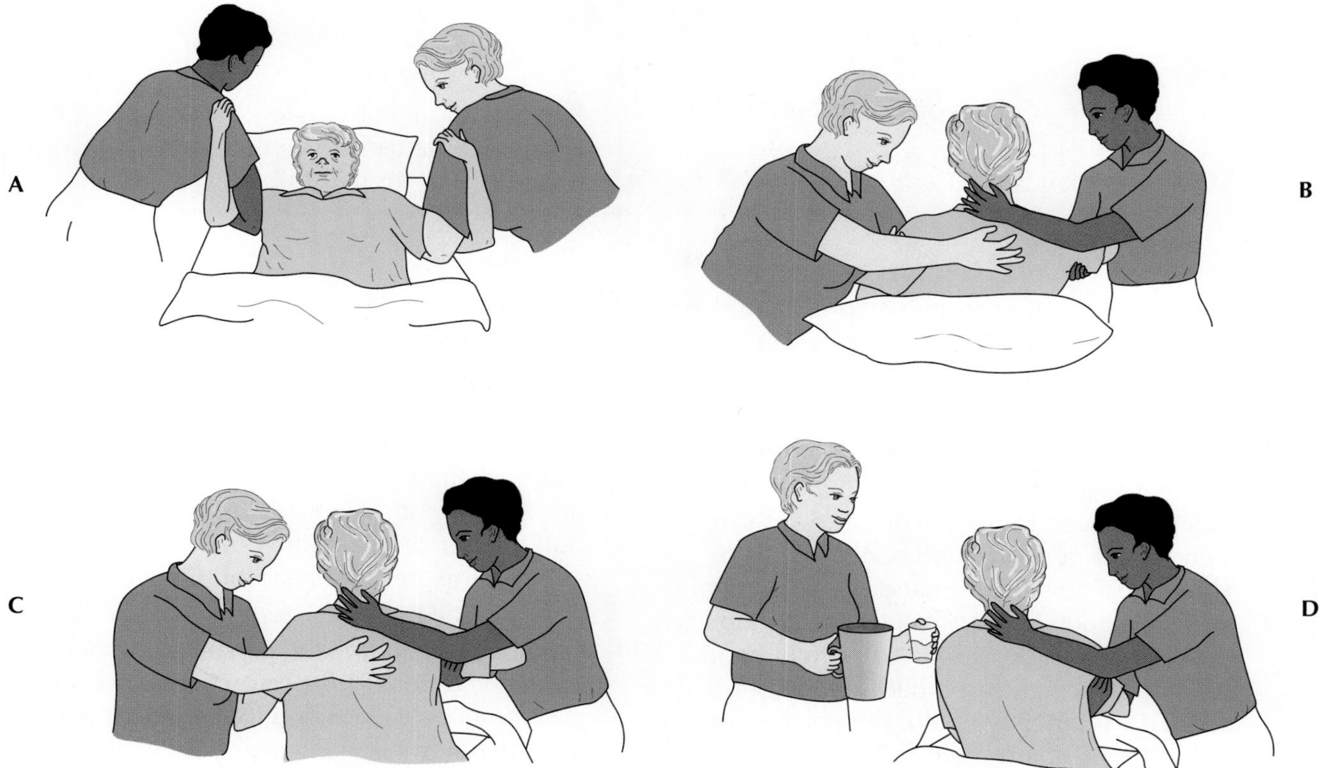

Figure 21-6 Raising the client's head and shoulders with a helper. **A,** You and your helper lock arms with the client. **B,** You and your helper have your arms under the client's head and neck. **C,** You and your helper raise the client to a semi-sitting position. **D,** Your helper supports the client in the semi-sitting position while you give care.

Raising the Person's Head and Shoulders

Compassionate Care

Remember to Promote:
- **Dignity**
- **Independence**
- **Preferences**
- **Privacy**
- **Safety**

Pre-Procedure

1 Identify the person according to employer policy.

2 Ask someone to help you if you need assistance.

3 Wash your hands.

4 Explain the procedure to the person.

5 Provide for privacy.

6 Raise bed to a comfortable working height. Make sure bed wheels are locked. Follow the care plan for bed rail use.*

Procedure

7 Position yourself near the person's shoulder and chest. Spread your feet about 30 cm (12 inches) apart for a good base of support.

8 Lower the bed rail near you if up.

9 If you have help, your helper does the same on the other side of the bed.

10 Ask the person to put his or her near arm under your near arm and behind your shoulder. The person's hand rests on top of your shoulder. If you are standing on the person's right side, the person's right hand rests on your right shoulder (see Figure 21-5, *A*). If you have help, the person does the same with your helper. The person's left hand rests on your helper's left shoulder (see Figure 21-6, *A*).

11 Put your arm nearest to the person under his or her arm. Put your hand on the person's shoulder. If you have help, your helper does the same.

12 Put your free arm under the person's neck and shoulders (see Figure 21-5, *B*). If you have help, your helper does the same (see Figure 21-6, *B*).

13 Help the person pull up to a sitting or semi-sitting position on the count of "3" (see Figure 21-5, *C*, and Figure 21-6, *C*). As you pull the person up, shift your weight from your foot nearest the head of the bed to your other foot.

14 Continue supporting the person with your arm locked under the person's shoulder. Use your other arm and hand to remove or adjust the pillows (see Figure 21-5, *D*). If you have help, your helper supports the person while you provide care (see Figure 21-6, *D*).

15 Help the person lie down. Provide support with your locked arms. Support the person's neck and shoulders with your other arm.

Post-Procedure

16 Provide for safety and comfort. Position the person in good body alignment according to the care plan (see page 284). Straighten linens.

17 Place the call bell within reach.*

18 Return bed to lowest position. Follow the care plan for bed rail use.*

19 Remove privacy measures.

20 Wash your hands.

21 Report and record your actions and observations according to employer policy.

*Steps marked with an asterisk may not apply in community settings.

Moving the Client Up in Bed

When sitting up in bed, it is easy for the client to slide down toward the middle and foot of the bed (Figure 21-7). The client is moved up in bed to maintain good body alignment and comfort. Moving the client up in bed is also usually done before providing bedside care.

You can move children and lightweight adults up in bed alone if they are able to help. The client helps by pushing with his or her hands or feet to move up in bed. Or, the client may have a *trapeze* to aid with moving. A trapeze is a device that attaches to the bed or to a frame over the bed. The client grasps the bars of the trapeze and pulls.

Clients who are very heavy or weak need two people to move them. Remember, check with your supervisor before attempting to move a client if you are unsure you can do it alone safely. Having someone help you protects you and the client from injury.

(text continues on page 274)

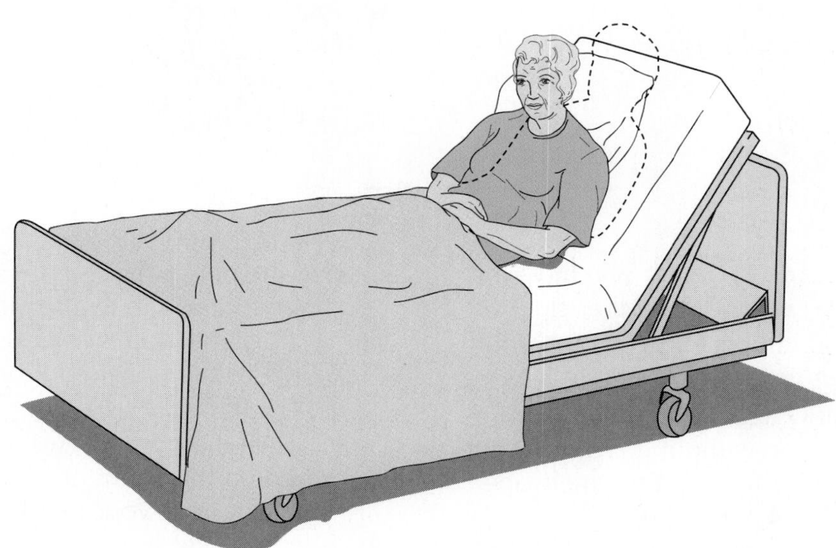

Figure 21-7 A client in poor alignment after sliding down in bed: shoulders are slouched, head and neck are forward, and the spine is curved.

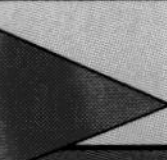

Moving the Person Up in Bed

Compassionate Care

Remember to Promote:
- **Dignity**
- **Independence**
- **Preferences**
- **Privacy**
- **Safety**

Pre-Procedure

1 Identify the person according to employer policy.
2 Ask someone to help you if you need assistance.
3 Wash your hands.
4 Explain the procedure to the person.
5 Provide for privacy.
6 Raise bed to a comfortable working height. Make sure bed wheels are locked. Follow the care plan for bed rail use. Lower the head of the bed to a level appropriate for the person. It should be as flat as possible.*

Procedure

7 Stand on one side of bed. If you have a helper, he or she stands on other side.
8 Lower the bed rail near you if up. If you have a helper, he or she does the same.
9 Place the pillow against the headboard if the person can be without it. This prevents the person's head from hitting the headboard when being moved up.
10 Stand with a wide base of support. Point your foot that is near the head of the bed toward the head of the bed. Face the head of the bed.
11 Bend your hips and knees. Keep your back straight.
12 *Method 1: Moving the person without a helper*
   a Place one arm under the person's shoulder and one arm under the thighs (Figure 21-8, *A*).
   b Have the person bend both knees and brace feet against the mattress.
   c Explain to the person that on the count of "3," he or she will push against the bed with feet and hands to help with the move (Figure 21-8, *B*).
   d If the person has a trapeze, ask the person to grasp it. Explain that on the count of "3," he or she will push against the bed with feet and pull on the trapeze, if able (Figure 21-9).
   e Move the person toward the head of the bed on the count of "3." Shift your weight from your rear leg to your front leg. Repeat if necessary.
13 *Method 2: Moving the person with a helper*
   a Place one arm under the person's shoulder and one arm under the thighs. Your helper does the same. You and your helper grasp each other's forearms (Figure 21-10).
   b Have the person flex both knees.
   c Explain that you will move on the count of "3."
   d Move the person toward the head of the bed on the count of "3." Shift your weight from your rear leg to your front leg. Your helper does the same. Repeat if necessary.
14 Reposition the pillow under the person's head and shoulders.

Post-Procedure

15 Follow steps 16 through 21 in *Raising the Person's Head and Shoulders,* page 270.

*Steps marked with an asterisk may not apply in community settings.

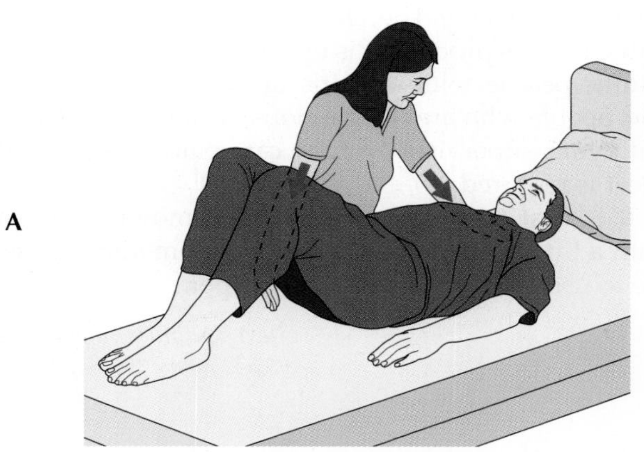

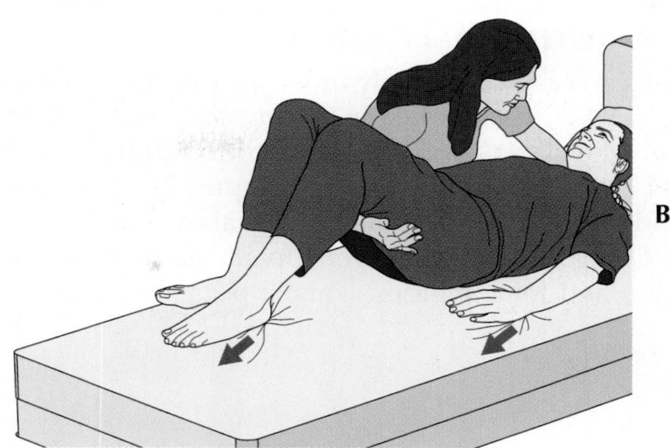

Figure 21-8 Moving the client up in bed without a helper. **A,** Place one arm under the client's shoulder and one arm under the thighs. The client's knees are flexed. **B,** The client pushes against the bed with feet and hands as you move the client up in bed. Shift your body weight from the rear leg to the front leg as you move the client. Note: Although you can move children and lightweight adults alone using this method, it is best to have help. Consult with you supervisor.

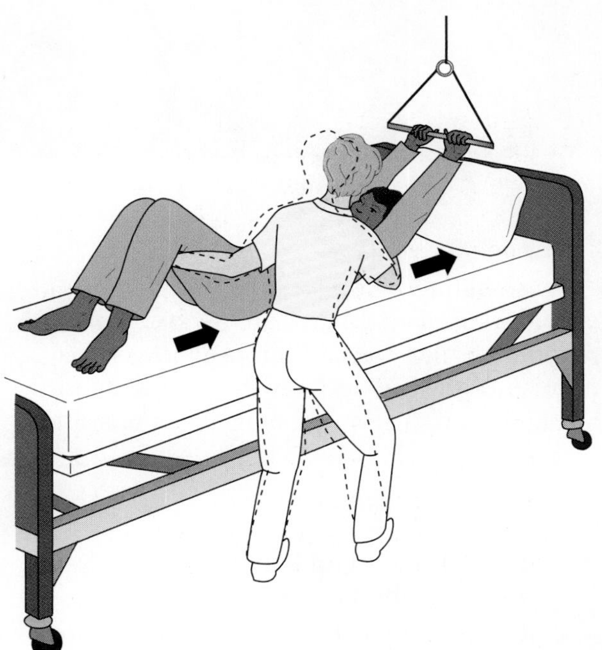

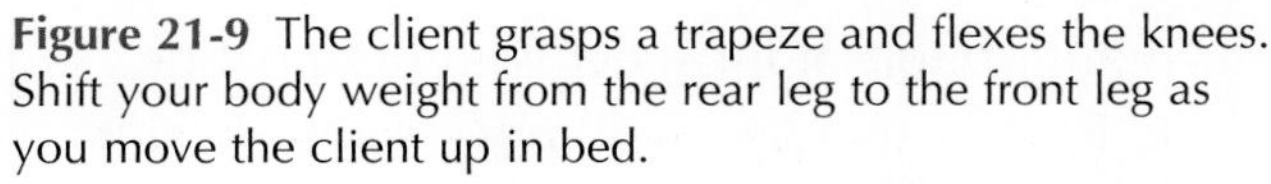

Figure 21-9 The client grasps a trapeze and flexes the knees. Shift your body weight from the rear leg to the front leg as you move the client up in bed.

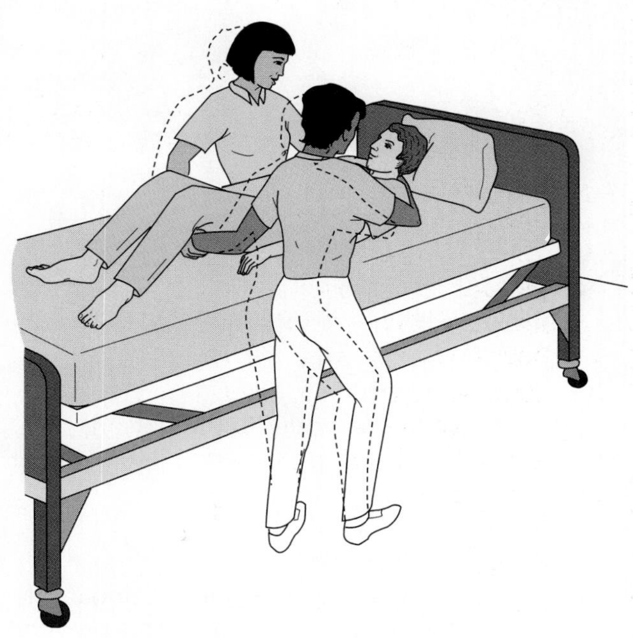

Figure 21-10 Moving the client up in bed with a helper. Place one arm under the client's shoulders and the other under the thighs. Your helper does the same. Lock arms with your helper under the client. The client's knees are flexed. Shift your weight from your rear leg to your front leg as you move the client. Your helper does the same.

Moving the Client Up in Bed with a Lift Sheet

You can easily and safely move a client up in bed with a *lift sheet*. (It is called a *turning sheet* when used to turn the client.) You can use a cotton drawsheet or a flat sheet folded in half (see Chapter 24). It is placed under the client from the head to above the knees.

Using a lift sheet prevents pain, skin damage, and bone and joint injuries. This is because the client is lifted more evenly. Therefore friction and shearing are reduced. This procedure is usually used to move older adults, people with arthritis or spinal cord injuries, and people who are unconscious or paralyzed. Check with your supervisor and the care plan to see if a lift sheet is required.

It is best to have a helper when moving a client with a lift sheet. However, it is also sometimes possible to use a lift sheet without a helper.

(text continues on page 276)

Moving the Person Up in Bed with a Lift Sheet

Compassionate Care

Remember to Promote:
- **Dignity**
- **Independence**
- **Preferences**
- **Privacy**
- **Safety**

Pre-Procedure

1. Identify the person according to employer policy.
2. Ask someone to help you if you need assistance.
3. Wash your hands.
4. Explain the procedure to the person.
5. Provide for privacy.
6. Raise bed to a comfortable working height. Make sure bed wheels are locked. Follow the care plan for bed rail use. Lower the head of the bed to a level appropriate for the person. It should be as flat as possible.*

Procedure

7. Fold back top sheet.
8. Place the pillow against the headboard if the person can be without it. This prevents the person's head from hitting the headboard when being moved up.
9. Make sure the turning sheet is in position under the person.
10. *Method 1: Moving the person without a helper*
    - a Keep bed rails up if used.
    - b Stand at the head of the bed. Use good body mechanics. Stand with a wide base of support. Place one foot slightly ahead of the other. Bend knees and hips. Keep back straight (Figure 21-11, *A*).
    - c Roll top of lift sheet toward the person's shoulders.
    - d Grasp top of lift sheet with both hands.
    - e Explain that you will move on the count of "3." The person pushes against the bed with the feet if able.
    - f On the count of "3," shift your weight from your front leg to your back leg while pulling the lift sheet and the person up toward the head of the bed. Use smooth movements, not sudden or jerky movements. Repeat if necessary.

Continued

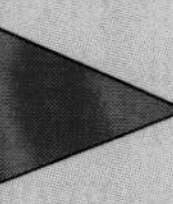

Moving the Person Up in Bed with a Lift Sheet—cont'd

Procedure

11 *Method 2: Moving the person with a helper*
- a Stand on one side of the bed. Your helper stands on the other.
- b Lower the bed rails if up.
- c Stand with a broad base of support. Point your foot that is near the head of the bed toward the head of the bed. Face that direction. Bend your hips and knees. Your helper does the same on the other side of the bed.
- d Roll the sides of the lift sheet up close to the person.
- e Grasp the rolled-up lift sheet firmly near the person's shoulders and buttocks (Figure 21-11, *B*). Make sure the person's head is supported.
- f Explain that you will move on the count of "3." The person pushes against the bed with the feet if able.
- g Slide the person up in bed on the count of "3." Shift your weight from your rear leg to your front leg. Your helper does the same. Repeat if necessary.

12 Unroll the lift sheet.

13 Put the pillow under the person's head and shoulders. Replace top sheet.

Post-Procedure

14 Follow steps 16 through 21 in *Raising the Person's Head and Shoulders,* page 270.

*Steps marked with an asterisk may not apply in community settings.

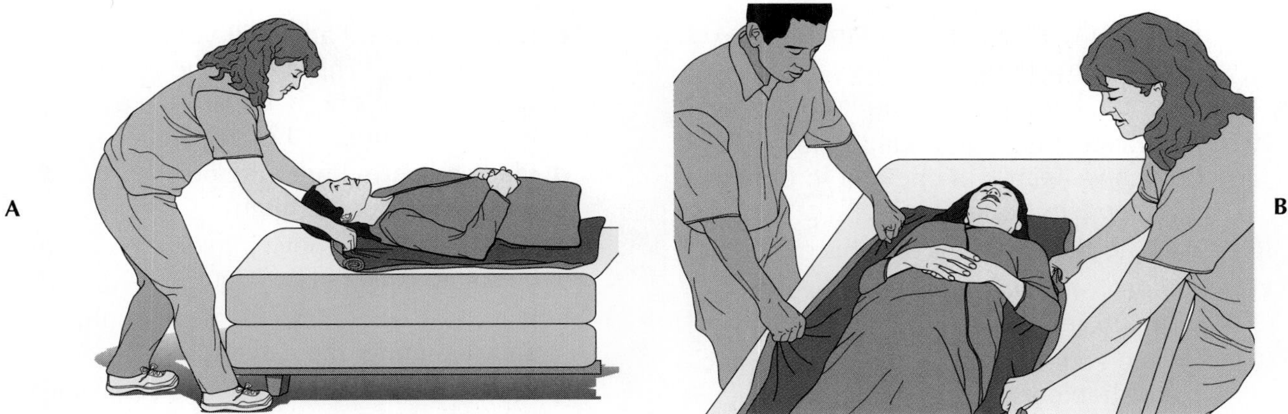

Figure 21-11 Using a lift sheet to move the client up in bed. The lift sheet extends from the client's head to above the knees. **A,** Without a helper, stand at the head of the bed and pull the lift sheet and client. **B,** With a helper, roll the lift sheet close to the client. Hold the lift sheet near the shoulders and buttocks. On the count of "3," you and your helper gently move the client toward the head of the bed.

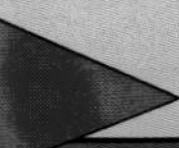

Moving the Client to the Side of the Bed

Many care procedures require moving the client to the side of the bed. Giving a bed bath is an example. When you move the client to the side of the bed, he or she is close to you. Therefore, you do not have to reach or stretch as much when doing the procedure. Also, you usually move clients to the side of the bed before repositioning or turning them.

One method involves moving the client in segments. You can usually do this method alone. Some clients cannot move in segments. Older adults, people with arthritis, and people with spinal cord injuries are examples. The lift sheet method is used for these clients. Using a lift sheet helps prevent pain, skin damage, and injury to the bones, joints, and spinal cord. When using a lift sheet to move a person to the side of the bed, it is best to have someone help you. Check with your supervisor for the correct procedure to use with each client.

(text continues on page 278)

Moving the Person to the Side of the Bed

Compassionate Care

Remember to Promote:
- Dignity
- Independence
- Preferences
- Privacy
- Safety

Pre-Procedure

1 Identify the person according to employer policy.
2 Ask someone to help you if you need assistance.
3 Wash your hands.
4 Explain the procedure to the person.
5 Provide for privacy.
6 Raise bed to a comfortable working height. Make sure bed wheels are locked. Follow the care plan for bed rail use. Lower the head of the bed to a level appropriate for the person. It should be as flat as possible.

Procedure

7 Stand on the side of the bed to which you will move the person.
8 Lower the bed rail near you if up.
9 Stand with your feet about 30 cm (12 inches) apart and one foot in front of the other. Flex your knees.
10 Cross the person's arms over his or her chest.
11 *Method 1: Moving the person without a helper (in segments)*
   - **a** Place your arm under the person's neck and shoulders. Grasp the far shoulder.
   - **b** Place your other arm under the middle of the person's back.
   - **c** Rock backward and shift your weight to your rear leg. This moves the upper part of the person's body toward the edge of the bed (Figure 21-12, *A*).
   - **d** Place one arm under the person's waist and one under the thighs.
   - **e** Rock backward, moving middle part of the person to edge of bed (Figure 21-12, *B*).
   - **f** Place one arm under the person's thighs and one under the calves.
   - **g** Rock backward, moving the person's legs to edge of bed (Figure 21-12, *C*).
   - **h** Repeat steps a through g as necessary.

Continued

Moving the Person to the Side of the Bed—cont'd

Procedure

12 *Method 2: Moving the person with a lift sheet*

a Roll the lift sheet up close to the person. Your helper does the same (see Figure 21-11, *B*).

b Grasp the rolled-up lift sheet near the person's shoulders and buttocks. Your helper does the same. Make sure you support the head.

c Rock backward on the count of "3," moving the person toward you. Your helper rocks backward slightly and then forward toward you while keeping the arms straight. Repeat if necessary.

d Unroll the lift sheet.

13 Reposition the pillow under the person's head and shoulders.

Post-Procedure

14 Follow steps 16 through 21 in *Raising a Person's Head and Shoulders,* page 270.

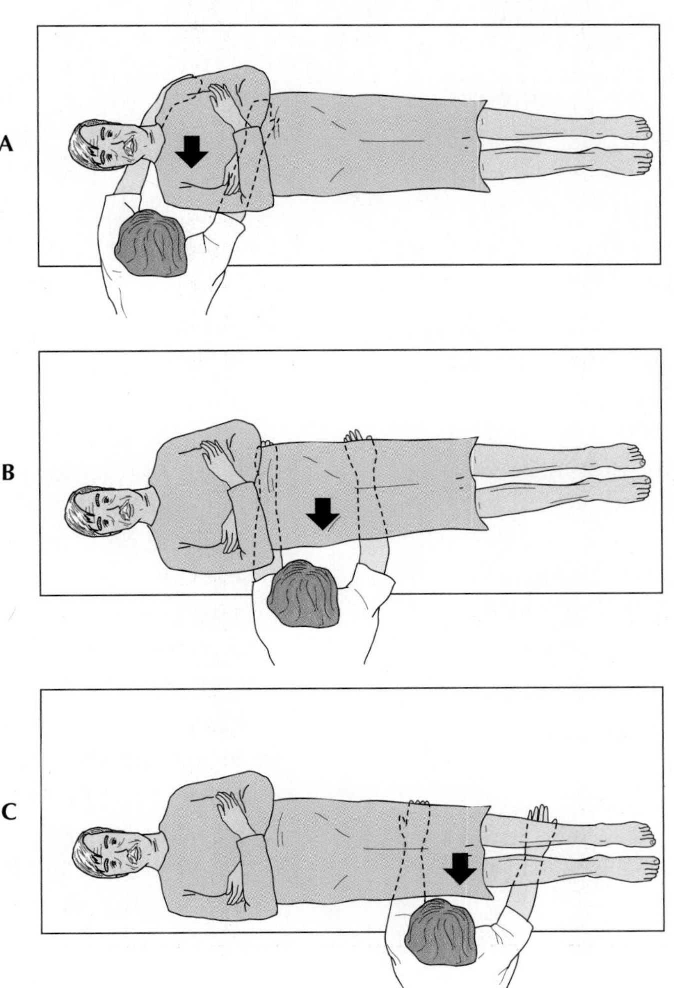

Figure 21-12 Move the client to the side of the bed in segments.

Turning the Client

Turning clients onto their sides helps prevent complications from bed rest. Certain care procedures require the side-lying position. Clients are turned toward or away from you. The direction depends on the client's condition and on the situation.

Many clients have conditions that make turning painful for them. People with arthritis in their spines or knees are examples. When turning these clients, it is best to logroll them using a turning sheet (lift sheet). Logrolling is less painful for them. Remember to check with your supervisor and the care plan to determine the correct procedure to use for each client.

(text continues on page 280)

Turning the Person

Compassionate Care

Remember to Promote:
- **Dignity**
- **Independence**
- **Preferences**
- **Privacy**
- **Safety**

Pre-Procedure

1. Identify the person according to employer policy.
2. Ask someone to help you if you need assistance.
3. Wash your hands.
4. Explain the procedure to the person.
5. Provide for privacy.
6. Raise bed to a comfortable working height. Make sure bed wheels are locked. Follow the care plan for bed rail use. Lower the head of the bed to a level appropriate for the person. It should be as flat as possible.*

Procedure

7. Stand on the side of the bed opposite to where you will turn the person.
8. Lower the bed rail near you if up. The far bed rail is left up if used.
9. Move the person to the side near you. (See *Moving the Person to the Side of the Bed,* page 276.)
10. Cross the person's arms over his or her chest. Cross the leg near you over the far leg.
11. *Method 1: Turning the person away from you*
    - **a** Stand with a wide base of support. Flex your knees.
    - **b** Place one hand on the person's shoulder and the other on the person's buttock that is near you.
    - **c** Roll the person gently toward the other side of the bed (Figure 21-13). Shift your weight from your rear leg to your front leg.
12. *Method 2: Turning the person toward you*
    - **a** Raise the bed rail if up.
    - **b** Go to the other side. Lower the bed rail if up.
    - **c** Stand with a wide base of support. Flex your knees.
    - **d** Place one hand on the person's far shoulder and the other on the far hip.
    - **e** Roll the person toward you gently (Figure 21-14).
13. Position the person. Follow the care plan and your supervisor's directions. The following position is common:
    - **a** Place a pillow under the head and neck.
    - **b** Adjust the shoulder. The person should not lie on an arm.
    - **c** Flex the upper knee. Position the upper leg in front of the lower leg.
    - **d** Support the upper leg and thigh with pillows.
    - **e** Place a small pillow under the upper hand and arm.
    - **f** Position a pillow against the back.

Continued

Turning the Person—cont'd

Post-Procedure

14 Provide for safety and comfort.

15 Place the call bell within reach.*

16 Return the bed to its lowest position. Raise or lower the bed rails according to the care plan.*

17 Remove privacy measures.

18 Wash your hands.

19 Report and record your actions and observations according to employer policy.

*Steps marked with an asterisk may not apply in community settings.

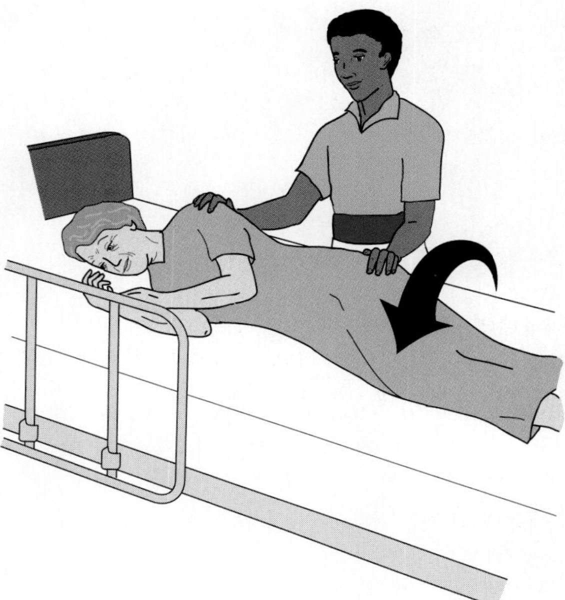

Figure 21-13 Turning the client away from you.

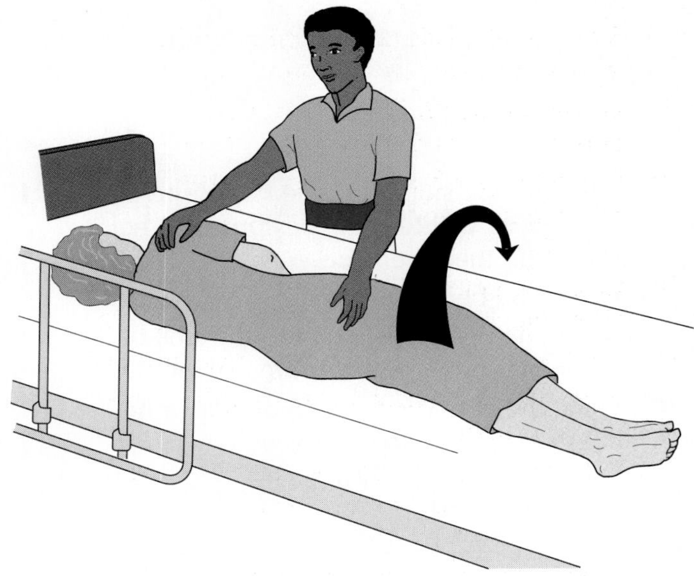

Figure 21-14 Turning the client toward you.

Logrolling

Logrolling involves turning the client as a unit, in alignment, with one motion. The spine is kept straight. The procedure is used to turn:

- Clients with arthritic spines or knees (common in older adults)
- Clients recovering from hip fractures
- Clients with spinal cord injuries (the spine must be kept straight at all times following spinal cord injury)
- Clients recovering from spinal surgery (the spine must be kept straight at all times following spinal cord surgery)

Two or three people are needed to logroll a client. Three are needed if the client is tall or heavy. Sometimes a turning sheet is used.

(text continues on page 282)

Logrolling the Person

Compassionate Care

Remember to Promote:
- **Dignity**
- **Independence**
- **Preferences**
- **Privacy**
- **Safety**

Pre-Procedure

1. Identify the person according to employer policy.
2. Ask someone to help you.
3. Wash your hands.
4. Explain the procedure to the person.
5. Provide for privacy.
6. Raise bed to a comfortable working height. Make sure bed wheels are locked. Follow the care plan for bed rail use. Make sure bed is flat.*

Procedure

7. Stand on the side of the bed opposite to where you will turn the person. Your helper stands on the other side.
8. Lower the bed rails if up.
9. Move the person as a unit to the side of the bed near you. Use the turning sheet.
10. Place the person's arms across his or her chest. Place a pillow between the knees.
11. Raise the bed rail if used.
12. Go to the other side of the bed next to your helper.
13. Stand near the shoulders and chest. Your helper stands near the buttocks and thighs.
14. Stand with a broad base of support. One foot is in front of the other.
15. Ask the person to hold his or her body rigid.
16. Roll the person toward you (Figure 21-15, *A*) or use a turning sheet (Figure 21-15, *B*). Turn the person as a unit.

Continued

Logrolling the Person—cont'd

Post-Procedure

17 Provide for safety and comfort. Position the person in good body alignment. Use pillows as directed by your supervisor and the care plan. The following is common:
   - a One pillow against the back for support
   - b One pillow under the head and neck if allowed
   - c One pillow or folded bath blanket between the legs
   - d A small pillow under the arm and hand

18 Place the call bell within reach.*

19 Return the bed to its lowest position. Follow the care plan for bed rail use.*

20 Remove privacy measures.

21 Wash your hands.

22 Report and record your actions and observations according to employer policy.

*Steps marked with an asterisk may not apply in community settings.

A

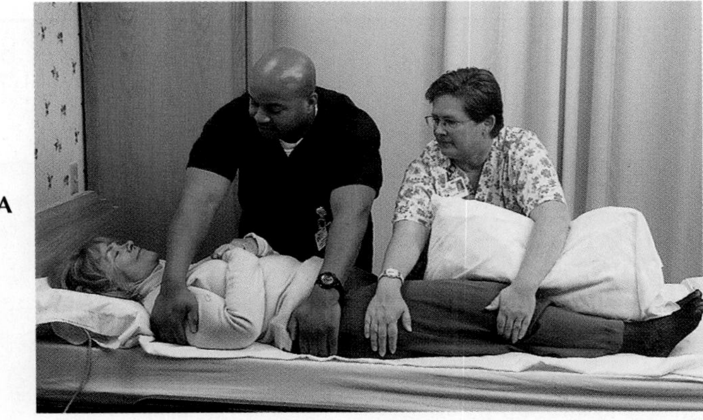

B

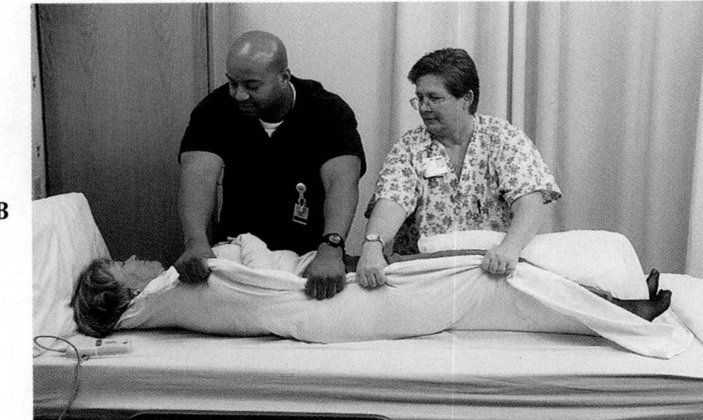

Figure 21-15 Logrolling. **A,** A pillow is between the client's legs, and the arms are crossed on the chest. The client is on the far side of the bed. **B,** A turning sheet is used to logroll the client. NOTE: If you plan on moving the client up in bed after logrolling him or her, place the pillow against the headboard.

SITTING ON THE SIDE OF THE BED (DANGLING)

Clients sit on the side of the bed (*dangle*) for many reasons. Many older adults become dizzy or faint when getting out of bed too fast. They need to sit on the side of the bed for 1 to 5 minutes before walking or transferring. Some clients increase activity in stages. They progress from resting in bed to sitting on the side of the bed and then to sitting in a chair. Walking is the next step.

Some clients sit on the side of the bed to perform their exercises. While dangling their legs, they cough and deep breathe. They also move their legs back and forth and in circles to stimulate circulation. The procedure is also part of preparing clients to walk or transferring them to a chair or wheelchair.

You might need a helper when assisting a client to sit on the side of the bed. Support the client if he or she has problems with balance or coordination. For example, people recovering from a stroke often have problems with sitting and balance. They must be supported when dangling to prevent falls and injuries. Check with your supervisor and the care plan for safety precautions necessary for each client.

Report and record the following after helping a client dangle:

- Pulse and respirations (if instructed to measure)
- Pale or bluish skin colour (cyanosis)
- Complaints of dizziness, light-headedness, or difficulty breathing
- How well the activity was tolerated
- The length of time the person dangled
- The amount of help needed
- Other observations or complaints

(text continues on page 284)

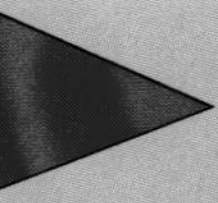

Helping the Person Sit on the Side of the Bed (Dangle)

COMPASSIONATE CARE

Remember to Promote:
- **Dignity**
- **Independence**
- **Preferences**
- **Privacy**
- **Safety**

Pre-Procedure

1 Identify the person according to employer policy.
2 Explain the procedure to the person.
3 Wash your hands.
4 Decide what side of the bed to use.
5 Move furniture to provide moving space.
6 Provide for privacy.
7 Position the person in a side-lying position facing you.
8 Make sure bed is in its lowest position and bed wheels are locked. Follow the care plan for bed rail use.*

Procedure

9 Help the person to a sitting position. (Raise the head of the bed or use pillows or a backrest.)
10 Stand near the person's waist on the side of the bed on which the person will be sitting.
11 Lower the bed rail if up.
12 Turn so you face the far corner of the foot of the bed. Stand with a broad base of support.
13 Slide one arm under the person's neck and shoulders. Grasp the far shoulder. Place your other arm over the person's thighs near the knees. Grasp under the thighs (Figure 21-16, *A*).

Continued

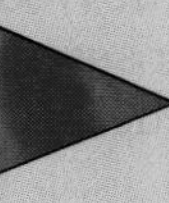

Helping the Person Sit on the Side of the Bed (Dangle)—cont'd

14 Pivot back toward the head of the bed while pulling the person's feet and lower legs over the edge of the bed.

15 Help the person sit upright. Do not pull the person too close to the edge of the bed. Only the person's knees should be at the edge, not the thighs or buttocks (Figure 21-16, *B*).

16 Ask the person to hold onto the edge of the mattress. This supports the person in the sitting position.

17 Do not leave the person alone. Remain in front of the person. Place both hands on the person's shoulders for support if necessary.

18 Check the person's condition:

a Ask how the person feels. Also ask if the person feels dizzy or light-headed.

b Check pulse and respirations.

c Check for difficulty breathing, pale skin, or *cyanosis* (bluish skin colour).

19 Help the person lie down if necessary.

20 Reverse the procedure to return the person to bed.

Post-Procedure

21 Provide for safety and comfort. Help the person move to the centre of the bed. Position the person in good body alignment according to the care plan.

22 Place the call bell within reach.*

23 Follow the care plan for bed rail use.*

24 Return furniture to its proper location.

25 Remove privacy measures.

26 Wash your hands.

27 Report and record your actions and observations according to employer policy.

*Steps marked with an asterisk may not apply in community settings.

A

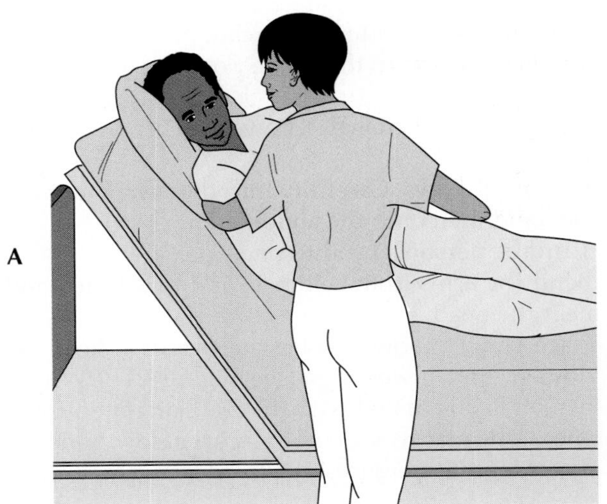

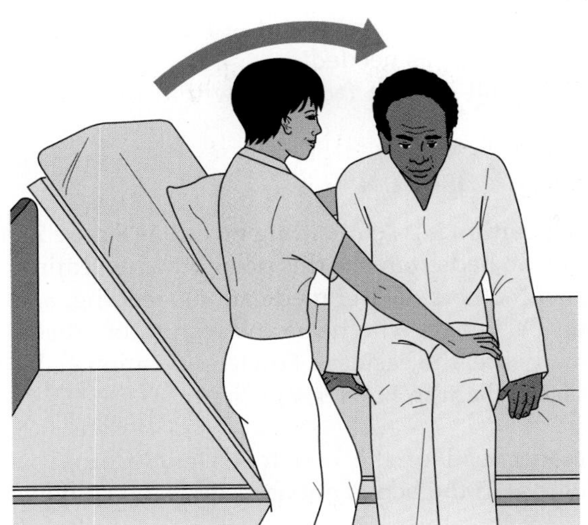

B

Figure 21-16 Helping the client sit on the side of the bed. **A,** Support the client under the shoulders and under the thighs. **B,** Pivot toward the foot of the bed while pulling the client's legs and feet over the edge of the bed. This brings the client to a sitting position.

Positioning the Client

The client must be properly positioned at all times. Regular position changes and good body alignment promote comfort and well-being. Breathing is easier. Circulation is promoted. Proper positioning also helps prevent many complications. These include pressure ulcers (see Chapter 41) and contractures (see Chapter 22).

Most clients can move and position themselves. Some need reminding to adjust their position. Others need help. Still others depend entirely on the health care team for position changes.

Comfort and Safety Measures

Whether in bed or a chair, clients are repositioned at least every 2 hours. Some are repositioned more often. Follow your supervisor's instructions and the care plan.

The physician may order certain positions or position limits. Every time you position a client, check the skin for signs of redness, paleness, or discolouration. Report any observations immediately.

Follow these guidelines to safely position a client:

- Check with your supervisor and the care plan about the best positions for each client
- Follow the scheduled times for repositioning the client
- Use good body mechanics
- Ask for help *before* beginning if necessary
- Explain the procedure to the client
- Be gentle when moving the client
- Provide for privacy
- Leave the client in good body alignment; use pillows as directed in the care plan for comfort and support
- Make sure linens are wrinkle-free; change or straighten them as needed
- Place the call bell (in facilities) within the client's reach

Fowler's Position

Fowler's position is a semi-sitting position (Figure 21-17). Clients in bed often use this position when eating, visiting with others, taking medications, reading, and watching TV. People with heart and respiratory disorders usually breathe easier in Fowler's position.

To place a client in Fowler's position:

- Raise the head of the bed to an angle of 45 to 60 degrees. If the bed is not adjustable, use pillows for support. You can use a backrest, foam wedge pillow, or sofa pillows. If using pillows for support, make sure the headboard is sturdy or the bed is pushed against the wall (see Chapter 24).
- Make sure the person is positioned in good alignment. The spine should be straight and the hips should be directly against the bend in the bed or the pillows.
- Place a small pillow behind the head and neck.
- Place small pillows under the arms and hands.
- Place small pillows under the lower back, thighs, and ankles if your supervisor tells you to do so.

Supine Position

The **supine (dorsal recumbent) position** is a back-lying position (Figure 21-18). It is used for sleeping and resting.

To place a client in the supine position:

- Make sure the bed is flat. Lower the head of the bed if necessary.
- Place a small pillow under the head and shoulders.
- Place the person's arms along the person's sides. Palms are facing down.
- Place a small pillow under the arms and hands.
- Place small pillows or rolled towels under the lower back, thighs, and ankles if your supervisor tells you to do so.

Prone Position

The **prone position** is a front-lying position on the abdomen, with the head turned to one side (Figure 21-19 and Figure 21-20 on page 286). Many people cannot tolerate the prone position. People with limited range of motion in their necks are examples. Use the prone position if it is called for in the care plan.

To place a client in the prone position:

- Make sure the bed is flat. Lower the head of the bed if necessary.
- Remove pillows. Carefully turn the person onto the side and then onto the abdomen.
- Turn the person's head to one side.
- Bend the arms at the elbows, and place the hands near the head.
- Place small pillows under the person's head, abdomen, and lower legs (see Figure 21-19). If the person is positioned with the feet hanging over the end of the mattress, do not place a pillow under the lower legs (see Figure 21-20).

(text continues on page 286)

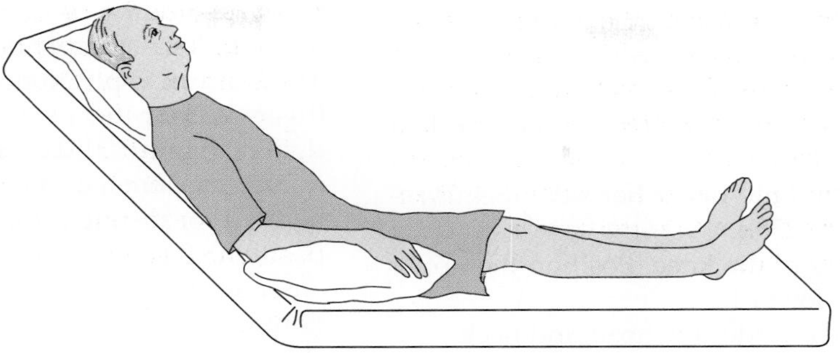

Figure 21-17 Fowler's position.

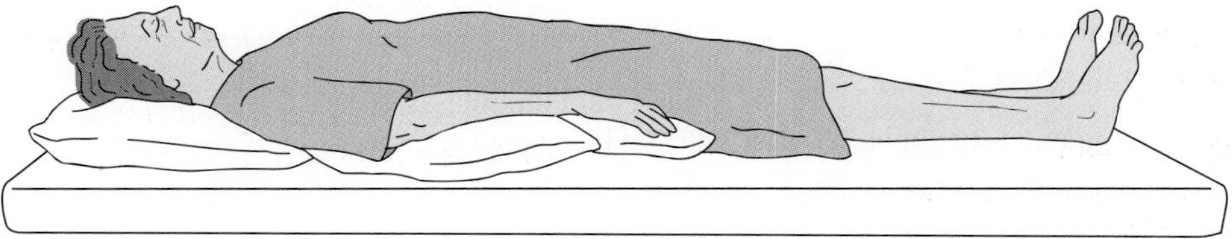

Figure 21-18 Supine position.

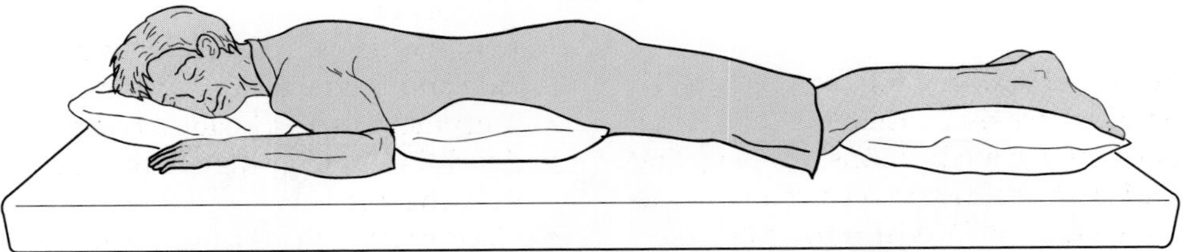

Figure 21-19 Prone position.

Lateral Position

The **lateral position** is a side-lying position (Figure 21-21). The person can lie on one side or the other. Check the client often to make sure he or she is not experiencing pain, numbness, or discomfort in this position.

To place a client in the lateral position:

- Make sure the bed is flat. Lower the head of the bed if necessary.
- Position the person onto his or her side. (See *Turning the Person*, page 278.)
- Bend the upper leg at the knee. Position the upper leg in front of the lower leg.
- Place a small pillow under the head and neck.
- Place small pillows under the upper leg and thigh.
- Place small pillows under the upper hand and arm.
- Position a small pillow against the person's back.

Sims' Position

Sims' position is a left side-lying position in which the right leg is sharply flexed so it is not on the left leg. The left arm is positioned along the person's back. In this position, the person is lying partly on the abdomen (Figure 21-22). This position is used for administering enemas and other procedures. It can also be used for resting if the person is comfortable in this position. This position is usually not comfortable for older adults. Check with your supervisor before positioning an older adult in Sims' position. Check the client frequently for good comfort and circulation in the lower arm and hand.

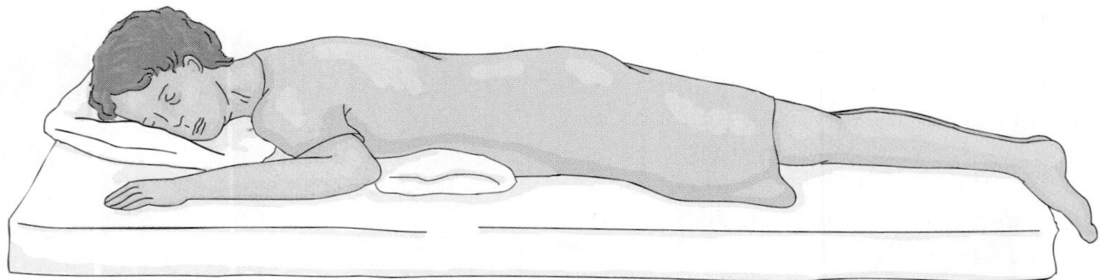

Figure 21-20 Prone position with feet hanging over the edge of the mattress.

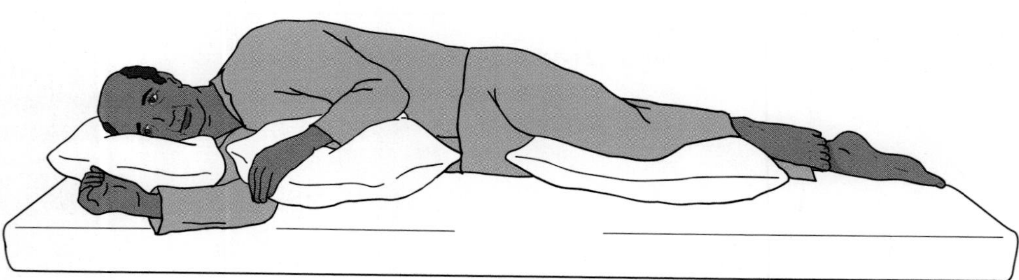

Figure 21-21 Lateral position.

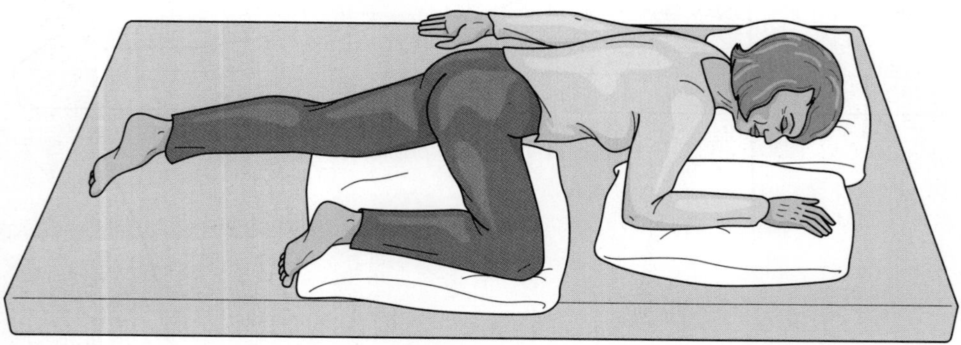

Figure 21-22 Sims' position.

To place a client in Sims' position:

- Make sure the bed is flat. Lower the head of the bed if necessary.
- Position the person onto his or her left side. (See *Turning the Person*, page 278.)
- Bend the upper (right) leg and position it so it does not lie on the lower (left) leg.
- Bend the upper (right) arm and position the hand, palm down, near the head.
- Place the lower (left) arm behind the person. The palm is facing up.
- Place a small pillow under the head and neck.
- Place small pillows under the upper arm and hand and under the upper leg.

Sitting Position

People in chairs or wheelchairs must hold their upper body and head erect (Figure 21-23). Otherwise poor alignment results. Some require postural supports if they cannot keep the upper body erect (Figure 21-24). Postural supports help maintain good alignment. The health care team selects the best product for the client's needs. The client's dignity, independence, preferences, and safety are considered. Assist with postural supports as needed.

To position a client in a chair or wheelchair:

- Position the person's back and buttocks against the back of the chair.
- Make sure the back is straight. The person should not be leaning to the side.
- Place the feet flat on the floor or on wheelchair footrests.
- Place the backs of the knees and calves slightly away from the edge of the seat.
- Support paralyzed arms on pillows. Follow the care plan. Some clients have special foam positioners (Figure 21-25 on page 288). Ask your supervisor about their proper use. Position the person's wrists at a slight upward angle.
- Place a small pillow between the person's lower back and the chair if your supervisor tells you to do so. *Remember, a pillow is not used behind the back if restraints are used* (see Chapter 17).

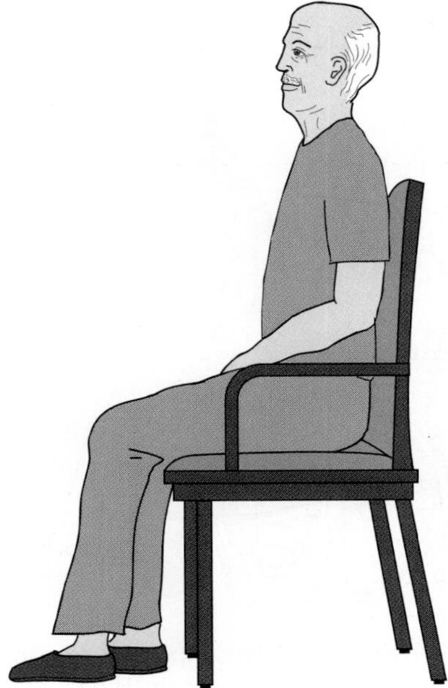

Figure 21-23 Client positioned in a chair. The client's feet are flat on the floor, the calves do not touch the chair, and the back is straight and against the back of the chair.

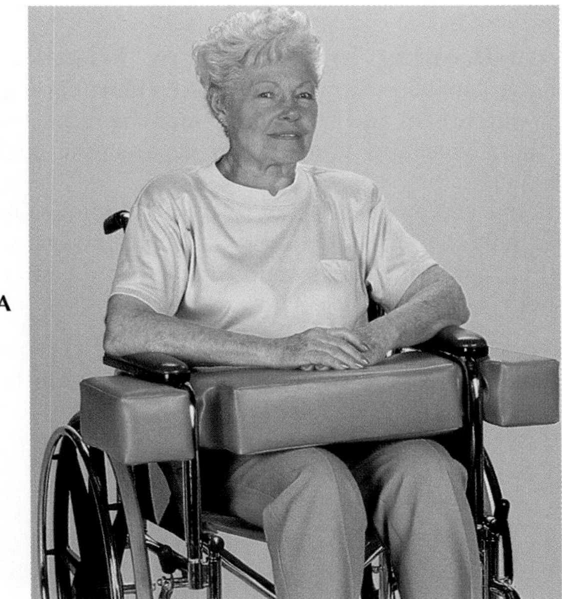

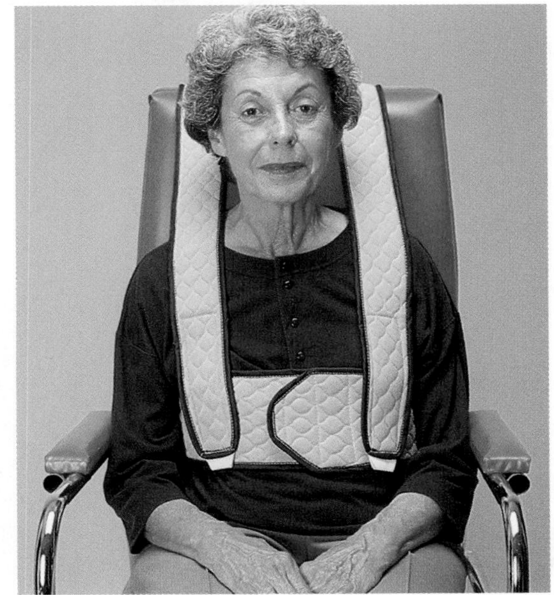

Figure 21-24 Postural supports. **A,** Pelvic holder. **B,** Torso support. *(Courtesy J.T. Posey Co., Aracadia, CA.)*

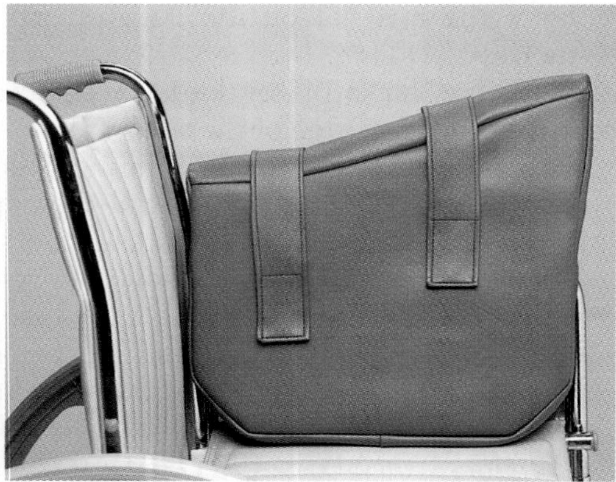
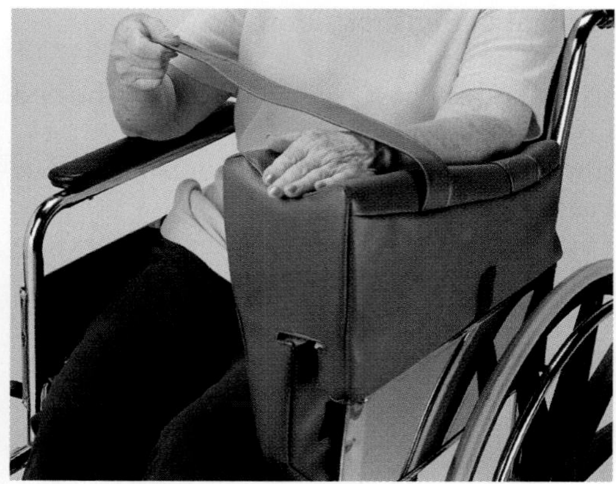

Figure 21-25 Elevated armrest. *(Courtesy J.T. Posey Co., Aracadia, CA.)*

Repositioning in a Chair or Wheelchair. Clients can slide down into their chairs. For good body alignment and safety, they must be repositioned so their back and buttocks are against the back of the chair.

Some clients can help with repositioning. Others need help. Use this method if the client is alert, cooperative, can follow instructions, and has the strength to help:

- Lock the wheelchair wheels.
- Stand in front of the client. Block his or her knees and feet with your knees and feet.
- Apply a transfer belt (see page 289).
- Position the client's feet flat on the floor.
- Position the client's arms on the armrests.
- Grasp the transfer belt on each side while the client leans forward. Or if a transfer belt is not available, put your arms under the client's arms and place your hands around the client's shoulder blades.
- Ask the client to push with his or her feet and arms on the count of "3."
- Lift the client back into the chair on the count of "3" as the client pushes with his or her feet and arms (Figure 21-26).

Use this method if the client cannot assist with repositioning. A helper is needed (Figure 21-27):

- Ask for a trained family member or co-worker to help you. Decide who is taller, you or your helper. The taller person stands behind the wheelchair. The other stands in front of the client.

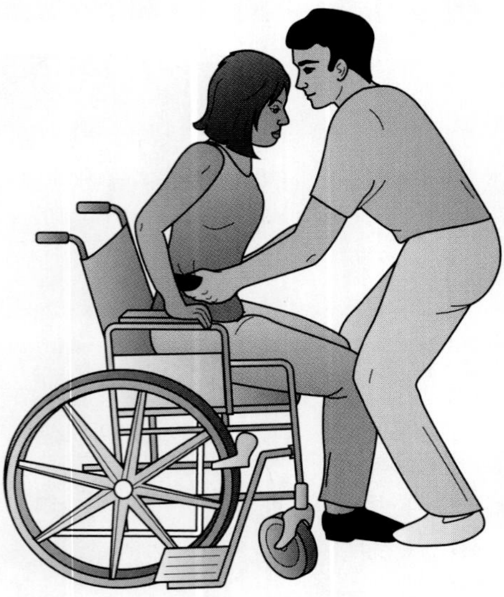

Figure 21-26 Repositioning the client in a wheelchair. Use a transfer belt to lift the client to the back of the chair.

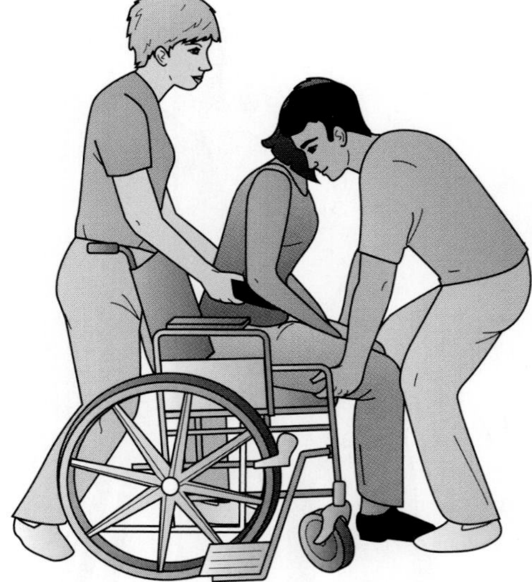

Figure 21-27 Two people (the support worker and a helper) repositioning a client in a wheelchair. The taller person stands behind the chair and lifts with the transfer belt. The other person stands in front of the client. Hands and arms are under the knees to support the legs during repositioning.

- Lock the wheelchair wheels.
- Apply a transfer belt.
- Ask the client to place folded hands in his or her lap.
- The person behind the wheelchair grasps the transfer belt on each side.
- The other person stands in front of the client. The hands and arms are placed under the client's knees.
- On the count of "3," lift the client to the back of the chair. Support the legs (person in front) and use the transfer belt (person in back).

TRANSFERRING THE CLIENT

Transfer means to move or help a client to move from one place to another. Clients are often moved from their beds to chairs, wheelchairs, commodes, toilets, or stretchers. Some clients need only minimal help with transferring. Others need two or three people to help them. Your supervisor and the care plan tell you how much help a client needs.

Always make sure that you have enough room for a safe transfer. Clear the area of potential hazards. You may have to move furniture to make room for a chair, wheelchair, or stretcher.

Before transferring a client, check the care plan or ask your supervisor if the person has one side of the body that is weaker than the other. The weak side (or *affected side*) is the side affected by disease or disability. The strong side (or *unaffected side*) is the side not affected by disease or disability. The strong side pulls the weak side along. Transfers from the weak side are awkward and unsafe. The weak arm and leg may not be able to bear the person's weight. For example, a client's left side is weak from a stroke. Her right side is the stronger side. Plan to move the client so her right side moves first.

The rules of good body mechanics apply to transfers. They will help you reduce the risk of injury to yourself and to the client. Also follow the same comfort and safety measures listed for lifting and moving clients (see page 266–267).

Report and record the following after transferring a client:

- Pulse rate (if instructed to measure) before and at the transfer
- Complaints of lightheadedness, pain, discomfort, difficulty breathing, weakness, or fatigue
- The amount of help needed to transfer the client
- How the client helped with the transfer

APPLYING TRANSFER BELTS

A **transfer belt** is used to transfer unsteady and disabled clients. It helps prevent falls and other injuries. The belt goes around the client's waist. Grasp the belt with your fingers pointing up to support the client during the transfer. The belt is called a **gait belt** when used for walking with a client. Many facilities require staff to use these belts when transferring or walking a client.

(text continues on page 291)

Applying a Transfer Belt

Compassionate Care

Remember to Promote:
- **Dignity**
- **Independence**
- **Preferences**
- **Privacy**
- **Safety**

Procedure

1 Identify the person according to employer policy.
2 Explain the procedure to the person.
3 Wash your hands.
4 Provide for privacy.
5 Assist the person to a sitting position.
6 Apply the belt around the person's waist over clothing. Do not apply it over bare skin.
7 Tighten the belt so it is snug. It should not cause discomfort or impair breathing. You should be able to slide your fingers under the belt.
8 Make sure that a woman's breasts are not caught under the belt.
9 Place the buckle off centre in the front or in the back for the person's comfort (Figure 21-28). The buckle should not be over the spine.
10 Grasp the transfer belt from underneath when using it to transfer a person.

A

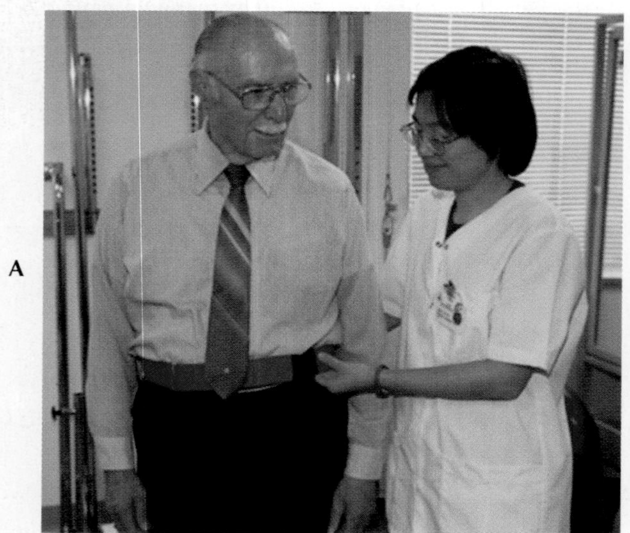

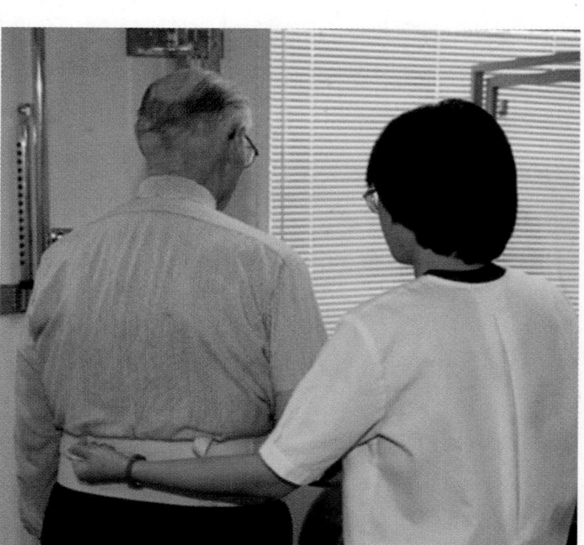

B

Figure 21-28 Transfer belt (gait belt). Note the different types of transfer belts. **A,** Position the belt buckle off centre in the front. **B,** Position the belt buckle off centre at the back. Grasp under the belt with your fingers pointing up.

Bed to Chair or Wheelchair Transfers

Safety is important for chair and wheelchair transfers. You must prevent falls and protect your back from injury. Always hold the client securely during the procedure. Make sure the client wears nonskid footwear to prevent sliding or slipping. The chair or wheelchair must support the client's weight.

The number of people needed for a transfer depends on the client's physical capabilities, condition, and size. You might be able to transfer a client alone. However, some transfers require one or more helpers. Most long-term care facilities require the use of transfer belts when residents are transferred to or from chairs or wheelchairs. Check with your supervisor and the care plan for instructions on how much assistance is needed.

If the client cannot assist with a transfer, a mechanical lift is used (see page 299). Never attempt a transfer without assistance if the client cannot help. Remember, some employers have a "no-lift" policy. Workers cannot lift clients to transfer them. If your employer has a "no-lift" policy, use a mechanical lift to transfer the client.

Also, remember to help the client out of the bed on his or her strong side. Place the chair or wheelchair with its back even with the head of the bed. Lock the bed and wheelchair wheels, and raise the footrests.

Most bedside chairs and wheelchairs have vinyl seats and backs. Vinyl holds body heat. To promote comfort, you can cover the back and seat with a folded blanket. Place small pillows or cushions behind the back if your supervisor tells you to do so. These are to promote comfort, prevent pressure ulcers, and maintain posture.

(text continues on page 296)

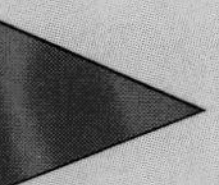

Transferring the Person to a Chair or Wheelchair

Compassionate Care

Remember to Promote:
- **Dignity**
- **Independence**
- **Preferences**
- **Privacy**
- **Safety**

Pre-Procedure

1. Identify the person according to employer policy.
2. Explain the procedure to the person.
3. Collect:
   - Wheelchair or arm chair
   - One or two bath blankets
   - Robe and nonskid footwear
   - Paper or sheet
   - Transfer belt if needed
   - Seat cushion if used by the person
4. Wash your hands.
5. Provide for privacy.
6. Decide which side of the bed to use. Move furniture to provide moving space.

Continued

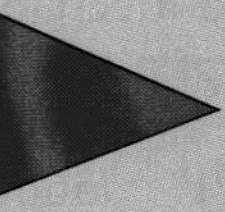

Transferring the Person to a Chair or Wheelchair—cont'd

Procedure

7 Place the chair back even with the headboard.

8 Place a folded bath blanket or cushion on the seat if needed.

9 Lock wheelchair wheels. Raise the footrests or swing them out of the way.

10 Lower the bed to its lowest position. Lock the bed wheels. Lower the bed rail near you if up.

11 Fanfold top linens to the foot of the bed.

12 Place the paper or sheet under the person's feet. Put nonskid footwear on the person.

13 Help the person dangle. (See *Helping the Person Sit on the Side of the Bed,* page 282.) Make sure his or her feet touch the floor.

14 Help the person put on a robe.

15 Apply the transfer belt if it will be used.

16 *Method 1: Using a transfer belt*

- a Stand in front of the person. Stand with your feet apart. Flex your hips and knees. Align your knees with the person's knees.
- b Have the person hold onto the mattress. Or ask the person to place his or her fists on the bed by the thighs.
- c Make sure the person's feet are flat on the floor.
- d Have the person lean forward.
- e Grasp the transfer belt at each side.
- f Brace your knees against the person's knees. Block his or her feet with your feet (Figure 21-29, *A*).
- g Tell the person to push down on the mattress and to stand on the count of "3." Pull the person into a standing position as you straighten your hips and legs. Keep your knees slightly flexed (Figure 21-29, *B*).

17 *Method 2: Without using a transfer belt*

- a Follow steps 16 a–c.
- b Place your hands under the person's arms. Your hands are around the person's shoulder blades (Figure 21-30, *A* on page 294).
- c Have the person lean forward.
- d Brace your knees against the person's knees. Block his or her feet with your feet.
- e Tell the person to push down on the mattress and to stand on the count of "3." Pull the person up into a standing position as you straighten your hips and legs. Keep your knees slightly flexed.

18 Support the person in the standing position. Hold the transfer belt, or keep your hands around the person's shoulder blades. Continue to block the person's feet and knees with your feet and knees.

19 Pivot on your foot and turn the person so he or she can grasp the far arm of the chair. The person's legs will touch the edge of the chair (Figure 21-30, *B* on page 294).

20 Continue to turn the person until he or she grasps the other armrest.

21 Lower the person into the chair as you bend your hips and knees. Keep your back straight. The person assists by leaning forward and bending the elbows and knees (Figure 21-30, *C* on page 294).

22 Make sure the person's buttocks are to the back of the seat. Position the person in good alignment.

23 Position the person's feet on the wheelchair footrests.

24 Cover the person's lap and legs with a bath blanket. Keep the blanket off the floor and the wheels.

25 Remove the transfer belt if used.

26 Position the chair as the person prefers. Lock the wheelchair wheels.

Continued

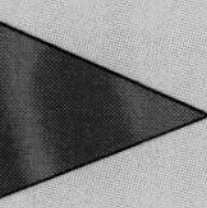

Transferring the Person to a Chair or Wheelchair—cont'd

Post-Procedure

27 Provide for safety and comfort.
28 Place the call bell within reach.*
29 Remove privacy measures.
30 Wash your hands.
31 Report and record your actions and observations according to employer policy.
32 Reverse the procedure to return the person to bed.

*Steps marked with an asterisk may not apply in community settings.

A 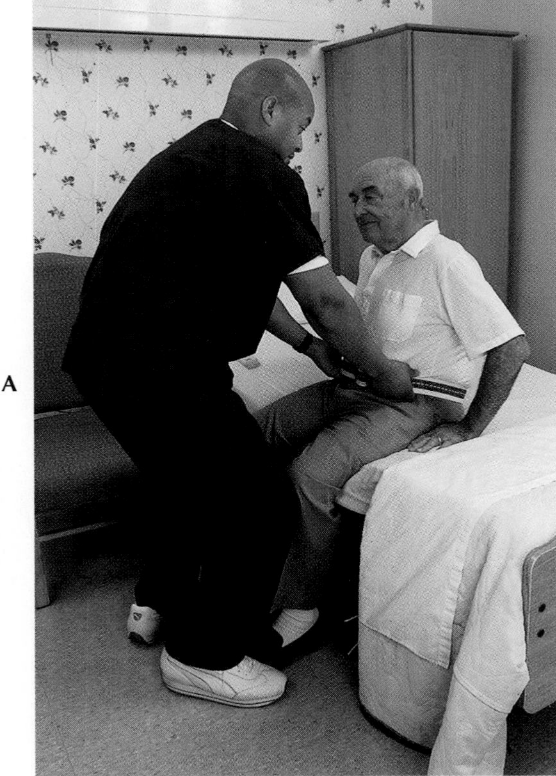

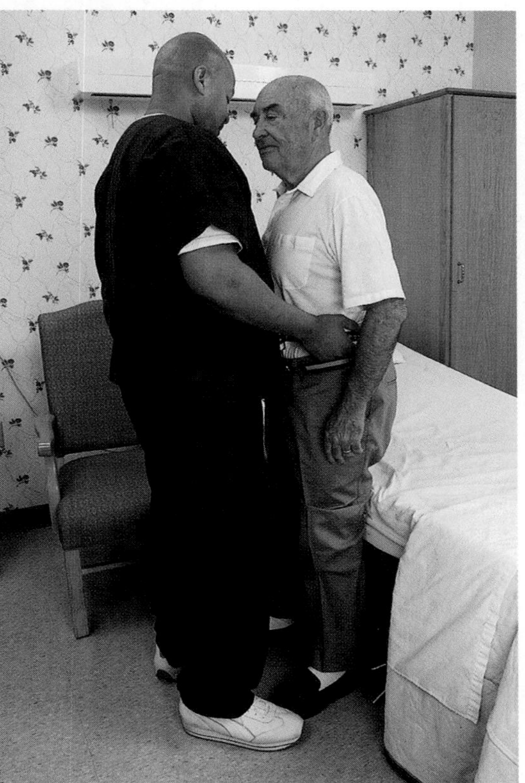 B

Figure 21-29 Transferring a client to a chair (or wheelchair) using a transfer belt. Position the chair next to and even with the headboard. **A,** Prevent the client from sliding or falling by blocking the client's knees and feet with your knees and feet. **B,** Pull the client up to a standing position. Support the client by holding the transfer belt and blocking the client's knees and feet.

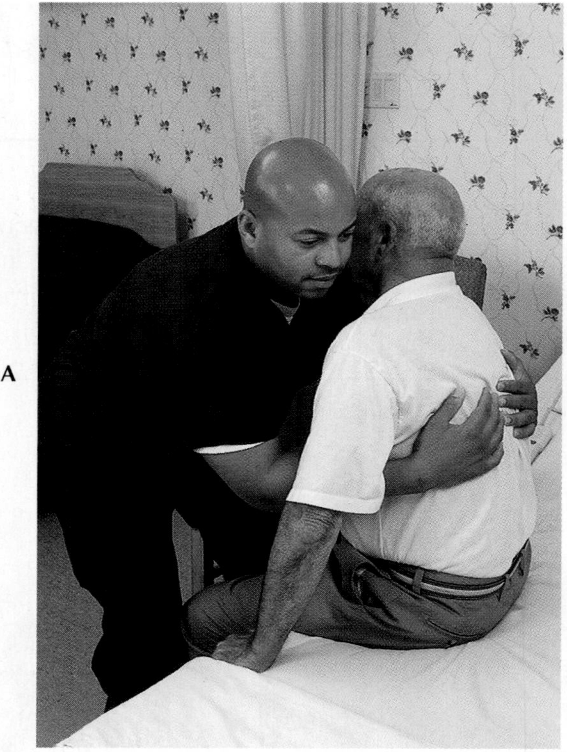

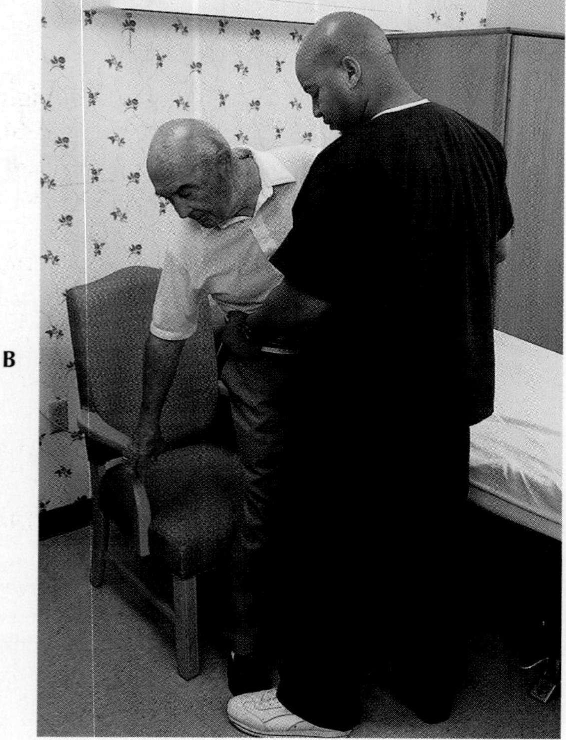

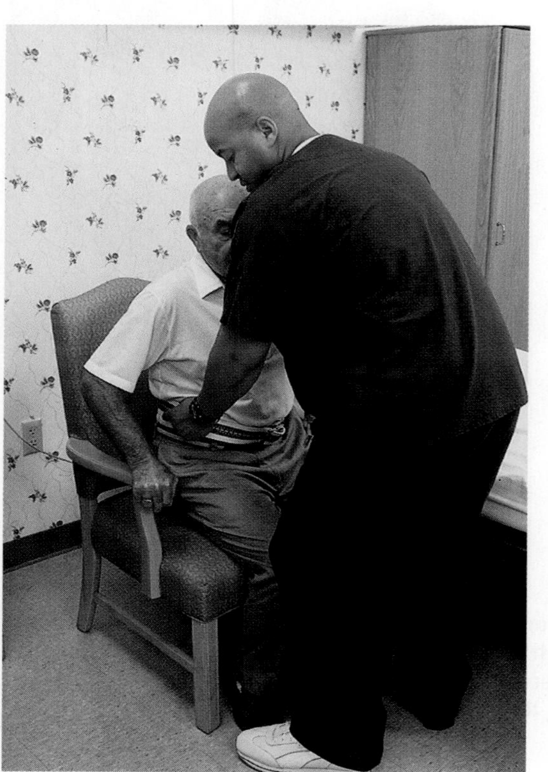

Figure 21-30 Transferring a client to a chair (or wheelchair) without a transfer belt. **A,** Place your hands under the client's arms and around the shoulder blades. **B,** Support the client as he or she grasps the far arm of the chair. The client's legs are against the chair. **C,** Lower the client into the chair while the client holds the armrests, leans forward, and bends the elbows and knees.

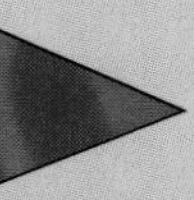

Transferring the Person to a Wheelchair with Assistance

Compassionate Care

Remember to Promote:
- **Dignity**
- **Independence**
- **Preferences**
- **Privacy**
- **Safety**

Pre-Procedure

1 Identify the person according to employer policy.
2 Ask someone to help you.
3 Explain the procedure to the person.
4 Collect:
- Wheelchair with removable armrests
- Bath blankets
- Footwear
- Cushion, if used

5 Wash your hands.
6 Provide for privacy.
7 Decide which side of the bed to use. Move furniture to provide moving space.

Procedure

8 Place the wheelchair at the side of the bed, even with the person's hips.
9 Place a folded bath blanket or cushion on the seat.
10 Remove the wheelchair armrest near the bed.
11 Lock wheelchair wheels and raise or remove the footrests.
12 Make sure the bed is in its lowest position and bed wheels are locked. Lower the bed rail if up.*
13 Fanfold top linens to the foot of the bed.
14 Help the person to the side of the bed near you. Help him or her to a sitting position by raising the head of the bed or using pillows for support.
15 Stand behind wheelchair, facing the person. Stand so your feet are shoulder-width apart. Flex your knees. Put your arms under the person's arms and grasp the person's forearms (Figure 21-31, *A* on page 296).
16 Have your helper grasp the person's thighs and calves (Figure 21-31, *B* on page 296).
17 Bring the person toward the chair on the count of "3." Lower him or her into the chair (Figure 21-31, *C* on page 296).
18 Make sure the person's buttocks are to the back of the seat. Position the person in good alignment.
19 Put the armrest and footrest back on the wheelchair.
20 Put the footwear on the person. Position the person's feet on the footrests.
21 Cover the person's lap and legs with a blanket. Keep the blanket off the floor and wheels.
22 Position the chair as the person prefers. Lock the wheelchair wheels.

Post-Procedure

23 Follow steps 27 through 32 of *Transferring the Person to a Chair or Wheelchair,* page 291.

*Steps marked with an asterisk may not apply in community settings.

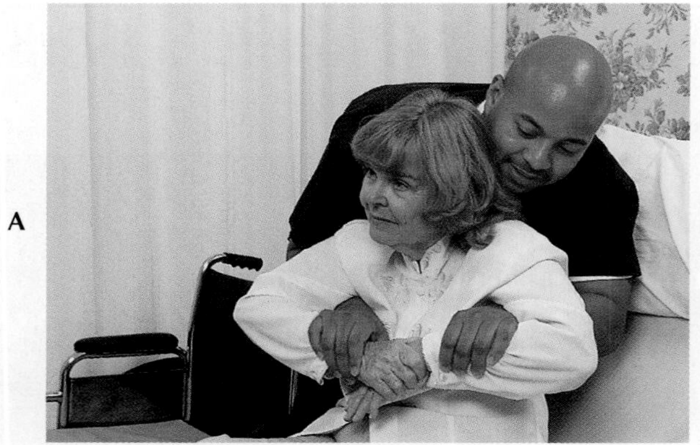

A

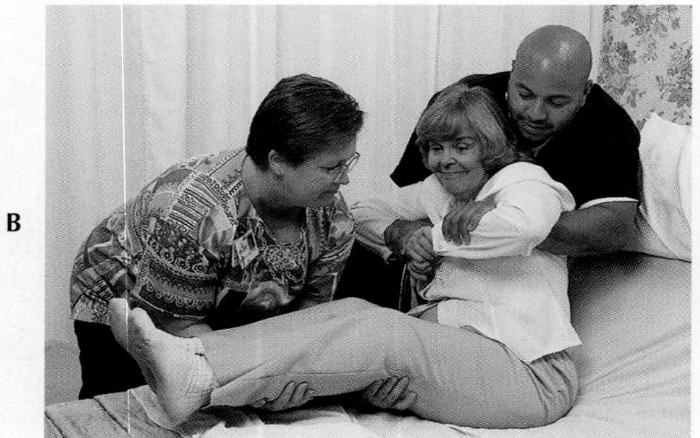

B

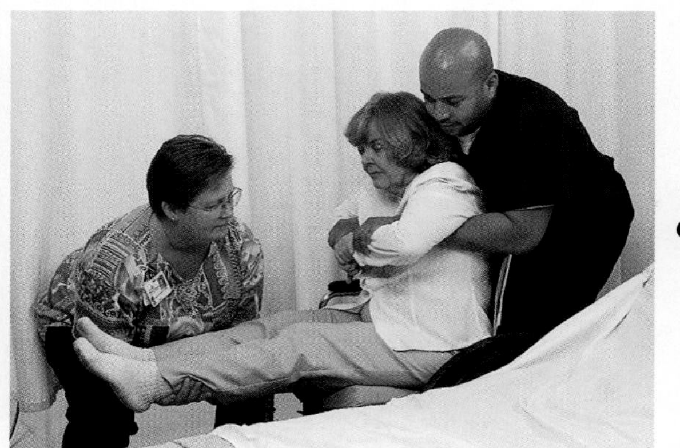

C

Figure 21-31 Transferring a client to a wheelchair with assistance. **A,** Put your arms under the client's arms and grasp the client's forearms. **B,** Your helper holds the thighs and calves to support the legs during the transfer. **C,** Lower the client into the chair. NOTE: This procedure involves lifting the client. Make sure the person does not weigh more than you can safely lift. Some employers have a "no lift" policy. Know your emplyer policy before attempting this transfer.

Other Transfers

The basic transfer from a bed to a chair or wheelchair can be modified for other situations. You can transfer a client from a wheelchair to a shower or bath chair. Or you can transfer a client to and from a toilet. Carefully consider how to proceed. First check with your supervisor and the care plan to determine the client's physical abilities and limitations. Also consider the client's environment. How much space do you have to move about? Are there assistive devices such as grab bars or sliding boards? Use good body mechanics and apply the general safety and comfort rules.

(text continues on page 299)

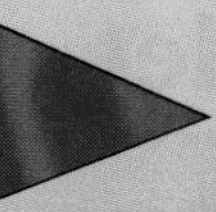

Transferring the Person from a Wheelchair to a Shower (or Bath) Chair

Compassionate Care

Remember to Promote:
- **Dignity**
- **Independence**
- **Preferences**
- **Privacy**
- **Safety**

Pre-Procedure

1 Identify the person according to employer policy.
2 Explain the procedure to the person.
3 Collect:
- Shower or bath chair
- Bath blanket
- Towel
- Transfer belt if used

4 Wash your hands.
5 Provide for privacy.
6 Check that the shower chair is securely positioned and locked in place. Do not transfer the person if the shower chair is not secure.
7 Check grab bars by the shower. If they are loose, report it to your supervisor. Do not transfer the person if the grab bars are not secure.

Procedure

8 Position the wheelchair at a 90-degree angle to the shower chair. The person's strong side is near the shower chair.
9 Lock the wheelchair wheels.
10 Raise the footrests. Remove or swing them out of the way.
11 Prepare the water.
12 Apply the transfer belt if used.
13 Help the person stand and turn to the shower chair. (See *Transferring the Person to a Chair or Wheelchair,* page 291, steps 16 and 17.) The person uses the grab bars or shower chair armrests for support.
14 Support the person while he or she undresses. Hold the transfer belt or keep your hands around the person's shoulder blades. Continue to block the person's feet and knees with your feet and knees. Or have the person hold onto the grab bars or armrests for support. Undress the person.
15 Lower the person onto the shower chair.
16 Remove the transfer belt if used.

Post-Procedure

17 Help the person dry off after the shower. Cover the person with a bath blanket.
18 Reverse the procedure to transfer the person from the shower chair to the wheelchair.
19 Help the person put on clean clothing.
20 Wash your hands.
21 Report and record your actions and observations according to employer policy.

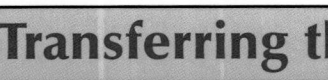

Transferring the Person to and from the Toilet

Compassionate Care

Remember to Promote:
- **Dignity**
- **Independence**
- **Preferences**
- **Privacy**
- **Safety**

Pre-Procedure

1 Explain the procedure to the person.

2 Wash your hands.

3 Provide for privacy.

4 Make sure the person has an elevated toilet seat. That way, the toilet seat and wheelchair are at the same level.

5 Check the grab bars by the toilet. If they are loose, tell your supervisor. Do not transfer the person to the toilet if the grab bars are not secure.

Procedure

6 Have the person wear nonskid footwear.

7 Position the wheelchair next to the toilet if there is enough room. If not, position the wheelchair at a right angle to the toilet (Figure 21-32). It is best if the person's strong side is near the toilet.

8 Lock the wheelchair wheels.

9 Raise the footrests. Remove or swing them out of the way.

10 Apply the transfer belt if used.

11 Help the person unfasten clothing.

12 Help the person stand and turn to the toilet. (See *Transferring the Person to a Chair or Wheelchair,* page 291, steps 16 and 17). The person uses the grab bars to turn to the toilet.

13 Support the person while he or she lowers clothing. Hold the transfer belt or keep your hands around the person's shoulder blades. Continue to block the person's feet and knees with your feet and knees. Or have the person hold onto the grab bars for support. Lower the person's pants and undergarments.

14 Lower the person onto the toilet seat.

15 Remove the transfer belt, if used.

16 Tell the person you will stay nearby. Remind the person to use the call bell (in facilities) or to call for you when help is needed.

17 Close the bathroom door to provide for privacy.

18 Stay near the bathroom. Complete other tasks in the person's room.

19 Knock on the bathroom door when the person calls for you.

20 Help with wiping, perineal care, flushing, and hand washing as needed. Wear gloves for this step.

21 Apply the transfer belt if used.

22 Help the person stand. Support the person in the standing position. Hold the transfer belt, or keep your hands around the person's shoulder blades. Continue to block the person's feet and knees with your feet and knees.

23 Help the person raise and secure clothing.

24 Transfer the person to the wheelchair. (See *Transferring the Person to a Chair or Wheelchair,* page 291, steps 19 through 26.)

Post-Procedure

25 Provide for safety and comfort.

26 Place the call bell within reach.*

27 Wash your hands.

28 Report and record your actions and observations according to employer policy.

*Step marked with an asterisk may not apply in community settings.

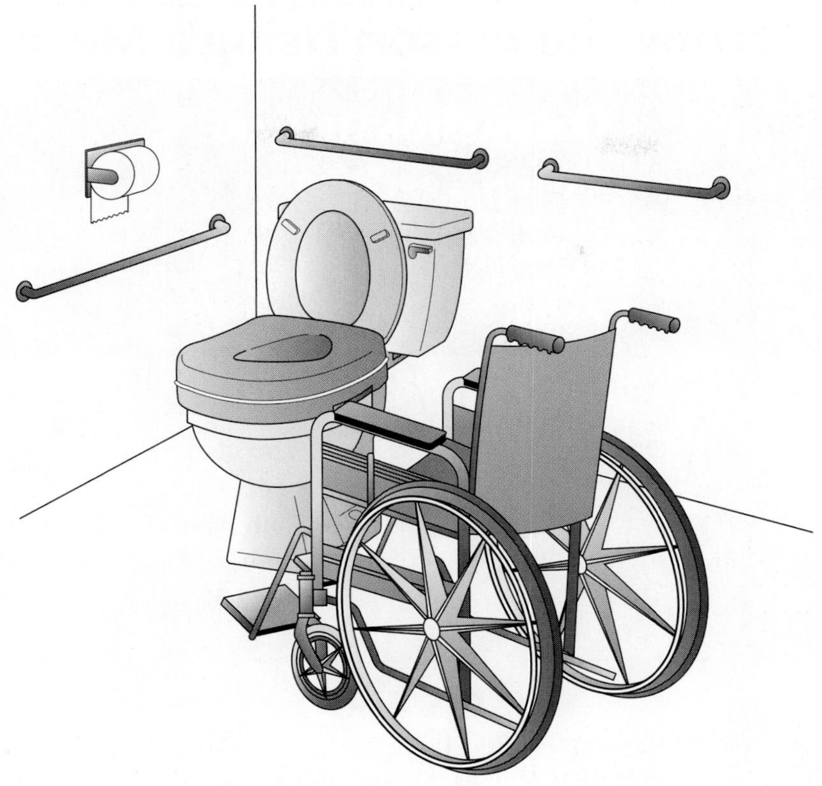

Figure 21-32 Position the wheelchair at a right angle to the toilet.

TRANSFERS USING A MECHANICAL LIFT

Clients who cannot help with a transfer are moved with a mechanical lift. Lifts are used for transfers to chairs, stretchers, tubs, shower chairs, toilets, whirlpools, and vehicles.

There are mechanical and electric mechanical lifts. Before using a lift:

- Make sure you are trained in its use.
- Make sure the lift works.
- Compare the client's weight and the lift's weight limit. Do not use the lift if a client's weight exceeds the lift's capacity.

At least two people are usually needed to work a mechanical lift. Get a co-worker or a trained family member to help you.

There are many different kinds of mechanical lifts. Knowing how to use one lift does not mean that you know how to use others. Always follow the manufacturer's instructions. Employers usually provide special training for the use of mechanical lifts. You may also be required to take yearly "refresher" courses to keep up your skills. If you have questions, ask your supervisor. If you have not used a certain lift before, ask your supervisor to show you how to use it safely. The following procedure is a guide.

(text continues on page 302)

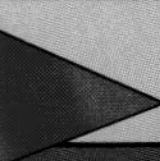

Transferring the Person Using a Mechanical Lift

Compassionate Care

Remember to Promote:
- **Dignity**
- **Independence**
- **Preferences**
- **Privacy**
- **Safety**

Pre-Procedure

1 Identify the person according to employer policy.
2 Ask someone to help you.
3 Explain the procedure to the person.
4 Collect:
- Mechanical lift
- Arm chair or wheelchair
- Footwear
- Bath blanket or cushion

5 Wash your hands.
6 Provide for privacy.

Procedure

7 Centre the sling under the person (Figure 21-33, *A*). Turn the person from side to side as if making an occupied bed to position the sling (see Chapter 24). Position the sling according to the manufacturer's instructions.
8 Place the chair at the head of the bed. It should be even with the headboard and about 30 cm (1 foot) away from the bed. Place a folded bath blanket or cushion in the chair, if needed.
9 Lock the bed wheels and lower the bed to its lowest position.*
10 Raise the lift so it can be positioned over the person.
11 Position the lift over the person (Figure 21-33, *B*).
12 Lock the lift wheels in position.
13 Attach the sling to the swivel bar (Figure 21-33, *C*).
14 Assist the person to a sitting position. Raise the head of the bed or use pillows for support.
15 Cross the person's arms over the chest. Let him or her hold onto the straps or chains, but not the swivel bar.
16 Raise the lift high enough until the person and sling are free of the bed (Figure 21-33, *D*).
17 Ask your helper to support the person's legs as you move the lift and person away from the bed (Figure 21-33, *E*).
18 Position the lift so that the person's back is toward the chair.
19 Position the chair so that you can lower the person into it.
20 Lower the person into the chair. (Follow the manufacturer's instructions.) Guide the person into the chair (Figure 21-33, *F*).
21 Lower the swivel bar to unhook the sling. Remove the sling from under the person unless instructed otherwise.
22 Put the footwear on the person. Position the person's feet on wheelchair footrests.
23 Cover the person's lap and legs with a blanket. Keep the blanket off the floor and wheels.
24 Position the chair as the person prefers. Lock the wheelchair wheels.

Continued

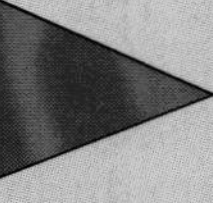

Transferring the Person Using a Mechanical Lift—cont'd

Post-Procedure

25 Provide for safety and comfort.
26 Place the call bell within reach.*
27 Wash your hands.
28 Report and record your actions and observations according to employer policy.
29 Reverse the procedure to return the person to bed.

*Steps marked with an asterisk may not apply in community settings.

A
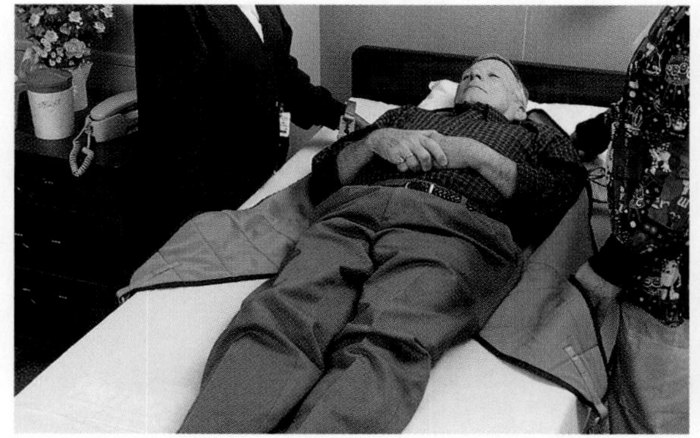

B
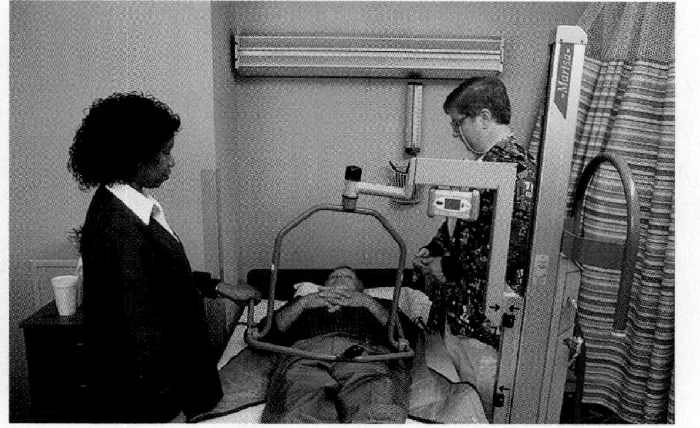

C
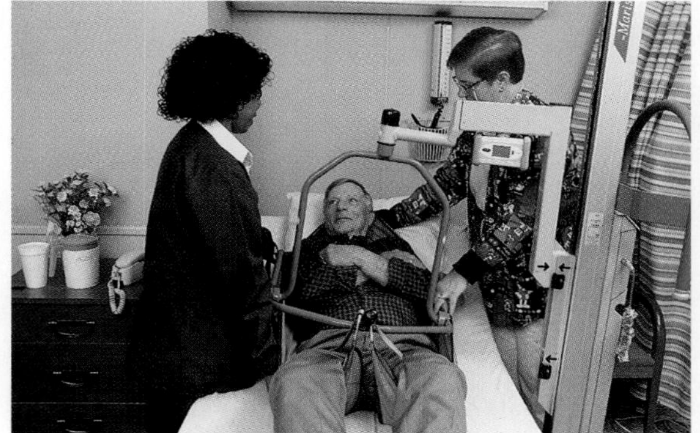

D
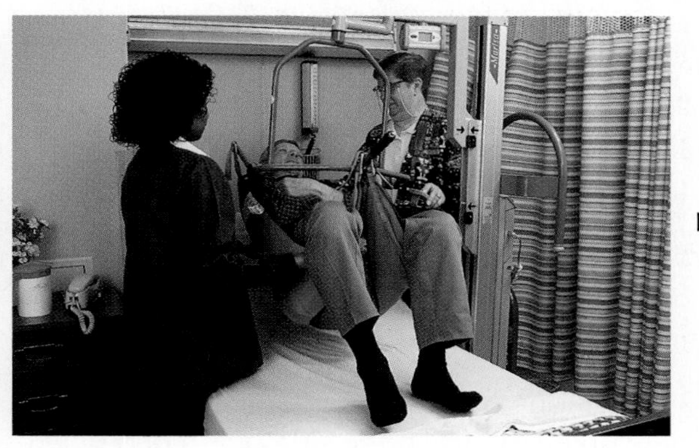

E
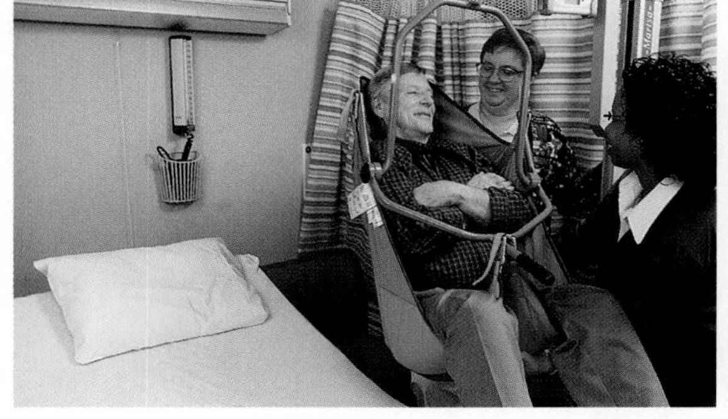

F
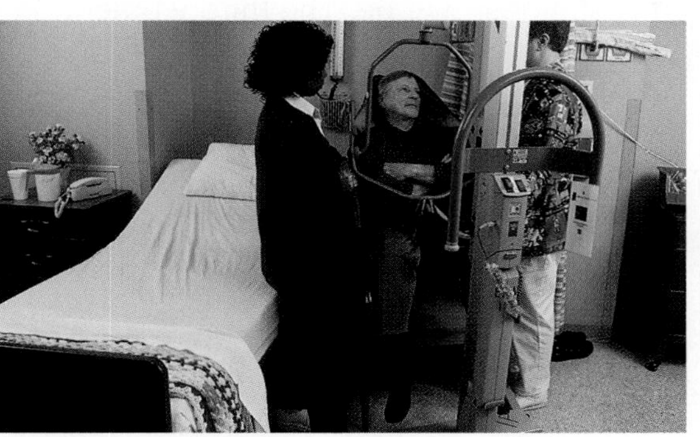

Figure 21-33 Using a mechanical lift. **A,** Position the sling under the client according to manufacturer's instructions. **B,** Position the lift over the client. The lift's legs are spread to widen the base of support. **C,** Attach the sling to the swivel bar. **D,** Raise the lift until the sling and client are off the bed. **E,** Your helper supports the client's legs as you move the lift and client away from the bed. **F,** Guide the client into the chair.

TRANSFERRING THE CLIENT TO A STRETCHER

Stretchers are sometimes used to transport clients to other areas in a facility. They are used for clients who:

- Cannot sit up
- Must stay in a lying position
- Are seriously ill
- Are waiting for or returning from surgery

The stretcher is covered with a folded flat sheet or bath blanket. A pillow and extra blankets are available. With your supervisor's permission, raise the head of the stretcher to Fowler's position. This increases the client's comfort.

Safety straps are used when the client is on the stretcher. The stretcher's side rails are kept up during the transport. Move the client's feet first so the worker at the head of the stretcher can watch the client's breathing and colour during the transport. Never leave a client on a stretcher unattended.

A drawsheet or lift sheet is used. At least three staff members are needed for a safe transfer. Remember, keep the client in good body alignment and use good body mechanics.

Transferring the Person to a Stretcher

COMPASSIONATE CARE

Remember to Promote:
- **Dignity**
- **Independence**
- **Preferences**
- **Privacy**
- **Safety**

Pre-Procedure

1. Identify the person according to employer policy.
2. Ask two co-workers to help you.
3. Explain the procedure to the person.
4. Collect:
   - Stretcher covered with a sheet or bath blanket
   - Bath blanket
   - Pillow(s) if needed
5. Wash your hands.
6. Provide for privacy.
7. Raise the bed to a height equal to the height of the stretcher.

Procedure

8. Position yourself and your co-workers. Two workers stand on the side of the bed where the stretcher will be. The third worker stands on the other side of the bed.
9. Cover the person with a bath blanket. Fan-fold top linens to foot of bed.
10. Loosen the cotton drawsheet on each side.
11. Lower head of bed so it is as flat as possible.
12. Lower bed rails if used.
13. Ask your co-workers to help move the person to the side of the bed. The drawsheet serves as your lift sheet.
14. Protect the person from falling by holding the far arm and leg.
15. Have your co-workers position the stretcher next to the bed. They stand behind the stretcher (Figure 21-34, *A*).
16. Lock the bed and stretcher wheels.
17. Roll up and grasp the drawsheet as shown in Figure 21-34, *B*. This supports the entire length of the person's body.
18. Transfer the person to the stretcher on the count of "3" by lifting and pulling him or her. Make sure the person is centred on the stretcher.

Continued

Transferring the Person to a Stretcher—cont'd

19 Place a pillow or pillows under the person's head and shoulders if allowed.

20 Cover the person. Provide for comfort.

21 Fasten safety straps. Raise the stretcher side rails.

22 Unlock the stretcher's wheels. Transport the person.

Post-Procedure

23 Wash your hands.

24 Report and record the following according to employer policy:
- The time of the transport
- Where the person was transported
- Who went with him or her
- How the transfer was tolerated

25 Reverse the procedure to return the person to bed.

A 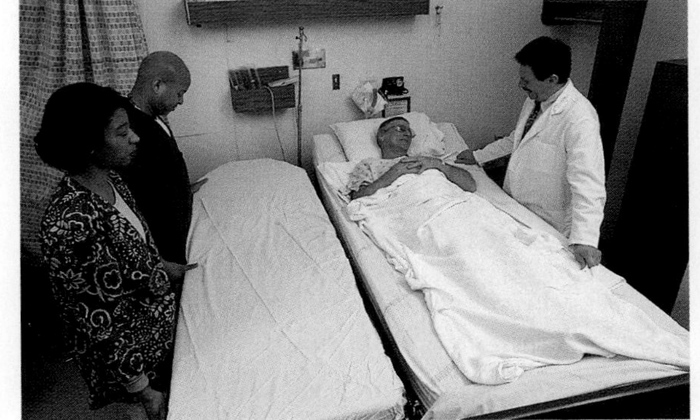

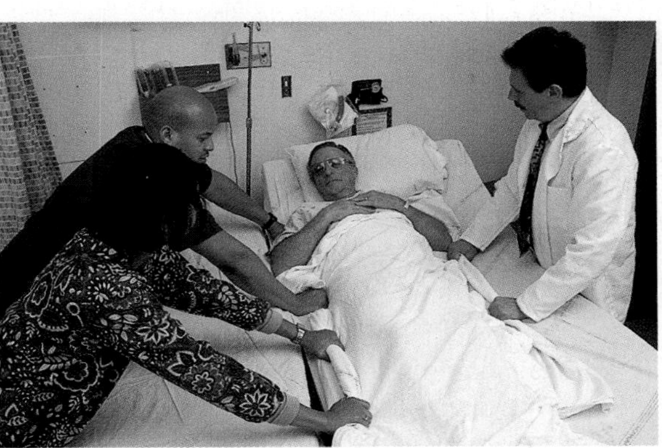 B

Figure 21-34 Transferring the client to a stretcher. **A,** Hold the stretcher in place against the bed. **B,** Use a drawsheet to transfer the client from the bed to the stretcher.

REVIEW

Circle T if the answer is true and F if it is false.

1. T F Body mechanics refers to the way in which body parts are positioned in relation to one another.
2. T F Good body mechanics helps protect you and the client from injury.
3. T F Body mechanics involves the use of small muscles.
4. T F Base of support is the area on which an object rests.
5. T F You should keep objects far away from the body when lifting, moving, or carrying them.
6. T F You should face the direction you are working to prevent unnecessary twisting.
7. T F You should push, slide, or pull heavy objects rather than lift them.
8. T F Sliding the client reduces friction and shearing.
9. T F You should ask your supervisor about limits or restrictions in positioning or moving a client.
10. T F The right to privacy should be protected when you are moving, lifting, or transferring clients.
11. T F A lift sheet should extend from below the shoulders to above the knees.
12. T F A client should be moved to the side of the bed before being turned to the side-lying position.
13. T F Logrolling is rolling the client in segments.
14. T F Clients with spinal cord injuries are logrolled.
15. T F Repositioning prevents deformities and pressure on body parts.
16. T F The head of the bed is elevated 45 to 60 degrees for the supine position.
17. T F The Sims' position is a left side-lying position.
18. T F A transfer belt is part of a mechanical lift.
19. T F A client is being transferred from the bed to a chair. He needs nonskid footwear.
20. T F You are going to transfer a client from the bed to a chair. You should move her from the direction of the weak side of her body.

Circle the BEST answer.

21. Good body alignment means
    A. The area on which an object rests
    B. Having the head, trunk, arms, and legs aligned with one another
    C. Using muscles, tendons, ligaments, joints, and cartilage correctly
    D. The back-lying or supine position
22. Support workers are at great risk for
    A. Friction and shearing
    B. Arm and hand injuries
    C. Back injuries
    D. Falls
23. A client's skin rubs against the sheet. This is called
    A. Shearing
    B. Friction
    C. Transferring
    D. Posture
24. Clients who are immobile must be repositioned at least every
    A. 30 minutes
    B. Hour
    C. 2 hours
    D. 3 hours
25. The back-lying position is called
    A. Fowler's position
    B. The supine position
    C. The prone position
    D. Sims' position

REVIEW

26. A client is positioned in a chair. The feet
    A. Must be flat on the floor
    B. Are crossed
    C. Dangle
    D. Must be positioned on pillows

27. When transferring a client to bed, a chair, or the toilet
    A. The client's strong side moves first
    B. The weak side moves first
    C. Pillows are used for support
    D. The transfer belt cannot be used

28. These statements are about transfers to and from a toilet. Which is *false*?
    A. The client wears nonskid footwear.
    B. Wheelchair brakes must be locked.
    C. The wheelchair is positioned so the client's strong side is near the toilet.
    D. The client uses the towel bars for support.

Answers to these questions are on page 824.

CHAPTER

22

Exercise and Activity

OBJECTIVES

- Define the key terms listed in this chapter
- Describe bed rest
- Describe the complications of bed rest and how to prevent them
- Describe the devices used to support and maintain body alignment
- Explain the purpose of a trapeze
- Describe range-of-motion exercises
- Explain how to help a falling client
- Describe four walking aids
- Learn the procedures described in this chapter

KEY TERMS

abduction Moving a body part away from the midline of the body

adduction Moving a body part toward the midline of the body

ambulation The act of walking

atrophy A decrease in size or a wasting away of tissue

brace An apparatus worn to support or align weak body parts or to prevent or correct problems with the muscoskeletal system; orthosis

contracture The lack of joint mobility caused by abnormal shortening of a muscle

deconditioning The loss of muscle strength from inactivity

dorsiflexion Bending the toes and foot up at the ankle

extension Straightening a body part

external rotation Turning the joint outward

flexion Bending a body part

footdrop The foot falls down at the ankle (permanent plantar flexion)

hyperextension Excessive straightening of a body part

internal rotation Turning the joint inward

orthosis A brace

orthostatic hypotension A drop in (*hypo*) blood pressure when the person stands (*ortho* and *static*); postural hypotension

plantar flexion The foot (*plantar*) is bent (*flexion*)

postural hypotension Orthostatic hypotension

pronation Turning downward

range of motion (ROM) The movement of a joint to the extent possible without causing pain

rotation Turning the joint

supination Turning upward

syncope A brief loss of consciousness; fainting

Being active is important for physical and mental well-being. Most people move about and function without help. However, illnesses, surgery, injuries, pain, and aging cause weakness and some activity limits. Some people are weak from chronic illnesses. Others are in bed for a long time. Some have permanent paralysis. Some disorders are progressive, causing decreases in activity. Examples include multiple sclerosis, Parkinson's disease, arthritis, and nervous system and muscular disorders (see Chapter 31). Inactivity, whether mild or severe, affects the normal function of every body system. Mental well-being also is affected.

Deconditioning is the loss of muscle strength from inactivity. When not active, older adults become deconditioned quickly. Each client is encouraged to be as active as possible. The care plan tells you about the client's activity level and what exercises to perform.

To help promote exercise and activity, you need to understand:

- Bed rest
- How to prevent complications from bed rest
- How to help clients exercise

Bed Rest

Bed rest is ordered by the physician to treat a health problem. Generally bed rest is ordered to:

- Reduce physical activity
- Reduce pain
- Encourage rest
- Regain strength
- Promote healing

You must know the activities allowed for each client. The care plan has this information. Check with your supervisor if you have questions. These types of bed rest are common:

- *Bed rest*—some activities of daily living (ADL) are allowed. Self-feeding, oral hygiene, bathing, shaving, and hair care are often allowed.
- *Strict bed rest*—everything is done for the client. No ADL are allowed.
- *Bed rest with commode privileges*—the client can use the bedside commode for elimination needs.
- *Bed rest with bathroom privileges (bed rest with BRP)*—the client can use the bathroom for elimination needs.

Always ask your supervisor what bed rest means for each client.

Complications of Bed Rest

Bed rest and lack of exercise and activity can cause serious complications. Every body system is affected. Pressure ulcers, constipation, and fecal impaction can result. Urinary tract infections, renal calculi (kidney stones), blood clots (thrombi), and pneumonia (infection of the lung) can occur (see Chapter 31).

Contractures and muscle atrophy occur in the musculoskeletal system. A **contracture** is the lack of joint mobility caused by the abnormal shortening of a muscle. The contracted muscle is fixed into position, is deformed, and cannot stretch (Figure 22-1). Common sites are the fingers, wrists, elbows, toes, ankles, knees, and hips. Contractures can occur also in the neck and spine. The person with a contracture is permanently deformed and disabled. **Atrophy** is the decrease in size or the wasting away of tissue. Muscle atrophy is a decrease in size or a wasting away of muscle (Figure 22-2). These complications must be prevented to maintain normal body movement.

Orthostatic hypotension and blood clots (see Chapter 45) occur in the cardiovascular system. **Orthostatic hypotension** (**postural hypotension**) is a drop in (*hypo*) blood pressure when the person stands (*ortho* and *static*). When a person moves from lying or sitting to a standing position, the blood pressure drops. The person experiences dizziness, weakness, and spots before the eyes. Syncope can occur. **Syncope** (fainting) is a brief loss of consciousness. (Syncope comes from the Greek word *synkoptein,* which means to cut short.) Box 22-1 lists the measures that prevent orthostatic hypotension. Slowly changing positions is an important measure.

You can help prevent complications from bed rest by providing good care. Make sure the client is in good body alignment. Reposition the client at least once every two hours following the care plan (see Chapter 21). Also help with range-of-motion exercises according to the care plan (see page 312).

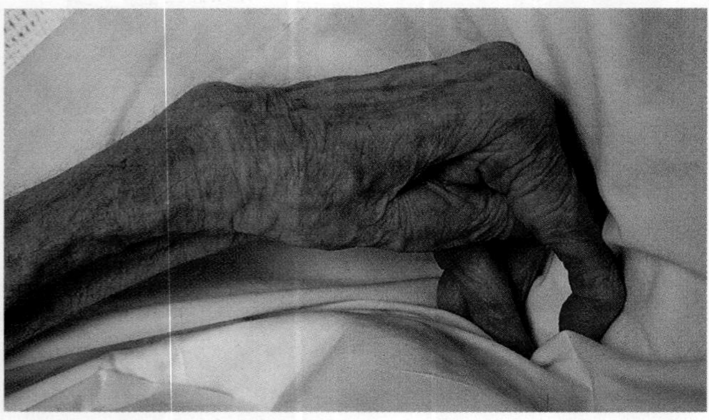

Figure 22-1 A contracture.

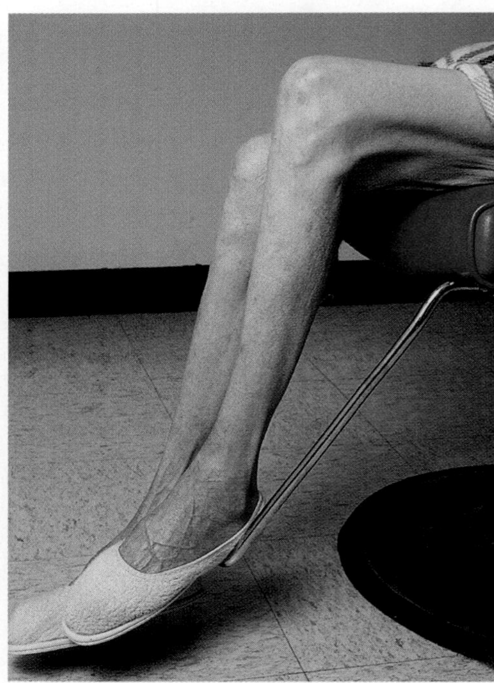

Figure 22-2 Muscle atrophy.

Box 22-1 Preventing Orthostatic Hypotension When Helping a Client from a Lying to a Standing Position

- Measure blood pressure, pulse, and respirations when the client is supine.*
- Position the client in Fowler's position. Raise the head of the bed slowly. Or, use pillows and backrests for positioning if the bed does not raise.
  - Ask the client about weakness, dizziness, or spots before the eyes. Lower the head of the bed or remove backrest if these symptoms occur.
  - Measure blood pressure, pulse, and respirations.*
  - Keep the client in Fowler's position for a short while. Ask the client about weakness, dizziness, or spots before the eyes.
- Help the client to sit on the side of the bed (see Chapter 21).
  - Ask the client about weakness, dizziness, or spots before the eyes. Assist the client to Fowler's position if any of these symptoms occur.
  - Measure blood pressure, pulse, and respirations.*
  - Have the client continue to sit on the side of the bed for a short while.
- Help the client to stand.
  - Ask the client about weakness, dizziness, or spots before the eyes. Help the client sit on the side of the bed if any of these symptoms occur.
  - Measure blood pressure, pulse, and respirations.*
- Help the client sit in a chair or walk as directed by the care plan.
  - Ask the client about weakness, dizziness, or spots before the eyes. If the client is walking, help the client to sit if symptoms occur.
  - Measure blood pressure, pulse, and respirations.*
- Report blood pressure, pulse, and respirations to your supervisor.* Also report other observations or complaints.

*Measure blood pressure, pulse, and respirations only if instructed (and allowed) to do so. Know your scope of practice and employer policy.

POSITIONING

Body alignment and positioning are discussed in Chapter 21. Supportive devices are often used to support and maintain the client in a certain position:

- *Bed boards*—are placed under the mattress. They prevent the mattress from sagging (Figure 22-3). They are usually made of plywood and are covered with canvas or other material. There are two sections so the head of the bed can be raised. One section is for the head of the bed and the other for the foot of the bed.
- *Foot boards*—are placed at the foot of mattresses (Figure 22-4). They prevent plantar flexion that can lead to footdrop. In **plantar flexion** the foot *(plantar)* is bent *(flexion)*. **Footdrop** occurs when the foot falls down at the ankle (permanent plantar flexion). The foot board is placed so the soles of the feet are flush against it. The feet are in good alignment as when standing. Foot boards also serve as bed cradles. They keep top linens off the feet.

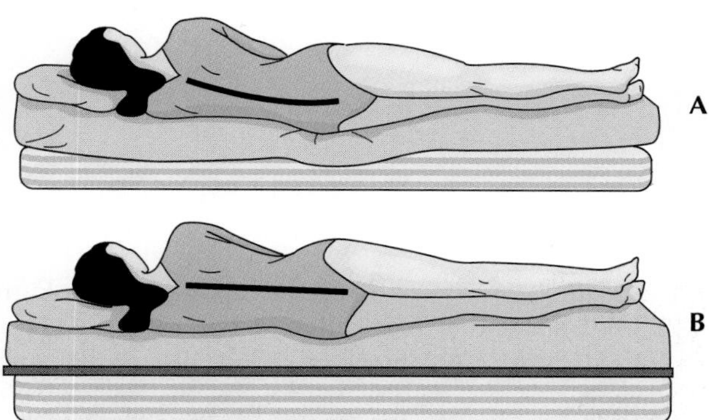

Figure 22-3 A, Mattress sagging without bed boards. **B,** Bed boards are placed under the mattress. No sagging occurs.

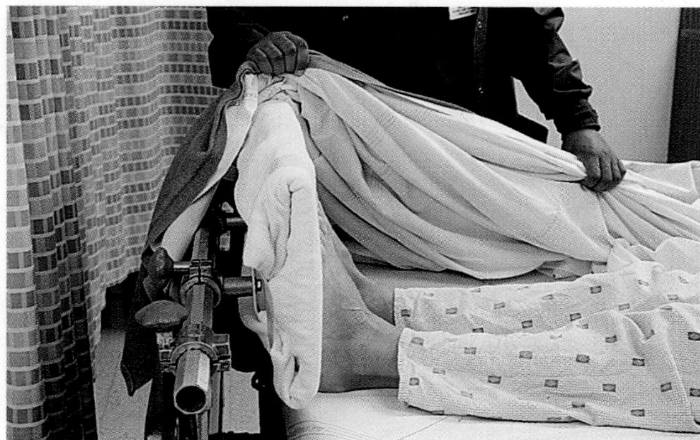

Figure 22-4 Foot board. Feet are flush with the board to keep them in normal alignment.

- *Trochanter rolls*—prevent the hips and legs from turning outward (external rotation) (Figure 22-5). They are made from bath blankets. A blanket is folded to the desired length and rolled up. The loose end is placed under the client from the hip to the knee. Then the roll is tucked alongside the body. Pillows or sandbags also are used to keep the hips and knees in alignment.

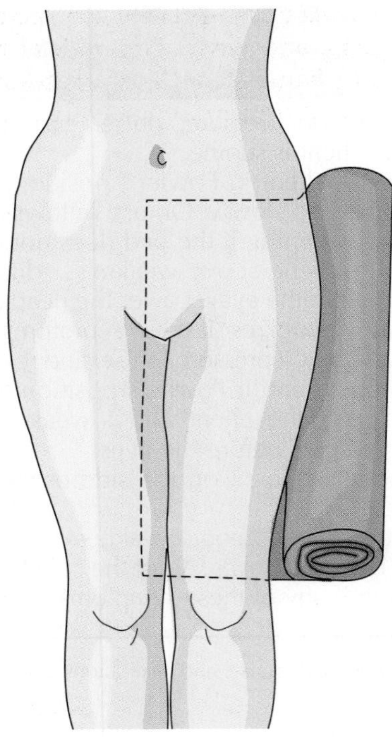

Figure 22-5 Trochanter roll made from a bath blanket. It extends from the hip to the knee.

- *Hip abduction wedges*—keep the hips abducted (Figure 22-6). The wedge is positioned between the client's legs. These are common after hip replacement surgery.

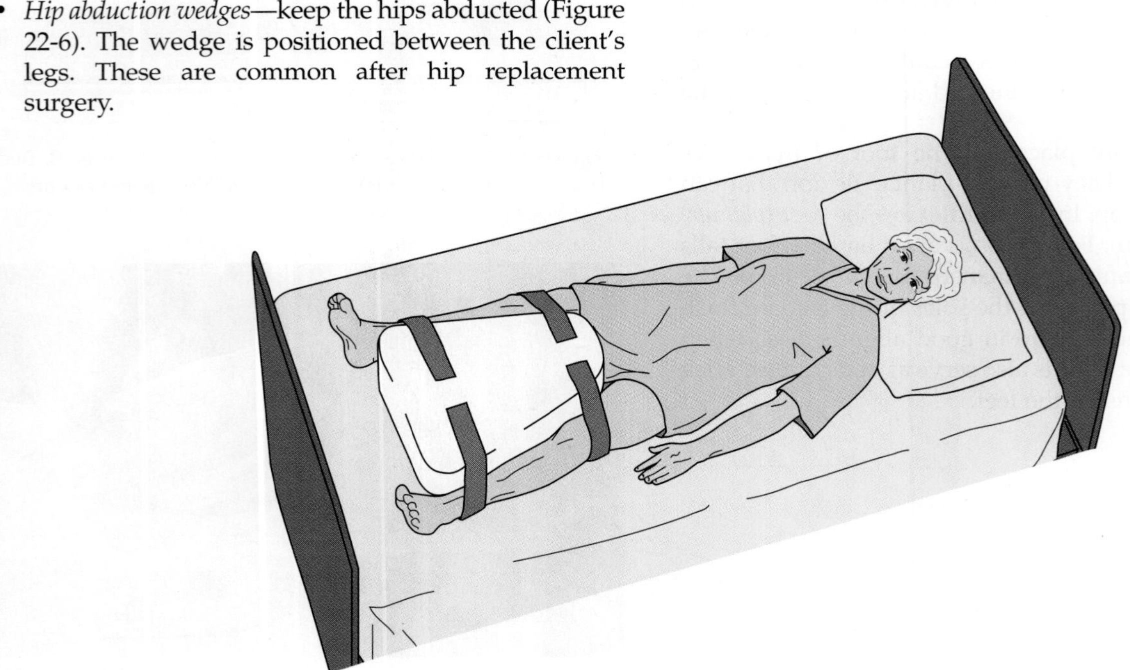

Figure 22-6 Hip abduction wedge.

- *Hand rolls or hand grips*—prevent contractures of the thumb, fingers, and wrist. Commercial hand rolls are common (Figure 22-7). Foam rubber sponges, rubber balls, and finger cushions (Figure 22-8) also are used.
- *Splints*—keep the wrist, thumb, and fingers in normal position. They are usually secured in place with Velcro. Some have foam padding (Figure 22-9).
- *Bed cradles*—keep the weight of top linens off the feet (see Figures 41-5 and 41-6 on page 684). The weight of top linens can cause footdrop and pressure ulcers.

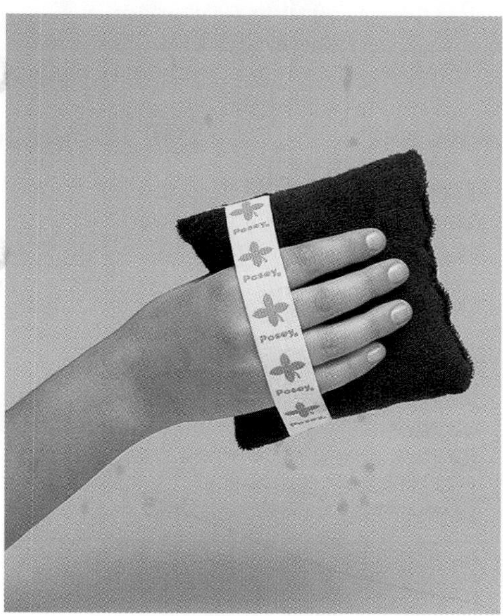

Figure 22-7 Hand grip. *(Courtesy J.T. Posey Co., Arcadia, CA.)*

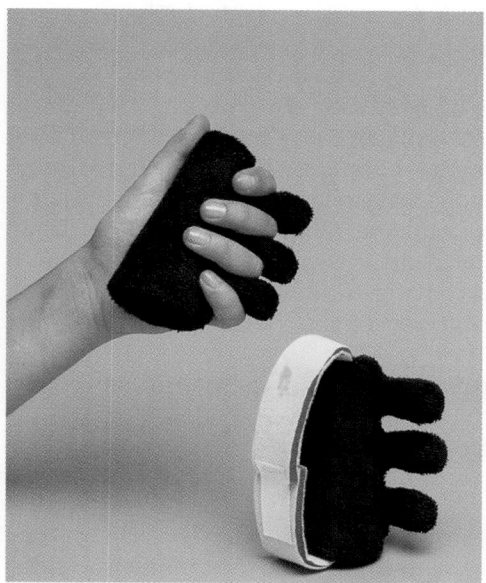

Figure 22-8 Finger cushion. *(Courtesy J.T. Posey Co., Arcadia, CA.)*

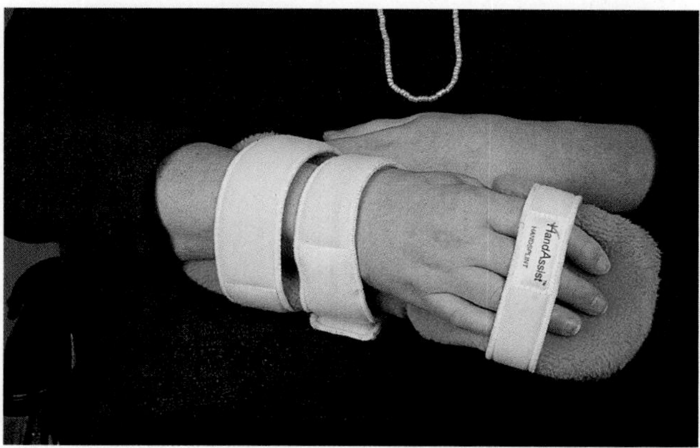

Figure 22-9 Splint.

EXERCISE

Exercise helps prevent contractures, muscle atrophy, and other complications of bed rest. Some exercise occurs with activities of daily living and from turning and moving in bed without assistance. Additional exercises are needed for muscles and joints.

A trapeze is used for exercises to strengthen arm muscles. The trapeze is suspended from an overbed frame (Figure 22-10). The client grasps the bar with both hands to lift the trunk off the bed. The trapeze is also used to move up and turn in bed (see Chapter 21).

Range-of-Motion Exercises. The movement of a joint to the extent possible without causing pain is the **range of motion (ROM)** of that joint. Range-of-motion exercises involve exercising the joints through their complete range of motion (Box 22-2). Clients who need these exercises usually do them at least twice a day. Range-of-motion exercises are active, passive, or active-assistive:

- *Active* range-of-motion exercises are done by the client.
- *Passive* range-of-motion exercises involve having another person move the joints through their range of motion.
- *Active-assistive* range-of-motion exercises are done by the client with some help from another person.

Range-of-motion exercises naturally occur during activities of daily living. Bathing, hair care, eating, reaching, and walking all involve joint movements. Clients on bed rest have little activity. So do clients who have mobility loss from illness or injury. Therefore, their care plans usually call for range-of-motion exercises. The care plan tells you which joints to exercise and whether the exercises are to be active, passive, or active-assistive. If you have questions, ask your supervisor. (See *Focus on Children: Play* and *Focus on Long-Term Care: Activity Programs* boxes.)

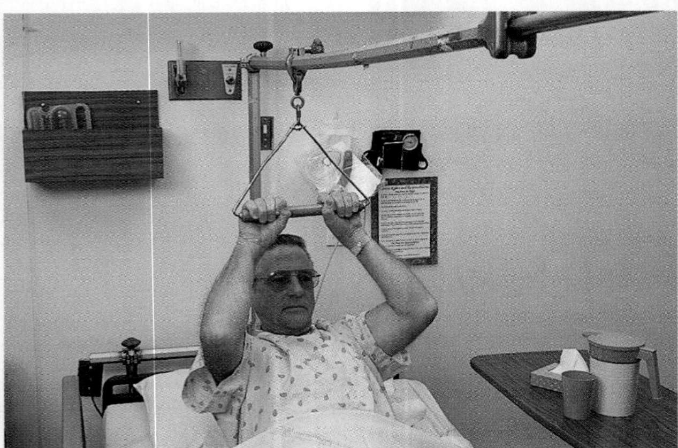

Figure 22-10 A trapeze is used to strengthen the arm muscles.

Box 22-2 Joint Movements

Abduction—moving a body part away from the midline of the body
Adduction—moving a body part toward the midline of the body
Extension—straightening a body part
Flexion—bending a body part
Hyperextension—excessive straightening of a body part
Dorsiflexion—bending the toes and foot up at the ankle
Rotation—turning the joint
Internal rotation—turning the joint inward
External rotation—turning the joint outward
Plantar flexion—bending the foot down at the ankle
Pronation—turning downward
Supination—turning upward

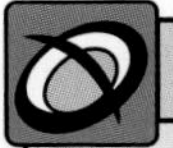

Focus on Children

PLAY

Depending on the child's activity limits, any play activity promotes active range-of-motion exercises in children. Some examples are:

- Kicking a Mylar balloon or foam rubber ball
- Playing "pat-a-cake" and having the child clap, kick, jump, or do other motions
- Playing basketball using a wastebasket and a foam rubber ball or wadded paper
- Playing video games for finger and hand movements
- Playing with finger paints, clay, or play dough
- Having tricycle or wheelchair races
- Playing "hide and seek" by hiding a toy in the bed or room

Always check the care plan for the child's activity limits. If you are still unsure, check with your supervisor.

Source: Adapted from D. L. Wong, *Whaley and Wong's Nursing Care of Infants and Children*, 6th ed. (St. Louis: Mosby, 1999).

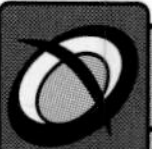

Focus on Long-Term Care

Activity Programs

Provincial and territorial long-term care legislation requires that long-term care facilities have an assessment and care planning process to prevent unnecessary reduction in a resident's range of motion. Prevention involves active, active-assistive, or passive range-of-motion exercises. Splints and braces are used if needed.

Long-term care legislation also requires activity programs for residents. Recreational activities are important for the physical and mental well-being of older adults. Joints and muscles are exercised, and circulation is stimulated. Recreational activities also provide social opportunities and are mentally stimulating.

The activities must meet the interests and physical and psychosocial needs of each resident. Bingo, movies, dances, exercise groups, shopping trips, museum trips, concerts, and guest speakers are often arranged. Some facilities have gardening activities.

The right to personal choice is protected. The resident chooses which activities to take part in. Activities should promote physical, intellectual, social, and emotional well-being. Well-being is promoted when the resident attends activities of personal choice. The resident must not be forced to take part in an activity that has no interest to him or her.

Residents may need help getting to an activity. Some also need help in participating. You must provide assistance as necessary.

Activity ideas are always welcome. Residents may share ideas with you or tell you about favourite pastimes. Or you may have ideas. Share these with the health care team. They are given to the resident group that plans activities.

Range-of-motion exercises can cause injury if not done properly. Muscle strain, joint injury, and pain are possible. Follow the guidelines in Box 22-3 when performing or assisting with range-of-motion exercises.

Report and record the following after performing range-of-motion exercises:

- The time the exercises were performed
- The joints exercised
- The number of times the exercises were performed on each joint
- Complaints of pain or signs of stiffness or spasm
- The degree to which the client took part in the exercises

(text continues on page 319)

Box 22-3 Guidelines for Performing Range-of-Motion Exercises

- Exercise only the joints you are instructed to exercise.
- Expose only the body part being exercised.
- Use good body mechanics.
- Support the part being exercised.
- Move the joint slowly, smoothly, and gently.
- Do not force a joint beyond its present range of motion or to the point of pain.
- *Perform range-of-motion exercises to the neck only if allowed by employer policy.* In some facilities and agencies, only physical or occupational therapists do neck exercises. This is because of the danger of neck injuries.

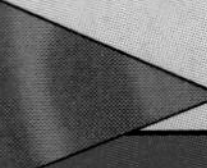

Performing Range-of-Motion Exercises

Compassionate Care

Remember to Promote:
- **Dignity**
- **Independence**
- **Preferences**
- **Privacy**
- **Safety**

Pre-Procedure

1 Identify the person according to employer policy.
2 Explain the procedure to the person.
3 Wash your hands.
4 Obtain a bath blanket.
5 Provide for privacy.
6 Raise bed to a comfortable working height. Follow the care plan for bed rail use.*

Procedure

7 Lower the bed rail near you if up.
8 Position the person supine.
9 Cover the person with a bath blanket. Fanfold top linens to the foot of the bed.
10 Exercise the neck *if allowed by your employer and if your supervisor instructs you to do so* (Figure 22-11, page 316):
- a Place your hands over the person's ears to support the head. Support the jaws with your fingers.
- b *Flexion*—bring the head forward. The chin touches the chest.
- c *Extension*—straighten the head.
- d *Hyperextension*—bring the head backward until the chin points up.
- e *Rotation*—turn the head from side to side.
- f *Lateral flexion*—move the head to the right and to the left.
- g Repeat b through f 5 times—or the number of times stated on the care plan.

11 Exercise the shoulder (Figure 22-12, page 316):
- a Grasp the wrist with one hand. Grasp the elbow with your other hand.
- b *Flexion*—raise the arm straight in front and over the head.
- c *Extension*—bring the arm down to the side.
- d *Hyperextension*—move the arm behind the body. (Do this if the person sits in a straight-backed chair or is standing.)
- e *Abduction*—move the straight arm away from the side of the body.
- f *Adduction*—move the straight arm to the side of the body.
- g *Internal rotation*—bend the elbow. Place it at the same level as the shoulder. Move the forearm down toward the body.
- h *External rotation*—Move the forearm toward the head.
- i Repeat b through h 5 times—or the number of times stated on the care plan.

12 Exercise the elbow (Figure 22-13, page 316):
- a Grasp the person's wrist with one hand. Grasp the elbow with your other hand.
- b *Flexion*—bend the arm so the hand touches the same-side shoulder.
- c *Extension*—Straighten the arm.
- d Repeat b and c 5 times—or the number of times stated on the care plan.

13 Exercise the forearm (Figure 22-14, page 316):
- a *Pronation*—turn the hand so the palm is down.
- b *Supination*—turn the hand so the palm is up.
- c Repeat a and b 5 times—or the number of times stated on the care plan.

Continued

Performing Range-of-Motion Exercises—cont'd

Procedure—cont'd

14 Exercise the wrist (Figure 22-15, page 317):
- a Hold the wrist with both of your hands.
- b *Flexion*—bend the hand down.
- c *Extension*—straighten the hand.
- d *Hyperextension*—bend the hand back.
- e *Radial flexion*—turn the hand toward the thumb.
- f *Ulnar flexion*—turn the hand toward the little finger.
- g Repeat b through f 5 times—or the number of times stated on the care plan.

15 Exercise the thumb (Figure 22-16, page 317):
- a Hold the person's hand with one hand. Hold the thumb with your other hand.
- b *Abduction*—move the thumb out from the inner part of the index finger.
- c *Adduction*—move the thumb back next to the index finger.
- d *Opposition*—touch each fingertip with the thumb.
- e *Flexion*—bend the thumb into the hand.
- f *Extension*—move the thumb out to the side of the fingers.
- g Repeat b through f 5 times—or the number of times stated on the care plan.

16 Exercise the fingers (Figure 22-17, page 317):
- a *Abduction*—spread the fingers and thumb apart.
- b *Adduction*—bring the fingers and thumb together.
- c *Extension*—straighten the fingers so the fingers, hand, and arm are straight.
- d *Flexion*—make a fist.
- e Repeat a through d 5 times—or the number of times stated on the care plan.

17 Exercise the hip (Figure 22-18, page 317):
- a Support the leg. Place one hand under the knee. Place your other hand under the ankle.
- b *Flexion*—raise the leg.
- c *Extension*—straighten the leg.
- d *Abduction*—move the leg away from the body.
- e *Adduction*—move the leg toward the other leg.
- f *Internal rotation*—turn the leg inward.
- g *External rotation*—turn the leg outward.
- h Repeat b through g 5 times—or the number of times stated on the care plan.

18 Exercise the knee (Figure 22-19, page 318):
- a Support the knee. Place one hand under the knee. Place your other hand under the ankle.
- b *Flexion*—bend the leg.
- c *Extension*—straighten the leg.
- d Repeat b and c 5 times—or the number of times stated on the care plan.

19 Exercise the ankle (Figure 22-20, page 318):
- a Support the foot and ankle. Place one hand under the foot. Place your other hand under the ankle.
- b *Dorsiflexion*—pull the foot forward. Push down on the heel at the same time.
- c *Plantar flexion*—turn the foot down. Or point the toes.
- d Repeat b and c 5 times—or the number of times stated on the care plan.

20 Exercise the foot (Figure 22-21, page 318):
- a Continue to support the foot and ankle.
- b *Pronation*—turn the outside of the foot up and the inside down.
- c *Supination*—turn the inside of the foot up and the outside down.
- d Repeat b and c 5 times—or the number of times stated on the care plan.

21 Exercise the toes (Figure 22-22, page 318):
- a *Flexion*—curl the toes.
- b *Extension*—straighten the toes.
- c *Abduction*—spread the toes apart.
- d *Adduction*—pull the toes together.
- e Repeat a through d 5 times—or the number of times stated on the care plan.

22 Cover the leg.

23 Raise the bed rail if used. Go to the other side. Lower the bed rail near you if up.

24 Repeat steps 11 through 21.

Continued

Performing Range-of-Motion Exercises—cont'd

Post-Procedure

25 Cover the person. Remove the bath blanket.
26 Provide for safety and comfort.
27 Place the call bell within reach.*
28 Return the bed to its lowest position. Follow the care plan for bed rail use.*
29 Remove privacy measures.
30 Return the bath blanket to its proper place.
31 Wash your hands.
32 Report and record your actions and observations according to employer policy.

*Steps marked with an asterisk may not apply in community settings.

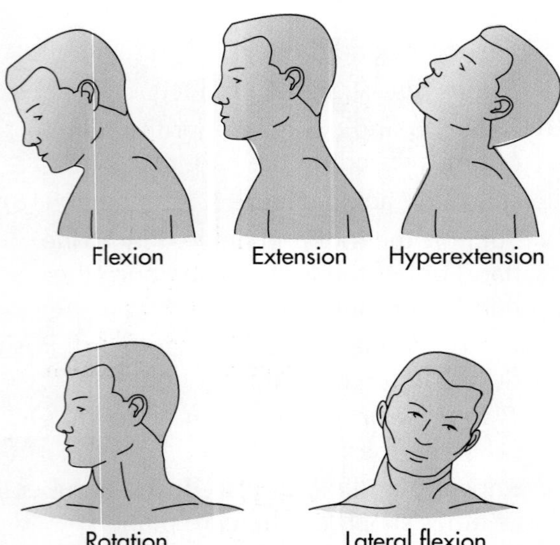

Figure 22-11 Range-of-motion exercises for the neck.

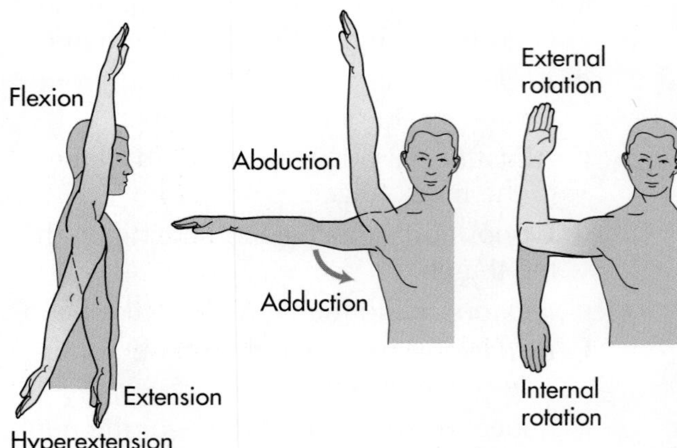

Figure 22-12 Range-of-motion exercises for the shoulder.

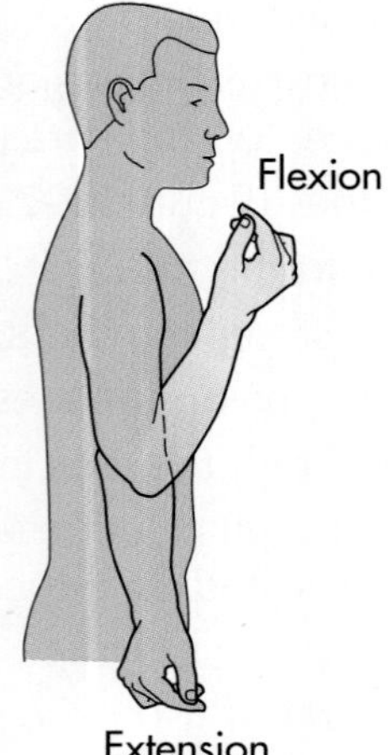

Figure 22-13 Range-of-motion exercises for the elbow.

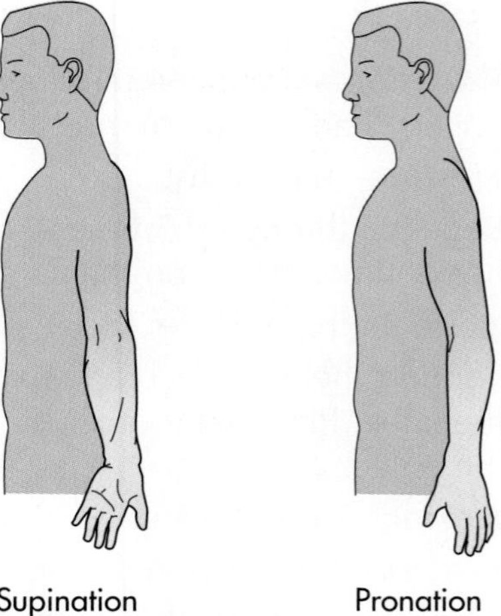

Figure 22-14 Range-of-motion exercises for the forearm.

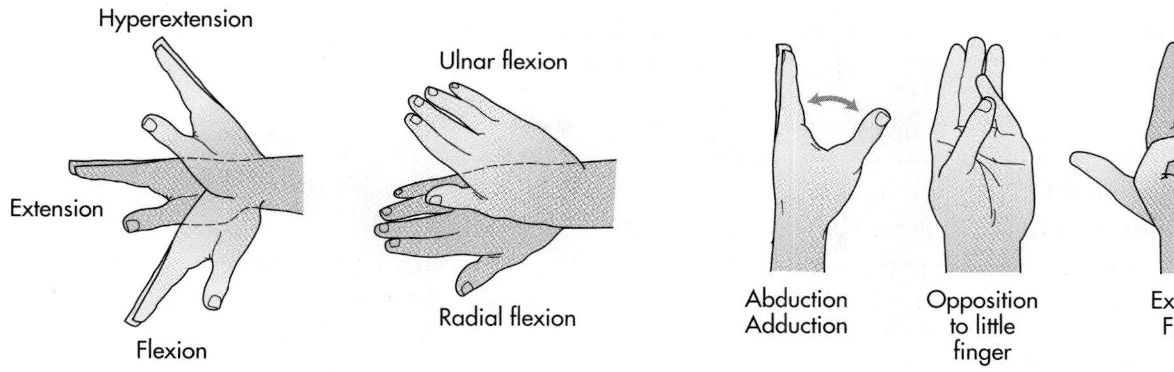

Figure 22-15 Range-of-motion exercises for the wrist.

Figure 22-16 Range-of-motion exercises for the thumb.

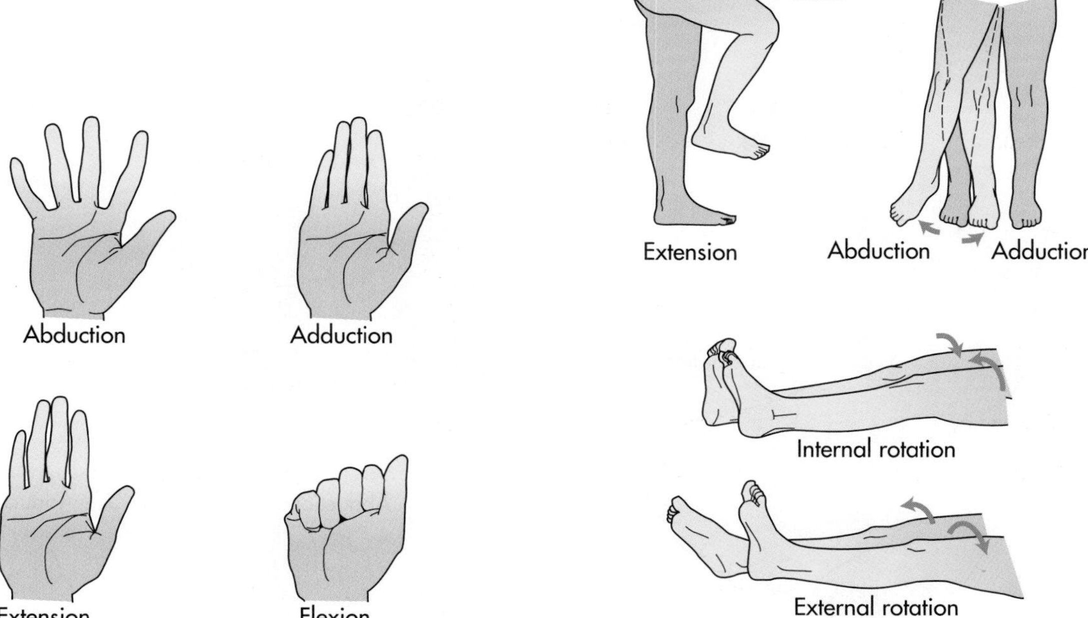

Figure 22-17 Range-of-motion exercises for the fingers.

Figure 22-18 Range-of-motion exercises for the hip.

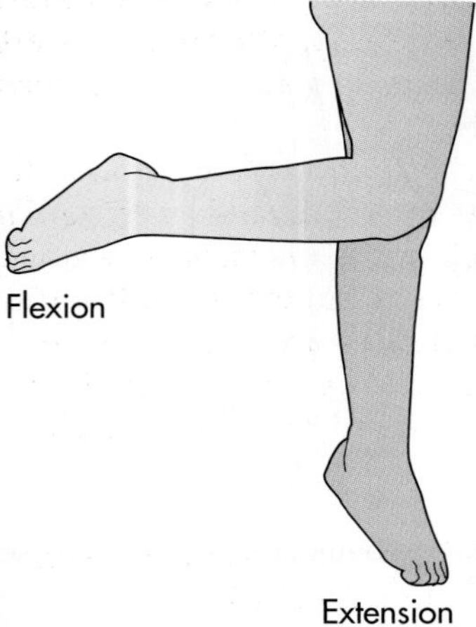

Figure 22-19 Range-of-motion exercises for the knee.

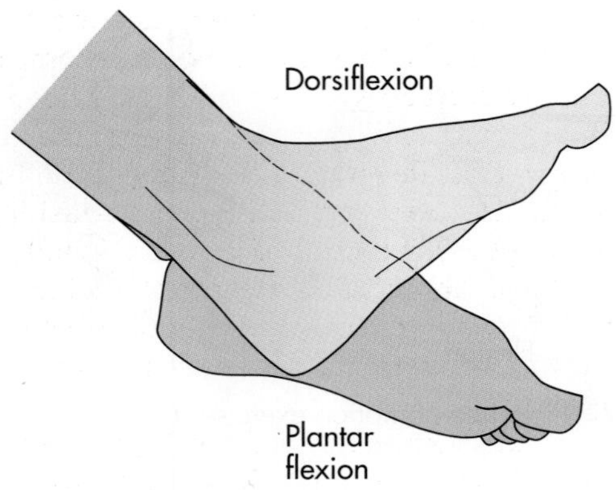

Figure 22-20 Range-of-motion exercises for the ankle.

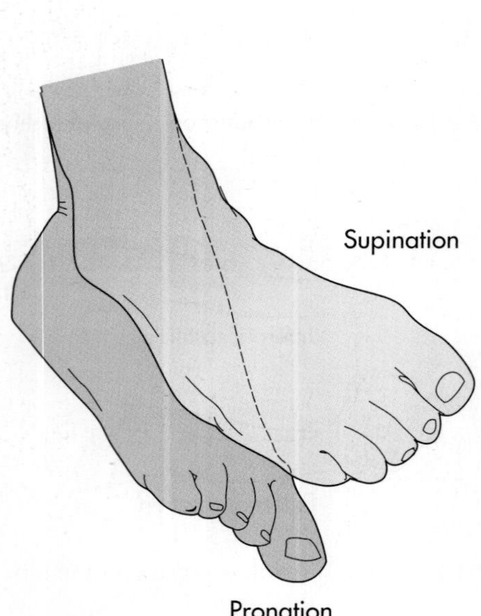

Figure 22-21 Range-of-motion exercises for the foot.

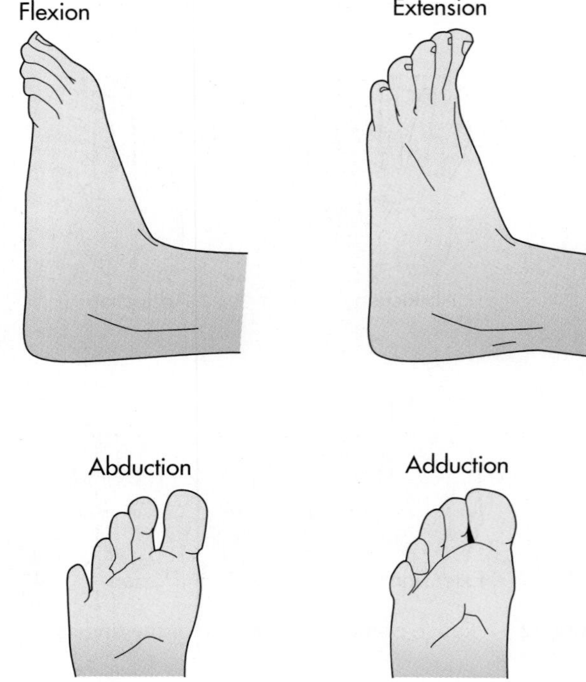

Figure 22-22 Range-of-motion exercises for the toes.

AMBULATION

Walking regularly helps prevent deconditioning. Many clients need help walking. Some become strong enough to walk alone. Others will always need help.

After bed rest, activity is usually increased slowly and in steps. First the person dangles (sits on the side of the bed). The next step is to sit in a bedside chair. Walking about in the room and then in the hallway are the next steps. **Ambulation**, the act of walking, is not a problem if complications (such as contractures and muscle atrophy) were prevented by proper positioning and exercise.

Some clients are weak and unsteady. Use a gait (transfer) belt when helping them walk (see Chapter 21). Encourage the client to use hand rails along the wall for additional support. Always check the client for orthostatic hypotension.

Before beginning the walk, remove any obstacles in your path. If necessary, place a chair nearby in case the client needs to rest. Make sure the client is wearing nonskid footwear.

Personal choice in walking should be encouraged. The client may want to walk outside. The client may prefer to walk in the morning, afternoon, or evening. Or the client may want to wait until a visitor arrives or leaves. Such choices are allowed whenever safe and possible. Be sure to get your supervisor's approval.

Report and record the following after helping with ambulation:

- How well the person tolerated the activity
- Complaints of pain or discomfort
- The distance walked

(text continues on page 321)

Helping the Person to Walk

COMPASSIONATE CARE

Remember to Promote:
- **Dignity**
- **Independence**
- **Preferences**
- **Privacy**
- **Safety**

Pre-Procedure

1 Identify the person according to employer policy.
2 Explain the procedure to the person.
3 Wash your hands.
4 Collect the following:
   - Robe and nonskid shoes
   - Paper or sheet to protect bottom linens
   - Gait (transfer) belt
5 Provide for privacy.

Procedure

6 Lower the bed to its lowest position. Lock the bed wheels. Lower the bed rail if used.*
7 Fanfold top linens to the foot of the bed.
8 Place the paper or sheet under the person's feet. This protects the bottom sheet from the shoes. Put the shoes on the person.
9 Help the person to dangle. (See *Helping the Person Sit on the Side of the Bed (Dangle),* page 282.)
10 Help the person put on the robe.
11 Apply the gait belt. (See *Applying a Transfer Belt,* page 290.)
12 Help the person stand. (See *Transferring the Person to a Chair or Wheelchair,* page 291.) Grasp the gait belt on each side. Or place your arms under the person's arms around to the shoulder blades.
13 Stand at the person's side while he or she gains balance. Hold the belt at the side and back. Or have one arm around the back to support the person.
14 Encourage the person to stand erect with the head up and back straight.

Continued

Helping the Person to Walk—cont'd

Procedure—cont'd

15 Help the person walk. Walk to the side and slightly behind the person. Provide support with the gait belt (Figure 22-23). Or have one arm around the back to support the person.

16 Encourage the person to walk normally. The heel strikes the floor first. Discourage shuffling, sliding, or walking on tiptoes.

17 Walk the required distance if the person can tolerate the activity. Do not rush the person.

18 Help the person return to bed:
- a Have the person stand at the side of the bed.
- b Pivot him or her a quarter turn. The backs of the knees should touch the bed.
- c Grasp the sides of the gait belt.
- d Lower the person onto the bed as you bend your knees. Remove gait belt and robe.
- e Help the person lie down. (See *Helping the Person Sit on the Side of the Bed (Dangle),* page 282.)

19 Help the person to the centre of the bed.

20 Remove footwear. Remove the paper or sheet over the bottom sheet.

Post-Procedure

21 Provide for safety and comfort.

22 Place the call bell within reach.*

23 Follow the care plan for bed rail use.*

24 Remove privacy measures.

25 Return the robe and shoes to their proper place.

26 Wash your hands.

27 Report and record your actions and observations according to employer policy.

*Steps marked with an asterisk may not apply in community settings.

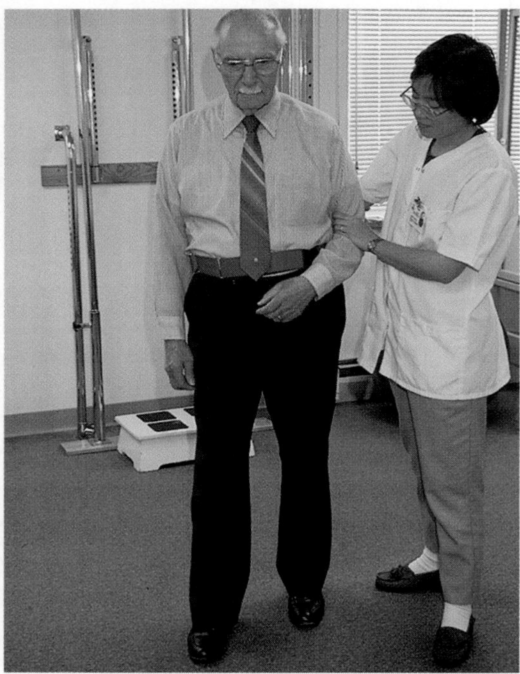

Figure 22-23 Assist with ambulation by walking slightly behind the client's side. Use a gait belt for the client's safety.

FALLS

A client may start to fall when standing or walking. The client may be weak, lightheaded, or dizzy. Fainting may occur. Falling may be caused by slipping or sliding on spills, waxed floors, throw rugs, or by wearing improper shoes (see Chapter 16).

When a client is falling, the tendency is to try to prevent the fall. However, trying to prevent a fall could cause greater harm. You could injure yourself and the client as you twist and strain to stop the fall. Or you could lose your balance. Thus both you and the client could fall. Head, hip, and knee injuries are common from falls.

If a client starts to fall, ease him or her to the floor. This lets you control the direction of the fall. You can also protect the person's head.

Your response after the fall will depend on whether you work in a facility with help readily available or in a private home where you will likely be working alone. (See *Focus on Home Care: When a Client Falls* box.)

If a client falls in a facility, do not move or allow him or her to get up. Remain calm and reassure the client. Call for a nurse to check the client for injuries. Afterwards, complete an incident report as required by facility policy.

(text continues on page 323)

Focus on Home Care

WHEN A CLIENT FALLS

When working in a private home, you will not have a nurse present to help if a client falls. Be aware of any procedures required by your employer before a fall occurs. Use the following as a guide.

If a client starts to fall, ease him or her to the floor (see *Helping the Falling Person* on page 322). After the fall, check for signs of a fracture, including the following:

- The client feels pain or tenderness.
- The client has swelling or bruising.
- The client is unable or has difficulty moving a limb.
- The client reports having felt or heard a bone snap or pop.

If you observe any of the above, or if you suspect the person has a head, neck, or back injury, *do not move the client.* Call your supervisor for help. Keep the client warm and calm, and stay with him or her until help arrives.

If the client is unhurt and is able to assist, help him or her up. Follow these steps:

- Place a chair beside the client. Have the client use the armrests for support.
- Support the client's hips and assist him or her into a kneeling position, facing the chair.
- Have the client rest his or her forearms on the chair.
- Tell the client to lift one knee and place the foot on the floor. Assist as required.
- On the count of "3," help the client push up, stand, and pivot into the chair, while holding onto the armrests.
- Once in the chair, let the client rest before assisting him or her up again.

Report the fall to your supervisor. Complete an occurrence (incident) report according to employer policy.

Helping the Falling Person

Procedure

1 Stand with your feet apart. Keep your back straight.

2 Bring the person close to your body as quickly as possible. Use the gait belt if one is worn. If not, wrap your arms around the person's waist. You can also hold the person under the arms (Figure 22-24, *A*).

3 Move your leg so the person's buttocks rest on it (Figure 22-24, *B*). Move the leg near the person.

4 Lower the person to the floor. Let him or her slide down your leg to the floor (Figure 22-24, *C*). Bend at your hips and knees as you lower the person.

5 After the fall:

a If you are in a facility, call for a nurse. Stay with the person.

b If you are in a home care setting, check for obvious signs of injury. *If you suspect injury, do not move the person.* Call your supervisor. Keep the person warm and calm until help arrives. If the person is not injured and can assist, help the person up.

6 Report and record the following according to employer policy:

- How the fall occurred
- How far the person walked
- How activity was tolerated before the fall
- Any complaints before the fall
- The amount of assistance needed by the person while walking

7 Complete an incident report.

A

B

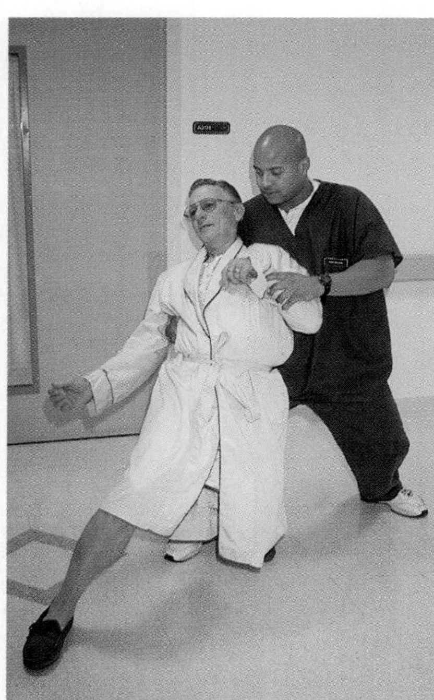

C

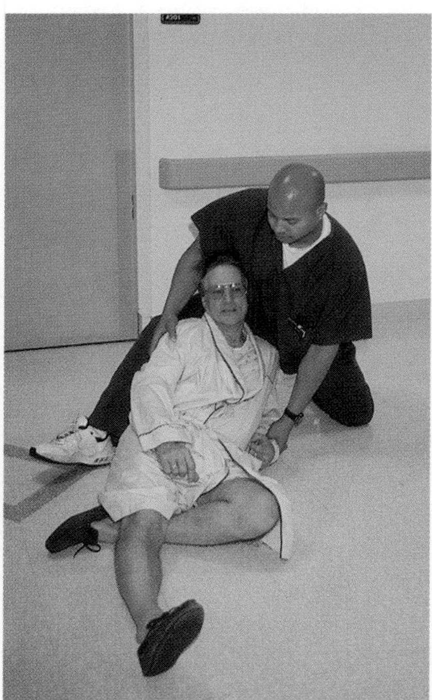

Figure 22-24 Helping a client who is falling. **A,** Hold the client close to your body. **B,** Move your leg to support the client's buttocks. **C,** Slide the client down your leg to the floor.

Walking Aids

Walking aids support the body. They are ordered by the physician, RN, or physical therapist. The type ordered depends on the client's physical condition, the amount of support needed, and the type of disability. The physical therapist or RN teaches the person to use the walking aid. Its use may be temporary or permanent.

Crutches. Crutches are used when the client cannot use one leg or when one or both legs need to gain strength. Some people with permanent leg weakness can use crutches. They usually use Lofstrand crutches (Figure 22-25). These crutches are made of metal. A metal band fits around the forearm. Axillary crutches extend from the underarm (*axilla*) to the ground (Figure 22-26). They are made of wood or metal.

The client learns to crutch walk, climb up and down stairs, and sit and stand. Safety is important. The person on crutches is at risk for falls. Follow these safety measures:

- Check the crutch tips. They must not be worn down, torn, or wet. Replace worn or torn crutch tips. Tell your supervisor. Dry wet tips with a towel or paper towels.
- Check crutches for flaws. Check wooden crutches for cracks and metal crutches for bends. All bolts must be tight.
- Make sure the client wears flat, nonskid street shoes.
- Ensure the client's clothing fits well. Loose clothing may get caught between the crutches and underarms. Loose clothing can also hang forward and block the person's view of the feet and crutch tips.
- Practise safety measures to prevent falls (see Chapter 16).
- Keep crutches within the client's reach. Place them next to the person's chair or against a wall.

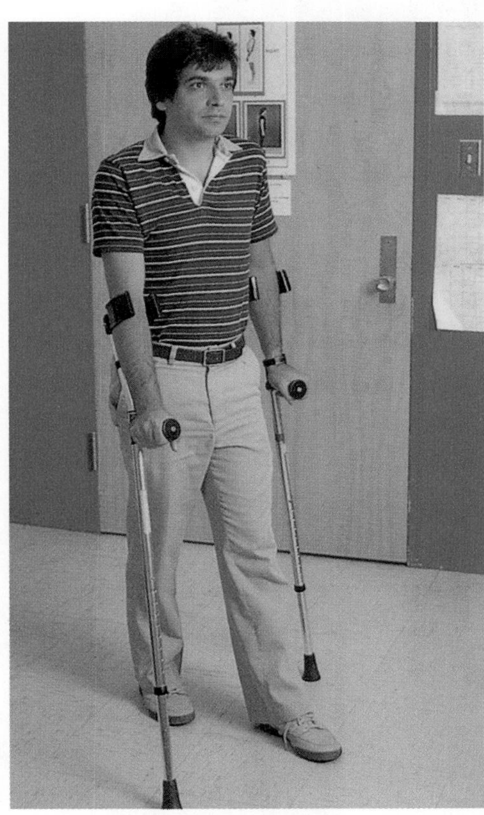

Figure 22-25 Lofstrand crutches. Source: M.K. Elkin, A.G. Perry, and P.A. Potter, *Nursing Interventions and Clinical Skills* (St. Louis: Mosby, 2000).

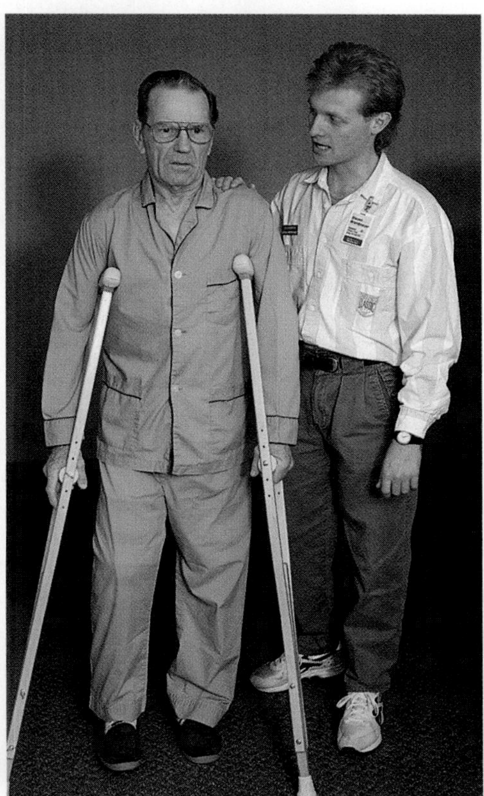

Figure 22-26 Axillary crutches. Source: M.K. Elkin, A.G. Perry, and P.A. Potter, *Nursing Interventions and Clinical Skills* (St. Louis: Mosby, 2000).

Canes. Canes are used for weakness on one side of the body. They help provide balance and support. There are single-tip and four-point (quad) canes (Figure 22-27). A cane is held on the *strong (unaffected) side* of the body. (If the left leg is weak, the cane is held in the right hand.) Four-point canes give more support than single-tip canes. However, they are harder to move.

The cane tip is about 15 to 25 cm (6 to 10 inches) to the side of the foot. It is about 15 to 25 cm (6 to 10 inches) in front of the foot on the strong side. The grip is level with the hip.

The person walks as follows:

Step A: The cane is moved forward 15 to 25 cm (6 to 10 inches) (Figure 22-28, *A*).

Step B: The weak leg (opposite the cane) is moved forward even with the cane (Figure 22-28, *B*).

Step C: The strong leg is brought forward and ahead of the cane and the weak leg (Figure 22-28, *C*).

A

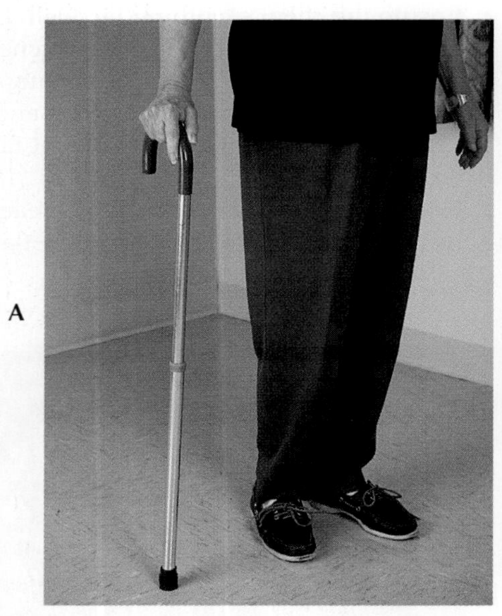

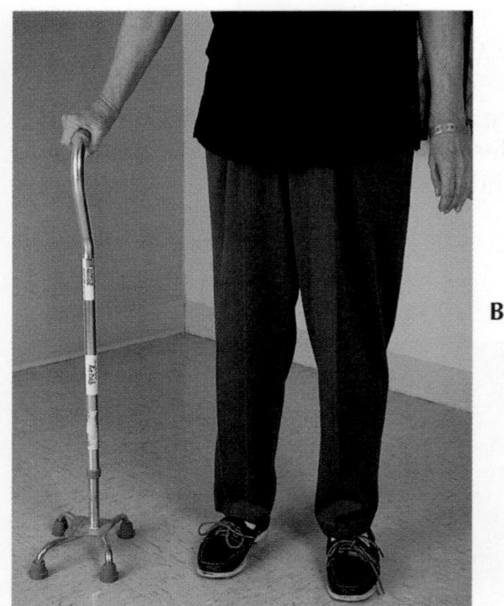

B

Figure 22-27 **A,** Single-tip cane. **B,** Four-point (quad) cane.

A

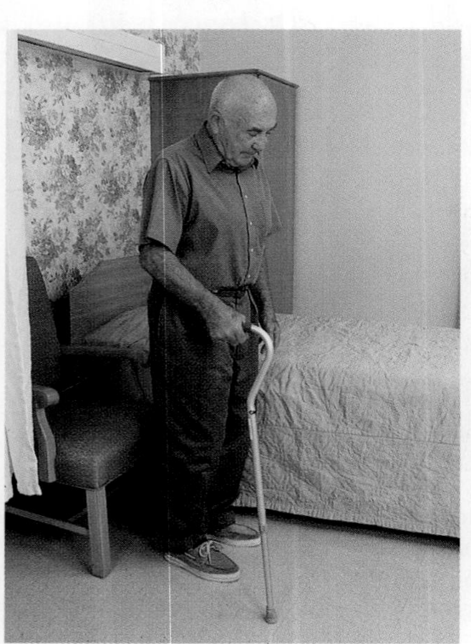

B

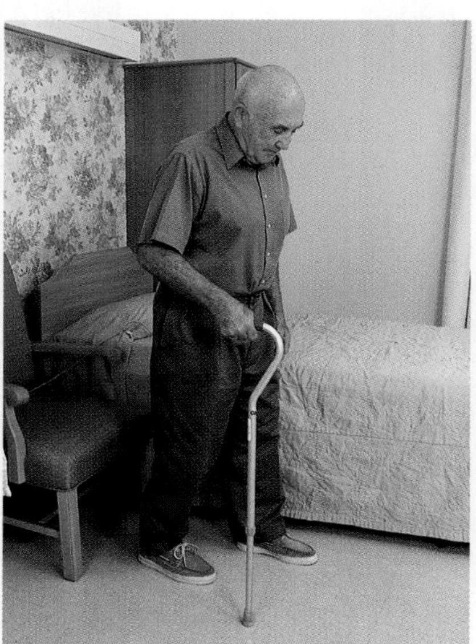

C

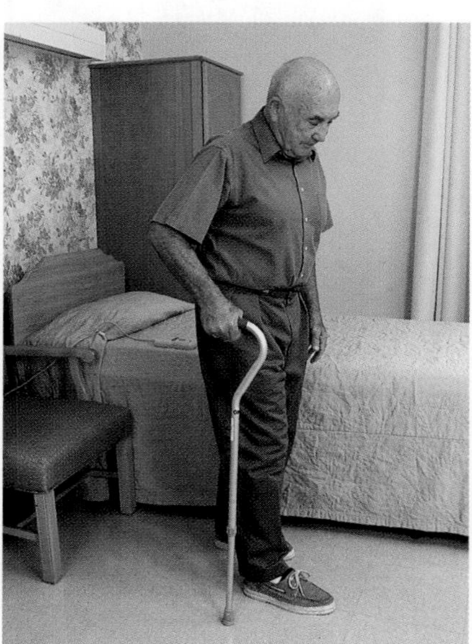

Figure 22-28 Walking with a cane. **A,** The cane is moved forward about 15 to 25 cm (6 to 10 inches). **B,** The leg opposite the cane (weak leg) is brought forward even with the cane. **C,** The leg on the cane side (strong leg) is moved ahead of the cane and the weak leg.

Walkers. A walker is a four-point walking aid (Figure 22-29). It gives more support than a cane. Many people feel safer and more secure with a walker than with a cane. There are many kinds of walkers. The standard walker is picked up and moved about 15 to 20 cm (6 to 8 inches) in front of the person. The person then moves the weak leg and foot and then the strong leg and foot up to the walker (Figure 22-30).

A wheeled walker has wheels on the front legs and rubber tips on the back legs (Figure 22-31). The person pushes the walker ahead about 15 to 20 cm (6 to 8 inches) and then walks up to it. The rubber tips on the back legs prevent the walker from moving while the person is walking or standing.

Baskets, pouches, and trays can be attached to walkers (see Figure 22-29). The attachment is used to carry needed items. The person is more independent and does not have to rely on others. The attachment also keeps the hands free to grip the walker.

The person uses the walker for support when moving from a standing to a sitting position. Assist clients with walkers as needed (Box 22-4 on page 326).

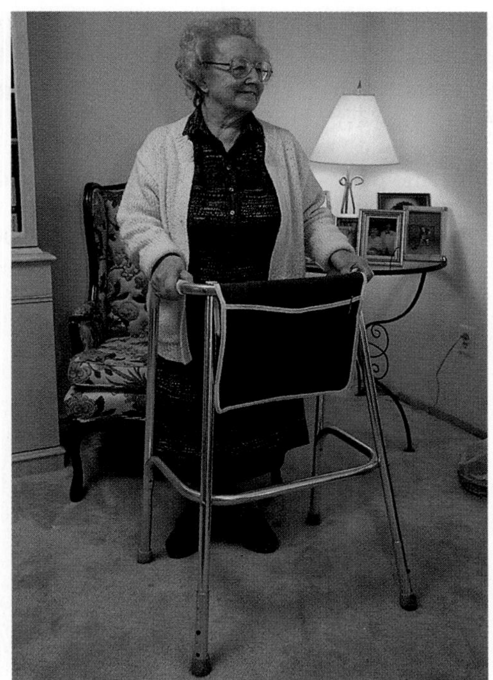

Figure 22-29 A walker.

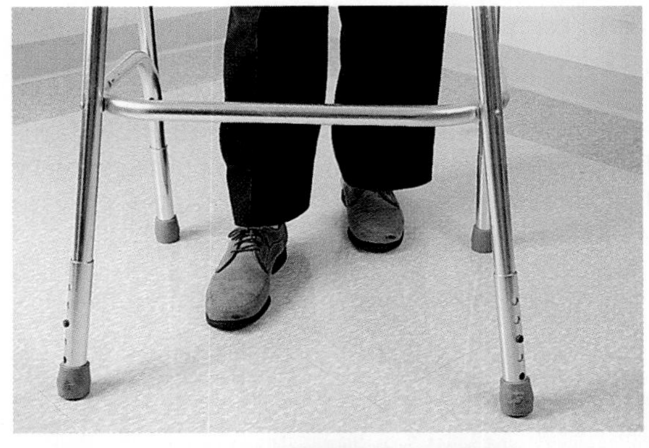

A

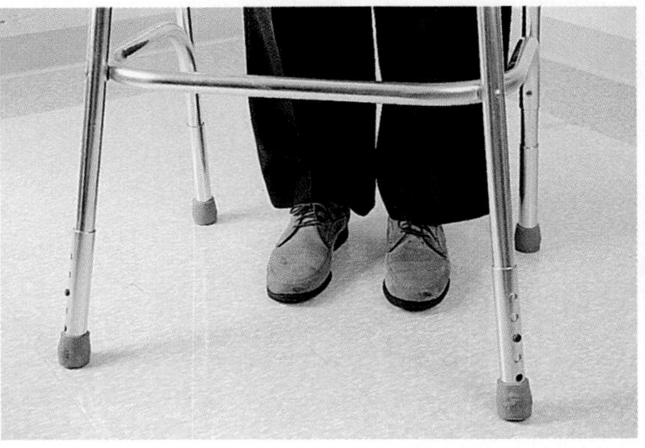

B

Figure 22-30 Walking with a walker. **A,** The walker is moved about 15 cm (6 inches) in front of the person. **B,** Both feet are moved up to the walker.

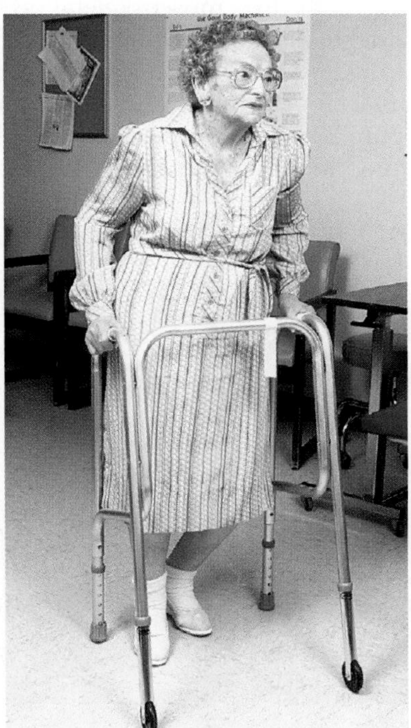

Figure 22-31 An older woman using a wheeled walker.

Box 22-4 Helping Clients with Walkers to Sit and Stand

HELPING THE CLIENT SIT ON A CHAIR, WHEELCHAIR, OR TOILET

- Lock the wheelchair wheels.
- Ask the person to stand with his or her back to the chair, wheelchair, or toilet.
- Ask the person to back up with the walker until his or her knees touch the seat.
- Ask the person to take one hand off the walker. Ask the person to use that hand to reach and grasp the armrest or grab bar.
- Help the person slowly sit down. His or her buttocks should be at the back of the seat.

If armrests and/or grab bars are not available, support the client as he or she sits down. (Use a transfer belt if the client is weak or unsteady.)

- Move the walker away from the person.
- Support the person in the standing position.
- Place your hands under the person's arms and over the shoulder blades.
- Block the person's feet and knees with your feet and knees.
- Lower the person onto the seat slowly.

HELPING THE CLIENT SIT ON A BED

- Use a transfer belt if the person is weak or unsteady.
- Raise the head of the bed to a sitting position.
- Ask the person to stand with his or her back to the bed. He or she should be near the middle of the bed.
- Ask the person to back up with the walker until his or her knees touch the bed.
- Ask the person to reach for the bed with one hand. Assist as necessary.
- Help the person sit down slowly.
- Provide for comfort.

HELPING THE CLIENT MOVE FROM SITTING TO STANDING

- Place the walker so the person can reach it with ease.
- Let the person position the walker.
- Ask the person to move to the edge of the seat or bed.
- Help the person rise to a standing position as needed.

Braces. A **brace (orthosis)** is an apparatus worn to support or align weak body parts or to prevent or correct problems with the muscoskeletal system (see Chapter 32). Metal, plastic, or leather is used for braces. A brace is applied over the ankle, knee, or back (Figure 22-32). An ankle–foot orthosis (AFO) is positioned in the shoe (Figure 22-33). Then the foot is inserted. The device is secured in place with a Velcro strap.

Skin and bony points under braces should be kept clean and dry to prevent skin breakdown. Report redness or signs of skin breakdown (see Chapter 41). Also report complaints of pain or discomfort. In facilities, the nurse assesses the skin under braces every shift. The care plan tells you when to apply and remove a brace.

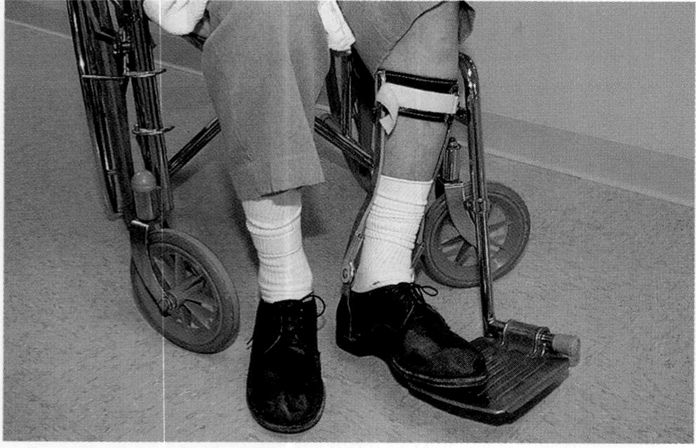

Figure 22-32 Leg brace.

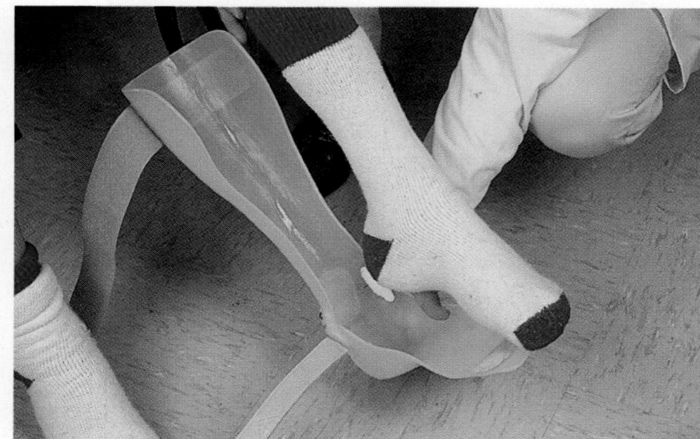

Figure 22-33 Ankle-foot orthosis (AFO).

REVIEW

Circle the BEST answer.

1. Ms. Porter is on bed rest. Which statement is *false?*
   A. She has orthostatic hypotension.
   B. Bed rest helps reduce pain and promotes healing.
   C. Complications of bed rest include pressure ulcers, constipation, and blood clots.
   D. Contractures and muscle atrophy can occur.

2. Which helps to prevent permanent plantar flexion?
   A. Bed boards
   B. A foot board
   C. Trochanter rolls
   D. Hand rolls

3. Which prevents the hip from turning outward?
   A. Bed boards
   B. A foot board
   C. Trochanter roll
   D. A leg brace

4. A contracture is
   A. The loss of muscle strength as a result of inactivity
   B. The lack of joint mobility caused by the shortening of a muscle
   C. A decrease in the size of a muscle
   D. A blood clot

5. Passive range-of-motion exercises are performed by
   A. The client
   B. A health care team member
   C. The client with the assistance of someone else
   D. The client with the use of a trapeze

6. ROM exercises are ordered for Ms. Porter. You should do the following *except*
   A. Support the body part being exercised
   B. Move the joint slowly, smoothly, and gently
   C. Force the joint through full range of motion
   D. Exercise only the joints indicated by your supervisor

7. Flexion involves
   A. Bending the body part
   B. Straightening the body part
   C. Moving the body part toward the body
   D. Moving the body part away from the body

8. Which statement about ambulation is *false?*
   A. A transfer belt is used if the client is weak or unsteady.
   B. The client can shuffle or slide when beginning to walk after bed rest.
   C. Walking aids may be needed.
   D. Crutches, canes, walkers, and braces are common walking aids.

9. You are getting a person ready to crutch walk. You should do the following *except*
   A. Check the crutch tips
   B. Have the person wear street shoes
   C. Get any pair of crutches from physical therapy
   D. Tighten the bolts on the crutches

10. A single-tip cane is used
    A. At waist level
    B. On the strong side
    C. On the weak side
    D. On either side

Circle T if the answer is true and F if it is false.

11. T F A single-tip cane and a four-point cane give equal support.

12. T F When a cane is used, the feet are moved first.

13. T F Mr. Jameel uses a walker. First he moves the walker in front of him. Then he moves his feet forward.

14. T F Mr. Jameel starts to fall. You should try to prevent the fall.

15. T F A client has a brace. Bony areas need protection from skin breakdown.

Answers to these questions are on page 824.

CHAPTER

23

HOME MANAGEMENT

OBJECTIVES

- Define the key terms listed in this chapter
- Explain why home management is important
- Explain your role in home management
- Explain how to use cleaning supplies safely
- Describe how to clean bedrooms, living rooms, bathrooms, and kitchens
- Explain how to do laundry

KEY TERMS

home management The cleaning and organizing of a home

laundry symbols Symbols on garment tags that indicate care for that garment

Some clients need help keeping their living environment clean, orderly, healthy, and safe. You might be assigned home management tasks. **Home management** is the cleaning and organizing of a home. Generally, your role in home management involves light housekeeping tasks. For example, you might straighten and clean parts of rooms. Or, you might be assigned to vacuum, dust, wash dishes, make beds, and/or do laundry. You will not be assigned heavy housecleaning tasks like washing windows or cleaning carpets.

You might do basic housekeeping tasks in a hospital or long-term facility. However, most facilities have a housekeeping staff. This chapter addresses home management in community care settings.

YOUR ROLE IN HOME MANAGEMENT

A clean and orderly setting is important for health and safety. Dust, dirt, and damp areas promote the growth of microbes. Clutter can cause falls and serious injury. Some people cannot do regular housekeeping. These include people who are ill, disabled, and recovering from surgery or injuries. New parents and caregivers tending to sick family members may need help with housekeeping. Older adults may also need help.

The client, family, and case manager decide what household tasks are required. These are listed in the care plan, along with other tasks. You must complete the tasks listed in the care plan. However, you need to be flexible. For example, your task is to straighten and clean the bathroom after you have helped Mrs. Jacob with personal care. However, Mrs. Jacob is incontinent of urine. You need to provide skin care, and help her change into clean clothes. The client's immediate personal care needs take priority.

Whatever the household task, remember the priorities of support work. (See *Providing Compassionate Care: Home Management* box.)

Providing Compassionate Care

HOME MANAGEMENT

Dignity. All people deserve a neat, clean, peaceful setting. Illness, disability, surgery, or injury may limit a person's ability to clean. Helping with home management promotes comfort, emotional well-being, and dignity. Treat your client's home and belongings with respect and care.

Independence. For some people, accepting help means a loss of control. Respect your client's wish for independence and control. As they recover, some people gradually assume responsibility for home management. Occupational therapists help some people learn new ways to perform household tasks. For example, Mr. Ho had an arm amputated. He is trying to make his bed using techniques he learned in occupational therapy. His progress is slow. Do not make the bed for him. Be patient. Praise him for trying and for the amount of work he has done.

Preferences. Follow your client's preferred methods for household tasks. These are listed in the care plan. Respect that all people have different preferences and standards. For example, Mrs. Neal shows no interest in having a neat bedroom. However, she cannot bear a tiny stain on her blouse.

Privacy. Some people may view you as an intrusion. Find out if there are any areas that the client considers private or "off limits" for you. There may be rooms, parts of rooms, or items that a client does not want touched or cleaned. Respect these wishes. Never judge or criticize a client's housekeeping skills. Never talk to others about the cleanliness of a client's house. This would be unprofessional and unethical.

Safety. Some cleaning solutions have WHMIS labels (see Chapter 16). Read these and other product labels carefully. Follow all use and storage instructions. Do not let people walk on mopped floors. They may be slippery and cause a fall. Put away buckets and cleaning solutions when finished with them. Store cleaning solutions out of reach of children and adults with dementia. Clear away clutter. If the client's safety is at risk, talk to your supervisor.

Dealing with Conflicting Demands

Many people have set routines. They want things done in a certain way. Because of time constraints or for health and safety reasons, this may not be possible. You may have to deal with conflicting demands. The care plan says one thing but the client wants something different. (See *Support Workers Solving Problems: Conflicting Home Management Demands* box.) Listen to your client. Discuss complaints with your supervisor.

Getting Organized

Usually, home management tasks are assigned in addition to personal care and other tasks. The key to completing home management tasks and your other duties is to use your time wisely. Review the time management skills described in Chapter 8. Follow the guidelines in Box 23-1 and these general points:

- *Set priorities*. Follow the care plan. Do the most important tasks first.
- *Set a routine*. Discuss the routine with your client. Agreeing about the routine will help you manage your time.
- *Use your time well*. Start with tasks that have waiting periods or that run automatically. For example, laundry and personal care activities are on your list. Start laundry first. Soak soiled linens while you help your client with his or her bath.
- *Finish tasks, and put items away*. Finish tasks that you have started. After finishing, put all items away in their proper place.
- *Set time limits for each task*. This helps you stay organized and finish on time.
- *Focus on the task*. Do not let your mind wander. For example, do not carelessly wipe a counter while talking to your client. Focus on the person. Then clean the counter properly.
- *Put the client's needs first*. Remember your first priority is to promote the person's comfort, well-being, and safety. Follow the care plan.

Box 23-1 Cleaning Guidelines

- **Clear away clutter.** Put items in their proper place. Nothing should be on the floor or counter unless it belongs there. Do not leave items on stairs or in high traffic areas. Ask the client where to put things. If the person does not know, place items neatly out of the way. Tell the client where you put things. Ask before throwing anything away. Even a scrap of paper may be important to the person.
- **Work from higher to lower.** Begin in high places. Work your way to the bottom. Dust and dirt from higher surfaces fall on lower surfaces. For example, when vacuuming stairs, start at the top of the stairs and work down to the bottom.
- **Work from far to near.** For example, when wiping a kitchen counter, make brisk strokes from the back to the front. When washing a floor, start at the far end of the room and work toward the door.
- **Work from dry to wet.** Begin with rooms and areas without sinks, tubs, showers, and toilets. Then clean bathrooms and kitchens. Sweep floors before washing them.
- **Work from cleanest to dirtiest.** This helps avoid contaminating clean areas with microbes from a dirtier area. For example, wipe the cleanest part of the counter first. Clean the part used for food preparation last.
- **Change cloths and water frequently.** Do not wait for these to become visibly dirty before changing them. Use fresh cloths for each task. For example, use one cloth for dusting and another for washing counters.
- **Use a damp cloth for dusting.** The moisture in a damp cloth picks up the dust. A dry cloth simply stirs the dust around.
- **Rinse and dry washed surfaces.** This removes soapy residue and dampness.
- **Avoid soiling a clean area.** For example, do not walk on a washed floor until it is dry.

Support Workers Solving Problems

Conflicting Home Management Demands

Scenario: Rosa's client, Mrs. Yeung, 67, is recovering from heart surgery. Mrs. Yeung asks Rosa to wash the bathroom floor. Rosa explains that the care plan does not specify washing the floor. Mrs. Yeung is upset because she wants the floor washed.

Discussion: Rosa sits down with Mrs. Yeung who says she feels too ill to clean her house. Rosa explains that she must be on time for her next appointment. She suggests that Mrs. Yeung talk to the case manager. Rosa shows that she cares by listening. This helps Mrs. Yeung regain her composure. Rosa reports the matter to her supervisor.

Equipment and Supplies

Some homes have enough cleaning equipment and supplies. Other homes do not. The following items are needed for cleaning. Clean and store items as appropriate after use.

Equipment

- *Clean rags, sponges, cloths, or paper towels.* Wash rags, sponges, and cloths after use in hot, soapy water. Hang them to air dry or dry them in a dryer.
- *Broom, dustpan, and brush.* Shake the broom and brush after use into a large, moistened bag. Wipe the dustpan with a damp cloth.
- *Mop and bucket.* Wash and rinse both after use.
- *Toilet brush.* Rinse in a bucket of cold water. Flush water down the toilet.
- *Utility gloves.* Wash in hot, soapy water, and hang to dry.
- *Vacuum cleaner.* Use the right attachments to clean carpets and upholstery. Follow manufacturer's instructions. Replace filter bags as needed. Make sure the cord and plug are in good repair.
- *Dish washing materials.* Clean cloths, sponges, scouring pads, and brushes.

Supplies

- *Detergents*—for laundry and dish washing
- *All-purpose cleaners*—for counters, floors, and other surfaces
- *Glass cleaners*—for mirrors
- *Special cleaners*—for bathrooms, toilets, mirrors, ovens, etc.
- *Cleansers and scouring powders*—for scrubbing
- *Disinfectants*—cleaners that destroy pathogens. Bleach can be used as a disinfectant, but must be used with caution because it can damage fabrics.
- *Baking soda*—for refrigerator odours, counter stains, etc.
- *White vinegar*—can be used as a disinfectant to clean toilets and commodes. Also can be used to clean mirrors. (Mix one part white vinegar to three parts water.)

If supplies and equipment are lacking, you may have to clean with what the client has on hand. Use problem-solving skills. (See *Support Workers Solving Problems: Substituting Household Products* box.)

Using Cleaning Products Safely

Cleaning products can cause harm if not used and stored properly. Remember the following points:

- Read all labels carefully. Follow manufacturers' instructions. Be familiar with WHMIS hazard labels (see Chapter 16).
- Never mix cleaning products. Some products contain chemicals that create poisonous fumes when mixed. Bleach and ammonia are examples.
- Wear utility gloves when using cleaning products. Do not use disposable gloves.
- Never use products in unlabelled containers.
- Store products in their original containers.
- Keep cleaning products away from food.
- Keep cleaning products out of reach of children and adults with dementia.
- Use products only for their intended purpose.
- Keep aerosol cans away from heat sources.
- Ask the client before using a strong cleaner on a surface.
- Rinse strong, abrasive cleaners immediately after use.
- Do not scrub vigorously. You could damage a delicate surface.

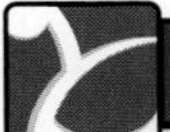

Support Workers Solving Problems

Substituting Household Products

Scenario: Ryan is assigned to help Mr. Saad with personal care and to clean the bathroom afterwards. Mr. Saad has cloths and paper towels, but he has no cleaners.

Discussion: Agency policy is to find cleaning substitutes before calling the office. Ryan finds white vinegar in the kitchen. He makes a cleaning solution with water and vinegar with which he cleans the bathroom. Ryan reports his actions and identifies needed supplies to his supervisor.

Cleaning Bedrooms

Some clients spend little time in bed. Others spend most or all of their time in bed. They may eat meals in their bedroom. The bedroom should be clean, orderly, and comfortable (Box 23-2). You need to:

- Make the bed
- Straighten bedding as needed
- Change the linens as needed

Box 23-2 Cleaning Bedrooms

Task	Supplies and equipment	Process
Making the bed/ straightening linens		• See Chapter 24
Changing the linens	• Sheets • Pillowcases • Protective sheets or pads • Blankets • Comforter or bedspread	• See Chapter 24
Straightening the room		• Straighten items on bedside table • Remove old magazines and newspapers, used tissues, drinking glasses, etc. (with permission from the client) • Place reading material and glasses within reach • Put away clothing, shoes, and other items (with permission from the client) • Look for items under and behind the bed • Empty the waste basket
Replenishing supplies	• Pitcher and glass • Tissues and toilet paper • Other supplies as necessary	• Discard stale water, wash pitcher and glass, and refill pitcher and glass • Replenish supplies as needed
Wiping surfaces	• Two cloths • Hot, soapy water	• Wipe doors, door knobs, and light switches • Dry with dry cloth
Dusting	• Damp cloth	• Dust all surfaces, including dressers, bookshelves, windowsills, bedside tables, lamps, etc.
Cleaning commodes	• Toilet bowl cleaner or disinfectant • Bucket of hot water • Utility gloves • Toilet brush or sponge • Fresh cloths or paper towels	• Wear gloves • Flush contents in the toilet; do not splash • Clean the commode bowl, under the bowl, and under and behind the seat (Figure 23-1) • Clean and dry commode surfaces with fresh cloths or paper towels
Cleaning floors	• Vacuum • Broom, dustpan, and brush • Mop and bucket of hot, soapy water • Damp mop	• Vacuum rugs • Sweep and damp mop floor • Use dry mop for hardwood • Shake and vacuum area rugs

Source: Adapted from J. Birchenall and E. Streight, *Mosby's Textbook for the Home Care Aide* (St. Louis: Mosby, 1997), pp. 93–94.

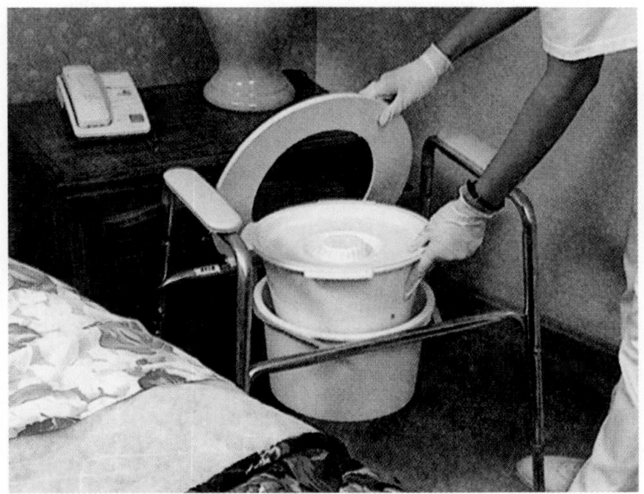

Figure 23-1 Clean commode surfaces thoroughly.

Cleaning Living Rooms

Some people use their living rooms infrequently. For others, the living room is the main living area. Some people eat and sleep in their living room. Whatever the situation, living rooms should be kept clean and comfortable (Box 23-3).

Box 23-3 Cleaning Living Rooms

Task	Supplies and equipment	Process
Straightening the room		• Remove clutter and items that could cause falls (with permission from the client) • Remove dirty dishes and ashtrays • Look under cushions and down furniture arms for food particles and other items • Sweep or vacuum crumbs off furniture • Plump cushions
Replenishing supplies	• Tissues • Other supplies	• Provide fresh water, tissues, reading materials, and other supplies
Wiping surfaces	• Two cloths • Hot, soapy water	• Wipe doors, door knobs, and light switches • Dry with dry cloth
Dusting	• Damp cloth	• Dust all furniture, including the television, VCR, etc.
Cleaning floors	• Vacuum cleaner • Broom, dustpan, and brush • Mop and bucket of hot, soapy water • Damp mop	• Vacuum rug • Sweep and damp mop floor • Use dry mop for hardwood • Shake and vacuum area rug

Source: Adapted from J. Birchenall and E. Streight, *Mosby's Textbook for the Home Care Aide* (St. Louis: Mosby, 1997), pp. 93–94.

Cleaning Bathrooms

Bathrooms need special attention because microbes easily grow and spread in damp places (Box 23-4). Family members must keep the bathroom clean. Toilets must be cleaned thoroughly with a disinfectant or toilet bowl cleaner. Wear utility gloves for cleaning toilets. Brushes or sponges used to clean the toilet must not be used for other cleaning jobs.

Since some cleaners scratch surfaces, use special cleaners for the bathroom. If not available, use laundry detergent and a cloth. Or use a vinegar and water solution.

Practise the following hygienic measures:

- Rinse and dry bar soaps after use.
- Flush the toilet with the seat down to prevent splashing and the spread of microbes.
- Rinse the sink after used for washing, shaving, or oral hygiene.
- Remove and dispose of hair from the sink, tub, or shower.
- Hang damp towels and bath mats out to dry. Or place them in a hamper.
- Wash bath mats, the wastebasket, and the laundry hamper every week.
- Put out clean towels.
- Wipe up water spills.
- Wipe out the bathtub or shower immediately after use.
- Provide enough toilet paper and tissue.
- Open shower doors to prevent mildew from developing inside the shower.
- Do not pour dirty or contaminated liquids in the sink. Flush them down the toilet.

Box 23-4 Cleaning Bathrooms

Task	Supplies and equipment	Process
Cleaning sinks	• Cloths or sponge • Utility gloves • Hot, soapy water • Disinfectant	• Wipe sink with hot, soapy water and disinfectant • Rinse and dry with dry cloth • Wipe and dry taps
Cleaning bathtubs, showers, and shower-curtains	• Cloths or sponge • Utility gloves • Hot, soapy water • Disinfectant	• Wipe with hot, soapy water and disinfectant (include shower curtain) • Rinse and dry with dry cloth • Wipe and dry taps
Replenishing supplies	• Toilet paper • Tissues • Soap and shampoo • Toothpaste • Other supplies as needed	• Check and replenish supplies
Cleaning surfaces	• Cloths or sponge • Utility gloves • Hot, soapy water • Disinfectant	• Wipe window sills, bathroom tiles, soap holders, and door handles with hot, soapy water and disinfectant • Rinse and dry all surfaces
Cleaning mirrors	• Glass cleaner or white vinegar and water • Paper towels	• Wipe with paper towels and cleaner • Dry with paper towels
Cleaning toilets	• Toilet bowl cleaner or disinfectant • Bucket of hot water • Utility gloves • Toilet brush or sponge • Fresh cloths or paper towels	• Wear gloves • Clean toilet tank • Clean the toilet bowl, outside and in; clean under the bowl, and under and behind the seat • Clean and dry the toilet seat and outer surfaces with fresh cloths or paper towels • Clean and dry toilet handle with fresh cloths or paper towels
Cleaning floors	• Bucket of hot, soapy water • Disinfectant • Utility gloves • Mop, cloths, or sponge	• Clean floor last • Dry floor to prevent falls • Vacuum carpeted floors

Source: Adapted from J. Birchenall and E. Streight, *Mosby's Textbook for the Home Care Aide* (St. Louis: Mosby, 1997), p. 93.

Some people are at high risk for infection. They include people recovering from surgery and those undergoing chemotherapy. Their bathrooms must be kept very clean. The care plan lists extra measures that may be needed for these clients. These may include instructions to:

- Clean the tub, shower, and sink with disinfectant before and after use.
- Use paper towels for hand drying.

Cleaning Kitchens

A clean kitchen is critical to preventing the spread of foodborne illnesses (see Chapter 25). Box 23-5 describes how to clean the kitchen. When cleaning kitchens, remember the following:

- Do not pour dirty or contaminated liquids down the kitchen sink. Flush them down the toilet.
- Use one cloth for counters, another for wiping floors, and another for dishes.

Box 23-5 Cleaning Kitchens

Task	Supplies and equipment	Process
Cleaning surfaces (counters, stove top, table)	• Hot, soapy water • Boiling water • Disinfectant • Baking soda • Cloth or sponge • Second cloth or paper towel to dry counter	• Wipe surfaces with cloth and hot, soapy water • Rinse and dry • Scrub with disinfectant and rinse with boiling water if the surfaces were in contact with raw poultry, meat, fish, or eggs; dry thoroughly with paper towels • Use baking soda to remove stubborn counter stains • Wipe table (and mats) with cloth and hot soapy water
Cleaning cutting boards	• Hot, soapy water • Boiling water • Disinfectant • Cloth and brush	• Wash with hot, soapy water • Rinse and pat dry with paper towels • Scrub with disinfectant and rinse with boiling water if the surfaces were in contact with raw poultry, meat, fish, or eggs; dry thoroughly with paper towels
Washing dishes	• Liquid detergent and hot water • Dish cloth, scouring pads, or brushes	• Scrape food remnants from dishes • Wash glassware and cups first, then utensils, plates, bowls, pots, and pans • Soak pots and pans in hot water if food is stuck on them • Rinse items well in hot water • Place items in a drainer to dry; air drying is cleaner than towel drying
Using automatic dishwashers	• Dishwasher detergent	• Read instructions or ask family member to demonstrate use • Scrape large food particles and rinse dishes before loading (Figure 23-2 on page 336) • Place glasses and cups in washer upside down • Do not stack items on top of one another, they will not clean properly • Do not put the following in a dishwasher: electrical appliances, delicate glasses, fine china, sharp knives, cast iron, wood, or most plastics • Check with the client before putting pots and pans in the dishwasher • Use only dishwasher detergent; other soaps or detergents will cause damage

Continued

Box 23-5 Cleaning Kitchens—cont'd

Task	Supplies and equipment	Process
Cleaning kitchen sinks	• Hot, soapy water • Scouring powder • Boiling water • Disinfectant • Paper towels	• Clean with hot, soapy water and scouring powder • Clean with disinfectant and paper towels if sink has been used for the preparation of poultry, raw meat, fish, or eggs; pour boiling water down sink after the sink has been cleaned; dry with paper towel • Wipe taps with hot, soapy water; dry with paper towel
Cleaning refrigerators	• Hot, soapy water • Baking soda • Cloth or paper towels	• Open all containers; discard food items that do not look fresh or are more than two days old (check with client) • Remove items one shelf at a time; remove shelves and wash with cloth and hot, soapy water; dry with paper towels or a clean cloth; replace items when shelf is cleaned • Clean drawers and inside of door • Clean interior (all surfaces) of the refrigerator • Place a small bowl of baking soda in the refrigerator to absorb odours • Wipe the door of refrigerator and handle
Disposing of waste	• Garbage bags • Utility gloves • Paper towels • Hot, soapy water	• Wear gloves • Remove and discard garbage in garage or apartment chute • Wash garbage can with paper towels and hot, soapy water • Place fresh bag in container • Check with client on recycling of newspapers, cans, and glass • Place appropriate items in recycling box
Cleaning kitchen floors	• Broom and dustpan and brush • Damp mop • Hot, soapy water	• Sweep kitchen floor • Damp mop kitchen floor

Source: Adapted from J. Birchenall and E. Streight, *Mosby's Textbook for the Home Care Aide* (St. Louis: Mosby, 1997), pp. 95–96.

- Use paper towels to dry your hands. Do not dry your hands on a towel used for dishes.
- Change cloths daily or as needed. Wash in bleach in hot water.
- Use paper towels when possible.
- Clean the microwave after every use.
- Do not put soiled diapers into the kitchen garbage.

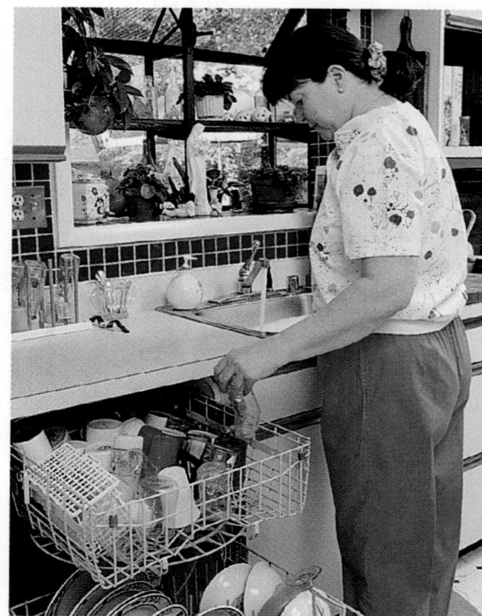

Figure 23-2 Rinse dishes before loading into the dishwasher.

Doing Laundry

When doing laundry, your goal is to clean items without damaging them. Many houses and apartments have laundry facilities. If not, a laundromat is used. Ask your client (or family member) about which detergent, bleach, and fabric softener to use. Also ask about special laundry instructions. For instance, are garments hung or placed in a dryer? Follow your client's preferences. Box 23-6 describes how to do laundry.

Box 23-6 Doing Laundry

Task	Process
Reading manufacturer's instructions	• Read instructions on the washer, dryer, and laundry product • Read garment's care label
Sorting items to be washed	• Separate by fabric • Separate heavily soiled or stained items • Sort by colour: whites, darks, and coloured fabrics • Close zippers, hooks, and buttons • Check pockets for tissue, change, and other items • If unsure about washing or dry cleaning, ask the client
Presoaking	• Presoak heavily soiled and stained items • Use the hottest water safe for the fabric • Soak in bleach or borax for 30 minutes • See Box 23-7 on page 338 for details about removing blood, urine, and feces stains
Prewashing	• Prewash heavily soiled items after presoaking • Use the recommended amount of detergent • Use the hottest water safe for the fabric
Selecting the water temperature and the cycle	• Use hot water (54–65° C; 130–150° F) and the regular cycle for heavily soiled clothes, cloth diapers, and whites • Use warm water (38–43° C; 100–110° F) and the permanent press cycle for moderately soiled clothes and permanent press fabrics; for example, nylon, polyester, and acrylic • Use cold water (26–38° C; 80–100° F) for bright colours, fabrics with colours that may run, fragile fabrics, and lightly soiled garments • Use the gentle cycle when the label recommends it • Wash garments with colours that may run (for example, bright reds) separately
Loading the machine	• Use a high water level for a full machine • Select the water level appropriate for wash size • Do not overload the washer • Wash large items alone • Use a measuring cup for the soap; follow directions on the package
Using the dryer	• Remove lint from the filter • Do not overload the dryer • Use cooler temperatures according to garment labels • Do not put woollen sweaters or garments that may shrink (see labels) in the dryer; lay these items flat to dry on a towel or clothes rack • Use a sheet of fabric softener (with permission from the client) • Remove garments when dryer stops to prevent wrinkling • Remove lint from the filter
Ironing	• Check garment labels before ironing • Use a steam iron for heavily wrinkled clothing • Make sure the iron is hot before using it

Source: Adapted from J. Birchenall and E. Streight, *Mosby's Textbook for the Home Care Aide* (St. Louis: Mosby, 1997), pp. 97–98.

Most garments have **laundry symbols** on inside labels. These symbols tell how to care for the garment (Figure 23-3). Common symbols include the following:

- ⊔ *The washtub symbol*—tells how to wash or not wash the garment. The water temperature is given in centigrade.
- △ *The triangle symbol*—tells if bleach can be used. A "Cl" inside the triangle means chlorine bleach can be used.
- ⊟ *The square symbol*—tells how to dry items.
- *The iron symbol*—tells if the garment can be ironed.
- ○ *The circle symbol*—tells if the garment needs to be dry cleaned.

Remember the following when doing laundry:

- Do not leave wet items in the washer. Moisture can cause mildew.
- If possible, dry items in a dryer rather than hanging them to dry. Quick drying helps eliminate microbes.
- Do not leave items in the dryer. Doing so can wrinkle or damage the fabric.
- Use the hottest water and the longest wash cycle allowed for the item (see Figure 23-3).

Laundry Soiled with Body Substances

Follow employer policy and Standard Precautions (see Chapter 18) when handling laundry soiled with blood, body fluids, secretions, or excretions. The policy describes how to handle, transport, and process soiled laundry. Do the following when handling laundry soiled with body substances:

- Wear gloves
- Place soiled laundry in leak-proof plastic bags. Secure bags to prevent spillage.
- Keep soiled laundry away from other laundry.
- Double bag laundry if the outside of the first bag becomes contaminated with body substances.

Removing Stains. When removing stains, handle chemicals carefully (Box 23-7). Follow label instructions. Both chlorine bleach and ammonia are poisonous. They can burn or irritate the eyes and skin. Never mix chlorine bleach and ammonia. Doing so creates a toxic gas. Do not inhale ammonia fumes. Open a window when using ammonia.

Make sure that clothes can be cleaned with bleach. Some people are allergic to chemicals in cleaning products. Check the care plan. If you are not sure, ask your supervisor.

The directions in Box 23-7 apply to white or colourfast clothes and linens. If possible, treat stains immediately before they become set in the fabric.

Box 23-7 Removing Stains

Urine Stains

- Rinse in cold water
- Soak in a solution of 1 L of warm water, 2 mL liquid (hand) dishwashing detergent, and 15 mL of ammonia for 30 minutes
- Rinse in cool water
- Soak in a solution of 1 L warm water and 15 mL of vinegar for 1 hour
- Machine wash with chlorine bleach and detergent; dry as usual

Blood Stains

- Rinse in cold water
- Soak in a solution of 1 L warm water, 2 mL liquid (hand) dishwashing detergent, and 15 mL ammonia for 15 minutes
- If fabric is strong, gently rub stain; continue as long as stain responds to treatment
- Soak another 15 minutes in the solution used above
- Soak in a solution of 1 L warm water and 15 mL enzyme product for 30 minutes
- Wash in machine using chlorine bleach and detergent; dry as usual

Fecal Stains

- Rinse in cold water
- Soak in a solution of 1 L warm water, 2 mL liquid (hand) dishwashing detergent, and 15 mL ammonia for 30 minutes
- Wash in machine using chlorine bleach and detergent; dry as usual

Source: Adapted from J. Birchenall and E. Streight, *Mosby's Textbook for the Home Care Aide* (St. Louis: Mosby, 1997), p. 99.

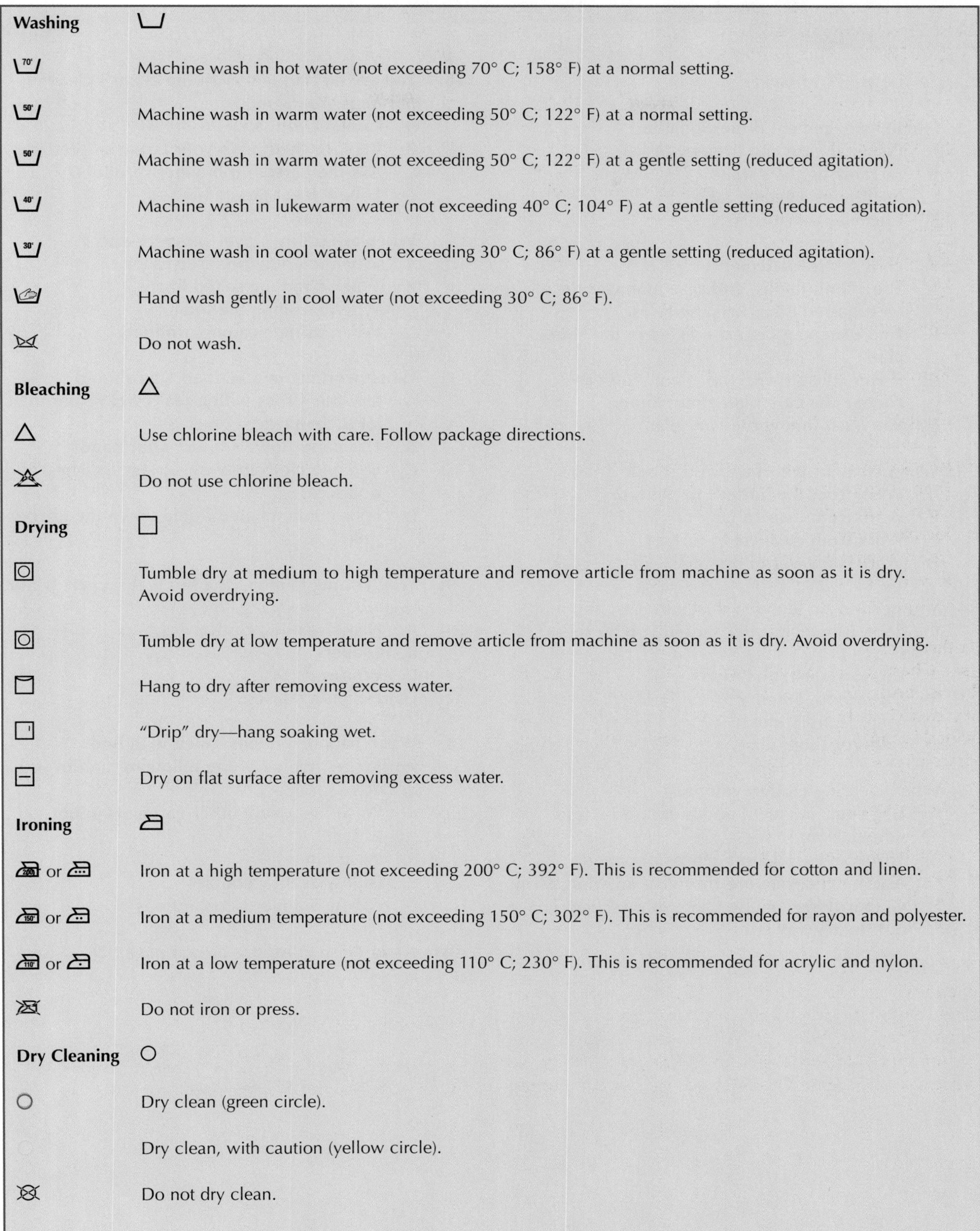

Symbol	Meaning
Washing	
	Machine wash in hot water (not exceeding 70° C; 158° F) at a normal setting.
	Machine wash in warm water (not exceeding 50° C; 122° F) at a normal setting.
	Machine wash in warm water (not exceeding 50° C; 122° F) at a gentle setting (reduced agitation).
	Machine wash in lukewarm water (not exceeding 40° C; 104° F) at a gentle setting (reduced agitation).
	Machine wash in cool water (not exceeding 30° C; 86° F) at a gentle setting (reduced agitation).
	Hand wash gently in cool water (not exceeding 30° C; 86° F).
	Do not wash.
Bleaching	
	Use chlorine bleach with care. Follow package directions.
	Do not use chlorine bleach.
Drying	
	Tumble dry at medium to high temperature and remove article from machine as soon as it is dry. Avoid overdrying.
	Tumble dry at low temperature and remove article from machine as soon as it is dry. Avoid overdrying.
	Hang to dry after removing excess water.
	"Drip" dry—hang soaking wet.
	Dry on flat surface after removing excess water.
Ironing	
200 or	Iron at a high temperature (not exceeding 200° C; 392° F). This is recommended for cotton and linen.
150 or	Iron at a medium temperature (not exceeding 150° C; 302° F). This is recommended for rayon and polyester.
110 or	Iron at a low temperature (not exceeding 110° C; 230° F). This is recommended for acrylic and nylon.
	Do not iron or press.
Dry Cleaning	
	Dry clean (green circle).
	Dry clean, with caution (yellow circle).
	Do not dry clean.

Figure 23-3 Laundry symbols. Source: Government of Canada, http://strategis.ic.bc.ca/SSG/cp01115e.html.

REVIEW

Circle the BEST answer.

1. Home management duties include
   A. Personal care and hygiene tasks
   B. Organizing the garage
   C. Light housekeeping tasks
   D. Cleaning the attic

2. Which is a *false* statement?
   A. The client, family, and case manager decide on required housekeeping tasks.
   B. Housekeeping tasks are listed in the care plan.
   C. If you consult with the client, you can change the care plan at any time.
   D. You must follow the care plan.

3. When cleaning a surface, you should
   A. Work from the bottom to the top
   B. Work from near to far
   C. Work from cleanest to dirtiest
   D. Work from wet to dry

4. You need to do laundry, dust surfaces, and mop the floor. In which order should you do these tasks?
   A. Laundry, dust, and mop
   B. Dust, mop, laundry
   C. Mop, laundry, dust
   D. Laundry, mop, dust

5. When clearing clutter, you must
   A. Use your judgment about important and unimportant items
   B. Throw away all stray pieces of paper
   C. Ask the client before throwing anything away
   D. Gather things in one place so the client can put them away later

6. You are not familiar with the client's cleaning products. You should
   A. Contact your supervisor
   B. Replace them with your brand of products
   C. Ask the person to buy new products
   D. Follow label directions

7. When are utility gloves *not* necessary?
   A. When loading the dishwasher
   B. When handling soiled linens
   C. When cleaning the toilet
   D. When using cleaning products

8. When working in a kitchen, you should
   A. Dry the dishes with a tea towel rather than let them air dry
   B. Use paper towels to dry your hands
   C. Use one cloth to wash surfaces, dishes, and floors
   D. Pour contaminated liquid down the kitchen sink

9. When doing laundry, the hot water cycle is *not* used for
   A. Heavily soiled clothes
   B. Diapers
   C. Whites
   D. Delicate fabrics

10. When handling linens soiled with body substances, which of the following should you *not* do
    A. Wash them with other garments in hot water
    B. Wear gloves
    C. Follow agency policies
    D. Follow Standard Precautions

Answers to these questions are on page 824.

CHAPTER

24

Beds and Bedmaking

OBJECTIVES

- Define the key terms listed in this chapter
- Know the basic bed positions
- Describe how to handle linens according to the rules of medical asepsis
- Explain the purposes of plastic drawsheets and cotton drawsheets
- Describe general rules for bedmaking
- Describe the differences between open, closed, occupied, and surgical beds
- Learn the procedures described in this chapter

KEY TERMS

drawsheet A small sheet placed over the middle of the bottom sheet; it helps keep the mattress and bottom linens clean and dry; can be used to turn and move the client in bed; the cotton drawsheet

plastic drawsheet A drawsheet placed between the bottom sheet and the cotton drawsheet to keep the mattress and bottom linens clean and dry

Many clients spend a great deal of time in bed. Some are recovering from illness, surgery, or injury. Others are on bed rest (see Chapter 22). Still others must stay in bed because of severe illness or disability.

It is important to know the different types of beds and how to position them for the client's comfort. It is also important to know how to make beds. A clean, dry, and wrinkle-free bed promotes the client's comfort and safety. It helps prevent skin breakdown and pressure ulcers (see Chapter 41).

In facilities, beds are usually made in the morning after baths. They are also made while the client is taking a shower or is out of the room. People usually like their beds made and rooms clean before visitors arrive. In homes, beds are made according to the care plan and the client's preferences.

Linens must be straightened whenever they are loose or wrinkled and at bedtime. Check linens for crumbs after meals, and remove the crumbs. Linens are changed whenever they become wet, soiled, or damp. Follow Standard Precautions when changing linens soiled with blood, body fluids, excretions, or secretions.

THE BED

Many home care clients use their regular beds. Hospital beds are used in hospitals and long-term care facilities. Some home care clients also use them. Hospital beds usually have bed rails. Chapter 16 describes bed rails and their use. Remember, bed rails have many safety hazards. Raise and lower them only as directed by your supervisor and the care plan.

REGULAR BEDS

You will see twin-, double-, queen-, and king-sized beds in homes. Waterbeds, sofa sleepers, cots, and recliners are also common.

Regular beds cannot be raised. The lower the bed, the more you will have to bend and reach when giving care or making the bed. Use good body mechanics to protect your back (see Chapter 21).

A good mattress is neither too hard nor too soft. A poor-quality mattress may not provide needed support or comfort. It could harm the client's back or skin. If you are concerned about the client's mattress, tell your supervisor.

HOSPITAL BEDS

Hospital beds have electrical or manual controls. Beds are raised horizontally to give care. This reduces bending and reaching. The lowest horizontal position lets the client get out of bed with ease (Figure 24-1). The head of the bed can be kept flat or raised to varying degrees for the client's comfort.

Most hospital beds are electric. Controls are on a side panel, bed rail, or panel at the foot of the bed (Figure 24-2). Clients are taught how to safely use the controls. They are warned not to raise the bed to the high position and not to adjust the bed to harmful positions. They are told of any position limits or restrictions.

Most electric beds can be "locked" into any position. This prevents the client from raising or lowering the head or foot of the bed. Clients restricted to certain positions may need to have their beds locked. The locking feature is useful for clients with dementia.

Manually operated beds are still in use in some places. They have cranks at the foot of the bed (Figure

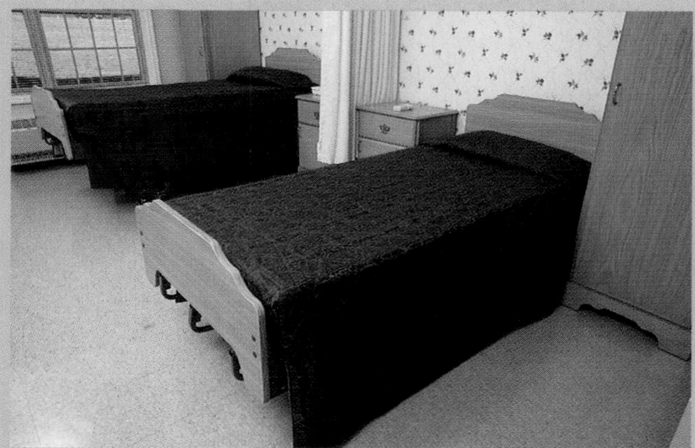

Figure 24-1 One bed in the highest horizontal position and the other bed in the lowest horizontal position.

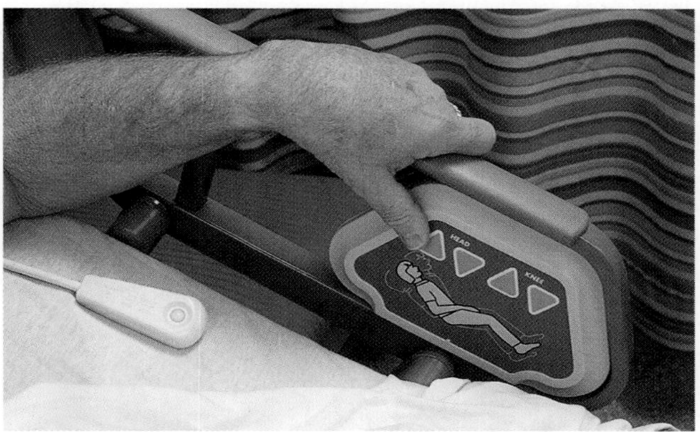

Figure 24-2 Controls for an electric bed.

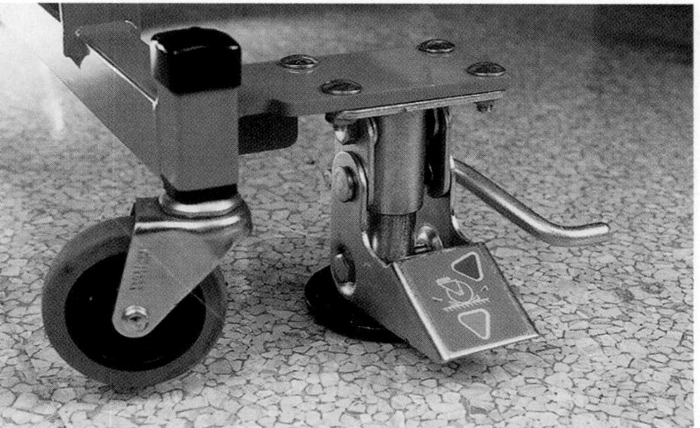

Figure 24-4 Lock on a bed wheel.

24-3). The left crank raises or lowers the head of the bed. The right crank adjusts the knee portion. The centre crank raises or lowers the entire bed. The cranks are pulled up for use. They are kept down at all other times. Cranks in the up position are safety hazards. Anyone walking past could bump into them.

Hospital beds should always be left in their lowest position. Only raise the bed immediately before giving care or when making the bed. As soon as you are finished, return the bed to its lowest position. Never leave the client alone when the bed is raised.

Hospital bed legs have wheels that let the bed move easily. Each wheel has a lock to prevent the bed from moving (Figure 24-4). Make sure bed wheels are locked when you are giving bedside care and when transferring a client to and from the bed. You or the client could be injured if the bed moves.

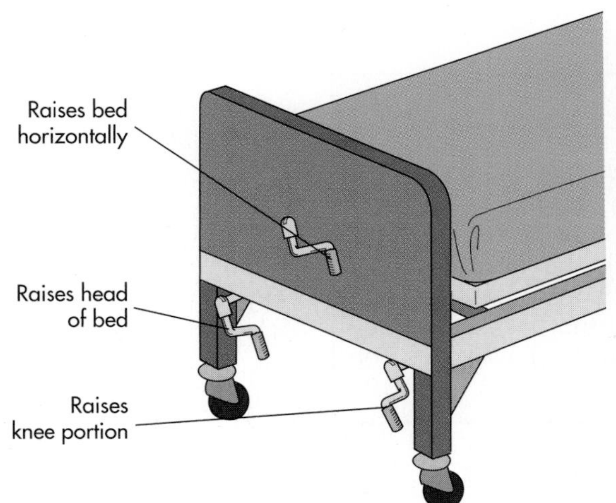

Figure 24-3 Manually operated hospital bed.

Bed Positions

There are five basic bed positions: flat, Fowler's, semi-Fowler's, Trendelenburg's, and reverse Trendelenburg's:

- *Flat*—the usual sleeping position. The position also is used after spinal cord injury or surgery and for cervical traction.
- *Fowler's position*—a semi-sitting position. The head of the bed is elevated 45 to 60 degrees (Figure 24-5 on page 344). The reasons for positioning a client in Fowler's position are described in Chapter 21.
- *Semi-Fowler's position*—the head of the bed is raised 45 degrees and the knee portion is raised 15 degrees (Figure 24-6 on page 344). This position is comfortable and prevents the client from sliding down in bed. However, raising the knee portion can interfere with leg circulation. Check with the care plan and your supervisor before positioning a client in semi-Fowler's position. Many employers define semi-Fowler's position as when the head of the bed is raised 30 degrees and the knee portion is *not* raised. You must know which definition your employer uses so you give safe care. (See *Focus on Home Care: Fowler's and Semi-Fowler's Positions* box on page 344.)
- *Trendelenburg's position*—the head of the bed is lowered, and the foot of the bed is raised (Figure 24-7 on page 344). A physician's order is required for this position. Blocks are placed under the legs at the foot of the bed. Some beds allow the entire bed frame to be tilted into Trendelenburg's position.
- *Reverse Trendelenburg's position*—the opposite of Trendelenburg's position. The head of the bed is raised, and the foot of the bed is lowered (Figure 24-8 on page 344). Blocks are put under the legs at the head of the bed, or the bed frame is tilted. This position requires a physician's order.

(text continues on page 345)

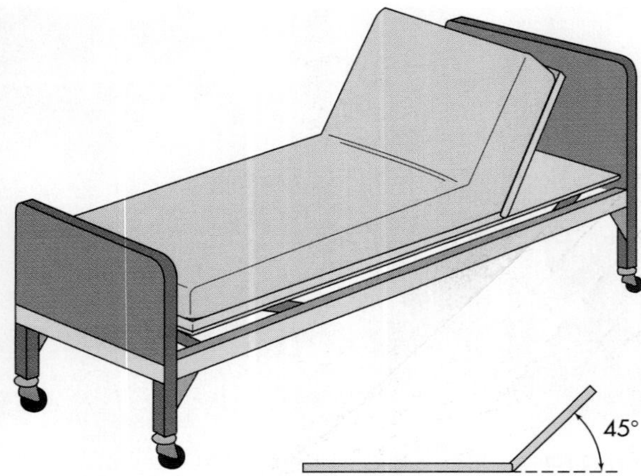

Figure 24-5 Fowler's position.

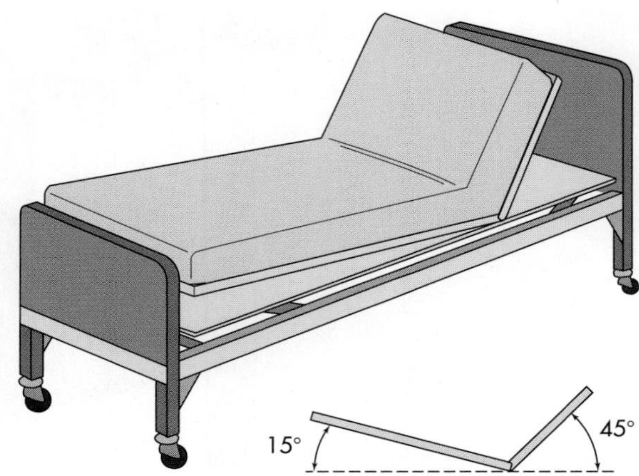

Figure 24-6 Semi-Fowler's position.

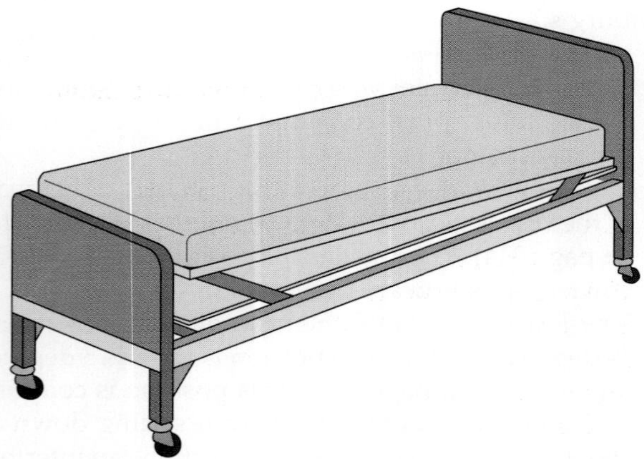

Figure 24-7 Trendelenburg's position.

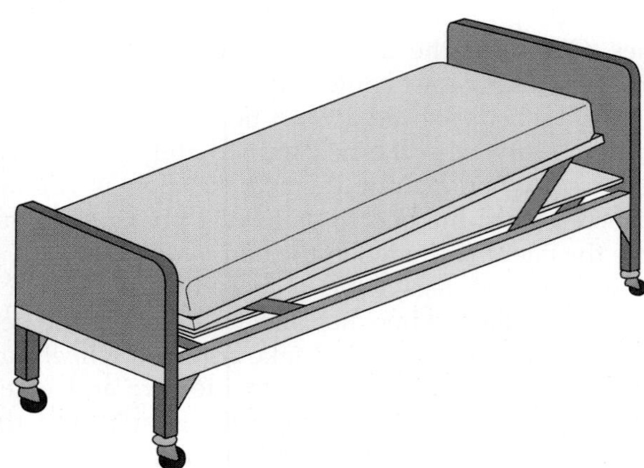

Figure 24-8 Reverse Trendelenburg's position.

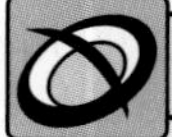

Focus on **Home Care**

FOWLER'S AND SEMI-FOWLER'S POSITIONS

Fowler's and semi-Fowler's positions can be achieved with regular beds by using backrests or pillows (Figure 24-9). Check the headboard to make sure it is sturdy. It needs to provide support when the client leans against the backrest. Large, sturdy, sofa pillows are useful if a backrest is not available.

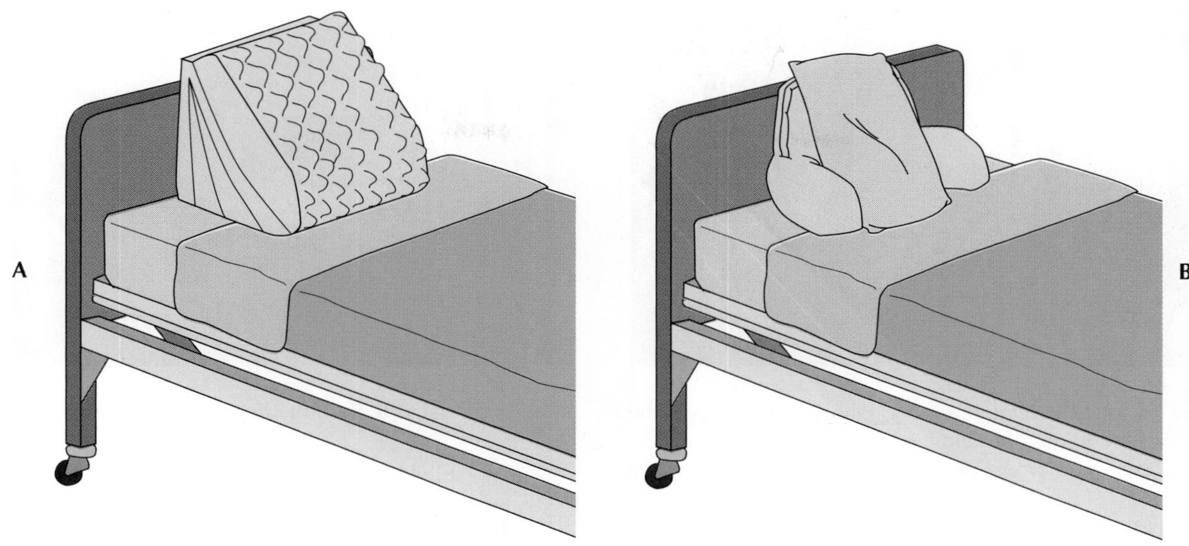

Figure 24-9 Backrests for regular beds. **A,** Wedge pillow. **B,** Study pillow with armrests.

LINENS

When handling linens and making beds, follow the rules of medical asepsis. Wash your hands before collecting clean linens. Your uniform is considered dirty. Therefore always hold linens away from your body and uniform (Figure 24-10). Never shake linens in the air. Shaking them spreads microbes. Clean linens are placed on a clean surface. Never put clean or dirty linens on the floor. If clean linen touches the floor, put it in the laundry.

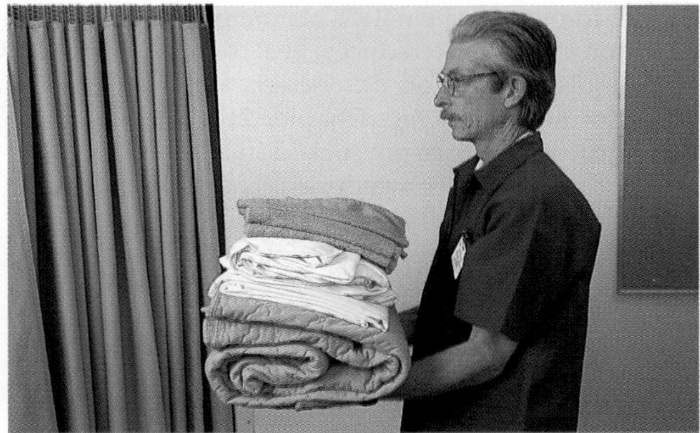

Figure 24-10 Hold linens away from your body and uniform.

Collect linens in the order you will use them:

- Mattress pad
- Bottom sheet (flat sheet or fitted sheet)
- Plastic drawsheet or disposable bed protector
- Cotton drawsheet
- Top sheet (flat sheet)
- Blanket
- Bedspread
- Pillowcase(s)
- Bath towel(s)
- Hand towel
- Washcloth
- Clean pyjamas or hospital gown (if needed)
- Bath blanket

Use one arm to hold the linens and the other hand to pick them up. Make sure the item you will use first is at the bottom of your stack. (You picked up the mattress pad first. It is at the bottom. The bath blanket is at the top.) You need the mattress pad first. To get it on top, place your arm over the bath blanket. Then turn the stack over onto the arm with the bath blanket (Figure 24-11 on page 346). The arm that held the linens is now free. Place the clean linens on a clean surface.

Follow Standard Precautions when removing linens. Used linen is considered dirty (contaminated with microbes). Wear gloves if the linens are soiled

A 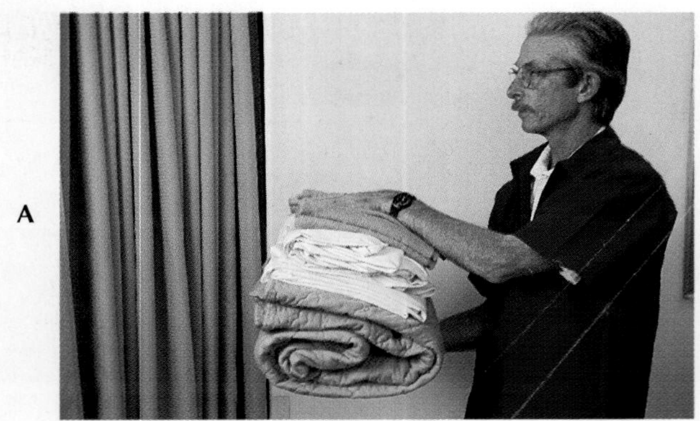

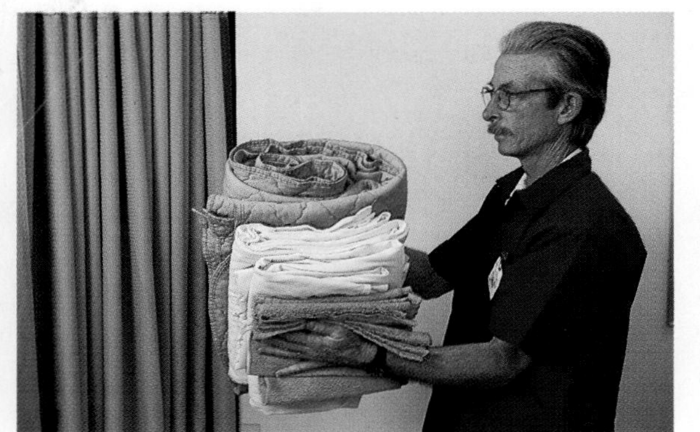 B

Figure 24-11 Collecting linens. **A,** Place your arm over the top of the linen stack. **B,** Turn the linen stack over onto your arm. Note that the linens are held away from the body.

with blood, body fluids, secretions, or excretions. Also check the linens for misplaced personal belongings. Some clients misplace dentures, hearing aids, eyeglasses, watches, or jewellery in their beds. Watch for stray needles in the linen. These are a risk when clients self-medicate.

Remove each piece of linen separately. Roll the linen away from you. The side that touched the client will be inside the roll. The side that has not touched the client is outside (Figure 24-12).

Immediately place used linens in a laundry container or special linen bag. Remove the bag from the client's room. Follow employer policy for soiled linen (see Chapter 18).

How often linen is changed varies among work settings (Table 24-1). Follow the care plan and employer policy. *In all settings, linens are changed when wet, damp, or soiled.*

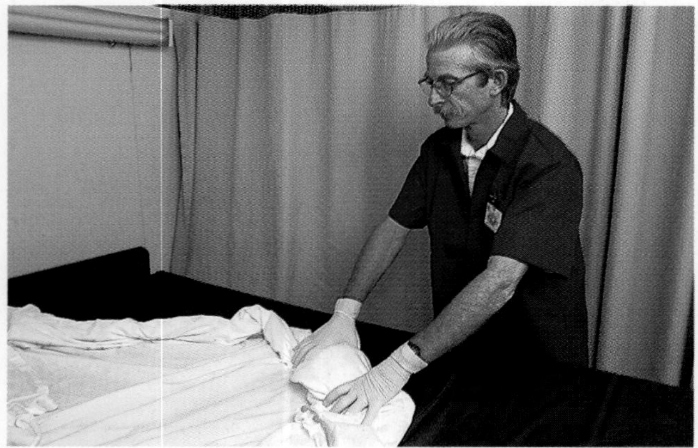

Figure 24-12 Roll dirty (used) linen away from you.

A **drawsheet** is a small sheet placed over the middle of the bottom sheet. It helps keep the mattress and bottom linens clean and dry. It is also called the cotton drawsheet because it is made of cotton. A **plastic drawsheet** is waterproof. It protects the mattress and bottom linens from dampness and soiling. It is placed between the bottom sheet and cotton drawsheet.

The cotton drawsheet protects the client from contact with the plastic and absorbs moisture. However, discomfort and skin breakdown may occur. The plastic retains heat, and plastic drawsheets are hard to keep tight and wrinkle-free.

Many employers use waterproof pads instead of plastic drawsheets. Plastic drawsheets are usually used only for clients with bowel or bladder control problems or those with excessive wound drainage.

Cotton drawsheets are often used without plastic drawsheets. Plastic-covered mattresses cause some people to perspire heavily. This increases discomfort. A cotton drawsheet reduces heat retention and absorbs moisture. Cotton drawsheets are often used as lift or turning sheets (see Chapter 21). When used for this purpose, they are not tucked in at the sides.

The bedmaking procedures that follow include plastic and cotton drawsheets. This is so you learn how to use them. Check with your supervisor if they are used with your clients. (See *Focus on Home Care: Drawsheets* box.)

BEDMAKING

Your job description will include making beds. No matter what type of bed you make, safety and medical asepsis are important. Practise Standard Precautions. Box 24-1 lists the guidelines for bedmaking. (See *Focus on Children: Crib Safety* box on page 348.)

(text continues on page 348)

Table 24-1 Linen Changes in Different Settings

Setting	How often	Special considerations
Home care	• Usually weekly • When wet, damp, or soiled	• Follow the client's preferences for linen choice. For example, some people want extra blankets. Others do not want any blankets.
Long-term care facilities	• Usually weekly. Pillowcases, top and bottom sheets, and drawsheets (if used) may be changed twice a week. • When wet, damp, or soiled	• Some residents bring their own bedspreads, pillows, blankets, or quilts from home. Use them when making the bed. Remember, these items are the resident's property. Handle them with care. Make sure they are labelled with the resident's name. • If the facility uses coloured linens, let the resident choose what colour to use. Also let the resident decide how many pillows or blankets to use. If possible, the resident also chooses the time when you make the bed.
Hospitals	• Daily • When a patient is discharged • When wet, damp, or soiled	• The mattress pad, plastic drawsheet, blanket, and bedspread are reused for the same patient. They are not reused if wet, damp, soiled, or very wrinkled.

KNOW THIS

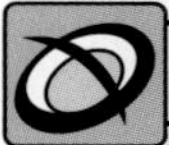

Focus on Home Care

DRAWSHEETS

A flat sheet folded in half can serve as a cotton drawsheet. Usually a twin-size sheet is easier to use for this purpose. Your supervisor and the care plan tell you what to use.

Medical supply stores sell plastic drawsheets and waterproof pads. The case manager discusses the need for these items with the client and family. Some clients place plastic mattress protectors on their beds. These do not protect the bottom linens (cotton drawsheet, bottom sheet, and mattress pad). Some place a piece of plastic under the drawsheet. Again, your supervisor and the care plan tell you what is safe to use for the client. Do not use plastic garbage bags or dry-cleaning bags. These are not strong enough to protect the linens and mattress. They slide easily and can move out of place. The danger of suffocation is great if the bag covers the client's nose and mouth.

Box 24-1 Guidelines for Bedmaking

- Use good body mechanics at all times.
- Follow the rules of medical asepsis.
- Practise Standard Precautions.
- Make the bed according to the client's wishes and the care plan. If the client's wishes are unsafe, tell your supervisor.
- Wash your hands before handling clean linen and after handling dirty linen.
- Bring enough linen to the client's room.
- Do not use torn linen.
- Never shake linens. Shaking linens spreads microbes.
- Extra linen in a client's room is considered contaminated. Do no use it for other clients (in facilities) or family members (in home care settings). Put it with the dirty laundry.
- Hold linens away from your uniform. Dirty linen and clean linen must not touch your uniform.
- Never put dirty linen on the floor or on clean linen. Handle and dispose of linen following employer policy (see Chapter 18).
- Keep bottom linens tucked in and wrinkle-free.
- Completely cover a plastic drawsheet with a cotton drawsheet. A plastic drawsheet must not touch the client's body.
- Straighten and tighten loose sheets, blankets, and bedspreads whenever necessary.
- Make as much of one side of the bed as possible before going to the other side. This saves time and energy.
- Change wet, damp, and soiled linens right away.

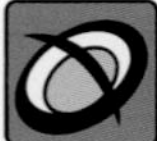

Focus on Children

Crib Safety

Cribs and crib linens present safety hazards. Mattresses, linens, and bumper pads pose many dangers. They can lead to strangulation and suffocation. Report any safety hazard to your supervisor. Always follow these safety rules:

- The crib mattress must be firm. A soft mattress can cover the baby's nose and mouth. This prevents breathing.
- The mattress must fit snugly in the crib frame. Otherwise the baby's head can get caught between the mattress and the frame. The baby can strangle.
- The space between the mattress and crib sides should be no more than 5 cm (2 inches). Only two adult fingers should fit in the space. If more than two fingers fit, the mattress does not fit.
- The mattress must be at least 65 cm (26 inches) lower than the top of the crib rails. This protects the baby from falling out of the crib. The mattress is lowered when the baby can stand in the crib.
- Plastic garbage bags and dry-cleaning bags must not be used to protect the mattress.
- Bumper pads must fit snugly against the slats. Otherwise the baby's head can get caught between the bumper pads and the slats. Strangulation can occur.
- Bumper pads must be secured in place with at least six ties.
- Bumper pad ties must be away from the baby. Avoid long ties. The baby can get entangled in the ties and strangle.
- Bumper pads must be removed when the baby can stand in the crib.
- Do not tuck blankets and top sheets under the crib. A baby can get caught in them.
- Do not place pillows, fluffy comforters, or heavy blankets in a crib with a baby. They can cause suffocation.
- Check linens for loose threads, stitching, and trim. These can cause strangulation.

The Closed Bed

A *closed bed* is made when the bed will be unoccupied for a period of time. Top linens are pulled up, and the bedspread is neatly pulled over the pillow (Figure 24-13). A closed bed is usually made when the client is up for most or all of the day. Clean linens are used as needed.

In facilities, a closed bed is also made after a client is discharged. It is made ready for a new patient or resident. The bed is made after the bed frame and mattress are cleaned and disinfected.

(text continues on page 354)

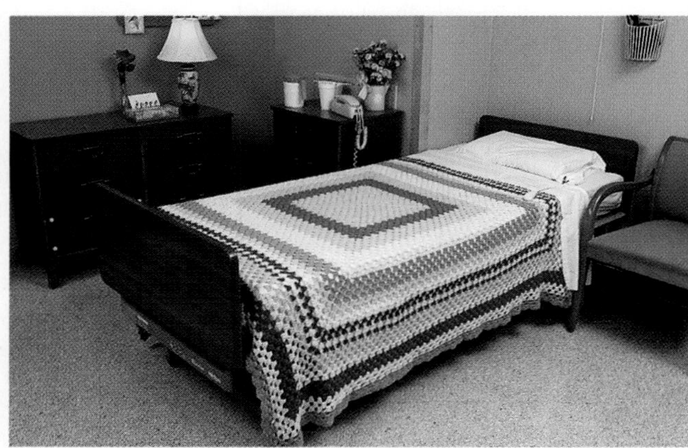

Figure 24-13 Closed bed.

Making a Closed Bed

Compassionate Care

Remember to Promote:
- **Dignity**
- **Independence**
- **Preferences**
- **Privacy**
- **Safety**

Pre-Procedure

1 Wash your hands.
2 Collect clean linen:
- Mattress pad
- Bottom sheet (flat or fitted sheet)
- Plastic drawsheet (if needed)
- Cotton drawsheet
- Top sheet
- Blanket
- Bedspread
- Two pillow cases
- Bath towel(s)*
- Hand towel*
- Wash cloth*
- Fresh pyjamas or hospital gown*
- Bath blanket*
- Gloves
- Laundry bag

3 Place linen on a clean surface.
4 Place laundry bag near the bed.
5 Make sure linens were removed and the bed and bed frame were cleaned if the person was discharged.*
6 Raise the bed to a comfortable working height.*

Procedure

7 Put on gloves if linens are soiled with blood, body fluids, secretions, or excretions.
8 Remove dirty linen. Roll each piece away from you. Place each piece in the laundry bag.
9 Remove and discard gloves. Wash your hands.
10 Move the mattress to the head of the bed.
11 Put the mattress pad on the mattress. Make sure the pad is even with the top of the mattress.
12 Place the bottom sheet on the mattress pad (Figure 24-14, page 351):
  a Unfold it lengthwise.
  b Place the centre crease in the middle of the bed.
  c Position the lower edge even with the bottom of the mattress.
  d Place the large hem at the top and the small hem at the bottom.
  e Face hem-stitching downward, away from the person.
13 Open the sheet. Fanfold it toward the other side of the bed (Figure 24-15, page 351).
14 Tuck the top of the sheet under the mattress. Make sure the sheet is tight and smooth.
15 Make a mitred corner if using a flat sheet (Figure 24-16, page 351).
16 Place the plastic drawsheet on the bed about 35 cm (14 inches) from the top of the mattress.
17 Open plastic drawsheet and fanfold it toward the other side of the bed.
18 Place a cotton drawsheet over the plastic drawsheet. It must cover the entire plastic drawsheet (Figure 24-17, page 352).
19 Open the cotton drawsheet. Fanfold it toward the other side of the bed.
20 Tuck both drawsheets under the mattress. Or tuck each in separately.

Continued

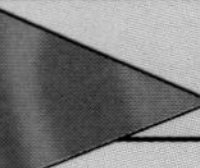

Making a Closed Bed—cont'd

Procedure—cont'd

21 Go to the other side of the bed.
22 Mitre the top corner of the bottom sheet.
23 Pull the bottom sheet tight so there are no wrinkles. Tuck in the sheet.
24 Pull the drawsheets tight so there are no wrinkles. Tuck both in together or separately (Figure 24-18, page 352).
25 Go to the other side of the bed.
26 Put the top sheet on the bed:
  a Unfold it lengthwise.
  b Place the centre crease in the middle.
  c Place the large hem even with the top of the mattress.
  d Open the sheet, and fanfold it to the other side.
  e Face hem stitching outward, away from the person.
27 Place the blanket on the bed:
  a Unfold it so the centre crease is in the middle.
  b Put the upper hem about 15 to 20 cm (6 to 8 inches) from the top of the mattress.
  c Open the blanket. Fanfold it to the other side.
  d If steps 33 and 34 are not done, turn the top sheet down over the blanket. Hem stitching is down.
28 Place the bedspread on the bed:
  a Unfold it so the centre crease is in the middle.
  b Place the upper hem even with the top of the mattress.
  c Open and fanfold the bedspread to the other side.
  d Make sure the bedspread facing the door is even and covers all the top linens.
29 Tuck in top linens together at the foot of the bed. They should be smooth and tight. Make a mitred corner.
30 Go to the other side.
31 Straighten all top linen. Work from the head of the bed to the foot.
32 Tuck in the top linens together. Make a mitred corner.
33 Turn the top hem of the bedspread under the blanket to make a cuff (Figure 24-19, page 352).
34 Turn the top sheet down over the spread. Hem stitching is down. *(Steps 33 and 34 are not done in some homes and facilities. The bedspread covers the pillow. If so, tuck the spread under the pillow.)*
35 Place the pillow on the bed.
36 Open the pillowcase so it is flat on the bed.
37 Put the pillowcase on the pillow (Figure 24-20, page 353). Fold extra material under the pillow at the seam end of the pillowcase.
38 Place the pillow on the bed. The open end is away from the door. The seam of the pillowcase is toward the head of the bed.

Post-Procedure

39 Attach the call bell to the bed.*
40 Lower the bed to its lowest position. Lock the bed wheels.*
41 Put towels, washcloth, pyjamas, and bath blanket in the bedside stand.*
42 Remove the laundry bag from the room. Follow employer policy for dirty linen.
43 Wash your hands.

*Steps marked with an asterisk may not apply in community settings.

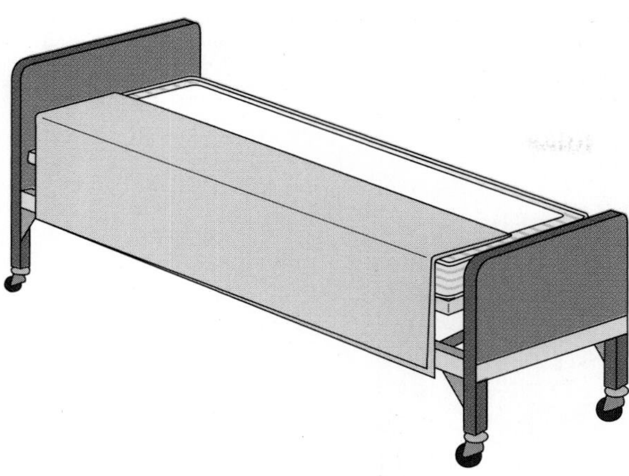

Figure 24-14 The bottom sheet is on the bed with the centre crease in the middle. The lower edge of the sheet is even with the bottom of the mattress.

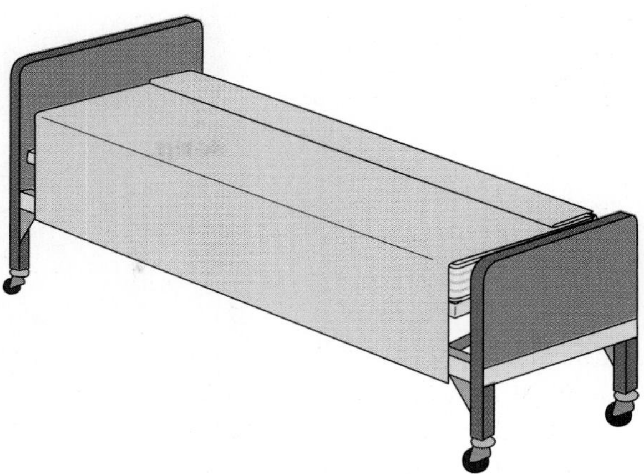

Figure 24-15 The bottom sheet is fanfolded to the other side of the bed.

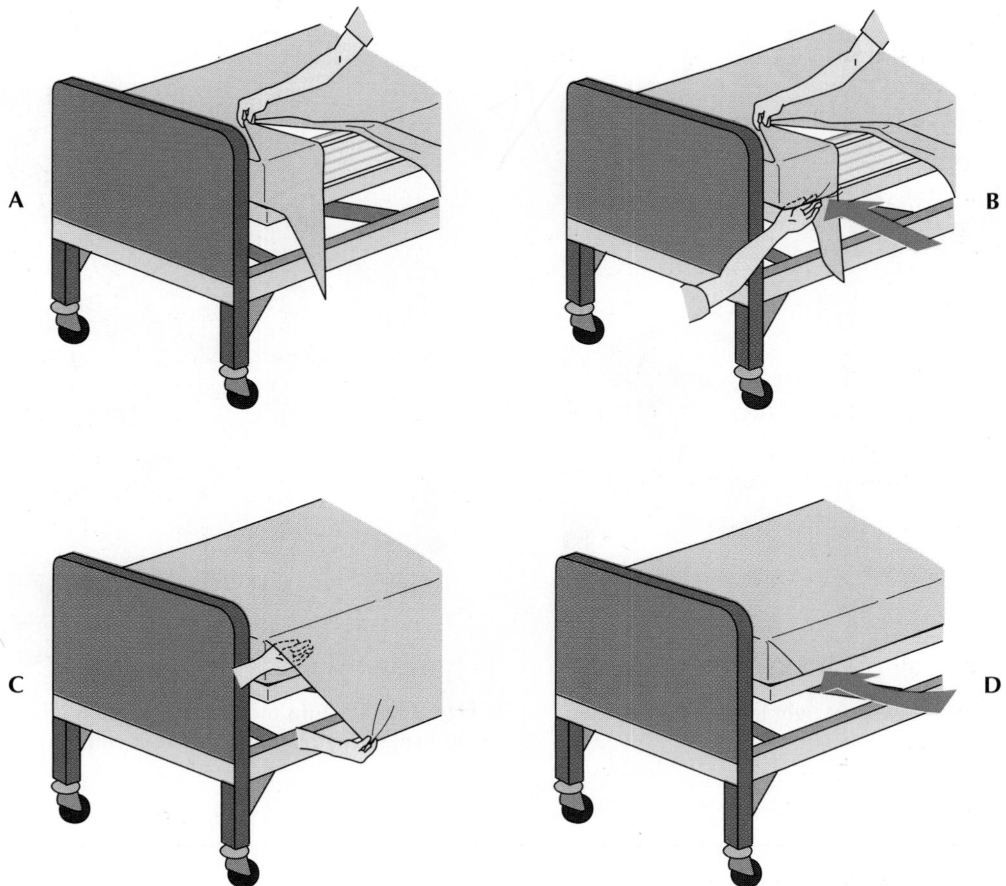

Figure 24-16 Making a mitred corner. **A,** Tuck the bottom sheet under the mattress. Raise the side of the sheet onto the mattress. **B,** Tuck the remaining portion of the sheet under the mattress. **C,** Bring the raised portion of the sheet off the mattress. **D,** Tuck the entire side of the sheet under the mattress.

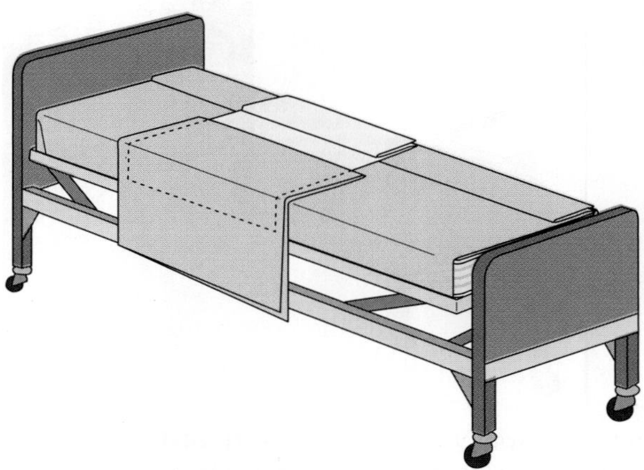

Figure 24-17 A cotton drawsheet completely covers the plastic drawsheet.

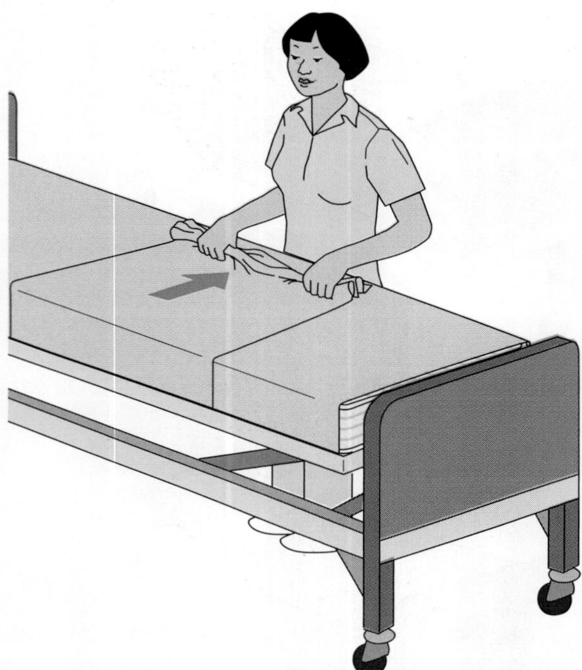

Figure 24-18 Pull the drawsheet tight to remove wrinkles.

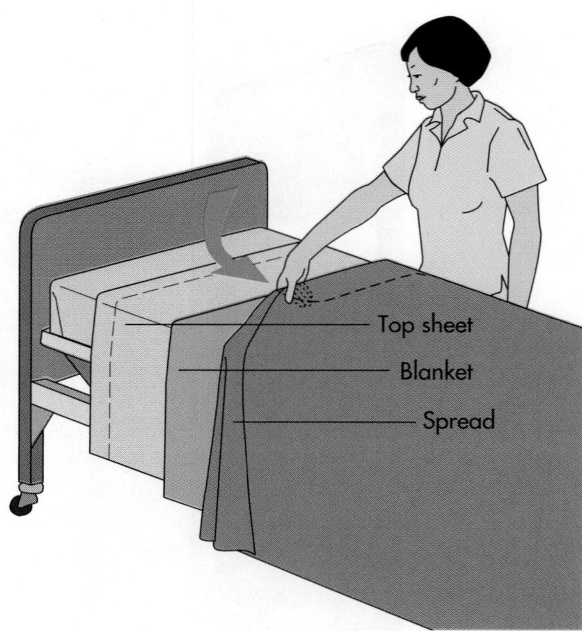

Figure 24-19 Turn the top hem of the bedspread under the top hem of the blanket to make a cuff.

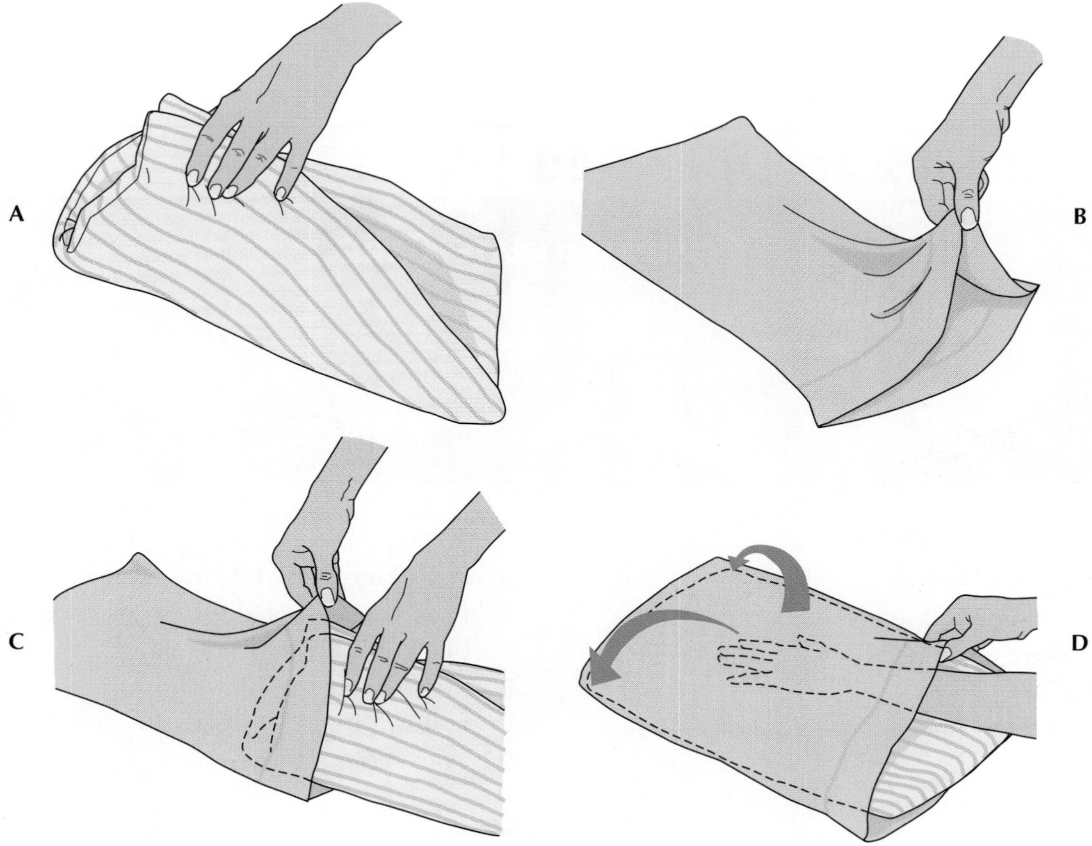

Figure 24-20 Putting a pillowcase on a pillow. **A,** Grasp the corners of the pillow at the seam end and form a "V" with the pillow. **B,** The pillowcase is flat on the bed; the pillowcase is opened with the free hand. **C,** The "V" end of the pillow is guided into the pillowcase. **D,** The "V" end of the pillow falls into the corners of the pillowcase.

THE OPEN BED

An *open* bed is made shortly before the bed is to be occupied. Top linens are folded back so the client can easily get into bed (Figure 24-21). An open bed is made when the client is out of bed for a short time only. Or it is made just before the client goes to bed.

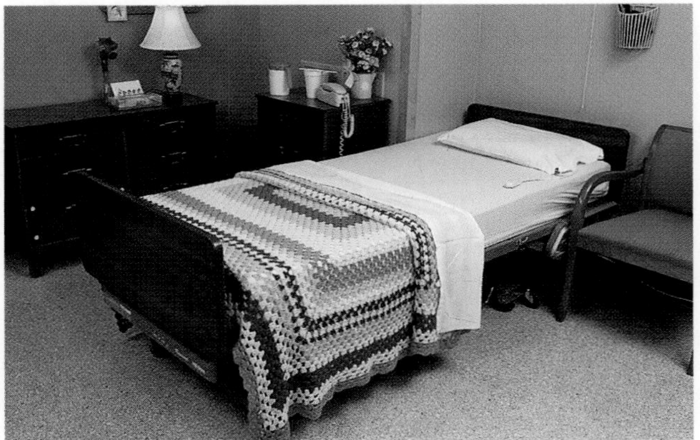

Figure 24-21 Open bed.

Making an Open Bed

COMPASSIONATE CARE

Remember to Promote:
- **Dignity**
- **Independence**
- **Preferences**
- **Privacy**
- **Safety**

Procedure

1. Wash your hands.
2. Collect linen for a closed bed.
3. Make a closed bed. (See *Making a Closed Bed*, page 349.)
4. Fanfold top linens to the foot of the bed (see Figure 24-21).
5. Attach the call bell to the bed.*
6. Lower the bed to its lowest position.*
7. Put towels, washcloth, pyjamas, and bath blanket in the bedside stand.*
8. Remove the laundry bag from the room. Follow employer policy for dirty linen.
9. Wash your hands.

*Steps marked with an asterisk may not apply in community settings.

The Occupied Bed

An *occupied bed* is made with the client in it (Figure 24-22). It is made when a client cannot get out of bed because of illness or injury. You must keep the client in good body alignment. You must know about restrictions or limits in the client's movement or positioning. Explain each step of the procedure to the client before it is done. Always explain what you are doing even if the client cannot respond to you or is in a coma.

(text continues on page 359)

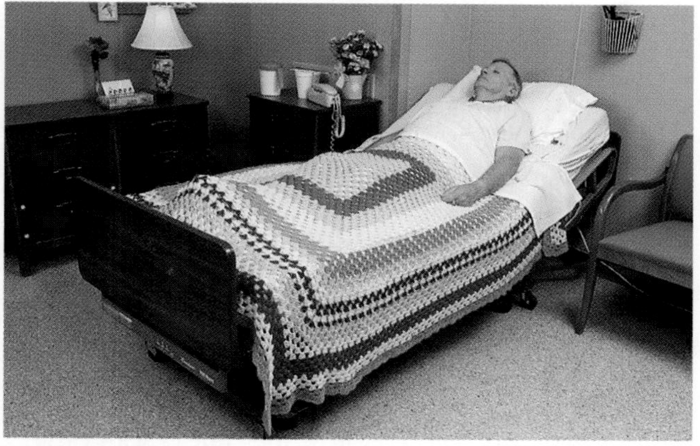

Figure 24-22 Occupied bed.

Making an Occupied Bed

Compassionate Care

Remember to Promote:
- **Dignity**
- **Independence**
- **Preferences**
- **Privacy**
- **Safety**

Pre-Procedure

1 Identify the person according to employer policy.
2 Explain the procedure to the person.
3 Wash your hands.
4 Collect the following:
- Gloves
- Laundry bag
- Clean linen (see *Making a Closed Bed*, page 349)

5 Place linen on a clean surface.
6 Provide for privacy.
7 Remove the call bell.*
8 Place the laundry bag near the bed.
9 Raise the bed to a comfortable working height. Follow the care plan for bed rail use.*
10 Lower the head of the bed. It should be as flat as possible. Lower the bed rail near you if up.*

Procedure

11 Put on the gloves if linens are soiled with blood, body fluids, secretions, or excretions.
12 Loosen top linens at the foot of the bed.
13 Remove the bedspread and blanket separately. Fold them as in Figure 24-23 on page 357 if you will reuse them. Place each over a chair.
14 Cover the person with a bath blanket to provide warmth and privacy:
a Unfold a bath blanket over the top sheet.
b Ask the person to hold on to the bath blanket. If he or she cannot, tuck the top part under the shoulders.

Continued

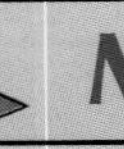

Making an Occupied Bed—cont'd

Procedure—cont'd

- **c** Grasp the top sheet under the bath blanket at the shoulders. Bring the sheet down to the foot of the bed. Remove the sheet from under the blanket (Figure 24-24, page 358).

15 Move the mattress to the head of the bed.

16 Position the person on the side of the bed away from you. Adjust the pillow for comfort.

17 Loosen bottom linens from the head to the foot of the bed.

18 Fanfold bottom linens one at a time toward the person. Start with the cotton drawsheet (Figure 24-25, page 358). If reusing the mattress pad, do not fanfold it.

19 Place a clean mattress pad on the bed. Unfold it lengthwise. The centre crease is in the middle. Fanfold the top part toward the person. If reusing the mattress pad, straighten and smooth any wrinkles.

20 Place the bottom sheet on the mattress pad. Hem stitching is away from the person. Unfold the sheet so the crease is in the middle. The small hem is even with the bottom of the mattress. Fanfold the top part toward the person.

21 Make a mitred corner at the head of the bed. Tuck the sheet under the mattress from the head to the foot.

22 Pull the plastic drawsheet toward you over the bottom sheet. Tuck excess material under the mattress. Do the following for a clean plastic drawsheet (Figure 24-26, page 358):

- **a** Place the plastic drawsheet on the bed. It is about 35 cm (14 inches) from the mattress top.
- **b** Fanfold the top part toward the person.
- **c** Tuck in the extra fabric.

23 Place the cotton drawsheet over the plastic drawsheet. It must cover the entire plastic drawsheet. Fanfold the top part toward the person. Tuck in extra fabric.

24 Raise the bed rail if used. Go to the other side and lower the bed rail.

25 Explain to the person that he or she will roll over a bump. Assure the person that he or she will not fall.

26 Help the person turn to the other side. Adjust the pillow for the person's comfort.

27 Loosen bottom linens. Remove one piece at a time. Place each piece in the laundry bag.

28 Remove and discard the gloves, if worn. Wash your hands.

29 Straighten and smooth the mattress pad.

30 Pull the clean bottom sheet toward you. Make a mitred corner at the top. Tuck the sheet under the mattress from the head to the foot of the bed.

31 Pull the drawsheets tightly toward you. Tuck both under together or separately.

32 Position the person supine in the centre of the bed. Adjust the pillow for comfort.

33 Put the top sheet on the bed. Unfold it lengthwise. The crease is in the middle, and the large hem is even with the top of the mattress. Hem stitching is on the outside.

34 Ask the person to hold on to the sheet so you can remove the bath blanket. Or tuck the top sheet under the person's shoulders. Remove the bath blanket.

35 Place the blanket on the bed. Unfold it so the crease is in the middle and it covers the person. The upper hem should be 15 to 20 cm (6 to 8 inches) from the top of the mattress.

36 Place the bedspread on the bed. Unfold it so the centre crease is in the middle and it covers the person. The top hem is even with the mattress top.

37 Turn the top hem of the bedspread under the blanket to make a cuff.

38 Bring the top sheet down over the bedspread to form a cuff.

39 Go to the foot of the bed.

40 Make a toe pleat. Make a 5-cm (2-inch) pleat across the foot of the bed. The pleat is about 15 to 20 cm (6 to 8 inches) from the foot of the bed.

Continued

Making an Occupied Bed—cont'd

Procedure—cont'd

41 Lift the mattress corner with one arm. Tuck all top linens under the mattress together. Make a mitred corner.

42 Raise the bed rail if used. Go to the other side, and lower the bed rail.

43 Straighten and smooth top linens.

44 Tuck the top linens under the mattress. Make a mitred corner.

45 Change the pillowcase(s).

46 Raise the head of the bed to a level appropriate for the person. Or use pillows to position the person.

Post-Procedure

47 Provide for safety and comfort.

48 Place the call bell within reach.*

49 Lower the bed to its lowest position. Follow the care plan for bed rail use.*

50 Put towels, washcloth, pyjamas, and bath blanket in the bedside stand.*

51 Remove privacy measures as needed.

52 Remove linen bag from the room. Follow employer policy for dirty linen.

53 Wash your hands.

*Steps marked with an asterisk may not apply in community settings.

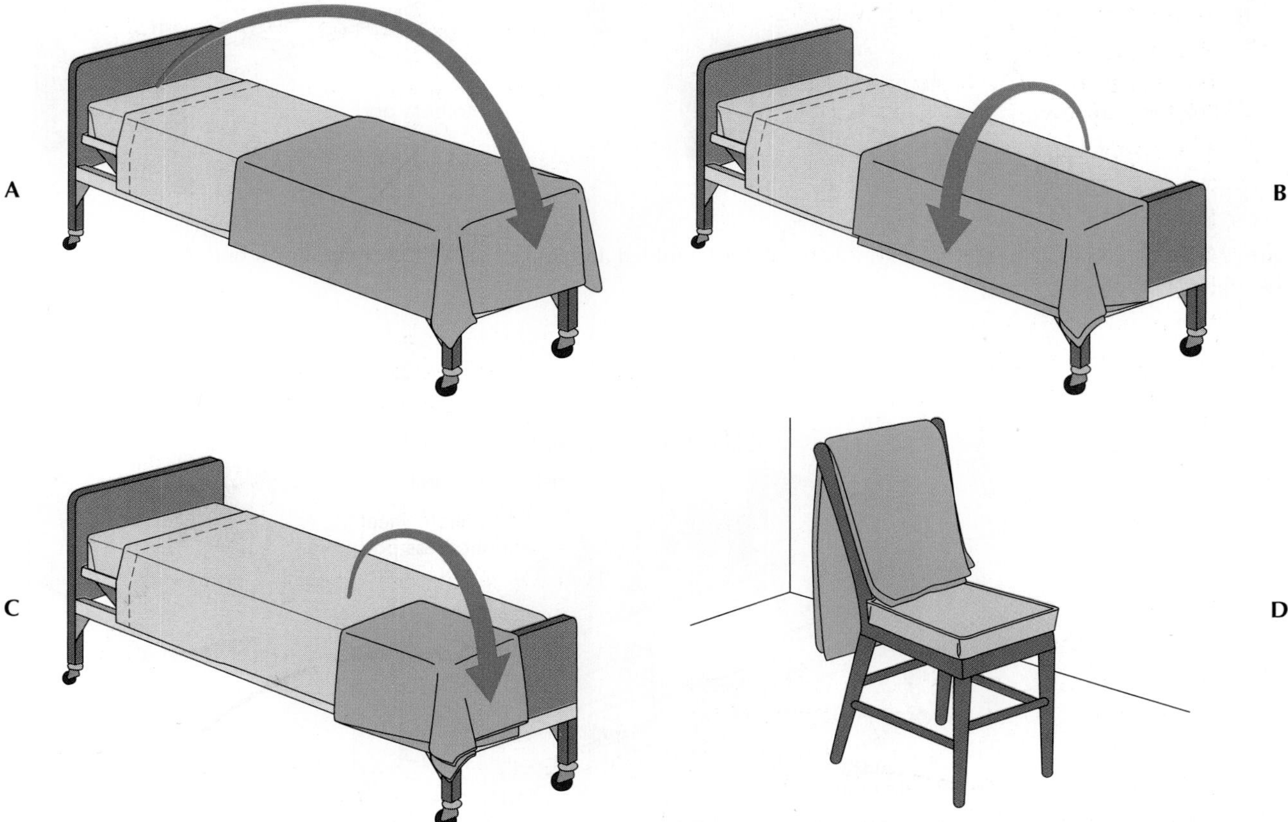

Figure 24-23 Folding linen for reuse. **A,** Fold the top edge of the blanket down to the bottom edge. **B,** Fold the blanket from the far side of the bed to the near side. **C,** Fold the top edge of the blanket down to the bottom edge again. **D,** Place the folded blanket over the back of a straight chair.

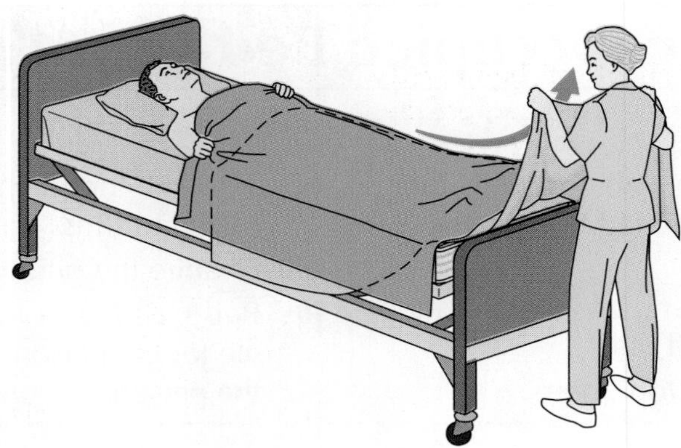

Figure 24-24 Ask the client to hold on to the bath blanket. Remove the top sheet from under the bath blanket.

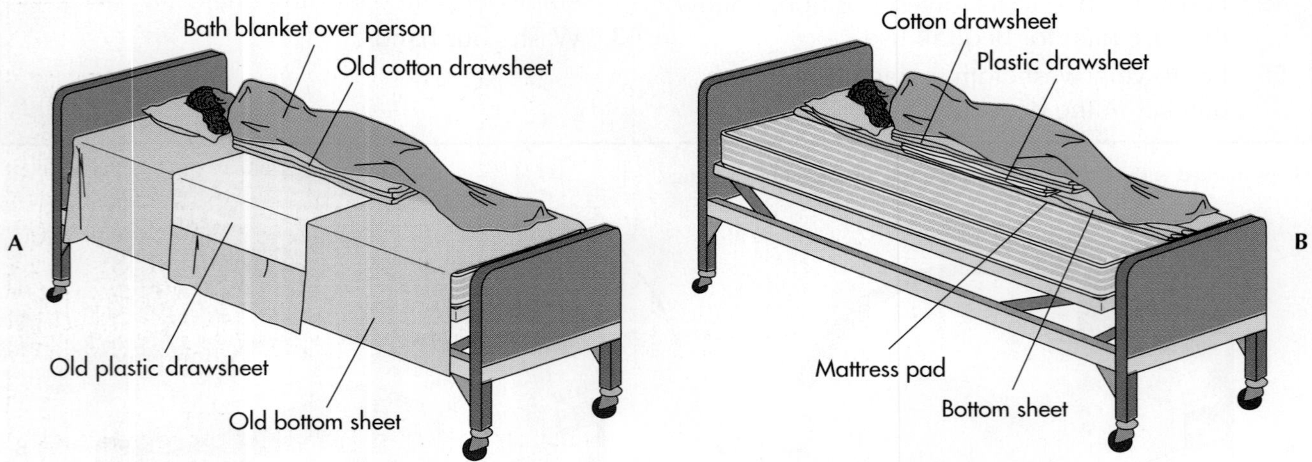

Figure 24-25 Occupied bed. **A,** The cotton drawsheet is fanfolded and tucked under the client. **B,** All bottom linens are tucked under the client.

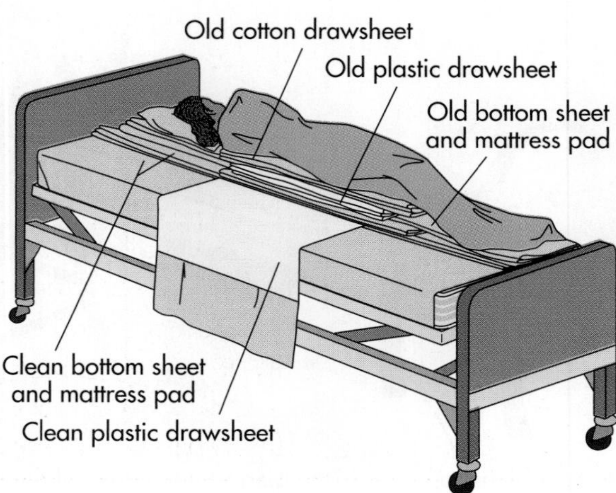

Figure 24-26 A clean bottom sheet and plastic drawsheet are on the bed, with both fanfolded and tucked under the client.

The Surgical Bed

A *surgical bed* is made so that a client can be moved from a stretcher to the bed. It also is called a postoperative bed, recovery bed, or anesthesia bed (Figure 24-27). It is a form of the open bed. Top linens are folded for transferring the client to or from a stretcher. If the bed is made for a postoperative (surgical) patient, a complete linen change is done. Surgical beds are only made in facilities.

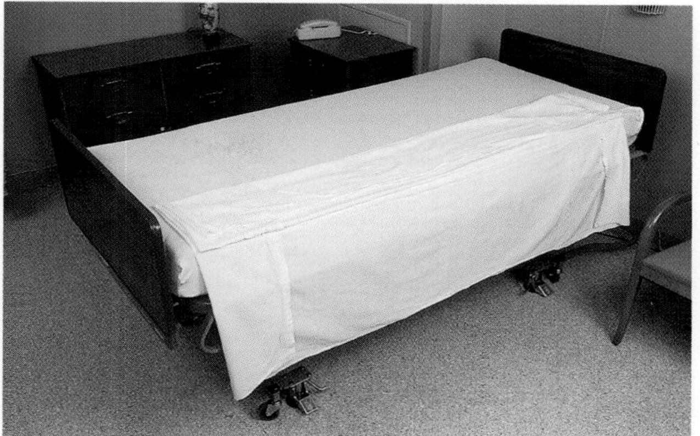

Figure 24-27 Surgical bed.

Making a Surgical Bed

Compassionate Care

Remember to Promote:
- **Dignity**
- **Independence**
- **Preferences**
- **Privacy**
- **Safety**

Procedure

1 Wash your hands.
2 Collect the following:
- Clean linen (see *Making a Closed Bed,* page 349)
- Gloves
- Laundry bag
- Equipment as requested by your supervisor

3 Place linen on a clean surface.
4 Remove the call bell.
5 Raise the bed to a comfortable working height.
6 Remove all linen from the bed. Wear gloves if contact with blood, body fluids, secretions, or excretions is likely.
7 Place removed linen in the laundry bag.
8 Make a closed bed (see *Making a Closed Bed,* page 349). Do not tuck the top linens under the mattress.
9 Fold all top linens at the foot of the bed back onto the bed. The fold is even with the edge of the mattress (Figure 24-28, page 360).
10 Fanfold linen lengthwise to the side of the bed farthest from the door (Figure 24-29, page 360).
11 Put the pillowcase(s) on the pillow(s).
12 Place the pillow(s) on a clean surface.
13 Leave the bed in its highest position.
14 Make sure both bed rails are down.
15 Put the towels, washcloth, gown, and bath blanket in the bedside stand.
16 Move all furniture away from the bed. Allow enough room for the stretcher and for the staff to move about.
17 Do not attach the call bell to the bed.
18 Remove the laundry bag from the room. Follow employer policy for dirty linen.
19 Wash your hands.

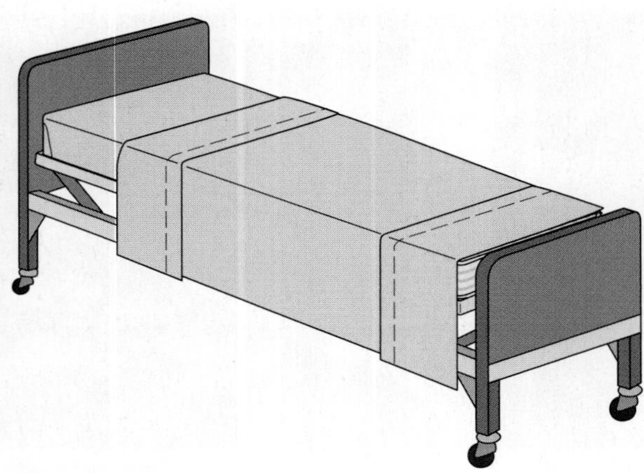

Figure 24-28 Surgical bed. The bottom of the top linens is folded back onto the bed. The fold is even with the edge of the mattress.

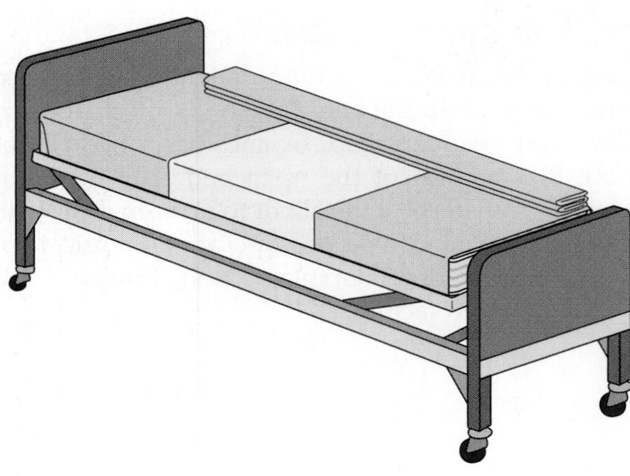

Figure 24-29 A surgical bed with the top linens fanfolded lengthwise to one side of the bed.

REVIEW

Circle the BEST answer.

1. A hospital bed
   A. Cannot be raised or lowered
   B. Cannot be controlled by the client
   C. Usually has bed rails
   D. Is kept in the highest position at all times

2. Trendelenburg's bed position is
   A. A semi-sitting position
   B. When the head of the bed is lowered, and the foot of the bed is raised
   C. A flat position for sleeping
   D. When the head of the bed is raised, and the foot of the bed is lowered

3. Which does *not* require a linen change?
   A. Soiled linen
   B. Wet linen
   C. A bed for a new patient or resident
   D. Wrinkled or loose linen

4. When handling linens
   A. Put dirty linens on the floor
   B. Hold linens away from your body and uniform
   C. Shake linens to remove crumbs
   D. Take extra linen to another client's room

5. A cotton drawsheet is
   A. Placed over the middle of the bottom sheet and over the plastic drawsheet
   B. Waterproof
   C. Placed under the bottom sheet
   D. Placed under the plastic drawsheet

6. You are using a plastic drawsheet. Which is *true*?
   A. A cotton drawsheet must completely cover the plastic drawsheet.
   B. Disposable bed protectors are needed.
   C. The client's consent is needed.
   D. The plastic must be in contact with the client's skin.

7. The following are crib safety rules. Which is *false*?
   A. Bumper pads must be removed when the baby can stand in the crib.
   B. The mattress must fit snugly in the crib frame.
   C. Plastic garbage bags and dry-cleaning bags may be used to protect the mattress.
   D. Pillows, fluffy comforters, and heavy blankets must not be in the crib with a baby.

8. An open bed is made
   A. When the bed will be unoccupied for a period of time
   B. Shortly before the bed is to be occupied
   C. With the client in it
   D. So that a client can be moved to or from a stretcher

9. When making an occupied bed, you do the following *except*
   A. Cover the client with a bath blanket
   B. Provide for privacy
   C. Raise the far bed rail if bed rails are used
   D. Fanfold top linens to the foot of the bed

10. A surgical bed is kept
    A. In Fowler's position
    B. In the lowest position
    C. In the highest position
    D. In semi-Fowler's position

Answers to these questions are on page 824.

CHAPTER 25

BASIC NUTRITION AND FLUIDS

OBJECTIVES

- Define the key terms listed in this chapter
- Describe the functions and major sources of protein, carbohydrates, fats, vitamins, minerals, and water
- Explain the principles of *Canada's Food Guide to Healthy Eating*
- Explain the purpose of food labels
- Explain how nutrient requirements change throughout the life cycle
- Explain factors that affect eating and nutrition
- Explain your role in meal planning and preparation
- Explain why food safety is important
- Describe special diets
- Explain your role in assisting clients to eat
- Explain how to feed clients
- Describe adult fluid requirements and the common causes of edema and dehydration
- Describe three common special fluid orders
- Explain the purpose of intake and output records
- Learn the procedures described in this chapter

KEY TERMS

allergy Sensitivity to a substance that causes the body to react with signs and symptoms

aspiration Inhaling fluid or an object into the lungs

calorie The amount of energy produced as the body burns food

cross-contamination The spread of pathogens from one source to another

Daily Value (DV) How a serving fits into the daily diet; expressed as a percentage based on recommended daily intake

dehydration A decrease in the amount of water in body tissues

dysphagia Difficulty (*dys*) swallowing (*phagia*)

edema Swelling of body tissues with water

foodborne illness An illness caused by improperly cooked or stored food

intake The amount of fluids taken in by the body

nutrient A substance that is ingested, digested, absorbed, and used by the body

nutrition The many processes involved in the ingestion, digestion, absorption, and use of foods and fluids by the body

output The amount of fluid lost by the body

pathogen Disease-causing microbe

Food and water are necessary for life and health. The amount and quality of foods and fluids in the diet are important. They affect a person's current and future health and well-being. A poor diet affects physical and mental function, increases the risk for disease, and slows healing. Poor physical and mental functioning increases the risk for accidents and injuries.

Food and drink contribute to social and emotional health. Eating and drinking are part of social activity with family and friends (Figure 25-1). Many people need a friendly, social setting for meals. Otherwise they eat poorly.

As a support worker, you will serve food and fluids to clients and assist them with eating. In home care settings, you may also prepare meals. This chapter introduces you to the basics of nutrition.

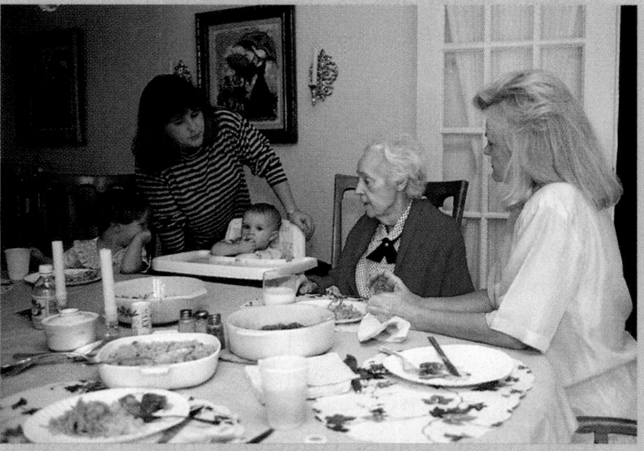

Figure 25-1 Meals are enjoyed when shared with family and friends.

BASIC NUTRITION

Nutrition refers to the many processes involved in the ingestion, digestion, absorption, and use of foods and fluids by the body. *Ingestion* is the process of taking food and fluids into the body. *Digestion* is the process of physically and chemically breaking down food so that it can be absorbed for use by the cells. *Absorption* is the process by which substances pass through the intestinal wall into the blood. Review the description of the digestive system in Chapter 13.

Good nutrition is needed for growth, healing, and the maintenance of body functions. Selected foods must provide a well-balanced diet and correct calorie intake. A diet high in fat and calories causes weight gain and obesity. Weight loss occurs when a person consumes fewer calories than needed.

NUTRIENTS

Foods and fluids contain nutrients. A **nutrient** is a substance that is ingested, digested, absorbed, and used by the body. Nutrients are grouped into proteins, carbohydrates, fats, vitamins, minerals, and water.

Proteins, fats, and carbohydrates give the body fuel for energy. The amount of energy provided by a nutrient is measured in calories. A **calorie** is the amount of energy produced as the body burns food.

- 1 gram of carbohydrate supplies the body with 4 calories
- 1 gram of protein supplies the body with 4 calories
- 1 gram of fat supplies the body with 9 calories

Protein. This nutrient is needed for tissue growth and repair. Protein sources include meat, fish, poultry, eggs, milk and milk products, cereals, beans, peas, and nuts. Animal products are the best sources of protein. People who do not eat animal products must consume sufficient protein from plant sources. Plant sources are best eaten in combination. For example, beans and rice eaten together are an excellent source of protein. Protein deficiency can result in severe malnutrition. Children and older adults who do not eat properly are at risk.

Carbohydrates. This nutrient provides energy for the body and fibre for bowel elimination. Most carbohydrates come from plants. There are three main kinds of carbohydrates:

- *Simple sugars* are in table sugar, fruit, and fruit juices.
- *Starches* are in bread, pasta, rice, and potatoes.
- *Fibre* is in bran, nuts, seeds, and raw fruits with skins. Fibre cannot be digested. It passes through the intestines undigested.

Most carbohydrates (except fibre) are broken down into sugars during digestion. The sugars are then absorbed into the blood stream.

Fats. These provide energy, help the body to use certain vitamins, and add flavour to food. Some fat is necessary in the diet. Dietary fat not needed by the body is stored as body fat. There are three main types of dietary fat:

- *Saturated fat* is in animal and dairy products (for example, meat, butter, milk, and cheeses).
- *Unsaturated fat* is in fish and many vegetable oils (for example, canola oil and olive oil).
- *Trans-fat* is in margarine, shortening, store-bought cookies, cakes, pies, doughnuts, and fried foods. Trans-fat is created when liquid oil is chemically altered to form a more solid substance. It is used to increase the flavour and shelf life of foods.

Unsaturated fat is healthier than saturated fat and trans-fat.

Vitamins. Vitamins are needed daily for normal function and growth. They do not provide calories. Each vitamin is needed for specific body functions (Table 25-1). For example, vitamin A is necessary for vision. Vitamins are an essential part of a healthy diet. The lack of a specific vitamin may result in illness. Older adults are at risk for developing vitamin deficiencies because the aging process affects the body's ability to absorb certain vitamins.

Minerals. These are chemical substances in both plant and animal foods. Each mineral is needed for specific body functions. For example, calcium and phosphorus are used to form strong bones and teeth. Table 25-2 lists the major functions and sources of minerals.

Water. Water is the most important nutrient for life. The body needs water for maintaining cell function, regulating body temperature, delivering nutrients, removing waste, and other body processes. Death can result from inadequate water intake or from excessive fluid loss. Water enters the body through fluids and foods. Water is lost through urine and feces, through the skin as perspiration, and through the lungs with expiration. There must be a balance between the amount of fluid taken in and the amount lost.

Canada's Food Guide to Healthy Eating

Canada's Food Guide to Healthy Eating was developed by Health Canada to promote wise food choices. Healthy eating is needed to:

- Ensure a daily diet of the essential nutrients
- Promote health and an overall sense of physical and mental well-being
- Reduce the risk of nutrient-related health problems

The Food Guide divides foods into four groups. Each contains different foods and nutrients.

- *Grain Products*—cereals, pasta, rice, and other foods made with flour
- *Vegetables & Fruit*—fresh, canned, frozen, and dried vegetables and fruit; fruit juices
- *Milk Products*—milk (fresh, powdered, or evaporated), cream, cheese, yogurt, and ice cream
- *Meat & Alternatives*—fresh and canned meat, poultry, fish, eggs, beans, lentils, dried peas, nuts, peanut butter, and tofu

A healthy diet contains foods from each food group. In the Food Guide, the four food groups are shown in a rainbow design (Figure 25-2 on page 366). The rainbow bands are of different lengths, indicating how much of the recommended diet should come from each food group. Most food servings should come from the yellow band, representing grains. Grains are rich in carbohydrates. Most Canadians eat too much fat. Eating more carbohydrates (whole bread, cereal, grains, vegetables, fruit, peas, beans, and lentils) helps reduce fat intake. Foods high in

(text continues on page 367)

Table 25-1 Vitamins: Major Functions and Sources

	Major functions	Sources
Vitamin A	Growth; vision; healthy hair, skin, and mucous membranes; resistance to infection	Liver, spinach, green leafy and yellow vegetables, yellow fruits, fish liver oils, egg yolk, butter, cream, whole milk
Vitamin B_1 (thiamin)	Muscle tone, nerve function, digestion, appetite, normal elimination, carbohydrate use	Pork, fish, poultry, eggs, liver, breads, pastas, cereals, oatmeal, potatoes, peas, beans, soybeans, peanuts
Vitamin B_2 (riboflavin)	Growth, vision, protein and carbohydrate metabolism, healthy skin and mucous membranes	Milk and milk products, liver, green leafy vegetables, eggs, breads, cereals
Vitamin B_3 (niacin)	Protein, fat, and carbohydrate metabolism; nervous system function; appetite; digestive system function	Meat, pork, liver, fish, peanuts, breads and cereals, green vegetables, dairy products
Vitamin B_{12}	Formation of red blood cells, protein metabolism, nervous system function	Liver, meats, poultry, fish, eggs, milk, cheese
Folic acid	Formation of red blood cells, intestinal function, protein metabolism	Liver, meats, fish, poultry, green leafy vegetables, whole grains
Vitamin C (ascorbic acid)	Formation of substances that hold tissues together; healthy blood vessels, skin, gums, bones, and teeth; wound healing; prevention of bleeding; resistance to infection	Citrus fruits, tomatoes, potatoes, cabbage, strawberries, green vegetables, melons
Vitamin D	Absorption and metabolism of calcium and phosphorous; healthy bones	Fish liver oils, milk, butter, liver, exposure to sunlight
Vitamin E	Normal reproduction, formation of red blood cells, muscle function	Vegetable oils, milk, eggs, meats, cereals, green leafy vegetables
Vitamin K	Blood clotting	Liver, green leafy vegetables, egg yolk, cheese

Table 25-2 Minerals: Major Functions and Sources

	Major functions	Sources
Calcium	Formation of teeth and bones, blood clotting, muscle contraction, heart function, nerve function	Milk and milk products, green leafy vegetables, whole grains, egg yolk, dried peas and beans, nuts
Phosphorus	Formation of bones and teeth; use of proteins, fats, and carbohydrates; nerve and muscle function	Meat, fish, poultry, milk and milk products, nuts, egg yolk, dried peas and beans
Iron	Allows red blood cells to carry oxygen	Liver, meat, eggs, green leafy vegetables, breads and cereals, dried peas and beans, nuts
Iodine	Thyroid gland function, growth, metabolism	Iodized salt, seafood, and shellfish
Sodium	Fluid balance, nerve and muscle function	Almost all foods
Potassium	Nerve function, muscle contraction, heart function	Fruits, vegetables, cereals, meats, dried peas and beans
Zinc	Growth process, healing process, immune system	Meat, poultry, whole grains, dried peas and beans, eggs

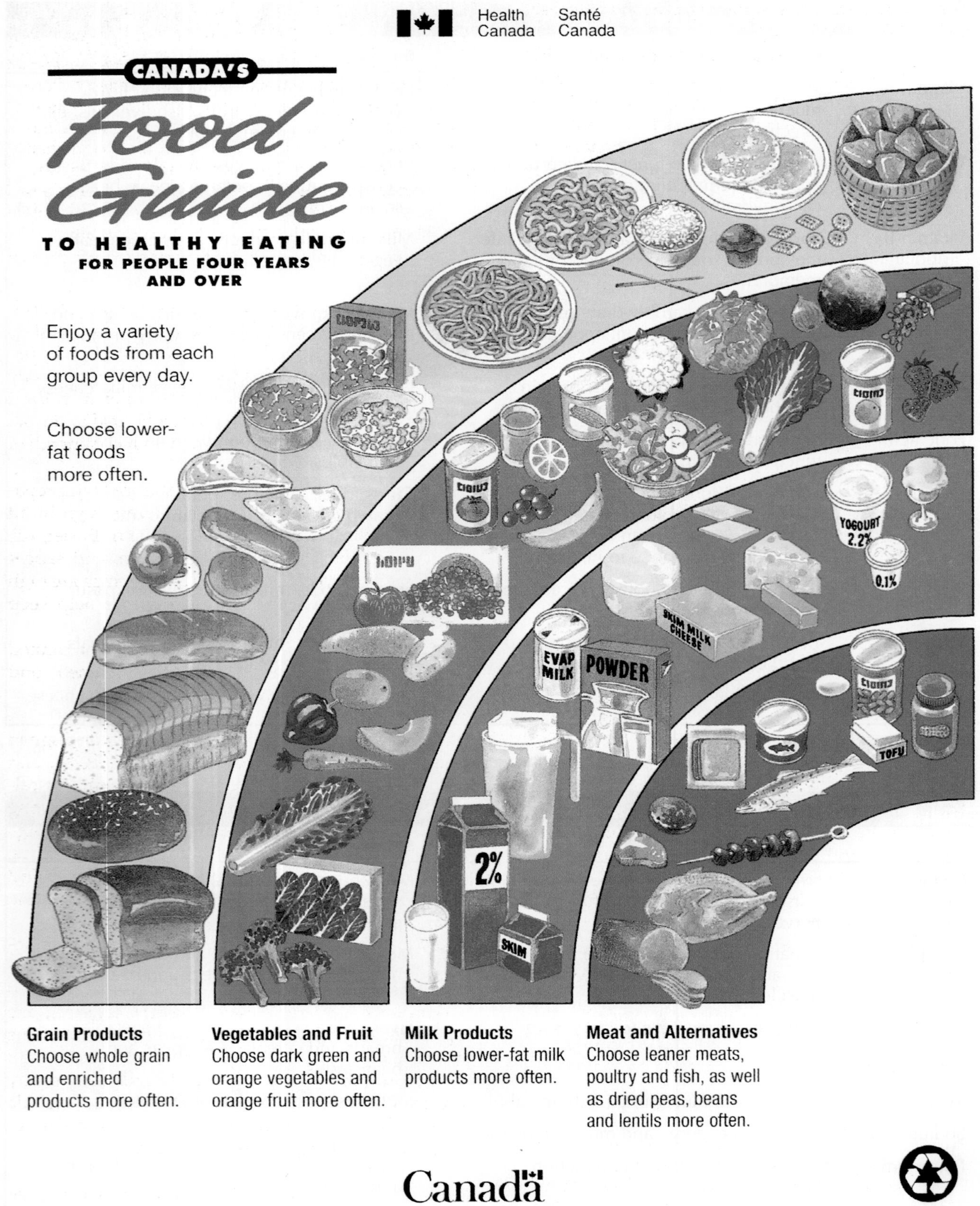

Health Canada
Santé Canada
CANADA'S
Food Guide
TO HEALTHY EATING
FOR PEOPLE FOUR YEARS AND OVER
Enjoy a variety of foods from each group every day.
Choose lower-fat foods more often.
YOGOURT 2.2%
0.1%
SKIM MILK CHEESE
EVAP MILK
POWDER
2%
SKIM
TOFU
Grain Products
Choose whole grain and enriched products more often.
Vegetables and Fruit
Choose dark green and orange vegetables and orange fruit more often.
Milk Products
Choose lower-fat milk products more often.
Meat and Alternatives
Choose leaner meats, poultry and fish, as well as dried peas, beans and lentils more often.
Canada

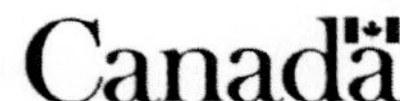

Figure 25-2 Canada's Food Guide to Healthy Eating. Source: Health Canada.

carbohydrates are filling, allowing a person to feel satisfied with less food.

The Food Guide contains a fifth category, called *Other Foods,* not included on the rainbow as a food group. Other foods include sugars, jam, honey, soft drinks, oils and fats, caffeine, and alcohol. Many of these foods are high in fat or sugar. Most have little nutritional value. These foods have been excluded from the rainbow to remind Canadians to use them in moderation.

The Food Guide is for everyone older than 4 years of age. Better health is the goal. Many diseases are related to diet and the kinds of foods eaten. They include heart disease, high blood pressure, stroke, diabetes, osteoporosis, and certain cancers. Following the guidelines in the Food Guide reduces the risk for such diseases. Box 25-1 lists the guidelines for healthy eating.

Servings from the Food Groups

The number of servings a person needs depends on age, size, gender, and activity level. The Food Guide gives a range for the number and size of servings for each food group. Children should choose the lowest number of servings. Women who are pregnant or breastfeeding, teenage boys, and very active individuals should choose the highest number. Most people should choose a number in between.

The Food Guide shows serving sizes as a guide. In the grain group, one serving is one slice of bread, $^{3}/_{4}$ cup of cereal, one bagel, or one cup of cooked pasta or rice (Figure 25-3 on page 368).

Grain Products. More servings are recommended from this group than from any other group. Health Canada recommends 5 to 12 servings per day. Carbohydrates (especially fibre), protein, iron, thiamin, niacin, riboflavin, folic acid, iron, and zinc are the main nutrients in this group. The Food Guide recommends whole-grain products, which are high in fibre. Enriched products are also recommended because they contain more iron and B vitamins than non-enriched products (Box 25-2).

Box 25-1 Guidelines for Healthy Eating

- Enjoy a variety of foods.
- Emphasize cereals, breads, other grain products, vegetables, and fruit.
- Choose lower-fat dairy products, leaner meats, and foods prepared with little or no fat.
- Achieve and maintain a healthy body weight by enjoying regular physical activity and healthy eating.
- Limit salt, alcohol, and caffeine.

Source: Health Canada, *Canada's Food Guide to Healthy Eating.*

Box 25-2 Fortified and Enriched Foods

Food processing removes valuable nutrients from food. To replace losses or enhance nutrient content, foods are *enriched* or *fortified.* In enriched foods, nutrients are replaced to their original level or higher. Examples are wheat flour, cereal, and pasta. In fortified foods, nutrients have been added. An example is milk, which is fortified with vitamin D. Food labels indicate whether a food is fortified or enriched.

Vegetables & Fruit. Vegetables and fruits (including juices) provide carbohydrates, vitamins C and A, iron, and magnesium. They are naturally low in fat. The Food Guide recommends 5 to 10 servings per day from this group. Some servings should contain dark green vegetables, which are rich in folic acid and iron. Orange fruits and vegetables are also recommended. They are rich in vitamin A.

Vegetables can become high in fat from food preparation. For example, french fries are very high in fat compared with a baked or boiled potato. Butter, oil, mayonnaise, salad dressing, sour cream, and sauces are often added to vegetables. These toppings are high in fat. Small amounts of low-fat toppings help keep vegetables low in fat.

Fresh fruits and juices are best. Frozen or canned fruit should be unsweetened. If sweetened and syrupy, they are high in sugar and calories.

Milk Products. Milk and milk products are high in protein, calcium, carbohydrates, fat, riboflavin, and vitamins A and D. They are the richest source of calcium, which is needed to form and maintain strong bones. The Food Guide recommends 2 to 4 servings per day from the milk products group—milk, cheese, and yogurt. Children 4–9 need 2 to 3 servings per day. Youths 10–16 as well as pregnant and breastfeeding women need 3 to 4 servings per day.

Lower-fat milk products have less fat than whole-milk products. Yet they provide the protein and calcium essential to a healthy diet. For example, one cup of skim milk has only a trace of fat (86 calories); one cup of whole milk has about 150 calories—72 of the calories come from fat. Choose products low in milk fat and butterfat. Skim, 1%, and 2% milk are healthy choices. Other low-fat foods in this group include cheeses made with skim milk, low-fat or non-fat yogurt, and ice milk rather than ice cream.

Meat & Alternatives. Protein, fat, thiamin, vitamin B_{12}, and iron are the main nutrients in this group. Health Canada recommends 2 to 3 servings of meat and alternatives per day.

(text continues on page 369)

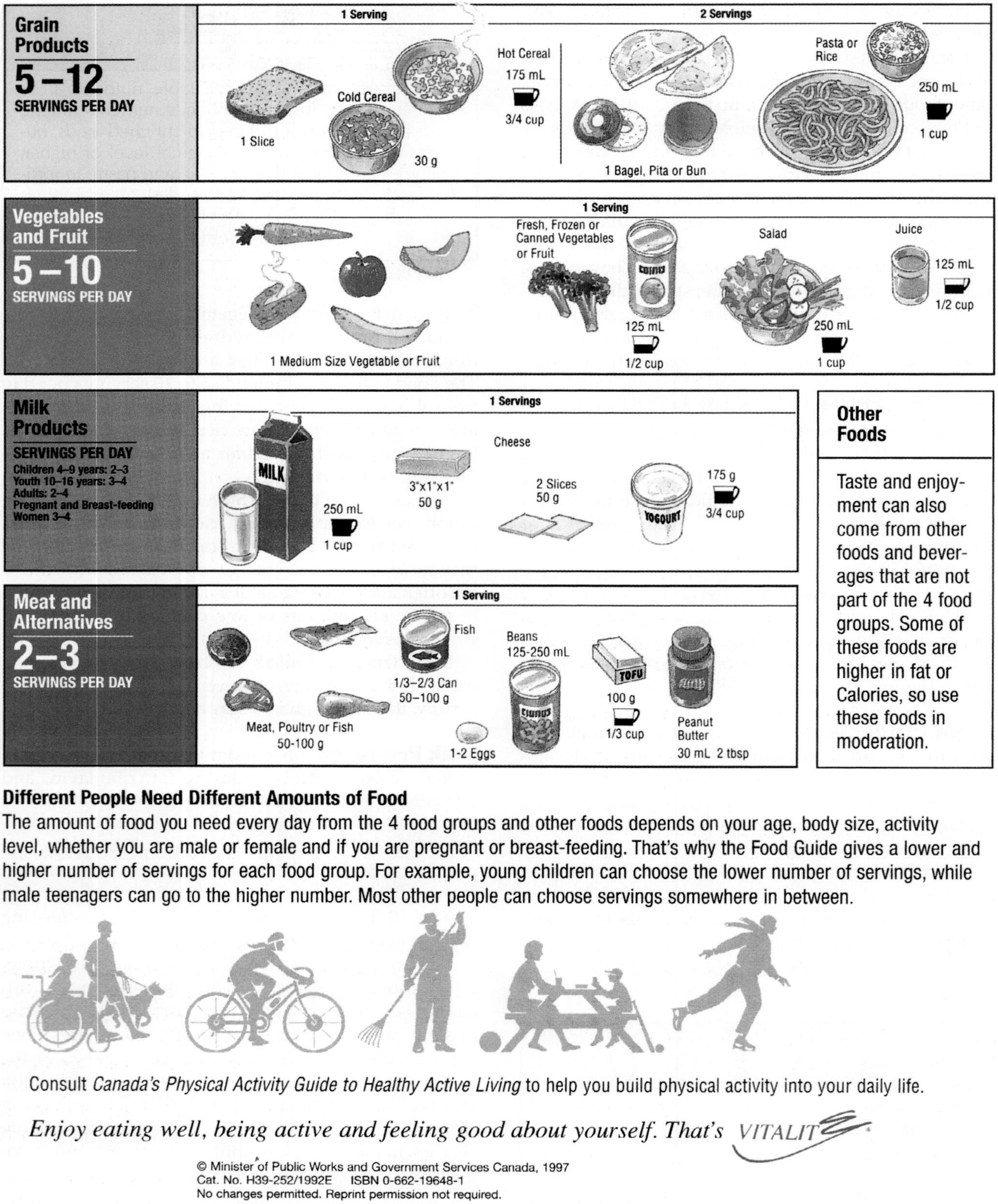

Grain Products
5–12
SERVINGS PER DAY

1 Serving: 1 Slice; Cold Cereal 30 g; Hot Cereal 175 mL 3/4 cup

2 Servings: 1 Bagel, Pita or Bun; Pasta or Rice 250 mL 1 cup

Vegetables and Fruit
5–10
SERVINGS PER DAY

1 Serving: 1 Medium Size Vegetable or Fruit; Fresh, Frozen or Canned Vegetables or Fruit 125 mL 1/2 cup; Salad 250 mL 1 cup; Juice 125 mL 1/2 cup

Milk Products
SERVINGS PER DAY
Children 4–9 years: 2–3
Youth 10–16 years: 3–4
Adults: 2–4
Pregnant and Breast-feeding Women 3–4

1 Servings: 250 mL 1 cup; Cheese 3"x1"x1" 50 g; 2 Slices 50 g; 175 g 3/4 cup

Meat and Alternatives
2–3
SERVINGS PER DAY

1 Serving: Meat, Poultry or Fish 50-100 g; Fish 1/3–2/3 Can 50–100 g; 1-2 Eggs; Beans 125-250 mL; 100 g 1/3 cup; Peanut Butter 30 mL 2 tbsp

Other Foods

Taste and enjoyment can also come from other foods and beverages that are not part of the 4 food groups. Some of these foods are higher in fat or Calories, so use these foods in moderation.

Different People Need Different Amounts of Food

The amount of food you need every day from the 4 food groups and other foods depends on your age, body size, activity level, whether you are male or female and if you are pregnant or breast-feeding. That's why the Food Guide gives a lower and higher number of servings for each food group. For example, young children can choose the lower number of servings, while male teenagers can go to the higher number. Most other people can choose servings somewhere in between.

Consult *Canada's Physical Activity Guide to Healthy Active Living* to help you build physical activity into your daily life.

Enjoy eating well, being active and feeling good about yourself. That's VITALIT

Cat. No. H39-252/1992E ISBN 0-662-19648-1

Figure 25-3 Serving Sizes. Source: Health Canada, *Canada's Food Guide to Healthy Eating.*

The foods in this group vary in fat content. Wise food choices lower fat intake from this group. Cold cuts and some luncheon meats are high in fat. Choose leaner meats, poultry, and fish. Chicken and turkey have less fat than veal, beef, pork, and lamb. Skinless chicken and turkey are even lower in fat. Veal is lower in fat than beef. Egg yolks have more fat than egg whites. Low-fat egg substitutes can be used for cooking and baking. Dried peas, lentils, and beans are recommended as meat alternatives. They are low in fat and provide fibre and protein.

Food preparation can help lower fat. Trim fat from meat and poultry. Baking, broiling, roasting, or microwaving are better than frying. Gravies and sauces also add fat.

Meat, poultry, and seafood contain many calories. Serving size is important. Restaurants frequently serve large servings of meat. For example, a 12-ounce steak equals 4 to 6 servings from this group.

Food Labels

Food labels are useful for planning a healthy diet and for following special diets ordered by physicians, dietitians, or RNs. Nutrition labels are required on packaged food. Food labels have three components: a list of ingredients, nutrition facts, and nutrition claims.

List of Ingredients

Ingredients are listed starting with the most plentiful ingredient. Use the list to compare two or more products. For example, Brand A lists sodium first, then wheat flour. Brand B lists wheat flour first, then sodium. Brand A has more sodium than Brand B. Use the list to check for ingredients that cause allergies or food intolerance (see page 370).

Nutrition Facts

The Nutrition Facts table (Figure 25-4) contains information on calories and 13 nutrients, including fat, carbohydrates, and protein. The **Daily Value (DV)** shows how a serving fits into the daily diet of an adult. It is expressed as a percentage based on recommended daily intake. Health Canada recommends the following daily intake of major nutrients:

- 60% of total calories per day should come from carbohydrates.
- 10% of total calories per day should come from protein.
- 30% (or less) of total calories per day should come from fat.
- 10% (or less) of total calories per day should come from saturated fat.

Nutrition Facts Per 125 mL (87 g)	
Amount	% DV*
Calories 80	
Fat 0.5 g	1 %
Saturated 0 g + Trans 0 g	0 %
Cholesterol 0 mg	
Sodium 0 mg	0 %
Carbohydrate 18 g	6 %
Fibre 2 g	8 %
Sugars 2 g	
Protein 3 g	
Vitamin A	2 %
Vitamin C	10 %
Calcium	0 %
Iron	2 %
* DV = Daily Value	

Valeur nutritive par 125 mL (87 g)	
Teneur	% VQ*
Calories 80	
Lipides 0,5 g	1 %
saturés 0 g + trans 0 g	0 %
Cholestérol 0 mg	
Sodium 0 mg	0 %
Glucides 18 g	6 %
Fibres 2 g	8 %
Sucres 2 g	
Protéines 3 g	
Vitamine A	2 %
Vitamine C	10 %
Calcium	0 %
Fer	2 %
* VQ = valeur quotidienne	

Figure 25-4 The Nutrition Facts Table. Source: Health Canada, *The Nutrition Facts.*

Nutrition Claims

Manufacturers' nutrition claims about foods (such as "low in fat," or "high in fibre") must meet government requirements. The following diet-related health claims are allowed:

- A healthy diet low in sodium and high in potassium may reduce the risk of high blood pressure.
- A healthy diet adequate in calcium and vitamin D may reduce the risk of osteoporosis.
- A healthy diet low in saturated fat and trans-fat may reduce the risk of heart disease.
- A healthy diet rich in vegetables and fruit may reduce the risk of some types of cancer.

Nutrition Throughout the Life Cycle

Nutritional requirements differ throughout the life cycle.

Infancy and Childhood

Infancy is a period of rapid growth and development. Mothers breastfeed or bottle-feed babies. Breastmilk provides the best source of nutrients and antibodies for the baby's first 6 months. Formula can provide adequate nourishment but lacks antibodies.

At 4 to 6 months, iron-fortified cereals are introduced. They are followed by puréed foods. Most babies are ready for finger foods and chopped foods at 10 months to a year. After the first year, the growth rate slows.

Children usually have strong likes and dislikes, which can make meal planning a challenge. Regular meals and physical activity are important. Children under 4 should not eat a low-fat diet. Fat is needed for brain development and energy.

When you care for infants and children, your supervisor will provide instructions about dietary requirements. Follow the care plan.

Adolescence

During puberty boys and girls have their biggest growth spurt since infancy. Increased nutrients are needed for this rapid growth. Many adolescents form unhealthy eating habits. They may skip meals, eat fast foods and soft drinks, diet, and drink alcohol. Poor eating habits can lead to eating disorders, iron deficiency, and poor health.

Young and Middle Adulthood

Nutritional requirements in young and middle adulthood depend on age, gender, body size, and activity levels. Unless extremely active, most adults have lower energy needs than adolescents. If their calorie intake exceeds energy needs, they gain weight. Energy needs continue to decline into the 40s and 50s. A healthy diet containing essential nutrients is extremely important.

Pregnancy. Pregnant women and their developing fetuses require nutrient-rich food. About 500 additional calories are needed per day.

Pregnant women are advised not to smoke, drink alcohol, or take drugs. Pregnant women who do not eat meat and dairy products need to discuss their diets with their physician.

Health Canada suggests that pregnant and breastfeeding women increase folic acid, iron, and calcium intake. Low folic acid intake before and during pregnancy increases the risk of spinal cord and brain abnormalities in infants (see Chapter 38).

Late Adulthood

Older adults vary widely in their health and nutritional status. Emotional, social, and physical factors affect their nutritional status.

Many older adults are used to eating with a family group. Preparing a meal for one may hold no interest. Some older adults do not drive. They may not be able to carry heavy grocery bags on public transit. Some may not have family or friends nearby who can help them with shopping and meal preparation. Many have low incomes. They may avoid buying high-protein foods like meat and cheese because of the expense. Those living in long-term care facilities may not like the food that is served.

Loss of hearing, smell, and taste affect appetite and social enjoyment of food. Poor vision may make shopping and meal preparation more challenging. Decreases in saliva may cause **dysphagia,** difficulty (*dys*) in swallowing (*phagia*). Secretion of digestive juices decreases. As a result, fried and fatty foods are hard to digest and may cause indigestion. Nutrients are not absorbed as easily. Medications may have side effects, such as nausea, constipation, and loss of appetite. Loss of teeth and ill-fitting dentures can affect chewing. Decreased peristalsis results in slower emptying of the stomach and colon. Flatulence and constipation are common because of decreased peristalsis.

Energy levels are lower in older adults. Fewer calories are needed to sustain weight. Yet, nutritional requirements remain high. High-protein foods are needed for tissue growth and repair. Foods high in calcium help keep bones strong. High-fibre foods such as raw vegetables help constipation problems. However, high-fibre foods can be hard to chew and can cause indigestion. Foods providing soft bulk such as cooked fruits and vegetables are often preferred for people with constipation or chewing problems. Drinking more fluids may aid digestion, kidney function, chewing, and swallowing.

Good oral hygiene and denture care can help prevent irritated gums and mouth sores. These practices can also improve the ability to eat and taste.

Factors that Affect Eating and Nutrition

Many factors affect nutrition and eating habits. Some begin during infancy and continue throughout life. Others develop later:

- *Personal choice*. The like or dislike of certain foods is a personal matter. Food preferences begin in childhood. They are influenced by the way the food tastes, smells, looks, and by how it is prepared.
- *Allergies*. An **allergy** is sensitivity to a substance that causes the body to react with signs and symptoms. Common reactions are swelling of the lips, throat, tongue, or face; skin rash; coughing or difficulty breathing; abdominal cramps; nausea; or diarrhea. In severe cases, *anaphylactic shock* occurs. This is a life-threatening sensitivity to a substance that can be fatal. For some people, food allergies are an annoyance. However, for others, avoiding certain foods is a matter of life and death. Nuts and shellfish cause the most severe reactions.
- *Food intolerances*. A food intolerance is a reaction to food that does not involve the immune system. It is not as serious as a food allergy. Common reactions are indigestion and diarrhea. For example, lactose intolerance occurs in people who lack the enzyme lactase. Lactase is needed to break down the sugar (lactose) in milk. Therefore, people who are lactose-intolerant cannot digest milk.
- *Culture*. Culture influences dietary practices, food choices, and food preparation. (See *Respecting*

Diversity: Food Practices box.) Frying, baking, smoking, and roasting food and eating raw food are cultural practices. The use of sauces and spices is also related to culture.

- *Religion*. The selection, preparation, and eating of food are often influenced by religious practices. Members of a religious group may follow all, some, or none of the dietary practices of their faith. You need to respect your clients' religious practices.
- *Finances*. People with limited incomes often buy cheaper foods. Their diets may lack protein and certain vitamins and minerals.
- *Appetite*. Appetite relates to the desire for food. When hungry, a person seeks food and eats until the appetite is satisfied. Aromas and thoughts of food can also stimulate the appetite. However, loss of appetite can occur. Illness, medications, anxiety, pain, and depression can cause loss of appetite. So can unpleasant sights, thoughts, and smells.
- *Illness*. Appetite usually decreases during illness and recovery from injuries. However, nutritional needs increase. The body must fight infection, heal tissues, and replace lost blood cells. Nutrients lost though vomiting and diarrhea need to be replaced. Some diseases and medications cause a sore mouth. This makes eating painful. Loss of teeth affects chewing, especially protein foods. Illness also affects the ability to prepare and serve meals. Poor nutrition is common among long-term care residents. They need good nutrition to correct or prevent health problems. (See *Focus on Long-Term Care: Food and Quality of Life* box.)
- *Age*. Age affects nutrition. See pages 369–370.

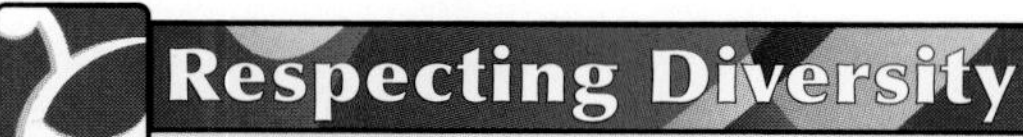

Respecting Diversity

Food Practices

Food practices vary among cultures. For example, rice and beans are common protein sources in Mexico. Rice is also common in the Philippines, China, and Japan. A diet high in starch and fat is common in Poland. A low-fat but high-sodium diet is common in China. In some countries (such as India) beef is not eaten.

Source: Adapted from E.M. Geissler, *Pocket Guide to Cultural Assessment*, 2nd ed. (St. Louis: Mosby, 1998).

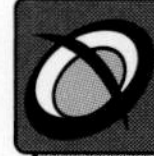

Focus on Long-Term Care

Food and Quality of Life

Food is important to a long-term care resident's quality of life. Legislation ensures that:

- Each resident's dietary and nutritional needs are met
- Nourishing, tasty, attractive, and well-balanced meals are served
- Hot food is served hot and cold food is served cold
- Special diets are provided as needed
- Special eating utensils are provided (Figure 25-5 on page 372) as needed. The resident's hands, wrists, and arms may be affected by disease or injury; the special eating utensils help the resident to eat independently

In some long-term care facilities, residents can dine with guests. The resident can have a meal with a spouse, partner, family members, or friends. The dietary department provides the meal or it is brought by the visitor.

Meal Planning and Preparation

Your role in meal planning and preparation depends on the care plan and on your client's needs. Most home care agencies expect clients' families to provide groceries and main meals. The case manager arranges for Meals on Wheels if desired by the family and client. Meals on Wheels provides clients with their main meal of the day. You might make a light meal for a client. For example, you might prepare toast for breakfast or make a sandwich for lunch. Sometimes, you might prepare several meals and freeze them for future use. Occasionally, you may plan menus and shop for groceries.

When preparing meals for clients, consider their dietary requirements, food preferences, and eating habits.

- *Dietary requirements*. The care plan includes special diets, mealtime instructions, dietary practices, and food allergies and intolerances. If there is no information in the care plan, ask your supervisor for guidance. A good cookbook is a helpful guide for planning and preparing meals.
- *Food preferences*. Many people have strong food preferences and definite ideas about preparing meals. Follow the client's wishes. Never give clients food that they are not allowed. If you have concerns about a client's diet, speak with your supervisor.
- *Eating habits*. Some people have their large meal in the evenings, others at noon. Some people eat several meals of the same size but never snack. Others snack between meals. Some people eat the same thing for breakfast or lunch every day.

(text continues on page 373)

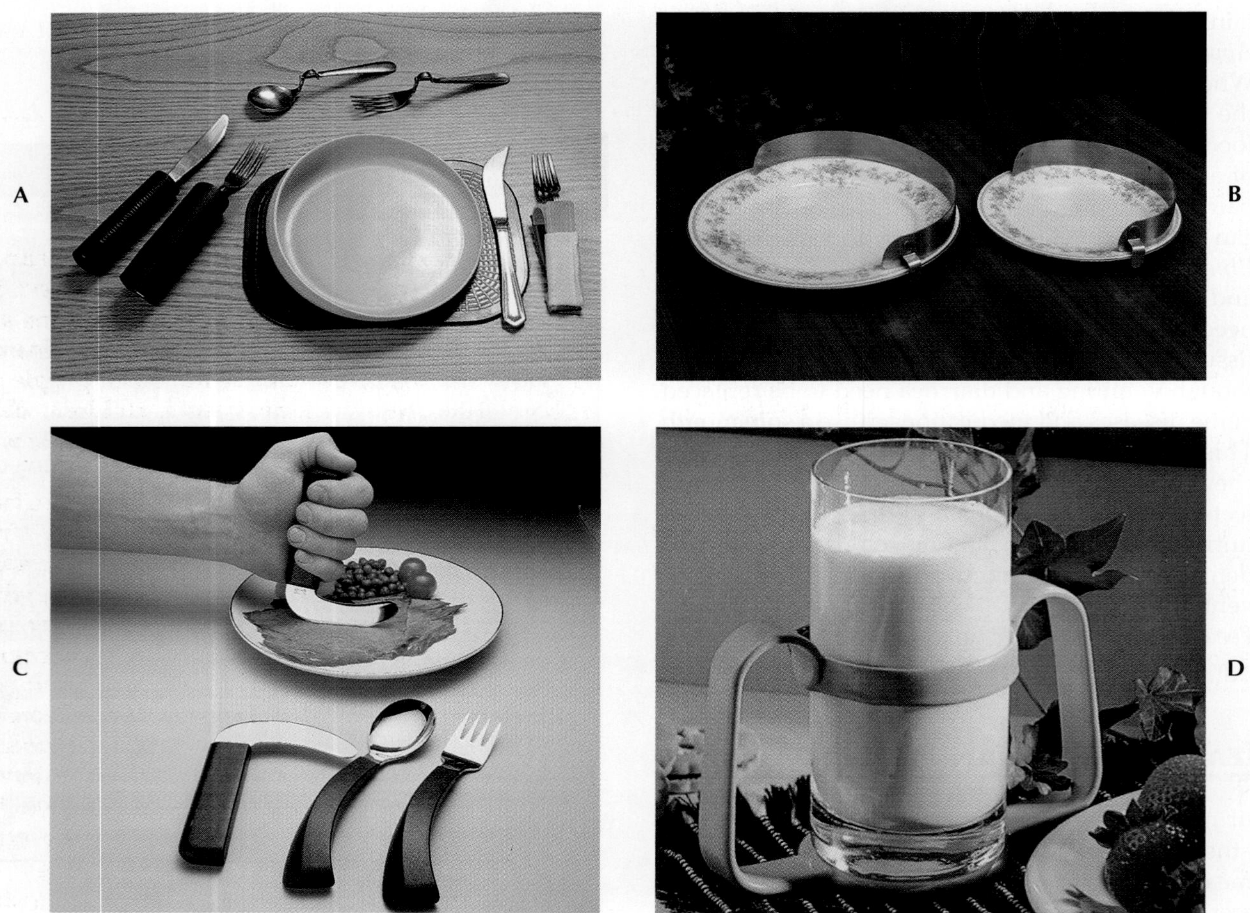

Figure 25-5 Eating utensils for people with special needs. **A,** The curved fork fits over the hand. The rounded plate helps keep food on the plate. Special grips and swivel handles are helpful for some people. **B,** Plate guards help keep food on the plate. **C,** Knives with rounded blades are rocked back and forth to cut food. The person does not need a fork in one hand and a knife in the other. **D,** Glass or cup holder. *(Courtesy of Sammons Preston; An AbilityOne Company, Bolingbrook, IL.)*

SHOPPING FOR GROCERIES

You may be expected to shop for a client's food. Use shopping lists to remember needed items. Keep a list in one place. Encourage the client to add to it throughout the week. Add personal care items as needed. On shopping day, rewrite the list.

Checking Expiry Dates. By law, expiry or "best before" dates must appear on products with a limited shelf life. If stored properly, the product can be safely used before the date listed. There are three commonly used dates:

- *Sell by* ...: This is the last recommended date of sale. Most products will keep at least 3 days beyond this date.
- *Best before* ...: This is the last date at which the manufacturer will guarantee freshness.
- *Expiry date* ...: This is the last date at which the product can be safely consumed.

Some products contain only the date on which the food was packaged. Select the product with the most recent dates. Packaged meats and fish usually list the date when the item was packaged. Choose items that were packaged most recently.

Handling Clients' Money. Some clients have grocery accounts. Others provide cash for groceries. Always handle someone else's money carefully. You must be honest, efficient, and organized. Keep a separate wallet or purse for the client's money, change, and receipts. Use the receipts to total the money spent. Return the right amount of change to the client. Most agencies have strict policies about handling clients' money. Be sure to follow these policies.

FOLLOWING RECIPES

Use a recipe to prepare meals. If necessary, consult a basic cookbook with key terms. You may have to substitute ingredients if your client does not have a recipe ingredient. For example, canola oil and margarine are usually substitutes for olive oil. Never substitute an ingredient without asking the client and checking the care plan. Do not use a substitute ingredient if the client is on a special diet or has a food allergy or intolerance. Consult your supervisor for guidance.

Canada uses the metric system, which has quantities such as millilitres and grams. However, household units of measure such as tablespoons or cups are common. Table 25-3 provides some common equivalents for metric units.

Table 25-3 Approximate Equivalent Measurements

LIQUIDS
1 cup = 250 millilitres
1 pint = 473 millilitres
1 quart = 1 litre
½ teaspoon = 2 millilitres
1 teaspoon = 5 millilitres
1 tablespoon = 15 millilitres
WEIGHTS
1 ounce = 30 grams
1 pound = 454 grams

FOOD SAFETY

Food safety is important. A **foodborne illness** is an illness caused by improperly cooked or stored food. Diarrhea, nausea, and vomiting are common signs and symptoms of a foodborne illness. Foodborne illnesses can cause serious illness and death. Some people are at high risk. These include infants, children, older adults, people with chronic illnesses, and people with weakened immune systems.

Pathogens are disease-causing microbes (see Chapter 18). They are also commonly called germs. When pathogens are in or on food, the food is *contaminated.* Many foods naturally have pathogens in them when they are raw. These include meat, fish, poultry, and eggs. When food is cooked properly, most pathogens are killed. However, raw food may spread pathogens to other, ready-to-eat food. **Cross-contamination** occurs when pathogens are passed from one source to another. For example, fluids from raw, contaminated chicken drip on to vegetables in the refrigerator. The vegetables are now contaminated. If they are eaten without being washed, they could cause illness.

It is usually hard to tell by sight, smell, or taste if something is contaminated. Safe food-handling practices and effective cooking can prevent cross-contamination and foodborne illness. Most pathogens die at temperatures below 4° C (40° F) and above 60° C (140° F). They thrive at room temperature. Therefore, it is important to cook foods well and keep them in the refrigerator. Never let foods sit out at room temperature for more than a few minutes.

If you prepare and serve meals to clients, you must know safe food-handling practices. Observe safety practices when grocery shopping, and when storing, cooking, reheating, and serving food (Box 25-3 on page 374).

(text continues on page 375)

Box 25-3 Guidelines for Safe Food Practices

Shopping
- Packaging should be secure. Do not buy ripped packages, broken seals, and dented cans.
- Check the "best before" date. Do not buy expired items.
- Select refrigerated and frozen foods last. Do not buy items with ice crystals on the package.
- Put meats, poultry, and seafood in bags to avoid cross-contamination.

Food Storages
- Do not leave groceries in a warm car. Freeze or refrigerate items promptly.
- Store raw meat, poultry, and seafood in plastic bags on the bottom shelf of the refrigerator. This prevents their fluids from dripping onto other foods.
- Store leftovers in small, shallow containers in the refrigerator. This allows rapid cooling and prevents the growth of pathogens. Cover the containers with lids, foil, or plastic wrap. Write the date you store the leftovers on the containers.
- Do not refreeze food.

Food Preparation
- Wash your hands before and after preparing food. Wash your hands immediately before and after handling raw meat, poultry, seafood, or eggs to avoid cross-contamination of other foods.
- Do not cough or sneeze over food. Wear a hair net.
- Wear bandages if you have cuts on your hands or wrists.
- Defrost foods in the refrigerator, in the microwave, or under cold running water. Do not defrost food at room temperature.
- Prevent contact between raw and ready-to-eat food.
- Wash vegetables and fruits to remove pathogens and pesticides.
- Discard food with expired "best before" dates. Discard food with mould on it. If in doubt about freshness, discard the product.
- Do not keep leftovers longer than 2–3 days.
- Use clean utensils to remove food from containers that will be refrigerated.
- Rinse raw meats, poultry, and seafood before use. Wash the sink thoroughly (see Chapter 23).
- Avoid recipes that call for raw eggs.
- Use two cutting boards: one for raw meats, poultry, and seafood; the other for cooked food and washed fruits and vegetables. For added safety, cut raw meats, poultry, and seafood on disposable waxed paper placed on top of the board. Wash the cutting board thoroughly (see Chapter 23).
- Wash and dry the tops of cans to remove pathogens. Wash can openers to prevent pathogens from entering cans when opening.
- Wash knives or scissors used to cut open food packages.
- Follow the guidelines for cleaning kitchens in Chapter 23.

Cooking and Reheating Food
- Cook foods to at least their minimum safe temperature (Table 25-4). Cooking foods to the right temperature kills pathogens.
- Cook food thoroughly, especially meat, poultry, seafood, and eggs. Use a meat thermometer to determine if the meat is cooked. Eggs should be firm when eaten.
- Reheat sauces and gravy to a rolling boil.
- Stir and rotate food reheated in microwaves to prevent cold or hot spots.

Serving Food
- Serve food immediately after cooking it or removing it from the refrigerator. Remember, pathogens grow at room temperature.
- Serve food on a clean plate. Wash plates, platters, or containers used for raw meats, poultry, seafood, or eggs immediately after use.
- Use clean table linens, plastic mats, and eating surfaces.
- Do not use chipped or cracked dishes.

Table 25-4 Minimum Safe Temperatures

Ground beef/pork	71° C (160° F)
Ground chicken/turkey	80° C (175° F)
Beef, lamb, and veal roasts/steaks	60° C (140° F) Rare 71° C (160° F) Medium 77° C (170° F) Well
Pork chops/roasts/fresh cured ham	71° C (160° F) Medium
Ham, ready-to-eat, fully cooked	Cold or 60° C (140° F)
Whole turkey (stuffed) or chicken (stuffed or not)	82° C (180° F)
Whole turkey (without stuffing)	77° C (170° F)
Stuffing	74° C (165° F)
Chicken/turkey pieces	77° C (170° F)
Rolled stuffed beef roasts or steaks (e.g., London Broil)	71° C (160° F)
Mechanically tenderized/delicated meats	71° C (160° F)
Egg dishes/casseroles	71° C (160° F)
Leftovers, reheated	74° C (165° F)

Source: Canadian Industry Standards *Food Safety at Home—You're in Control,* in Kraft Canada Inc. *FightBac!: Keep Food Safe From Bacteria.* p. 10.

Special Diets

Physicians may order special diets. They are ordered because of a nutritional deficiency or a disease, to eliminate or decrease certain substances in the diet, or for weight control (Table 25-5 on page 376). Special diets are common before and after surgery and for people with diabetes. People with diseases of the heart, kidneys, gallbladder, liver, stomach, or intestines may receive special diets. Allergies, food intolerances, obesity, and other disorders also require special diets.

When a special diet is ordered, the RN and dietitian work together to plan the client's nutritional needs. The plan is influenced by the client's preferences, culture, religion, and food allergies and intolerances. The RN and dietitian also consider eating problems. For example, some people have dysphagia (difficulty swallowing). Their nutritional plan takes these problems into account (see page 378).

In facilities, the terms *regular diet*, *general diet*, and *house diet* mean there are no dietary limits or restrictions. Two common special diets are the sodium-controlled diet and diabetes meal planning.

The Sodium-Controlled Diet

The average amount of sodium in the daily diet is 3000 to 5000 mg. The body needs half this amount daily. Physically healthy people excrete excess sodium in the urine. Heart and kidney diseases cause the body to retain the extra sodium. So do some drugs and some complications of pregnancy.

Sodium causes the body to retain water. If there is too much sodium, the body retains more water. Tissues swell with water and there are excess amounts of fluid in the blood vessels. The heart has to work harder. The extra workload for the heart can cause serious complications or death. Restricting sodium in the diet decreases the amount of sodium in the body. The body retains less water. Less water in the tissues and blood vessels reduces the amount of work for the heart.

The client's physician orders sodium control (restriction) for the client. Many low-salt or salt-free foods can be bought. Food labels are used to determine salt content.

- *2000 to 3000 mg sodium diet*—this is called the *low-salt diet* or *no added salt diet*. Sodium restriction is mild. All high-sodium foods are omitted. A minimum amount of salt is used for cooking. Salt is not added to foods at the table.
- *1000 mg sodium diet*—sodium restriction is moderate. Food is cooked without salt. Foods high in sodium are omitted. Vegetables high in sodium are restricted in amount. Salt-free products, such as salt-free bread, are used. Diet planning is necessary.
- *500 mg sodium diet*—sodium restriction is severe. Restrictions for the mild and moderate sodium diets are followed. In addition, vegetables high in sodium are omitted. Milk is limited to 1 cup per day. Only 1 egg per day is allowed. Meat is limited to 120 grams (4 ounces) per day. Diet planning is essential.

Diabetes Meal Planning

Diabetes meal planning is for people with diabetes. *Diabetes* is a chronic condition resulting from a lack of insulin (see Chapter 31). In physically healthy people the pancreas produces and secretes insulin, which lets the body use sugar. In people who lack insulin, sugar builds up in the bloodstream rather than being used by cells for energy. Diabetes is usually treated with insulin or medication, diet, and exercise.

(text continues on page 378)

Table 25-5 Special Diets

Diet	Use	Foods allowed
Clear-liquid: foods that are liquid at body temperature and that leave small amounts of residue; nonirritating and non-gas-forming	Postoperatively, for acute illness, infection, nausea and vomiting, and in preparation for gastrointestinal exams	Water, tea, and coffee (without milk or cream); carbonated beverages; gelatin; clear fruit juices (apple, grape, and cranberry); fat-free clear broth; hard candy, sugar, and Popsicles
Full-liquid: foods that are liquid at room temperature or that melt at body temperature	Advance from clear-liquid diet postoperatively; for stomach irritation, fever, nausea, and vomiting; and for people unable to chew, swallow, or digest solid foods	Foods on the clear-liquid diet; custard; eggnog; strained soups; strained fruit and vegetable juices; milk and milk-shakes; strained, cooked cereals; plain ice cream and sherbet; pudding; yogurt
Mechanical soft: semisolid foods that are easily digested	Advance from full-liquid diet; for chewing problems, gastrointestinal disorders, and infections	All liquids; eggs (not fried); broiled, baked, or roasted meat, fish, or poultry that is chopped or shredded; mild cheeses (American, Swiss, cheddar, cream, and cottage); strained fruit juices; refined bread (no crust) and crackers; cooked cereal; cooked or puréed vegetables; cooked or canned fruit without skin or seeds; pudding; plain cakes and soft cookies without fruit or nuts
Fibre and residue restricted: food that leaves a small amount of residue in the colon	Diseases of the colon and diarrhea	Coffee, tea, milk, carbonated beverages, strained fruit juices; refined bread and crackers; creamed and refined cereal; rice; cottage and cream cheese; eggs (not fried); plain puddings and cakes; gelatin; custard; sherbet and ice cream; strained vegetable juices; canned or cooked fruit without skin or seeds; potatoes (not fried); strained, cooked vegetables; plain pasta; *no raw fruits and vegetables*
High-fibre: foods that increase the amount of residue and fibre in the colon to stimulate peristalsis	Constipation and GI disorders	All fruits and vegetables; whole wheat bread; whole grain cereals; fried foods; whole grain rice; milk, cream, butter, and cheese; meats

Continued

Table 25-5 Special Diets—cont'd

Diet	Use	Foods allowed
Bland: foods that are mechanically and chemically nonirritating and low in roughage; foods served at moderate temperatures; no strong spices or condiments	Ulcers, gallbladder disorders, and some intestinal disorders; after abdominal surgery	Lean meats; white bread; creamed and refined cereals; cream or cottage cheese; gelatin, plain puddings, cakes, and cookies; eggs (not fried); butter and cream; canned fruits and vegetables without skin and seeds; strained fruit juices; potatoes (not fried); pastas and rice; strained or soft cooked carrots, peas, beets, spinach, squash, and asparagus tips; creamed soups from allowed vegetables; no fried foods
High-calorie: calorie intake is increased to about 3000 to 4000; includes 3 full meals and between-meal snacks	Weight gain and some thyroid imbalances	Dietary increases in all foods; large portions of a regular diet with 3 between-meal snacks
Calorie-controlled: provides adequate nutrients while controlling calories to promote weight loss and reduction of body fat	Weight reduction	Foods low in fats and carbohydrates and lean meats; avoid butter, cream, rice, gravies, salad oils, noodles, cakes, pastries, carbonated and alcoholic beverages, candy, potato chips, and similar foods
High-iron: foods that are high in iron	Anemia; following blood loss; for women during the reproductive years	Liver and other organ meats; lean meats; egg yolks; shellfish; dried fruits; dried beans; green leafy vegetables; lima beans; peanut butter; enriched breads and cereals
Fat-controlled (low-cholesterol): foods low in fat and foods prepared without adding fat	Heart disease, gallbladder disease, disorders of fat digestion, liver disease, diseases of the pancreas	Skim milk or buttermilk; cottage cheese (no other cheeses allowed); gelatin; sherbet; fruit; lean meat, poultry, and fish (baked, broiled, or roasted); fat-free broth; soups made with skim milk; margarine; rice, pasta, breads, and cereals; vegetables; potatoes
High-protein: aids and promotes tissue healing	For burns, high fever, infection, and some liver diseases	Meat; milk, eggs, and cheese; fish and poultry; breads and cereals; green leafy vegetables
Sodium-controlled: a certain amount of sodium is allowed	Heart disease, fluid retention, liver disease, and some kidney diseases	Fruits and vegetables and unsalted butter are allowed; adding salt at the table is not allowed; highly salted foods and foods high in sodium are not allowed; the use of salt during cooking may be restricted
Diabetes meal planning: the same amount of carbohydrates, protein, and fat are eaten at the same time each day	Diabetes	Determined by nutritional and energy requirements

The dietitian and client develop a meal plan. Consistency is the key. It involves:

- *The client's food preferences.* It may be necessary to limit amounts or change the way food is prepared.
- *The calories needed.* The same amount of carbohydrates, protein, and fat are eaten each day.
- *Eating meals and snacks at regular times.* The client eats at the same time every day.

Meal and snack times are the same from day to day. You must serve the client's meal and snack on time. The client must eat at regular times to maintain a certain blood sugar level. If all food was not eaten, a between-meal nourishment is needed. The nourishment makes up for what was not eaten at the regular meal. The amount of insulin given also depends on the client's daily food intake. Report to your supervisor any changes in the client's eating habits.

Assisting Clients with Eating

Weakness and illness can affect a person's appetite and ability to eat. So can odours, unpleasant equipment, an uncomfortable position, the need for oral hygiene, the need to eliminate, and pain. You can help control some of these factors by helping your clients prepare for meals.

- Assist with oral hygiene, elimination, and hand washing.
- Change clothing and provide clean linens for incontinent clients.
- Be sure dentures, eyeglasses, and hearing aids are in place.
- Help clients get to the dining room.
- Position clients for eating. Help people transfer from beds to chairs. Or help people in bed move to a sitting position.

Making Meals Enjoyable

Some people lose interest in eating because of illness or other factors. Small details can help a person enjoy a meal. Some of the following may not apply to clients on special diets. Check the care plan.

- *Assist with menu choices.* Help home care clients choose from the Meals on Wheels menu. Help long-term care residents select a meal from the facility menu. If planning and preparing meals, involve the client.
- *Make the setting attractive.* In home care settings, let the client choose table linens and utensils.
- *Serve hot meals immediately.* Lukewarm meals lack appeal.
- *Serve moderate portions.* Some people lose their appetite when faced with too much food. Ask the client how much food he or she wants. Place that amount on the plate.
- *Make mealtimes social occasions.* Mealtimes can be lonely. Encourage long-term care residents to dine with others. In home care settings, keep the client company. Do quiet tasks, such as folding laundry, where the client is eating.

Assisting Clients with Eating Problems

Changes resulting from aging, illness, and disabilities can cause eating problems. These include chewing and swallowing problems, weakness, and vision loss.

Chewing Problems. Foods that provide soft bulk are served (see soft diet, page 376). A food processor or blender is used to purée foods. Follow the care plan. To help ease chewing problems:

- Offer plenty of fluids
- Offer small mouthfuls
- Give the person time to chew

Swallowing Problems (Dysphagia). People have trouble swallowing for many reasons. Certain medications (including chemotherapy) decrease saliva production. Dry mouth is the result. People with paralysis may have trouble swallowing because throat muscles are affected. Thick, soft, moist foods are served. The care plan may include the following measures to help a client swallow:

- Help the client to sit upright, leaning slightly forward
- Ask the client to lower the chin while swallowing
- Offer plenty of fluids
- Give the client time to chew and swallow before offering more food
- Ask the client to remain sitting for at least 30 minutes after the meal

People with swallowing problems are at risk for choking and aspiration. **Aspiration** is inhaling fluid or an object into the lungs. A client who cannot talk or cough may be choking. Call for help immediately if this happens. If no help is available, follow the emergency measures for choking (foreign-body airway obstruction) in Chapter 47.

Weakness. Some clients are too weak to chew and swallow. People who do not eat become even weaker. They have even less energy to eat. Never force a client to eat. If the person cannot eat, tell your supervisor. To encourage a person to eat, offer frequent, small, high-calorie meals. Serve nutritious drinks. These may include liquid dietary supplements. Soft foods that do not need much chewing are preferred. Follow the care plan and do the following:

- Let the client rest before and after meals.
- Provide a straw so the client does not need to lift a glass (if allowed).
- Provide cups, glasses, and utensils that are light and easy to handle.

Vision Loss. People with vision loss are often keenly aware of food aromas. Often they can identify foods served. Most clients with vision loss can eat independently with some guidance. To assist these clients to eat:

- Identify the location of foods and fluids on the tray or table
- Use the numbers on a clock to identify the location of foods and fluids (Figure 25-6)
- If you are feeding the person, describe what you are offering

SERVING MEAL TRAYS

Most hospital patients eat their meals in their rooms. Long-term care residents are encouraged to eat in the dining room. (See *Focus on Long-Term Care: Dining Programs* box.) Residents who are too ill to move about eat in their rooms. Other residents may also choose to eat in their rooms. Home care clients usually eat in their dining room or kitchen. If they are weak or ill, they may eat in bed or in a chair in their bedroom. Meals served in beds and bedrooms are delivered on trays. Food is served in containers that keep hot and

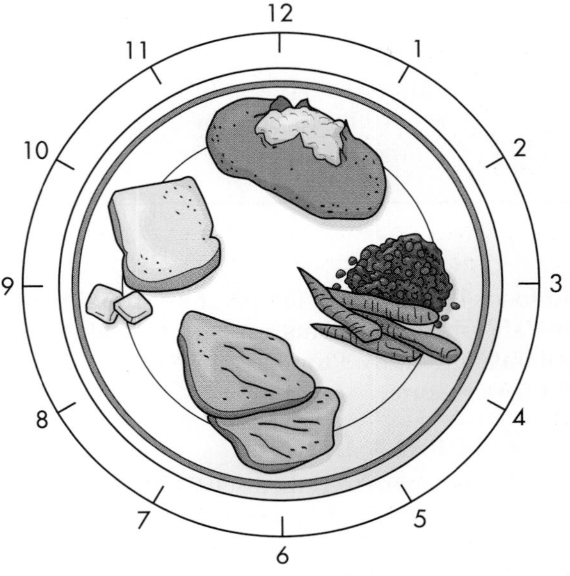

Figure 25-6 The numbers on a clock are used to help a client with vision loss locate food on a plate.

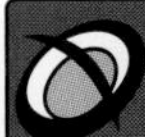

***Focus on* Long-Term Care**

DINING PROGRAMS

Many long-term care facilities have special dining programs:

- Social dining—residents eat in a dining room. Each table has four to six residents (Figure 25-7). Food is served as in a restaurant.
- Family dining—food is placed in bowls and on platters. Residents serve themselves as they would at home.
- Assistive dining—the dining room has circular or horseshoe-shaped tables. Residents who need assistance with eating are seated around the tables. You sit at the centre of the table and feed as many as four residents (Figure 25-8).

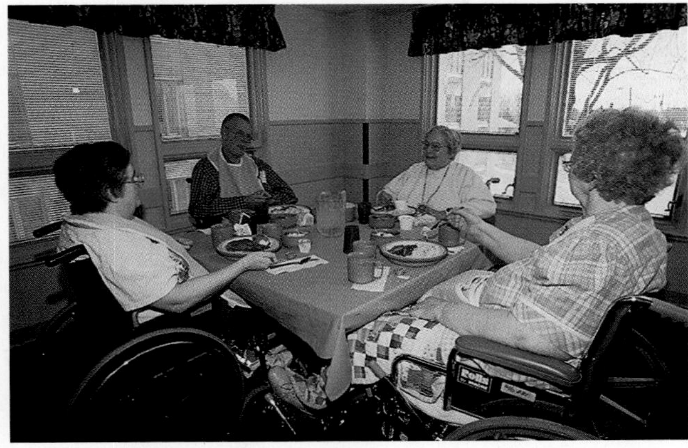

Figure 25-7 Residents enjoy a pleasant meal in the dining room.

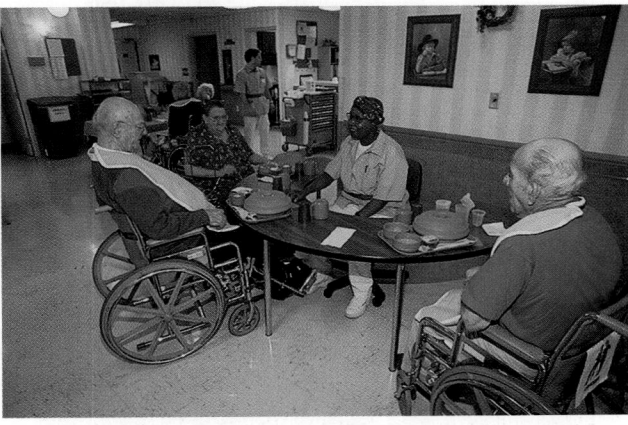

Figure 25-8 Special tables are used for assistive dining programs. A support worker feeds three residents at one time. Residents are in the company of others.

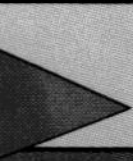

Serving Meal Trays

Compassionate Care

Remember to Promote:
- **Dignity**
- **Independence**
- **Preferences**
- **Privacy**
- **Safety**

Pre-Procedure

1 Identify the person according to employer policy.
2 Wash your hands.
3 Prepare the person for the meal. Assist with hand washing.
4 Provide for privacy.
5 Make sure the tray is complete. Make sure special utensils are included if needed.

Procedure

6 Help person to a sitting position.
7 Place tray on the overbed or other table. If the person is in bed and there is no overbed table, position the tray on the person's lap.
8 Remove food covers. Open milk cartons and cereal boxes, cut meat, and butter bread if indicated (Figure 25-9).
9 Place the napkin, clothes protector, if needed, and utensils within reach.
10 Measure and record intake if ordered (see page 383). Note the amount and type of foods eaten.
11 Check for and remove any food in the mouth (pocketing). Wear gloves.
12 Remove the tray.
13 Assist with hand washing. Offer oral hygiene.
14 Clean any spills and change soiled linen.
15 Help the person to return to bed if indicated.

Post-Procedure

16 Provide for safety and comfort.
17 Place the call bell within reach.*
18 Follow the care plan for bed rail use.*
19 Remove privacy measures.
20 Wash your hands.
21 Report and record your actions and observations according to employer policy. Include the amount and kind of food eaten.

*Steps marked with an asterisk may not apply in community settings.

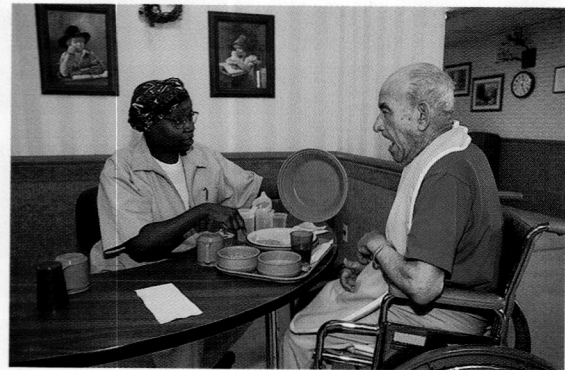

Figure 25-9 Open cartons and other containers for the client.

cold foods at the correct temperature. You serve meal trays after helping clients prepare for eating. Serve meal trays promptly. Prompt service keeps food at the right temperature.

Feeding a Client

Some clients cannot feed themselves. Weakness, paralysis, casts, and other physical limits may make self-feeding impossible. These people are fed. Depending on others for feeding is difficult for the client. You need to be kind and supportive when feeding people. (See *Providing Compassionate Care: Feeding A Client* box.)

BETWEEN-MEAL NOURISHMENTS

Many special diets involve between-meal nourishments. Commonly served nourishments are crackers, milk, juice, a milkshake, cake, wafers, a sandwich, gelatin, and custard. Provide nourishments according to the care plan. In home care settings, you may prepare between-meal nourishments. In facilities these are brought to the unit. Provide eating utensils, a straw, and a napkin. Follow the procedures for serving meals and feeding clients.

CALORIE COUNTS

For some clients, it is important to keep track of calorie intake. A flow sheet is provided for this purpose. You must note what the client ate and how much. For example, a client is served a chicken breast, a baked potato, green beans, a roll, pudding, and two pats of butter. You note that the person ate all the chicken, half the potato, the roll, and one pat of butter, but did not eat the beans and pudding. You note these on the form. The care plan tells you which clients require calorie counts.

FLUID BALANCE

Fluid balance is needed for health. Death can result from too much or too little water. The amount of fluid taken in (**intake**) and the amount lost (**output**) must be equal. If fluid intake exceeds fluid output, tissues swell with water. This is called **edema.** Edema is common in people with heart and kidney diseases. **Dehydration** is a decrease in the amount of water in body tissues. It results when fluid output exceeds intake. Common causes are low fluid intake, vomiting, diarrhea, bleeding, excess sweating, and increased urine production.

NORMAL FLUID REQUIREMENTS

An adult needs 1500 mL of water daily to survive. About 2000 to 2500 mL of fluid per day is needed for normal fluid balance. Water requirements increase with hot weather, exercise, fever, illness, and excessive fluid loss. Minimum water requirements vary with age. (See *Focus on Children: Fluid Requirements* and *Focus on Older Adults: Fluid Requirements* boxes on page 383.)

(text continues on page 383)

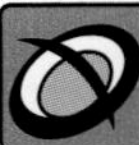

Providing **Compassionate Care**

FEEDING A CLIENT

Dignity. People who cannot feed themselves may feel embarrassed, humiliated, or angry. Some people are depressed or resentful. Some may refuse to eat. Be gentle, patient, and encouraging. Provide for comfort. Sit so you face the client. Sitting is more relaxing. It also shows that you have time to spend with the person. Standing communicates that you are in a hurry. Clients should never feel rushed. Clean up dribbles and spills discretely to save the person from embarrassment.

Independence. Encourage the client to participate in some aspect of the meal. Allow the client to set the pace. The person may be able to gesture or nod to show preferences.

Preferences. The client may want to pray before eating. Provide time and privacy for a prayer. Describe the food on the tray. Ask the client the order in which foods and fluids should be served. Ask questions and use paraphrasing (see Chapter 12) to make sure that you understand the person's feelings and wishes. Engage the person in pleasant conversation.

Privacy. Some people do not like others to see them being fed. Be sensitive to your client's needs and feelings. Provide for privacy if desired by the client.

Safety. Follow the care plan. Use spoons not forks as they are less likely to cause injury. The spoon should be only 1/3 full (Figure 25-10). This portion is easy to chew and swallow. Some people need smaller portions. Sit facing the client so you can observe for choking and for problems with eating, chewing, or swallowing. Offer small amounts of food so the client can easily chew and swallow. Give the person enough time to chew and swallow. Remember to offer fluids during the meal as they help with chewing and swallowing.

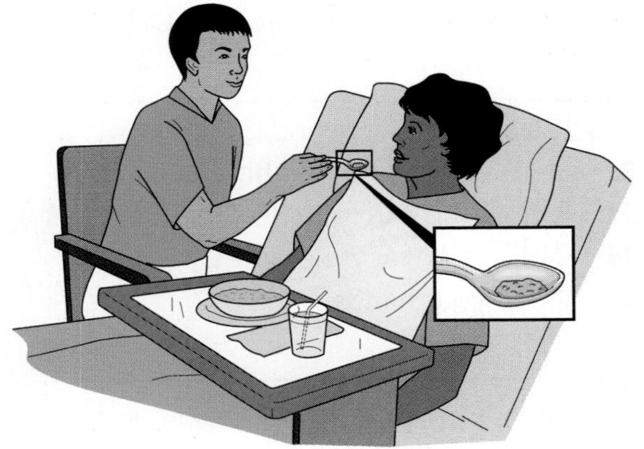

Figure 25-10 A spoon is used to feed a client. The spoon is no more than 1/3 full.

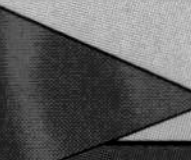

Feeding the Person

Compassionate Care

Remember to Promote:
- **Dignity**
- **Independence**
- **Preferences**
- **Privacy**
- **Safety**

Pre-Procedure

1 Identify the person according to employer policy.
2 Explain the procedure to the person.
3 Wash your hands.
4 Prepare the person for mealtime. Assist with hand washing.
5 Provide for privacy.
6 Help the person to a comfortable sitting position.
7 Place the tray on the overbed table, other table, or the person's lap.

Procedure

8 Drape a napkin across the person's chest and under the chin.
9 Prepare the food for eating.
10 Tell the person what foods are on the tray.
11 Serve foods in the order the person prefers. Alternate between solid and liquid foods. Use a spoon for safety (see Figure 25-10). Allow time for chewing. Do not rush.
12 Use straws if the person cannot drink out of a glass or cup. Use one straw for each liquid. Use a short straw for weak people.
13 Follow the care plan if the person has dysphagia. (Some people with dysphagia do not use straws.) Give thickened liquids with a spoon.
14 Talk with the person.
15 Encourage the person to eat.
16 Wipe the person's mouth with a napkin.
17 Note how much and which foods were eaten.
18 Measure and record intake if ordered.
19 Remove the tray.
20 Assist with oral hygiene (if in the care plan) and hand washing. Wear gloves for this step.

Post-Procedure

21 Provide for safety and comfort.
22 Place the call bell within reach.*
23 Follow the care plan for bed rail use.*
24 Remove privacy measures.
25 Wash your hands.
26 Report and record your actions and observations according to employer policy. Include:
- The amount of food eaten and the kind of food eaten
- Complaints of nausea or dysphagia
- Signs of aspiration

*Steps marked with an asterisk may not apply in community settings.

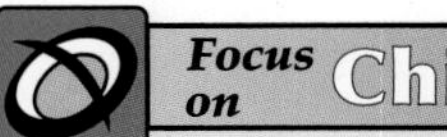

Focus on Children

FLUID REQUIREMENTS
Infants and young children have more body water than adults. They need more fluids. Excessive fluid loss can quickly cause death in infants and children.

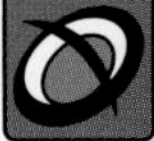

Focus on Older Adults

FLUID REQUIREMENTS
Older adults are at risk for diseases that affect fluid balance. These include heart disease, kidney disease, cancer, and diabetes. Many older adults also take medications that cause the body to lose fluids or retain water. Older adults are at risk for edema and dehydration.

Older adults may have a decreased sense of thirst. Their bodies need water, but they may not feel thirsty. Offer water often to your older clients.

SPECIAL ORDERS

The physician may order the amount of fluid that a client can have in a 24-hour period. This is done to maintain fluid balance. Common orders in the care plan are:

- *Encourage fluids*—The client needs to drink more fluids. The order states the amount to ingest. Intake records are kept. A variety of allowed fluids are provided. Fluids are kept within the person's reach. They are offered regularly to clients who cannot feed themselves.
- *Restrict fluids*—Fluids are restricted to a certain amount. They are offered in small amounts and in small containers. The water pitcher is removed or kept out of sight. Intake records are kept. The person needs frequent oral hygiene. It helps keep the mucous membranes of the mouth moist.
- *Nothing by mouth*—The client cannot eat or drink anything. NPO is the abbreviation for the Latin term *nil per os*. It means nothing (*nil*) by (*per*) mouth (*os*). Clients are usually NPO before and after surgery, before some laboratory tests and X-ray procedures, and in the treatment of certain illnesses. Clients who are tube fed may be NPO. An NPO sign is posted above the bed. The water pitcher and glass are removed. Frequent oral hygiene is important, but the client must not swallow any fluid.

INTAKE AND OUTPUT RECORDS

The physician or RN may want a client's fluid intake and output measured. This means keeping intake and output (I&O) records. They are used to evaluate fluid balance and kidney function. They help in evaluating and planning medical treatment. They also are kept when the client has special fluid orders.

All fluids taken by mouth are measured and recorded. So are fluids given in IV therapy and tube feedings (see Chapter 26). The obvious fluids are measured—water, milk, coffee, tea, juices, soups, and soft drinks. So are soft and semisolid foods such as ice cream, sherbet, custard, pudding, gelatin, and Popsicles. Output measured includes urine, vomitus, diarrhea, and wound drainage.

Measuring Intake and Output. Intake and output are measured in millilitres (mL) or in cubic centimetres (cc). These metric system measurements are equal in amount.

- 30 mL equals 1 ounce
- 500 mL is about 1 pint
- 1000 mL is about 1 quart

You need to know the serving size of bowls, cups, glasses, and other containers. The information may be on the I&O record.

A container called a *graduate* is used to measure fluids. These include leftover fluids, urine, vomitus, and drainage from suction (see Chapter 41). Like a measuring cup, the graduate is marked in millilitres or cubic centimetres and in ounces (Figure 25-11). Plastic urinals and kidney basins are often marked.

When intake or output is measured, the amount is recorded in the correct column on the I&O record (Figure 25-12 on page 384). Amounts are totalled at the end of the shift and recorded in the client's chart. In facilities, totals are shared during end-of-shift report.

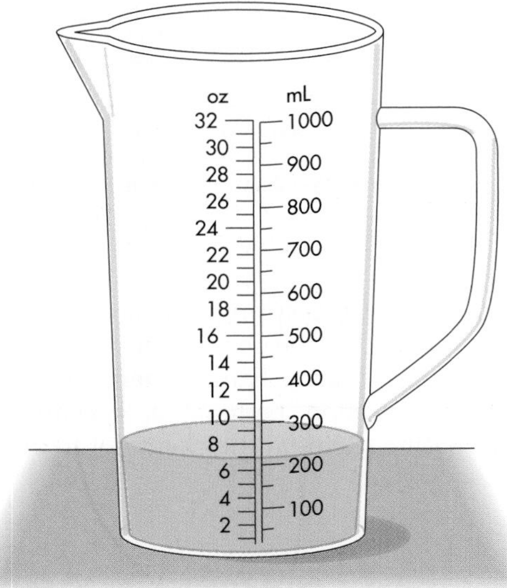

Figure 25-11 A graduate marked in millilitres and ounces.

CODE
O - Oral NG - Nasogastric
IV - Intravenous GT - Gastrostomy Tube

CODE
U - Urine
E - Emesis

	INTAKE										OUTPUT									
DATE	NIGHT	CODE	INIT.	DAY	CODE	INIT.	EVE	CODE	INIT.	24 HR TOTAL	NIGHT	CODE	INIT.	DAY	CODE	INIT.	EVE	CODE	INIT.	24 HR TOTAL

Initials	NURSE'S SIGNATURE	Initials	NURSE'S SIGNATURE	Initials	NURSE'S SIGNATURE	Initials	NURSE'S SIGNATURE
1		3		5		7	
2		4		6		8	

Name ______ Birthdate ______

Admission Date ______ Medical Rec. # ______

Physician ______

GSS #242

INTAKE & OUTPUT RECORD

Rev. 2-12-82

Figure 25-12 An intake and output record.

The purpose of measuring I&O and how they can help are explained to the client. Some clients measure and record their intake. Family members may help. The urinal, commode, bedpan, or specimen pan is used for voiding. Remind the client not to void in the toilet. Also remind the person not to put toilet tissue into the container.

Follow medical asepsis and Standard Precautions when measuring intake and output.

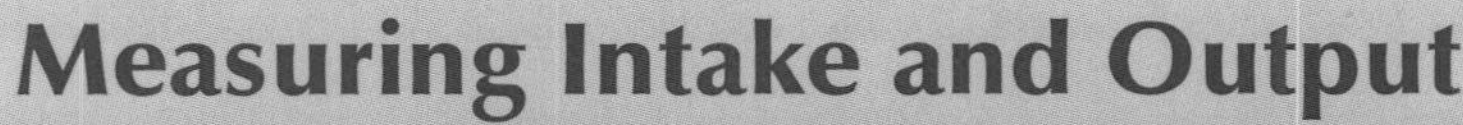

Measuring Intake and Output

Compassionate Care

Remember to Promote:
- **Dignity**
- **Independence**
- **Preferences**
- **Privacy**
- **Safety**

Pre-Procedure

1 Identify the person according to employer policy.
2 Explain the procedure to the person.
3 Wash your hands.
4 Collect the following:
  - Intake and output (I&O) record
  - Graduates
  - Gloves
5 Provide for privacy.

Procedure

6 Put on gloves.
7 Measure intake as follows:
  a Pour liquid remaining in a container into the graduate.
  b Measure the amount at eye level. Keep the container level.
  c Check the serving amount on the I&O record.
  d Subtract the remaining amount from the full serving amount. Record the amount.
  e Repeat steps 7a through d for each liquid.
  f Add the amounts from each liquid together.
  g Record the time and amount on the I&O record.
8 Measure output as follows:
  a Pour the fluid into the graduate used to measure output.
  b Measure the amount at eye level. Keep the container level.
9 Dispose of fluid in the toilet. Avoid splashes.
10 Clean and rinse the graduate. Dispose of rinse into the toilet. Return the graduate to its proper place.
11 Clean and rinse the bedpan, urinal, kidney basin, or other drainage container. Discard the rinse into the toilet. Return the item to its proper place.
12 Remove gloves. Wash your hands.
13 Record the amount on the I&O record.
14 Remove privacy measures.

Post-Procedure

15 Report and record your actions and observations according to employer policy.

REVIEW

Circle the BEST answer.

1. Nutrition is
   A. Fats, proteins, carbohydrates, vitamins, minerals, and water
   B. The many processes involved in the ingestion, digestion, absorption, and use of foods and fluids by the body
   C. The Food Guide Rainbow
   D. The balance between calories taken in and used by the body

2. Protein is needed for
   A. Tissue growth and repair
   B. Energy and fibre
   C. Body heat and the protection of organs from injury
   D. Improving the taste of food

3. *Canada's Food Guide to Healthy Eating* encourages
   A. A low-carbohydrate diet
   B. A high-fat diet
   C. A low-fibre diet
   D. A low-fat diet

4. How many daily servings of grain product does the Food Guide recommend?
   A. 5 to12
   B. 4 to 8
   C. 2 to 4
   D. 2 to 3

5. Which food groups contain the most fat?
   A. Grain Products and Milk Products
   B. Grain Products and Meat & Alternatives
   C. Milk Products and Meat & Alternatives
   D. Grain Products and Vegetables & Fruit

6. The Daily Value (DV) is an amount that indicates
   A. The number of calories an adult of average weight should consume daily
   B. Intake and output measured in millilitres (mL) or in cubic centimetres (cc)
   C. The nutrients in each meal served in hospitals and long-term care facilities
   D. Whether there is a little or a lot of a nutrient in a serving of food

7. Older adults
   A. Have lower nutrient requirements than younger adults
   B. Should eat a high-fat diet
   C. Should eat foods high in protein and calcium
   D. Should eat at least 3000 calories per day

8. Which is an acceptable food safety practice?
   A. Washing your hands immediately after handling raw chicken
   B. Defrosting frozen chicken on the kitchen counter
   C. Cutting raw chicken and vegetables on the same cutting board
   D. Serving chicken that is crisp on the outside and pink on the inside

9. Which of the following conditions does *not* usually require a sodium-restricted diet?
   A. Diabetes
   B. Heart disease
   C. Kidney disease
   D. Liver disease

10. People with diabetes must
    A. Restrict their intake of fluids
    B. Eat a diet high in saturated fat and protein
    C. Eat a high-fibre diet
    D. Eat the same amount of carbohydrates, protein, and fat each day

11. Which of the following is *not* suggested for clients who are weak and fatigued?
    A. A straw for liquids
    B. Large portions
    C. Foods that are high in calories
    D. Soft foods

12. Which statement about feeding a client is *false*?
    A. Ask if he or she wants to pray before eating
    B. Use a fork
    C. Ask the person the order in which to serve foods
    D. Engage the person in pleasant conversation

13. Adult fluid requirements for normal fluid balance are about
    A. 1000 to 1500 mL daily
    B. 1500 to 2000 mL daily
    C. 2000 to 2500 mL daily
    D. 2500 to 3000 mL daily

14. A person is NPO. You should
    A. Provide a variety of fluids
    B. Offer fluids in small amounts and small containers
    C. Remove the water pitcher and glass
    D. Prevent the person from having oral hygiene

Answers to these questions are on page 824.

CHAPTER

26

ENTERAL NUTRITION AND IV THERAPY

OBJECTIVES

- Define the key terms listed in this chapter
- Explain the purpose of enteral nutrition and necessary comfort measures
- Explain how to prevent aspiration and regurgitation
- Identify the signs and symptoms of aspiration
- Identify the solutions, equipment, and complications involved in IV therapy
- Explain the safety measures necessary for IV therapy and your role in maintaining the flow rate

KEY TERMS

aspiration Inhaling fluid or an object into the lungs

enteral nutrition Giving nutrients through the gastrointestinal tract (*enteral*)

flow rate The number of drops per minute (gtt/min)

gastrostomy tube A tube inserted through an opening (*stomy*) into the stomach (*gastro*)

gavage Tube feeding

intravenous (IV) therapy Fluids given through a needle or catheter inserted into a vein; IV, IV therapy, and IV infusion

jejunostomy tube A tube inserted into the intestines through an opening (*stomy*) into the middle part of the small intestine (*jejunum*)

nasogastric (NG) tube A tube inserted through the nose (*naso*) into the stomach (*gastro*)

nasointestinal tube A tube inserted through the nose (*naso*) into the small intestine (*intestinal*)

percutaneous endoscopic gastrostomy (PEG) tube A tube inserted into the stomach (*gastro*) through a stab or puncture wound (*stomy*) made through (*per*) the skin (*cutaneous*); a lighted instrument (*scope*) allows the physician to see inside the body cavity or organ (*endo*)

regurgitation The backward flow of food from the stomach into the mouth

Some clients have special requirements for nutrition and fluids. Because of illness, injury, or surgery, some cannot eat or drink. Others cannot chew or swallow. Methods are used to provide nutrition and fluids though tubes. Medications may also be delivered through a tube. A physician orders these procedures. An RN or other qualified professional administers the procedures. You care for clients who have had these procedures.

ENTERAL NUTRITION

People who cannot chew or swallow often require enteral nutrition. **Enteral nutrition** is giving nutrients through the gastrointestinal tract (*enteral*). A nurse gives formula through a feeding tube. (**Gavage** is another term for tube feeding.)

- A **nasogastric (NG) tube** is inserted through the nose (*naso*) into the stomach (*gastro*) (Figure 26-1). A physician or an RN performs the procedure.
- A **nasointestinal tube** is inserted through the nose (*naso*) into the small intestine (*intestinal*) (Figure 26-2). A physician or an RN performs the procedure.
- A **gastrostomy tube** is inserted into the stomach. A surgically created opening (*stomy*) in the stomach (*gastro*) is needed (Figure 26-3).
- A **jejunostomy tube** is inserted into the intestines. A surgically created opening (*stomy*) in the middle part of the small intestine (*jejunum*) is needed (Figure 26-4).
- A **percutaneous endoscopic gastrostomy (PEG) tube** is inserted with an endoscope. An endoscope is a lighted instrument (*scope*). It allows the physician to see inside a body cavity or organ (*endo*). The endoscope allows the physician to see inside the stomach. The physician inserts the endoscope through the person's mouth and esophagus and into the stomach. A stab or puncture wound (*stomy*) is made through (*per*) the skin (*cutaneous*) and into the stomach (*gastro*). A tube is inserted into the stomach through the stab wound (Figure 26-5 on page 390).

Feeding tubes are used when food cannot pass normally from the mouth into the esophagus and then into the stomach. Cancers of the head, neck, and esophagus are common causes. So is trauma or surgery to the face, mouth, head, or neck. Coma is another reason for tube feedings. So is dysphagia caused by paralysis. Some people with dementia no longer know how to eat and may require tube feedings. Gastrostomy, jejunostomy, and PEG feedings are used for long-term enteral nutrition. The ostomy may be temporary or permanent.

(text continues on page 390)

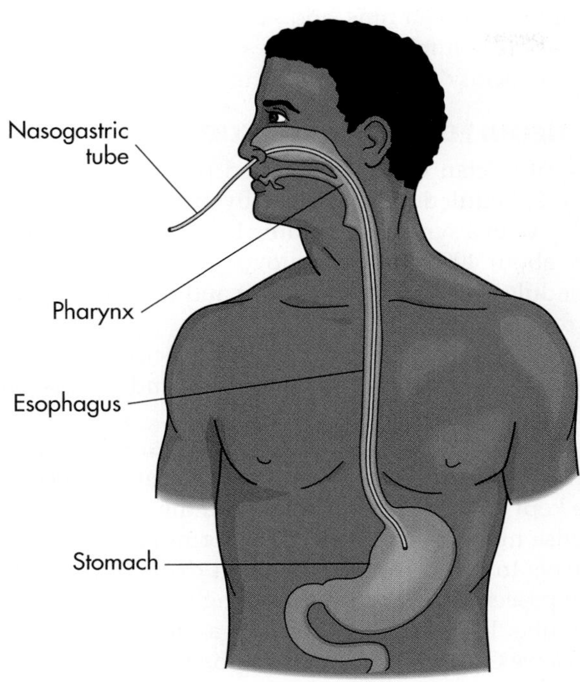

Figure 26-1 A nasogastric tube is inserted through the nose and esophagus into the stomach.

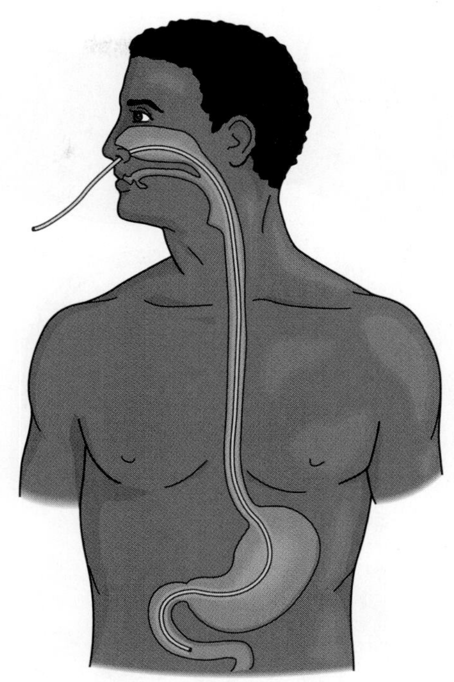

Figure 26-2 A nasointestinal tube is inserted through the nose into the duodenum or jejunum of the small intestine.

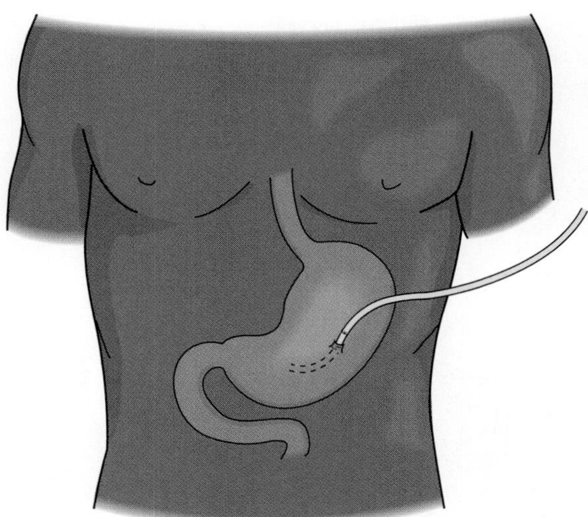

Figure 26-3 A gastrostomy tube.

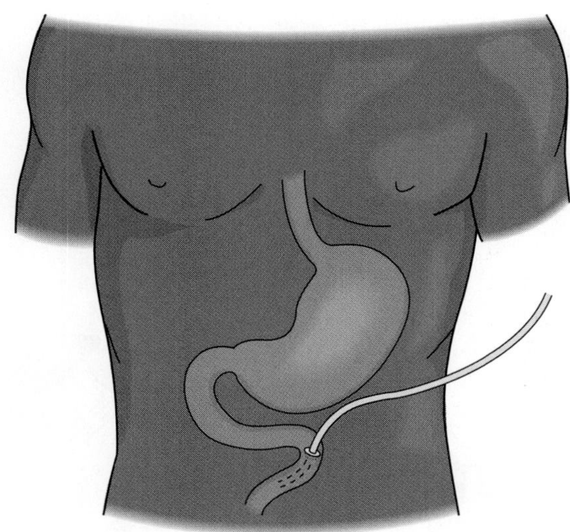

Figure 26-4 A jejunostomy tube.

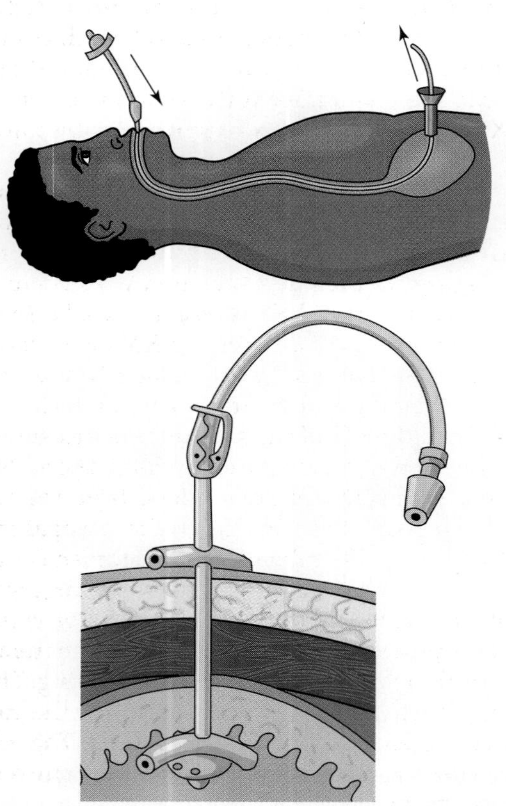

Figure 26-5 A percutaneous endoscopic gastrostomy.

Formulas

The physician orders the type of formula and the amount to give. Most formulas contain protein, carbohydrates, fat, vitamins, and minerals. Commercial formulas are common. Sometimes formulas are prepared by the facility's dietary department.

Scheduled and Continuous Feedings

The physician orders scheduled or continuous feedings. Scheduled feedings usually are given four times a day with a syringe or feeding bag (Figure 26-6). Usually about 400 mL is given over 20 minutes during a scheduled feeding. The amount and rate are the same as regular meals.

Continuous feedings require electronic feeding pumps (Figure 26-7). Nasointestinal and jejunostomy tube feedings are always continuous.

Formula is given at room temperature. Cold fluids can cause cramping. Sometimes continuous feedings are kept cold with ice chips around the container. Otherwise microbes grow in warm formula. The formula warms to room temperature as it drips from the bag and passes through the connecting tubing to the feeding tube. The nurse adds formula as needed. (See *Focus on Home Care: Enteral Nutrition* box.)

Preventing Aspiration

Aspiration is a major complication of nasogastric and nasointestinal tubes. **Aspiration** is inhaling fluid or an

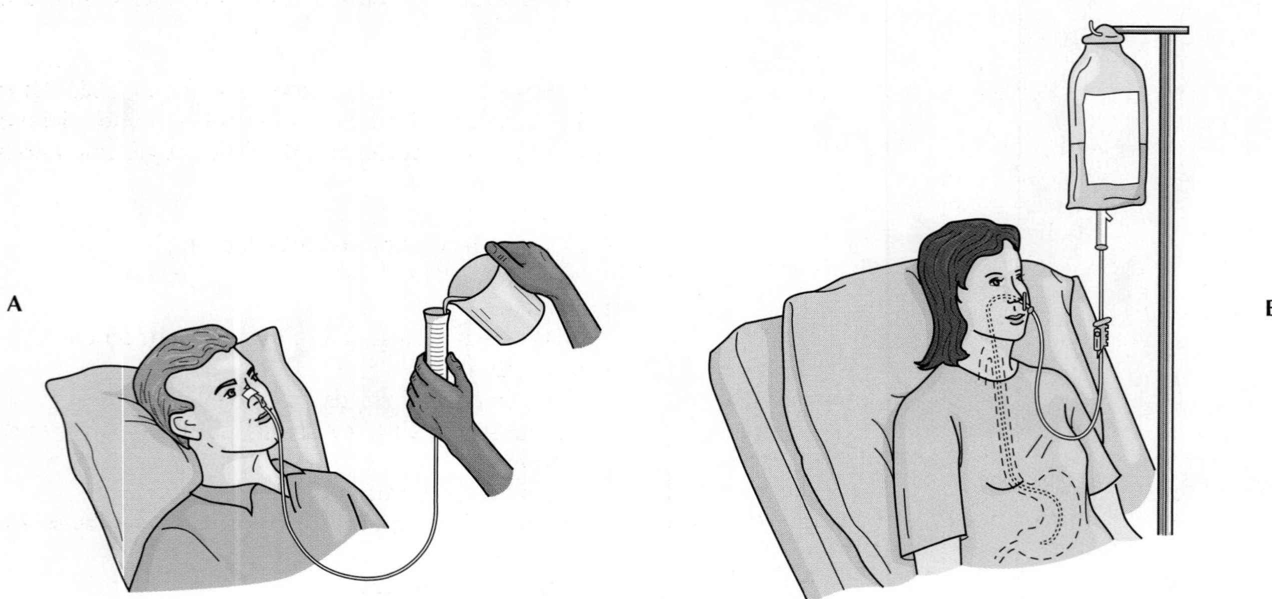

Figure 25-6 A, A tube feeding is given with a syringe. **B,** Formula drips from a feeding bag into the feeding tube.

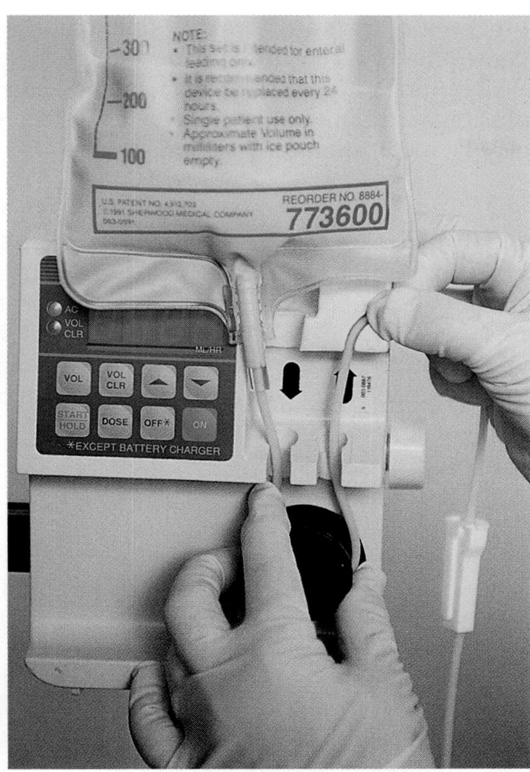

Figure 26-7 Feeding pump. Source: P.A. Potter and A.G. Perry, *Fundamentals of Nursing: Concepts, Process, and Practice,* 4th ed. (St Louis: Mosby, 1997).

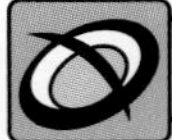

Focus on Home Care

ENTERAL NUTRITION

You care for clients who are being fed by tubes at home. You may assist the nurse with a tube feeding. You never:

- Insert feeding tubes
- Test the position of the tube
- Give the first dose of a tube feeding

However, some home care agencies do permit support workers to start feeding pumps and pour formula into feeding bags. This is done only with gastrostomy tubes and jejunostomy tubes and only if the tube is established. These tasks are *always* delegated by an RN. The nurse in the home will either teach you the task or will teach your supervisor the task. Your supervisor will then teach you. Another method of teaching may be to attend a course given by an RN in your agency. The agency supervises and monitors your performance closely. In most circumstances for each new client you work with, you will need to be retaught the task. This process is needed to ensure competency in the delegated task. The person who teaches you the task has full responsibility for the tube feeding.

object into the lungs. It can cause pneumonia and death. Nasogastric and nasointestinal tubes are passed through the esophagus and then into the stomach or small intestine. During insertion, the tube can slip into the respiratory tract. This causes aspiration. An X-ray is the best way to determine tube placement. One is taken after insertion.

The tube can move out of place from coughing, sneezing, vomiting, suctioning, and poor positioning. It can move from the stomach or intestines into the esophagus and then into the airway. *Therefore the RN checks tube placement before every scheduled tube feeding. With continuous tube feedings, the RN checks tube placement every 4 to 8 hours.* To do so, the RN attaches a syringe to the tube and aspirates gastrointestinal secretions. Then the pH of the secretions is measured.

Aspiration also occurs from regurgitation. **Regurgitation** is the backward flow of food from the stomach into the mouth. This can occur with nasogastric, gastrostomy, and PEG tubes. Delayed stomach emptying and overfeeding are common causes of regurgitation. To prevent regurgitation, the client sits or is in semi-Fowler's position for the feeding. The client remains in this position for 1 to 2 hours after the feeding. This promotes movement of the formula through the gastrointestinal system and prevents aspiration. The left side-lying position is avoided. This position prevents the stomach from emptying.

The risk of regurgitation is less with nasointestinal and jejunostomy tubes. Formula passes directly into the small intestine. Also, formula is given at a slow rate. Remember, during digestion, food slowly passes from the stomach to the small intestine. The stomach handles larger amounts of food at one time than does the small intestine.

Observations. Aspiration is a major risk. Other risks include diarrhea, constipation, and delayed stomach emptying. Report the following immediately:

- Nausea
- Discomfort during the tube feeding
- Vomiting
- Diarrhea
- Distended (enlarged and swollen) abdomen
- Coughing
- Complaints of indigestion or heart burn
- Redness, swelling, drainage, odour, or pain at the ostomy site
- Elevated temperature
- Signs and symptoms of respiratory distress (see Chapter 43)
- Increased pulse rate
- Complaints of flatulence (see Chapter 30)

Comfort Measures

The client with a feeding tube is usually NPO. (*NPO* is the abbreviation for the Latin term *nil per os,* which means nothing by mouth.) Dry mouth, dry lips, and sore throat cause discomfort. Some clients can have hard candy or gum. The client's needs include frequent oral hygiene, lubricant for the lips, and mouth rinses. The nose and nostrils also are cleaned every 4 to 8 hours. Give care as directed by your supervisor and the care plan.

Nasogastric and nasointestinal tubes can irritate and cause pressure on the nose. Sometimes they alter the shape of the nostrils or cause pressure ulcers. Securing the tube helps prevent these problems. Use tape or a tube holder to secure the tube to the nose (Figure 26-8). Tube holders have foam cushions that prevent pressure on the nose. They also eliminate the need for retaping, which irritates the nose. The tube also is secured to the client's gown. Loop a rubber band around the tube. Then pin the rubber band to the person's gown with a safety pin. Or tape the tube to the gown.

IV Therapy

Intravenous (IV) therapy involves giving fluids through a needle or catheter inserted into a vein. *IV* and *IV infusion* also refer to IV therapy. Physicians order IV therapy to:

- Provide needed fluids when a person cannot take fluids by mouth
- Replace minerals and vitamins lost because of illness or injury
- Provide sugar for energy
- Administer medications and blood
- Provide *hyperalimentation*—a solution highly concentrated with nutrients

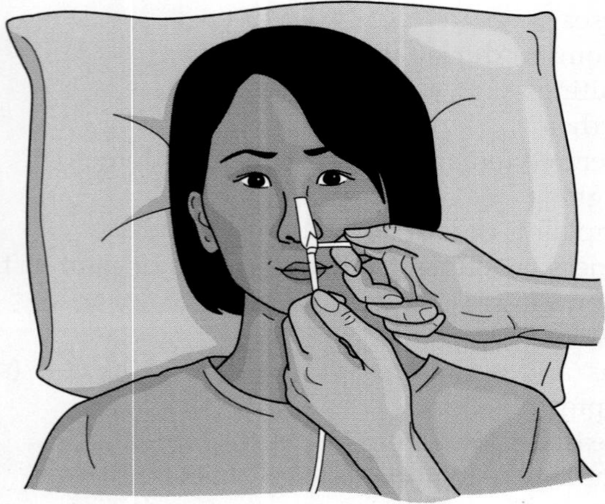

Figure 26-8 The feeding tube is taped to the nose.

IV therapy is given in hospital, outpatient, subacute care, long-term care, and home settings. RNs are responsible for IV therapy. They start and maintain the infusion according to the physician's orders. RNs also give IV medications and administer blood.

Sites

Peripheral and central venous sites are used. Periphery means around (*peri*) a boundary (*phery*). The boundary is the centre of the body near the heart. *Peripheral IV sites* are away from the centre of the body. In adults, the back of the hand, forearm, and crease of the elbow are used (Figure 26-9). (See *Focus on Children: IV Sites* box.)

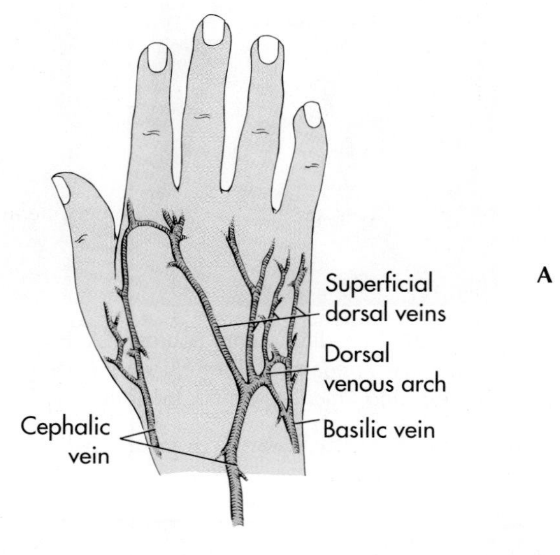

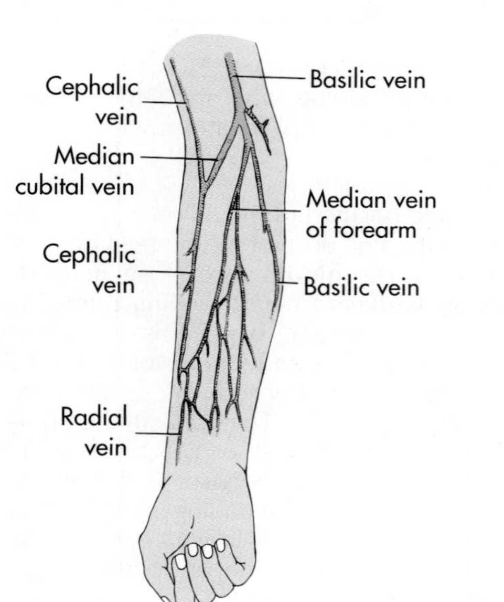

Figure 26-9 Peripheral IV sites for adults. **A,** Back of the hand. **B,** Forearm and crease of the elbow. Source: P.A. Potter and A.G. Perry, *Fundamentals of Nursing: Concepts, Process, and Practice,* 4th ed. (St Louis: Mosby, 1997).

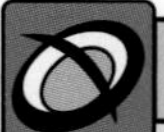

Focus on Children

IV Sites

The hand, wrist, foot, and crease of the elbow are peripheral sites used for infants and children. Sometimes scalp veins are used in infants (Figure 26-10).

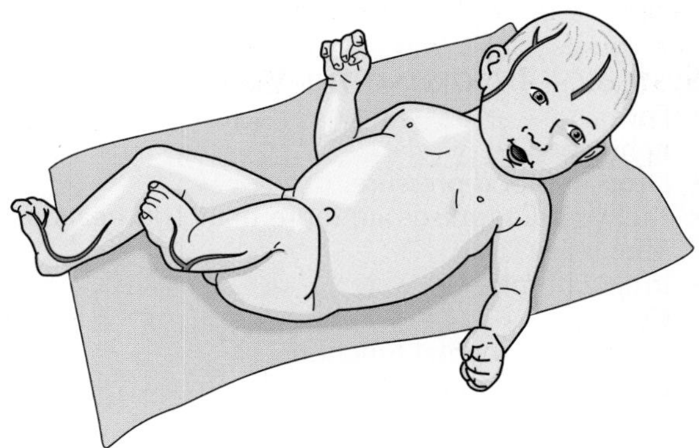

Figure 26-10 The scalp and foot provide peripheral IV sites in infants.

The subclavian vein and the internal jugular vein are *central venous sites.* They are close to the heart. A physician inserts a long catheter into a central vein. The catheter tip is then threaded into the superior vena cava or right atrium (Figure 26-11, *A* and *B*). The catheter is called a *central venous catheter* or *central line.* The cephalic and basilic veins in the arm also are used. Catheters inserted into these sites are called *peripherally inserted central catheters (PICC).* The catheter tip is threaded into the subclavian vein or the superior vena cava (Figure 26-11, *C*). Physicians and specially trained RNs insert PICCs.

Central venous sites are used to give large amounts of fluid and for long-term IV therapy. They also are used for IV medications that irritate the peripheral veins. Sometimes surgery is necessary to insert a central venous catheter. (See *Focus on Home Care: IV Therapy* box on page 394.)

Assisting with IV Therapy

You help meet the hygiene and activity needs of clients with IVs. You are never responsible for starting or maintaining IV therapy. However, you provide safe care. Follow the safety measures in Box 26-1 on page 394. Complications can occur from IV therapy. Report at once any of the signs and symptoms listed in Box 26-2 on page 394.

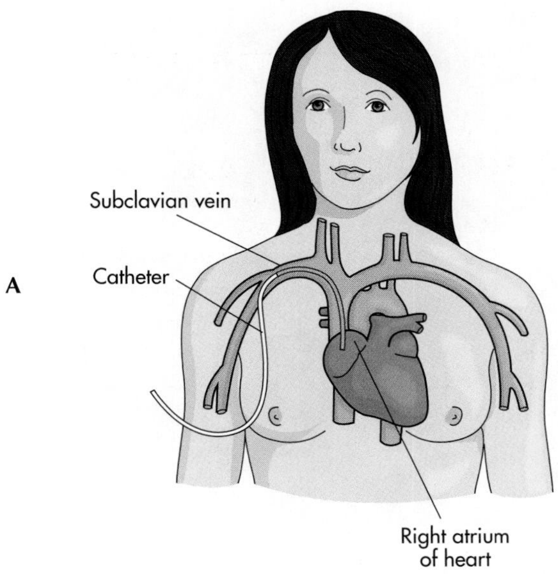

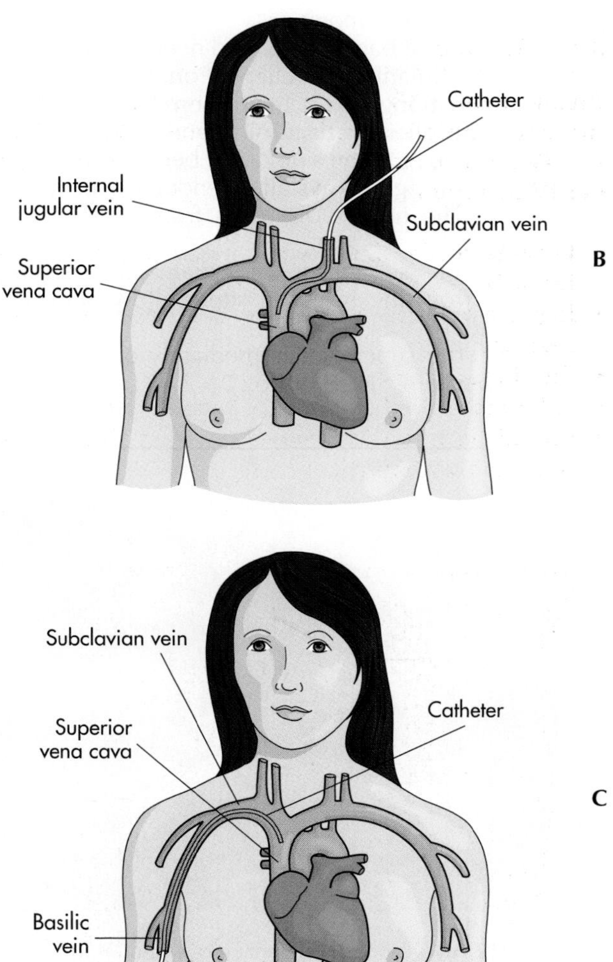

Fig. 26-11 Central venous sites. **A,** Subclavian vein. The catheter tip is in the right atrium. **B,** Internal jugular vein. The catheter tip is in the superior vena cava. **C,** Basilic vein. This is a peripherally inserted central catheter (PICC).

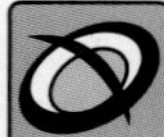

Focus on Home Care

IV Therapy

Clients can receive IV therapy in their homes. These people often have central venous catheters. The RN teaches the client and family about giving medications and managing the catheter.

Box 26-1 Safety Measures for IV Therapy

- Practise Standard Precautions.
- Do not move the needle or catheter. The position of the IV needle or catheter must be maintained. If the needle or catheter is moved, it may come out of the vein. Then fluid flows into the tissues (infiltration) or the flow stops.
- Follow the safety measures for restraints (see Chapter 17). Sometimes the nurse splints or restrains the extremity to prevent movement of the part (Figure 26-12). This helps prevent the needle or catheter from moving.
- Protect the IV bag, tubing, and needle or catheter when ambulating the client. Portable IV stands are rolled along next to the person (Figure 26-13).
- Assist the client with turning and repositioning. Move the bag to the side of the bed on which the person is lying. Always allow enough slack in the tubing. The needle dislodges from pressure on the tube.
- Notify your supervisor immediately if bleeding occurs from the insertion site. Follow Standard Precautions.
- Notify your supervisor immediately of any signs and symptoms listed in Box 26-2.

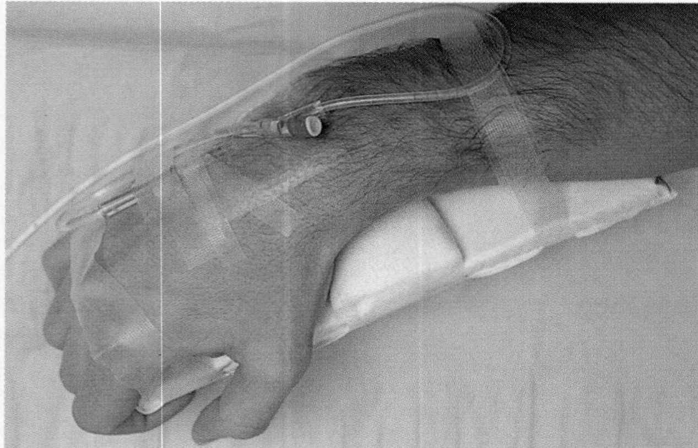

Figure 26-12 An armboard prevents movement at an IV site. Source: M.K. Elkin, A.G. Perry, and P.A. Potter, *Nursing Interventions and Clinical Skills,* 2nd ed. (St Louis: Mosby, 2000).

Box 26-2 Signs and Symptoms of IV Therapy Complications

Local—At the IV Site

- Bleeding
- Puffiness or swelling
- Pale or reddened skin
- Complaints of pain at or above the IV site
- Hot or cold skin near the site

Systemic—Involving the Whole Body

- Fever
- Itching
- Drop in blood pressure
- Tachycardia (pulse rate more than 100 beats per minute)
- Irregular pulse
- Cyanosis
- Changes in mental function
- Loss of consciousness
- Difficulty breathing (dyspnea)
- Shortness of breath
- Decreasing or no urine output
- Chest pain
- Nausea
- Confusion

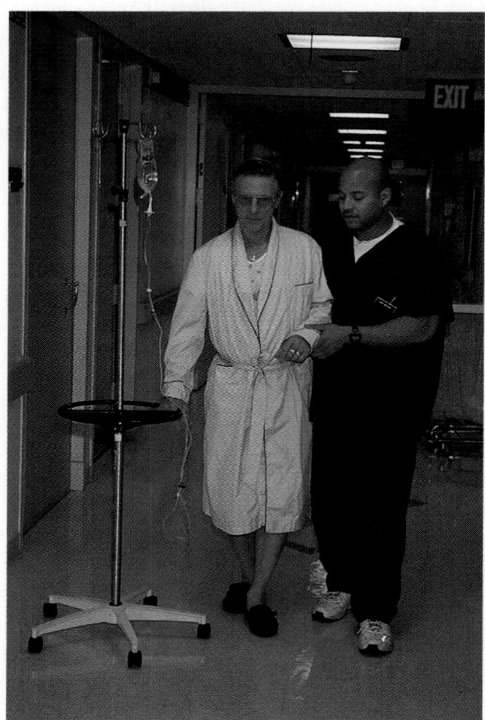

Figure 26-13 A client ambulating with an IV.

REVIEW

Circle the BEST answer.

1. A gastrostomy tube is inserted into the
   A. Small intestine
   B. Stomach
   C. Colon
   D. Nose

2. Which is *not* a common reason for tube feedings?
   A. Cancer of the esophagus
   B. Surgery to the mouth
   C. Dysphagia
   D. Pneumonia

3. Continuous feedings require
   A. Electronic feeding pumps
   B. IV bags
   C. Catheters
   D. Syringes

4. Aspiration is a major complication of
   A. Hyperalimentation
   B. IV therapy
   C. Nasogastric and nasointestinal tubes
   D. Central venous catheters

5. A client with a feeding tube is usually
   A. NPO
   B. On bed rest
   C. Allowed a regular diet
   D. In a coma

6. Care of a person with NPO does *not* include
   A. Frequent oral hygiene
   B. Lubricant for the lips
   C. Mouth rinses
   D. Frequent drinks of water

7. Which is *not* a common IV site for adults?
   A. Back of the hand
   B. Upper arm
   C. Crease of the elbow
   D. Forearm

8. A person is bleeding from an IV site. You should
   A. Remove the IV catheter or needle
   B. Apply direct pressure
   C. Call your supervisor at once
   D. Apply a dressing to the site

9. Which is *not* a sign of IV therapy complications?
   A. Swelling at the IV site
   B. Changes in mental function or confusion
   C. Polyuria
   D. Changes in blood pressure, pulse, and respirations

Answers to these questions are on page 825.

CHAPTER

27

PERSONAL HYGIENE

OBJECTIVES

- Define the key terms listed in this chapter
- Explain the importance of personal hygiene
- Describe oral hygiene and the observations to report
- Describe the guidelines for bathing and the observations to report
- Identify the safety precautions for clients taking tub baths or showers
- Explain the purposes of a back massage
- Identify the purposes of perineal care
- Describe menstrual care
- Learn the procedures described in this chapter

KEY TERMS

afternoon care Routine care given in a facility after lunch and the evening meal

AM care Routine care given in a facility before breakfast; early morning care

aspiration Inhaling fluid or an object into the lungs

early morning care AM care

evening care HS care or PM care

HS care Routine care given in a facility in the evening at bedtime (HS means hour of sleep); evening care or PM care

morning care Routine care given in a facility after breakfast; hygiene measures are more thorough at this time

oral hygiene Measures performed to keep the mouth and teeth clean; mouth care

pericare Perineal care

perineal care Cleansing the genital and anal areas

plaque A thin film that sticks to the teeth; it contains saliva, microbes, and other substances

PM care HS care or evening care

tartar Hardened plaque on teeth

Personal hygiene promotes comfort, safety, and health. It involves activities that clean the skin, teeth, and the mucous membranes of the mouth, genital area, and anus.

Good hygiene helps keep teeth, skin, and mucous membranes intact and healthy. Microbes can enter the body through breaks in the skin or mucous membranes. Infections can result. Therefore, intact skin and mucous membranes are the body's first line of defence against disease. As well as keeping the body clean and healthy, personal hygiene prevents body and breath odours, promotes relaxation, and increases circulation.

Support workers often help clients with personal hygiene. Some clients need only minimal help. Others need you to do hygiene care for them. Illness, disability, and changes associated with aging affect the ability to practise hygiene. Many factors affect hygiene and skin care needs—perspiration, elimination, vomiting, drainage from wounds or body openings, bed rest, and activity.

Culture and personal choice also affect hygiene practices. (See *Respecting Diversity: Personal Hygiene Practices of East Indian Hindus* box.) Most people have hygiene routines and habits. For example, some people bathe at bedtime. Others bathe in the morning. Many people brush their teeth and wash their face and hands on awakening. These and other hygiene measures often are done before and after meals and at bedtime. The care plan lists what personal hygiene measures are needed and when to provide them. You assist with personal hygiene whenever needed. If you have questions, check with your supervisor. (See *Focus on Long-Term Care: Daily Care* box on page 398.)

Clients may feel frustrated, angry, or embarrassed because they need help with such personal care. Remember the priorities of support work when assisting with hygiene. Promote the client's dignity, independence, preferences, privacy, and safety. Doing so will help the client feel more at ease during hygiene procedures. (See *Providing Compassionate Care: Assisting with Personal Hygiene* box on page 398.)

(text continues on page 399)

Respecting Diversity

PERSONAL HYGIENE PRACTICES OF EAST INDIAN HINDUS

Personal hygiene is very important to East Indian Hindus. Their religion requires at least one bath a day. Some Hindus believe that bathing after a meal causes injury. It is also believed that eye injuries can occur from a bath that is too hot. When preparing a bath, hot water can be added to cold water. However, cold water is not added to hot water. After bathing, the body is carefully rubbed dry with a towel.

Remember, individuals may not follow every belief and practice of their culture and religion. Each person is unique.

Source: Adapted from J.N. Giger and R.E. Davidhizar, *Transcultural Nursing: Assessment and Intervention*, 3rd ed. (St. Louis: Mosby, 1999).

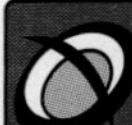

Focus on Long-Term Care

Daily Care

Most facilities provide routine hygiene care at certain times of the day.

- **AM care (early morning care)**—routine care provided before breakfast or morning tests. AM care usually includes the following hygiene measures: cleaning incontinent residents, assisting with face and hand washing, and assisting with oral hygiene.
- **Morning care**—routine care given after breakfast. Hygiene measures are more thorough. They usually involve bathing and providing back massage and perineal care. The client is also assisted with grooming—hair care, shaving, and dressing.
- **Afternoon care**—routine care given after lunch and the evening meal. Many clients like to complete afternoon care before taking a nap, having visitors, or attending activity programs. Afternoon care usually includes assisting with oral hygiene, face and hand washing, and hair care.
- **HS care (evening care** or **PM care)**—care provided at bedtime. (*HS* means hour of sleep.) HS care is relaxing and increases comfort. It includes face and hand washing, oral hygiene, and back massages. The client is helped into sleepwear, and the bed linens and units are straightened.

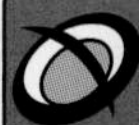

Providing Compassionate Care

Assisting with Personal Hygiene

Dignity. Hygiene is a very personal and private matter. People often are embarrassed when others provide hygiene care. This is especially true when the caregiver and client are opposite sexes. Remember, personal hygiene is necessary for the person's health and well-being. Never be embarrassed or hesitant when assisting with hygiene procedures. The client is likely to sense your discomfort. Talk to the client before and during the procedure. Let him or her know what will happen next. Listen to what the client has to say about the procedure and address any concerns or questions. If appropriate, chat with the client about anything he or she is interested in. Your calm, professional manner will help put the person at ease.

Independence. Allow and encourage clients to do as much self-care as possible. Sometimes you only need to assist with a task. Give the client enough time to do what he or she can independently. Check with your supervisor and the care plan to determine the person's abilities and limitations.

Preferences. People usually have hygiene preferences and routines. Routines provide a sense of order and control. Clients have a say about when and how a hygiene procedure is done. Personal choice is allowed in such matters as bath times and products used. The care plan should reflect the person's preferences and cultural practices. If there is a conflict between the care plan and the client's wishes, tell your supervisor.

Privacy. Protecting privacy is very important when assisting with hygiene. All procedures must be done in a private area. Close doors, privacy curtains, and drapes before giving care. Ask family members or visitors to leave the room. A family member or friend may want to help. The client must consent to this. Do not unnecessarily expose the client's body when bathing. Cover clients when taking them to and from tub or shower rooms.

Safety. Some clients have easily damaged skin. Always be gentle. Never scrub the skin or use rough sponges or cloths. Make sure your fingernails are trimmed. Remove rings before giving skin care. This prevents scratching or tearing the client's skin. Remember to wash your hands with soap and warm water before and after every procedure. Wear gloves when giving perineal care, oral care, and whenever you may have contact with blood, body fluids, secretions, or excretions. Gloves are also worn when you have cuts or rashes on your hands. Always check the water temperature before bathing the client.

Oral Hygiene

Oral hygiene (mouth care) keeps the mouth and teeth clean. This prevents mouth odours and infections. It also increases comfort and makes food taste better. *Cavities* (*dental caries*) are prevented. So is *periodontal disease* (*gum disease, pyorrhea*). Periodontal disease is an inflammation of the tissues around the teeth. Poor oral hygiene allows the build-up of plaque and tartar. **Plaque** is a thin film that sticks to teeth. It contains saliva, microbes, and other substances. Plaque leads to tooth decay, or cavities. When plaque hardens it is called **tartar.** Tartar builds up at the gum line near the neck of the tooth. Tartar build-up leads to periodontal disease. The gums are red, swollen, and bleed easily. As the disease progresses, bone is destroyed and teeth loosen. Tooth loss is common.

Illness and disease often cause a bad taste in the mouth. Some medications and diseases cause a whitish coating on the mouth and tongue. Others cause redness and swelling of the mouth and tongue. Dry mouth is common from oxygen, smoking, decreased fluid intake, and anxiety. Some medications cause dry mouth.

Your supervisor and the care plan tell you the type of mouth care and assistance needed. Oral hygiene is given on awakening, after each meal, and at bedtime. Many people also practise oral hygiene before meals.

Equipment

A toothbrush, toothpaste, dental floss, and mouthwash are needed. The toothbrush should have soft bristles. Clients with dentures need a denture cleaner, denture cup, and denture brush or regular toothbrush. Use only those products that are recommended for cleaning dentures. Otherwise you could damage the dentures.

You also need a kidney basin or small bowl, water glass, straw, tissue, towels, and gloves.

Sponge swabs are used for clients with sore, tender mouths and for unconscious clients. Be careful when using sponge swabs. Always check the foam pad to make sure it is tight on the stick. The client could choke on the foam pad if it comes off the stick.

When giving oral hygiene you have contact with the client's mucous membranes. Gums may bleed during oral hygiene. Also, the mouth contains many microbes. Therefore wear gloves and follow Standard Precautions when giving oral hygiene.

Observations

Report and record the following if observed when assisting with oral hygiene:

- Dry, cracked, swollen, or blistered lips
- Redness, swelling, irritation, sores, or white patches in the mouth or on the tongue
- Bleeding, swelling, or redness of the gums
- Loose teeth
- Rough, sharp, or chipped areas on dentures
- Complaints of pain or discomfort

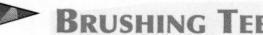

Brushing Teeth

Many clients perform oral hygiene themselves. Others need help gathering and setting up equipment. Encourage the client to be as independent as possible according to his or her abilities and the care plan. The person may choose to brush his or her teeth in the bathroom, at the kitchen sink, or at the bedside.

You may have to brush the teeth of clients who are very weak, who cannot use or move their arms, or who are too confused to brush their own teeth. (See *Focus on Children: Brushing Teeth* box.)

(text continues on page 403)

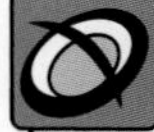

Focus on Children

Brushing Teeth

Children learn to brush their teeth around 3 years of age. However, they may not be thorough. They need help brushing. Older children can do a thorough job. Reminding them to brush is often necessary.

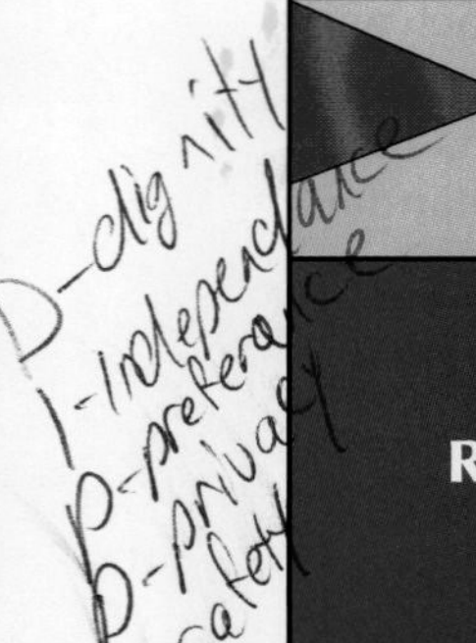

Assisting the Person to Brush Teeth at the Bedside

Compassionate Care

Remember to Promote:
- **Dignity**
- **Independence**
- **Preferences**
- **Privacy**
- **Safety**

Pre-Procedure

1 Identify the person according to employer policy.
2 Explain the procedure to the person.
3 Wash your hands.
4 Collect the following:
- Toothbrush
- Toothpaste
- Mouthwash (or solution specified in the care plan)
- Dental floss (if used)
- Water glass with cool water
- Straw
- Kidney basin or small bowl
- Face towel
- Paper towels
- Gloves

5 Place paper towels on the overbed table (in facilities) or on a work area that the person can easily reach from the bedside. Arrange items on top of paper towels.
6 Provide for privacy.
7 Raise bed to a comfortable working height. Follow the care plan for bed rail use.*

Procedure

8 Lower the bed rail near you if up.
9 Position the person so he or she can brush with ease.
10 Place the towel over the person's chest. This protects garments and linens from spills.
11 Adjust the overbed table in front of the person.*
12 Let the person perform oral hygiene. This includes brushing teeth, rinsing the mouth, flossing, and using mouthwash or other solution. The person spits into the kidney basin or small bowl.
13 Remove the towel when the person is done.
14 Adjust the overbed table next to the bed.*

Post-Procedure

15 Provide for safety and comfort.
16 Place the call bell within reach.*
17 Return bed to its lowest position. Follow the care plan for bed rail use.*
18 Clean and return equipment to its proper place. Wear gloves for this step.
19 Wipe off the overbed table or work area with the paper towels. Discard the paper towels.
20 Remove privacy measures.
21 Follow employer policy for dirty linen.
22 Wash your hands.
23 Report and record your actions and observations according to employer policy.

*Steps marked with an asterisk may not apply in community settings.

Brushing the Person's Teeth

Compassionate Care

Remember to Promote:
- **Dignity**
- **Independence**
- **Preferences**
- **Privacy**
- **Safety**

Pre-Procedure

1 Identify the person according to employer policy.
2 Explain the procedure to the person.
3 Wash your hands.
4 Collect gloves and items listed in *Assisting the Person to Brush Teeth at the Bedside,* page 400.
5 Place paper towels on the overbed table (in facilities) or on a work area within easy reach. Arrange items on top of paper towels.
6 Provide for privacy.
7 Raise bed to a comfortable working height. Follow the care plan for bed rail use.*

Procedure

8 Lower the bed rail near you if up.
9 Assist the person to a sitting or side-lying position facing you.
10 Place the towel over the person's chest.
11 Adjust the overbed table so you can reach it with ease.*
12 Put on gloves.
13 Apply toothpaste to the toothbrush.
14 Hold the toothbrush over the kidney basin or bowl. Pour some water over the brush.
15 Brush the person's teeth gently (Figure 27-1 on page 402).
16 Brush the person's tongue gently, if needed.
17 Let the person rinse the mouth with water. Hold the kidney basin or bowl under the person's chin (Figure 27-2 on page 402). Repeat this step as needed.
18 Floss the person's teeth (see *Flossing the Person's Teeth,* page 403).
19 Let the person use mouthwash or other solution. Hold the kidney basin or bowl under the chin.
20 Remove the towel when done.
21 Remove and discard gloves. Wash your hands.
22 Adjust the overbed table next to the bed.*

Post-Procedure

23 Follow steps 15 through 23 for *Assisting the Person to Brush Teeth at the Bedside,* page 400.

*Steps marked with an asterisk may not apply in community settings.

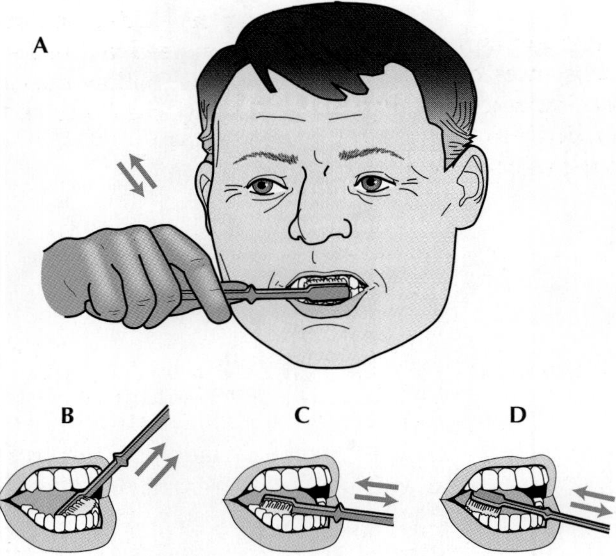

Figure 27-1 Brushing teeth. **A,** Position the brush at a 45-degree angle to the gums. Brush with short strokes. **B,** Position the brush at a 45-degree angle against the inside of the front teeth. Brush from the gum to the crown of the tooth with short strokes. **C,** Hold the brush horizontally against the inner surfaces of the teeth. Brush back and forth. **D,** Position the brush on the biting surfaces of the teeth. Brush back and forth.

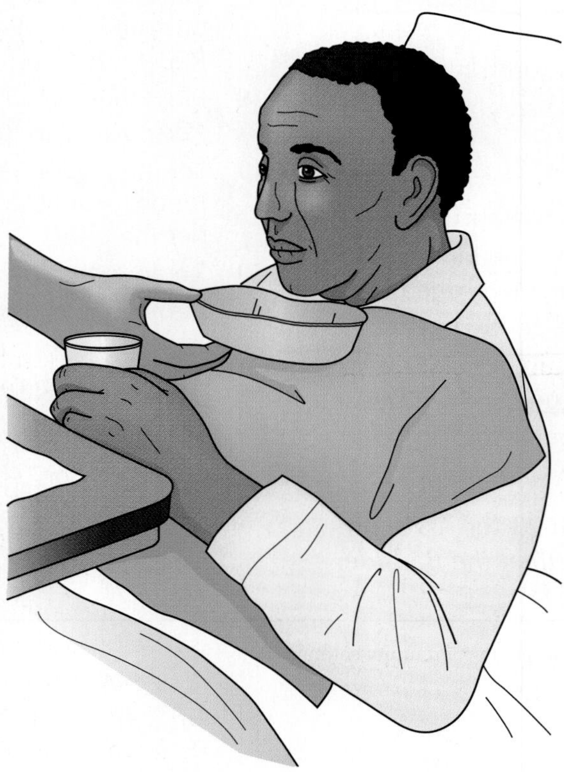

Figure 27-2 Hold a kidney basin under the client's chin.

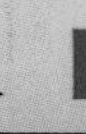

Flossing

Flossing is a preventive measure. It removes plaque and tartar from the teeth. These substances cause serious gum disease that leads to loosening and loss of teeth. Flossing also removes food from between the teeth. It is usually done after brushing but can be done at other times. Some people floss after meals. If flossing is done only once a day, bedtime is the best time to floss.

You need to floss for clients who cannot tend to oral hygiene. Follow the care plan. (See *Focus on Children: Flossing* and *Focus on Older Adults: Flossing* boxes on page 404.)

(text continues on page 405)

Flossing the Person's Teeth

Compassionate Care

Remember to Promote:
- **Dignity**
- **Independence**
- **Preferences**
- **Privacy**
- **Safety**

Pre-Procedure

1 Identify the person according to employer policy.
2 Explain the procedure to the person.
3 Wash your hands.
4 Collect the following:
- Kidney basin or small bowl
- Water glass with cool water
- Dental floss
- Face towel
- Paper towels
- Gloves

5 Place paper towels on the overbed table (in facilities) or on a work area within easy reach. Arrange items on top of paper towels.
6 Provide for privacy.
7 Raise bed to a comfortable working height. Follow the care plan for bed rail use.*

Procedure

8 Lower the bed rail near you if up.
9 Assist the person to a sitting or side-lying position facing you.
10 Place the towel over the person's chest.
11 Adjust the overbed table so you can reach it with ease.*
12 Put on gloves.
13 Break off a 45 cm (18 inch) piece of floss from the dispenser.
14 Hold the floss between the middle fingers of each hand (Figure 27-3, *A* on page 404).
15 Stretch the floss with your thumbs.
16 Start at the upper back tooth on the right side. Work around to the left side.
17 Move the floss gently up and down between the teeth (Figure 27-3, *B* on page 404). Move the floss up and down from the top of the tooth to the gum line.
18 Move to a new section of floss after every second tooth.
19 Floss the lower teeth. Hold the floss with your index fingers (Figure 27-3, *C* on page 404). Use up-and-down motions and go under the gums as for the upper teeth. Start on the right side. Work around to the left side.
20 Let the person rinse his or her mouth. Hold the kidney basin or bowl under the chin. Repeat rinsing as necessary.
21 Remove the towel when done.
22 Remove and discard gloves. Wash your hands.
23 Adjust the overbed table next to the bed.*

Continued

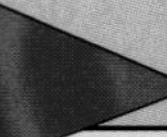

Flossing the Person's Teeth—cont'd

Post-Procedure

24 Follow steps 15 through 23 for *Assisting the Person to Brush Teeth at the Bedside*, page 400.

*Steps marked with an asterisk may not apply in community settings.

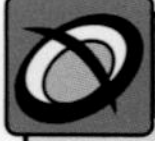

Focus on Children

FLOSSING
Preschoolers and older children need to floss. You need to floss for preschoolers. Older children can floss themselves. However, they need reminding and some supervision.

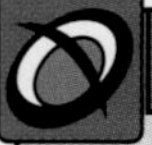

Focus on Older Adults

FLOSSING
Flossing was not a common oral hygiene practice many years ago. Therefore some older adults have never flossed their teeth. A client may refuse to floss or to let you do it. Respect the person's wishes, and tell your supervisor. The client's care plan may be changed as needed.

A

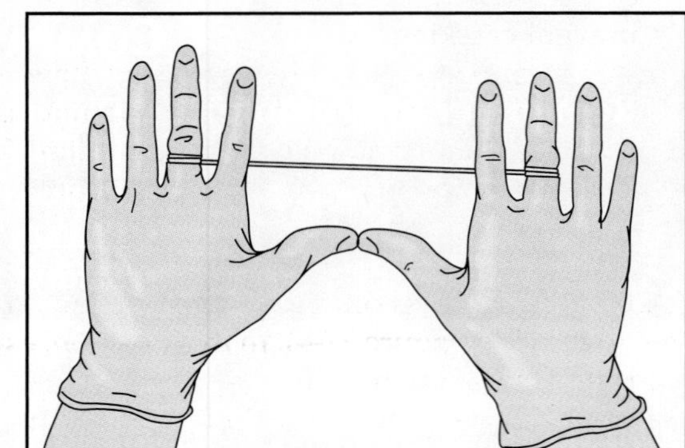

B

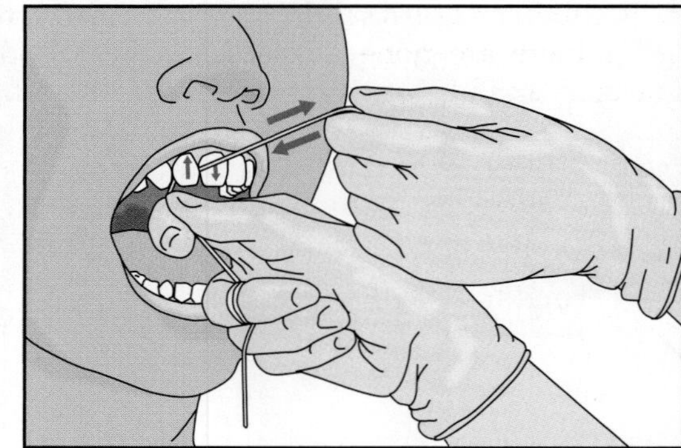

C

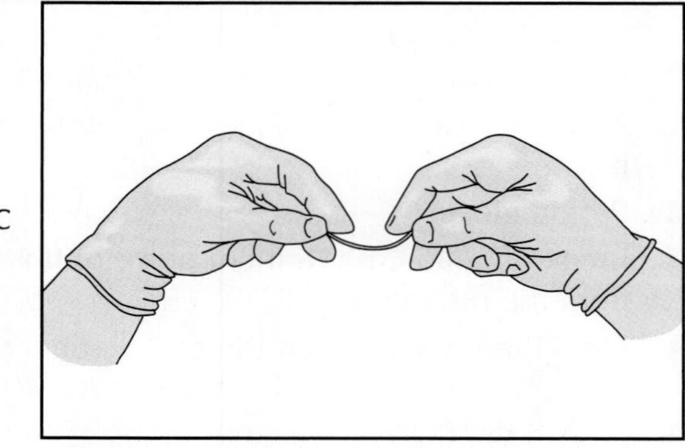

Figure 27-3 Flossing. **A,** Hold dental floss between the middle fingers to floss the upper teeth. **B,** Move floss in up-and-down motions between the teeth. Move floss up and down from the top of the tooth to the gum line. **C,** Hold floss with the index fingers to floss the lower teeth.

Mouth Care for an Unconscious Client

Unconscious clients need special mouth care. They cannot eat or drink, and they may breathe with their mouths open. Many receive oxygen (see Chapter 43). These factors cause mouth dryness. They also cause crusting on the tongue and mucous membranes. Oral hygiene helps keep the mouth clean and moist. It also prevents infection.

The care plan tells you what cleaning agent to use. Use sponge swabs to apply the cleaning agent. Apply a lubricant (check the care plan) to the lips after cleaning to prevent cracking.

Unconscious people usually cannot swallow. Protect them from choking and aspiration. **Aspiration** is the inhaling of fluid or an object into the lungs. It increases the risk of pneumonia and death. To prevent aspiration:

- Position the client on one side with the head turned well to the side (Figure 27-4). In this position, excess fluid runs out of the mouth.
- Use only a small amount of fluid. Sometimes oral suctioning is needed (see Chapter 43).

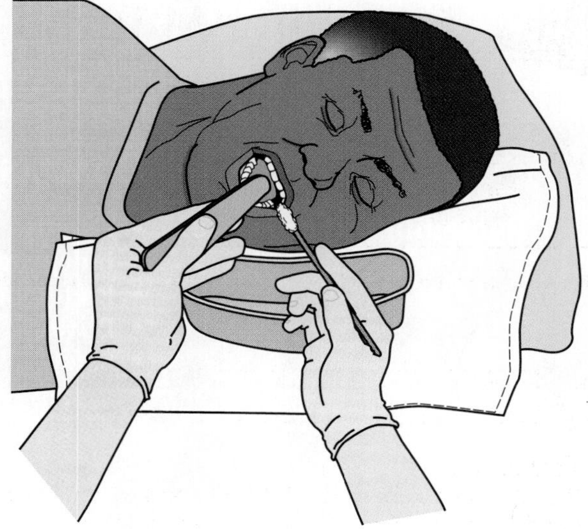

Figure 27-4 Turn the head of the unconscious client well to the side to prevent aspiration. Use a padded tongue blade to keep the mouth open while cleaning the mouth with swabs.

Keep the client's mouth open with a padded tongue blade. If there are none available, make a padded tongue blade as in Figure 27-5. Do not use your fingers to hold the mouth open. The person could bite down on them. Remember, breaks in the skin create a portal of entry for microbes. An infection could develop.

Unconscious people cannot speak or respond to what is happening. However, many can hear. Always assume that unconscious clients can hear. Explain what you are doing step by step. Also tell the client when you are done and when you are leaving the room.

Mouth care is given at least every 2 hours. Follow your supervisor's directions. Check with your supervisor and the care plan. They tell you how often to do oral hygiene and what to use. Unconscious clients are also repositioned at least every 2 hours. Combining mouth care, skin care, and other comfort measures increases their comfort and safety.

(text continues on page 407)

A

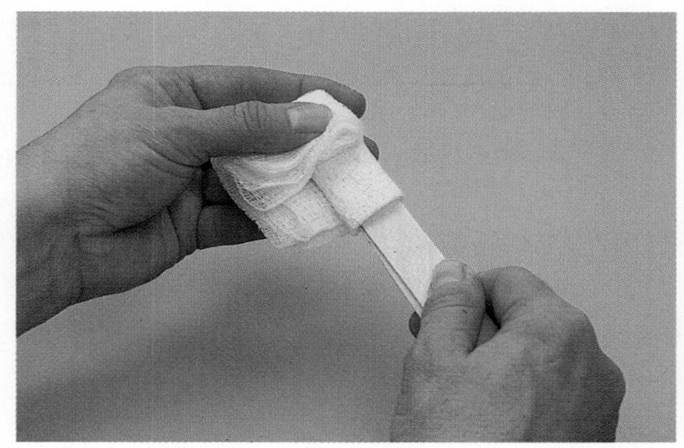

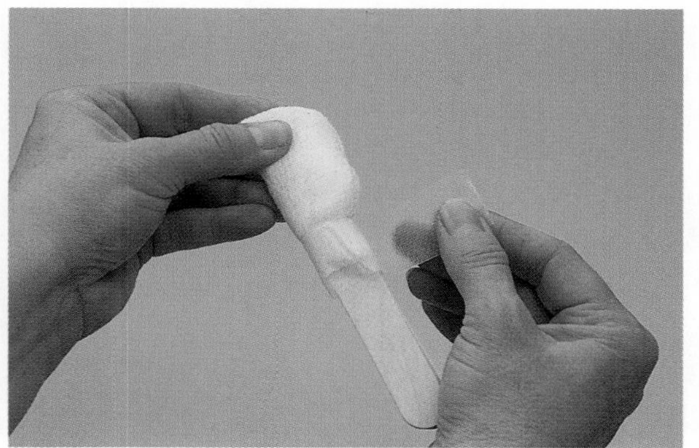

B

Figure 27-5 Making a padded tongue blade. **A,** Place two wooden tongue blades together and wrap gauze around the top half. **B,** Tape the gauze in place.

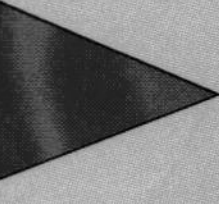

Providing Mouth Care for an Unconscious Person

Compassionate Care

Remember to Promote:
- **Dignity**
- **Independence**
- **Preferences**
- **Privacy**
- **Safety**

Pre-Procedure

1 Identify the person according to employer policy.
2 Explain the procedure to the person.
3 Wash your hands.
4 Collect the following:
- Cleaning agent (check the care plan)
- Sponge swabs
- Padded tongue blade
- Water glass with cool water
- Face towel
- Kidney basin or small bowl
- Lubricant for lips
- Paper towels
- Gloves

5 Place paper towels on the overbed table (in facilities) or on a work area within easy reach. Arrange items on top of paper towels.
6 Provide for privacy.
7 Raise bed to a comfortable working height. Follow the care plan for bed rail use.*

Procedure

8 Lower the bed rail near you if up.
9 Position the person in a side-lying position facing you. Turn his or her head well to the side.
10 Place the towel under the person's chin.
11 Place the kidney basin or bowl under the person's chin.
12 Adjust the overbed table so you can reach it with ease.*
13 Put on gloves.
14 Separate the upper and lower teeth with the padded tongue blade. Be gentle. Do not use force.
15 Clean the mouth with sponge swabs moistened with the cleaning agent (see Figure 27-4 on page 405):
a Clean the chewing and inner surfaces of the teeth.
b Clean the outer surfaces of the teeth.
c Swab the roof of the mouth, inside of the cheeks, and the lips.
d Swab the tongue.
e Moisten a clean swab with water, and swab the mouth to rinse.
f Place used swabs in the kidney basin or bowl.

16 Dry the person's mouth with the towel.
17 Apply lubricant to the lips.
18 Remove the towel.
19 Remove gloves. Wash your hands.

Continued

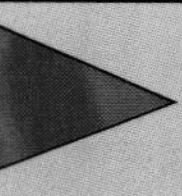

Providing Mouth Care for an Unconscious Person—cont'd

Post-Procedure

20 Explain to the person that you will reposition him or her.

21 Reposition the person, and provide for safety and comfort.

22 Place the call bell within reach.*

23 Return bed to its lowest position. Follow the care plan for bed rail use.*

24 Clean and return equipment to its proper place. Discard disposable items. Wear gloves for this step.

25 Wipe off the overbed table or work area with the paper towels. Discard the paper towels.

26 Remove privacy measures.

27 Tell the person that you are leaving the room.

28 Follow employer policy for dirty linen.

29 Wash your hands.

30 Report and record your actions and observations according to employer policy.

*Steps marked with an asterisk may not apply in community settings.

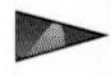

Denture Care

Dentures are artificial teeth. A client may have a complete set of dentures or a partial set. Mouth care is given and dentures are cleaned as often as natural teeth. Dentures are very costly. Handle them carefully. They are slippery when wet. They easily break or chip if dropped onto a hard surface (floors, sinks). During cleaning, firmly hold dentures over a basin of water lined with a towel. Use gauze or a clean cloth to grasp the dentures. Wear gloves when handling dentures.

The cleaning agent has the manufacturer's instructions. They explain how to use the cleaning agent and what water temperature to use. Very hot water causes warping. If dentures are not worn after cleaning, store them in a container of cool water. Otherwise, they can dry out and warp.

Dentures are usually removed at bedtime. Some clients do not wear their dentures. Others wear dentures for eating and remove them after meals. Remind them to not wrap dentures in tissues or napkins. Otherwise they can easily be discarded.

Many clients clean their own dentures. Some need help collecting and cleaning items. They also may need help getting to the bathroom. You clean dentures for clients who cannot do so themselves.

Many people do not like being seen without their dentures. If you clean dentures, return them to the client as quickly as possible. Provide privacy for clients who clean their own dentures.

(text continues on page 410)

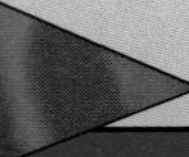

Providing Denture Care

Compassionate Care

Remember to Promote:
- **Dignity**
- **Independence**
- **Preferences**
- **Privacy**
- **Safety**

Pre-Procedure

1 Identify the person according to employer policy.
2 Explain the procedure to the person.
3 Wash your hands.
4 Collect the following:
- Denture brush or toothbrush (soft bristle)
- Denture cup
- Denture cleaner agent
- Water glass with cool water
- Straw
- Mouthwash (or other specified solution)
- Kidney basin or small bowl
- Two face towels
- Paper towels
- Gauze squares
- Gloves

5 Provide for privacy.

Procedure

6 Lower the bed rail near you if up.
7 Place a towel over the person's chest.
8 Put on gloves.
9 Ask the person to remove the dentures. Carefully place them in the kidney basin or bowl.
10 Remove the dentures using gauze if the person cannot do so. (The gauze lets you get a good grip on the slippery dentures.)
   a Grasp the upper denture with your thumb and index finger (Figure 27-6). Move the denture up and down slightly to break the seal. Gently remove the denture once the seal is broken. Place it in the kidney basin or bowl.
   b Remove the lower denture by grasping it with your thumb and index finger. Turn it slightly, and lift it out of the person's mouth. Place it in the kidney basin or bowl.
11 Raise the bed rail if used.
12 Take the kidney basin, denture cup, brush, and cleaning agent to the sink.
13 Line the sink with a towel, and fill it with water.
14 Rinse each denture under warm running water. Return them to the denture cup.
15 Apply the cleaning agent to the brush.
16 Brush the dentures as in Figure 27-7.
17 Rinse dentures under running water. Use warm or cool water as directed by the cleaning agent manufacturer.
18 Place them in the denture cup. Fill it with cool water until the dentures are covered.
19 Clean the kidney basin or bowl.
20 Bring the denture cup and kidney basin to the client.
21 Lower the bed rail if up.
22 Position the person for oral hygiene.
23 Assist the person to rinse his or her mouth with mouthwash or specified solution. Hold the kidney basin under the chin.
24 Ask the person to insert the dentures. If the person cannot do this, insert them in the following manner:
   a Grasp the upper denture firmly with your thumb and index finger. Raise the upper lip with the other hand, and insert the denture. Use your index fingers to gently press on the denture to make sure it is securely in place.

Continued

Providing Denture Care—cont'd

Procedure—cont'd

b Grasp the lower denture securely with your thumb and index finger. Pull down slightly on the lower lip, and insert the denture. Gently press down on it to make sure it is in place.

25 Store the dentures in a safe location if they are not worn.

26 Remove the towel.

27 Remove gloves. Wash your hands.

Post-Procedure

28 Provide for safety and comfort.

29 Place the call bell within reach.*

30 Follow the care plan for bed rail use.*

31 Clean and return equipment to its proper place. Discard disposable items. Wear gloves for this step.

32 Remove privacy measures.

33 Follow employer policy for dirty linen.

34 Wash your hands.

35 Report and record your actions and observations according to employer policy.

*Steps marked with an asterisk may not apply in community settings.

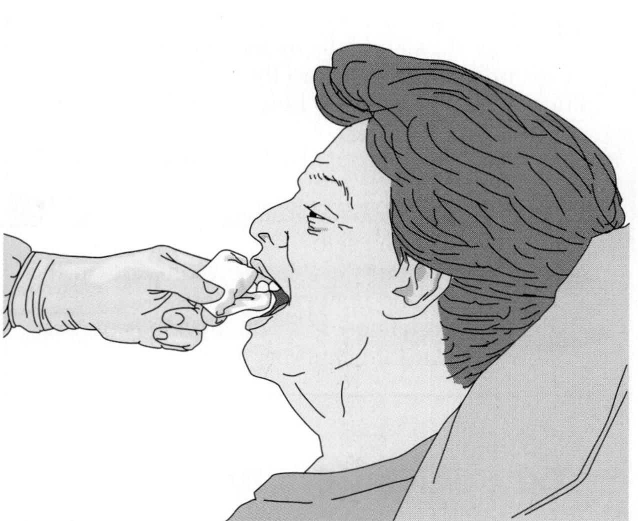

Figure 27-6 Remove the upper denture. Grasp it with the thumb and index finger of one hand. Use a piece of gauze to grasp the slippery denture.

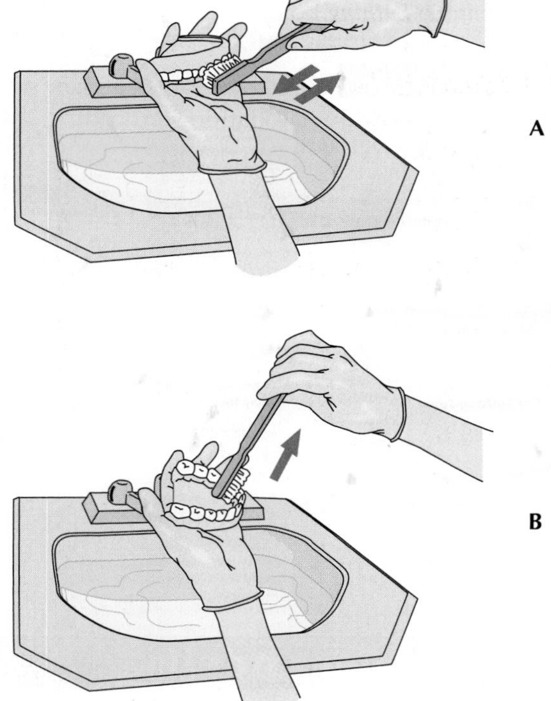

Figure 27-7 Cleaning dentures. **A,** Brush the outer surfaces of the upper denture with back-and-forth motions. Note that the denture is held over the sink, which is filled halfway with water and lined with a towel. **B,** Position the brush vertically to clean the inner surfaces of the denture. Use upward strokes.

Bathing

Bathing cleans the skin. It also cleans the mucous membranes of the genital and anal areas. Microbes, dead skin, perspiration, and excess oils are removed. A bath also is refreshing and relaxing. Circulation is stimulated and body parts exercised. You make observations during the bath. The bath also gives you time to get to know the client.

A client may require a complete or partial bed bath, a tub bath, or a shower. The method depends on the person's condition, self-care abilities, and personal choice. In facilities, bathing usually occurs after breakfast or the evening meal. The client's choice of bath time is respected whenever possible.

Bathing frequency is a personal matter. Some people bathe daily. Others take a complete bath only once or twice a week. Personal choice, weather, physical activity, and illness affect bathing frequency. Illness usually increases the need for bathing because of fever and increased perspiration. Other illnesses and dry skin may limit bathing to every 2 or 3 days.

Guidelines to observe when assisting with bed baths, showers, and tub baths are listed in Box 27-1. Table 27-1 describes common skin care products. (See *Focus on Older Adults: Bathing* box.)

Observations

Observe the skin during bathing procedures. Report and record the following:

- The colour of the skin, lips, nail beds, and sclera (whites of the eyes)
- The location and description of rashes
- Dry skin
- Bruises or open skin areas
- Pale or reddened areas, particularly over bony parts
- Drainage or bleeding from wounds or body openings
- Swelling of the feet and legs
- Corns or calluses on the feet
- Skin temperature
- Complaints of pain or discomfort

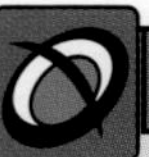

Focus on Older Adults

Bathing

Dry skin occurs with aging. Soap also dries the skin. Dry skin is easily damaged. Therefore older adults usually need a complete bath or shower only 2 times a week. Partial baths are taken the other days. Some bathe daily but do not always use soap. Thorough rinsing is needed when using soap. Lotions and oils help keep the skin soft.

Box 27-1 Guidelines for Bathing Clients

- Follow the care plan for bathing method and skin care products. Allow personal choice whenever possible.
- Follow Standard Precautions.
- Make sure the person fully understands the procedure before you begin. Talk with your supervisor if you are not sure the client fully understands and agrees to the procedure.
- Collect needed items before starting the procedure.
- Provide for privacy. Close doors, shades, drapes, or privacy curtains.
- Cover the person for warmth and privacy.
- Reduce drafts. Close doors and windows.
- Protect the person from falling.
- Use good body mechanics at all times (see Chapter 21).
- Protect the person from burns and scalds. Make sure water is not too hot, particularly for older adults. Check water temperature with a bath thermometer, the inside of your wrist, or your elbow. Water temperature for a complete bed bath is usually 43.3° to 46.1° C (110° to 115° F) for adults. However, older adults may need lower temperatures. Follow the care plan.
- Keep bar soap in the soap dish between latherings. This prevents soapy water. It reduces the chance of slips and falls in showers and tubs.
- Wash from the cleanest to the dirtiest areas.
- Encourage the person to help as much as is safely possible.
- Rinse the skin thoroughly. You must remove all soap.
- Pat the skin dry to avoid irritating or breaking the skin. Never rub the skin.
- Dry under the breasts, between skinfolds, in the perineal area, and between the toes.
- Bathe the skin whenever stool or urine is present. Follow Standard Precautions.

The Complete Bed Bath

The *complete bed bath* involves washing the client's entire body in bed. You give complete bed baths to clients who cannot bathe themselves. Bed baths are usually needed by clients who are unconscious, paralyzed, in casts or traction, or weak from illness or surgery.

Ask your supervisor about the client's ability to assist with the bath. Also ask about any activity or position limits. Remember to follow Standard Precautions. Also, remember to allow personal choice during the bath.

A bed bath is a new experience for some clients. Some are embarrassed to have another person see their bodies. Some fear exposure. Explain to the client how a bed bath is given. Also explain how you cover the body for privacy.

Table 27-1 Common Skin Care Products

Type	Purpose	Considerations
Soaps	Clean the skin Remove dirt, dead skin, skin oil, some microbes, and perspiration	Tend to dry and irritate the skin Dry skin is easily injured and causes itching and discomfort Skin must be rinsed well to remove all soap Not needed for every bath; plain water can clean the skin Plain water is often used for older adults and clients with very dry skin
Bath oils	Keep the skin soft and prevent drying	Some soaps contain bath oil Liquid bath oil can be added to bathwater Showers and tubs become slippery from bath oils; safety precautions are necessary to prevent falls
Creams and lotions	Protect the skin from the drying effect of air and evaporation	Do not feel greasy but leave an oily film on the skin Most are scented Lotion is used for back massage; applying lotion to bony points helps prevent skin breakdown Apply lotion to the back, elbows, knees, and heels after bathing
Powders	Absorb moisture and prevent friction when two skin surfaces rub together	Usually applied under the breasts, under the arms, in the groin area, and sometimes between the toes To apply powder, turn away from the person and sprinkle a small amount onto your hands or a cloth; apply in a thin, even layer Excessive amounts cause caking and crusts that can irritate the skin Do not shake or sprinkle powder onto the person; inhaling powder can irritate the airway and lungs Not used near clients with respiratory diseases Check the care plan before applying powder
Deodorants and antiperspirants	Deodorants mask and control body odours Antiperspirants reduce the amount of perspiration	Applied to the axillae (underarms) Not applied to irritated skin Do not take the place of bathing

The bed bath procedure on page 412 is for adults. See Chapter 37 for bathing infants. Follow the adult procedure for bathing toddlers and older children. Infants, young children, and older adults have fragile skin. Lower water temperatures must be used. Ask your supervisor about what water temperature to use. Always remember to test bathwater before bathing a client.

Towel Baths. With the *towel bath*, a large bath towel is saturated with a cleaning solution. Usually the towel is oversized. This is so it covers the body from the neck to the feet. The solution contains water, a cleaning agent, and a skin-softening agent. It also has a drying agent so the client's body dries quickly. The towel bath is quick, soothing, and relaxing. Clients with dementia often respond well to this type of bath. Your supervisor and the care plan tell you when to use the towel bath. To give a towel bath, follow employer policies and procedures.

Bag Baths. *Bag baths* are commercially prepared or prepared by the employer. Eight to ten washcloths are in a plastic bag. The washcloths are moistened with a cleaning agent that does not require rinsing. The washcloths are warmed in the microwave. Check with your supervisor and manufacturer's instructions for the microwave setting to use. A new washcloth is used for each body part. The skin air dries. Towels are not needed.

(text continues on page 417)

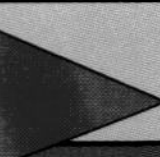

Giving a Complete Bed Bath

Compassionate Care

Remember to Promote:
- **Dignity**
- **Independence**
- **Preferences**
- **Privacy**
- **Safety**

Pre-Procedure

1 Identify the person according to employer policy.
2 Explain the procedure to the person.
3 Offer the bedpan or urinal (see Chapter 29). Provide for privacy.
4 Wash your hands.
5 Collect the following:
- Washbasin
- Soap
- Bath thermometer
- Orange stick, nail file, or soft nail brush
- Washcloth
- Two bath towels and two face towels
- Bath blanket
- Clean gown, pyjamas, or clothing of the person's choice
- Items for oral hygiene
- Lotion
- Powder
- Deodorant or antiperspirant
- Brush and comb
- Other grooming items if requested
- Paper towels
- Gloves (wear when contact with blood, body fluids, secretions, or excretions is likely; gloves are not necessary for bathing a continent person with intact skin. However, wear gloves when bathing the genital and rectal [perineal] area.)

6 Place paper towels on the overbed table (in facilities) or on a work area within easy reach. Arrange items on top of paper towels.
7 Close doors and windows to prevent drafts.
8 Provide for privacy.
9 Raise bed to a comfortable working height. Follow the care plan for bed rail use.*

Procedure

10 Lower the bed rail near you if up. Remove the call bell.*
11 Provide oral hygiene if necessary. (See *Brushing the Person's Teeth*, page 401.)
12 Cover the person with a bath blanket. Remove top linens (see *Making an Occupied Bed*, page 335).
13 Lower the head of the bed until flat.* Ensure the person has at least one pillow.
14 Raise the bed rail near you if bed rails are used. Fill the washbasin ⅔ (two-thirds) full with water. Check the care plan for water temperature to use. Water temperature is usually 43.3° to 46.1° C (110° to 115° F) for adults. Measure the water temperature. (Use a bath thermometer. Or test the bath water by dipping your elbow or inner wrist into the basin.)
15 Place the basin on the overbed table or work area.
16 Lower the bed rail if up.
17 Help the person to move to the side of the bed near you.
18 Place a face towel over the person's chest.
19 Make a mitt with the washcloth (Figure 27-8 on page 414). Use a mitt for the entire bath.
20 Wash around the person's eyes with water. Do not use soap. Gently wipe from the inner part of the eye to the outer with a corner of the mitt (Figure 27-9 on page 415). Clean around the far eye first. Repeat this step for around the near eye, using a clean part of the mitt.

Continued

Giving a Complete Bed Bath—cont'd

Procedure—cont'd

21 Ask the person if you should use soap on the face.
22 Wash the face, ears, and neck. Rinse and pat dry with the towel on the chest.
23 Remove the person's garments. Do not expose the person. (Waiting to remove garments at this time helps the person feel less exposed and more comfortable with the bath.)
24 Place a bath towel lengthwise under the far arm.
25 Support the arm with your palm under the person's elbow. His or her forearm rests on your forearm.
26 Wash the arm, shoulder, and underarm (axilla). Use long, firm strokes (Figure 27-10 on page 415). Rinse and pat dry.
27 Place the basin on the towel. Place the person's hand into the water (Figure 27-11 on page 415). Wash it well. Clean under fingernails with an orange stick, nail file, or soft nail brush.
28 Have the person exercise the hand and fingers.
29 Remove the basin, and dry the hand well. Cover the arm with the bath blanket.
30 Repeat steps 24 to 29 for the near arm.
31 Place basin back on the bedside work area.
32 Place a bath towel over the chest crosswise. Hold the towel in place. Pull the bath blanket from under the towel to the waist.
33 Lift the towel slightly, and wash the chest (Figure 27-12 on page 416). Do not expose the person. Rinse and pat dry, especially under breasts.
34 Move the towel lengthwise over the chest and abdomen. Do not expose the person. Pull the bath blanket down to the pubic area.
35 Lift the towel slightly, and wash the abdomen (Figure 27-13 on page 416). Rinse and pat dry.
36 Pull the bath blanket up to the shoulders, covering both arms. Remove the towel.
37 Change soapy or cool water. Measure temperature as in step 14. If bed rails are used, raise the bed rail before leaving the bedside. Lower it when you return.
38 Uncover the far leg. Do not expose the genital area. Place a towel lengthwise under the foot and leg.
39 Bend the knee, and support the leg with your arm. Wash it with long, firm strokes. Rinse and pat dry.
40 Place the basin on the towel near the foot.
41 Lift the leg slightly. Slide the basin under the foot.
42 Place the foot in the basin (Figure 27-14 on page 416). Use an orange stick, nail file, or soft nail brush to clean under toenails if necessary. If the person cannot bend the knees:
  a Wash the foot. Carefully separate the toes. Rinse and pat dry.
  b Clean under toenails with an orange stick, nail file, or soft nail brush, if necessary.
43 Remove the basin. Dry the leg and foot. Cover the leg with the bath blanket. Remove the towel.
44 Repeat steps 38 to 43 for the near leg.
45 Change the water. Measure temperature as in step 14. If bed rails are used, raise the bed rail near you before leaving the bedside. Lower it when you return.
46 Turn the person onto his or her side facing away from you. Keep him or her covered with the bath blanket.
47 Uncover the back and buttocks. Do not expose the person. Place a towel lengthwise on the bed along the back.
48 Wash the back. Work from the back of the neck to the lower end of the buttocks. Use long, firm, continuous strokes (Figure 27-15 on page 417). Rinse and dry well.
49 Give a back massage (see *Giving a Back Massage*, page 425). The person may want a back massage after the bath.
50 Turn the person onto his or her back.
51 Change the water for perineal care. Measure water temperature as in step 14. If bed rails are used, raise the bed rail near you before leaving the bedside. Lower it when you return.

Continued

Giving a Complete Bed Bath—cont'd

Procedure—cont'd

52 Let the person wash the genital area. Place the washbasin, soap, and towels within easy reach. Place the call bell (in facilities) within reach. Ask the person to call you when finished. Make sure the person understands what to do. Answer calls for assistance promptly. If the person cannot do self-care, put on gloves and provide perineal care for the person (see *Perineal Care,* page 427).

53 Give a back massage if you have not already done so.

54 Apply deodorant or antiperspirant, lotion, and powder as directed by the care plan or person.

55 Put clean garments on the person.

56 Comb and brush the hair (see Chapter 28).

57 Make the bed.

Post-Procedure

58 Provide for safety and comfort.

59 Return the bed to its lowest position. Attach the call bell. Follow the care plan for bed rail use.*

60 Empty and clean the washbasin. Return it and other supplies to their proper place.

61 Wipe off the overbed table or work area with the paper towels. Discard the paper towels.

62 Remove privacy measures.

63 Follow employer policy for dirty linen.

64 Wash your hands.

65 Report and record your actions and observations according to employer policy.

*Steps marked with an asterisk may not apply in community settings.

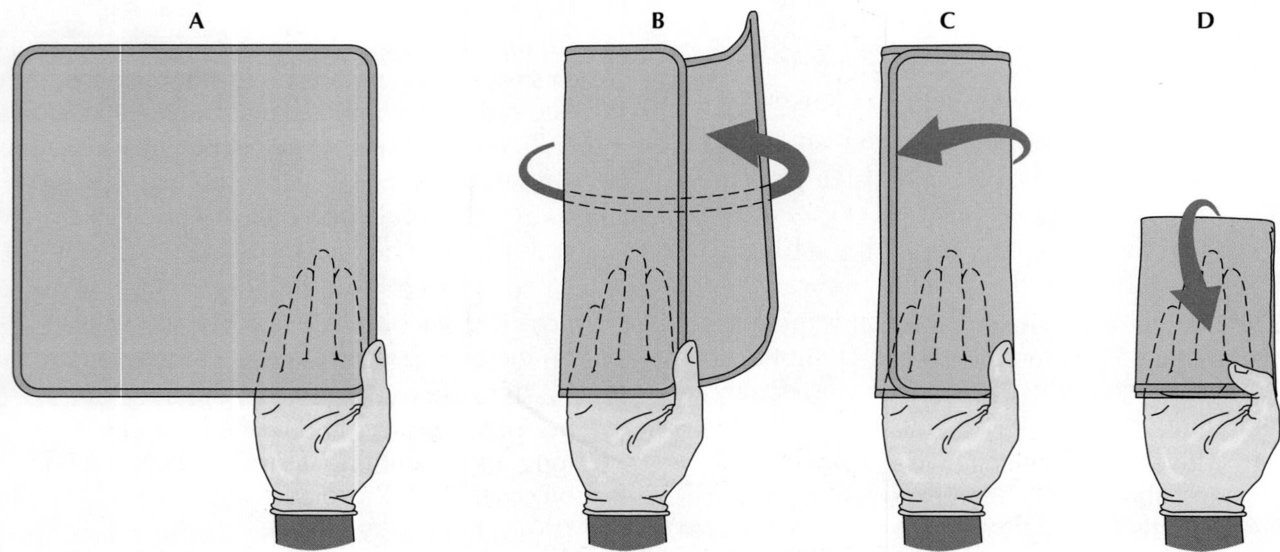

Figure 27-8 Making a mitted washcloth. **A,** Grasp the near side of the washcloth with your thumb. **B,** Bring the washcloth around and behind your hand. **C,** Fold the side of the washcloth over your palm as you grasp it with your thumb. **D,** Fold the top of the washcloth down and tuck it under next to your palm.

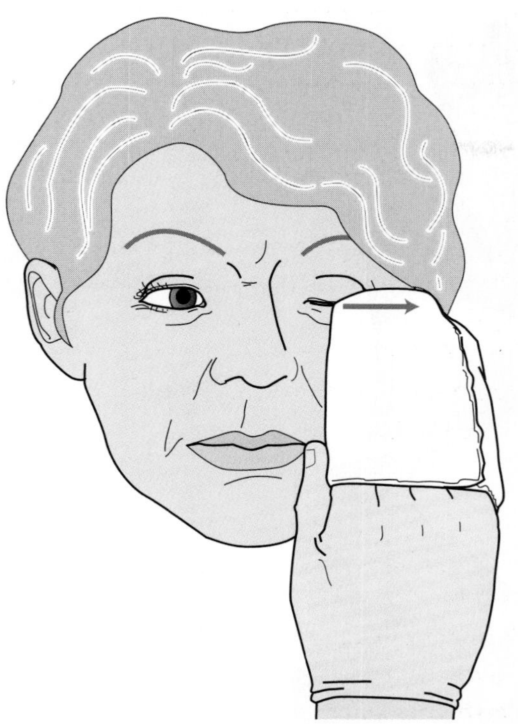

Figure 27-9 Wash around the client's eyes with a mitted washcloth. Wipe from the inner to the outer part of the eye.

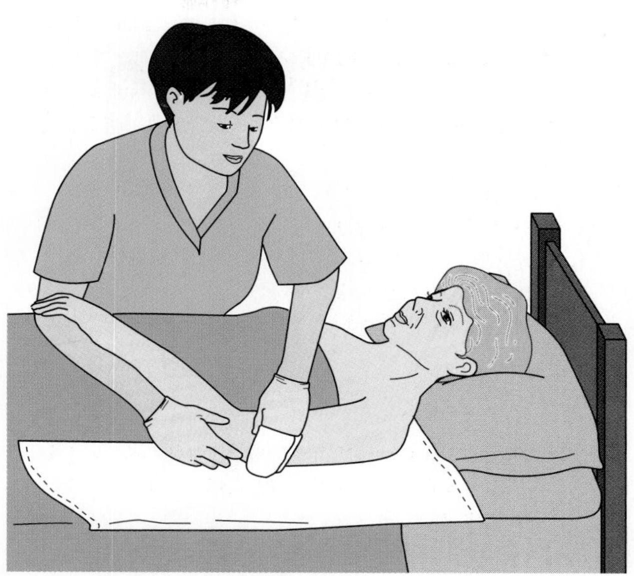

Figure 27-10 Wash the client's arm with firm, long strokes using a mitted washcloth.

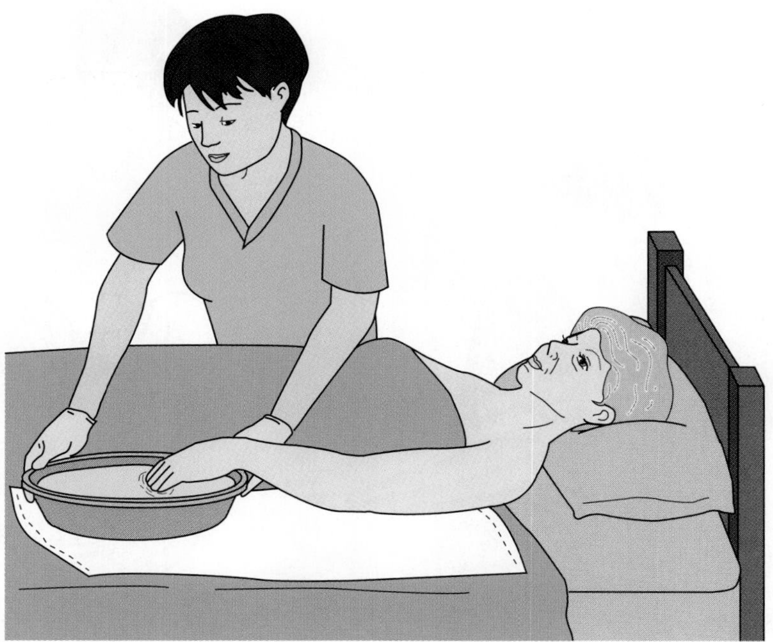

Figure 27-11 Place the wash basin on the bed. Wash the client's hands in it.

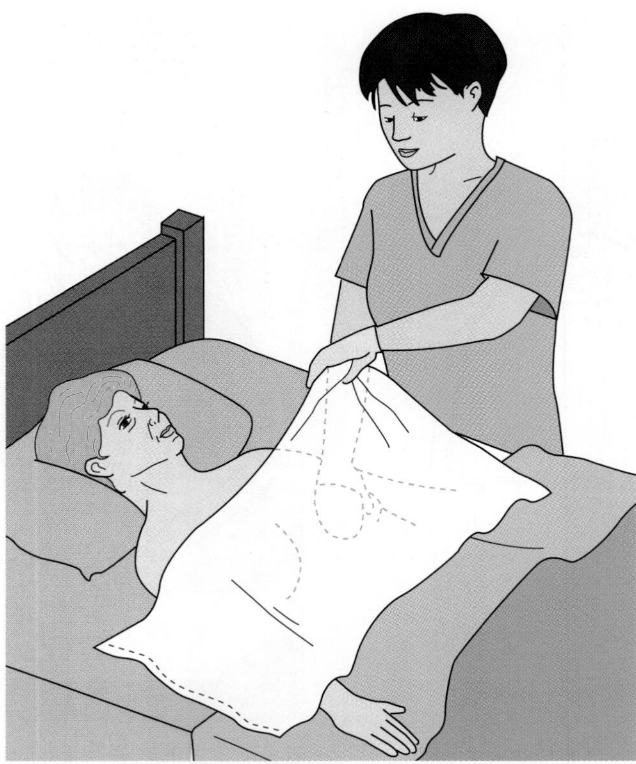

Figure 27-12 Do not expose the client's breasts during the bath. Place a bath towel horizontally over the chest area. Lift the towel slightly to reach under to wash the breasts and chest.

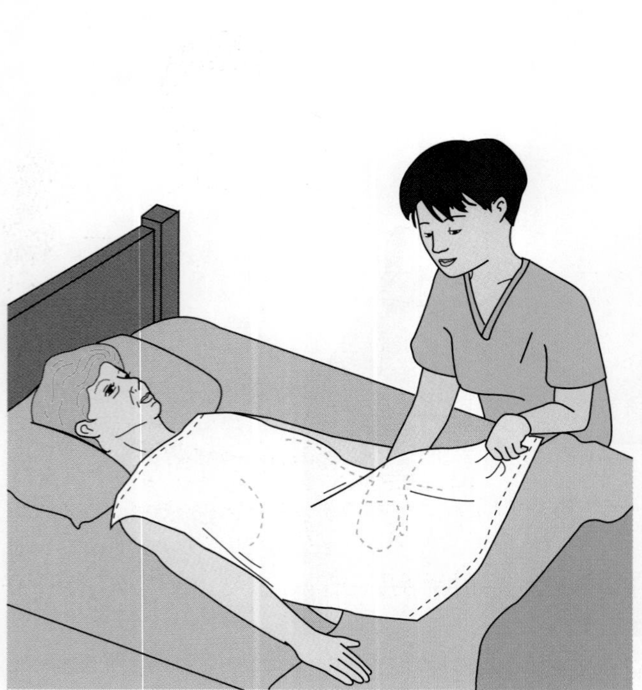

Figure 27-13 Turn the bath towel vertically to cover the breasts and abdomen. Lift the towel slightly to bathe the abdomen. The bath blanket covers the pubic area.

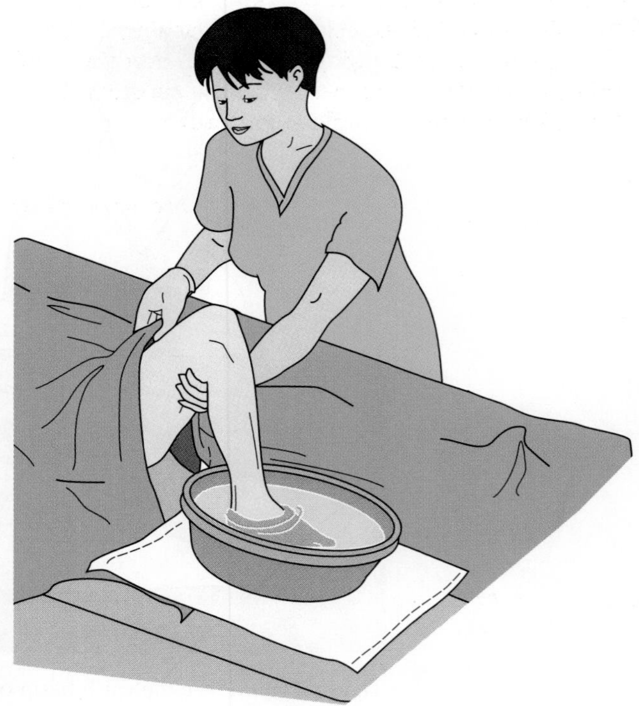

Figure 27-14 Wash the foot by placing it in the washbasin on the bed.

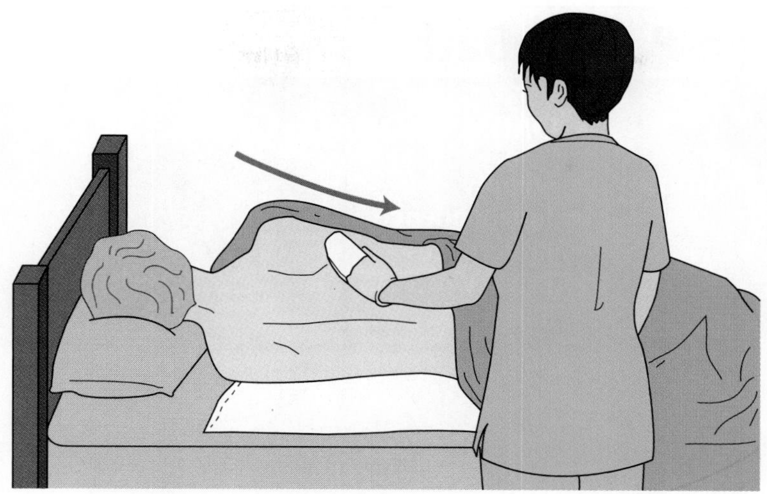

Figure 27-15 Wash the back with long, firm, continuous strokes. Note that the client is in a side-lying position. A towel is placed lengthwise on the bed to protect the linens from water.

The Partial Bath

The *partial bath* involves bathing the face, hands, axillae (underarms), back, buttocks, and perineal area. These areas develop odours or cause discomfort if not clean. You give partial bed baths to clients who cannot bathe themselves. Clients who are able bathe themselves in bed or at the bathroom sink (Figure 27-16). You assist as needed, especially with washing the back.

The guidelines for bathing (see Box 27-1 on page 410) apply for partial bed baths. So do the considerations involved in giving a complete bed bath.

(text continues on page 419)

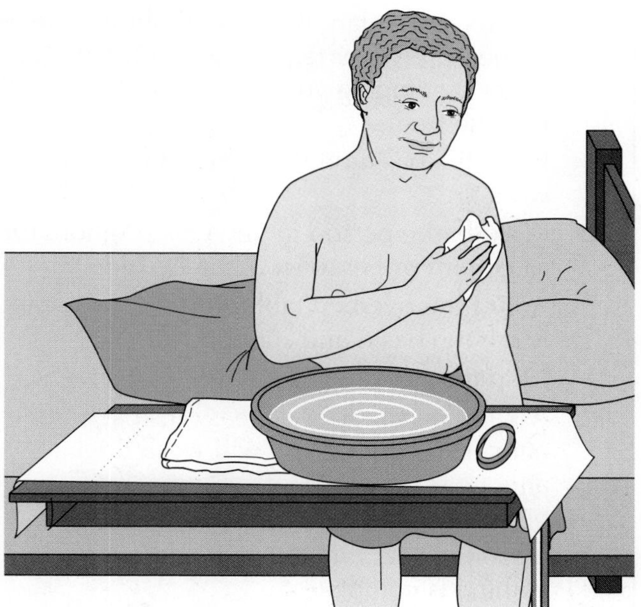

Figure 27-16 The client is bathing himself in bed. Necessary equipment is within his reach.

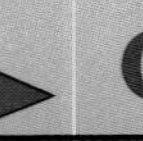

Giving a Partial Bath

Compassionate Care

Remember to Promote:
- **Dignity**
- **Independence**
- **Preferences**
- **Privacy**
- **Safety**

Pre-Procedure

1 Follow steps 1 through 8 in *Giving a Complete Bed Bath* (page 412). Put on gloves.

Procedure

2 Make sure the bed is in the lowest position.*

3 Assist with oral hygiene.

4 Remove top linen. Cover the person with a bath blanket.

5 Place paper towels on the overbed table (in facilities) or on a work area that the person can easily reach from the bedside.

6 Fill the washbasin with water. Water temperature should be 43.3° to 46.1° C (110° to 115° F) or as directed by your supervisor and the care plan. (Use a bath thermometer to measure water temperature. Or test bathwater by dipping your elbow or inner wrist into the basin.)

7 Place the basin on the overbed table or work area.

8 Position the person in Fowler's position. Or assist him or her to sit at the bedside.

9 Adjust the overbed table so the person can reach the basin and supplies.*

10 Help the person undress.

11 Ask the person to wash easy-to-reach body parts. Explain that you will wash the back and areas the person cannot reach.

12 Place the call bell within reach. Ask the person to use it if help is needed or when bathing is complete.*

13 Wash your hands. Leave the room if it is safe to do so. Stay within hearing distance.

14 Return when the person calls for assistance. Knock before entering.

15 Change the bath water. (Measure bath water temperature as in step 6.)

16 Raise the bed to a comfortable working height. Adjust the overbed table as needed.*

17 Ask what was washed. Wash and dry areas the person could not reach. The face, hands, underarms, back, buttocks, and genital and rectal areas (perineal area) are washed for the partial bath. Wear gloves for this step.

18 Give a back massage.

19 Apply deodorant or antiperspirant as requested.

20 Help the person put on clean garments.

21 Assist with hair care.

22 Assist the person to a chair. (See *Transferring the Person to a Chair or Wheelchair,* page 291.) Otherwise, turn the person onto the side away from you.

23 Make the bed.

24 Return the bed to its lowest position.*

Continued

Giving a Partial Bath—cont'd

Post-Procedure

25 Provide for safety and comfort.
26 Place the call bell within reach.*
27 Follow the care plan for bed rail use.*
28 Empty and clean the basin. Return the basin and supplies to their proper place.
29 Wipe off the overbed table or work area with the paper towels. Discard the paper towels.
30 Remove privacy measures.
31 Follow employer policy for dirty linen.
32 Wash your hands.
33 Report and record your actions and observations according to employer policy.

*Steps marked with an asterisk may not apply in community settings.

Tub Baths and Showers

Many people like tub baths. Others prefer showers. However, falls and burns from hot water are risks. Safety is important (Box 27-2). You must prevent slipping, falls, chills, and burns. *Only give a tub bath or shower if it is written in the care plan.* Check with your supervisor and the care plan for special instructions.

Tub Baths. Tub baths are relaxing for many people. However, a tub bath can cause a client to feel faint, weak, or tired. These are greater risks for clients who are on bed rest. A bath should last no longer than 20 minutes.

In a facility, you reserve the tub room for the client. The tub is cleaned before and after use. This prevents the spread of microbes and infection.

Box 27-2 Safety Guidelines for Assisting Clients with Tub Baths and Showers

- Know what water temperature to use. Check with your supervisor and the care plan. Usually the temperature is 40.5° C (105° F).
- Clean the tub or shower before and after use. This prevents the spread of microbes and infection.
- Dry the bathroom or shower room floor.
- Check hand rails, grab bars, hydraulic lifts, and other safety aids. They must be in working order.
- Place a bath mat in the tub or on the shower floor. This is not needed if there are nonskid strips or a nonskid surface.
- Cover the person for warmth and privacy. This includes during transport to and from the shower room or tub.
- Place needed items within the person's reach.
- Place the call bell (in facilities) within the person's reach. Show the person how to use the call bell in the shower or tub room.
- Have the person use safety bars when getting in and out of the tub or shower. The person must not use towel bars for support.
- Use good body mechanics when transferring clients to and from tubs and showers (see Chapter 21). If necessary, ask for help with the transfer before beginning.
- Turn cold water on first, then the hot water. Turn hot water off first, then the cold water.
- Adjust water temperature and pressure to prevent chilling or burns. Do this before the person gets into the shower. If a shower or bath chair is used, position the chair first.
- Direct water away from the person while adjusting water temperature and pressure.
- Fill the tub before the person gets into it.
- Measure the water temperature. Use a bath thermometer. Or for showers and tub baths in facilities, use the digital display (see Figure 27-23 on page 424).
- Keep the water spray directed toward the person during the shower. This helps keep him or her warm.
- Avoid using bath oils. They make tub and shower surfaces slippery.
- Keep bar soap in the soap dish. This prevents soapy water. It also reduces the chance of slips and falls in the tub or shower.
- Do not leave weak or unsteady people unattended in the tub or shower.
- Stay within hearing distance if the person can be left alone. Wait outside the door or shower curtain. You will be nearby if the person calls for you or has an accident.
- Drain the tub before the person gets out of the tub.

Some facilities have portable tubs. The sides are lowered to transfer the person from bed to the tub (Figure 27-17). The sides are raised after the transfer. The person is transported to the tub room in the portable tub. There the tub is filled and the person bathed in the usual manner. Remember to cover the client with a blanket for privacy and warmth during the transfers and transports.

Whirlpool tubs have hydraulic lifts (Figure 27-18). The client is transported to the tub room in a special wheelchair or stretcher. The client and the chair or stretcher are lifted into the tub (Figure 27-19). The whirlpool action cleans the person's lower body. You wash the upper body. Carefully wash under breasts, between skinfolds, and in the perineal area. Dry the person after the bath.

In a client's home, the bathroom should be as safe as possible. Make sure there is a rubber bath mat or nonskid strips on the tub floor. Safety devices like grab bars, transfer boards, and bath or shower chairs are helpful for some clients (Figure 27-20). The case manager and other members of the health care team arrange for these devices. Make sure they are in place and used when necessary. Bring a straight chair into the bathroom so the client can sit when preparing for the bath or shower. Make sure the bathroom is warm, well lit, and the floor is free of clutter and water spills.

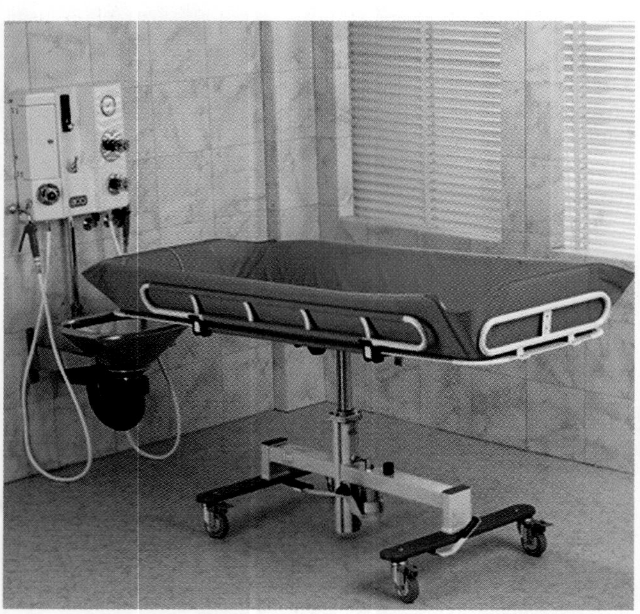

Figure 27-17 Portable tub. *(Courtesy Arjo, Inc, Morton Grove, IL.)*

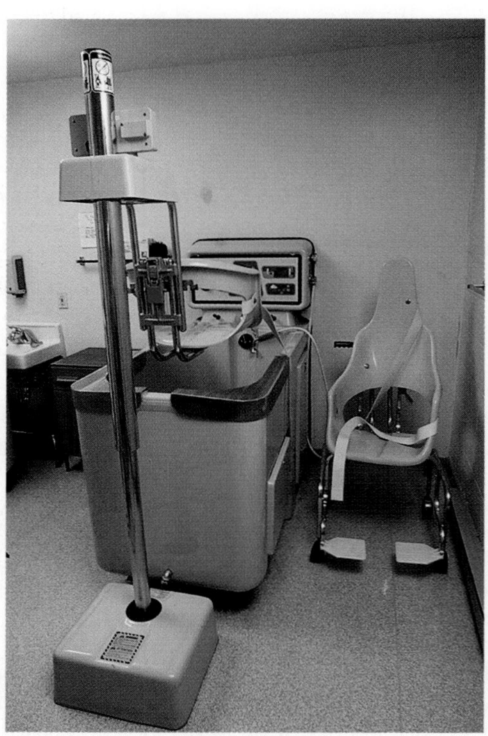

Figure 27-18 Whirlpool tub with a hydraulic lift.

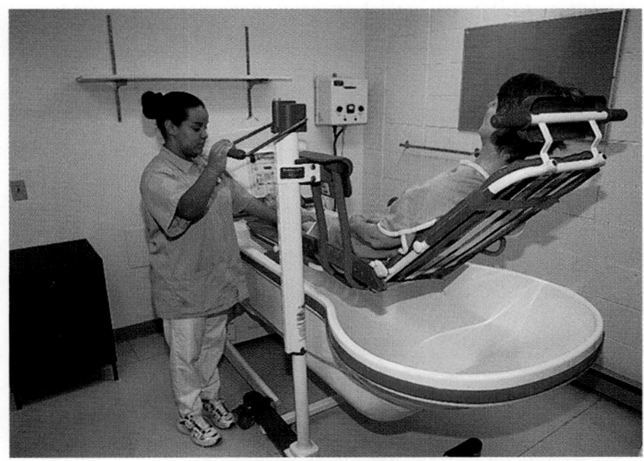

Figure 27-19 The stretcher and client are lowered into the tub.

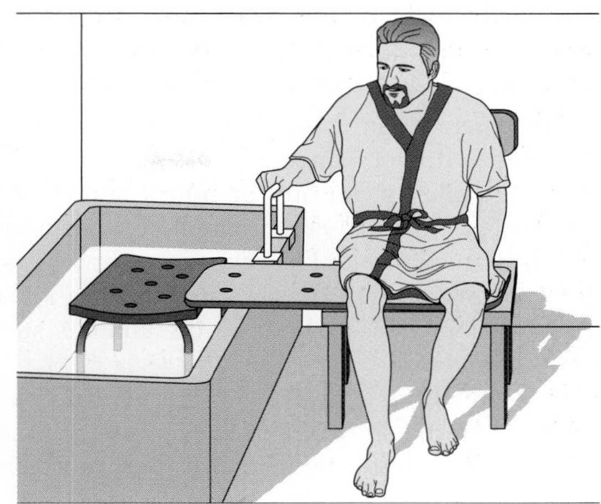

Figure 27-20 A client using a transfer board, bath chair, and grab bar when taking a bath at home.

Showers. Some facilities provide private baths or showers in the person's room. Other facilities have common baths or shower rooms that must be reserved before use. Shower rooms have shower stalls or shower cabinets (Figure 27-21). The client walks into the stall or cabinet or is wheeled in on a shower chair. An open area on the plastic seat lets water drain off the chair. The chair can be used to transport the client to and from the shower room. The wheels are locked during the shower. This prevents the chair from moving.

The shower room may have more than one stall or cabinet. Protect the client's right to privacy. The client has the right to not have his or her body seen by others. Properly screen and cover the client. Also close doors and the shower curtain.

A

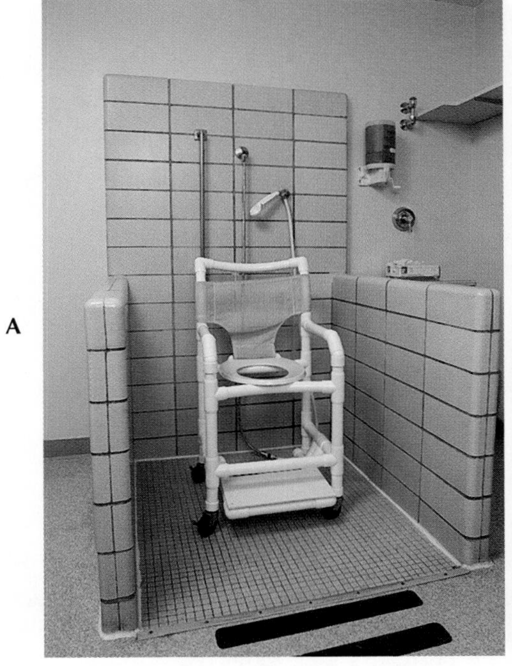

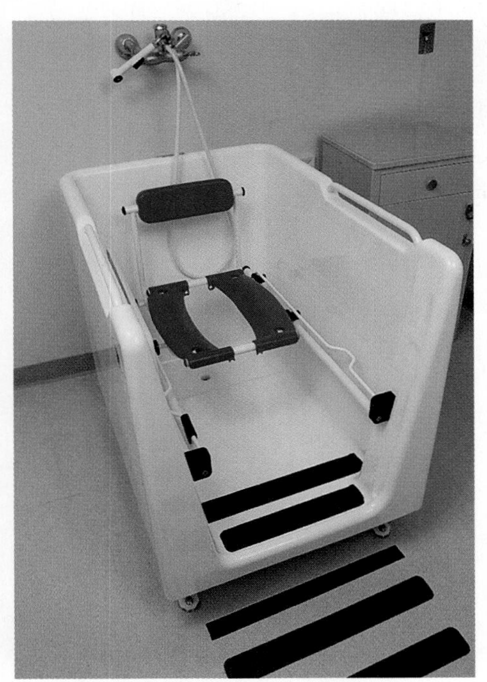

B

Figure 27-21 Common showers in facilities. **A,** Shower chair in a shower stall. **B,** Shower cabinet.

Shower stalls are common in most homes. So are bathtub-shower units. If the client has to step into the bathtub to take a shower, make sure there are safety bars for the client's use. Assist the client in getting into and out of the shower as needed.

Home care clients can buy or rent a shower chair for home use. Or a sturdy chair can be used. A sturdy lawn chair is an example. The case manager will assist the client or family in finding a safe chair for shower use. Before every use, make sure the chair is steady and will not slide.

Turn on the water and test its temperature before the client enters the shower. Some clients can stand in the shower. Encourage them to use the grab bars, if available, for support during the shower. Like tubs, showers floors should have nonskid surfaces. If not, a rubber bath mat is used. Make sure the bath mat does not cover the drain. Never let weak or unsteady clients stand in the shower. They need to use a shower chair. Contact your supervisor if you are concerned about the client's safety. (See *Focus on Children: Showers* box.)

(text continues on page 424)

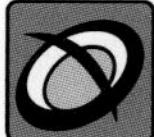

Focus on Children

SHOWERS

Many older children enjoy showers. Your supervisor tells you how much help and supervision to give the child. Remember, independence and privacy are important to older children.

Assisting with a Tub Bath or Shower

Compassionate Care

Remember to Promote:

- **Dignity**
- **Independence**
- **Preferences**
- **Privacy**
- **Safety**

Pre-Procedure

1. Reserve the bathtub or shower.*
2. Identify the person according to employer policy.
3. Explain the procedure to the person.
4. Wash your hands.
5. Collect the following:
   - Washcloth and two bath towels
   - Soap
   - Bath thermometer (for a tub bath)
   - Straight chair (optional)
   - Bath or shower chair as necessary
   - Transfer board if necessary
   - Clean garments
   - Grooming items as requested
   - Robe and nonskid footwear
   - Rubber bath mat if needed
   - Disposable floor mat if needed
   - Gloves

Procedure

6. Place items in the bathroom or shower room. Use the space provided or a chair.
7. Clean the tub or shower.*
8. Place a rubber bath mat in the tub or on the shower floor. Do not block the drain.
9. Place bath mat on the floor in front of the tub or shower.
10. Place bath or shower chair in position. Lock the wheels. Position the transfer board if one is used.
11. Put the *Occupied* sign on the door.*
12. Return to the person's room. Provide for privacy.
13. Help the person sit on the side of the bed.
14. Help the person put on a robe and nonskid footwear.

Continued

Assisting with a Tub Bath or Shower—cont'd

Procedure—cont'd

15 Assist the person to the bathroom or shower room. Use a wheelchair if necessary.

16 *For a tub bath:*

- **a** Have the person sit on the chair by the tub.
- **b** Fill the tub halfway with warm water (40.5° C; 105° F). See Figure 27-22 on page 424. Measure water temperature with the bath thermometer, or check the digital display (Figure 27-23 on page 424).

For a shower:

- **a** Turn on the shower.
- **b** Adjust water temperature and pressure.

17 Help the person undress and remove footwear.

18 Assist the person into the tub or shower (see Chapter 21). Have the person use grab bars for support.

19 Assist with washing if necessary (a bath lasts no longer than 20 minutes).

20 Place a towel across the chair.

21 Turn off the shower or drain the tub. Cover the person while the tub drains.

22 Help the person out of the tub or shower and onto the chair. Encourage the person to use the grab bars.

23 Help the person dry off. Pat gently. Dry under breasts, between skinfolds, in the perineal area, and between toes.

24 Assist with lotion and other grooming items as needed.

25 Help the person dress and put on footwear.

26 Help the person return to the room. Assist the person into bed or to a chair.

27 Provide for privacy.

28 Give a back massage if the person returns to bed.

29 Assist with hair care and other grooming needs.

Post-Procedure

30 Provide for safety and comfort.

31 Place the call bell within reach.*

32 Follow the care plan for bed rail use.*

33 Return to bathroom or shower room. Remove soiled linen. Discard disposable items. Wear gloves for this step.

34 Put the *Unoccupied* sign on the door.*

35 Return supplies to their proper place.

36 Follow employer policy for dirty linen.

37 Wash your hands.

38 Report and record your actions and observations according to employer policy.

*Steps marked with an asterisk may not apply in community settings.

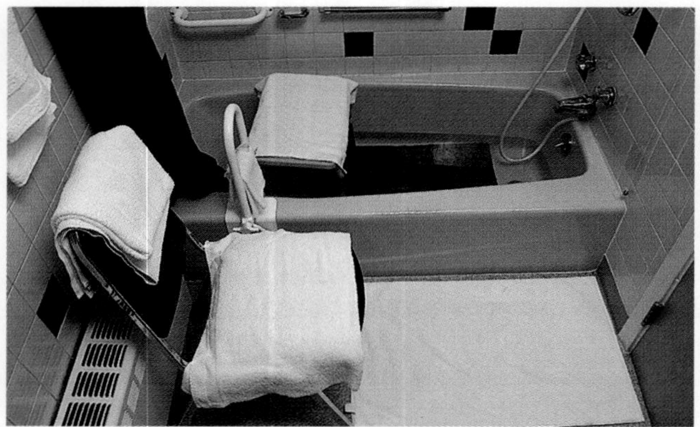

Figure 27-22 A bath mat is in the tub, the tub is filled halfway with water, a floor mat is in front of the tub, and a straight chair is next to the tub.

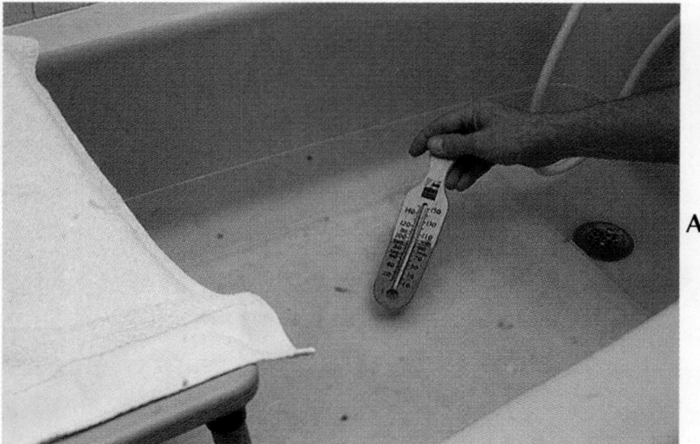

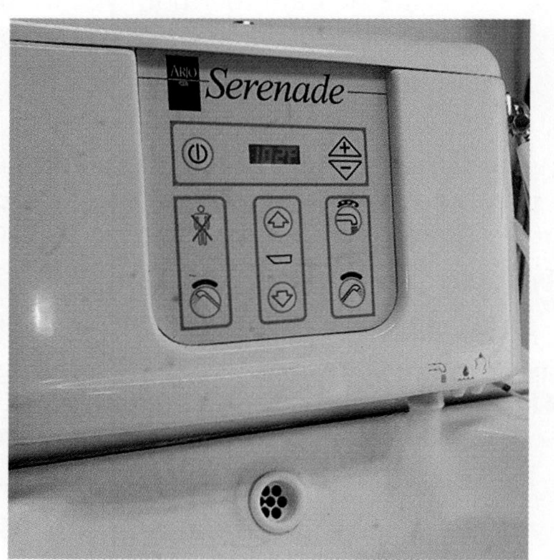

Figure 27-23 Measuring bathwater temperature. **A,** A bath thermometer is used to measure water temperature. **B,** The digital display shows water temperature.

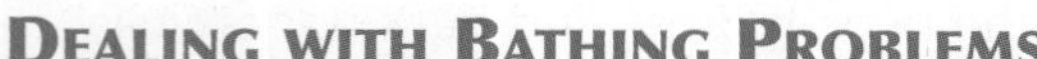

Dealing with Bathing Problems

Problems can arise when bathing a client. The client may refuse the bath. Bathing procedures can frighten clients with dementia. The client may urinate or have a bowel movement during the procedure. You need to be prepared for these and other problems.

The Client Refuses the Bath. As with all procedures, the client has a right to refuse a bath. You cannot perform a bathing procedure without the client's informed consent. Sometimes people feel too ill or weak to bathe. Some are afraid of falling or getting chilled. Some are too embarrassed. Listen carefully to the client to learn how you can provide reassurance. Did the person get cold during the last bath? If so, offer to raise the room temperature before you start. Does the person think a bath is not needed? If so, remind the person that bathing promotes hygiene, comfort, and relaxation. If the client continues to refuse the bath, talk to your supervisor. Do not bathe the client against his or her wishes.

The Client Has Dementia. People with dementia are often frightened by bathing procedures. They do not understand what is happening or why. They may fear harm or danger. Therefore clients with dementia may resist care and become agitated and combative. They may shout at you and cry for help.

The guidelines in Box 27-1 on page 410 apply when you are bathing clients with dementia. The client's care plan lists measures to help him or her through the bathing procedure. Such measures include:

- Not rushing the client
- Using a calm, pleasant voice
- Diverting the client's attention (see Chapter 34)
- Calming the client and trying the bath later

The Client Cannot Tolerate the Bathing Position. Some people cannot sit or lie on their backs or sides for long periods of time. Disease, injury, surgery, and shortness of breath are common causes. You must adapt the procedure to meet the client's needs. Follow your supervisor's directions and the care plan. Perhaps you will give a partial bath. Perhaps you will need to ask for help to bathe the client quickly.

You may have to adapt your technique to whatever position the client finds more comfortable.

The Client Urinates or Has a Bowel Movement. Some people cannot control urination or bowel movements (see Chapters 29 and 30). If this happens during a bed bath, put on gloves if you are not wearing them. Turn the client away from you, and clean the client with toilet tissue. Put the used toilet tissue in a bedpan. Change the soiled linens. Then clean the bedpan. Remove your gloves, wash your hands, and put on clean gloves. Change the bathwater and washcloths to prevent contamination of other body areas.

If the client is taking a tub bath, drain the bath. Cover the client with a towel to prevent chilling. Help the client out of the tub. Remove stool with toilet tissue, and dispose in the toilet. Clean and refill the tub. Then help the client back into the tub. Use a clean washcloth for the bath. Remember to control your verbal and nonverbal reactions. Do not embarrass the client.

Hardened Secretions or Stool on the Client's Body. To remove hardened secretions or stool, use unscented lotion or petroleum jelly. Place some on a clean, damp washcloth. Gently clean the area. Repeat this step as needed. Use a clean washcloth and more lotion or petroleum jelly. Do not rub or scratch. You can irritate the skin and cause skin breakdown.

A Client Has an Erection. Privacy is important when a male has an erection. In a professional and calm manner, tell him that you will give him some time alone. Provide for safety, leave the room, and close the door. When you return, knock on the door before entering the room. Identify yourself, and ask if you can enter the room. Continue with the bath.

An erection is a normal reaction to physical contact, especially to the genital area. Try not to show embarrassment. Remember, the client is probably embarrassed too. A professional manner will help both of you.

The Back Massage

The back massage (back rub) relaxes muscles and stimulates circulation. A massage is normally given after the bath and before bedtime. It should last 3 to 5 minutes. Observe the skin before giving the massage. Look for breaks in the skin, bruises, reddened areas, and other signs of skin breakdown.

Lotion reduces friction during the massage. Before applying lotion, warm it by placing the bottle in the bathwater or holding it under warm water. Or rub some lotion between your hands.

The prone position is best for a massage. Older or disabled people may find the side-lying position more comfortable. Use firm strokes, and always keep your hands in contact with the person's skin. After the massage, apply some lotion to the elbows, knees, and heels to keep the skin soft. These bony areas are at risk for skin breakdown. Report any reddened areas or signs of skin breakdown at once. Do not massage bony areas that are reddened.

Some clients should not have back massages as described in this procedure. They are dangerous for those with certain heart diseases, back injuries, back surgeries, skin diseases, and some lung disorders. Check with the care plan and your supervisor before giving back massages.

(text continues on page 427)

Giving a Back Massage

Compassionate Care

Remember to Promote:

- Dignity
- Independence
- Preferences
- Privacy
- Safety

Pre-Procedure

1 Identify the person according to employer policy.
2 Explain the procedure to the person.
3 Wash your hands.
4 Collect the following:
- Bath blanket
- Bath towel
- Lotion

5 Provide for privacy.
6 Raise the bed to a comfortable working height. Follow the care plan for bed rail use.*

Continued

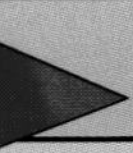

Giving a Back Massage—cont'd

Procedure

7 Lower the bed rail near you if up.

8 Position the person in the prone or side-lying position. The back is toward you.

9 Expose the back, shoulders, upper arms, and buttocks. Cover the rest of the body with the bath blanket.

10 Lay the towel on the bed along the back.

11 Warm the lotion.

12 Explain that the lotion may feel cool and wet.

13 Apply lotion to the lower back area.

14 Stroke up from the buttocks to the shoulders. Then stroke down over the upper arms. Stroke up the upper arms, across the shoulders, and down the back to the buttocks (Figure 27-24). Use firm strokes. Keep your hands in contact with the person's skin.

15 Repeat step 14 for at least 3 minutes, unless the person asks you to stop sooner.

16 Knead by grasping skin between your thumb and fingers (Figure 27-25). Knead half of the back, starting at the buttocks and moving up to the shoulder. Then knead down from the shoulder to the buttocks. Repeat on the other half of the back.

17 Apply lotion to bony areas. Use circular motions with the tips of your index and middle fingers. (Do not massage bony areas that are reddened. See Chapter 41.)

18 Use fast movements to stimulate. Use slow movements to relax the person.

19 Stroke with long, firm movements to end the massage. Tell the person you are finishing.

20 Cover the person. Remove the towel and bath blanket.

Post-Procedure

21 Provide for safety and comfort.

22 Place the call bell within reach.*

23 Return bed to its lowest position. Follow the care plan for bed rail use.*

24 Return lotion to its proper place.

25 Remove privacy measures.

26 Follow employer policy for dirty linen.

27 Wash your hands.

28 Report and record your actions and observations according to employer policy.

*Steps marked with an asterisk may not apply in community settings.

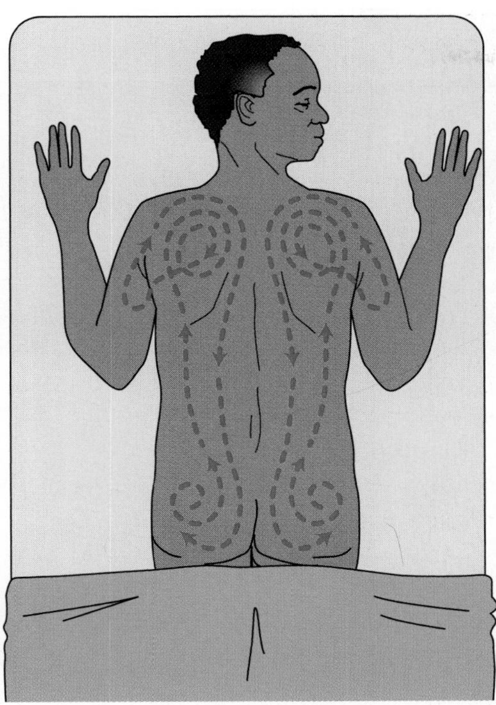

Figure 27-24 The client lies in the prone position for a back massage. Stroke upward from the buttocks to the shoulders, down over the upper arms, back up the upper arms, across the shoulders, and down the back to the buttocks.

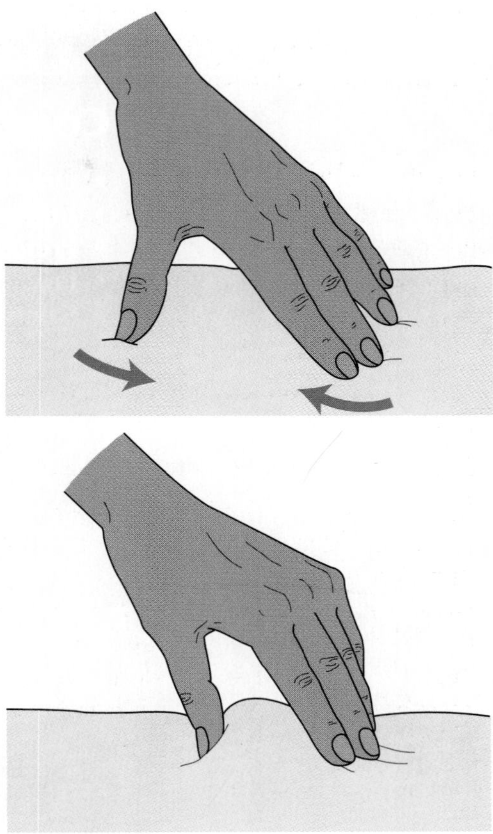

Figure 27-25 Kneading is done by grasping skin between the thumb and fingers.

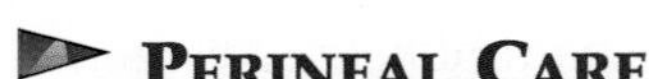

Perineal Care

Perineal care (**pericare**) involves cleaning the genital and anal areas. These areas provide a warm, moist, and dark place for microbes to grow. Cleaning prevents infection and odours and promotes comfort.

Perineal care is done at least daily during the bath. The procedure is also done whenever the area is soiled with urine or stool. People with certain disorders need perineal care more often. Your supervisor and the care plan tell you when the client needs perineal care.

Clients do their own perineal care if able. Some need assistance with perineal care. Clients may not know the terms *perineum* and *perineal*. Most understand *privates, private parts, crotch, genitals,* or the *area between your legs*. Use terms the client understands. The term must also be in good taste professionally.

Follow Standard Precautions and medical asepsis when providing perineal care. Wear gloves. Work from the cleanest area to the dirtiest. The urethral area is the cleanest, the anal area the dirtiest. Therefore clean from the urethra to the anal area. The perineal area is very delicate and easily injured. Use warm water, not hot. Test water temperature according to employer policy. Use washcloths, towelettes, cotton balls, or swabs according to employer policy. Rinse the area thoroughly. Pat dry after rinsing to reduce moisture and promote comfort. (See *Focus on Children: Perineal Care* box.)

Report and record the following if observed when providing perineal care:

- Odours
- Redness, swelling, discharge, or irritation
- Complaints of pain, burning, or other discomfort
- Signs of urinary or fecal incontinence (see Chapters 29 and 30)

(text continues on page 432)

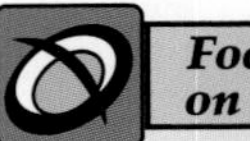

Focus on Children

Perineal Care

Children of all ages need perineal care. In children who wear diapers, the perineal area is often exposed to urine and stool. Inadequate wiping after urinating and bowel movements is a common problem in younger children. Older children may hesitate to clean the genital and anal areas.

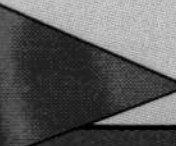

Giving Female Perineal Care

Compassionate Care

Remember to Promote:
- **Dignity**
- **Independence**
- **Preferences**
- **Privacy**
- **Safety**

Pre-Procedure

1 Identify the person according to employer policy.

2 Explain the procedure to the person.

3 Wash your hands.

4 Collect the following:
- Washbasin
- Soap
- At least four washcloths
- Bath towel
- Bath blanket
- Bath thermometer
- Waterproof pad
- Gloves
- Paper towels

5 Place paper towels on an overbed table (in a facility) or on a work area within easy reach from the bedside. Arrange items on top of the paper towels.

6 Provide for privacy.

7 Raise the bed to a comfortable working height. Follow the care plan for bed rail use.*

Procedure

8 Lower the bed rail near you if up.

9 Cover the person with a bath blanket. Move top linens to the foot of the bed.

10 Position the person on her back. Remove garments from the waist down.

11 Position waterproof pad under person's buttocks.

12 Drape the person as in Figure 27-26.

13 Raise the bed rail if used.

14 Fill the washbasin. Water temperature must be 40.5° to 42.7° C (105° to 109° F). Measure water temperature according to employer policy.

15 Place the basin on the overbed table or work area.

16 Lower the bed rail if up.

17 Help the person flex her knees and spread her legs. If she cannot flex her knees, help her spread her legs as much as possible with her knees straight.

18 Put on gloves.

19 Fold the corner of the bath blanket between the person's legs onto her abdomen.

20 Wet the washcloths. Squeeze out excess water from washcloths before using them.

21 Apply soap to a washcloth.

22 Separate the labia. Clean downward from front to back with one stroke (Figure 27-27 on page 430).

23 Repeat steps 21 and 22 until the area is clean. Use a clean part of the washcloth for each stroke. Use more than one washcloth if needed.

24 Rinse the perineum with a clean washcloth. Separate the labia. Stroke downward from front to back. Repeat as necessary. Use a clean part of the washcloth for each stroke. Use more than one washcloth if needed.

25 Pat the area dry with the towel.

26 Fold the blanket back between the person's legs.

27 Help the person lower her legs and turn onto her side away from you.

Continued

Giving Female Perineal Care—cont'd

Procedure—cont'd

28 Apply soap to a washcloth.
29 Clean the rectal area. Separate buttocks and clean from the vagina to the anus with one stroke (Figure 27-28 on page 430).
30 Repeat steps 28 and 29 until the area is clean. Use a clean part of the washcloth for each stroke. Use more than one washcloth if needed.
31 Rinse the rectal area with a washcloth. Stroke from the vagina to the anus. Repeat as necessary using a clean part of the washcloth for each stroke. Use more than one washcloth if needed.
32 Pat the area dry with the towel.
33 Remove the waterproof pad.
34 Remove gloves. Wash your hands.

Post-Procedure

35 Provide for safety and comfort.
36 Cover the person.
37 Remove the bath blanket.
38 Place the call bell within reach.*
39 Return the bed to its lowest position. Follow the care plan for bed rail use.*
40 Empty and clean the washbasin.
41 Return the basin and supplies to their proper place.
42 Wipe off the overbed table or work area with the paper towels and discard the paper towels.
43 Remove privacy measures.
44 Follow employer policy for dirty linen.
45 Wash your hands.
46 Report and record your actions and observations according to employer policy.

*Steps marked with an asterisk may not apply in community settings.

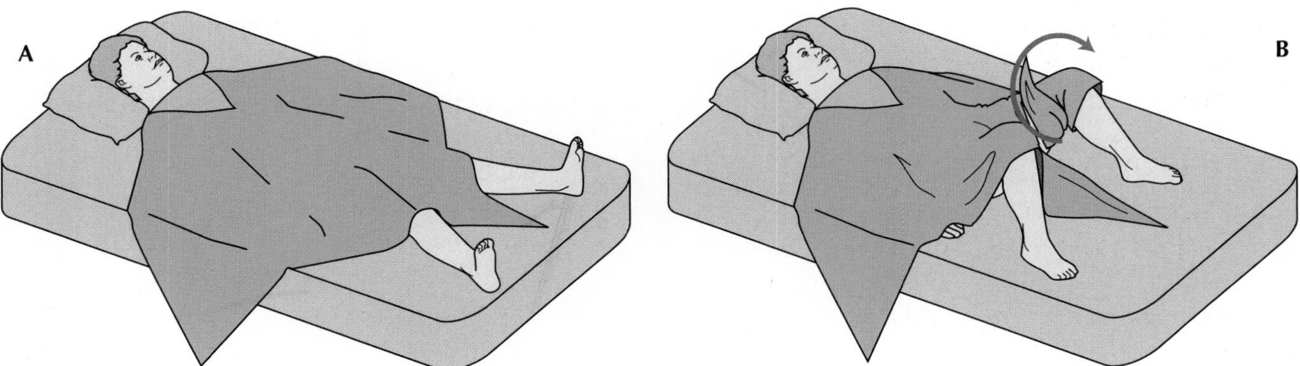

Figure 27-26 Draping for perineal care. **A,** Position the bath blanket like a diamond: one corner is at the neck, one corner is at each side, and one corner is between the client's legs. **B,** Wrap the blanket around the leg by bringing the corner around under the leg and over the top. Tuck the corner under the hip.

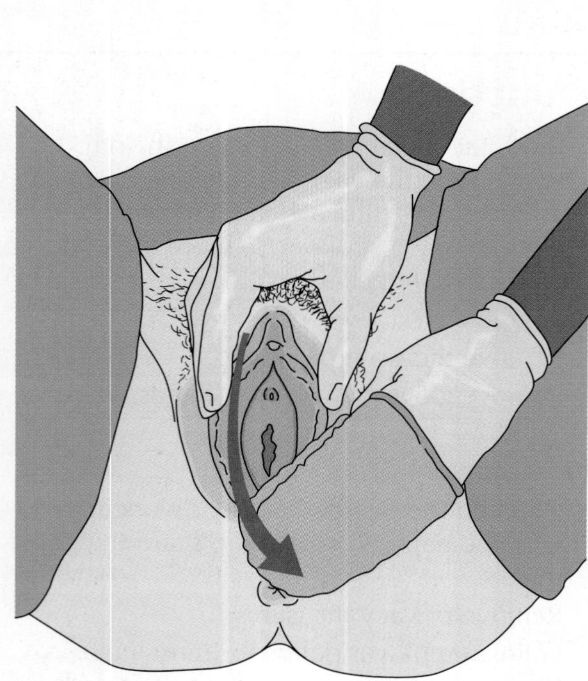

Figure 27-27 Female perineal care. Separate the labia with one hand. Use a mitted washcloth to cleanse between the labia with downward strokes.

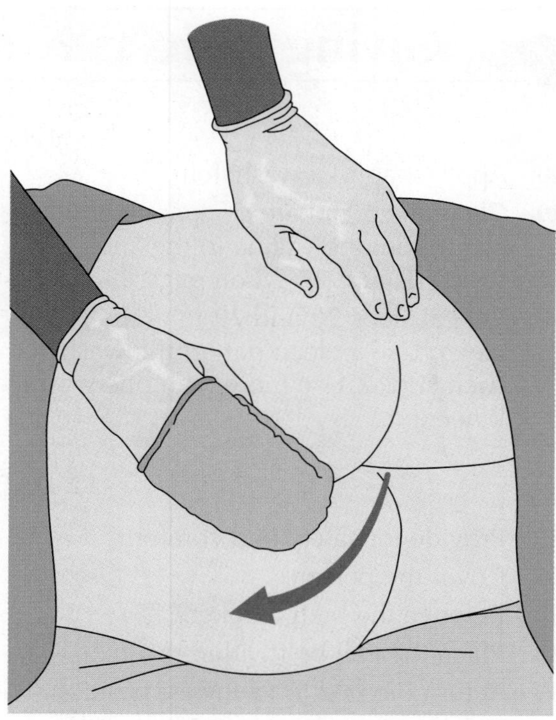

Figure 27-28 Cleaning the rectal area. Wipe from the vagina to the anus. The side-lying position allows thorough cleaning of the anal area.

Giving Male Perineal Care

Compassionate Care

Remember to Promote:
- **Dignity**
- **Independence**
- **Preferences**
- **Privacy**
- **Safety**

Pre-Procedure

1 Follow steps 1 through 21 in *Giving Female Perineal Care* on page 428.

Procedure

2 Retract the foreskin if the person is uncircumcised (Figure 27-29 on page 432).

3 Grasp the penis.

4 Clean the tip using a circular motion. Start at the urethral opening, and work outward (Figure 27-30 on page 432). Repeat this step as necessary. Use a clean part of the washcloth each time.

5 Rinse the area with another washcloth.

6 Return the foreskin to its natural position.

7 Clean the shaft of the penis with firm downward strokes. Rinse the area.

8 Help the person flex his knees and spread his legs. If he cannot flex his knees, help him spread his legs as much as possible with his knees straight.

9 Clean the scrotum and rinse well. Observe for redness and irritation in the skinfolds.

10 Pat dry the penis and scrotum.

11 Fold the bath blanket back between his legs.

12 Help him lower his legs and turn onto his side away from you.

13 Clean the rectal area (see steps 28 to 32 of *Giving Female Perineal Care*). Rinse and dry well.

14 Remove the waterproof pad.

15 Remove and discard the gloves. Wash your hands.

Post-Procedure

16 Follow steps 35 through 46 in *Giving Female Perineal Care.*

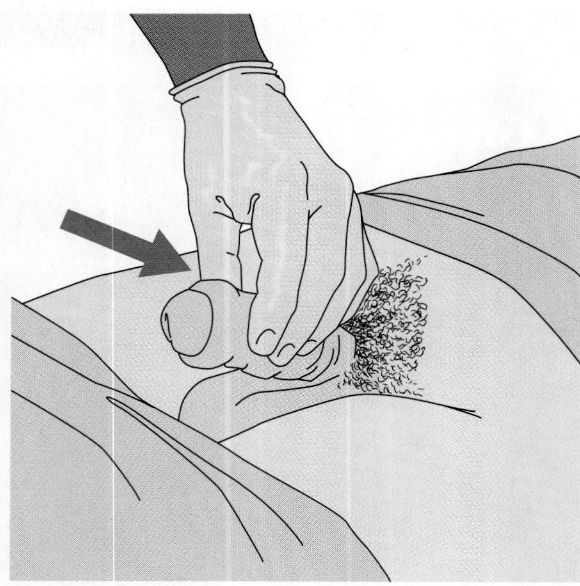

Figure 27-29 Male perineal care. Pull back the foreskin of the uncircumcised male. Return the foreskin to its normal position immediately after cleaning.

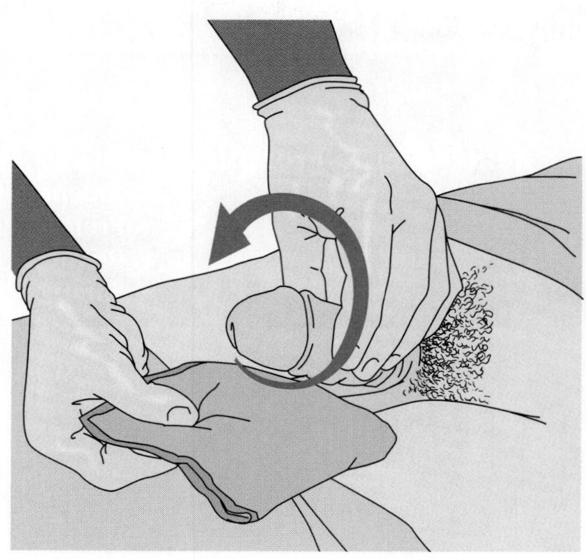

Figure 27-30 Clean the penis with circular motions starting at the urethra.

Menstrual Care

Menstruation is a woman's monthly bleeding. Blood flows from the uterus through the vaginal opening (see Chapter 13). Sanitary pads absorb menstrual blood. Most menstrual periods last 3 to 5 days. Some clients need assistance with menstrual care. They may be too ill or weak to change their sanitary pads.

Usually women use disposable sanitary pads. These have an adhesive strip to hold them in place in the woman's undergarments. Sanitary pads containing perfumes can irritate the skin and should be avoided. In some hospitals, female patients may use disposable sanitary pads that are held in place with sanitary belts or reusable mesh undergarments.

Sanitary pads should be changed often. This promotes good hygiene and prevents odours and infection. It also promotes comfort. Follow the care plan for when to change the woman's sanitary pad. Frequency depends on the amount of menstrual flow. Usually they need to be changed at least every 3 to 5 hours. However, they should be changed before the pad is soaked with blood.

Contact with the client's blood and mucous membranes is likely. Therefore always wear gloves when removing or applying sanitary pads. Wash your hands, and help the client wash her hands after menstrual care. Dispose of sanitary pads according to employer policy. Also follow employer policy for soiled sanitary belts and mesh undergarments.

Record and report the following if observed while providing menstrual care:

- Odours
- Fever
- Redness, swelling, or irritation in the perineum
- Complaints of pain, burning, difficulty urinating, or other discomforts
- Heavy bleeding; for example, the sanitary pad is soaked within one hour of application (report this at once)
- Large number of blood clots on the pad (report this at once)

REVIEW

Circle T if the answer is true and F if it is false.

1. T F Hygiene is needed for comfort, safety, and health.
2. T F Culture and personal choice affect hygiene practices.
3. T F Mrs. Lam's toothbrush has hard bristles. They are good for oral hygiene.
4. T F Unconscious clients are supine for mouth care.
5. T F You use your fingers to keep an unconscious client's mouth open for oral hygiene.
6. T F Mrs. Lam has a lower denture. It is washed in warm water over a hard surface.
7. T F Bath oils cleanse and soften the skin.
8. T F Powders absorb moisture and prevent friction.
9. T F Deodorants reduce the amount of perspiration.
10. T F The care plan says that Mrs. Lam can have a tub bath. You can let her take a 30-minute bath.
11. T F Weak clients can be left alone in the shower if they are sitting.
12. T F A back massage relaxes muscles and stimulates circulation.
13. T F Perineal care helps prevent infection.
14. T F Foreskin is returned to its normal position after cleaning.
15. T F Sanitary pads should be changed at least every 3 to 5 hours.

Circle the BEST answer.

16. When brushing Mrs. Lam's teeth, which of the following does *not* need to be reported?
    A. Bleeding, swelling, or redness of the gums
    B. Irritations, sores, or white patches in the mouth or on the tongue
    C. Lips that are dry, cracked, swollen, or blistered
    D. Food between the teeth
17. Which is *not* a purpose of bathing?
    A. Increasing circulation
    B. Promoting drying of the skin
    C. Preventing odours and cleansing skin
    D. Refreshing and relaxing the person
18. Soaps do the following *except*
    A. Remove dirt and dead skin
    B. Remove pigment
    C. Remove skin oil and perspiration
    D. Dry the skin
19. Which action is *wrong* when bathing Mrs. Lam?
    A. Cover her for warmth and privacy.
    B. Rinse her skin thoroughly to remove all soaps.
    C. Wash from the dirtiest to the cleanest area.
    D. Pat her skin dry.
20. Water for Mrs. Lam's complete bed bath should be approximately
    A. 37.8° C (100° F)
    B. 40.5° C (105° F)
    C. 43.4° C (110° F)
    D. 48.9° C (120° F)
21. You are going to give Mrs. Lam a back massage. Which is *false*?
    A. The massage should last 3 to 5 minutes.
    B. Lotion is warmed before being applied.
    C. Your hands are always in contact with the skin.
    D. The side-lying position is best.

Answers to these questions are on page 825.

CHAPTER

28

Grooming and Dressing

OBJECTIVES

- Define the key terms listed in this chapter
- Explain the importance of hair care and shaving
- Identify the factors that affect hair care
- Explain how to care for matted and tangled hair
- Describe how to shampoo hair
- Describe how to shave a client
- Explain why nail and foot care is important
- Describe how to dress and undress clients
- Explain the purpose of elastic stockings and bandages and when you assist with them
- Learn the procedures described in this chapter

KEY TERMS

alopecia Hair loss

dandruff Excessive amount of dry, white flakes on the scalp

hirsutism Excessive body hair in women and children

pediculosis (lice) Infestation with lice

pediculosis capitis Infestation of the scalp (*capitis*) with lice

pediculosis corporis Infestation of the body (*corporis*) with lice

pediculosis pubis Infestation of the pubic (*pubis*) hair with lice

Clean hair, nails, and clothes are important to many clients. Like hygiene, grooming measures prevent infection and promote comfort. They also help emotional well-being.

People vary in how much attention they give to their grooming. Some want only clean hair. Others want hair styled in a certain way. Clean hands are enough for some people. Others want nails clean, manicured, and polished. Shaving and beard grooming are important to many men. Many women shave their legs and underarms. Some women have facial hair. They may shave or use other means to remove this hair.

HAIR CARE

How one's hair looks and feels affects emotional well-being. People generally feel better about themselves when they are well groomed. Illness and disability can interfere with hair care. Some clients cannot care for their hair. You help with hair care whenever needed.

The care plan addresses the client's hair care needs. Culture, personal choice, skin and scalp condition, physical and mental health, and self-care abilities are considered. The following terms are common in care plans:

- **Alopecia** means hair loss. Hair loss may be complete or partial. Male pattern baldness occurs with aging and is the result of heredity. Hair also thins in some women with aging. Cancer treatments (radiation therapy to the head and chemotherapy) often cause alopecia in both men and women. Skin disease is another cause. Stress, poor nutrition, pregnancy, some medications, and hormone changes are other causes. Except for hair loss from aging, the hair grows back in many cases.
- **Hirsutism** is excessive body hair in women and children. It is the result of heredity and abnormal amounts of male hormones.
- **Dandruff** is the excessive amount of dry, white flakes on the scalp. Itching often occurs. Sometimes the eyebrows and ear canals are involved. Medicated shampoos correct the problem.
- **Pediculosis (lice)** is the infestation with lice. Lice are parasites. Lice bites cause severe itching in the affected body area. **Pediculosis capitis** is the infestation of the scalp (*capitis*) with lice. **Pediculosis pubis** is the infestation of the pubic (*pubis*) hair with lice. Both head and pubic lice attach their eggs to hair shafts. **Pediculosis corporis** is the infestation of the body (*corporis*) with lice. Lice eggs attach to clothing and furniture. Lice easily spread to other people through clothing, furniture, bed linen, and physical contact. Lice is also spread by sharing combs and brushes. Medicated shampoos, lotions, and creams are used to treat lice. Thorough bathing is necessary. So is washing clothing and linen in hot water. Report signs of lice to your supervisor immediately.

BRUSHING AND COMBING HAIR

Brushing and combing hair are part of the daily routine. Usually a client's hair is groomed in the morning (after the bath or shower) and at bedtime. However, assist with brushing and combing as needed during the day. For example, some clients want their hair styled before visitors arrive.

Encourage clients to do their own hair care. Assist as needed. You perform hair care for those who cannot do so on their own. The client chooses how to brush, comb, and style hair (see *Focus on Children: Grooming Preferences* box on page 436.)

Never cut a client's hair. Only a professional barber or hairstylist should cut hair. Some make home visits or provide their services in long-term care facilities.

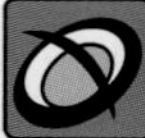

Focus on Children

Grooming Preferences

Hairstyles are important to adolescents. Many school-age children also are concerned about hairstyles. Do not make judgments about the child's hairstyle. Style hair in a manner that pleases the child and parents. Remember not to style hair according to your standards or customs.

Some facilities have barber or beauty shops, where residents or patients can have their hair shampooed, cut, and styled.

When giving hair care, place a towel across the client's shoulders to protect the garments. If the client is in bed, give hair care before changing the pillowcase. If done after a linen change, place a towel across the pillow to collect falling hair. When brushing and combing hair, start at the scalp. Then brush or comb to the hair ends. Handle hair gently to avoid hurting the person or damaging the hair. Brush slowly. Do not tug or pull.

Talk to your supervisor if the client has matted or tangled hair. You may be told to comb or brush through the matting and tangling. To do this, take a small section of hair near the ends. Then gently comb or brush through to the hair ends. Working up to the scalp, add small sections of hair. Comb or brush through each longer section to the hair ends. Finally, brush or comb from the scalp to the hair ends. *Never cut hair to remove tangles.*

Special measures are needed for curly, coarse, and dry hair. Use a wide-toothed comb for curly hair. Start at the neckline. Work upward, lifting and fluffing hair outward. Continue until you reach the forehead. Wetting the hair or applying a conditioner or petroleum jelly makes combing easier.

The client may have certain practices or use special hair care products. These become part of the client's care plan. The client can guide you when giving hair care. (See *Respecting Diversity: Braiding Hair* box.)

Report and record the following if observed when brushing or combing:

- Scalp sores
- Flaking
- The presence of lice (check for tiny, white oval-shaped specks in the hair; these are the nits, or egg cases)
- Patches of hair loss
- Very dry or very oily hair

(text continues on page 438)

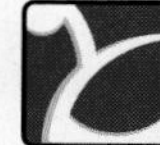

Respecting Diversity

Braiding Hair

Styling hair in small braids is a common practice in some cultural groups. The braids are left intact for shampooing. Your supervisor obtains consent to undo these braids. You do not braid hair or remove braids without the client's consent.

Brushing and Combing Hair

Compassionate Care

Remember to Promote:
- **Dignity**
- **Independence**
- **Preferences**
- **Privacy**
- **Safety**

Pre-Procedure

1 Identify the person according to employer policy.
2 Explain the procedure to the person. Ask the person how to style his or her hair.
3 Wash your hands.
4 Collect the following:
- Comb and brush
- Bath towel
- Other grooming items as requested

5 Arrange items on a work area within easy reach.
6 Provide for privacy.

Procedure

7 Position the person:
  a If the person can get out of bed, provide a comfortable chair. Help the person to the chair (see *Transferring the Person to a Chair or Wheelchair,* page 291). The person puts on a robe and footwear when up.
  b If the person remains in bed, raise the bed to a comfortable working height. Follow the care plan for bed rail use. Lower the bed rail near you if up. Assist the person to semi-Fowler's position if allowed.

8 Place the towel across the person's shoulders or the pillow.
9 Ask the person to remove eyeglasses. Put them in the eyeglass case. Put the case in a safe location.
10 Part the hair into 2 sections (Figure 28-1, *A* on page 438). Divide one side into 2 sections (Figure 28-1, *B* on page 438).
11 Brush the hair. Start at the scalp, and brush toward the hair ends (Figure 28-2 on page 438).
12 Style the hair as the person prefers.
13 Remove the towel.
14 Help the person put on eyeglasses.

Post-Procedure

15 Provide for safety and comfort.
16 Place the call bell within reach.*
17 Return the bed to its lowest position. Follow the care plan for bed rail use.*
18 Remove privacy measures.
19 Clean and return equipment to its proper place.
20 Follow employer policy for dirty linen.
21 Wash your hands.
22 Report and record your actions and observations according to employer policy.

*Steps marked with an asterisk may not apply in community settings.

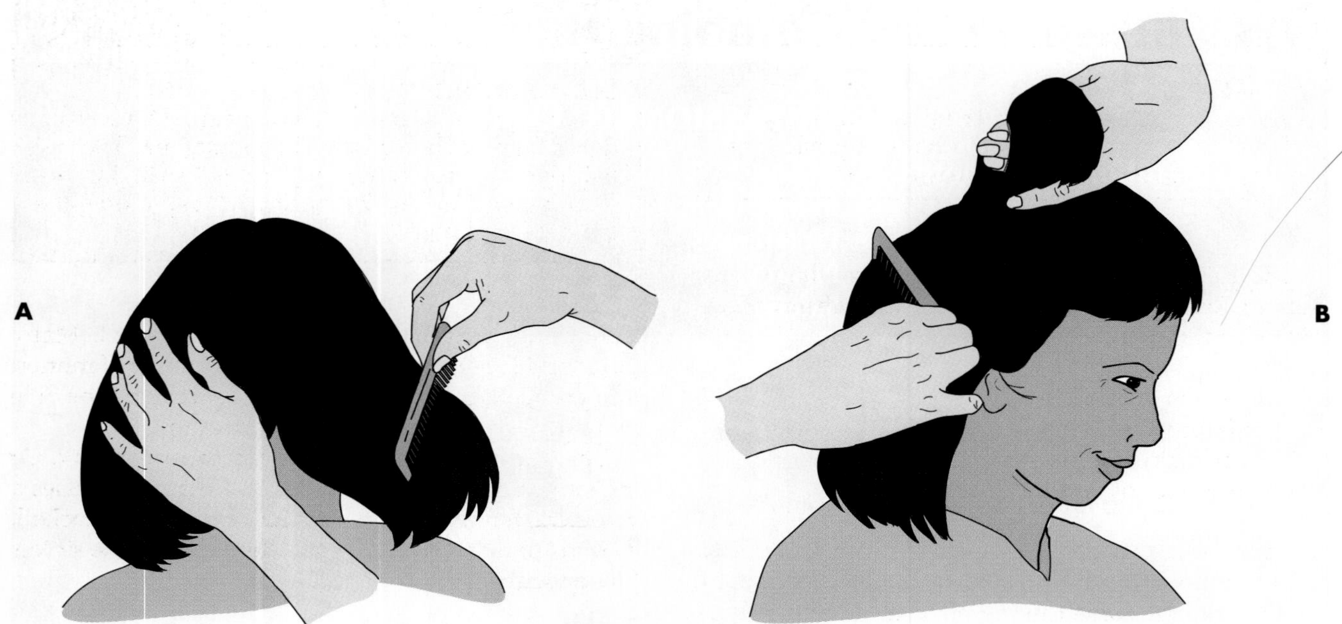

Figure 28-1 Parting hair. **A,** Part hair down the middle. Divide it into two sections. **B,** Then part the sections into two smaller sections.

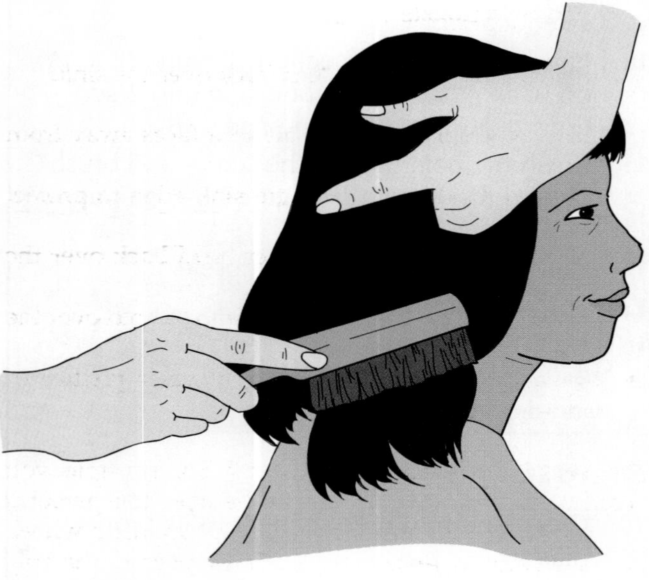

Figure 28-2 Brush hair by starting at the scalp. Then brush down to the hair ends.

Shampooing

Most people shampoo at least once a week. Some shampoo two or three times a week. Others shampoo every day. Many factors affect frequency. These include the condition of the hair and scalp, hairstyle, and personal choice. Shampoo and hair conditioner also involve personal choice. (See *Focus on Children: Shampooing* box.)

Clients often need help shampooing. Personal choice is followed whenever possible. However, safety is important and your supervisor's approval is needed. Tell your supervisor if your client requests a shampoo. Do not wash a client's hair unless your supervisor or the care plan instructs you to do so.

The shampooing method depends on the client's condition, safety factors, and personal choice if possible. Follow the care plan. Dry and style hair as quickly as possible after shampooing. Women may want hair curled or rolled up before drying. Consult with your supervisor before curling or rolling up a client's hair. (See *Focus on Long-Term Care: Shampooing* box.)

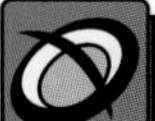

Focus on Children

SHAMPOOING

Oil gland secretion increases during puberty. Therefore, adolescents tend to have oily hair. Frequent shampooing is often necessary.

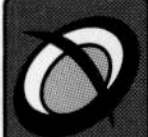

Focus on Long-Term Care

SHAMPOOING

Shampooing is usually done weekly on the resident's bath or shower day. If a woman has had her hair done in the beauty shop, do not shampoo her hair. Protect her hair with a shower cap during the tub bath or shower.

The guidelines listed in Box 28-1 apply when shampooing. Report and record the following observations after shampooing:

- Scalp sores
- Hair falling out in patches
- How the client tolerated the procedure
- The presence of lice

Shampooing during the Shower or Tub Bath. Clients who shower or bathe in a tub can usually shampoo at the same time. A hand-held shower nozzle is used. The client tips his or her head back to keep shampoo and water out of the eyes. Support the back of the client's head with one hand. Shampoo with your other hand. Some people cannot tip their head back. They should lean forward and hold a folded washcloth over the eyes. Support the forehead with one hand as you shampoo with the other. Be sure that the client can breathe easily.

Shampooing at the Sink. Clients who can sit up may have their hair washed at a sink. They must be able to tilt their head forward or backward. Many older or disabled people have limited range of motion in their necks and upper backs. They may not be able to use this method. Follow the care plan.

The person can sit facing away from the sink. Or the person can sit facing the sink. If the person uses a wheelchair, make sure the wheels are securely locked.

If the person chooses to face the sink and the sink is low enough:

- Have the person lean forward over the sink
- Place a towel over the shoulders
- Give the person a folded washcloth to hold over the eyes
- Wet and rinse the hair using a water pitcher or hand-held nozzle

If the person prefers to lean back over the sink:

- Place the chair or wheelchair so it faces away from the sink
- Place a folded towel over the sink edge to protect the neck
- Help the person tilt his or her head back over the edge of the sink
- Give the person a folded washcloth to hold over the eyes
- Wet and rinse the hair using a water pitcher or hand-held nozzle

Assistive devices may be useful. For example, you could use a plastic cape to drape over the person's shoulders and into the sink. Or, you may use a wheelchair shampoo rinse tray. Made of plastic, the tray clamps onto the back of the wheelchair. The client's head rests directly on it. The tray extends over the sink. The tray sides keep the water from spilling over the edges. The water runs across the tray and into the sink (Figure 28-3 on page 440).

Some clients lie on a stretcher when having their hair shampooed at the sink:

- Place the stretcher in front of the sink; lock the stretcher wheels and use the safety straps; follow the care plan for side rail use
- Place a folded towel over the edge of the sink

Box 28-1 Guidelines for Shampooing a Client's Hair

- Shampoo hair only if instructed to do so by your supervisor.
- Ask your supervisor and check the care plan about what method to use (shampooing during the shower or tub bath, at the sink, or in bed).
- Check if the person has position restrictions or limits.
- Return medicated shampoos to their place or give them to your supervisor. Do not leave them at the bedside unless instructed to do so.
- Wear gloves and follow Standard Precautions if the person has scalp lesions.
- Check what water temperature to use. Usually water temperature should be 40.5° C (105° F). Measure water temperature according to employer policy.
- Keep shampoo out of the person's eyes. Have the person hold a face towel or wash cloth over the eyes.
- Cup your hand against the person's forehead when rinsing. This keeps soapy water from running down the person's forehead and into the eyes.

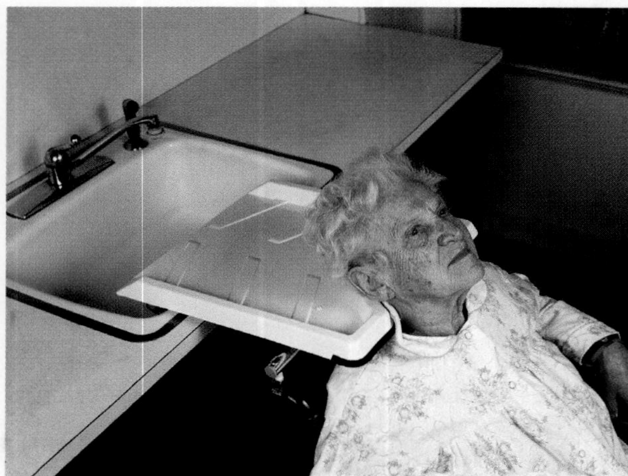

Figure 28-3 Shampooing at the sink. The wheelchair is in front of the sink, with its wheels locked in place. A wheelchair shampoo rinse tray may be useful.

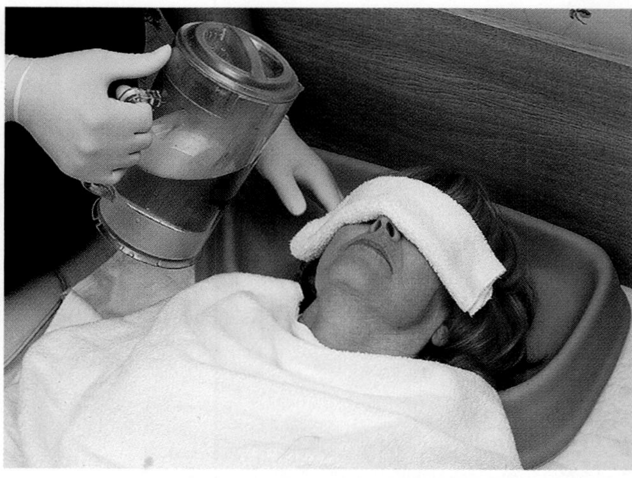

Figure 28-4 Shampooing tray is used when shampooing a client in bed. The tray is directed to the side of the bed so water drains into a collecting basin.

- Help the person tilt his or her head over the edge of the sink
- Place a folded washcloth over the person's eyes
- Wet and rinse the hair using a water pitcher or hand-held nozzle

Shampooing in Bed. This method is for those who cannot be out of bed. The client's head and shoulders are moved to the edge of the bed if possible. A shampoo tray is placed under the client's head to protect the linens and mattress from water. The tray also drains water into a basin placed on a chair next to the bed (Figure 28-4). Use a water pitcher to wet and rinse the hair. (See *Focus on Home Care: Shampoo Trays* box.)

(text continues on page 442)

Shampooing the Person's Hair

Compassionate Care

Remember to Promote:

- **Dignity**
- **Independence**
- **Preferences**
- **Privacy**
- **Safety**

Pre-Procedure

1 Identify the person according to employer policy.
2 Explain the procedure to the person.
3 Wash your hands.
4 Collect the following:
- Two bath towels
- Face towel or washcloth
- Shampoo
- Hair conditioner (if requested)
- Bath thermometer
- Pitcher or nozzle (if needed)
- Shampoo tray (if needed)
- Basin or pail (if needed)
- Waterproof pad (if needed)
- Gloves (if needed)
- Comb and brush
- Hair dryer

5 Arrange items nearby.
6 Provide for privacy.

Continued

Shampooing the Person's Hair—cont'd

Procedure

7 Position the person for the method you will use. Place the waterproof pad and shampoo tray under the head and shoulders if needed.
8 Place a bath towel across the shoulders or across the pillow.
9 Brush and comb hair to remove snarls and tangles.
10 Raise the bed rail if used.
11 Obtain water. Water temperature should be about 40.5° C (105° F). Test temperature according to employer policy.
12 Lower the bed rail if used.
13 Put on gloves if needed.
14 Ask the person to hold a dampened face towel or washcloth over the eyes. It should not cover the nose or mouth. (A wet cloth will not slip off as easily as a dry cloth.)
15 Use the pitcher or nozzle to wet the hair.
16 Use a small amount of shampoo.
17 Work up lather with both hands. Start at the hairline. Work toward the back of the head. Or, if the person is leaning forward, start at the back of the head and work toward the hairline.
18 Massage the scalp with your fingertips. Do not scratch the scalp with your fingernails.
19 Rinse the hair.
20 Repeat steps 15 through 18.
21 Rinse the hair completely.
22 Apply conditioner. Follow directions on the container.
23 Squeeze water from the person's hair.
24 Cover hair with a bath towel.
25 Dry the person's face with the towel.
26 Help the person raise the head if appropriate.
27 Rub the hair and scalp with the towel. Use the second towel if the first is wet.
28 Comb hair to remove snarls and tangles.
29 Dry and style the hair as quickly as possible.
30 Remove gloves if used. Wash your hands.

Post-Procedure

31 Provide for safety and comfort.
32 Place the call bell within reach.*
33 Follow the care plan for bed rail use.*
34 Remove privacy measures.
35 Clean and return equipment to its proper place. Discard disposable items.
36 Follow employer policy for dirty linen.
37 Wash your hands.
38 Report and record your actions and observations according to employer policy.

*Steps marked with an asterisk may not apply in community settings.

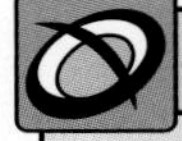

Focus on Home Care

SHAMPOO TRAYS

You can make a shampoo tray from a plastic shower curtain or tablecloth. A plastic drop cloth for painting is also useful. Avoid plastic garbage bags. They slip and slide easily and are not sturdy. To make a shampoo tray, place the plastic under the client's head. Make a raised edge around the plastic to prevent water from spilling over the sides. Direct the ends of the plastic into the basin. This directs water into the basin. Check the care plan and consult with your supervisor.

Shaving

Many men shave for comfort and a sense of well-being. Younger women usually shave their legs and underarms. Some older women with coarse facial hair want it shaved off. Most clients are able to shave themselves. Some require your assistance. Shaving may be done at the sink, bedside, or in bed. Shaving guidelines are listed in Box 28-2.

Some clients use electric shavers. These shavers are cleaned between each use. Make sure the shaver is in good working order before each use. Follow the safety rules for electrical equipment (see Chapter 16).

Other clients use blade shavers. Razor blades can cause nicks or cuts. Follow Standard Precautions to prevent contact with blood. Handle razor blades and disposable shavers very carefully to prevent cutting yourself. Discard them in the sharps container (see Chapter 18).

Soften the client's skin before shaving with a blade. Apply a warm washcloth or face towel to the face for a few minutes. Then lather the face with soap and water or shaving cream. Take care not to cut or irritate the skin while shaving.

Some clients have conditions that make shaving dangerous:

- Blade shavers are not used on clients receiving medications that slow down blood clotting (*anticoagulants*). For these clients, a nick or cut can cause serious bleeding problems. Electric shavers are used for clients taking such medications.
- Blade shavers are also not used on clients with dementia. Clients with dementia may not understand what you are doing. They may resist care and move suddenly. This increases the risk for serious nicks and cuts. Electric shavers are used for these clients.
- Electric shavers are not used on clients receiving oxygen. A spark from the electric shaver could cause a fire.

Your supervisor and the care plan tell you the safest way to shave the client.

Caring for Mustaches and Beards

Beards and mustaches need daily care. Food can collect in hair. So can mouth and nose drainage. Daily washing and combing usually are enough. Ask the person how to groom his beard or mustache. *Never trim or shave a beard or mustache without the client's consent.*

Shaving Female Legs and Underarms

Many women shave their legs and underarms. This practice varies among cultures. Some women shave only the lower legs. Others shave to mid-thigh, and others shave the entire leg.

Women's legs and underarms are shaved after bathing, when the skin is soft. Soap and water or a shaving cream is used for lather. Collect shaving items with bath items. Rinse the razor in a kidney basin. Do not rinse in the bathwater.

The guidelines in Box 28-2 apply when shaving underarms and legs.

(text continues on page 445)

Box 28-2 Guidelines for Shaving Clients

- Follow Standard Precautions. Wear gloves when shaving clients.
- Follow the care plan for the type of shaver used for each person.
- Protect bed linens. Place a towel under the part being shaved. Or place a towel across the shoulders to protect clothing.
- Soften the skin before shaving. Apply a warm, damp cloth onto the skin.
- Encourage the person to do as much as safely possible.
- Hold the skin taut as needed.
- Shave in the direction of hair growth when shaving the face and underarms.
- Shave up from the ankles when shaving legs. This is against hair growth.
- Do not cut, nick, or irritate the skin.
- Rinse the body part completely.
- Apply direct pressure to nicks or cuts (wear gloves).
- Report nicks, cuts, or irritation to your supervisor at once.
- Discard used disposable razors and blades in the sharps container. Handle them carefully. Follow employer policy for disposing of sharps.

Shaving the Person

Compassionate Care

Remember to Promote:
- **Dignity**
- **Independence**
- **Preferences**
- **Privacy**
- **Safety**

Pre-Procedure

1 Identify the person according to employer policy.
2 Explain the procedure to the person.
3 Wash your hands.
4 Collect the following:
- Washbasin
- Bath towel
- Face towel
- Washcloth
- Blade razor or electric shaver, according to the care plan
- Mirror
- Shaving cream, soap, or lotion
- Shaving brush (optional)
- Aftershave lotion (men only)
- Tissues
- Paper towels
- Gloves

5 Arrange paper towels and supplies on the overbed table (in facilities) or on a work area within easy reach.
6 Provide for privacy.
7 Raise the bed to a comfortable working height. Follow the care plan for bed rail use.*

Procedure

8 Fill the basin with warm water.
9 Place the basin on the overbed table or work area.
10 Lower the bed rail near you if up.
11 Assist the person to semi-Fowler's position if allowed. Or assist the person to the supine position.
12 Adjust lighting to clearly see the person's face.
13 Place the bath towel over the chest.
14 Adjust the overbed table for easy reach.*
15 If using a blade shaver:
- **a** Tighten the razor blade to the shaver.
- **b** Wash the person's face. Do not dry.
- **c** Wet a washcloth or face towel. Wring it out.
- **d** Apply the washcloth or towel to the face for a few minutes.
- **e** Put on gloves.
- **f** Apply shaving cream with your hands. Or use a shaving brush to apply lather.
- **g** Hold the skin taut with one hand.
- **h** Shave in the direction of hair growth. Use shorter strokes around the chin and lips (Figure 28-5 on page 444).
- **i** Rinse the razor often. Shake off excess water and lather.
- **j** Apply direct pressure to any bleeding area.
- **k** Wash off remaining shaving cream or soap. Dry with a towel.

16 If using an electric shaver:
- **a** Put on gloves
- **b** Make sure the face is dry. Do not apply shaving cream or a warm cloth to the face.
- **c** Hold skin taut with one hand.
- **d** Turn on the razor.

Continued

Shaving the Person—cont'd

Procedure—cont'd

e Place the razor over the hair growth. Move the razor back and forth or in a circular pattern.

f Apply direct pressure to any bleeding area.

17 Apply aftershave lotion if requested.

18 Remove the towel and gloves. Wash your hands.

19 Move the overbed table to the side of the bed.*

Post-Procedure

20 Provide for safety and comfort.

21 Place the call bell within reach.*

22 Return the bed to its lowest position. Follow the care plan for bed rail use.*

23 Clean and return equipment and supplies to their proper place. Discard disposable items. Wear gloves for this step.

24 Wipe off the overbed table or work area with paper towels. Discard paper towels.

25 Remove privacy measures.

26 Follow employer policy for dirty linen.

27 Wash your hands.

28 Report nicks or bleeding to your supervisor.

*Steps marked with an asterisk may not apply in community settings.

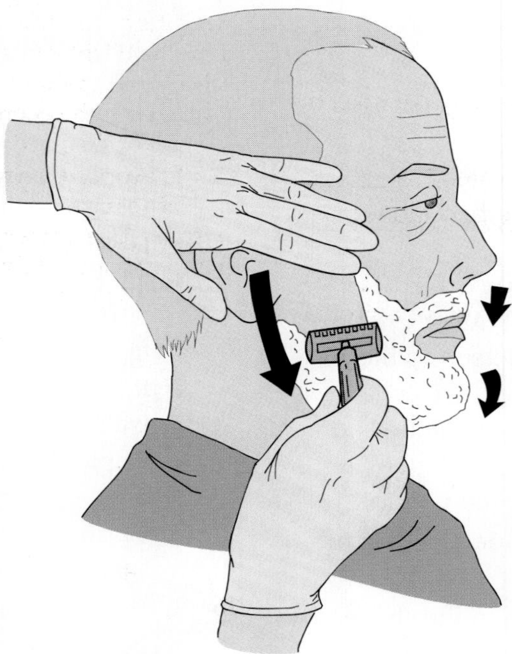

Figure 28-5 Shave in the direction of hair growth. Use longer strokes on the larger areas of the face. Use short strokes around the chin and lips.

Care of Nails and Feet

Foot and nail care is a very important part of daily personal care. Nails and feet need special attention to prevent infection, injury, and odours. Hangnails, ingrown nails (nails that grow in at the side), and nails torn away from the skin cause skin breaks. Microbes could enter these breaks. Long or broken nails can scratch skin or snag clothing.

The feet are easily infected and injured. Dirty or moist feet, socks, and stockings harbour microbes and cause odours. Shoes and socks provide a warm, moist environment for the growth of microbes. Injuries occur from stubbing toes, stepping on sharp objects, or being stepped on. Shoes that fit poorly cause blisters or ingrown nails.

Poor circulation in the feet prolongs healing. Diabetes and vascular disease are common causes of poor circulation. Infections or foot injuries are particularly serious for older adults and people with circulatory disorders. Gangrene and amputation are serious complications (see Chapter 31).

Check the client's feet every day. This is very important if the client has a circulatory disorder or diabetes, or takes medications that affect blood clotting. Notify your supervisor if you observe any of the following:

- Very dry skin
- Foot odours
- Cracks or breaks in the skin, especially between the toes
- Ingrown nails
- Loose nails
- Reddened, irritated, or calloused areas on the feet, heels, or ankles
- Drainage or bleeding
- Change in colour or texture of nails, especially black, thick, or brittle nails
- Corns, bunions, or blisters

Trimming and clipping toenails can easily cause injuries. Support workers do not cut or trim toenails if the client:

- Has diabetes
- Has poor circulation to the legs and feet
- Takes medications that affect blood clotting
- Has very thick or ingrown nails

Some employers do not allow support workers to cut or trim toenails under any circumstances. Follow employer policy. If a client needs toenails trimmed, tell your supervisor. Do not assume you can trim them. Also, support workers do not treat corns, bunions, or blisters. These foot problems may require a podiatrist. A *podiatrist* is a professional who provides foot care.

Fingernail and foot soaks may be part of the client's care plan. Nails are easier to trim and clean right after soaking or bathing. Check with your supervisor about the correct water temperature for foot soaks. Feet are easily burned. You must be very careful when preparing soaks for people with decreased sensation or circulatory problems. They may not feel hot temperatures and are at risk for scalding or burning their feet.

Tub baths are a good time for soaking feet and fingernails. If soaking is done at other times, the client can sit on the side of the tub and soak the feet. Make sure the client can step into and out of the tub. Otherwise, soak the feet in a basin. If the position is comfortable for the client, fingers can soak in the sink or in a small basin or bowl. Usually fingernail or foot soaks last for 15 to 20 minutes.

Nail clippers are used to cut fingernails. *Never use scissors.* Use extreme caution to prevent damage to nearby tissue. Only cut fingernails if instructed to do so by your supervisor and the care plan.

(text continues on page 448)

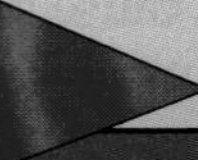

Giving Nail and Foot Care

Compassionate Care

Remember to Promote:
- **Dignity**
- **Independence**
- **Preferences**
- **Privacy**
- **Safety**

Pre-Procedure

1 Identify the person according to employer policy.
2 Explain the procedure to the person.
3 Wash your hands.
4 Collect the following:
- Washbasin
- Soap
- Bath thermometer
- Bath towel
- Face towel
- Washcloth
- Kidney basin
- Nail clippers
- Orange stick
- Emery board or nail file
- Lotion or petroleum jelly
- Paper towels
- Disposable bath mat
- Gloves

5 Arrange paper towels and other items on the overbed table (in facilities) or on a work area within easy reach.
6 Provide for privacy.
7 Help the person to a bedside chair. Place the call bell (in facilities) within reach.

Procedure

8 Place the bath mat under the person's feet.
9 Fill the wash basin. The care plan tells you what temperature to use. Measure water temperature according to employer policy.
10 Place the basin on the bath mat.
11 Help the person remove shoes and socks.
12 Help the person put the feet into the basin.
13 Adjust the overbed table or work area in front of the person. It should be low and close to the person.
14 Fill the kidney basin. Measure water temperature according to employer policy.
15 Place the kidney basin on the overbed table or work area.
16 Put the person's fingers into the basin. Position the arms for comfort (Figure 28-6).
17 Let the feet and fingernails soak for 15 to 20 minutes. Rewarm water as needed.
18 Remove the kidney basin. Dry the hands and between the fingers thoroughly.
19 Put on gloves.
20 Clean under fingernails with the orange stick. Use a towel to wipe the orange stick after each nail.
21 Clip fingernails straight across with nail clippers (Figure 28-7).
22 Shape nails with an emery board or nail file.
23 Push cuticles back with a washcloth or orange stick (Figure 28-8).
24 Move the overbed table to the side.*
25 Wash the feet with soap and a washcloth. Wash between the toes.
26 Rinse the feet and between the toes.
27 Remove the feet from the basin. Dry thoroughly, especially between the toes.
28 Apply lotion or petroleum jelly to the tops and soles of the feet. Do not apply between the toes. Warm lotion before applying it.
29 Remove gloves. Wash your hands.
30 Help the person put on socks and shoes.

Continued

Giving Nail and Foot Care—cont'd

Post-Procedure

31 Provide for safety and comfort.
32 Place the call bell within reach.*
33 Follow the care plan for bed rail use.*
34 Clean and return equipment and supplies to their proper places. Discard disposable items. Wear gloves for this step.
35 Remove privacy measures.
36 Follow employer policy for soiled linen.
37 Wash your hands.
38 Report and record your actions and observations according to employer policy.

*Steps marked with an asterisk may not apply in community settings.

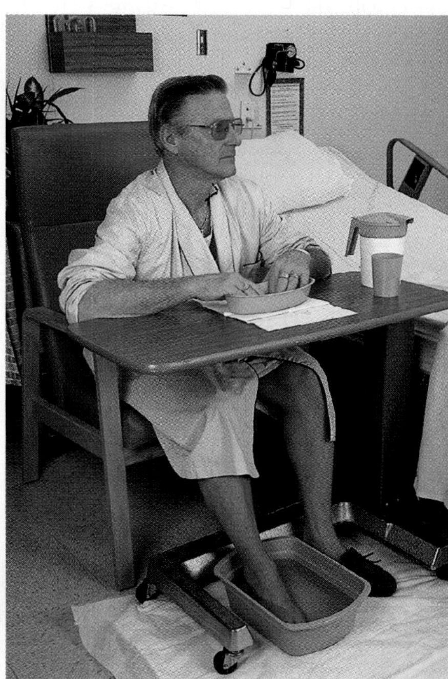

Figure 28-6 Nail and foot care. The feet soak in a foot basin, and the fingers soak in a kidney basin.

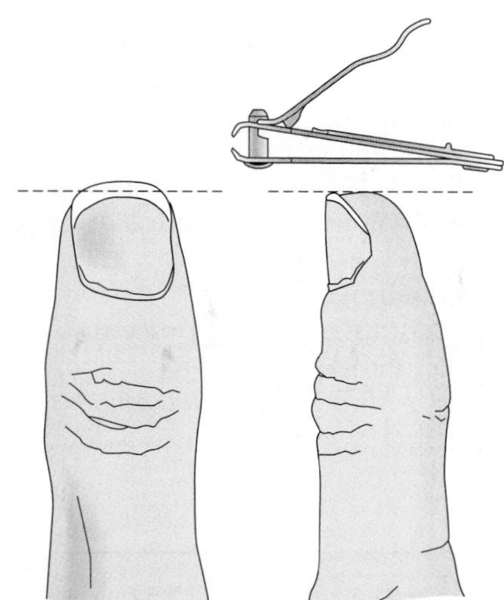

Figure 28-7 Clip fingernails straight across. Use a nail clipper.

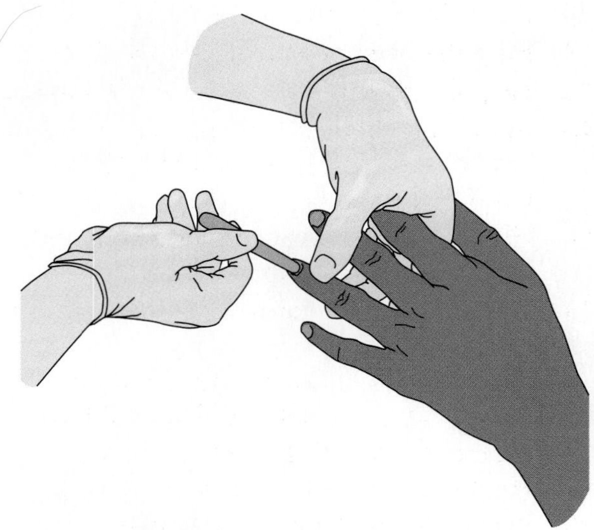

Figure 28-8 Push the cuticle back with an orange stick.

Changing Clothing and Hospital Gowns

Dressing and undressing occur at least daily. Most clients living in the community or in long-term care facilities wear street clothes during the day. They undress and put on sleepwear at bedtime. Incontinent clients may change clothing more often. Some clients choose to wear sleepwear and robes during the day if they are ill or confined to bed. Hospital patients usually change clothes on admission and discharge.

Some clients wear hospital gowns. Gowns usually are worn for IV therapy. Hospital gowns are put on and removed in a certain way when the person is receiving IV therapy (see page 455).

Some clients need help dressing and undressing. Changing is easier for those who can move their arms and legs. Arm or leg injuries or paralysis require special measures.

Follow the guidelines in Box 28-3 when dressing and undressing clients. Report and record the following observations after helping a client dress or undress:

- How much help was given
- How the client tolerated the procedure
- Any complaints from the client

(text continues on page 455)

Box 28-3 Guidelines for Changing Clients' Clothing or Hospital Gowns

- Provide for privacy. Do not expose the person.
- Encourage the person to do as much as possible.
- Let the person choose what to wear. Make sure the right undergarments are chosen.
- Support the arm or leg when removing or putting on a garment.
- Put clothing on the weak side first. The weak side is often called the *affected side*. It is the side affected by disease or disability. Never call the affected side the "bad" side. When dressing a person, remember the acronym DAF—**D**ress **A**ffected side **F**irst.
- Remove clothing from the strong side first. The strong side is often called the *unaffected side*. It is the side not affected by disease or disability. When undressing a person, remember the acronym RUF—**R**emove from **U**naffected side **F**irst.

Undressing the Person

Compassionate Care

Remember to Promote:
- **Dignity**
- **Independence**
- **Preferences**
- **Privacy**
- **Safety**

Pre-Procedure

1 Identify the person according to employer policy.
2 Explain the procedure to the person.
3 Wash your hands.
4 Collect a bath blanket.
5 Provide for privacy.
6 Raise the bed to a comfortable working height. Follow the care plan for bed rail use.*
7 Lower the bed rail (if up) on the person's weak side.
8 Position the person supine.
9 Cover the person with the bath blanket. Fanfold linens to the foot of the bed. Do not expose the person during the procedure.

Continued

Undressing the Person—cont'd

Procedure

10 Remove garments that open in the back:
- **a** Raise the head and shoulders (see *Raising the Person's Head and Shoulders,* page 270). Or turn him or her onto the side away from you.
- **b** Undo buttons, zippers, ties, or snaps.
- **c** Bring the sides of the garment to the person's sides (Figure 28-9, page 450). If he or she is in a side-lying position, tuck the far side under the person. Fold the near side onto the chest (Figure 28-10, on page 450).
- **d** Position the person supine.
- **e** Slide the garment off the shoulder on the strong side. Remove the garment from the arm (Figure 28-11, page 450).
- **f** Repeat step 10 e for the weak side.

11 Remove garments that open in the front.
- **a** Undo buttons, zippers, snaps, or ties.
- **b** Slide the garment off the shoulder and arm on the strong side.
- **c** Raise the person's head and shoulders. Bring the garment over to the weak side (Figure 28-12, page 451). Lower the person's head and shoulders.
- **d** Remove the garment from the weak side.
- **e** If you cannot raise the person's head and shoulders:
  - **(1)** Turn the person toward you. Tuck the removed part of the garment under the person.
  - **(2)** Turn him or her onto the side away from you.
  - **(3)** Pull the side of the garment out from under the person. Make sure he or she will not lie on it when supine.
  - **(4)** Return the person to the supine position.
  - **(5)** Remove the garment from the weak side.

12 Remove pullover garments.
- **a** Undo any buttons, zippers, ties, or snaps.
- **b** Remove the garment from the person's strong side.
- **c** Raise the person's head and shoulders. Or turn him or her onto the side away from you. Bring the garment up to the person's neck (Figure 28-13, page 451).
- **d** Remove the garment from the weak side.
- **e** Bring the garment over the person's head.
- **f** Position the person supine.

13 Remove pants or slacks.
- **a** Remove footwear.
- **b** Position the person supine.
- **c** Undo buttons, zippers, ties, snaps, or buckles.
- **d** Remove the belt if one is worn.
- **e** Ask the person to lift the buttocks off the bed. Slide the pants down over the hips and buttocks (Figure 28-14, page 451). Have the person lower the hips and buttocks.
- **f** If the person cannot raise the hips off the bed:
  - **(1)** Turn the person toward you.
  - **(2)** Slide the pants off the hip and buttock on the strong side (Figure 28-15, page 452).
  - **(3)** Turn the person away from you.
  - **(4)** Slide the pants off the hip and buttock on the weak side (Figure 28-16, page 452).
- **g** Slide the pants down the legs and over the feet.

14 Dress the person (see *Dressing the Person,* page 453).

15 Help the person get out of bed if he or she is to be up. If the person will stay in bed:
- **a** Cover the person and remove the bath blanket.
- **b** Provide for safety and comfort.
- **c** Return the bed to its lowest position. Follow the care plan for bed rail use.*

Continued

Undressing the Person—cont'd

Post-Procedure

16 Place the call bell within reach.*
17 Remove privacy measures.
18 Follow employer policy for dirty linen.
19 Wash your hands.
20 Report and record your actions and observations according to employer policy.

*Steps marked with an asterisk may not apply in community settings.

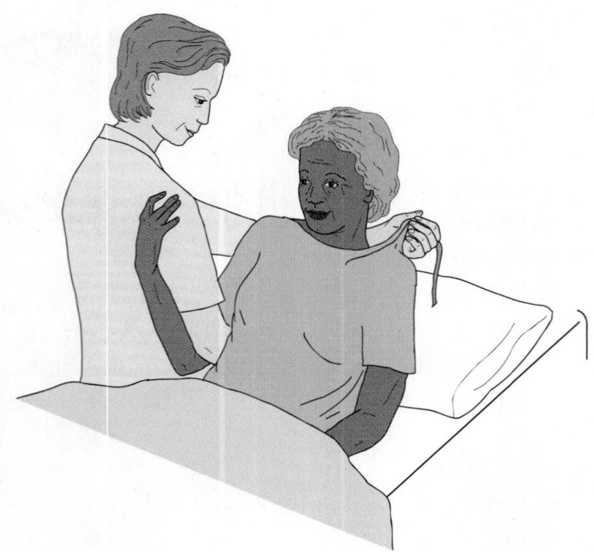

Figure 28-9 Bring the sides of the garment from the back to the sides of the client.

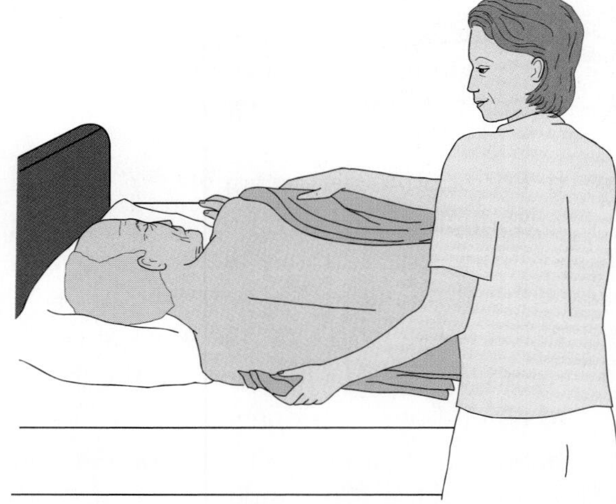

Figure 28-10 Assist the client to a side-lying position to remove a garment that opens in the back. Tuck the far side of the garment under the client. Fold the near side onto the client's chest.

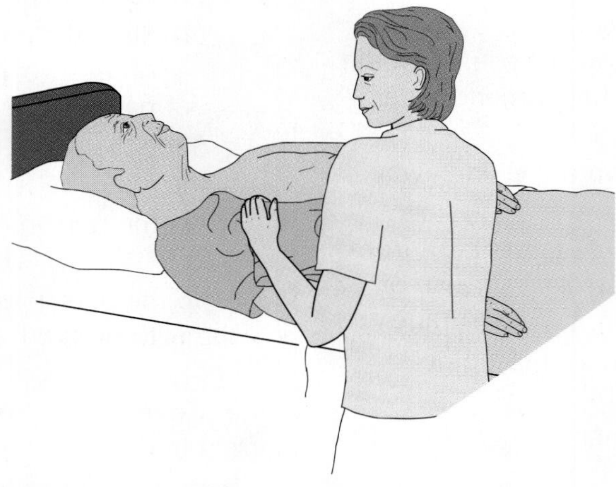

Figure 28-11 Remove the garment from the strong side first.

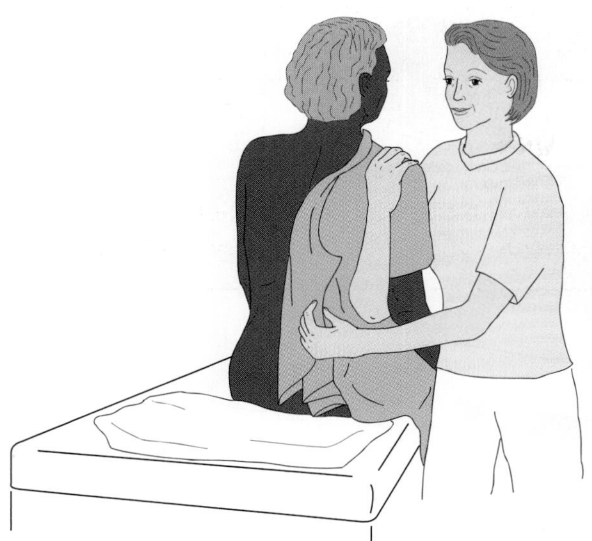

Figure 28-12 Raise the client's head and shoulders to remove a front-opening garment. Remove the garment from the strong side first. Then bring it around the back to the weak side.

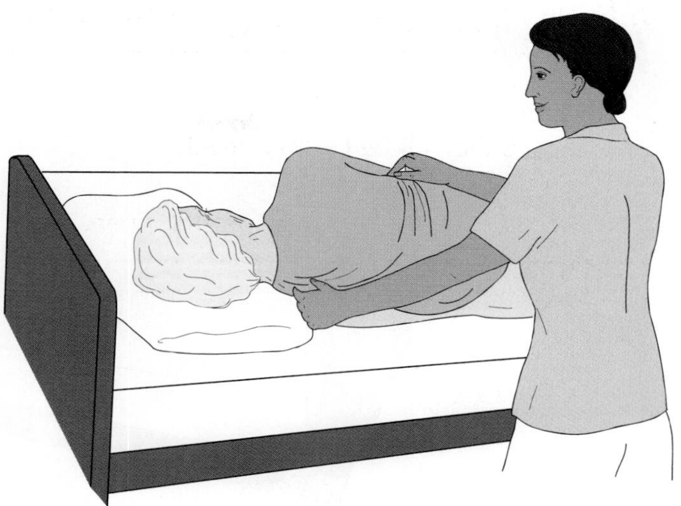

Figure 28-13 Remove a pullover garment from the strong side first. Then bring the garment up the client's neck to remove it from the weak side.

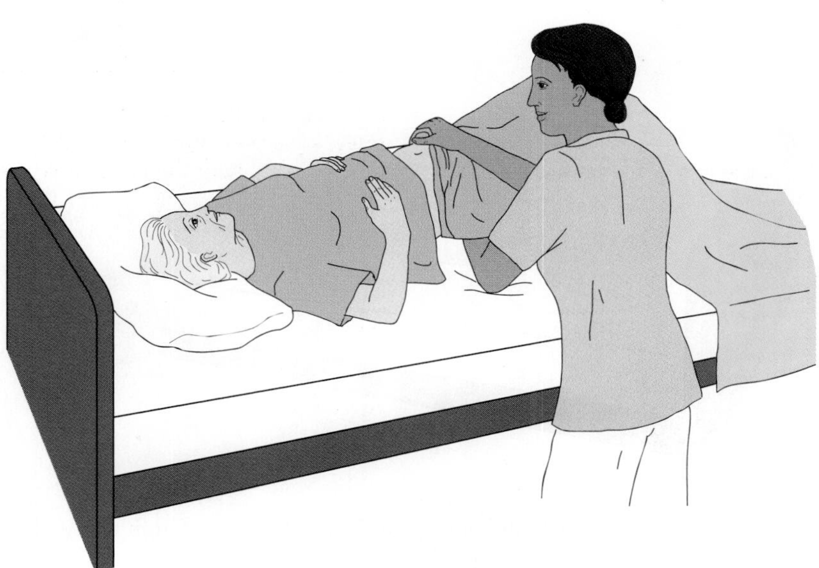

Figure 28-14 The client lifts the hips and buttocks for removing the pants. Slide the pants down over the hips and buttocks.

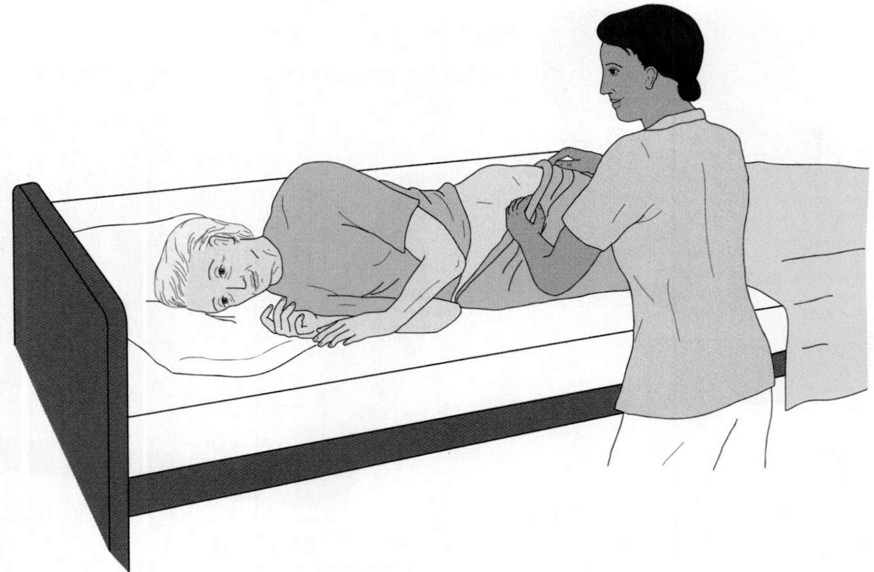

Figure 28-15 Pants are removed in the side-lying position. Remove them from the strong side first. Slide them over the hips and buttocks.

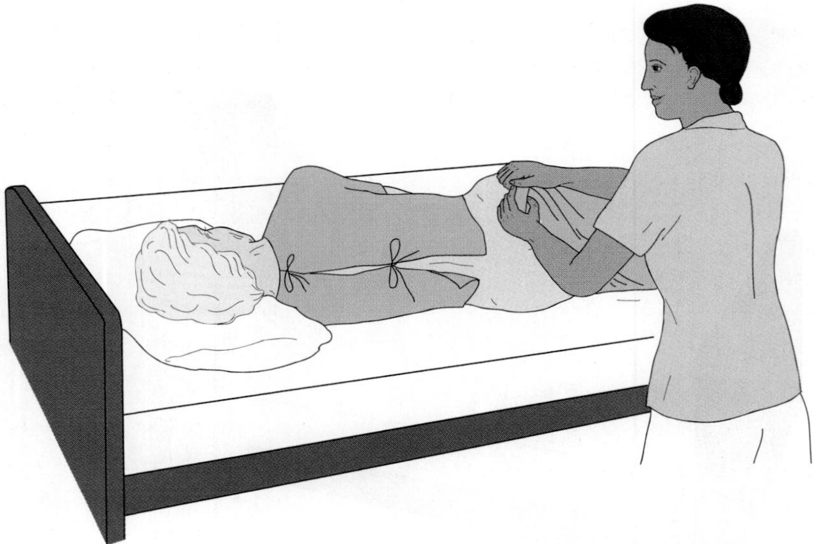

Figure 28-16 Turn the client onto the other side. Remove the pants from the weak side.

Dressing the Person

Compassionate Care

Remember to Promote:
- **Dignity**
- **Independence**
- **Preferences**
- **Privacy**
- **Safety**

Pre-Procedure

1 Identify the person according to employer policy.
2 Explain the procedure to the person.
3 Wash your hands.
4 Collect a bath blanket and clothing requested by the person.
5 Provide for privacy.
6 Raise the bed to a comfortable working height. Follow the care plan for bed rail use.*
7 Undress the person (see *Undressing the Person,* page 448).
8 Lower the bed rail (if up) on the person's strong side.
9 Position the person supine.

Procedure

10 Cover the person with the bath blanket. Fanfold linens to the foot of the bed. Do not expose the person during the procedure.
11 Put on garments that open in the back:
  a Slide the garment onto the arm and shoulder of the weak side.
  b Slide the garment onto the arm and shoulder of the strong side.
  c Raise the person's head and shoulders.
  d Bring the sides of the garment to the back.
  e If the person is in a side-lying position:
    (1) Turn the person toward you.
    (2) Bring one side of the garment to the person's back (Figure 28-17, *A*, page 455).
    (3) Turn the person away from you.
    (4) Bring the other side of the garment to the person's back (Figure 28-17, *B*, page 455).
  f Fasten buttons, snaps, ties, or zippers.
  g Position the person supine.
12 Put on garments that open in the front:
  a Slide the garment onto the arm and shoulder on the weak side.
  b Raise the person's head and shoulders. Bring the side of the garment around to the back. Lay the person down. Slide the garment onto the arm and shoulder of the strong arm.
  c If the person cannot raise the head and shoulders:
    (1) Turn the person toward you.
    (2) Tuck the garment under him or her.
    (3) Turn the person away from you.
    (4) Pull the garment out from under the person.
    (5) Turn the person back to the supine position.
    (6) Slide the garment over the arm and shoulder of the strong arm.
  d Fasten buttons, snaps, ties, or zippers.
13 Put on pullover garments:
  a Position the person supine.
  b Bring the neck of the garment over the head.

Continued

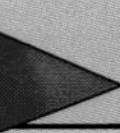

Dressing the Person—cont'd

Procedure—cont'd

- c Slide the arm and shoulder of the garment onto the person's weak side.
- d Raise the person's head and shoulders.
- e Bring the garment down.
- f Slide the arm and shoulder of the garment onto the strong side.
- g If the person cannot assume a semi-sitting position:
  - (1) Turn the person toward you.
  - (2) Tuck the garment under the person.
  - (3) Turn the person away from you.
  - (4) Pull the garment out from under him or her.
  - (5) Position the person supine.
  - (6) Slide the arm and shoulder of the garment onto the strong side.
- h Fasten buttons, snaps, ties, or zippers.

14 Put on pants or slacks:
- a Slide the pants over the feet and up the legs.
- b Ask the person to raise the hips and buttocks off the bed.
- c Bring the pants up over the buttocks and hips.
- d Ask the person to lower the hips and buttocks.
- e If the person cannot raise the hips and buttocks:
  - (1) Turn the person onto the strong side.
  - (2) Pull the pants over the buttock and hip on the weak side.
  - (3) Turn the person onto the weak side.
  - (4) Pull the pants over the buttock and hip on the strong side.
  - (5) Position the person supine.
- f Fasten buttons, ties, snaps, zipper, and belt buckle.

15 Put socks and footwear on the person.

16 Help the person get out of bed. If the person will stay in bed:
- a Cover the person. Remove the bath blanket.
- b Provide for safety and comfort.
- c Return the bed to its lowest position. Follow the care plan for bed rail use.*

Post-Procedure

17 Place the call bell within reach.*

18 Remove privacy measures.

19 Follow employer policy for dirty linen.

20 Wash your hands.

21 Report and record your actions and observations according to employer policy.

*Steps marked with an asterisk may not apply in community settings.

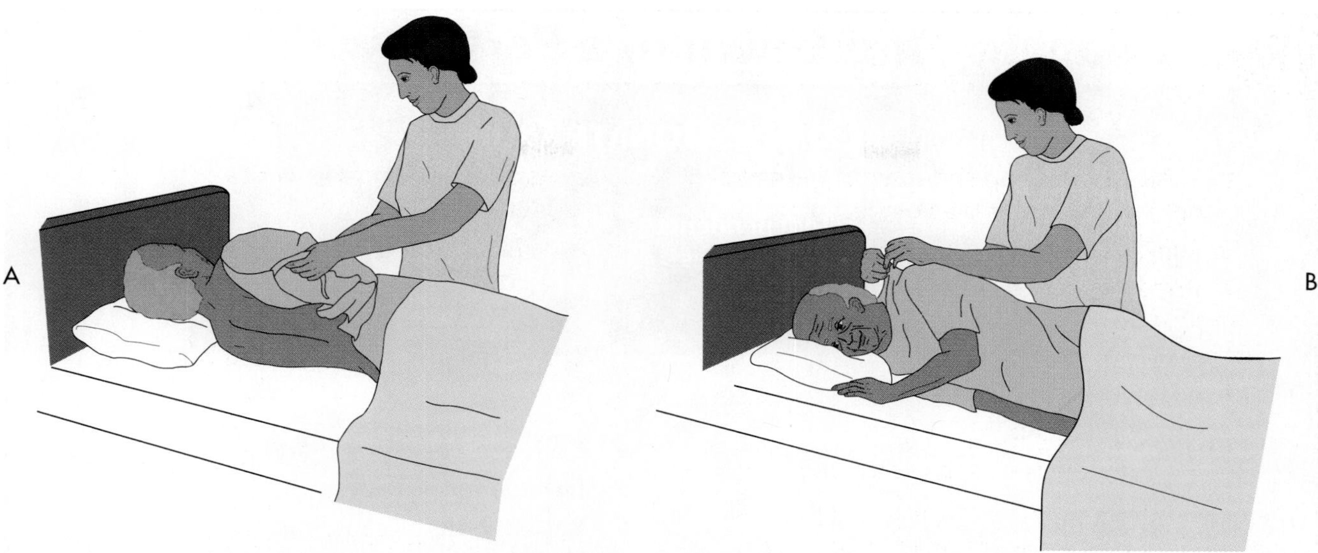

Figure 28-17 Putting on garments that open in the back. **A,** The side-lying position can be used to put on garments that open in the back. Turn the client toward you after the garment is put on the arms. Bring the side of the garment to the client's back. **B,** Then turn the client away from you. Bring the other side of the garment to the back. Fasten the garment.

Changing Hospital Gowns

Some clients wear hospital gowns. Gowns are usually worn for IV therapy. Some facilities and agencies have special gowns for IV therapy. The gowns open along the sleeve and close with ties, snaps, or Velcro. Some facilities and agencies use standard hospital gowns. If so, use the following procedure. However, some clients have IV pumps that control the infusions. If the client has an IV pump and a standard hospital gown, do not use the following procedure. The arm with the IV is not put through the sleeve.

(text continues on page 458)

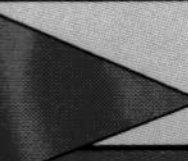

Changing the Gown of a Person with an IV

Compassionate Care

Remember to Promote:
- **Dignity**
- **Independence**
- **Preferences**
- **Privacy**
- **Safety**

Pre-Procedure

1 Identify the person according to employer policy.
2 Explain the procedure to the person.
3 Wash your hands.
4 Collect a clean gown and a bath blanket.
5 Provide for privacy.
6 Raise the bed to a comfortable working height. Follow the care plan for bed rail use.*

Procedure

7 Lower the bed rail near you if up.
8 Cover the person with a bath blanket. Fan-fold linens to the foot of the bed.
9 Untie the gown. Free parts that the person is lying on.
10 Remove the gown from the arm with no IV.
11 Gather up the sleeve of the arm with the IV. Slide it over the IV site and tubing. Remove the arm and hand from the sleeve (Figure 28-18, *A*).
12 Keep the sleeve gathered. Slide your arm along the tubing to the bag (Figure 28-18, *B*).
13 Remove the IV bag from the pole. Slide the bag and tubing through the sleeve (Figure 28-18, *C*). Do not pull on the tubing. Keep the bag above the person.
14 Hang the IV bag on the pole.
15 Gather the sleeve of the clean gown that will go on the arm with the IV infusion.
16 Remove the bag from the pole. Slip the sleeve over the bag at the shoulder part of the gown (Figure 28-18, *D*). Hang the bag.
17 Slide the gathered sleeve over the tubing, hand, arm, and IV site. Then slide it onto the shoulder.
18 Put the other side of the gown on. Fasten the back.
19 Cover the person. Remove the bath blanket.

Post-Procedure

20 Provide for safety and comfort.
21 Place the call bell within reach.*
22 Return the bed to its lowest position. Follow the care plan for bed rail use.*
23 Remove privacy measures.
24 Follow employer policy for dirty linen.
25 Wash your hands.
26 Report and record your actions and observations according to employer policy. (In facilities, ask your supervisor to check the flow rate.)

*Steps marked with an asterisk may not apply in community settings.

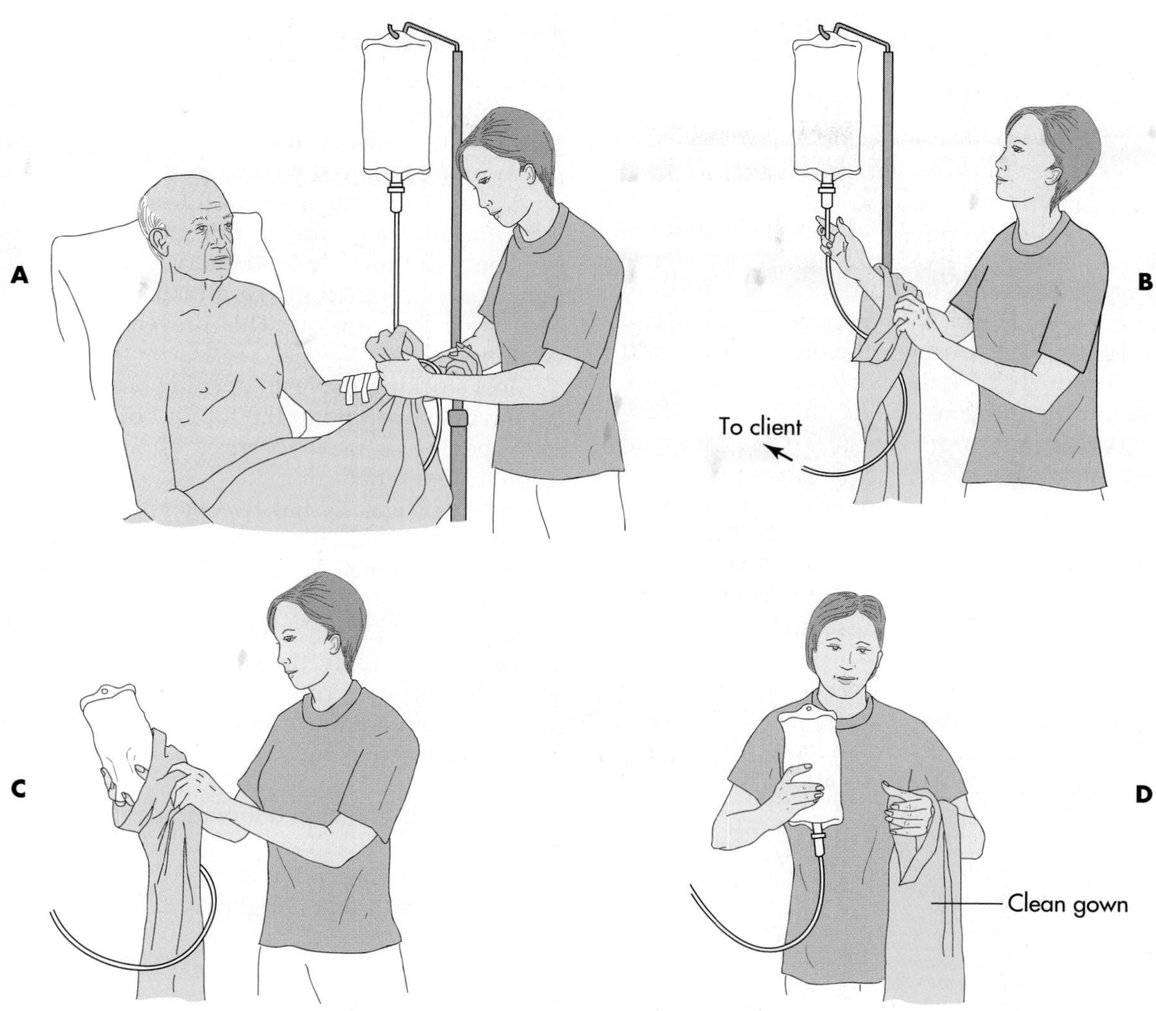

Figure 28-18 Changing a hospital gown. **A,** Remove the gown from the arm with no IV. Gather up the sleeve on the arm with the IV, slide it over the IV site and tubing, and remove it from the arm and hand. **B,** Slip the gathered sleeve along the IV tubing to the bag. **C,** Remove the IV bag from the pole and pass it through the sleeve. **D,** Slip the gathered sleeve of the clean gown over the IV bag at the shoulder part of the gown.

Applying Elastic Stockings and Bandages

Some clients must wear elastic stockings or bandages on their legs. They must be applied as part of their daily dressing routine.

A physician orders elastic stockings and bandages for the client. They are used to help prevent blood clots (thrombi). A blood clot (thrombus) can form in deep leg veins (see Figure 45-6 on page 755). The clot can break loose, travel through the bloodstream, and lodge in a distant vessel. If the clot lodges in the lungs, severe respiratory problems and death can result. People with circulatory disorders and heart disease are at risk for blood clots. So are people on bed rest.

Elastic stockings and bandages help prevent thrombi. The elastic exerts pressure on the veins. The pressure promotes venous blood flow to the heart. They also provide support and reduce swelling from injuries. However, elastic stockings and bandages can harm the client if applied incorrectly. Therefore, most hospitals do not allow support workers to apply them to acute care patients. You may be asked to apply them on clients in stable condition. Some employers do not allow support workers to apply them at all. Know your employer's policy.

Applying Elastic Stockings

Elastic stockings come in a variety of sizes. They also come in thigh-high or knee-high lengths. The care plan lists the correct size to use. They are applied in the morning before the client gets out of bed. Otherwise, the client's legs can swell from sitting or standing. Stockings are hard to put on when the legs are swollen. They are removed every 8 hours for 30 minutes or according to the care plan. The client lies in bed while they are off. This prevents the legs from swelling.

Most stockings have an opening near the toes. Others have an opening in the top or bottom of the foot. The opening is used to check circulation and skin colour and temperature.

The client usually has two pairs of stockings. One pair is washed while the client wears the other pair. Wash the stockings by hand with a mild soap. Hang them to dry.

Stockings should not have twists, creases, or wrinkles after you apply them. Twists can affect circulation. Creases and wrinkles can cause skin breakdown. Report and record the following observations after applying elastic stockings:

- Skin colour and skin temperature
- Leg and foot swelling
- Signs of skin breakdown
- Complaints of pain, tingling, or numbness

(text continues on page 460)

Applying Elastic Stockings

Compassionate Care

Remember to Promote:
- **Dignity**
- **Independence**
- **Preferences**
- **Privacy**
- **Safety**

Pre-Procedure

1 Identify the person according to employer policy.
2 Explain the procedure to the person.
3 Wash your hands.
4 Collect elastic stockings in the correct size and length.
5 Provide for privacy.
6 Raise the bed to a comfortable working height. Follow the care plan for bed rail use.*

Continued

Applying Elastic Stockings—cont'd

Procedure

7 Lower the bed rail near you if up.
8 Position the person supine.
9 Expose the legs. Fanfold top linens toward the person's thighs.
10 Turn the stocking inside out down to the heel (Figure 28-19, *A*).
11 Slip the foot of the stocking over the toes, foot, and heel (Figure 28-19, *B*).
12 Grasp the stocking top. Slip it over the foot and heel. Pull it up the leg. It turns right side out as it is pulled up. The stocking must be even and snug (Figure 28-19, *C*).
13 Remove twists, creases, or wrinkles.
14 Repeat steps 10 through 13 for the other leg.

Post-Procedure

15 Cover the person.
16 Provide for safety and comfort.
17 Place the call bell within reach.*
18 Return the bed to its lowest position. Follow the care plan for bed rail use.*
19 Remove privacy measures.
20 Wash your hands.
21 Report and record your actions and observations according to employer policy.

*Steps marked with an asterisk may not apply in community settings.

A

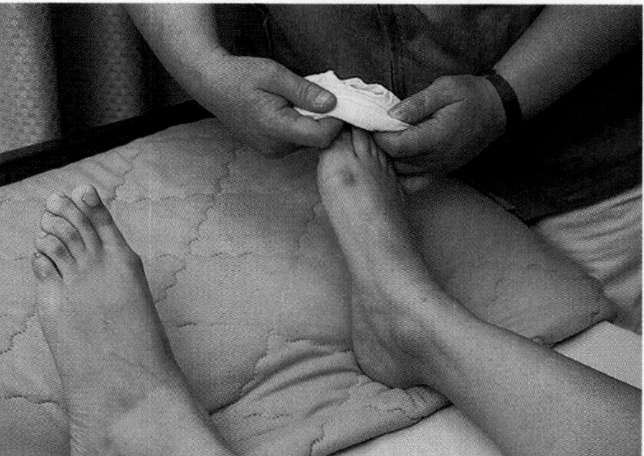

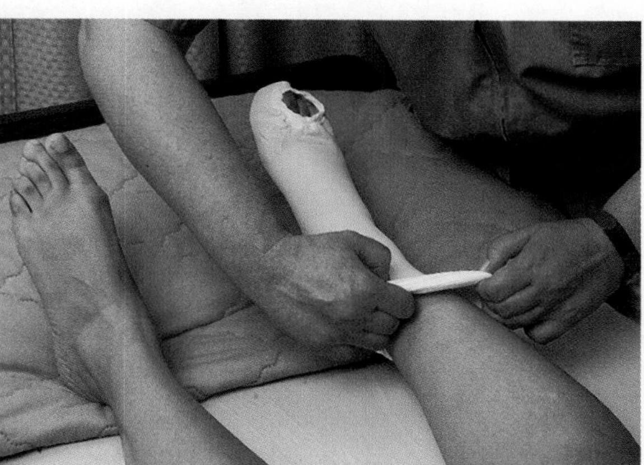

B

C

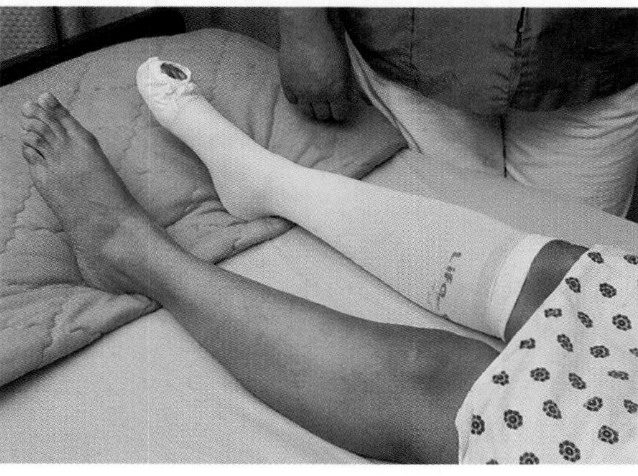

Figure 28-19 Applying elastic stockings. **A,** Turn the stocking inside out down to the heel. **B,** Slip the stocking over the toes, foot, and heel. **C,** The stocking turns right side out as it is pulled up over the leg.

Applying Elastic Bandages

Elastic bandages have the same purposes as elastic stockings. They also hold dressings in place. They are applied to the upper or lower extremities.

The bandage is applied from the lower (distal) part of the extremity to the top (proximal) part. Your supervisor and the care plan tell you what area to bandage. Elastic bandages are removed every 8 hours for 30 minutes.

Follow these guidelines when applying elastic bandages:

- Use the correct length and width
- Position the body part in good alignment
- Face the client during the procedure
- Expose fingers or toes if possible. This allows circulation checks.
- Apply the bandage with firm, even pressure.
- Make sure the bandage is firm and snug. It must not be tight. A tight bandage can affect circulation.
- Check the colour and temperature of the extremity every hour.
- Reapply a loose, wrinkled, moist, or soiled bandage.

Report and record the following observations after applying elastic bandages:

- Skin colour and skin temperature
- Leg and foot swelling
- Signs of skin breakdown
- Complaints of pain, tingling, or numbness

(text continues on page 462)

Applying Elastic Bandages

Compassionate Care

Remember to Promote:
- **Dignity**
- **Independence**
- **Preferences**
- **Privacy**
- **Safety**

Pre-Procedure

1 Identify the person according to employer policy.
2 Explain the procedure to the person.
3 Wash your hands.
4 Collect the following:
   - Elastic bandage as directed by the care plan
   - Tape or metal clips (unless the bandage has Velcro)
5 Provide for privacy.
6 Raise the bed to a comfortable working height. Follow the care plan for bed rail use.*

Continued

Applying Elastic Bandages—cont'd

Procedure

7 Lower the bed rail near you if up.

8 Help the person to a comfortable position. Expose the part you will bandage.

9 Make sure the area is clean and dry.

10 Hold the bandage so that the roll is up. The loose end must be on the bottom (Figure 28-20, *A*).

11 Apply the bandage to the smallest part of the wrist, foot, ankle, or knee.

12 Make two circular turns around the part (Figure 28-20, *B*).

13 Make overlapping spiral turns in an upward direction. Each turn overlaps about ⅔ (two-thirds) of the previous turn (Figure 28-20, *C*).

14 Apply the bandage smoothly with firm, even pressure. It must not be tight.

15 Secure the bandage in place with Velcro, tape, or a clip. The clip must not be under the body part.

16 Check the fingers or toes for coldness or cyanosis (bluish colour). Ask about pain, itching, numbness, or tingling. Remove the bandage if any are noted. Report it to your supervisor.

Post-Procedure

17 Follow steps 16 through 21 of *Applying Elastic Stockings,* page 458.

*Steps marked with an asterisk may not apply in community settings.

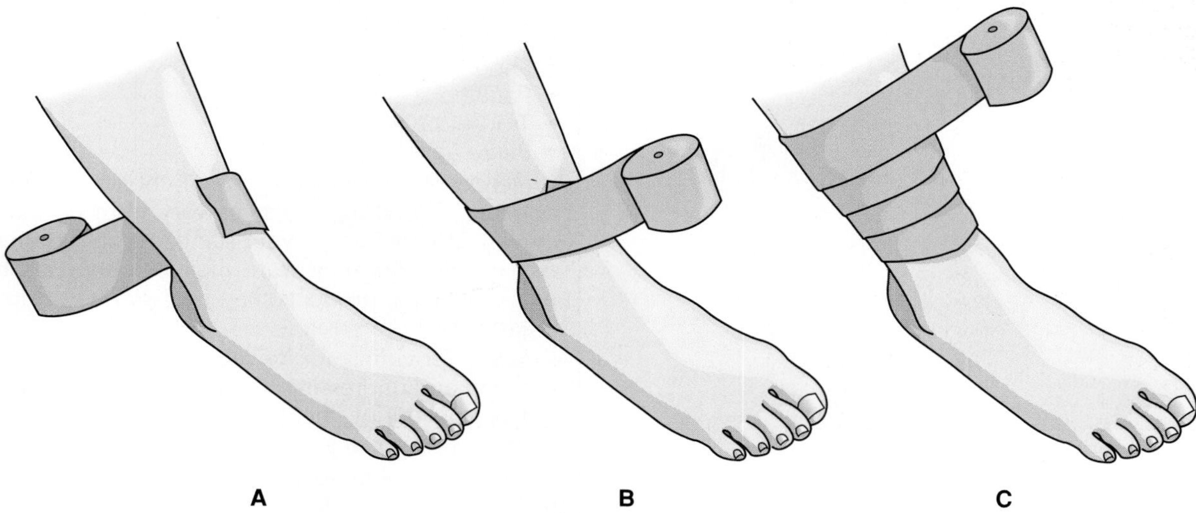

Figure 28-20 Applying an elastic bandage. **A,** The roll of the bandage is up, and the loose end is at the bottom. **B,** Apply the bandage to the smallest part with two circular turns. **C,** Apply the bandage with spiral turns in an upward direction.

Compassionate Care

When helping with grooming and dressing, remember to focus on the whole person rather than only on the task. Promote the person's dignity, independence, preferences, privacy, and safety (see *Providing Compassionate Care: Assisting Clients with Grooming and Dressing* box).

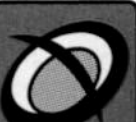

Providing Compassionate Care

Assisting Clients with Grooming and Dressing

D*ignity.* Being clean and well-groomed helps the person maintain dignity. People often feel good about themselves when they have a neat appearance and clean clothing. When assisting with grooming, carefully handle the person's hygiene products, shaver, hair dryer, brush and comb, perfumes, and other personal care items. Clothing also needs your attention. Do not break zippers, tear clothing, lose buttons, or cause other damage. Treat the person's property with care and respect. If damage occurs, notify your supervisor.

I*ndependence.* Encourage the person to be as independent as possible. Only assist when needed. Like other activities of daily living, dressing and undressing stimulate circulation and increase muscle strength and flexibility. They also increase the person's confidence and self-esteem. Sometimes having clients do what they can for themselves requires patience and understanding. Allow the client extra time to dress and undress independently.

If the person has self-care devices, encourage him or her to use them. There are many self-care devices available (see Chapter 32). Devices that promote independence with dressing and undressing include:

- Button hooks (see Figure 32-3, *A* on page 559)
- Sock pullers (see Figure 32-3, *B*)
- Shoe removers (see Figure 32-3, *C*)
- Pantyhose aids
- Trouser pulls
- Pant clips

P*references.* Encourage personal choice whenever possible. Grooming practices vary from person to person. Do not impose your standards on the client. Ask clients how they want their hair styled, what hair or shaving products they use, and what clothing they want to wear.

P*rivacy.* Providing for privacy is important when dressing and undressing the person. Do not expose the person during the procedures in this chapter. Also provide privacy when assisting with grooming.

S*afety.* Remember to dress the affected side first (DAF) and remove clothing from the unaffected side first (RUF). Also remember to check clients with elastic stockings and bandages often. Check for signs of reduced circulation, swelling, or skin breakdown. Report your observations to your supervisor. This information is needed to meet the person's needs.

REVIEW

Circle the BEST answer.

1. Mr. Lee has alopecia. This is
   A. Excessive body hair
   B. Dry, white flakes on the scalp
   C. An infestation of lice
   D. Hair loss

2. When brushing hair that is not matted or tangled, start at
   A. The forehead and brush backward
   B. The hair ends
   C. The scalp
   D. The back of the neck and brush forward

3. Brushing is important to keep the hair
   A. Soft and shiny
   B. Clean
   C. Free from lice
   D. Long

4. Mr. Lee wants his hair washed. You should
   A. Wash his hair during his shower
   B. Wash his hair at the sink
   C. Shampoo him in bed
   D. Follow the care plan

5. When shaving Mr. Lee with a blade razor, you need to do the following *except*
   A. Practise Standard Precautions
   B. Moisten the skin before shaving to soften it
   C. Shave in the opposite direction of hair growth
   D. Shave when the skin is dry

6. Mr. Lee is nicked during shaving. Your first action should be to
   A. Wash your hands
   B. Apply direct pressure
   C. Tell your supervisor
   D. Apply a bandage

7. Fingernails are cut with
   A. Toenail clippers
   B. Scissors
   C. A nail file
   D. Nail clippers

8. Fingernails are trimmed
   A. Before soaking
   B. After soaking
   C. Before trimming toenails
   D. After trimming toenails

9. Elastic stockings are used for these reasons *except*
   A. To reduce swelling in the legs
   B. To prevent blood clots
   C. To exert pressure on the veins
   D. To reduce circulation

10. Elastic stockings are applied
    A. Before the client gets out of bed
    B. When the client is standing
    C. After the client's shower or tub bath
    D. For 30 minutes and then removed

11. When applying an elastic bandage
    A. The body part needs to be in good alignment
    B. The fingers or toes are covered
    C. It is applied from the largest to the smallest part of an extremity
    D. It is applied from the upper to the lower part of the extremity

Circle T if the answer is true and F if it is false.

12. T F Mr. Lee has a mustache and beard. You think he would be more comfortable without facial hair. You can shave his beard and mustache.

13. T F You can cut and trim toenails when a client has diabetes.

14. T F Clothing is removed from the strong side first.

15. T F The client chooses what to wear.

Answers to these questions are on page 825.

CHAPTER

29

URINARY ELIMINATION

OBJECTIVES

- Define the key terms listed in this chapter
- Identify the characteristics of normal urine
- Describe the guidelines for maintaining normal urinary elimination
- List the observations to make about urine
- Describe urinary incontinence and the care required
- Explain why catheters are used
- Explain the differences between straight, indwelling, suprapubic, and condom catheters
- Describe the guidelines for caring for clients with indwelling catheters
- Describe two methods of bladder training
- Describe the guidelines for collecting urine specimens
- Explain how to care for a client with a ureterostomy
- Learn the procedures described in this chapter

KEY TERMS

acetone A compound that appears in the urine from the rapid breakdown of fat for energy; ketone body

catheter A tube used to drain or inject fluid through a body opening

catheterization The process of inserting a catheter

condom catheter A sheath that slides over the penis; tubing connects the catheter and drainage bag

dysuria Painful or difficult (*dys*) urination (*uria*)

Foley catheter A retention or indwelling catheter

functional incontinence The loss of urine that occurs when the person has bladder control but cannot use the toilet in time

glucosuria Sugar (*glucos*) in the urine (*uria*); glycosuria

glycosuria Glucosuria

hematuria Blood (*hemat*) in the urine (*uria*)

indwelling catheter A catheter that is left in place in the bladder so urine drains constantly into a drainage bag; Foley or retention catheter

ketone body Acetone

micturition Urination

nocturia Frequent urination (*uria*) at night (*noct*)

oliguria Scant amount (*olig*) of urine (*uria*); usually less than 500 mL in 24 hours

ostomy Surgical creation of an artificial opening

overflow incontinence The leaking of urine when the bladder is too full

polyuria The production of abnormally large amounts (*poly*) of urine (*uria*)

reflex incontinence The loss of urine at predictable intervals

retention catheter A Foley or indwelling catheter

stoma An artificial opening

straight catheter A catheter that drains the bladder and is removed

stress incontinence The leaking of urine during exercise and certain movements

suprapubic catheter A catheter that is surgically inserted into the bladder through the abdomen

ureterostomy An artificial opening (*stomy*) between the ureter (*uretero*) and the abdomen

urge incontinence The loss of urine in response to a sudden, urgent need to void

urinary frequency Voiding at frequent intervals

urinary incontinence The inability to contol the loss of urine from the bladder; the loss of bladder control

urinary urgency The need to void immediately

urination The process of emptying urine from the bladder; micturition or voiding

voiding Urination

Eliminating waste is a physical need. The respiratory, digestive, integumentary, and urinary systems all remove body wastes. The digestive system rids the body of solid wastes. The lungs rid the body of carbon dioxide. Sweat contains water and other substances. Blood contains waste products from body cells burning food for energy. The urinary system removes waste products from the blood and maintains the body's water balance. See Chapter 13 to review the urinary system.

When assisting a client with elimination, you may be exposed to urine, stool (feces), and soiled linen and clothing. Protect yourself and your client by following the rules of medical asepsis and Standard Precautions (see Chapter 18). Follow the infection control precautions in Box 29-1 on page 466 when assisting with elimination.

Normal Urination

The healthy adult excretes about 1500 mL (millilitres) (3 pints) of urine a day. Many factors affect urine production. They include age, disease, the amount and kinds of fluid ingested, dietary salt, and medications. Some substances increase urine production. Examples are coffee, tea, alcohol, and some medications. A diet high in salt causes the body to retain water. When water is retained, less urine is produced.

Box 29-1 Infection Control Precautions When Assisting with Elimination

- Wash hands before and after wearing gloves.
- Wear gloves whenever there is a risk of contact with urine, feces, secretions, or mucous membranes. Examples include:
  - Assisting clients who have diarrhea, urinary incontinence (page 474), or fecal incontinence (see Chapter 30)
  - Handling or cleaning bedpans, urinals, commodes, toilets, or bathroom floors
  - Handling soiled clothing or linens
  - Changing incontinence products
  - Measuring client's output or collecting specimens
- Change gloves between procedures on the same client if the gloves might be contaminated. For example, change gloves after perineal care and before cleaning an indwelling catheter.
- Remove contaminated gloves before touching a clean surface. For example, remove soiled gloves before raising a bed rail.
- Wear a protective apron or gown if you might be sprayed or splashed with blood, body fluids, secretions, or excretions. This could occur when you are emptying bedpans or commodes.
- Cover bedpans and tightly cap urinals when carrying them. Avoid splashing when disposing bedpan, urinal, or commode contents. If splashing occurs, clean area immediately. Dispose of body wastes immediately and carefully. Clean and disinfect bedpans, urinals, and commodes immediately after use.
- Place soiled disposable materials in leak-proof plastic bags. Seal tightly. Immediately discard the bag following employer policy.
- Place soiled linen and clothing in a leak-proof plastic bag. Launder as soon as possible according to employer policy. In a client's home, wash soiled linen separately from other laundry.

Source: Adapted from J. Birchenall and E. Streight, *Mosby's Textbook for the Home Care Aide* (St. Louis: Mosby Lifeline, 1997), p. 262.

Urination, micturition, and **voiding** mean the process of emptying urine from the bladder. The amount of fluid intake, personal habits, and available toilet facilities affect frequency. So do activity, work, and illness. People usually void at bedtime, after getting up, and before meals. Some people void every 2 to 3 hours. The need to void at night disturbs sleep.

Clients often need help with urinary elimination. Some need help getting to the bathroom. Others use bedpans, urinals, or commodes. Follow the guidelines listed in Box 29-2 to help maintain normal elimination. Also follow the care plan.

Box 29-2 Guidelines for Maintaining Normal Elimination

- Practise medical asepsis and Standard Precautions.
- Provide fluids as instructed by the care plan.
- Follow the client's normal voiding routines and habits. Check with your supervisor and the care plan.
- Help the client to the bathroom when the request is made. Or provide the commode, bedpan, or urinal. The need to void may be urgent.
- Help the client assume a normal position for voiding if possible. Women sit or squat; men stand.
- Warm the bedpan or urinal.
- Cover the client for warmth and privacy.
- Provide for privacy. Pull the curtain around the bed, close room and bathroom doors, and pull drapes or window shades. Leave the room if the client can be alone.
- Tell the client that running water, flushing the toilet, or playing music can mask urination sounds. Some people are embarrassed about voiding with others close by.
- Remain nearby if the client is weak or unsteady.
- Place the call bell (in facilities) and toilet tissue within reach.
- Allow the client enough time to void. Do not rush the client. However, do not let the client lie on a bedpan for a long time. Pressure ulcers are a risk.
- Promote relaxation. Some people like to read when eliminating.
- Run water in a nearby sink if the client has difficulty starting the stream. Or place the person's fingers in some warm water.
- Provide perineal care as needed.
- Assist with hand washing after voiding. Provide a wash basin, soap, washcloth, and towel.
- Assist the client to the bathroom or offer the bedpan, urinal, or commode at regular times. Some people are embarrassed or are too weak to ask.

Observations

Urine is normally pale yellow, straw coloured, or amber. It is clear with no particles. A faint odour is normal. Observe urine for colour, clarity, odour, amount, and particles.

Some foods normally affect urine colour. Red food dyes, beets, blackberries, and rhubarb cause red-coloured urine. Carrots and sweet potatoes cause bright yellow urine. Certain medications cause changes in urine colour. Asparagus causes a change in urine odour.

Report to your supervisor if you observe urine that looks or smells abnormal. Report complaints of urgency, burning on urination, or dysuria. **Dysuria** means painful or difficult (*dys*) urination (*uria*). Urinary tract infection is a common cause. Also report the problems described in Table 29-1.

Table 29-1 Common Urinary Elimination Problems

	Definition	Causes
dysuria	Painful or difficult (*dys*) urination (*uria*)	Urinary tract infection, trauma, urinary tract obstruction
hematuria	Blood (*hemat*) in the urine (*uria*)	Kidney disease, urinary tract infection, trauma
nocturia	Frequent urination (*uria*) at night (*noct*)	Excessive fluid intake, kidney disease, disease of the prostate
oliguria	Scant amount (*olig*) of urine (*uria*), usually less than 500 mL in 24 hours	Inadequate fluid intake, shock, burns, kidney disease, heart failure
polyuria	The production of abnormally large amounts (*poly*) of urine (*uria*)	Medications, excessive fluid intake, diabetes, hormone imbalance
urinary frequency	Voiding at frequent intervals	Excessive fluid intake, bladder infections, pressure on the bladder, medications
urinary incontinence	Inability to control the loss of urine from the bladder	Trauma, disease, urinary tract infections, reproductive or urinary tract surgeries, aging, fecal impaction, constipation, not getting to the bathroom
urinary urgency	The need to void immediately	Urinary tract infection, fear of incontinence, full bladder, stress

Bedpans

Bedpans are used when people cannot be out of bed. Women use bedpans for voiding and bowel movements. Men use them only for bowel movements. Bedpans are made of plastic or stainless steel. Stainless steel bedpans are often cold. Warm the bedpan before use by holding it under warm tap water. Wipe it dry with a paper towel.

With your supervisor's permission, you can lightly dust the bedpan rim with talcum powder. When you remove the bedpan, it will not stick to the client's skin. Powder is not used if a urine specimen is needed. You may also want to protect the bed and linen by placing a waterproof or incontinence pad under the bedpan before use.

A *fracture pan* has a thinner rim and is only about 1 cm deep at one end (Figure 29-1). The smaller end is placed under the buttocks (Figure 29-2 on page 468). Fracture pans are used:

- By clients in casts
- By clients in traction
- By clients with limited back motion
- By clients with fragile bones or painful joints
- After a hip fracture

Follow medical asepsis and Standard Precautions when handling bedpans and their contents. Bedpans must be thoroughly cleaned after each use. Follow employer policy.

(text continues on page 471)

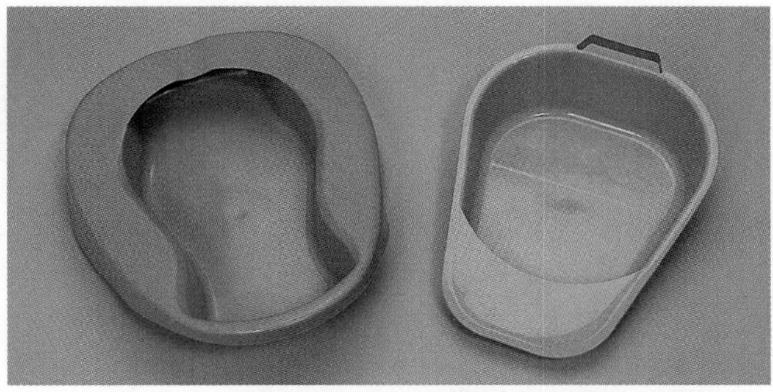

Figure 29-1 The regular bedpan and the fracture pan.

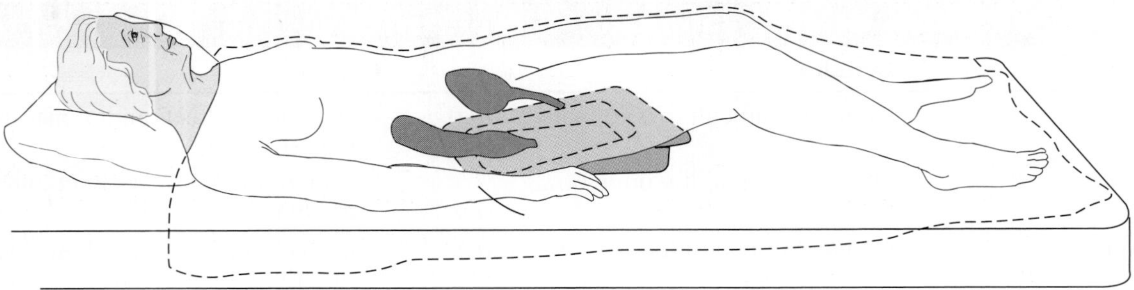

Figure 29-2 A client positioned on a fracture pan. The smaller end is placed under the buttocks.

Giving the Bedpan

Compassionate Care

Remember to Promote:
- **Dignity**
- **Independence**
- **Preferences**
- **Privacy**
- **Safety**

Pre-Procedure

1 Identify the person according to employer policy.
2 Explain the procedure to the person.
3 Provide for privacy.
4 Wash your hands. Put on gloves.
5 Collect the following:
- Bedpan
- Bedpan cover
- Toilet tissue
- Talcum powder (optional)
- Extra gloves

6 Arrange equipment on the chair or bed.

Procedure

7 Warm and dry the bedpan if necessary. Lightly dust the rim of the bedpan with talcum powder (optional).
8 Lower the bed rail near you if up.
9 Position the person supine. Raise the head of the bed slightly. Or, use pillows to raise the person's head and shoulders.
10 Fold the top linens and gown out of the way. Keep the lower body covered.
11 Ask the person to flex the knees and raise the buttocks by pushing against the mattress with the feet.
12 Slide your hand under the lower back, and help raise the buttocks.
13 Slide the bedpan under the person (Figure 29-3 on page 470).
14 If the person cannot assist in getting on the bedpan:
a Turn the person onto the side away from you.
b Place the bedpan firmly against the buttocks (Figure 29-4, *A* on page 470).
c Push the bedpan down and toward the person (Figure 29-4, *B* on page 470).
d Hold the bedpan securely. Turn the person onto the back.
e Make sure the bedpan is centred and under the person.
15 Cover the person.
16 Raise the head of the bed so the person is

Continued

Giving the Bedpan—cont'd

Procedure—cont'd

in a sitting position. If the bed is not adjustable, assist the person into a sitting position, using pillows for support.

17 Make sure the person is correctly positioned on the bedpan (Figure 29-5 on page 471).

18 Raise the bed rail if used.

19 Place the toilet tissue and call bell (in facilities) within reach.

20 Ask the person to call when done or when help is needed.

21 Remove gloves. Wash your hands.

22 Leave the room, and close the door.

23 Return when the person calls. Knock before entering.

24 Wash your hands. Put on gloves.

25 Raise the bed to a comfortable working height. Lower the bed rail (if used) and the head of the bed.* Or, remove the pillows and position the person supine.

26 Ask the person to raise the buttocks. Remove the bedpan. Or hold the bedpan securely and turn the person onto the side away from you.

27 Clean the genital area if the person cannot do so. Clean from the front (urethra) to back (anus) with toilet tissue. Use fresh tissue for each wipe. Provide perineal care if necessary.

28 Cover the bedpan. Take it to the bathroom. Lower the bed and raise the bed rail (if used) before leaving the bedside.

29 Note the colour, amount, and character of urine or stool.

30 Empty and rinse the bedpan with cold water. Clean it with a disinfectant.

31 Remove soiled gloves. Wash your hands. Put on clean gloves.

32 Put bedpan and cover away.

33 Help the person wash hands.

34 Remove gloves. Wash your hands.

Post-Procedure

35 Provide for safety and comfort.

36 Place the call bell within reach.*

37 Follow the care plan for bed rail use.*

38 Remove privacy measures.

39 Follow employer policy for soiled linen.

40 Wash your hands.

41 Report and record your actions and observations according to employer policy.

*Steps marked with an asterisk may not apply in community settings.

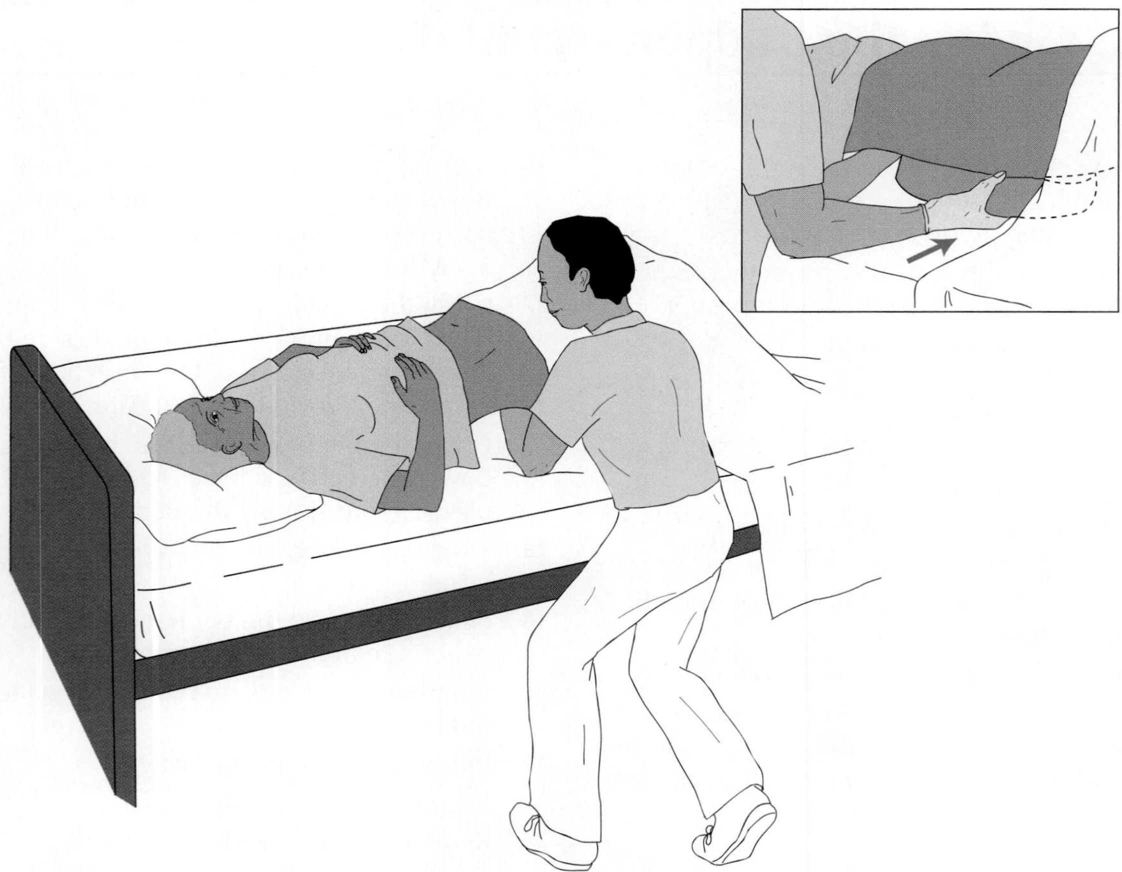

Figure 29-3 The client raises the buttocks off the bed with help. Slide the bedpan under the client.

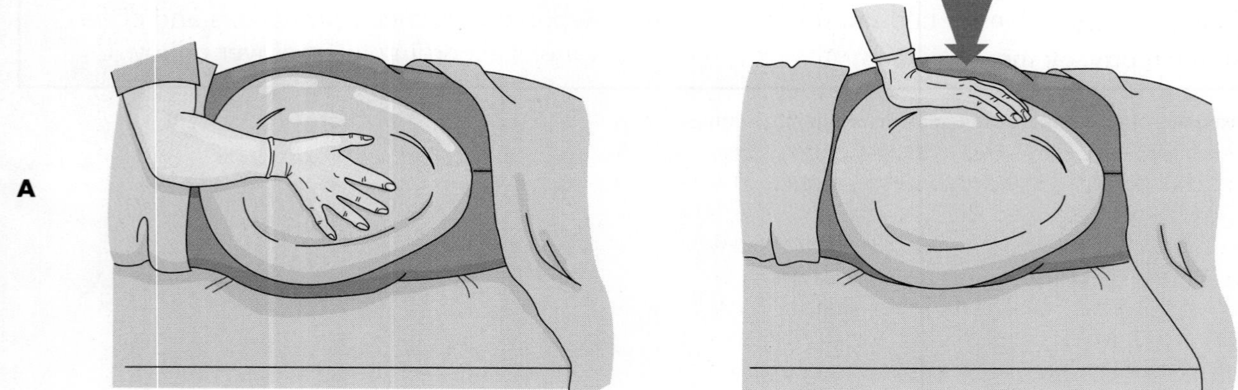

Figure 29-4 Giving a bedpan. **A,** Position the client on one side, and place the bedpan firmly against the buttocks. **B,** Push downward on the bedpan and toward the client.

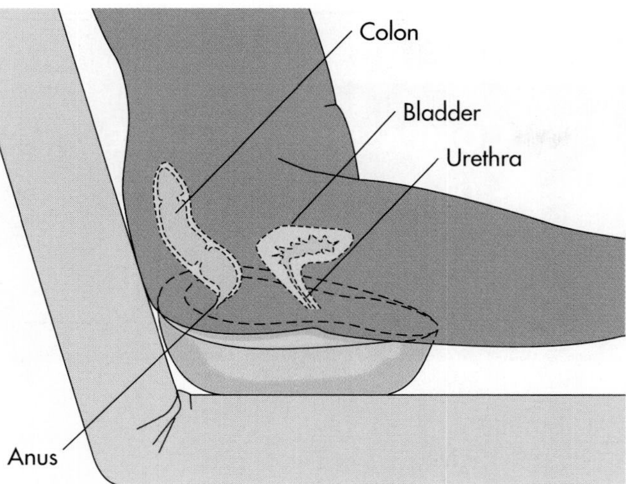

Figure 29-5 Position the client on the bedpan so the urethra and anus are directly over the opening.

URINALS

Men use urinals to void (Figure 29-6). Plastic urinals have caps at the top and hook-type handles. The urinal hooks to the bed rail, the back of a chair, or any place within the client's reach that is sturdy enough to support a filled urinal. Follow employer policy for where to place urinals.

The man stands to use the urinal if possible. Otherwise, he sits on the side of the bed or lies in bed. Some men stand with the support of one or two people. You may have to place and hold the urinal for some men.

Remind clients to cap the urinal after voiding. This prevents urine spills. Remind clients to hang used urinals on bed rails or the backs of chairs. They are to call you when urinals need emptying. Also remind them not to place urinals on bedside tables or stands. These are used as work areas, for eating, or for storing personal items. Table surfaces must not be contaminated with urine.

Follow medical asepsis and Standard Precautions when handling urinals and their contents. Empty urinals promptly to prevent odours and the spread of microbes. A filled urinal spills easily, causing safety hazards. Also, it may be embarrassing for the client to see the filled urinal sitting out. Urinals are cleaned like bedpans.

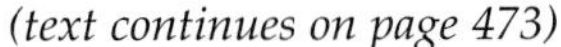
(text continues on page 473)

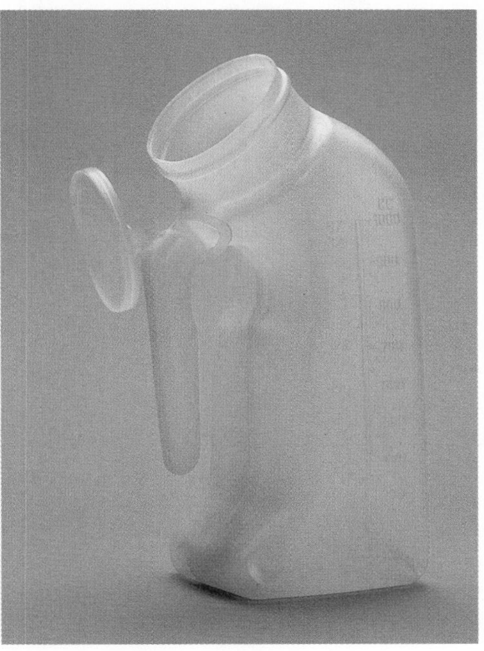

Figure 29-6 A urinal.

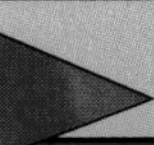

Giving the Urinal

Compassionate Care

Remember to Promote:
- **Dignity**
- **Independence**
- **Preferences**
- **Privacy**
- **Safety**

Pre-Procedure

1. Provide for privacy.
2. Determine if the person will stand, sit, or stay in bed.
3. Wash your hands. Put on gloves.

Procedure

4. Give the person the urinal if he is in bed. Remind him to tilt the bottom down to prevent spills.
5. If the person is going to stand:
   - **a** Help him sit on the side of the bed.
   - **b** Help him put on nonskid footwear.
   - **c** Help him stand. Provide support if he is unsteady.
   - **d** Give him the urinal.
6. Position the urinal if necessary. Position his penis in the urinal if he cannot do so.
7. Provide for privacy.
8. Place the call bell within reach.
9. Ask the person to call when done or when he needs help.
10. Remove gloves. Wash your hands.
11. Leave the room, and close the door.
12. Return when he calls for you. Knock before entering.
13. Wash your hands. Put on gloves.
14. Close the cap on the urinal. Take it to the bathroom.
15. Note the colour, amount, and character of the urine.
16. Empty the urinal, and rinse it with cold water. Clean it with disinfectant.
17. Return urinal to its proper place.
18. Remove gloves. Wash your hands. Put on clean gloves.
19. Help the person wash his hands.
20. Remove gloves. Wash your hands.

Post-Procedure

21. Provide for safety and comfort.
22. Place the call bell within reach.*
23. Follow the care plan for bed rail use.*
24. Remove privacy measures.
25. Follow employer policy for soiled linen.
26. Wash your hands.
27. Report and record your actions and observations according to employer policy.

*Steps marked with an asterisk may not apply in community settings.

Commodes

A commode is a portable chair or wheelchair with an opening for a bedpan or container (Figure 29-7). People unable to walk to the bathroom often use commodes. The commode allows a normal position for elimination. The commode arms and back provide support and help prevent falls. The bedpan or container is cleaned after use like the regular bedpan. Follow Standard Precautions.

Some commodes are wheeled into the bathroom and placed over the toilet. They provide privacy and safety for clients unable to walk to the bathroom. Such commodes are useful for clients who cannot sit unsupported on the toilet. The container is removed if the commode is used with the toilet. Make sure the commode wheels are locked and that the commode is positioned over the toilet.

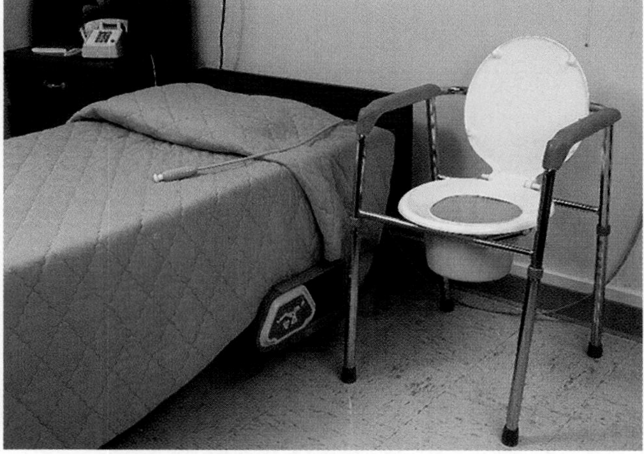

Figure 29-7 The bedside commode has a toilet seat with a container. The container slides out from under the toilet seat for emptying.

Helping the Person to the Commode

Compassionate Care

Remember to Promote:
- **Dignity**
- **Independence**
- **Preferences**
- **Privacy**
- **Safety**

Pre-Procedure

1 Explain the procedure to the person.
2 Provide for privacy.
3 Wash your hands. Put on gloves.
4 Collect the following:
- Commode
- Toilet tissue
- Bath blanket
- Extra gloves
- Transfer belt (optional)

Procedure

5 Bring the commode next to the bed. Remove the cushion and lift the container lid.
6 Help the person sit on the side of the bed.
7 Help the person put on a robe and nonskid footwear.
8 Assist the person to the commode. Use a transfer belt if necessary.
9 Cover the person with a bath blanket for warmth.
10 Place the call bell (in facilities) and toilet tissue within reach.
11 Ask the person to call when done or when help is needed. (Stay with the person if necessary. Be respectful. Provide as much privacy as possible.)
12 Remove gloves. Wash your hands.
13 Leave the room, and close the door.
14 Return when the person calls. Knock before entering.

Continued

Helping the Person to the Commode—cont'd

Procedure

15 Wash your hands. Put on gloves.
16 Help the person clean the genital area as needed. Remove gloves. Wash your hands.
17 Help the person back to the bed. Remove the robe and footwear. Follow the care plan for bed rail use.
18 Put on clean gloves. Remove and cover the commode container. Clean the commode.
19 Take the container to the bathroom.
20 Check urine and stool for colour, amount, and character.
21 Empty, then clean and disinfect the container.
22 Return the container to the commode. Return other supplies to their proper place.
23 Return the commode to its proper place.
24 Remove soiled gloves. Wash your hands. Put on clean gloves.
25 Help the person with hand washing.
26 Remove gloves. Wash your hands.

Post-Procedure

27 Provide for safety and comfort.
28 Place the call bell within reach.*
29 Follow the care plan for bed rail use.*
30 Remove privacy measures.
31 Follow employer policy for soiled linen.
32 Wash your hands.
33 Report and record your actions and observations according to employer policy.

*Steps marked with an asterisk may not apply in community settings.

URINARY INCONTINENCE

Urinary incontinence is the loss of bladder control. It may be temporary or permanent. There are different types of incontinence:

- **Stress incontinence**—the leaking of urine during exercise and certain movements. Urine loss is small (less than 50 mL). Often called *dribbling*, it occurs with laughing, sneezing, coughing, lifting, or other activities. Late pregnancy and obesity are other causes. The problem is common in women. Pelvic muscles weaken from pregnancies and with aging.
- **Urge incontinence**—the loss of urine in response to a sudden, urgent need to void. The person cannot get to a toilet in time. Urinary frequency, urinary urgency, and nighttime voidings are common. Causes include urinary tract infections, nervous system disorders, bladder cancer, and an enlarged prostate.
- **Overflow incontinence**—the leaking of urine when the bladder is too full. The person feels like the bladder is never completely empty. The person only dribbles or has a weak urine stream. Diabetes, enlarged prostate, and some medications are causes.
- **Functional incontinence**—the loss of urine that occurs when the person has bladder control but cannot use the toilet in time. Immobility, restraints, unanswered calls for help, lack of a call bell within reach, and not knowing where to find the bathroom are causes. So are confusion, disorientation, and difficulty removing clothing.
- **Reflex incontinence**—the loss of urine at predictable intervals. Urine is lost when the bladder is full. The person does not feel the need to void. Nervous system disorders and injuries are common causes.

Sometimes incontinence results from intestinal, rectal, and reproductive system surgeries. More than one type of incontinence can be present. This is called *mixed incontinence.*

Incontinence is embarrassing for the client. Clothing and linens get wet, and odours develop. The client is uncomfortable. Skin irritation, breakdown, and infection can occur. Falling is a risk for clients who rush to the bathroom. The client's pride, dignity, and self-esteem are affected. Some people avoid participating in activities, leaving the home, or visiting with others because they fear being incontinent in public. The client who is incontinent needs your support, understanding, and compassion.

Check with your supervisor and consult the care plan for the best ways to meet the client's needs. Care measures depend on the type of incontinence. The client's care plan may include some of the measures listed in Box 29-3. *Providing good skin care and dry garments and linens is essential.* Failing to do so is a form of neglect. Following the guidelines for normal urination prevents incontinence in some clients. Others need bladder training (page 487). Sometimes catheters are ordered.

A variety of incontinence products are available. The client selects products best suited to his or her needs. A nurse may provide advice if needed. Some clients use garment protectors or incontinence pads (Figure 29-8). Keeping skin and clothing clean and dry is important even when the client uses incontinence products. Check the products often for wetness. Change the products as needed following the manufacturer's instructions. Check the skin for signs of redness or rash.

Incontinence drawsheets keep bed linens dry. Placed over the bottom sheet, the drawsheet has two layers and a waterproof back. Fluid passes through the first layer and is absorbed by the lower layer. When the drawsheet becomes wet or soiled, change it and any damp linens. Do not place a dry drawsheet over wet bed linen to save time. This could be considered neglect.

Caring for people with incontinence is stressful. Family caregivers who cannot cope with incontinence often seek long-term care for the person. Professional caregivers also may find caring for these clients stressful. These clients may need frequent care and may wet again just after you changed wet garments and linens and gave skin care. Do not lose patience. Their needs are great, and your role is to meet their needs. If you find yourself short-tempered and impatient, discuss the problem with your supervisor immediately. Remember, the client has the right to be free from abuse, mistreatment, and neglect. The incontinence is beyond the client's control. It is not something he or she chooses to let happen. Kindness, empathy, understanding, and patience are very important.

Box 29-3 Care Measures for Clients with Urinary Incontinence

- Record the person's voidings. This includes incontinent episodes and successful use of the toilet, commode, bedpan, or urinal.
- Answer all calls for assistance promptly. The person may have an urgent need to void.
- Promote normal urinary elimination (see Box 29-2 on page 466).
- Promote normal bowel elimination (see Chapter 30).
- Encourage urination at scheduled intervals.
- Follow the person's bladder training program (page 487).
- Encourage the person to wear clothing that is easy to remove. Incontinence can occur as the person is trying to deal with buttons, zippers, and undergarments.
- Encourage the person to do pelvic muscle exercises as instructed by the care plan.
- Help prevent urinary tract infections:
  - Encourage adequate fluid intake as directed by the care plan.
  - Encourage the person to wear cotton undergarments.
  - Provide perineal care as needed (see Chapter 27). Keep the perineal area clean and dry.
- Decrease fluid intake before bedtime.
- Provide good skin care (see Chapter 27).
- Provide dry garments and linens.
- Observe for signs of skin breakdown (see Chapter 41).
- Use incontinence products as directed by the care plan. Follow manufacturer's instructions. Remove when wet.

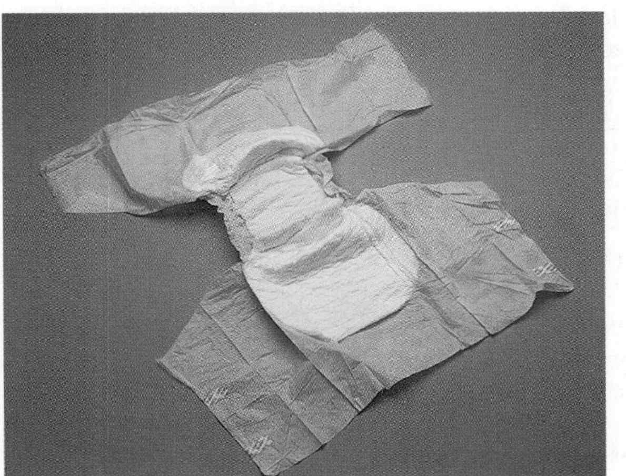
A

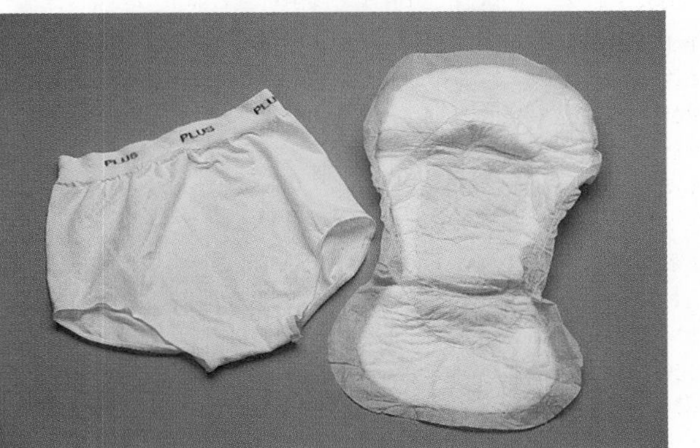

B

Figure 29-8 Garment protectors. **A,** Complete incontinence brief. **B,** Pant liner and undergarment.

CATHETERS

A **catheter** is a tube used to drain or inject fluid through a body opening. A *urinary catheter* is a tube inserted into the bladder to drain urine.

- A **straight catheter** drains the bladder and is removed. It is inserted through the urethra into the bladder.
- An **indwelling catheter** (**retention** or **Foley catheter**) is left in the bladder. Most indwelling catheters are inserted through the urethra into the bladder. Urine drains constantly into a drainage bag. A balloon near the tip is inflated after the catheter is inserted. The balloon prevents the catheter from slipping out of the bladder (Figure 29-9). Tubing connects the catheter to the drainage bag.
- A **suprapubic catheter** is a catheter that is surgically inserted into the bladder through the abdomen. It is inserted above the pubic bone. It is a type of indwelling catheter, meaning it is left in the bladder and is attached to a drainage bag by tubing. Suprapubic catheters may be used by people needing long-term catheterization or after some surgeries. The insertion site (the opening on the abdomen) and the tubing must be cleaned daily with soap and water and covered with dry gauze. Follow the care plan and your assignment sheet.

Catheter insertion (**catheterization**) is done by a nurse or physician. Catheters often are used before, during, and after surgery to keep the bladder empty. This reduces the risk of accidental bladder injury during surgery. After surgery, a full bladder causes pressure on nearby organs.

Catheters also allow hourly urinary output measurements in critically ill people. Catheters are a last resort for incontinence. Catheters do not treat the cause of incontinence, and the risk of infection is high. However, some people have wounds and pressure ulcers that need protection from urine. Catheters can protect the wounds and pressure ulcers from contamination with urine.

Some people are too weak or disabled to use the bedpan, commode, or toilet. Dying people are an example. For them, catheters can promote comfort. Also, the person is protected from incontinence.

Catheters also have diagnostic uses. They are used to collect sterile urine specimens. Another test involves inserting a catheter to see how much urine is left in the bladder (*residual urine*). The catheter is inserted after the person voids.

You will care for clients with indwelling catheters. Follow the guidelines listed in Box 29-4 to promote comfort and safety.

(text continues on page 480)

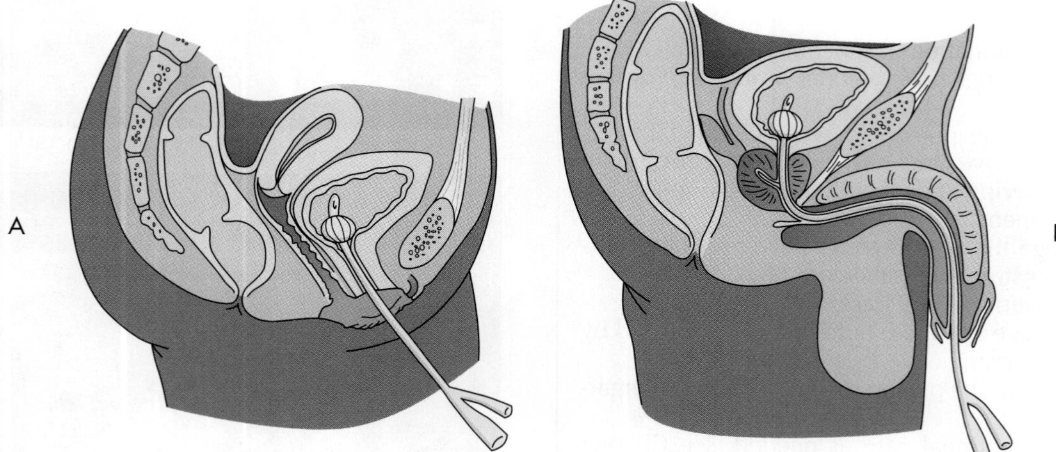

Figure 29-9 A, Indwelling catheter in the female bladder. The inflated balloon at the top prevents the catheter from slipping out through the urethra. **B,** Indwelling catheter with the balloon inflated in the male bladder.

Box 29-4 Guidelines for Caring for Clients with Indwelling Catheters

- Follow the rules of medical asepsis and Standard Precautions.
- Make sure urine flows freely through the catheter or tubing. Tubing should not have kinks. The client should not lie on the tubing.
- When the client is being moved, the catheter tube must remain slack, never taut or pulled.
- Make sure the catheter is connected to the drainage tubing. Follow the measures on page 480 if the catheter and drainage tube are disconnected.
- Keep the drainage bag below the bladder. This prevents urine from flowing backward into the bladder.
- Attach the drainage bag to the bed frame, to the back of a chair, or to the lower part of an IV pole. *Never attach the drainage bag to the bed rail.* Otherwise the drainage bag is higher than the bladder when the bed rail is raised.
- Move the drainage bag to the side of the bed to which the person will be turned. Move the drainage bag before turning the person.
- Do not let the drainage bag rest on the floor. This can contaminate the system.
- Coil the drainage tubing on the bed. Secure it to the bottom linen (Figure 29-10). Follow employer policy. Use a clip, tape, or a safety pin and rubber band. Tubing must not loop below the drainage bag.
- Secure the catheter to the inner thigh for women as in Figure 29-10, *A*. Or secure it to the abdomen for men (Figure 29-10, *B*). This prevents excessive movement of the catheter and reduces friction at the insertion site. Secure the catheter with tape or other devices as ordered by the care plan.
- Check for leaks. Check the site where the catheter connects to the drainage bag. Report any leaks immediately.
- Provide catheter care if ordered. Catheter care is done daily or twice a day. It includes cleaning the part of the tube that extends outside of the body. This helps to prevent bladder or urethra infections (see *Giving Catheter Care* on page 478). Some employers consider perineal care to be sufficient. Catheter care is sometimes needed after bowel movements and when there is vaginal drainage. Follow the care plan.
- Provide perineal care daily, after bowel movements, and when vaginal drainage is present. Follow the care plan.
- Empty the drainage bag at the end of the shift or at time intervals as directed by the care plan. Measure and record the amount of urine (see *Emptying a Urinary Drainage Bag* on page 483). Report increases or decreases in the amount of urine.
- Use a separate measuring container for each client. This prevents the spread of microbes from one client to another.
- Do not let the drain on the drainage bag touch any surface.
- Immediately report any complaints of pain, burning, need to urinate, or irritation. Also report the colour, clarity, and odour of urine and the presence of particles.
- Encourage fluid intake as instructed by the care plan.

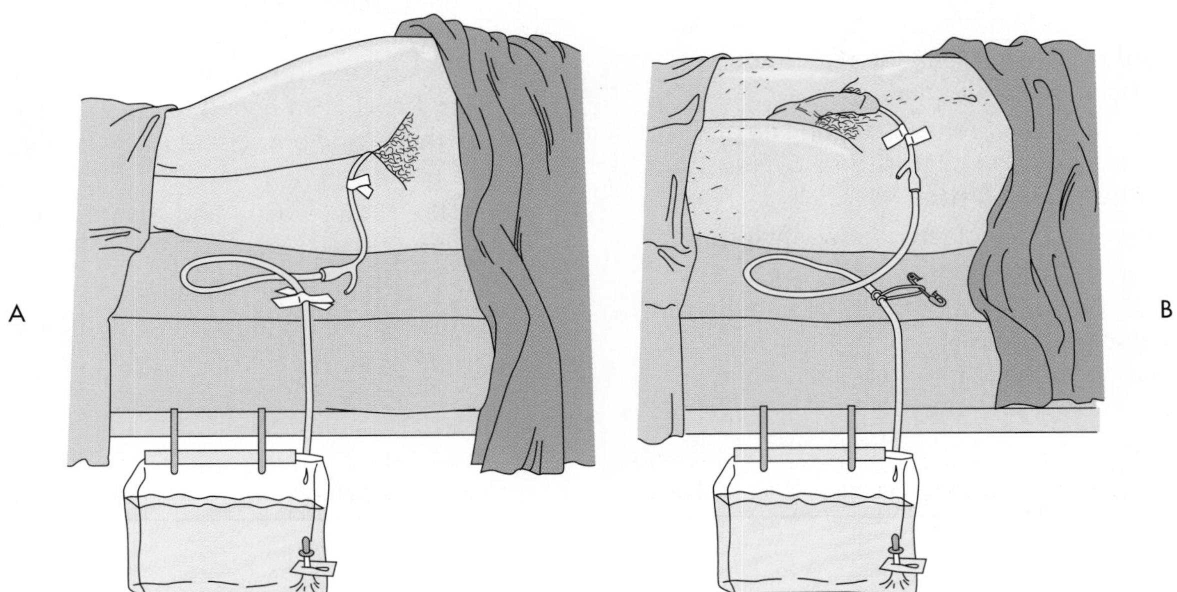

Figure 29-10 Securing catheters. **A,** The drainage tubing is coiled on the bed and secured to the bottom linens so urine flows freely. The catheter is taped to the inner thigh. Enough slack is left on the catheter to prevent friction at the urethra. **B,** The catheter is secured to the man's abdomen.

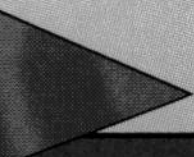

Giving Catheter Care

Compassionate Care

Remember to Promote:
- **Dignity**
- **Independence**
- **Preferences**
- **Privacy**
- **Safety**

Pre-Procedure

1 Identify the person according to employer policy.
2 Explain the procedure to the person.
3 Wash your hands.
4 Collect the following:
- Items for perineal care (page 428)
- Gloves
- Bed protector
- Bath blanket

5 Provide for privacy.
6 Raise bed to a comfortable working height. Follow the care plan for bed rail use.

Procedure

7 Lower the bed rail near you if up.
8 Put on gloves.
9 Cover the person with a bath blanket. Fanfold top linens to the foot of the bed.
10 Drape the person for perineal care (see Figure 27-26 on page 429).
11 Fold back the bath blanket to expose the genital area.
12 Place the bed protector under the buttocks. Ask the person to flex the knees and raise the buttocks off the bed.
13 Give perineal care (see *Giving Female Perineal Care* on page 428 or *Giving Male Perineal Care* on page 431).
14 Apply soap to a clean, wet washcloth.
15 Separate the labia (female) as in Figure 27-27 on page 430. Or retract the foreskin (uncircumcised male) as in Figure 27-29 on page 432. Check for crusts, abnormal drainage, or secretions.
16 Hold the catheter near the meatus (insertion point).
17 Clean the catheter from the meatus down the catheter about 10 cm (4 inches) (Figure 29-11). Clean downward, away from the meatus with one stroke. Do not tug or pull on the catheter. Repeat as needed with a clean area of the washcloth. Use a clean washcloth if needed.
18 Rinse the catheter. Rinse from the meatus down the catheter about 10 cm (4 inches). Rinse downward, away from the meatus with one stroke. Do not tug or pull on the catheter. Repeat as needed with a clean area of the washcloth. Use a clean washcloth if needed.
19 Secure the catheter. Coil and secure tubing (see Figure 29-10).
20 Remove the bed protector.
21 Cover the person. Remove the bath blanket.
22 Remove gloves. Wash your hands.

Continued

Giving Catheter Care—cont'd

Post-Procedure

23 Provide for safety and comfort.
24 Place the call bell within reach.*
25 Return the bed to its lowest position. Follow the care plan for bed rail use.*
26 Clean and return equipment to its proper place. Discard disposable items. (Wear gloves for this step.)
27 Remove privacy measures.
28 Follow employer policy for soiled linen.
29 Wash your hands.
30 Report and record your actions and observations according to employer policy.

*Steps marked with an asterisk may not apply in community settings.

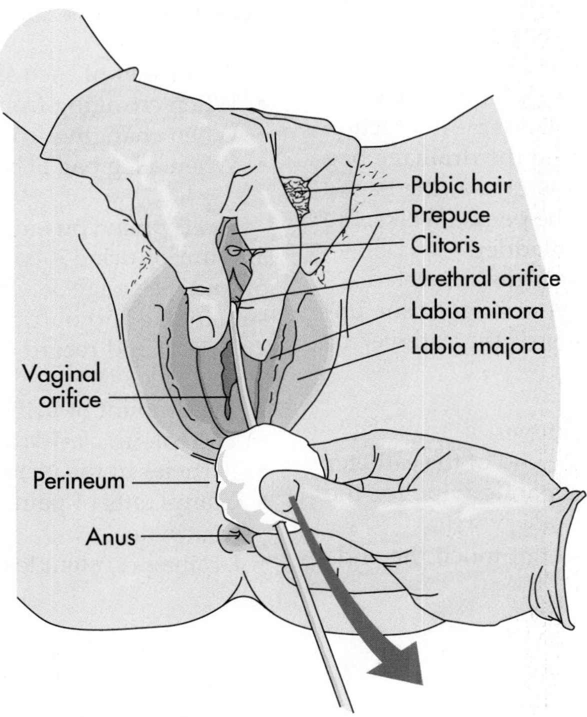

Figure 29-11 Hold the catheter near the meatus (insertion point). Clean the catheter starting at the meatus and moving down about 10 cm (4 inches).

Drainage Systems

A closed drainage system is used for indwelling catheters (including suprapubic catheters). Nothing can enter the system from the catheter to the drainage bag. The urinary system is sterile. Infection can occur if microbes enter the drainage system and travel up the tubing or catheter into the bladder and kidneys. A urinary tract infection can threaten health and life.

The drainage system consists of tubing and a drainage bag. Tubing attaches at one end to the catheter. At the other end, it attaches to the drainage bag.

The bag hangs from the bed frame, chair, or wheelchair. It must not touch the floor. The bag must always be lower than the client's bladder (see Figure 29-10 on page 477). Clients may be embarrassed if visitors can see the drainage bag. Carefully drape a bed sheet or robe over it when visitors are present. Some clients wear leg bags when up. The bag is attached to the thigh or calf (page 485). A pant leg or robe can cover it.

Urine provides an environment for the growth of microbes. If the drainage bag is higher than the bladder, urine can flow back into the bladder. An infection can develop. Therefore do not hang the drainage bag on a bed rail. When the bed rail is raised, the bag is higher than bladder level. When the person walks, the bag must be held lower than the bladder.

Sometimes drainage systems are disconnected accidentally. If that happens, tell your supervisor immediately. Do not touch the ends of the catheter or tubing. Do the following:

- Wash your hands, and put on gloves.
- Wipe the end of the tube and the end of the catheter with antiseptic wipes. Use a separate wipe for the tube end and catheter end.
- Do not put the ends down. Do not touch the ends after you clean them.
- Connect the tubing to the catheter.
- Discard the wipes into a biohazard plastic bag.
- Remove the gloves, and wash your hands.

Leg bags are switched to drainage bags when the client is in bed. This is so that the drainage bag is kept lower than bladder level. You will have to open the closed drainage system. You must prevent microbes from entering the system. Review the principles of surgical asepsis in Chapter 18.

Some employers do not allow support workers to change leg bags to drainage bags. The risk of infection is high. If you are delegated to change a leg bag to a drainage bag, make sure this procedure is in your job description. You must be formally trained, supervised, and monitored. Follow employer policy and procedures.

Drainage bags are emptied according to the care plan. Usually this occurs

- At the end of each shift
- When changing from a leg bag to a drainage bag
- When changing from a drainage bag to a leg bag
- When a leg bag is becoming full

Every time you empty a drainage bag, measure the amount of urine it contains. This is called measuring output. See page 383 for a description of how to measure intake and output (I&O).

Report and record the following:

- The amount of urine measured
- The colour, clarity, and odour of urine
- Particles in the urine
- Complaints of pain, burning, irritation, or the need to urinate
- Drainage system leaks

(text continues on page 485)

Changing a Leg Bag to a Drainage Bag

Compassionate Care

Remember to Promote:
- Dignity
- Independence
- Preferences
- Privacy
- Safety

Pre-Procedure

1 Identify the person according to employer policy.
2 Explain the procedure to the person.
3 Wash your hands.
4 Collect the following:
- Gloves
- Drainage bag and tubing
- Antiseptic wipes
- Bed protector
- Sterile cap and plug
- Catheter clamp
- Paper towels
- Bedpan
- Bath blanket

5 Arrange paper towels and equipment on the work area.
6 Provide for privacy.

Procedure

7 Have the person sit on the side of the bed.
8 Put on gloves.
9 Expose the catheter and leg bag.
10 Clamp the catheter (Figure 29-12 on page 482). This prevents urine from draining from the catheter into the drainage tubing.
11 Let urine drain from below the clamp site into the drainage tubing. This empties the lower end of the catheter.
12 Help the person lie down.
13 Raise the bed to a comfortable working height.*
14 Cover the person with a bath blanket. Expose the catheter and leg bag.
15 Place the bed protector under the leg.
16 Open the antiseptic wipes. Set them on the paper towels.
17 Open the package with the sterile cap and plug. Set the package on the paper towels. Do not let anything touch the sterile cap or plug (Figure 29-13 on page 483).
18 Open the package with the drainage bag and tubing.
19 Attach the drainage bag to the bed frame.
20 Disconnect the catheter from the drainage tubing. Do not let anything touch the ends.
21 Insert the sterile plug into the catheter end (Figure 29-14 on page 483). Touch only the end of the plug. Do not touch the part that goes inside the catheter. (If you contaminate the end of the catheter, wipe the end with an antiseptic wipe. Do so before you insert the sterile plug.)
22 Place the sterile cap on the end of the leg bag drainage tube (see Figure 29-14). (If you contaminate the tubing end, wipe it with an antiseptic wipe. Do so before you put on the sterile cap.)
23 Remove the cap from the new drainage tubing.
24 Remove the sterile plug from the catheter.
25 Insert the end for the drainage tubing into the catheter.

Continued

Changing a Leg Bag to a Drainage Bag—cont'd

Procedure—cont'd

26 Remove the clamp from the catheter.
27 Loop drainage tubing on the bed. Secure the tubing to the mattress.
28 Remove the leg bag. Place it in the bedpan.
29 Remove and discard the bed protector.
30 Cover the person. Remove the bath blanket.
31 Take the bedpan to the bathroom.
32 Remove gloves. Wash your hands.

Post-Procedure

33 Provide for safety and comfort.
34 Place the call bell within reach.*
35 Return the bed to its lowest position. Follow the care plan for bed rail use.*
36 Remove privacy measures.
37 Put on clean gloves. Discard disposable items.
38 Empty drainage bag (see *Emptying a Urinary Drainage Bag* on page 483).
39 Discard the drainage tubing and bag following employer policy. Or, clean the bag following employer policy.
40 Clean the bedpan. Place it in a clean cover.
41 Return the bedpan and other supplies to their proper place.
42 Remove gloves. Wash your hands.
43 Report and record your actions and observations according to employer policy.
44 Reverse the procedure to attach a leg bag to the catheter.

*Steps marked with an asterisk may not apply in community settings.

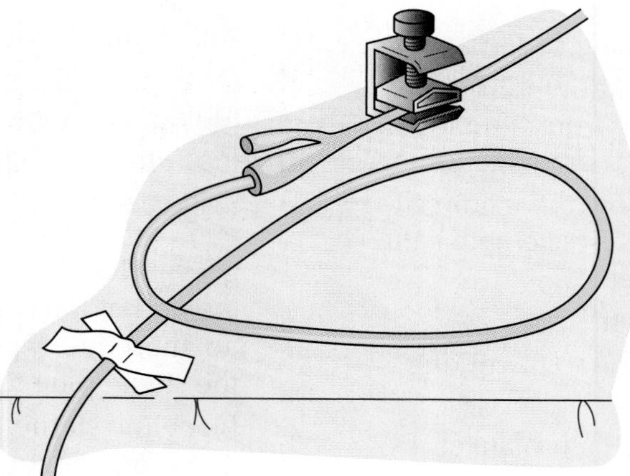

Figure 29-12 The catheter is clamped. The clamped catheter prevents urine from draining out of the bladder. The clamp is applied to the catheter, not to the drainage tubing.

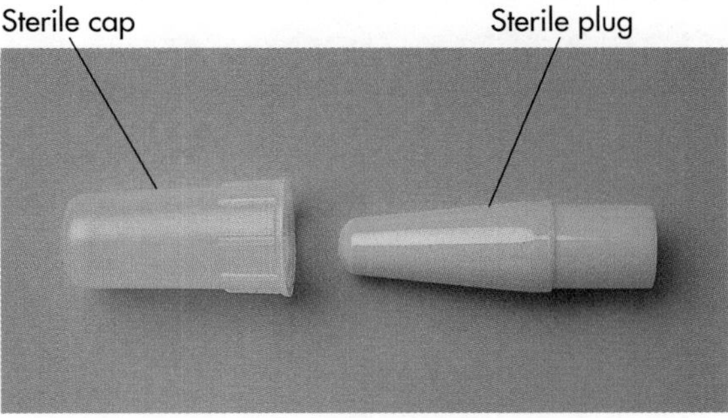

Figure 29-13 Sterile cap and catheter plug. The inside of the cap is sterile. It is inserted into the catheter. Touch only the end of the plug.

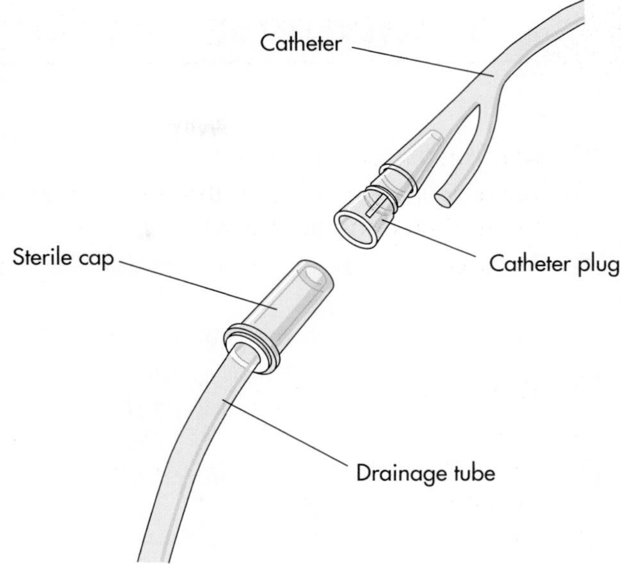

Figure 29-14 Sterile plug inserted into the end of the catheter. A sterile cap is on the end of the drainage tube.

Emptying a Urinary Drainage Bag

Compassionate Care

Remember to Promote:
- **Dignity**
- **Independence**
- **Preferences**
- **Privacy**
- **Safety**

Pre-Procedure

1. Identify the person according to employer policy.
2. Explain the procedure to the person.
3. Wash your hands.
4. Collect the following:
   - Graduate (measuring container)
   - Gloves
   - Paper towels
5. Provide for privacy.

Continued

Emptying a Urinary Drainage Bag—cont'd

Procedure

6 Put on gloves.

7 Place the paper towel on the floor. Place the graduate on top of the paper towel.

8 Position the graduate under the drainage bag drain.

9 Open the clamp on the drainage bag.

10 Let all urine drain into the graduate. Do not let the drain touch the graduate (Figure 29-15).

11 Close and position the clamp (see Figure 29-10 on page 477).

12 Measure urine.

13 Remove and discard the paper towel.

14 Dispose of the urine in the toilet.

15 Rinse the graduate and dispose of the graduate rinse in the toilet.

16 Return the graduate to its proper place.

17 Remove gloves. Wash your hands.

18 Record the time and amount on the intake and output (I&O) record (see Chapter 25).

Post-Procedure

19 Remove privacy measures.

20 Report and record the amount and other observations (Figure 29-16). Follow employer policy.

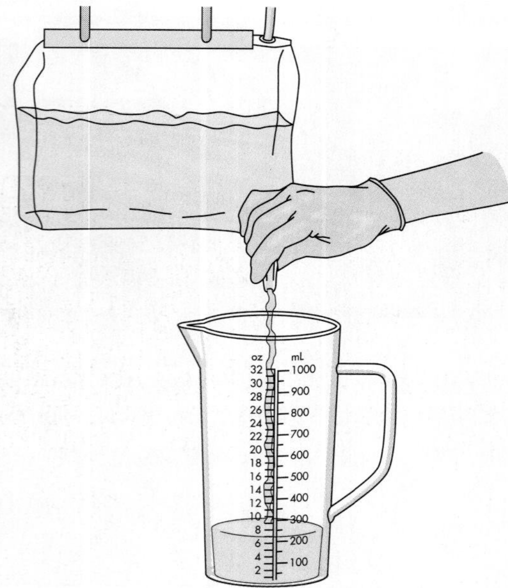

Figure 29-15 Open the clamp on the drainage bag, and direct the drain into the measuring container. The drain must not touch the inside of the container.

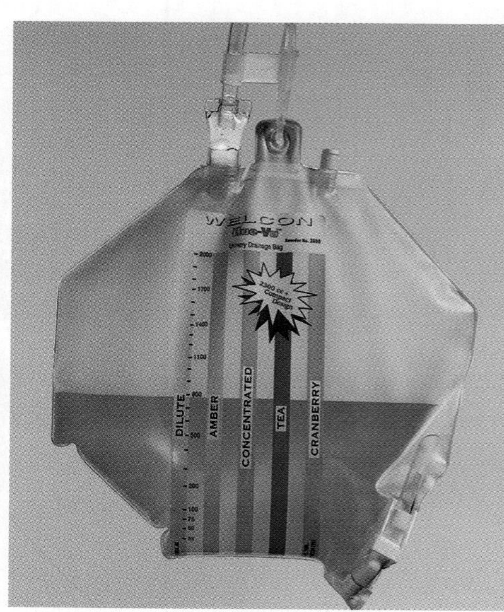

Figure 29-16 This urinary drainage bag has a comparison chart for the urine colour. *(Courtesy of Welcon, Inc., Fort Worth, TX.)*

The Condom Catheter

Condom catheters are often used for incontinent men. They are also called *external catheters* and *urinary sheaths*. A **condom catheter** is a soft sheath that slides over the penis. Tubing connects the condom catheter and the drainage bag. Many men use leg bags (Figure 29-17).

To apply a condom catheter, follow the manufacturer's instructions. Thoroughly wash the penis with soap and water. Then dry it before applying the condom catheter. A new condom catheter is usually applied daily or every few days. Follow the care plan.

Elastic tape secures the catheter in place. Use the elastic tape packaged with the condom catheter. Elastic tape expands when the penis changes size. This allows blood flow to the penis. *Never use adhesive tape to secure condom catheters. Adhesive tape does not expand. Blood flow to the penis would be cut off, injuring the penis.* Follow medical asepsis and Standard Precautions when removing and applying condom catheters.

Report and record the following:

- Reddened or open areas on the penis
- Swelling of the penis
- Colour, clarity, and odour of urine
- Particles in the urine

(text continues on page 487)

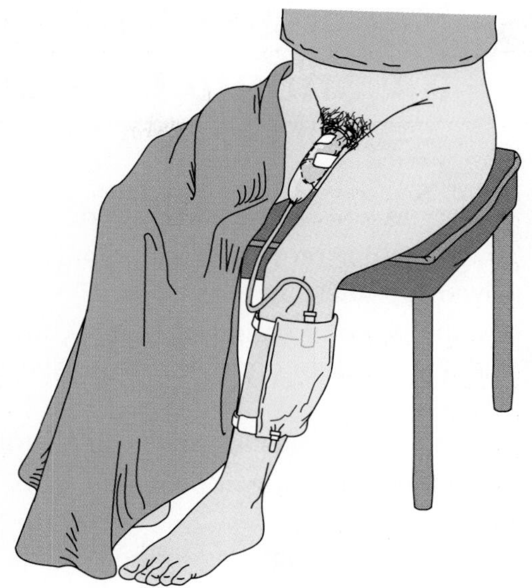

Figure 29-17 A condom catheter attached to a leg bag.

Removing and Applying a Condom Catheter

Compassionate Care

Remember to Promote:

- **Dignity**
- **Independence**
- **Preferences**
- **Privacy**
- **Safety**

Pre-Procedure

1 Identify the person according to employer policy.
2 Explain the procedure to the person.
3 Wash your hands.
4 Collect the following:
  - Condom catheter
  - Elastic tape
  - Drainage bag or leg bag
  - Cap for the drainage bag
  - Basin of warm water
  - Soap
  - Towel and washcloths
  - Bath blanket
  - Gloves
  - Bed protector
  - Paper towels
5 Place paper towels on the work area. Arrange equipment on top of the paper towels.
6 Provide for privacy.
7 Raise the bed to a comfortable working height. Follow the care plan for bed rail use.*

Continued

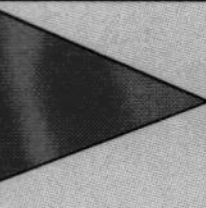

Removing and Applying a Condom Catheter—cont'd

Procedure

8 Lower the bed rail near you if up.
9 Cover the person with a bath blanket. Lower top linens to the knees.
10 Ask the person to raise his buttocks off the bed. Or turn him onto his side away from you.
11 Slide the bed protector under his buttocks.
12 Have the person lower his buttocks, or turn him onto his back.
13 Secure the drainage bag to the bed frame, or have a leg bag ready. Close the drain.
14 Expose the genital area.
15 Put on gloves.
16 Remove the condom catheter:
  a Remove the tape. Roll the sheath off the penis.
  b Disconnect the drainage tubing from the condom. Cap the drainage tube.
  c Discard the tape and condom.
17 Provide perineal care (see *Giving Male Perineal Care* on page 431). Observe the penis for skin breakdown or irritation.
18 Remove the protective backing from the condom. This exposes the adhesive strip.
19 Hold the penis firmly. Roll the condom onto the penis. Leave a 2.5 cm (1 inch) space between the penis and the catheter end (Figure 29-18).
20 Secure the condom with elastic tape. Apply tape in a spiral (see Figure 29-18). Do not apply tape completely around the penis.
21 Connect the condom to the drainage tubing. Coil excess tubing on the bed (see Figure 29-10 on page 477). Or attach a leg bag.
22 Remove the bed protector.
23 Remove gloves. Wash your hands.
24 Cover the person. Remove the bath blanket.

Post-Procedure

25 Provide for safety and comfort.
26 Place the call bell within reach.*
27 Return the bed to its lowest position. Follow the care plan for bed rail use.*
28 Remove privacy measures.
29 Wash your hands. Put on clean gloves.
30 Measure and record the amount of urine in the bag. Clean or discard the drainage bag.
31 Discard disposable items.
32 Clean and return the washbasin and other equipment. Return items to their proper place.
33 Remove gloves. Wash your hands.
34 Report and record your actions and observations according to employer policy.

*Steps marked with an asterisk may not apply in community settings.

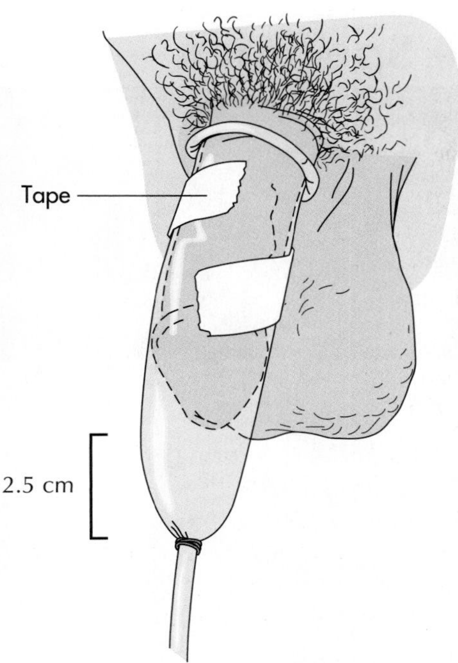

Figure 29-18 A condom catheter applied to the penis. There is a 2.5 cm (1 inch) space between the penis and the end of the catheter. Apply tape in a spiral fashion to secure the condom catheter to the penis.

Bladder Training

Bladder training programs are developed for people with urinary incontinence. Some people need bladder training after indwelling catheter removal. Voluntary control of urination is the goal. The bladder training program is part of the care plan. You assist with bladder training as directed by your supervisor and the care plan.

There are two basic methods for bladder training:

- The client uses the toilet, commode, bedpan, or urinal at scheduled times. The client is given 15 or 20 minutes to start voiding. The guidelines for maintaining normal urination are followed. The normal position for voiding is assumed if possible. Privacy is important. Help the client relax and provide encouragement. This can help the client succeed.
- The client has a catheter. The catheter is clamped to prevent urine from draining out of the bladder (see Figure 29-12 on page 482). Usually the catheter is clamped for 1 hour at first. Eventually it is clamped for 3 to 4 hours at a time. Urine drains from the bladder when the catheter is unclamped. When the catheter is removed, voiding is encouraged every 3 to 4 hours or as directed by your supervisor and the care plan.

Collecting Urine Specimens

Urine specimens (samples) are collected for urine tests. Physicians use test results to make a diagnosis or evaluate treatment. Follow the guidelines in Box 29-5 when collecting specimens.

The Random Urine Specimen

The random urine specimen is collected for a urinalysis. No special measures are needed. It is collected at any time. Many clients can collect the specimen themselves. Weak and very ill clients need assistance.

(text continues on page 489)

Box 29-5 Guidelines for Collecting Urine Specimens

- Follow the rules of medical asepsis and Standard Precautions. Wear gloves when collecting specimens.
- Use a clean container for each specimen.
- Use a container appropriate for the specimen.
- Label the container accurately. Write the client's full name, address or room and bed number, date, and time the specimen was collected. If preprinted labels are used, place a label on the container.
- Do not touch the inside of the container or lid.
- Collect the specimen at the time specified.
- Ask the client not to have a bowel movement during specimen collection. The specimen must not contain feces.
- Ask the client to put used toilet tissue in the toilet. The specimen must not contain tissue.
- Put the lid on the specimen container.
- Place the specimen container in a plastic bag for transportation. In a facility, take the specimen and requisition slip to the laboratory or storage area. In community settings, follow your supervisor's instructions for storing the specimen. Tell the client or family members where the specimen is stored. Follow your supervisor's instructions for sending the specimen to the laboratory.
- Report and record the following observations:
  - Difficulty in obtaining the specimen
  - Colour, clarity, and odour of urine
  - Particles in the urine
  - Complaints of pain, burning, urgency, dysuria, or other problems

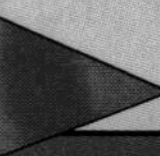

Collecting a Random Urine Specimen

Compassionate Care

Remember to Promote:
- **Dignity**
- **Independence**
- **Preferences**
- **Privacy**
- **Safety**

Pre-Procedure

1 Identify the person according to employer policy.
2 Explain the procedure to the person.
3 Wash your hands.
4 Collect the following:
- Bedpan and cover, urinal, or specimen pan (Figure 29-19)
- Specimen container and lid
- Label
- Gloves
- Plastic bag

Procedure

5 Label the container.
6 Put the container and lid in the bathroom.
7 Provide for privacy.
8 Put on gloves.
9 Ask the person to urinate in the receptacle (the bedpan, urinal, or specimen pan). Remind him or her to put toilet tissue into the wastebasket or toilet, not in the bedpan or specimen pan.
10 Take the receptacle to the bathroom.
11 Measure urine if intake and output (I&O) is ordered.
12 Pour about 120 mL (4 oz) of urine into the specimen container. Dispose of excess urine.
13 Place the lid on the specimen container. Put the container in the plastic bag.
14 Clean and return the receptacle to its proper place.
15 Help the person with hand washing.
16 Remove gloves. Wash your hands.

Post-Procedure

17 Provide for safety and comfort.
18 Place the call bell within reach.*
19 Follow the care plan for bed rail use.*
20 Remove privacy measures.
21 Wash your hands.
22 Report and record your actions and observations according to employer policy.
23 Follow your supervisor's instructions for storage and transportation of the specimen.

*Steps marked with an asterisk may not apply in community settings.

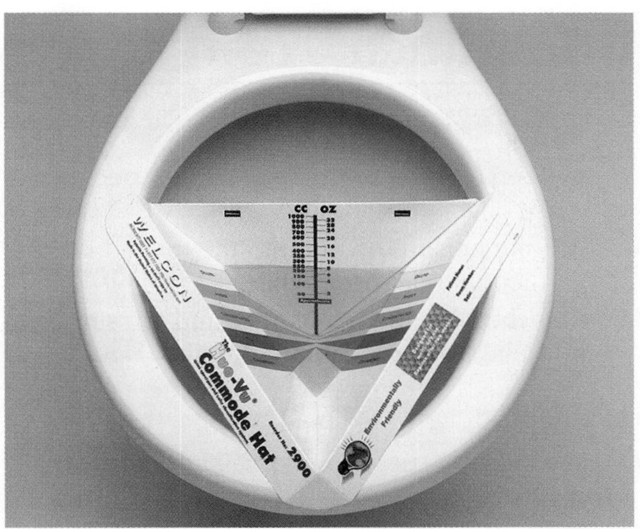

Figure 29-19 The specimen pan is placed on the rim of the toilet. It has a colour chart for urine. *(Courtesy Welcon, Inc., Fort Worth, TX.)*

THE MIDSTREAM SPECIMEN

The midstream specimen is also called a *clean-voided specimen* or a *clean-catch specimen.* The perineal area is cleaned before collecting the specimen. This reduces the number of microbes in the urethral area. The client starts to void into the toilet, bedpan, urinal, or commode. Then the stream is stopped and a sterile specimen container is positioned. The client voids into the container until the specimen is obtained.

Stopping the stream of urine is hard for many people. You may need to position and hold the specimen container in place after the client starts to void.

(text continues on page 491)

Collecting a Midstream Specimen

COMPASSIONATE CARE

Remember to Promote:
- **Dignity**
- **Independence**
- **Preferences**
- **Privacy**
- **Safety**

Pre-Procedure

1 Identify the person according to employer policy.
2 Explain the procedure to the person.
3 Wash your hands.
4 Collect the following:
- Clean-voided specimen kit (with antiseptic solution)
- Label
- Disposable gloves
- Sterile gloves (if not in the kit)
- Bedpan, urinal, or commode if needed
- Plastic bag
- Supplies for perineal care

5 Provide for privacy.

Continued

Collecting a Midstream Specimen—cont'd

Procedure

6 Label the container.

7 Provide perineal care. Wear gloves for this step. Remove gloves. Wash your hands.

8 Open the sterile kit. Use sterile technique (see Chapter 18).

9 Put on the sterile gloves.

10 Pour the antiseptic solution over the cotton balls.

11 Open the sterile specimen container. Do not touch the inside of the container or lid. Set the lid down so the inside is up.

12 *For a female:* clean the perineum with cotton balls:

- **a** Spread the labia with your thumb and index finger. Use your non-dominant hand. (This hand is now contaminated. It must not touch anything sterile.)
- **b** Clean down the urethral area from front to back. Use a clean cotton ball for each stroke.
- **c** Keep the labia separated to collect the urine specimen (steps 14 to 17).

13 *For a male:* clean the penis with cotton balls:

- **a** Hold the penis with your non-dominant hand. (This hand is now contaminated. It must not touch anything sterile.)
- **b** Clean the penis starting at the urethral opening. Use a cotton ball and clean in a circular motion.
- **c** Keep holding the penis until the specimen is collected (steps 14 to 17).

14 Ask the person to void into the toilet, bedpan, commode, or urinal.

15 Pass the specimen container into the stream of urine. Keep the labia separated (Figure 29-20).

16 Collect about 30 to 60 mL of urine (1 to 2 oz).

17 Remove the specimen container before the person stops voiding.

18 Release the labia or penis.

19 Let the person finish voiding into the toilet, bedpan, commode, or urinal.

20 Put the lid on the specimen container. Touch only the outside of the container or lid.

21 Wipe the outside of the container.

22 Place the container in a plastic bag.

23 Provide toilet tissue after the person finishes voiding.

24 Remove and empty the bedpan, commode container, or urinal.

25 Clean the bedpan, urinal, or commode container and other items. Return equipment to its proper place.

26 Remove gloves. Wash your hands.

27 Put on clean gloves.

28 Help the person with hand washing.

29 Remove gloves. Wash your hands.

Post-Procedure

30 Follow steps 17-23 in *Collecting a Random Urine Specimen* on page 488.

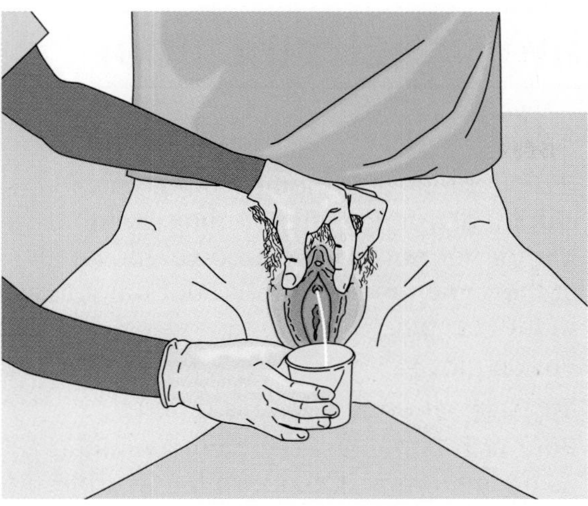

Figure 29-20 The labia are separated to collect a midstream specimen.

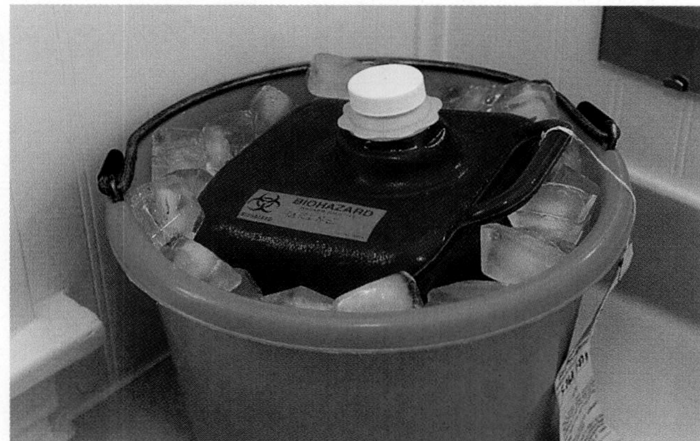

Figure 29-21 For the 24-hour urine specimen, the urine container may be stored in a bucket of ice.

The 24-Hour Urine Specimen

All urine voided during a 24-hour period is collected for a 24-hour urine specimen. Urine is chilled on ice or refrigerated during the collection period (Figure 29-21). This prevents the growth of microbes. A preservative is added to the collection container for some tests.

The client voids to begin the test; this voiding is discarded. *All* voidings during the next 24 hours are collected. The client and staff must clearly understand the procedure and test period. In home care settings, the client and primary caregiver need to collect some of the specimen on their own. Make sure they understand what to do. Contact your supervisor if they are unsure. Follow the guidelines for collecting urine specimens.

Collecting a 24-Hour Urine Specimen

Compassionate Care

Remember to Promote:
- **Dignity**
- **Independence**
- **Preferences**
- **Privacy**
- **Safety**

Pre-Procedure

1 Identify the person according to employer policy.
2 Explain the procedure to the person.
3 Wash your hands.
4 Collect the following:
   - 24-hour urine container (with preservative if needed)
   - Bucket with ice if needed
   - Two 24-hour urine specimen labels
   - Funnel
   - Bedpan, urinal, commode, or specimen pan
   - Gloves
   - Measuring container

Continued

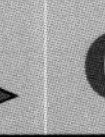

Collecting a 24-Hour Urine Specimen—cont'd

Procedure

5 Label the specimen container.
6 Arrange equipment in the person's bathroom.
7 Place one 24-hour specimen label in the bathroom. Place the other near the bed.
8 Put on gloves.
9 Offer the bedpan or urinal. Or, assist the person to the bathroom or commode.
10 Ask the person to void.
11 Discard the specimen, and note the time. This starts the 24-hour collection period.
12 Clean the bedpan, urinal, commode, or specimen pan.
13 Remove gloves. Wash your hands.
14 Mark the time the test began and the time it ends on the room and bathroom labels. Also mark the specimen container.
15 Ask the person to use the bedpan, urinal, commode, or specimen pan when voiding during the next 24 hours. Tell the person to call for assistance after voiding. Remind him or her not to have a bowel movement at the same time and not to put toilet tissue in the receptacle.
16 Put on gloves.
17 Measure all urine if I&O is ordered.
18 Pour urine into the specimen container, using the funnel. Do not spill any urine. Restart the test if you spill or discard urine. Store the specimen container in a refrigerator or in a bucket filled with ice.
19 Clean the bedpan, urinal, commode, or specimen pan. Remove gloves. Wash your hands.
20 Add ice to the bucket as necessary.
21 Ask the person to void at the end of the 24-hour period. Pour the urine into the specimen container. Wear gloves for this step.

Post-Procedure

22 Provide for safety and comfort.
23 Place the call bell within reach.*
24 Follow the care plan for bed rail use.*
25 Remove the labels from the room and bathroom.
26 Clean and return equipment to its proper place. Discard disposable items. (Wear gloves for this step.)
27 Remove gloves. Wash your hands.
28 Report and record your actions and observations according to employer policy.
29 Follow your supervisor's instructions for storage and transportation of the specimen.

*Steps marked with an asterisk may not apply in community settings.

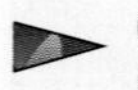

Collecting a Specimen from an Infant or Child

Sometimes specimens are needed from infants and children who are not toilet trained. A collection bag is applied over the urethra. A parent or another staff member assists if the child is agitated. This procedure may also be adapted for clients who are in wheelchairs or who are incontinent.

(text continues on page 494)

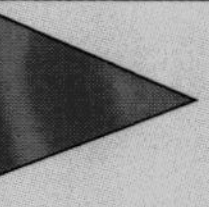

Collecting a Urine Specimen from an Infant or Child

Compassionate Care

Remember to Promote:
- **Dignity**
- **Independence**
- **Preferences**
- **Privacy**
- **Safety**

Pre-Procedure

1 Identify the child according to employer policy.
2 Explain the procedure to the child and parents.
3 Wash your hands.
4 Collect the following:
- Collection bag
- Washbasin
- Cotton balls
- Bath towel
- Two diapers
- Specimen container
- Gloves
- Plastic bag
- Scissors

5 Provide for privacy.

Procedure

6 Remove and dispose of the diaper.
7 Clean the perineal area. Use a new cotton ball for each stroke. Rinse and dry the area.
8 Wash your hands.
9 Position the child on the back. Flex the child's knees, and separate the legs.
10 Remove the adhesive backing from the collection bag.
11 Apply the bag to the perineum. Do not cover the anus (Figure 29-22 on page 494).
12 Cut a slit in the bottom of a new diaper.
13 Diaper the child.
14 Pull the collection bag through the slit in the bottom of the diaper.
15 Wash your hands.
16 Raise the head of the crib if allowed. This helps urine to collect in the bottom of the bag.
17 Raise the crib rail.
18 Return to the room periodically. Check the bag to see if the child has voided. (Wear gloves, and provide for privacy.)
19 Provide privacy if the child has urinated.
20 Put on gloves.
21 Lower the crib rail.
22 Remove the diaper.
23 Remove the collection bag gently.
24 Press the adhesive surfaces of the bag together. Or transfer urine to the specimen container through the drainage tab.
25 Clean the perineal area, rinse, and dry well.
26 Diaper the child.
27 Remove gloves. Wash your hands.

Continued

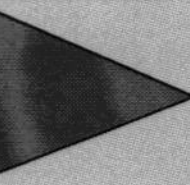

Collecting a Urine Specimen from an Infant or Child—cont'd

Post-Procedure

28 Provide for safety and comfort. Raise the crib rail.

29 Remove privacy measures.

30 Write the requested information on the specimen container. Place the container in the plastic bag.

31 Clean and return equipment to its proper place. Discard disposable items. (Wear gloves for this step.)

32 Wash your hands.

33 Report and record your actions and observations according to employer policy.

34 Follow your supervisor's instructions for storage and transportation of the specimen.

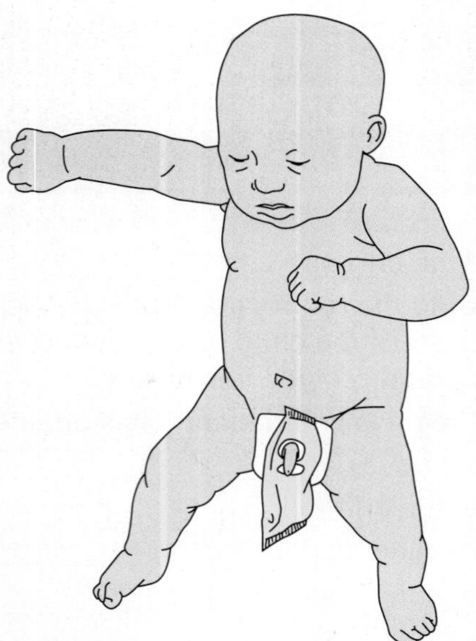

Figure 29-22 A disposable collection bag is applied to the perineal area of the infant. Urine collects in the bag for a specimen.

TESTING URINE

You may be asked to do simple urine tests. You can test for pH, glucose, ketones, and blood using reagent strips. Straining urine for stones is another simple test. A physician orders the type and frequency of urine tests. You must be accurate when testing urine. Promptly report the results according to employer policy.

- *Testing pH*—Urine pH measures if urine is acidic or alkaline. Changes in normal pH (4.6 to 8.0) occur from illness, foods, and medications. A routine urine specimen is needed.
- *Testing for glucose and ketones*—In diabetes, the pancreas does not secrete enough insulin (see Chapter 31). The body needs insulin to use sugar for energy. If not used, sugar builds up in the blood. Some sugar appears in the urine. **Glucosuria** or **glycosuria** means sugar (*glucos, glycos*) in the urine (*uria*). The diabetic person may also have **acetone (ketone bodies)** in the urine. These appear in urine because of the rapid breakdown of fat for energy. The body uses fat for energy if it cannot use sugar. Urine is also tested for ketones. These tests are usually done four times a day: 30 minutes before each meal (ac) and at bedtime (hs). The physician uses the test results to regulate the person's medication and diet.
- *Testing for blood*—Normal urine is free of blood. Injury and disease can cause blood (*hemat*) to appear in the urine (*uria*). This is called **hematuria.** Sometimes blood is seen in the urine. At other times it is unseen (*occult*). A routine urine specimen is needed.

Using Reagent Strips

Reagent strips are chemically treated "dipsticks." They have different sections that change colour when they react with urine. To use a reagent strip, dip the strip into urine. Then compare the strip with the colour chart on the bottle (Figure 29-23). Instructions vary depending on the test. Your supervisor tells you how to do the urine test ordered. You must read the manufacturer's instructions before you begin. Always check the date on the container. Do not use if it is expired.

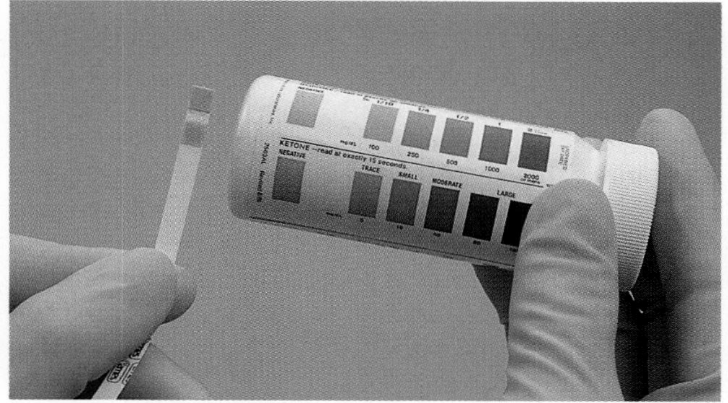

Figure 29-23 Reagent strip for sugar and ketones.

Testing Urine with Reagent Strips

Compassionate Care

Remember to Promote:
- **Dignity**
- **Independence**
- **Preferences**
- **Privacy**
- **Safety**

Pre-Procedure

1 Identify the person according to employer policy.
2 Explain the procedure to the person.
3 Wash your hands.
4 Put on gloves.
5 Collect the following:
- Urine specimen (check with your supervisor for method to obtain)
- Reagent strip as ordered
- Gloves

Procedure

6 Remove a strip from the bottle. Recap the bottle immediately. The cap must be on tight.
7 Dip the reagent strip into the specimen.
8 Remove the strip after the correct amount of time (see manufacturer's instructions).
9 Tap the strip gently against the container to remove excess urine.
10 Wait the required amount of time (see manufacturer's instructions).
11 Compare the strip with the colour chart on the bottle. Read the results.
12 Discard disposable items and the specimen.

Post-Procedure

13 Clean and return equipment to its proper place.
14 Remove gloves. Wash your hands.
15 Report and record the results and other observations according to employer policy.

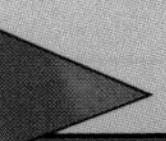

Straining Urine

Stones (*calculi*) can develop in the kidneys, ureters, or bladder. Stones vary in size. Some are pinhead size; others are the size of an orange. Stones causing severe pain and damage to the urinary system may require surgical removal. Some stones exit the body through urine. When the care plan calls for the client's urine to be strained, all the urine is poured through a disposable strainer. If any stones are found, they are sent to the laboratory for examination.

(text continues on page 498)

Straining Urine

Compassionate Care

Remember to Promote:
- **Dignity**
- **Independence**
- **Preferences**
- **Privacy**
- **Safety**

Pre-Procedure

1. Identify the person according to employer policy.
2. Explain the procedure to the person. Also explain that the urinal, bedpan, commode, or specimen pan is used for voiding.
3. Wash your hands.
4. Collect the following:
   - Strainer or 4 × 4 gauze
   - Specimen container
   - Urinal, bedpan, commode, or specimen pan
   - Two labels stating that all urine is strained
   - Gloves
   - Plastic bag

Procedure

5. Arrange items in the person's bathroom. Place the specimen pan in the toilet.
6. Place one label in the bathroom. Place the other near the bed.
7. Put on gloves.
8. Offer the bedpan or urinal. Or assist the person to the bedside commode or bathroom.
9. Provide for privacy.
10. Tell the person to call after voiding.
11. Remove gloves. Wash your hands.
12. Return when the person calls for you. Knock before entering the room.
13. Wash your hands. Put on gloves.
14. Place the strainer or gauze over the specimen container.
15. Pour urine into the specimen container. Urine passes through the strainer or gauze (Figure 29-24).
16. Discard the urine.
17. Place the strainer or gauze in the container if any crystals, stones, or particles appear.
18. Provide perineal care if needed.
19. Clean and return equipment to its proper place.
20. Remove soiled gloves. Wash your hands. Put on clean gloves.
21. Help the person with hand washing.
22. Remove gloves. Wash your hands.

Continued

Straining Urine—cont'd

Post-Procedure

23 Provide for safety and comfort.

24 Place the call bell within reach.*

25 Follow the care plan for bed rail use.*

26 Remove privacy measures.

27 Label the specimen container with the requested information. Put the container in the plastic bag. (Wear gloves for this step.)

28 Wash your hands.

29 Report and record your actions and observations according to employer policy.

30 Follow your supervisor's instructions for storage and transportation of the specimen.

*Steps marked with an asterisk may not apply in community settings.

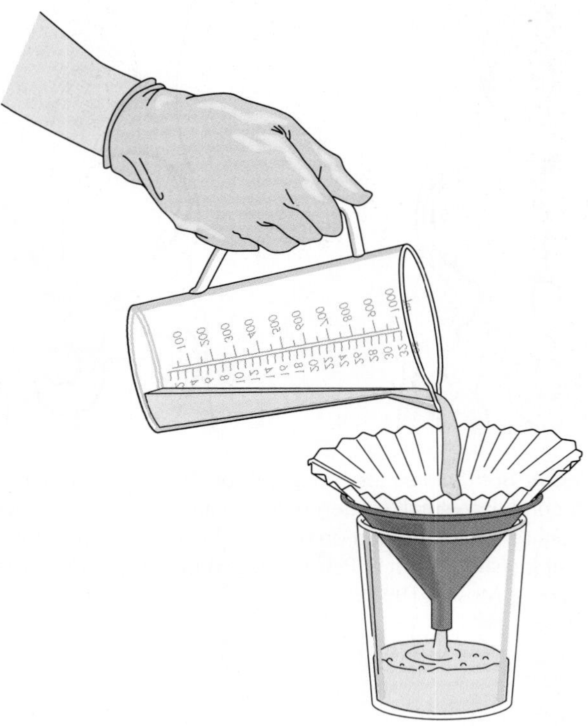

Figure 29-24 Place a disposable strainer in a specimen container. Pour urine through the strainer into the specimen container.

The Person with a Ureterostomy

Sometimes the bladder is surgically removed. Cancer and bladder injuries are common causes. When the bladder is removed, urine must still leave the body. A new pathway is created. It is called a *urinary diversion*.

There are many types of urinary diversions. Often an ostomy is involved. An **ostomy** is the surgical creation of an artificial opening. A **ureterostomy** is an artificial opening (*stomy*) between the ureter (*uretero*) and the abdomen. The artificial opening is called a **stoma** (Figure 29-25). Stomas do not have nerve endings and are not painful.

A pouch is applied over the stoma (Figure 29-26). The pouch is a disposable plastic bag. Urine drains through the stoma into the pouch. The pouch is replaced anytime it leaks. Leakage can cause skin irritation, breakdown, and infection. Clients often worry about odours and leaking pouches. A nurse provides care after surgery. You may care for clients with long-standing ureterostomies. The client assists with care as able.

The client needs good skin care. Skin breakdown must be prevented. Report changes in the skin around the stoma.

(text continues on page 501)

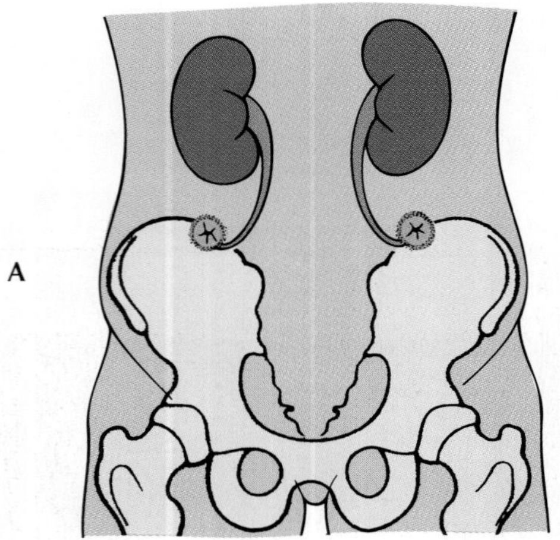

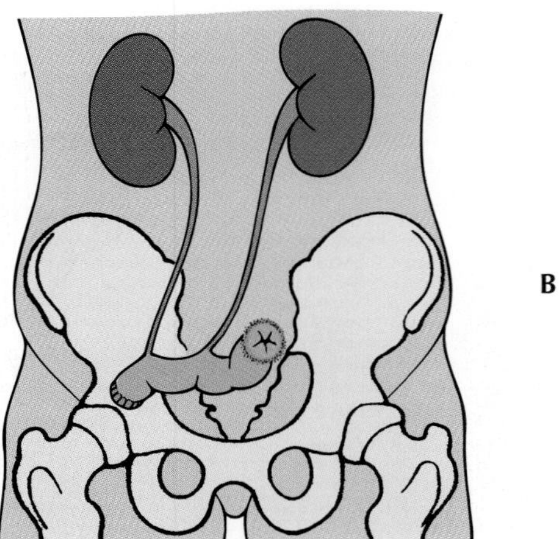

Figure 29-25 Ureterostomies. **A,** Both ureters are brought through the skin onto the abdomen. The person has two stomas. **B,** The ileal conduit. A small section of the small intestine is removed. One end is sutured closed. The other end is brought through the skin onto the abdomen to form a stoma. The ureters are attached to this part of the small intestine. Source: P.A. Beare and J.L. Myers, *Principles and Practices of Adult Health Nursing,* 3rd ed. (St. Louis: Mosby, 1998).

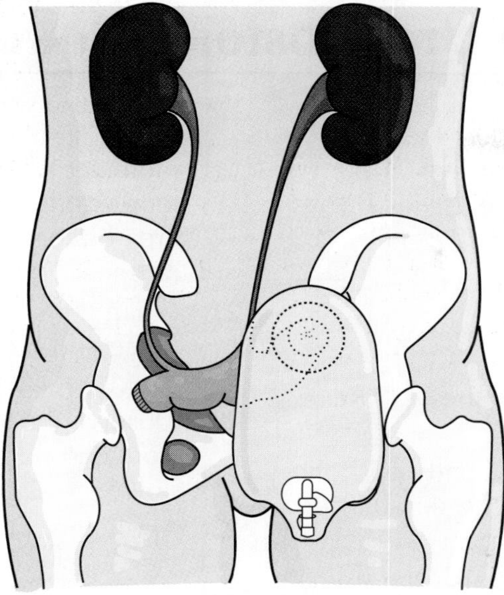

Figure 29-26 Ureterostomy pouch.

Changing a Ureterostomy Pouch

COMPASSIONATE CARE

Remember to Promote:
- **Dignity**
- **Independence**
- **Preferences**
- **Privacy**
- **Safety**

Pre-Procedure

1. Identify the person according to employer policy.
2. Explain the procedure to the person.
3. Wash your hands.
4. Collect the following:
   - Clean pouch with skin barrier
   - Skin barrier (if not part of pouch)
   - Pouch clamp, clip, or wire closure
   - Clean ostomy belt (if used)
   - Skin barrier as ordered
   - 4 to 8 gauze squares
   - Adhesive remover
   - Cotton balls
   - Bedpan with cover
   - Waterproof pad
   - Bath blanket
   - Toilet tissue
   - Washbasin
   - Bath thermometer
   - Soap or cleansing agent, according to the care plan
   - Pouch deodorant
   - Paper towels
   - Gloves
   - Disposable bag
5. Arrange paper towels on a work area. Place items on top of paper towels.
6. Provide for privacy.
7. Raise bed to a comfortable working height. Follow the care plan for bed rail use.*

Continued

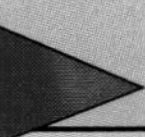

Changing a Ureterostomy Pouch—cont'd

Procedure

8 Lower the bed rail near you if up.
9 Cover the person with a bath blanket. Fan-fold linens to the foot of the bed.
10 Place the waterproof pad under the person's buttocks.
11 Put on gloves.
12 Disconnect the pouch from the belt. Remove the belt.
13 Remove the pouch gently. Gently push the skin down and away from the skin barrier. Place the pouch in the bedpan.
14 Place 1 or 2 gauze squares over the stoma to absorb urine.
15 Wipe around the stoma with toilet tissue or a gauze square. Place soiled tissue in the bedpan. Discard gauze squares into the disposable bag.
16 Moisten a cotton ball with adhesive remover. Clean around the stoma to remove any remaining skin barrier. Clean from the stoma outward.
17 Cover the bedpan, and take it to the bathroom. (If the person uses bed rails, raise the bed rails before leaving the bedside.)
18 Measure urine. Report any abnormal urine. Then empty the pouch and bedpan into the toilet. Note the colour, clarity, and odour of the urine. Put the pouch in the disposable bag.
19 Remove gloves. Wash your hands. Put on clean gloves.
20 Fill the washbasin with warm water. (Measure temperature of water with bath thermometer. Check the care plan for correct temperature.) Place the basin on the work area on top of paper towels. Lower the bed rail near you if up.
21 Clean the skin around the stoma with water. Rinse and pat dry. Use soap or other cleansing agent.
22 Observe the stoma and skin around the stoma. Report any irritation or skin breakdown.
23 Apply the skin barrier if it is a separate device.
24 Put a clean ostomy belt on the person (if a belt is worn).
25 Add deodorant to the new pouch.
26 Remove adhesive backing on the pouch.
27 Remove the gauze square used to absorb urine from the stoma.
28 Centre the pouch over the stoma. The drain points downward.
29 Press around the skin barrier so the pouch seals to the skin. Apply gentle pressure from the stoma outward.
30 Maintain pressure for 1 to 2 minutes.
31 Connect the belt to the pouch (if a belt is worn).
32 Remove the waterproof pad.
33 Remove gloves. Wash your hands. (If the person uses bed rails, raise the bed rails before leaving the bedside.)
34 Cover the person. Remove the bath blanket.

Post-Procedure

35 Provide for safety and comfort.
36 Place the call bell within reach.*
37 Return the bed to its lowest position. Follow the care plan for bed rail use.*
38 Remove privacy measures.
39 Clean the bedpan, washbasin, and other equipment. (Put on gloves for this step.)
40 Return equipment to its proper place.
41 Discard the disposable bag according to employer policy. Follow employer policy for soiled linen.
42 Remove gloves. Wash your hands.
43 Report and record your actions and observations according to employer policy.

*Steps marked with an asterisk may not apply in community settings.

COMPASSIONATE CARE

Elimination is a very personal and private act. Be sensitive to the client's feelings. The client may feel embarrassed or uncomfortable. Try to make the person feel better about accepting your help. Tell your supervisor if the client refuses care. Promote the client's dignity, independence, preferences, privacy, and safety. (See *Providing Compassionate Care: Assisting Clients with Elimination* box.)

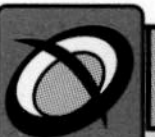

Providing Compassionate Care

ASSISTING CLIENTS WITH ELIMINATION

Dignity. Never add to the person's embarrassment. Always be encouraging and positive when providing care. Do not act offended by the sights or odours associated with elimination and ostomy care. Remember that your nonverbal gestures and expressions reveal your feelings. For example, do not wrinkle your nose or grimace while you are assisting.

Independence. Respond promptly to all requests for help with elimination. The need may be urgent. Believe clients when they ask for help, even if they just used the toilet, bedpan, urinal, or commode. Responding promptly gives the client some control.

Preferences. Respect the client's preferences whenever possible. For example, some people want to use the urinal while sitting up. Others prefer to lie down. The client decides.

Privacy. Provide as much privacy as possible. Lack of privacy may inhibit the person and interfere with elimination. Pull privacy curtains and close doors, shades, and drapes. Ask visitors or family members to step out of the room. If allowed by the care plan, leave the room after assisting the client to the bathroom or providing a bedpan, urinal, or commode. Stand just outside the door in case the client needs you. Or stand on the other side of the privacy curtain or look away if safe to do so. Ask your supervisor for advice on ways to protect the client's privacy.

Safety. Do not leave clients who are weak or dizzy. If you can leave the client and a call bell is available, make sure it is always within reach. Stay close enough so you can hear the person call for help. Remember to follow Standard Precautions.

REVIEW

Circle the BEST answer.

1. Which is *false*?
   A. Urine is normally clear and yellow or amber in colour.
   B. Urine normally has a foul odour.
   C. Micturition usually occurs before going to bed and on rising.
   D. A person normally voids about 1500 mL a day.

2. Which will *not* help normal elimination?
   A. Help the client assume a normal position for urination.
   B. Provide for privacy.
   C. Help the client to the bathroom or commode, or provide the bedpan or urinal as soon as requested.
   D. Always stay with the client who is on a bedpan.

3. The best position for using a bedpan is
   A. Fowler's position
   B. The supine position
   C. The prone position
   D. The side-lying position

4. After using the urinal, the man should
   A. Put the urinal on the bedside stand
   B. Call for assistance
   C. Put the urinal on the overbed table
   D. Empty the urinal

5. Urinary incontinence
   A. Is always permanent
   B. Requires good skin care
   C. Is always treated with an indwelling catheter
   D. Requires urine tests

6. A person has an indwelling catheter. Which is *incorrect*?
   A. Tape any leaks at the connection site.
   B. Keep the drainage bag below the level of the bladder.
   C. Make sure the tubing is free of kinks.
   D. Report complaints of pain, burning, the need to void, or irritation immediately.

7. Mr. Powers has a condom catheter. You apply elastic tape
   A. Completely around the penis
   B. To the inner thigh
   C. To the abdomen
   D. In a spiral fashion

8. The goal of bladder training is to
   A. Remove the catheter
   B. Allow the person to walk to the bathroom
   C. Gain voluntary control of urination
   D. Heal the stoma

9 When collecting a random urine specimen, you should do the following *except*
   A. Label the container with the requested information
   B. Use the correct container
   C. Collect the specimen at the time specified
   D. Ask the client to put toilet tissue in the specimen container

10. The perineum is cleaned immediately before collecting
   A. Random specimens
   B. Midstream specimens
   C. 24-hour urine specimens
   D. Random and 24-hour urine specimens

11. A 24-hour urine specimen involves
   A. Collecting all urine voided by a client during a 24-hour period
   B. Collecting a random specimen every hour for 24 hours
   C. A catheterization
   D. Testing the urine for sugar and blood

12. Straining urine is done to find
   A. Hematuria
   B. Stones
   C. Nocturia
   D. Urgency

13. A client has a ureterostomy. You must do the following *except*
   A. Provide good skin care
   B. Change the pouch whenever it leaks
   C. Report any changes in the skin around the stoma
   D. Provide incontinent briefs

Answers to these questions are on page 825.

CHAPTER

30

Bowel Elimination

OBJECTIVES

- Define the key terms listed in this chapter
- Describe normal stools and the normal pattern and frequency of bowel movements
- List the observations to make about bowel movements
- Identify the factors that affect bowel elimination
- Describe common bowel elimination problems
- Describe the measures that promote comfort and safety during defecation
- Describe bowel training
- Explain why enemas are given
- Know the common enema solutions
- Describe the comfort and safety measures for giving enemas
- Explain the purpose of rectal tubes
- Describe how to care for a client with an ostomy pouch
- Explain why stool specimens are collected
- Learn the procedures described in this chapter

KEY TERMS

anal incontinence Fecal incontinence

colostomy An artificial opening (*stomy*) between the colon (*colo*) and abdominal wall

constipation A condition in which bowel movements are less frequent than usual; the stool is hard, dry, and difficult to pass

defecation The process of excreting feces from the rectum through the anus; a bowel movement

dehydration The excessive loss of water from tissues

diarrhea The frequent passage of liquid stools

enema The introduction of fluid into the rectum and lower colon

fecal impaction The prolonged retention and accumulation of feces in the rectum

fecal incontinence The inability to control the passage of feces and gas through the anus; anal incontinence

feces The semisolid mass of waste products in the colon

flatulence The excessive formation of gas in the stomach and intestines

flatus Gas or air from the stomach or intestines passed through the anus

ileostomy An artificial opening (*stomy*) between the ileum (small intestine; *ileo*) and the abdominal wall

melena A black, tarry stool

ostomy The surgical creation of an artificial opening

peristalsis The alternating contraction and relaxation of intestinal muscles

stoma An artifical opening; see colostomy and ileostomy

stool Excreted feces

suppository A cone-shaped, solid medication that is inserted into a body opening; it melts at body temperature

Like urinary elimination, bowel elimination is a basic physical need. It is the excretion of wastes from the digestive system (see Chapter 13). Many factors affect bowel elimination. They include privacy, personal habits, age, diet, exercise and activity, fluids, and medications. Problems easily occur. Promoting normal bowel elimination is important. You will assist clients in meeting their elimination needs.

Bowel elimination problems and treatments may be uncomfortable, frustrating, embarrassing, and humiliating for the client. Be sensitive and offer emotional support. (See *Providing Compassionate Care: Assisting Clients with Elimination* on page 501.) Also follow Standard Precautions and the infection control guidelines listed in Box 29-1 on page 466.

NORMAL BOWEL MOVEMENTS

Foods and fluids are partially digested in the stomach. The partially digested foods and fluids are called *chyme*. Chyme passes from the stomach into the small intestine. Then it enters the large intestine (large bowel or colon) where fluid is absorbed. Chyme becomes less fluid and more solid in consistency. **Feces** is the semisolid mass of waste products in the colon.

Feces move through the intestine by **peristalsis**, the alternating contraction and relaxation of intestinal muscles. Feces move through the colon to the rectum, where they are stored until excreted from the body. **Defecation** (bowel movement [BM]) is the process of excreting feces from the rectum through the anus. **Stool** is the term for excreted feces.

Some people have a bowel movement every day. Others have one every 2 to 3 days. Some people have 2 or 3 bowel movements a day. Many people defecate after breakfast. Others do so in the evening. Many older adults expect a bowel movement every day. The slightest irregularity concerns them. The nurse teaches them about normal elimination.

Stools are normally brown. Bleeding in the stomach and small intestine causes black or tarry stools. Bleeding in the lower colon and rectum causes red-coloured stools. So do beets. A diet high in green vegetables can cause green stools. Diseases and infection can also cause clay-coloured or white, pale, orange-coloured, or green-coloured stools.

Stools are normally soft, formed, moist, and shaped like the rectum. They have a characteristic odour. The odour is from bacterial action in the intestines. Certain foods and medications also cause odours.

Observations

Your observations are important for the care planning process. Carefully observe stools before disposing of them. In a facility setting, ask the nurse to observe abnormal stools. In a community setting, call your supervisor. You need to observe stools and report abnormalities in the following: colour, amount, consistency, odour, shape, size, frequency, and any complaints of pain.

Factors Affecting Bowel Elimination

Normal, regular defecation is affected by many factors. The following factors affect the frequency, consistency, colour, and odour of stools:

- *Privacy*—Like voiding, bowel elimination is a private act. Lack of privacy prevents many people from defecating despite having the urge. Bowel movement odours and sounds are embarrassing. Some people ignore the urge to defecate when others are present. This can lead to constipation.
- *Personal habits*—Many people routinely have a bowel movement after breakfast. Some drink a hot beverage, read a book or newspaper, or take a walk. These activities relax the person. Defecation is easier when a person is relaxed, not tense.
- *Diet*—A well-balanced diet and bulk are needed. High-fibre foods leave a residue that provides needed bulk. Fruits, vegetables, and whole grain cereals and breads are high in fibre. Many older adults do not eat enough fruits and vegetables. Some do not have teeth. Or their dentures fit poorly. Therefore they cannot chew these foods. Some people think they cannot digest fruits and vegetables, so they refuse to eat them. Bran, prunes, and juices help prevent constipation. Certain foods can cause diarrhea or constipation. Milk causes constipation in some people and diarrhea in others. Other foods and chocolate can cause similar reactions. Spicy foods can irritate the intestines. Frequent stools or diarrhea can result. Gas-forming foods stimulate peristalsis. Increased peristalsis results in defecation. Gas-forming foods include onions, beans, cabbage, cauliflower, radishes, and cucumbers. Many people avoid gas-forming foods because they cause stomachaches or bloating.
- *Fluids*—Feces contain water. Stool consistency depends on the amount of water absorbed in the colon. The amount of fluid ingested, urine output, and vomiting are factors. Feces become hard and dry when large amounts of water are absorbed and when fluid intake is poor. Hard, dry feces move through the intestines at a slower rate. Constipation can occur. Drinking 6 to 8 glasses of water every day promotes normal bowel elimination. Warm fluids—coffee, tea, hot cider, and warm water—increase peristalsis.
- *Activity*—Exercise and activity maintain muscle tone and stimulate peristalsis. Irregular elimination and constipation often occur from inactivity and bed rest. Inactivity may result from disease, surgery, injury, and aging.
- *Medications*—Medications can prevent constipation or control diarrhea. Other medications have diarrhea or constipation as side effects. Medications for pain relief often cause constipation. Antibiotics, used to fight or prevent infection, often cause diarrhea. Diarrhea occurs when the antibiotics kill normal flora in the large intestine. Normal flora is necessary in forming stools.
- *Aging*—With aging, feces pass through the intestines at a slower rate. Constipation results. Some people lose bowel control. Older adults may not completely empty the rectum. They often need to defecate 30 to 45 minutes after the first bowel movement.
- *Disability*—Some people cannot control bowel movements. They defecate whenever feces enter the rectum. A bowel training program is needed (page 507). The goal is to have a bowel movement at the same time each day.

Comfort and Safety

The care plan lists comfort and safety measures to meet the client's elimination needs. They may involve diet, fluids, and exercise. The actions in Box 30-1 on page 506 are routinely practised. They promote comfort and safety during bowel elimination.

Box 30-1 Comfort and Safety during Bowel Elimination

- Assist the client to the toilet or commode, or provide the bedpan as soon as requested.
- Wheel the client into the bathroom on the commode if possible. Place the commode over the toilet. This provides privacy.
- Provide for privacy. Ask visitors or family members to leave the room. Close doors, pull privacy curtains, and close window curtains, blinds, or shades.
- Make sure the bedpan is warm.
- Position the client in a normal sitting or squatting position.
- Cover the client for warmth and privacy when using a bedpan.
- Allow enough time for defecation. Do not rush the client.
- Place the call bell (in facilities) and toilet tissue within the client's reach.
- Stay with the client if he or she is weak or unsteady.
- Leave the room if the client can be alone. Stay within hearing distance.
- Provide perineal care.
- Dispose of stool promptly. This reduces odours and prevents the spread of microbes.
- Assist the client with hand washing after elimination.
- Follow the care plan if the client has fecal incontinence. The care plan tells you when to assist with elimination.
- Follow Standard Precautions.

Common Problems

Many factors affect normal bowel elimination. Common problems include constipation, fecal impaction, diarrhea, fecal incontinence, and flatulence.

Constipation

Constipation is a condition in which bowel movements are less frequent than usual and the stool is hard, dry, and difficult to pass. The person usually strains to have a bowel movement. Stools are large or marble-size. Large stools cause pain as they pass through the anus. Constipation occurs when feces move through the intestine slowly. This allows more time for water absorption. Common causes include a low-fibre diet, ignoring the urge to defecate, decreased fluid intake, inactivity, medications, aging, and certain diseases.

A person may be too embarrassed to tell you he or she is constipated. If the person is having fewer bowel movements than normal, notify your supervisor. Common measures used to prevent or relieve constipation include changing the diet (increasing fibre, increasing fluids, and encouraging physical activity). The physician may order medications or enemas.

Fecal Impaction

A **fecal impaction** is the prolonged retention and accumulation of feces in the rectum. Feces are hard or puttylike in consistency. Fecal impaction results if constipation is not relieved. The person cannot defecate. More water is absorbed from already hard feces. If left untreated, a fecal impaction can lead to complete bowel obstruction and require surgery to correct.

The person tries many times to have a bowel movement. If a client shows any of the following signs or symptoms of a fecal impaction, report it at once:

- Abdominal discomfort and swelling
- Cramping
- A feeling of fullness or pain in the rectum
- Nausea or vomiting
- Fever
- Increased need or decreased ability to urinate
- Liquid feces seeping from the anus. Seepage may look like diarrhea. However, it is feces that is passing around the hardened fecal mass.

A physician or nurse performs a digital (finger) exam to check for an impaction. This is done by inserting a gloved finger into the rectum and feeling for a hard mass. The person may feel uncomfortable after the procedure. The physician may order medications and enemas to remove the impaction. Sometimes the physician or nurse removes the fecal mass with a gloved finger. This is called *digital removal of an impaction.*

Diarrhea

Diarrhea is the frequent passage of liquid stools. Feces move through the intestines rapidly. This reduces the time for fluid absorption. The need to defecate is urgent. Some people cannot get to a bathroom in time. Abdominal cramping, nausea, and vomiting may also occur.

Causes of diarrhea include infections, certain medications, irritating foods, and microbes in food and water. Diet and medications reduce peristalsis. You need to:

- Assist with elimination needs promptly.
- Dispose of stools promptly. This prevents odours and the spread of microbes.
- Give good skin care. Liquid feces irritate the skin. So does frequent wiping with toilet tissue. Skin breakdown and pressure ulcers are risks.

Fluid lost through diarrhea must be replaced. Otherwise dehydration occurs. **Dehydration** is the excessive loss of water from tissues. Signs and symptoms include pale or flushed skin, dry skin, coated tongue, oliguria (scant amount of urine), cracked lips, sunken eyes, dark urine, thirst, weakness, dizziness, and confusion. Falling blood pressure and increased pulse and respirations are serious signs. Death can occur. The care plan tells you how to meet the client's fluid needs. The physician orders intravenous fluids in severe cases.

Microbes often cause diarrhea. Preventing the spread of infection is important. Always practise Standard Precautions when in contact with stools.

See *Focus on Children: Dehydration* and *Focus on Older Adults: Dehydration* boxes.

Fecal Incontinence

Fecal incontinence (anal incontinence) is the inability to control the passage of feces and gas through the anus. Causes include intestinal and nervous system diseases, injuries, fecal impaction, diarrhea, and some medications. Fecal incontinence can also occur when requests for help to use the bathroom, commode, or bedpan are unanswered.

People with mental health problems, dementia, or cognitive disorders (see Chapters 33 and 34) may not recognize the need to defecate. Some may smear stool on themselves, furniture, and walls. In such situations, resisting care is a common problem. It may be hard to keep the person clean. Follow the person's care plan. Also talk to your supervisor if you have problems keeping the person clean.

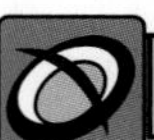

Focus on Children

Dehydration

The bodies of infants and young children contain large amounts of water. Infants and children are at risk for dehydration. Death can occur quickly. Report any liquid or watery stool immediately. Note the number of wet diapers in 24 hours. Infants wet less when dehydrated. Fewer than 6 wet diapers in 24 hours may indicate that an infant is dehydrated. Report any concerns immediately.

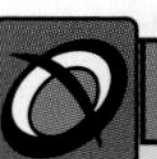

Focus on Older Adults

Dehydration

Older adults also are at risk for dehydration. The amount of body water decreases with aging. Therefore diarrhea is very serious in older adults. Report any signs of diarrhea immediately. Death is a risk from unrecognized and untreated dehydration.

Flatulence

Gas and air are normally found in the stomach and intestines. They are expelled through the mouth (belching, eructating) and anus. Gas and air passed through the anus is called **flatus**. **Flatulence** is the excessive formation of gas or air in the stomach and intestines. Common causes are:

- Swallowing air while eating and drinking. This includes chewing gum, eating fast, drinking through a straw, and drinking carbonated beverages. Tense or anxious people may swallow large amounts of air when drinking.
- Bacterial action in the intestines
- Gas-forming foods (onions, beans, cabbage, cauliflower, radishes, cucumbers)
- Constipation
- Bowel and abdominal surgeries
- Medications that decrease peristalsis

If flatus is not expelled, the intestines distend. That is, they swell or enlarge from the pressure of the gases. Abdominal cramping or pain (sometimes severe), shortness of breath, and a swollen abdomen occur. "Bloating" is a common complaint. Exercise, walking, and the left side-lying position often produce flatus. Physicians may order enemas, medications, or rectal tubes to relieve flatulence.

Bowel Training

Bowel training has two goals:

- To gain control of bowel movements
- To develop a regular pattern of elimination. Fecal impaction, constipation, and fecal incontinence are prevented.

The urge to defecate is usually felt after a meal, usually breakfast. The client's usual time of day for a bowel movement is noted on the care plan. Toilet, commode, or bedpan use is offered at this time. Factors that promote elimination are part of the care plan and bowel training program. These include a high-fibre diet, increased fluids, warm fluids, activity, and privacy. Your supervisor tells you about a client's bowel training program.

The physician may order a suppository to stimulate defecation. A **suppository** is a cone-shaped, solid medication that is inserted into a body opening. It melts at body temperature. A nurse inserts a rectal suppository into the rectum. Or the client self medicates. Assist as needed (see Chapter 39). A bowel movement occurs about 30 minutes later.

ENEMAS

An **enema** is the introduction of fluid into the rectum and lower colon. Enemas are ordered by physicians. They are given to remove feces and to relieve constipation or fecal impaction. People with poor mobility or who are paralyzed are at risk for these problems. Enemas also are ordered to clean the bowel of feces before certain surgeries or X-ray procedures. Sometimes enemas are ordered to relieve flatulence and intestinal distension.

Enemas are usually safe procedures. Many people give themselves enemas at home. However, enemas are dangerous for older adults and those with certain heart and kidney diseases. Enemas involve inserting a tube into a body opening. Therefore, giving an enema is a delegated task (see Chapter 5). You may or may not be allowed to give enemas. If you are delegated to give one, make sure that:

- Provincial or territorial laws and your employer allow you to perform the procedure
- The procedure is in your job description
- You have the necessary education and training
- You review the procedure with a nurse
- A nurse is available to answer questions and to supervise you

Comfort and safety measures are practised when giving an enema. Follow the guidelines in Box 30-2.

ENEMA SOLUTIONS

A physician orders the enema solution. The kind of solution ordered depends on the enema's purpose:

- *Tap-water enema*—obtained from a faucet.
- *Soapsuds enema (SSE)*—add 3 to 5 mL (½ to 1 teaspoon) of castile soap to 500 to 1000 mL of tap water.
- *Saline enema*—add 5 to 10 mL (1 to 2 teaspoons) of table salt to 500 to 1000 mL of tap water.
- *Oil-retention enema*—mineral oil or a commercial oil-retention enema is used.
- *Commercial enema*—contains about 120 mL (4 oz) of solution.

Other enema solutions may be ordered. Consult with your supervisor and your employer's procedure manual to safely prepare and give enemas. Do not administer enemas that contain medications. Nurses give these enemas.

THE CLEANSING ENEMA

Cleansing enemas clean the bowel of feces and flatus. They relieve constipation and fecal impaction. They are also needed before certain surgeries and diagnostic procedures.

Box 30-2 Comfort and Safety Measures for Giving Enemas

- Measure solution temperature with a bath thermometer—usually 40.5° C (105° F) for adults. Your supervisor and the care plan tell you what temperature to use.
- Give the amount of solution ordered by the physician and written in the care plan—usually 500 to 1000 mL.
- Position the client as directed by your supervisor and the care plan. Sims' position is usually preferred.
- Ask your supervisor and check your employer's policies for how far to insert the enema tubing. In adults, the tube is usually inserted 7.5 to 10 cm (3 to 4 inches). Stop if you feel resistance, the client complains of pain, or bleeding occurs.
- Lubricate the enema tip before inserting it.
- Ask your supervisor how high to raise the enema bag. For adults, it is usually held 30 cm (12 inches) above the anus.
- Force air out of the enema tubing before inserting into the anus. Do this by dribbling a small amount of water from the tubing into a bedpan before insertion.
- Give the enema solution slowly. Usually it takes 10 to 15 minutes to give 750 to 1000 mL.
- Hold the enema tube in place while giving the solution.
- Ask your supervisor how long the client should retain the enema solution. The length of time depends on the amount and type of solution.
- Make sure the bathroom will be vacant when the client needs to defecate.
- A nurse observes the enema results.
- Follow Standard Precautions.

The physician orders a soapsuds, tap-water, or saline enema. The physician may order *enemas until clear*. This means that enemas are given until the return solution is clear and free of feces. Ask your supervisor how many enemas to give. Employer policy may allow repeating cleansing enemas only 2 or 3 times.

Tap-water enemas can be dangerous. The large intestine may absorb some of the water into the bloodstream. This creates a fluid imbalance in the body. Only one tap-water enema is given. Do not repeat the enema. Repeated enemas increase the risk of excessive fluid absorption. The tap-water enema takes effect in 15 to 20 minutes.

Soapsuds enemas irritate the bowel's mucous lining. Repeated enemas can damage the bowel, as can using more than 3 to 5 mL (1 teaspoon) of castile soap or stronger soap. The soapsuds enema takes effect in about 10 to 15 minutes.

The saline enema solution is similar to body fluid. However, some of the salt solution may be absorbed. This too can cause a fluid imbalance. When there is excess salt in the body, the body retains water. The saline enema takes effect in about 15 to 20 minutes. (See *Focus on Children: Saline Enemas* box.)

(text continues on page 511)

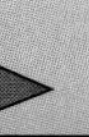
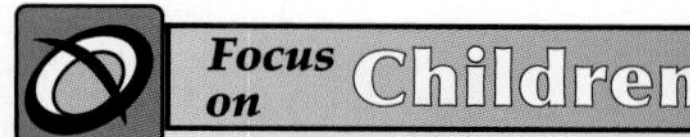

Focus on Children

SALINE ENEMAS

Only saline enemas are used for children. The amount of enema solution varies for infants and children. If you are delegated to give an enema to a child, your supervisor will give you the necessary instructions.

Giving a Cleansing Enema to an Adult

COMPASSIONATE CARE

Remember to Promote:
- **Dignity**
- **Independence**
- **Preferences**
- **Privacy**
- **Safety**

Pre-Procedure

1 Identify the person according to employer policy.
2 Explain the procedure to the person.
3 Wash your hands.
4 Collect the following:
   - Disposable enema kit as directed by your supervisor (enema bag, tube, clamp, and waterproof pad)
   - Bath thermometer
   - Waterproof pad
   - Water-soluble lubricant
   - Gloves
   - Material for enema solution: 3 to 5 mL (1 teaspoon) castile soap or 5 to 10 mL (1 to 2 teaspoons) salt
   - Toilet tissue
   - Bath blanket
   - IV pole
   - Robe and nonskid footwear
   - Bedpan or commode
   - Paper towels
5 Provide for privacy.
6 Raise the bed to a comfortable working height. Follow the care plan for bed rail use.*

Procedure

7 Lower the bed rail near you if up.
8 Cover the person with a bath blanket. Fan-fold top linens to the foot of the bed.
9 Position the IV pole so the enema bag is 30 cm (12 inches) above the anus. Or it is at a height directed in the care plan.
10 Raise the bed rail if used.
11 Prepare the enema:
   a Close the clamp on the tube.
   b Adjust water flow until it is lukewarm.
   c Fill enema bag for the amount ordered.
   d Measure water temperature. For adults it is usually 40.5° C (105° F).
   e Prepare the enema solution as directed in the care plan.
      (1) Saline enema: add 5 to 10 mL (1 to 2 teaspoons) of salt
      (2) Soapsuds enema: add 3 to 5 mL (1 teaspoon) of castile soap
      (3) Tap-water enema: add nothing to the water

Continued

Giving a Cleansing Enema to an Adult—cont'd

Procedure—cont'd

- **f** Stir the solution with the bath thermometer. Scoop off any suds (SSE).
- **g** Seal the bag.
- **h** Hang the bag on the IV pole.

12 Lower the bed rail near you if up.

13 Position the person in the Sims' position or in a comfortable left side-lying position.

14 Put on gloves.

15 Place waterproof pad under the buttocks.

16 Expose the anal area.

17 Place the bedpan behind the person.

18 Position the enema tube in the bedpan.

19 Remove the cap from the enema tubing.

20 Open the clamp. Let solution flow through the tube to remove air. Clamp the tube.

21 Lubricate the tube 7.5 to 10 cm (3 to 4 inches) from the tip.

22 Separate the buttocks to see the anus.

23 Ask the person to take a deep breath through the mouth.

24 Insert the tube gently 7.5 to 10 cm (3 to 4 inches) into the rectum when the person is exhaling (Figure 30-1). Stop if the person complains of pain, if you feel resistance, or if bleeding occurs.

25 Check the amount of solution in the bag.

26 Unclamp the tube. Administer the solution slowly (Figure 30-2).

27 Ask the person to take slow, deep breaths. This helps the person relax.

28 Clamp the tube if the person needs to defecate, has cramping, or starts to expel solution. Unclamp when symptoms subside.

29 Give the amount of solution ordered. Stop if the person cannot tolerate the procedure.

30 Clamp the tube before it is empty. This prevents air from entering the bowel.

31 Hold toilet tissue around the tube and against the anus. Remove the tube.

32 Discard the toilet tissue into the bedpan.

33 Wrap the tubing tip with paper towels. Place it inside the enema bag.

34 Help the person onto the bedpan. Raise the head of the bed, or help the person into a sitting position. Raise the bed rail if used. Or assist the person to the bathroom or commode. The person wears a robe and nonskid footwear when up. The bed is in the lowest position.

35 Place the call bell (in facilities) and toilet tissue within reach. Remind the person not to flush the toilet.

36 Discard disposable items.

37 Remove gloves. Wash your hands.

38 Leave the room if the person can be left alone. Stay within hearing distance.

39 Return when the person calls. Knock before entering.

40 Wash your hands. Put on gloves. Lower the bed rail if up.

41 Observe enema results for amount, colour, consistency, and odour. Call your supervisor to observe the results (in a facility).

42 Provide perineal care as needed.

43 Remove the bed protector.

44 Empty, clean, and disinfect the bedpan or commode. Flush the toilet. Return items to their proper place.

45 Remove gloves. Wash your hands.

46 Help the person with hand washing. Wear gloves if needed.

47 Return top linens, and remove the bath blanket.

Continued

Giving a Cleansing Enema to an Adult—cont'd

Post-Procedure

48 Provide for safety and comfort.
49 Place the call bell within reach.*
50 Return the bed to its lowest position. Follow the care plan for bed rail use.*
51 Remove privacy measures.
52 Follow employer policy for soiled linen and used supplies. Wear gloves for this step.
53 Wash your hands.
54 Report and record your actions and observations according to employer policy.

*Steps marked with an asterisk may not apply in community settings.

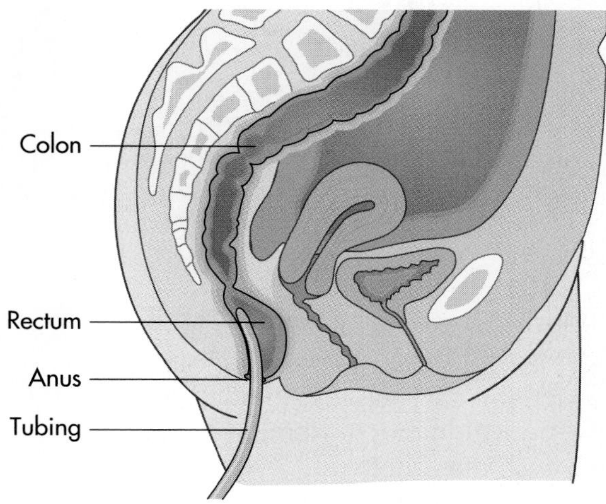

Figure 30-1 Enema tubing inserted into the adult rectum.

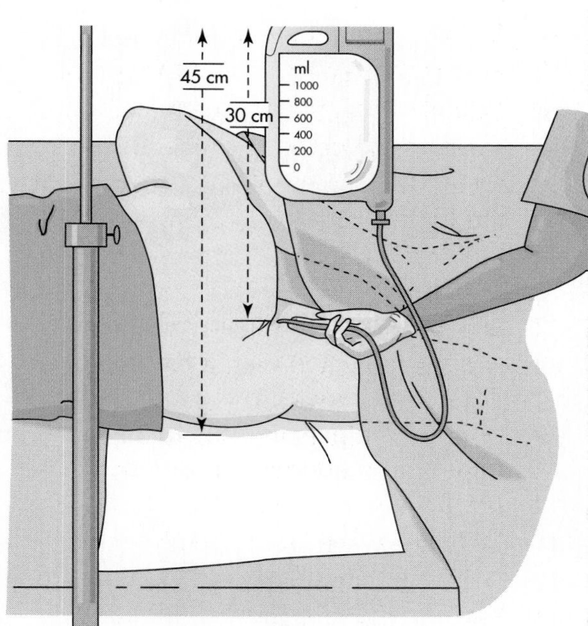

Figure 30-2 Giving an enema. The client is in the Sims' position. The enema bag hangs from an IV pole. The enema bag is 30 cm (12 inches) above the anus and 45 cm (18 inches) above the mattress.

The Commercial Enema

Commercial enemas irritate and distend the rectum. This causes defecation. They are often ordered for constipation or when complete cleansing of the bowel is not needed.

Manufacturers prepare and package the commercial enema. It is ready to give. The solution is usually given at room temperature. To give the enema, squeeze and roll up the plastic bottle from the bottom. Do not release pressure on the bottle. Otherwise solution is drawn from the rectum back into the bottle.

Encourage the client to retain the solution until he or she feels the urge to defecate. It usually takes 5 to 10 minutes to take effect. Remaining in the Sims' or left side-lying position helps the person retain the enema longer.

(text continues on page 513)

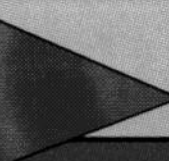

Giving a Commercial Enema to an Adult

Compassionate Care

Remember to Promote:
- **Dignity**
- **Independence**
- **Preferences**
- **Privacy**
- **Safety**

Pre-Procedure

1 Identify the person according to employer policy.
2 Explain the procedure to the person.
3 Wash your hands.
4 Collect the following:
- Commercial enema
- Bedpan or commode
- Waterproof pad
- Toilet tissue
- Gloves
- Robe and nonskid footwear
- Bath blanket

5 Provide for privacy.
6 Raise the bed to a comfortable working height. Follow the care plan for bed rail use.*

Procedure

7 Lower the bed rail near you if up.
8 Cover the person with a bath blanket. Fanfold top linens to the foot of the bed.
9 Position the person in the Sims' or a comfortable left side-lying position.
10 Put on gloves.
11 Place the waterproof pad under the buttocks.
12 Expose the anal area.
13 Position the bedpan near the person.
14 Remove the cap from the enema tip.
15 Separate the buttocks to see the anus.
16 Ask the person to take a deep breath through the mouth.
17 Insert the enema tip 5 cm (2 inches) into the rectum when the person is exhaling (Figure 30-3). Stop if the person complains of pain, you feel resistance, or bleeding occurs.
18 Squeeze and roll the bottle gently. Release pressure on the bottle *after* removing the tip from the rectum.
19 Put the bottle into the box, tip first.
20 Help the person onto the bedpan; raise the head of the bed, or help the person into a sitting position. Raise the bed rail if used. Or assist the person to the bathroom or commode. The person wears a robe and nonskid footwear when up. The bed is in the lowest position.
21 Place the call bell (in facilities) and toilet tissue within reach. Remind the person not to flush the toilet.
22 Discard used disposable items.
23 Remove gloves. Wash your hands.
24 Leave the room if the person can be left alone. Stay within hearing distance.
25 Return when the person calls. Knock before entering.
26 Wash your hands. Put on gloves.
27 Lower the bed rail if up.
28 Observe enema results for amount, colour, consistency, and odour. Call your supervisor to observe the results (in a facility).
29 Help the person clean the perineal area.
30 Remove the bed protector.
31 Empty, clean, and disinfect the bedpan or commode. Flush the toilet.
32 Return equipment to its proper place.
33 Remove gloves. Wash your hands.
34 Help the person with hand washing. Wear gloves if necessary.
35 Return top linens, and remove the bath blanket.

Continued

Giving a Commercial Enema to an Adult—cont'd

Post-Procedure

36 Follow steps 48 through 54 in *Giving a Cleansing Enema to an Adult* on page 511.

*Steps marked with an asterisk may not apply in community settings.

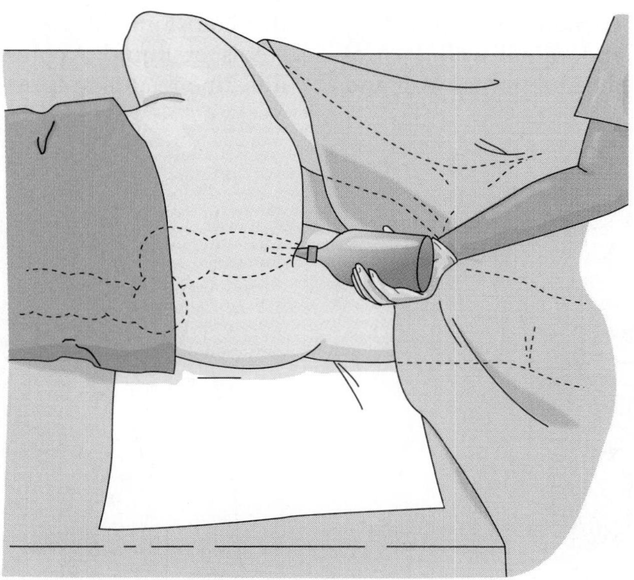

Figure 30-3 Insert the commercial enema tip 5 cm (2 inches) into the rectum.

Rectal Tubes

A nurse inserts a rectal tube into the rectum to relieve flatulence and intestinal distention. Flatus is passed without effort or straining.

The rectal tube is usually inserted 10 cm (4 inches) into the adult rectum. It is left in place for 20 to 30 minutes. This helps prevent rectal irritation. It can be reinserted every 2 to 3 hours.

Often the tube is connected to a flatus bag or to a water container (Figure 30-4). The bag inflates as gas passes into it. If the tube is connected to a container with water, the water bubbles as gas passes through the tube into the water. For this system, the rectal tube is attached to connecting tubing. The connecting tubing attaches to the water container.

Feces may be expelled along with flatus. If a flatus bag is not used, the open end of the tube is placed in a folded, waterproof pad.

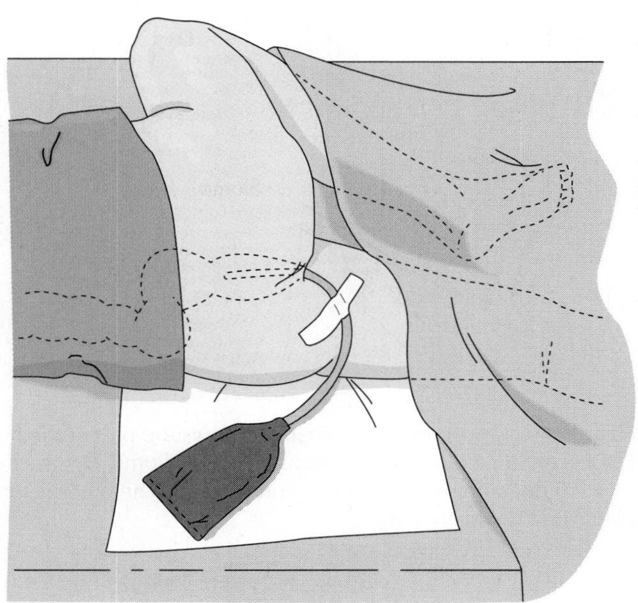

Figure 30-4 A rectal tube. A nurse inserts the rectal tube 10 cm (4 inches) into the adult rectum. The rectal tube is taped to the buttocks. The flatus bag rests on the bed.

The Person with an Ostomy

Sometimes surgical removal of part of the intestines is necessary. Cancer, diseases of the bowel, and trauma (such as stab or bullet wounds) are common reasons for intestinal surgery. An ostomy is sometimes necessary. An **ostomy** is the surgical creation of an artificial opening. The opening is called a **stoma.** The person wears a pouch over the stoma to collect feces and flatus.

Colostomy

A **colostomy** is the surgically created opening (*stomy*) between the colon (*colo*) and abdominal wall. Part of the colon is brought out onto the abdominal wall and a stoma is made. Feces and flatus pass through the stoma, not the anus. Colostomies are permanent or temporary. If the colostomy is permanent, the diseased part of the colon is removed. A temporary colostomy gives the diseased or injured bowel time to heal. After healing, surgery is done to reconnect the bowel.

The colostomy site depends on the site of colon disease or injury (Figure 30-5). Stool consistency ranges from liquid to formed. The more colon remaining to absorb water, the more solid and formed the stool. If the colostomy is near the beginning of the colon, stools are liquid. A colostomy near the end of the large intestine results in formed stools.

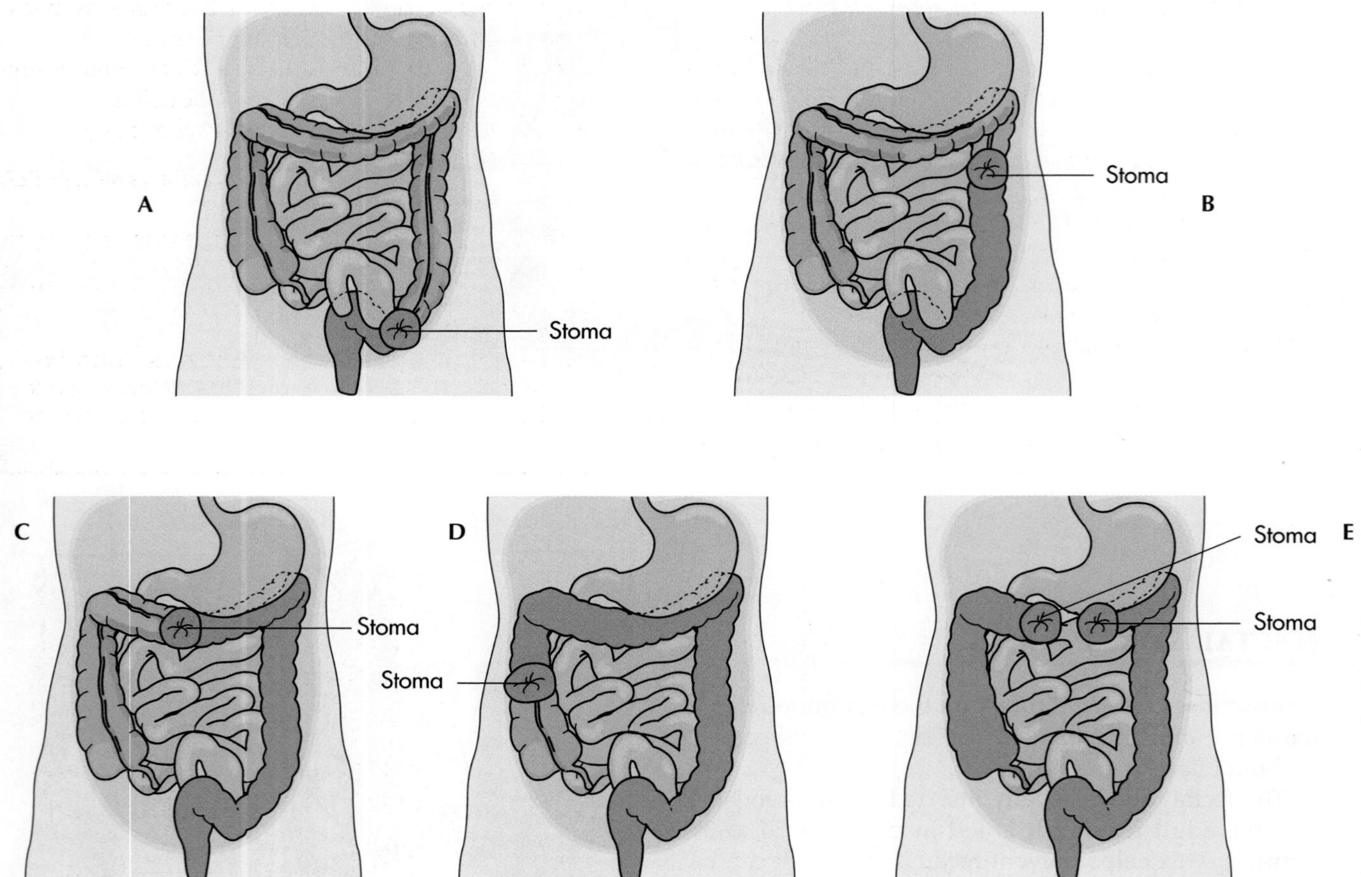

Figure 30-5 Colostomy sites. *Shading* shows the part of the bowel that was surgically removed. **A,** Sigmoid colostomy. **B,** Descending colostomy. **C,** Transverse colostomy. **D,** Ascending colostomy. **E,** Double-barrel colostomy. Two stomas are created: one allows for the excretion of feces. The other is for the introduction of medicine to help the bowel heal. This type of colostomy is usually temporary.

Feces irritate the skin. Skin care prevents skin breakdown around the stoma. The skin is washed and dried when the pouch is removed. Then a skin barrier is applied around the stoma. The skin barrier prevents feces from coming in contact with the skin. The skin barrier may be part of the pouch or a separate device.

ILEOSTOMY

An **ileostomy** is the surgically created opening (*stomy*) between the ileum (small intestine [*ileo*]) and the abdominal wall. Part of the ileum is brought out onto the abdominal wall and a stoma is made. The entire colon is removed (Figure 30-6). Liquid feces drain constantly from an ileostomy. Water is not absorbed because the colon was removed. Feces in the small intestine contain digestive juices that are very irritating to the skin. The ileostomy pouch must fit well so feces do not touch the skin. Good skin care is essential.

 **Ostomy Pouches.** The pouch has an adhesive backing that is applied to the skin. Sometimes pouches are secured to ostomy belts (Figure 30-7). Many pouches have a drain at the bottom that is closed with clips, clamps, or wire closures. The drain is opened to empty the pouch (see Figure 30-7). The pouch is emptied when feces are present. It is opened when the bag balloons or bulges with flatus. The drain is wiped with toilet tissue before it is closed.

The pouch is changed every 3 to 7 days and when it leaks. Some clients want the pouch changed daily or whenever soiling occurs. However, frequent pouch changes can damage the skin. Many clients manage their ostomy pouches without help.

Odours are prevented by the following:

- Good hygiene
- Emptying the pouch
- Avoiding gas-forming foods
- Putting deodorants into the pouch. The care plan tells you what to use.

The client can wear normal clothes with an ostomy pouch. However, tight undergarments can prevent feces from entering the pouch. Also, bulging from feces and flatus can be seen with tight clothes.

Peristalsis increases after eating. Therefore stomas are usually quiet before breakfast. That is, expelling feces is less likely at this time. If the client showers or bathes with the pouch off, it is best done before breakfast. Showers and baths are delayed 1 or 2 hours after applying a new pouch. This gives the adhesive backing on the pouch time to stick to the skin.

Do not flush pouches down the toilet. Follow employer policy for disposing of used pouches.

(See *Focus on Children: Ostomy Pouches* box.)

(text continues on page 517)

Focus on Children

OSTOMY POUCHES

Children of all ages can have ostomies, even premature infants. If changing a child's ostomy pouch is assigned to you, your supervisor will give you the necessary instructions.

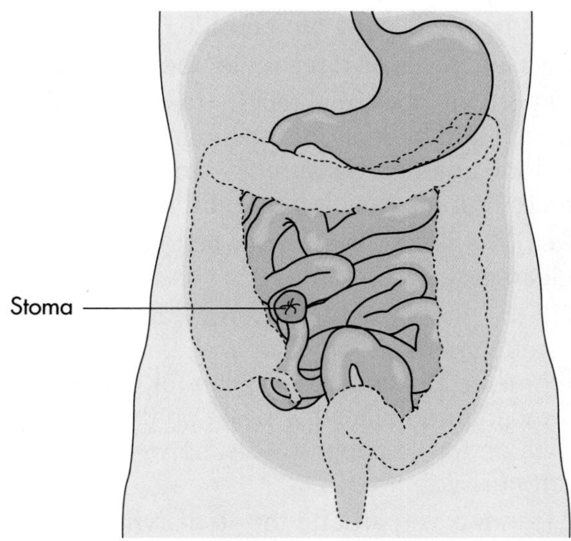

Figure 30-6 An ileostomy. The entire colon is surgically removed.

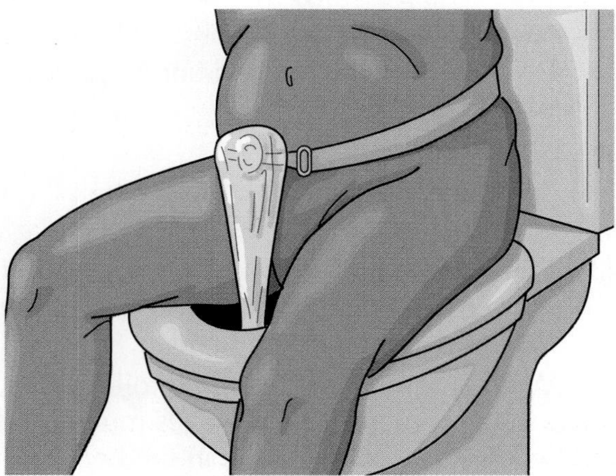

Figure 30-7 The ostomy pouch is secured to an ostomy belt. The pouch is emptied by directing it into the toilet and unclamping the end.

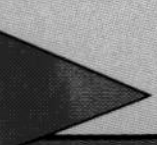

Changing an Ostomy Pouch

Compassionate Care

Remember to Promote:
- **Dignity**
- **Independence**
- **Preferences**
- **Privacy**
- **Safety**

Pre-Procedure

1. Identify the person according to employer policy.
2. Explain the procedure to the person.
3. Wash your hands.
4. Collect the following:
   - Clean pouch with skin barrier
   - Skin barrier as ordered (if not part of pouch)
   - Pouch clamp, clip, or wire closure
   - Clean ostomy belt (if used)
   - 4 to 8 gauze squares
   - Adhesive remover
   - Cotton balls
   - Bedpan with cover
   - Waterproof pad
   - Bath blanket
   - Toilet tissue
   - Washbasin
   - Bath thermometer
   - Soap or cleansing agent, according to the care plan
   - Pouch deodorant
   - Paper towels
   - Gloves
   - Disposable bag
5. Arrange paper towels on a work area. Place items on top of paper towels.
6. Provide for privacy.
7. Raise bed to a comfortable working height. Follow the care plan for bed rail use.*

Procedure

8. Lower the bed rail near you if up.
9. Cover the person with a bath blanket. Fan-fold linens to the foot of the bed.
10. Place the waterproof pad under the person's buttocks.
11. Put on gloves.
12. Disconnect the pouch from the belt if one is worn. Remove the belt.
13. Remove the pouch gently. Gently push the skin down and away from the skin barrier. Place the pouch in the bedpan.
14. Wipe around the stoma with toilet tissue or a gauze square. This removes mucus and feces. Place soiled tissue in the bedpan. Discard gauze squares into the disposable bag.
15. Moisten a cotton ball with adhesive remover. Clean around the stoma to remove any remaining skin barrier. Clean from the stoma outward.
16. Cover the bedpan. Take it to the bathroom. (If the person uses bed rails, raise the bed rails before leaving the bedside.)
17. Measure feces as directed by the care plan.
18. Report any abnormal feces. Then empty the pouch and bedpan into the toilet. Note the colour, amount, consistency, and odour of feces. Put the pouch in the disposable bag.
19. Remove gloves. Wash your hands. Put on clean gloves.
20. Fill the washbasin with warm water. (Measure temperature of water with bath thermometer. Check the care plan for correct temperature.) Place the basin on the work area on top of paper towels. Lower the bed rail near you if up.
21. Clean the skin around the stoma with water. Rinse and pat dry. Use soap or other cleansing agent.

Continued

Changing an Ostomy Pouch—cont'd

Procedure—cont'd

22 Observe the stoma and skin around the stoma. Report any irritation or skin breakdown.
23 Apply the skin barrier if it is a separate device.
24 Put a clean ostomy belt on the person (if a belt is worn).
25 Add deodorant to the new pouch.
26 Remove adhesive backing on the pouch.
27 Centre the pouch over the stoma. The drain points downward.
28 Press around the skin barrier so the pouch seals to the skin. Apply gentle pressure from the stoma outward.
29 Maintain pressure for 1 to 2 minutes.
30 Connect the belt to the pouch (if a belt is worn).
31 Remove the waterproof pad.
32 Remove gloves. Wash your hands. (If the person uses bed rails, raise the bed rails before leaving the bedside.)
33 Cover the person. Remove the bath blanket.

Post-Procedure

34 Provide for safety and comfort.
35 Place the call bell within reach.*
36 Return the bed to its lowest position. Follow the care plan for bed rail use.*
37 Remove privacy measures.
38 Clean the bedpan, washbasin, and other equipment. (Put on gloves for this step.)
39 Return equipment to its proper place.
40 Discard the disposable bag according to employer policy. Follow employer policy for soiled linen.
41 Remove gloves. Wash your hands.
42 Report and record your actions and observations according to employer policy.

*Steps marked with an asterisk may not apply in community settings.

STOOL SPECIMENS

When internal bleeding is suspected, feces are checked for blood. Stools are also studied for fat, microbes, worms, and other abnormal contents. The guidelines for collecting urine specimens (see Chapter 29) apply when collecting stool specimens. Follow Standard Precautions.

The stool specimen must not be contaminated with urine. Some tests require a warm stool. The specimen is taken to the laboratory immediately if a warm stool is needed.

(text continues on page 519)

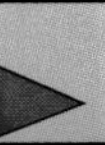

Collecting a Stool Specimen

Compassionate Care

Remember to Promote:
- **Dignity**
- **Independence**
- **Preferences**
- **Privacy**
- **Safety**

Pre-Procedure

1 Identify the person according to employer policy.
2 Explain the procedure to the person.
3 Wash your hands.
4 Collect the following:
- Bedpan and cover or bedside commode
- Urinal (or bedpan with cover) for voiding
- Specimen pan for the toilet or commode
- Specimen container and lid
- Tongue blade
- Disposable bag
- Gloves
- Toilet tissue
- Laboratory requisition slip
- Plastic bag

5 Label the container.
6 Provide for privacy.

Procedure

7 Ask the person to void. Provide the bedpan, commode, or urinal if the person does not use the bathroom. Empty and clean the device. Wear gloves.
8 Place the specimen pan under the toilet seat (Figure 30-8) if the person uses the bathroom.
9 Assist the person onto the bedpan or to the toilet or commode. The person wears a robe and nonskid footwear when up.
10 Ask the person not to put toilet tissue in the bedpan, commode, or specimen pan. Provide a disposable bag for toilet tissue.
11 Place the call bell (in facilities) and toilet tissue within reach. Raise or lower bed rails according to the care plan.
12 Wash your hands, and leave the room, if safe to do so. Stay within hearing distance.
13 Return when the person calls. Knock before entering. Wash your hands.
14 Lower the bed rail near you if up.
15 Put on gloves. Provide perineal care if needed.
16 Use a tongue blade to take about 30 mL (2 tablespoons) of feces from the bedpan, commode, or specimen pan to the specimen container (Figure 30-9). Take the sample from the middle of a formed stool. If required by employer policy, take stool from two different places on the specimen.
17 Put the lid on the specimen container. Do not touch the inside of the lid or container. Place the container in the plastic bag.
18 Wrap the tongue blade in toilet tissue.
19 Empty, clean, and disinfect the equipment.
20 Remove gloves. Wash your hands.
21 Return equipment to its proper place.
22 Assist the person with hand washing. Wear gloves if needed.

Continued

Collecting a Stool Specimen

Post-Procedure

23 Provide for safety and comfort.
24 Place the call bell within reach.*
25 Return the bed to its lowest position. Follow the care plan for bed rail use.*
26 Remove privacy measures.
27 Follow your supervisor's instructions for specimen storage and transportation.
28 Wash your hands.
29 Report and record your actions and observations according to employer policy.

*Steps marked with an asterisk may not apply in community settings.

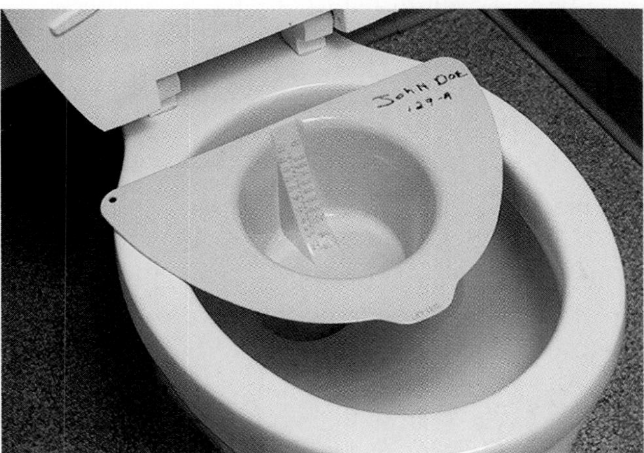

Figure 30-8 A specimen pan is placed in the toilet for a stool specimen.

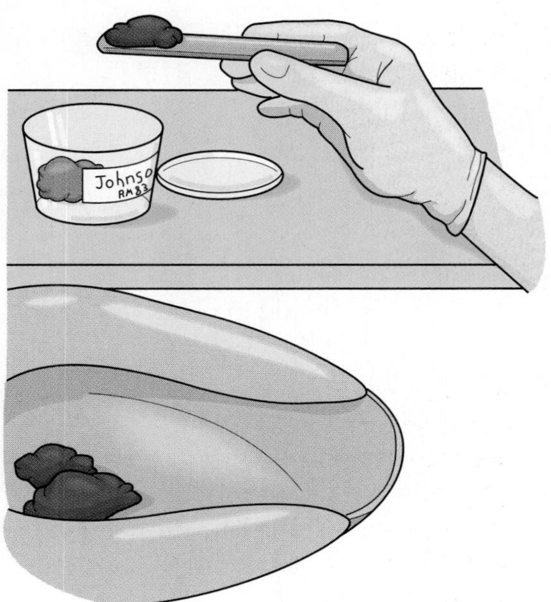

Figure 30-9 A tongue blade is used to transfer a small amount of stool from the bedpan to the specimen container.

Testing Stools for Blood

Blood can appear in stools for many reasons. Ulcers, colon cancer, and hemorrhoids are common causes. Often blood is visible. Blood can usually be seen if bleeding is low in the gastrointestinal tract. Stools are black and tarry if there is bleeding in the stomach or upper GI tract. **Melena** is a black, tarry stool.

Sometimes bleeding occurs in very small amounts. It is difficult to detect such bleeding by just observing the stools. Therefore stools are tested for the presence of *occult blood.* Occult means *hidden* or *unseen*. The test is often done to screen for colon cancer.

There are many types of tests. Follow the manufacturer's instructions for the test ordered. Also follow Standard Precautions. The care plan and your assignment sheet tell you when to collect the specimen. Many factors can affect the test results. One is eating red meat. Therefore the person cannot eat red meat for 3 days before the test. Bleeding from hemorrhoids and menstrual periods also affects test results.

Testing a Stool Specimen for Blood

Compassionate Care

Remember to Promote:
- **Dignity**
- **Independence**
- **Preferences**
- **Privacy**
- **Safety**

Pre-Procedure

1 Explain the procedure to the person.
2 Wash your hands.
3 Collect a stool specimen (see *Collecting a Stool Specimen* on page 518).
4 Collect the following:
- Paper towel
- Hemoccult test kit (includes developer)
- Tongue blades
- Gloves

5 Put on gloves.

Procedure

6 Open the test kit.
7 Use a tongue blade to obtain a small amount of stool.
8 Apply a thin smear of stool on box A on the test paper (Figure 30-10, *A*).
9 Use another tongue blade to obtain some stool from another part of the specimen.
10 Apply a thin smear of stool on box B on the test paper (Figure 30-10, *B*).
11 Close the test packet.
12 Turn the test packet to the other side. Open the flap. Apply developer to boxes A and B. Follow the manufacturer's instructions (Figure 30-10, *C*).
13 Wait the amount of time noted in the manufacturer's instructions. Time varies from 10 to 60 seconds.
14 Note and record the colour changes (Figure 30-10, *D*). Follow the manufacturer's instructions.
15 Dispose of the test packet.
16 Wrap the tongue blades in toilet tissue, then discard them.
17 Dispose of the specimen.
18 Remove gloves. Wash your hands.
19 Report and record your actions and observations according to employer policy.

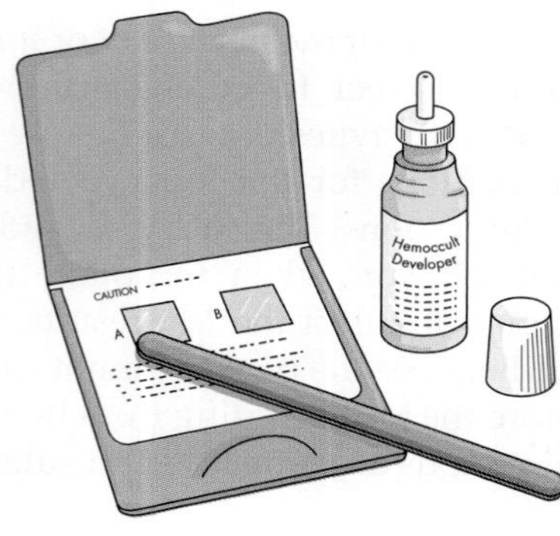

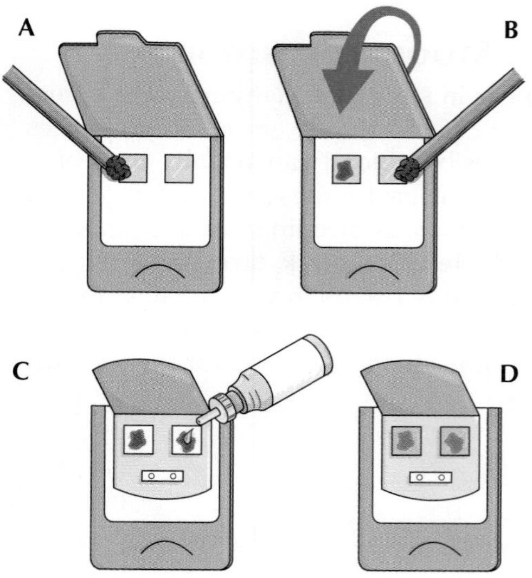

Figure 30-10 Testing for occult blood. **A,** Stool is smeared on box A. **B,** Stool is smeared on box B. **C,** Developer is applied to boxes A and B. **D,** Colour changes are noted.

REVIEW

Circle the BEST answer.

1. Which is *false*?
   A. A person must have a bowel movement every day.
   B. Stools are normally brown, soft, and formed.
   C. Diarrhea occurs when feces move through the intestines rapidly.
   D. Constipation results when feces move through the large intestine slowly.

2. The prolonged retention and accumulation of feces in the rectum is called
   A. Constipation
   B. Fecal impaction
   C. Diarrhea
   D. Anal incontinence

3. Which will *not* promote comfort and safety in relation to bowel elimination?
   A. Asking visitors to leave the room
   B. Helping the client assume a sitting position
   C. Offering the bedpan after meals
   D. Telling the client to hurry

4. Bowel training is aimed at
   A. Gaining control of bowel movements and developing a regular elimination pattern
   B. Ostomy control
   C. Preventing fecal impaction, constipation, and anal incontinence
   D. Preventing bleeding

5. Which is *not* used for a cleansing enema?
   A. Soapsuds
   B. Saline
   C. Oil
   D. Tap water

6. Which is *false*?
   A. Enema solutions should be 40.5° C (105° F).
   B. The Sims' position is used for an enema.
   C. The enema bag is held 30 cm (12 inches) above the anus.
   D. The enema solution is given rapidly.

7. In adults, the cleansing enema tube is inserted
   A. 5 cm (2 inches)
   B. 7.5 to 10 cm (3 to 4 inches)
   C. 13 to 15 cm (5 to 6 inches)
   D. 20 cm (8 inches)

8. The commercial enema
   A. Must be prepared before it is given
   B. Is ordered when complete cleansing of the bowel is needed
   C. Is retained until the person feels the urge to defecate
   D. Is retained for 60 to 90 minutes

9. Rectal tubes are left in place no longer than
   A. 60 minutes
   B. 30 minutes
   C. 20 minutes
   D. 10 minutes

10. Which statement about ostomies is *false*?
    A. Good skin care around the stoma is essential.
    B. Deodorants can control odours.
    C. The person wears a pouch.
    D. Feces are always liquid.

11. A client wears an ostomy pouch. It is usually emptied
    A. Every 4 to 6 hours
    B. Every morning
    C. Every 3 to 7 days
    D. When feces are present

12. You note a black, tarry stool. This is called
    A. Melena
    B. Feces
    C. Hemostool
    D. Occult blood

Answers to these questions are on page 825.

CHAPTER

31

Common Diseases and Conditions

OBJECTIVES

- Define the key terms listed in this chapter
- Describe cancer and its treatment
- Describe common cardiovascular disorders and the care required
- Describe common respiratory disorders and the care required
- Describe common neurological disorders and the care required
- Identify the causes and effects of brain and spinal cord injuries and the care required
- Describe common musculoskeletal disorders and the care required
- Explain how to care for clients in casts, in traction, and with hip fractures
- Describe the effects of amputation
- Describe common endocrine disorders and the care required
- Describe common digestive disorders and the care required
- Explain what to do when a client vomits
- Describe common urinary disorders and the care required
- Describe common communicable diseases and the care required

KEY TERMS

acquired brain injury Damage to brain tissue caused by disease, medical condition, accident, or violence

acquired immunodeficiency syndrome (AIDS) Immune system disease caused by the human immunodeficiency virus (HIV)

amputation The removal of all or part of an extremity

amyotrophic lateral sclerosis (ALS) A neurological disorder that results in the loss of all muscle control but does not affect intelligence; Lou Gehrig's disease

angina pectoris Chest (*pectoris*) pain (*angina*) due to coronary artery disease

arrhythmia Abnormal (*a*) heart rhythm (*rhythmia*)

arthritis Joint (*arthr*) inflammation (*itis*)

arthroplasty Surgical replacement (*plasty*) of a joint (*arthro*)

asthma Respiratory disease characterized by narrowed air passages; episodes of difficulty breathing (asthma attacks) occur

benign Noncancerous

cancer A group of diseases characterized by out of control cell division and growth

cerebral vascular accident (CVA) Stroke

chronic obstructive pulmonary disease (COPD) A chronic lung disorder that obstructs (blocks) the airways; refers to chronic bronchitis and emphysemia

communicable disease A disease caused by microbes that spread easily

congestive heart failure (CHF) Condition occurring when the heart cannot pump blood normally; causes a build up (congestion) of fluid in the tissues

coronary artery disease (CAD) A condition in which the coronary arteries are narrowed or blocked

diabetes A disorder in which the body cannot produce or use insulin properly; causes sugar (glucose) to build up in the blood

diverticulosis The condition (*osis*) of having small pouches in the colon that bulge outward (*diverticulum*)

fibromyaliga A condition associated with aching, stiffness, and fatigue in muscles, ligaments, and tendons

fracture A broken bone

gangrene A condition in which there is tissue death

heart attack Myocardial infarction

hemiplegia Paralysis (*plegia*) of one side (*hemi*) of the body; the right arm and leg or left arm and leg could be affected

hepatitis Inflammation (*itis*) of the liver (*hepat*) caused by a viral infection

Huntington's disease An inherited neurological disorder; causes uncontrolled movements, emotional disturbances, and cognitive losses

hypertension High blood pressure

influenza Respiratory tract infection; the "flu"

malignant Cancerous

metastasis The spread of cancer to other parts of the body

multiple sclerosis (MS) Progressive neurological disease in which nerve impulses are not sent to and from the brain in a normal manner

myocardial infarction (MI) Death (*infarction*) of heart tissue (*myocardium*) caused by lack of oxygen to the heart; heart attack

osteoporosis A bone disorder (*osteo*) in which the bone becomes porous and brittle (*poros*)

paralysis Complete or partial loss of ability to move a limb or muscle group

paraplegia Paralysis (*plegia*) from the waist down

Parkinson's disease Neurological disorder in which cells in certain parts of the brain are gradually destroyed; causes tremors, muscle stiffness, slow movement, and poor balance

pneumonia Infection of the lung tissue

quadriplegia Paralysis (*plegia*) of all four (*quad*) limbs and the trunk; paralysis from the neck down

renal calculi Kidney (*renal*) stones (*calculi*)

sexually transmitted disease (STD) A disease that is spread by sexual contact

stroke Sudden loss of brain function; cerebral vascular accident (CVA)

tuberculosis (TB) A bacterial infection, usually affecting the lungs

tumour An abnormal lump or mass caused by cells growing out of control; tumours are benign or malignant

This chapter gives basic information about common diseases and conditions. Some diseases and conditions are acute. Others are chronic. Many diseases are progressive—that is, they gradually get worse over time. Some clients become immobile and confined to bed. Others have physician's orders to stay in bed. Follow the guidelines listed in Box 31-1 when caring for clients confined to bed. These measures prevent complications of bed rest.

Understanding the disease or health condition is important when providing care. Your supervisor gives you more information as needed. A good attitude is important. Many diseases and health conditions are very disabling or life-threatening. Be positive when with clients. Remember the priorities of support work. (See *Providing Compassionate Care: Caring for Clients with Diseases or Conditions* box.)

A review of Chapter 13 (Body Structure and Function) will help you study this chapter. See Chapters 33 through 36 and 38 for descriptions of other health problems.

Box 31-1 Guidelines for Caring for Clients Confined to Bed

- Practise safety precautions. Check with your supervisor and the care plan about the use of bed rails.
- Give good skin care. Skin breakdown can occur rapidly (see Chapter 27).
- Turn and reposition the person as directed by the care plan. The person must be repositioned at least every 2 hours.
- Keep the person in good body alignment. Use pillows, trochanter rolls, foot boards, and other devices as needed (see Chapter 21).
- Make sure the person can call for assistance. In facilities, keep the call bell within easy reach. In private homes, stay within hearing distance. Or provide a tap bell, horn, or other device with which the person can call for you. Answer calls for assistance promptly.
- Meet food, fluid, and elimination needs.
- Change damp, soiled, or wet linen and garments immediately.
- Straighten wrinkled linen as needed.
- Perform range-of-motion exercises as directed by the care plan (see Chapter 22). These and other exercises maintain muscle function and prevent contractures.
- Encourage coughing and deep breathing exercises as directed by the care plan. These prevent respiratory complications (see Chapter 43).

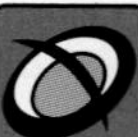

Providing Compassionate Care

Caring for Clients with Diseases or Conditions

D*ignity.* The care you give impacts the person's life. The physical support you provide is very important. But clients also need emotional support. Providing emotional support promotes the person's dignity. It shows that you care about the whole person, not just his or her physical needs. Remember, many people dealing with serious health problems are coping with change, loss, and fear. Imagine what life must be like for the person. The person may need someone to talk to. Being there when needed is important. You may not have to say anything. Just be a good listener when the person needs to talk. Use touch, if appropriate. Do not avoid the person out of fear of getting the disease. Do not judge the person or assume that he or she "deserves" the disease. This is very important, especially for people with communicable diseases.

Many people with health problems rely on their spiritual faith to help them cope. Respect all expressions of spirituality. Tell your supervisor if the person asks to speak with a spiritual adviser.

I*ndependence.* The more people can do for themselves, the better off they are. Always encourage clients to do what they can for themselves. This includes clients with advanced stages of disease.

P*references.* Protect the right to personal choice. Always explain what you are going to do. The client's consent is necessary. Also involve the person in deciding when to begin care or procedures. Always ask clients about their preferences. Respect them. If they conflict with the care plan, notify your supervisor.

P*rivacy.* Protect the right to privacy and confidentiality. Remember to close doors and privacy curtains before procedures. Expose only the body part involved in the procedure. Always keep your conversations private. Discuss the client's health problems only with your supervisor and the health team members involved in the client's care. Do not give information to families and visitors. Do not discuss clients with your family and friends.

S*afety.* Clients with health problems are at high risk for falls, choking, and other accidents (see Chapter 16). Know the safety measures required for the client. Also follow the guidelines listed in Box 31-1. Always remember to practise Standard Precautions. They protect you and others.

CANCER

Cells reproduce for tissue growth and repair. Cells usually divide in an orderly and controlled way. **Cancer** is a group of diseases characterized by out of control cell division and growth. A lump or mass of cells develops. This new growth of abnormal cells is called a **tumour**. Tumours are **benign** (noncancerous) or **malignant** (cancerous). Benign tumours grow slowly and are contained in one area. They do not usually cause death. Malignant tumours grow rapidly and invade other tissues (Figure 31-1).

Metastasis is the spread of cancer to other body parts (Figure 31-2). Cancer cells break off the tumour and travel to other body parts. New tumours grow in other body parts. Death occurs if the cancer is not treated and controlled.

Cancer can occur in almost any body part. Common cancer sites are the lungs, breast, prostate, colon and rectum, uterus, urinary tract, and skin. Cancer is the second leading cause of death in Canada.[1] It occurs in all age groups. *Leukemia* (a type of blood cancer) is the most common cancer in children.

The exact causes of cancer are unknown. However, certain factors contribute to its development. They include:

- A family history of cancer
- Smoking
- Overuse of alcohol
- High-fat, high-calorie, low-fibre diet
- Exposure to radiation (including the sun)
- Exposure to certain chemicals (carcinogenic agents)
- Hormones
- Viruses

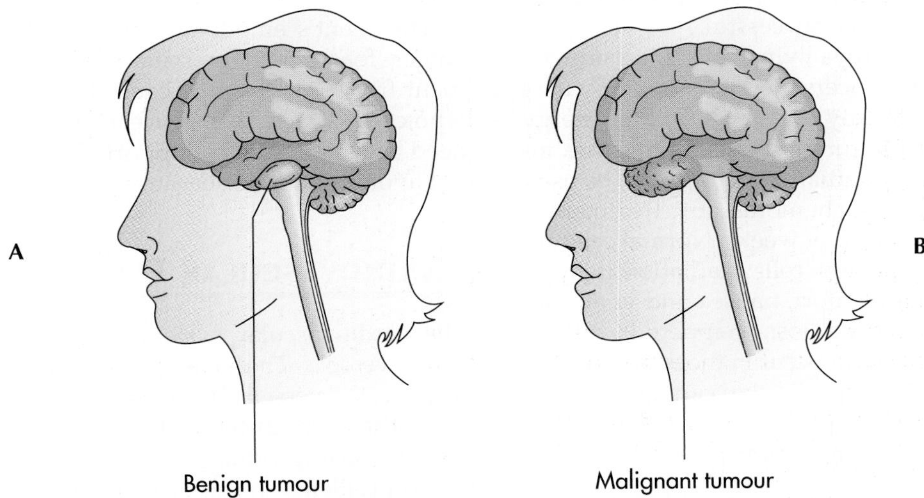

Figure 31-1 A, Benign tumours grow within a localized area. **B,** Malignant tumours invade other tissues.

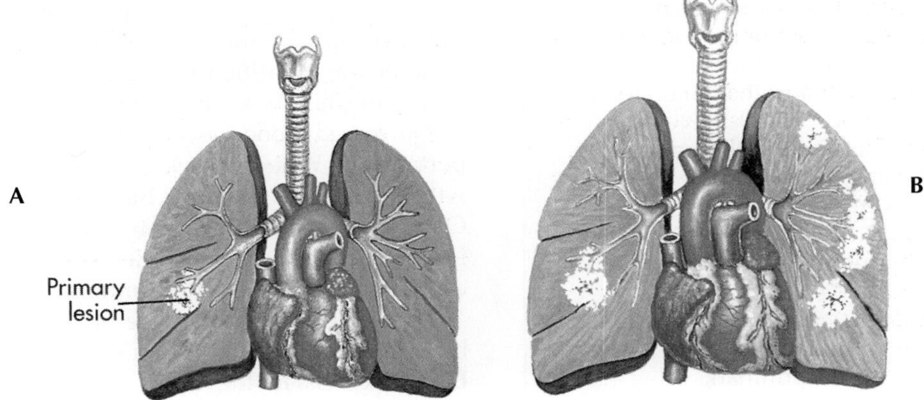

Figure 31-2 A, A tumour in the lung. **B,** The tumour has metastasized to the other lung. Source: A.E. Belcher, *Cancer Nursing* (St. Louis: Mosby, 1992).

Treatment is most successful when the cancer is detected as early as possible. The warning signs identified by the Canadian Cancer Society are listed in Box 31-2.

Treatment depends on the type of tumour, its location and size, and whether it has spread. One or a combination of treatments is used. The treatment can be used to:

- Cure the cancer
- Keep the cancer from spreading
- Slow the cancer's growth
- Relieve symptoms caused by the cancer

The three major cancer treatments are surgery, radiation therapy, and chemotherapy.

Surgery is often the first treatment if the cancer is localized (contained to one area). Malignant tissue and surrounding tissue that might contain cancer cells are removed. If the tumour has not spread to other areas, surgery is more likely to be successful.

Radiation therapy destroys living cells. Like surgery, it is used for localized cancers. Radiation therapy uses high-energy rays to destroy cancer cells. High-energy rays are directed at the tumour. Or implants are inserted near the tumour. Radiation therapy can be used alone or with surgery and chemotherapy. Treatment is usually given over a period of weeks. Normal cells are destroyed along with cancer cells. Radiation therapy side effects include discomfort, nausea and vomiting, fatigue (tiredness), anorexia (loss of appetite), and diarrhea. Skin breakdown can occur in the exposed area. The physician may order special skin care procedures.

Chemotherapy involves powerful drugs that kill cells. Like radiation, chemotherapy affects normal cells and cancer cells. Side effects can be severe. The digestive tract may be irritated. Nausea, vomiting, and diarrhea may result. An inflammation of the mouth (*stomatitis*) may develop. Hair loss (*alopecia*) may occur. Decreased production of blood cells occurs. As a result, the person may tire easily and is at risk for bruising, bleeding, and infection.

Clients with cancer have many needs. Their care often includes:

- Providing pain relief or control
- Ensuring adequate rest and exercise
- Providing fluids and good nutrition
- Preventing skin breakdown
- Preventing bowel elimination problems (constipation occurs from pain medications; diarrhea occurs from chemotherapy)
- Managing the side effects of radiation therapy and chemotherapy

The client's emotional and social needs are great. Anger, fear, and depression are common. Disfigurement from surgery may cause the person to feel unwhole, unattractive, or unclean. The client and family need much emotional support. Talk to the client. Do not avoid him or her because you are uncomfortable.

Box 31-2 Warning Signs of Cancer

- A cough that goes on for more than two weeks
- Blood in the stool
- Any change in bowel habits (constipation or diarrhea) that continues for more than a few days
- Indigestion that continues for more than 2 weeks
- Unexplained aches and pains that go on for more than 2 weeks
- Difficulty urinating or blood in the urine
- Unexplained bleeding of any sort
- Any lump or mass, especially in the breasts or testicles
- Any sore that does not heal
- Any new growth on the skin
- Patches of skin that bleed, itch, or become red
- Any change in the colour, shape, surface appearance, or size of moles or birthmarks

Source: Canadian Cancer Society, 2003.

CARDIOVASCULAR DISORDERS

The cardiovascular system involves the heart and blood vessels. The heart pumps blood continuously through the vessels. Blood delivers oxygen, nutrients, and other substances to the body's cells. It also removes waste products. Cardiovascular disorders involve problems in the heart or in the blood vessels. They are the leading causes of death in Canada.[2]

HYPERTENSION

Hypertension is abnormally high blood pressure. The systolic pressure is 140 mm Hg or higher. Or the diastolic pressure is 90 mm Hg or higher (see Chapter 40). Elevated measurements must occur on two occasions. Risk factors identified by the Heart and Stroke Foundation of Canada are listed in Box 31-3.

Narrowed blood vessels are a common cause of hypertension. When vessels narrow, the heart pumps with more force to move blood through the vessels. Other causes of hypertension include underlying medical problems. Kidney disorders, head injuries, complications of pregnancy, and tumours are examples.

Hypertension can damage other body organs. The heart may enlarge so it can pump with more force. Blood vessels in the brain may burst and cause a stroke. Blood vessels in the eyes, kidneys, and other organs may be damaged.

Box 31-3 Risk Factors for Hypertension

- *Age*—Blood pressure tends to rise with age, beginning at about age 35.
- *Ethnicity*—The incidence of hypertension is higher among Canadians of South Asian, Aboriginal, and African descent.
- *Family history*—If a parent has hypertension, the adult child has a greater chance of also developing it. The risk increases if both parents have hypertension.
- *Obesity*—The risk increases if the weight is stored around the abdomen.
- *Diabetes*—People with diabetes are at increased risk for hypertension.
- *Stress*—Repeated exposure to stress may raise blood pressure levels.
- *Alcohol*—Excessive alcohol consumption increases blood pressure.
- *Smoking*—Cigarette smoking may contribute to hypertension in some people.

Source: Heart and Stroke Foundation of Canada, 2002.

At first, hypertension may not cause signs or symptoms. Many people have hypertension but do not know it. Usually it is discovered when blood pressure is measured. Signs and symptoms develop as the disorder progresses. Headache, blurred vision, and dizziness may be reported. Complications of hypertension include stroke, heart attack, kidney (renal) failure, and blindness.

Certain medications can lower blood pressure. The person needs to quit smoking and get enough exercise and rest. A sodium-restricted diet (low-salt diet) may also be ordered. If the person is overweight, a low-calorie diet is ordered.

Coronary Artery Disease

The coronary arteries are in the heart. They supply the heart with oxygen- and nutrient-rich blood. **Coronary artery disease (CAD)** is a condition in which the coronary arteries are narrowed or blocked. The thickening and narrowing of the artery walls is called *atherosclerosis*. This is caused by a build-up of cholesterol (a soft, waxy substance) and other fatty substances along their inside walls (Figure 31-3). When the coronary arteries are narrowed or blocked, blood flow to the heart is slowed or stopped. The heart muscle does not get enough oxygen and nutrients. It cannot work properly. CAD may lead to chest pain and heart attack.

Risk factors for CAD include:

- Hypertension
- High blood cholesterol

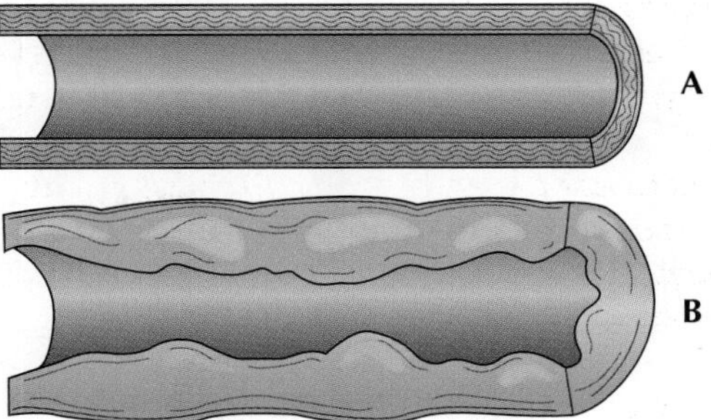

Figure 31-3 A, Normal artery. **B,** Fatty deposits on the walls of arteries with atherosclerosis.

- Lifestyle factors (lack of exercise, obesity, smoking, excessive alcohol, stress)
- Uncontrolled diabetes
- Age (more common in older adults)
- Sex (more common in men)
- Family history of CAD

Treatment for CAD involves reducing risk factors. Nothing can be done about the person's sex, age, and family history. However, efforts are directed at weight loss, regular exercise, no smoking, and a healthy diet. Controlling blood pressure and diabetes also is important.

Angina Pectoris. **Angina pectoris** means chest (*pectoris*) pain (*angina*) due to coronary artery disease. It occurs when the heart muscle does not get enough oxygen. People with angina are at risk for a heart attack. Physical exertion is the most common trigger for angina. Other triggers include emotional stress, extreme cold or heat, heavy meals, alcohol, and smoking.

The chest pain associated with angina has been described as a feeling of heaviness, tightness, or pressure. Usually the pain occurs on the left side. Some people feel severe pain, lasting 2 to 15 minutes. Pain may travel (radiate) to the jaw, neck, shoulders, back, and/or arms (Figure 31-4 on page 528). Sometimes, angina is mistaken for indigestion or heartburn when felt in the upper abdominal area. Besides pain, the person may have shortness of breath, nausea, sweating, dizziness or light-headedness, fatigue, or palpitations (quick heartbeats). These signs and symptoms cause the person to stop activity and rest. Rest often relieves the symptoms in 3 to 15 minutes. Rest reduces the heart's need for oxygen. Therefore normal blood flow is achieved and heart damage is prevented.

Besides resting and avoiding common triggers, *nitroglycerin* often is prescribed to relieve angina. Nitroglycerin is taken in tablet, ointment, patch, or spray form. The medication is kept near the client at all times. The person takes a dose when an angina attack occurs.

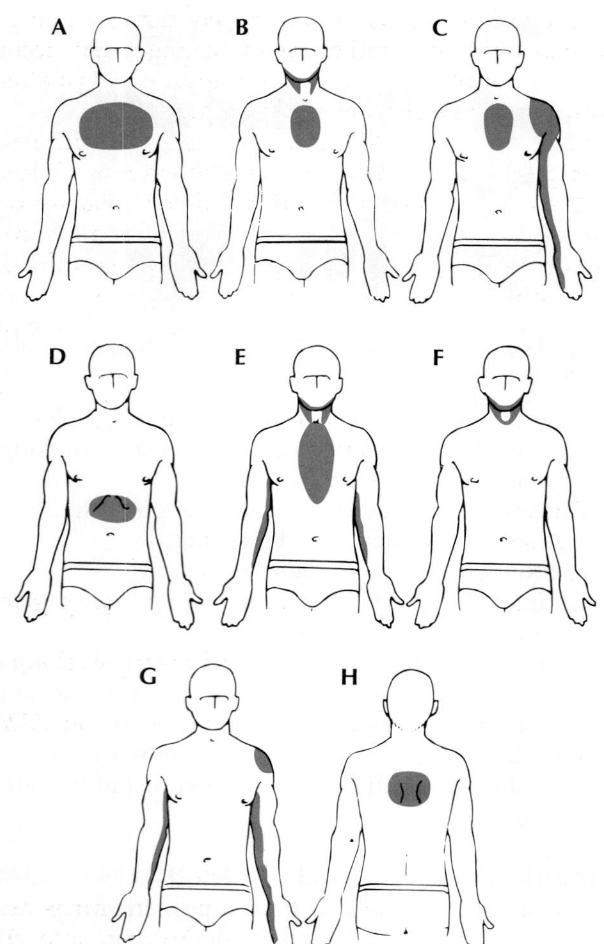

Figure 31-4 Shaded areas show where the pain of angina pectoris is located. Source: W.J. Phipps, V.L. Cassmeyer, J.K. Sands, and M.K. Lehman, *Medical-Surgical Nursing: Concepts and Clinical Practice*, 5th ed. (St. Louis: Mosby, 1995).

Some people need coronary artery bypass surgery. The surgery bypasses the diseased part of the artery and increases blood flow to the heart. Many people with angina eventually have heart attacks (myocardial infarctions).

Myocardial Infarction. A **myocardial infarction (MI)** is death (*infarction*) of heart tissue (*myocardium*) caused by lack of oxygen to the heart. Common terms for MI are *heart attack, coronary, coronary thrombosis,* and *coronary occlusion.* Blood flow to the heart is suddenly interrupted. Atherosclerosis or a thrombus (blood clot) obstructs blood flow through an artery. The area of damage may be small or large (Figure 31-5). Sudden cardiac death (*cardiac arrest*) can occur (see Chapter 47).

The person has one or more of the signs and symptoms listed in Box 31-4. Often, the person denies that he or she is having an MI. The average person waits almost 5 hours before getting help. Myocardial infarction is an emergency. Efforts are directed at relieving pain, stabilizing vital signs, giving oxygen, and calming the person. Many medications are given. The person is treated in a hospital coronary care unit (CCU). The unit has emergency equipment and medications needed to prevent life-threatening complications.

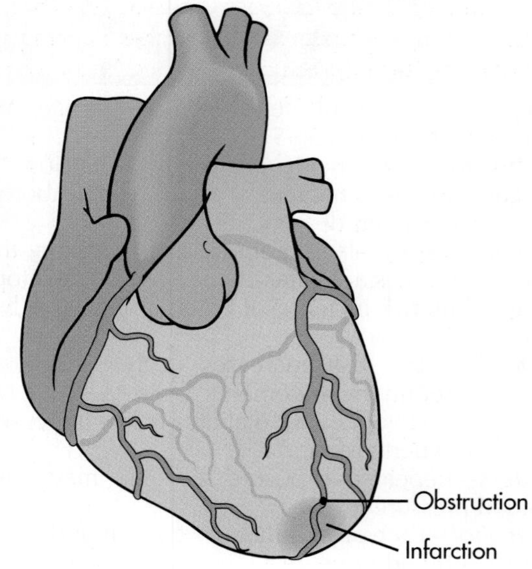

Figure 31-5 Myocardial infarction. Source: S.M. Lewis, M.M. Heitkemper, and S.R. Dirkson, *Medical-Surgical Nursing: Assessment and Management of Clinical Problems*, 5th ed. (St. Louis: Mosby, 2000).

Box 31-4 Signs and Symptoms of Myocardial Infarction

- Sudden, severe chest pain, usually on the left side
- Pain described as crushing, stabbing, or squeezing; most people complain of feelings of tightness, heaviness, pressure, fullness, or burning in the chest
- Pain that radiates to the neck and jaw, and down the arm or to other sites
- Pain that is more severe and lasts longer than angina
- Pain that is not relieved by rest and nitroglycerin
- Indigestion
- Shortness of breath
- Nausea or vomiting
- Dizziness
- Perspiration
- Cyanosis (bluish lips and nail beds from lack of oxygen in the blood)
- Cold and clammy skin
- Low blood pressure
- Weak and irregular pulse

The person is in the CCU for 2 to 3 days. When stable, the person is transferred to another nursing unit. Activity is increased gradually. Medications and measures to prevent complications are continued. Rehabilitation is planned and continues when the person returns home. The goal is to prevent another heart attack. The program includes an exercise program and teaching about medications, dietary changes, and activity. Lifestyle changes may be necessary. Normal activities are increased slowly, including normal sexual activity. The person returns to work when advised by the physician.

Arrhythmias

Arrhythmias are abnormal (*a*) heart rhythms (*rhythmias*). They happen when the heart's electrical system malfunctions. Sometimes heartbeats are skipped. Or there are extra beats. Usually the person's health is not affected. Other arrhythmias are more serious. They can cause dizziness, shortness of breath, fainting, or death. Sometimes avoiding caffeine (coffee, tea, colas, and chocolate) or alcohol may prevent arrhythmias. Medications are needed for severe arrhythmias.

Pacemakers are used to treat some arrhythmias. Pacemakers are medical devices that are implanted in the person's body. They monitor heart rates. When necessary, they give small electric shocks to stimulate the heartbeat. Pacemakers run on batteries for several years. Clients with pacemakers should avoid any areas or equipment that have strong electrical or magnetic fields.

Congestive Heart Failure

Congestive heart failure (CHF), or heart failure, occurs when the heart cannot pump blood normally. Blood backs up and causes an abnormal amount (congestion) of fluid in the tissues. CHF may affect the right side, left side, or both sides of the heart.

The right side of the heart receives blood from the body tissue and pumps it into the lungs to get oxygen. With right-sided heart failure, blood backs up into the veins. Fluid collection in the body produces weight gain. There is swelling in the feet and ankles and enlarged neck veins. The liver becomes engorged and liver function is impaired. Congestion in the abdomen may cause digestive problems including loss of appetite, abdominal pain, and (eventually) loss of weight.

The left side of the heart receives blood from the lungs and pumps it into the rest of the body. With left-sided heart failure, the blood collects in the lung tissue. This results in difficulty breathing (dyspnea), increased sputum (mucus in the lungs), cough, and gurgling sounds in the lungs. Dyspnea is worse during activity and when the person is lying down. It disrupts sleep. The person may wake up with a suffocating feeling. Fatigue and limb weakness are common.

In advanced CHF, the brain may not get enough oxygen. Confusion and behaviour changes may occur. Poor blood flow to the kidneys results in impaired kidney function and low urine output.

CHF can be treated and controlled. Medications strengthen the heart and reduce the amount of fluid in the body. A sodium-restricted diet is usually ordered. Oxygen may be given. Weight is measured daily to check for weight gain, an early sign of fluid build-up. Most clients with CHF prefer semi-Fowler's or Fowler's position for breathing. You may be involved with:

- Maintaining bed rest (see Box 31-1 on page 524)
- Measuring intake and output
- Measuring daily weight
- Restricting fluids as ordered by the physician
- Assisting with transfers or ambulation
- Assisting with self-care activities
- Maintaining good positioning and body alignment according to the care plan
- Applying elastic stockings to reduce leg swelling

(See *Focus on Children: CHF* and *Focus on Older Adults: CHF* boxes.)

Respiratory Disorders

The respiratory system is made up of the lungs and their airways. The airways bring oxygen into the lungs and remove carbon dioxide from the body. Respiratory disorders interfere with this function and threaten life.

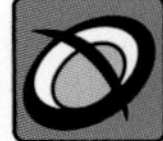

Focus on Children

CHF

Congenital heart defects can cause congestive heart failure in children. (Congenital comes from the Latin word *congenitus*. It means *to be born with*.)

Focus on Older Adults

CHF

Many older adults have CHF. They may need home care or long-term care. The older adult is at risk for skin breakdown. Tissue swelling, poor circulation, and fragile skin combine to increase the risk of pressure ulcers. Good skin care and regular position changes are essential.

Chronic Obstructive Pulmonary Disease

Chronic obstructive pulmonary disease (COPD) is the fourth leading cause of death for Canadian men and the seventh for Canadian women.[3] It is a chronic lung disorder that obstructs (blocks) the airways. Breathing is difficult. COPD refers to chronic bronchitis and emphysema. Chronic bronchitis and emphysema often occur together. COPD is a progressive disease. That is, it worsens over time.

Smoking is the most common cause of COPD. Long-time exposure to chemical fumes and to certain dusts is another cause.

COPD cannot be cured, but it can be controlled. The person must quit smoking and avoid second-hand smoke. Medications are ordered to open the airways. They are usually delivered by metered dose inhalers, or "puffers" (see Chapter 39). Breathing exercises and oxygen therapy may be ordered. Fluid intake is encouraged to decrease the thickness of secretions. Efforts are made to prevent respiratory tract infections. If one occurs, prompt treatment is necessary.

Chronic Bronchitis. Chronic bronchitis is a chronic inflammation of the bronchi, the large airway passages entering the lungs. Large amounts of mucus are produced in the bronchi. The bronchial walls swell. The mucus is thick and difficult to cough up. The mucus cannot be cleared completely and obstructs the airways. This makes airflow into and out of the lungs difficult. Therefore the body cannot get normal amounts of oxygen. The excess mucus also provides a place for the growth of microbes. Infection is a risk. Coughing is the first and most common symptom of chronic bronchitis. The person also has difficulty breathing and tires easily. Eventually, breathing becomes difficult even while the person is resting.

Emphysema. Emphysema occurs when the walls of the alveoli (tiny air sacs within the lungs) are damaged. The alveoli are less elastic than normal. They do not expand and shrink normally when the person inhales and exhales. As a result, when the person breathes out, air is trapped in some of the alveoli and not exhaled. As the disease progresses, more alveoli are involved. Therefore more air is trapped. The normal exchange of oxygen and carbon dioxide cannot occur in affected alveoli. As more air is trapped in the lungs, the person develops a *barrel chest* (Figure 31-6).

Breathing is very difficult for people with emphysema. Sometimes they lose weight because eating is difficult when they are out of breath. Clients with emphysema usually prefer to sit upright and slightly forward. Breathing is easier in this position.

Asthma

Asthma is a respiratory disease characterized by narrowed air passages. Sudden episodes of difficulty breathing (asthma attacks) occur. The person becomes short of breath, produces wheezing sounds, and may be very frightened. The person may also have a rapid pulse, perspiration, and cyanosis. Allergies, exercise, cold air, and emotional stress are common causes of asthma attacks.

Medications are used to treat asthma. Emergency room treatment may be necessary for severe attacks. The person and family are taught how to prevent asthma attacks. Repeated attacks can damage the respiratory system.

Pneumonia

Pneumonia is an infection of the lung tissue. Alveoli in the affected area fill with pus, mucus, and other liquid. Oxygen and carbon dioxide are not exchanged properly. There is not enough oxygen in the blood.

Bacteria and viruses cause pneumonia. People who are immobile or aspirate are at higher risk for developing pneumonia. The onset can be gradual or sudden. Signs and symptoms include: shaking, chills, severe

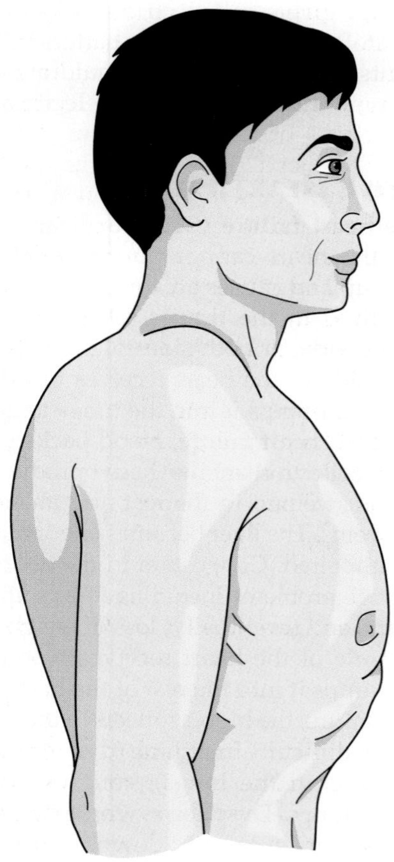

Figure 31-6 Barrel chest from emphysema.

chest pain, a cough that produces rust-coloured or greenish sputum, high temperature, rapid breathing and pulse rate, cyanosis, and confusion. Follow Standard Precautions. Isolation Precautions may also be ordered to prevent the spread of pneumonia.

Treatments include:

- Antibiotics to fight the infection
- Medications to ease chest pain, cough, and fever
- Proper diet
- Proper fluid and hydration
- Fowler's or semi-Fowler's position to make breathing easier
- Oxygen therapy

Influenza

Influenza ("the flu") is a respiratory tract infection caused by a virus. In Canada, the flu season is from November or December through April or May. Millions of people suffer from the flu. Influenza is highly contagious. It spreads when an infected person coughs or sneezes. It can also be spread by indirect contact—for example, by touching an object like a doorknob or telephone that was recently handled by an infected person.

Onset is usually sudden, with headache, chills, and cough. Fever, appetite loss, muscle aches, and tiredness also occur. Coldlike symptoms occur, including runny nose, sneezing, watery eyes, and throat irritation. Nausea, vomiting, or diarrhea may occur, especially in children. Recovery is usually complete in 1 to 2 weeks. However, some people develop serious and life-threatening complications. Pneumonia is an example.

Good hygiene and Standard Precautions reduce the risk of infection. Washing your hands before and after client contact is essential. The most effective method of prevention is the flu vaccine. People at high risk need yearly flu vaccinations. At-risk people include:

- People 65 years of age and older
- Residents of long-term care facilities
- People who have chronic disease
- Caregivers and people who live with someone in a high-risk group

Your employer may request or require that you get a yearly flu vaccination. This protects you and your clients.

Tuberculosis

Tuberculosis (TB) is a bacterial infection, usually affecting the lungs. However, TB can also occur in the brain, kidneys, bones, lymph nodes, and urinary and digestive systems.

TB was a major cause of death in the early 1900s. TB medications were introduced in the 1940s. A dramatic decline in the number of TB cases resulted. However, TB still occurs and is a major health problem. In the late 1980s, the number of cases began to increase.

The bacteria causing TB are spread by airborne droplets (see Chapter 18). Bacteria are spread when the infected person coughs, sneezes, or speaks. Others in the environment can inhale the bacteria. Anyone who has close, frequent contact with an infected person is at risk. TB is more likely to occur in close, crowded areas such as inner-city neighbourhoods. People with HIV infection are also at risk.

Sometimes bacteria do not cause an infection until many years later. The person may not have symptoms at first. The disease is found during a routine chest X-ray or a TB skin test. Early signs and symptoms are tiredness, loss of appetite, weight loss, fever, and night sweats. Coughing occurs. The cough is more frequent as the disease progresses. Sputum production also increases. Chest pain occurs.

People with active TB may need hospital care for treatment. When they return home, they must continue taking TB medications daily for several months.

Clients with TB need to cover their noses and mouths with tissues when coughing or sneezing. Tissues are flushed down the toilet. In health care facilities, tissues are placed in a biohazard bag and disposed of following facility policy. Standard Precautions and Airborne Precautions are practised (see Chapter 18).

Neurological Disorders

Neurological disorders involve problems in the nervous system. The nervous system communicates signals between the brain and the body. Nervous system disorders affect physical and cognitive functions. *Physical functions* include tasks such as moving, touching, seeing, hearing, and controlling the bowel and bladder. *Cognitive functions* include tasks controlled by the mind. (The word *cognitive* is related to knowledge.) Cognitive functions include thinking, reasoning, understanding, remembering, learning, reading, and problem solving.

Stroke

Stroke, or *cerebral vascular accident (CVA)*, is the fourth leading cause of death in Canada.[4] It is also the leading cause of nervous system disabilities in adults.

The Heart and Stroke Foundation of Canada defines **stroke** as a sudden loss of brain function. It is caused by one of the following:

- An interruption of blood flow to the brain, often caused by a blood clot
- The rupture of a blood vessel in the brain

When a vessel to the brain is blocked or bursts, blood supply to a part of the brain is suddenly obstructed. Brain cells in the affected area do not get oxygen and nutrients. Brain injury occurs. Functions controlled by that part of the brain are lost or impaired.

Temporary interruption of blood flow to the brain is called a *transient ischemic attack (TIA)*. There is no permanent brain injury. However, a TIA is an important warning sign. Sometimes a TIA occurs before a stroke. The person having a TIA needs medical attention.

The risk of stroke increases with age. Most strokes affect people aged 65 or older. Men are at slightly higher risk than women. However, more women than men die from stroke. Other risk factors include high blood pressure, smoking, diabetes, heart disease, high blood cholesterol, lack of exercise, and high alcohol intake.

Common warning signs of a stroke are listed in Box 31-5. Stroke is a medical emergency. The person needs immediate medical attention.

If the person survives the stroke, some brain injury is likely. The injured area in the brain cannot send messages to control certain parts of the body. Normal function is affected. The functions lost depend on the area of brain injury (Figure 31-7). The effects of stroke include:

- **Hemiplegia**—paralysis (*plegia*) of one side (*hemi*) of the body; the right arm and leg or the left arm and leg could be affected
- Weakness on one side of the body
- Loss of face control
- Changing emotions (the person may cry easily, sometimes for no apparent reason)
- Difficulty swallowing (dysphagia)
- Dimmed vision or loss of vision
- Loss of ability to speak or understand others (see Chapter 35)
- Changes in sight, touch, movement, and thought
- Impaired memory
- Urinary frequency, urgency, or incontinence

The person's behaviour is affected. The person may forget about or ignore the weaker side. This is from loss of movement and feeling on that side. If vision is affected, the person may not see one side of the visual field. For example, this can cause the person to see and therefore eat food only on one side of the plate. Or, he or she might be able to read only one side of a page.

Box 31-5 Warning Signs of a Stroke

- Sudden weakness, numbness, or tingling in the face, arm, or leg
- Sudden loss of speech or trouble understanding speech
- Sudden vision problems, particularly in one eye
- Sudden, severe headache with no known cause
- Sudden, unexplained dizziness

Source: Heart and Stroke Foundation of Canada, 2003.

After a stroke, people may no longer recognize familiar objects or know how to use them. Telling time may be hard. They may not recognize people. Memory problems or difficulty learning and remembering new information are common. The person may forget what to do or how to do it. Or if the person does know, the body may not respond. This makes it difficult to carry out activities of daily living (see Chapter 34).

Depression is common after a stroke. This can be a result of the brain injury. Depression is also often caused by illness and disability. Clients should be encouraged to share their feelings during this difficult period. Sometimes their emotional responses may seem exaggerated or inappropriate. Outbursts of anger, moaning, laughing, or crying for little or no reason are common. Remember, these reactions are beyond the client's control. Be patient and kind. Report to your supervisor any changes in the client's behaviour or mood.

Rehabilitation starts immediately after a stroke. Many clients can regain or improve lost functions. Speech, physical, and occupational therapies are usually ordered. Self-help devices may be necessary (see Chapter 32). The client may depend partially or totally on others for care. Many stroke survivors return home. They may require home care. Other stroke survivors need subacute or long-term care. Care depends on the client's needs and condition. Many clients require assistance with activities of daily living. The client is encouraged to do as much as possible. Clients who are immobile need good skin care to prevent pressure ulcers. They also may require a bladder or bowel training program and range-of-motion exercises. Communication methods are established for clients with language disorders (see Chapter 35).

Parkinson's Disease

Parkinson's disease is a neurological disorder in which cells in certain parts of the brain are gradually destroyed. It is progressive, with no cure. The disease is usually seen in people over 50 years of age. Signs and symptoms become worse over time. They include:

- *Tremors*—often start in one finger and spread to the whole arm. Pill-rolling movements (rubbing of the thumb and index finger) may occur. Tremors may occur in the legs, jaw, and face.
- *Stiff muscles*—in the arms, legs, neck, and trunk
- *Masklike expression*—the person cannot blink or smile. A fixed stare is common.
- *Slow movement*—the person has a slow, shuffling walk.
- *Stooped posture and impaired balance*—it is hard to walk. Falls are a risk.

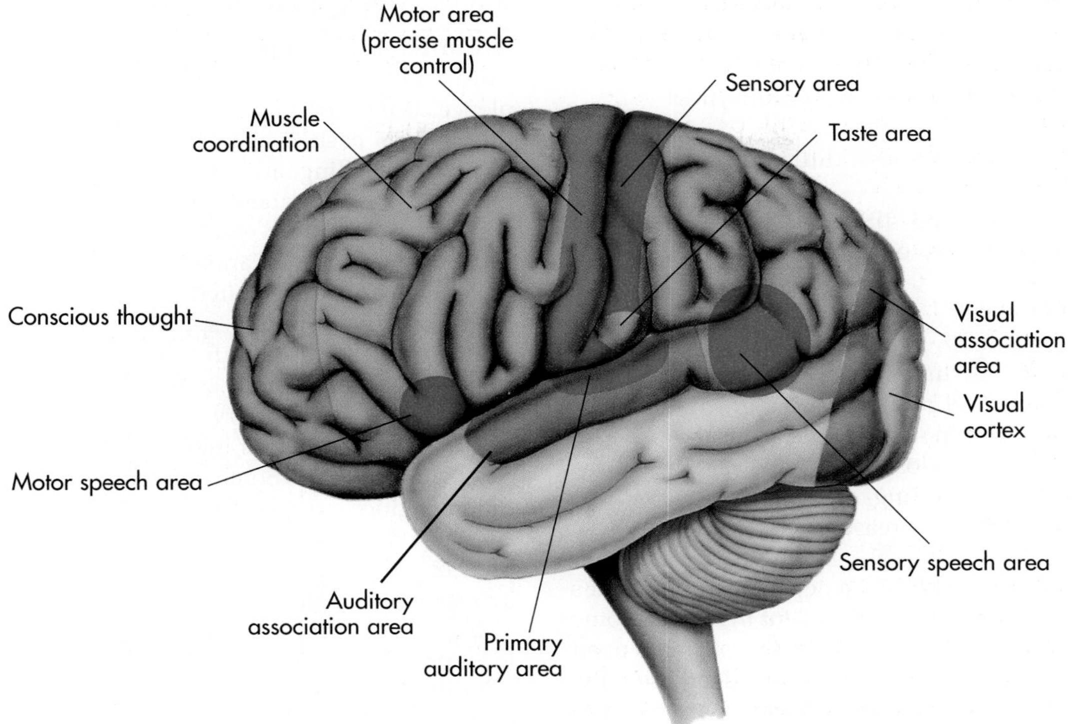

Figure 31-7 Functions lost from a stroke depend on the area of brain injury. Source: G.A. Thibodeau and K.T. Patton, *The Human Body in Health and Disease*, 2nd ed. (St. Louis: Mosby, 1997).

Other signs and symptoms can also develop over time. They include swallowing and chewing problems, constipation, and bowel and bladder problems. Sleep problems and depression can occur. So can dementia—memory loss, slow thinking, and emotional changes (see Chapter 34). Speech changes occur. They include slurred, monotone, and soft speech. Some people talk too fast or repeat what they say.

The physician orders medications specific for Parkinson's disease. Exercise and physical therapy are ordered. These help improve or maintain strength, posture, balance, and mobility. The client needs to have regular rest periods and to avoid stress. Tiredness and stress can make the symptoms worse. The client may need help with activities of daily living. Measures to promote normal elimination are practised. Safety practices are followed to prevent falls and choking. The client is treated with dignity and respect. Remember, the person's masklike facial expression does not show the person's true feelings.

Huntington's Disease

Huntington's disease is an inherited neurological disorder. It destroys brain cells and causes uncontrolled movements, emotional disturbances, and cognitive losses. Signs and symptoms usually appear between the ages of 20 and 60. They begin with twitching, fidgeting, and clumsiness. Over time, the person's arms and legs constantly move, making walking impossible. The person may have difficulty eating and swallowing. The person cannot perform many activities of daily living.

People with Huntington's disease also may have slurred speech, depression, irritability, and apathy. Cognitive losses include intellectual speed, attention, and short-term memory. Concentration on intellectual tasks becomes increasingly difficult as the disease progresses. Currently, there is no cure. There are no treatments to prevent or control the disease.

Care depends on the client's needs. Safety practices are followed to prevent falls, choking, and other accidents.

Multiple Sclerosis

Multiple sclerosis (MS) is a progressive neurological disease in which nerve impulses are not sent to and from the brain in a normal manner. Functions are impaired or lost.

Canadians have one of the highest rates of MS in the world. It is the most common neurological disease affecting young adults in Canada.[5] Symptoms usually start between the ages of 20 and 40 years. Women are affected more often than men. The onset is gradual. Symptoms vary greatly from person to person. A person can also have different symptoms at different times. Often, symptoms improve during periods of remission. Common symptoms are:

- Blurred vision, double vision, or blindness
- Extreme fatigue
- Loss of balance, dizziness, difficulty walking, and clumsiness
- Muscle weakness and stiffness
- Tingling, numbness, or a burning feeling in one area of the body
- Sensitivity to heat
- Difficulty speaking
- Difficulty swallowing
- Bladder and bowel problems
- Impotence or diminished sexual arousal
- Short-term memory loss
- Difficulties concentrating
- Impaired judgment or reasoning

There is no cure for MS. Care depends on the client's needs and condition. At first, the client may need home care to avoid fatigue. For example, some clients need help with housekeeping. As mobility decreases, the client depends more on others. Measures are taken to prevent injury and to promote bowel and bladder elimination. Eventually, the client may require long-term care. If the client is confined to bed, follow the measures in Box 31-1 on page 524.

Amyotrophic Lateral Sclerosis

Amyotrophic lateral sclerosis (**ALS**) is also known as Lou Gehrig's disease. ALS is a neurological disorder that results in the loss of all muscle control but does not affect intelligence. In Canada, about 2000 people are currently living with this disease.[6] It most commonly occurs between the ages of 40 and 70. Nerve cells in the brain and spinal cord are destroyed. This disease is progressive.

The first sign of the disease is usually difficulty using the fingers and hands. The person may not be able to pick up a cup, lace shoes, pull up zippers, or do buttons. The person then has difficulty walking. Stumbling and falling are common. Eventually, all muscle control is lost. The person cannot speak, swallow, move, or breathe independently. Eventually death occurs.

The person is alert and can think clearly. If your client cannot speak, remember that he or she can understand what you and others say. The speech therapist may recommend new communication methods. Follow the care plan.

The person eventually is confined to bed. The client is usually placed in a side-lying position. Follow the guidelines for caring for clients who are confined to bed (see Box 31-1 on page 524).

Acquired Brain Injuries

Acquired brain injury is damage to brain tissue caused by disease, medical condition, accident, or violence. When the head is subjected to violent forces, the brain is bashed against the skull. This results in bleeding, swelling, and bruising of brain tissue. Brain injury can be permanent. Most acquired brain injuries are caused by motor vehicle accidents. Other common causes are falls, sports and recreational injuries, acts of violence, and work-related accidents. Other injuries often occur. For example, spinal cord injuries are likely. Brain injury can also occur without any signs of physical damage. For example, babies who are shaken sometimes acquire brain injury.

Some acquired brain injuries are caused by lack of oxygen to the brain. Some accidents, diseases, and conditions reduce oxygen to the brain. This destroys brain cells and can cause permanent brain injury. For example, conditions during birth, near drowning, choking, suffocation, and stroke can cause acquired brain injury.

Signs and symptoms depend on the severity and location of the injury. Confusion, poor coordination, personality changes, headache, dizziness, fatigue, problems with vision, sensitivity to noise or light, or problems with sleep may occur. Behavioural changes include moodiness, irritability, or an inability to sit still. Cognitive problems include difficulty making decisions, problems with attention or concentration, or problems recalling simple words. Severe brain injury can result in intellectual disability, speech problems, breathing difficulties, and loss of bowel and bladder control. Rehabilitation is required (see Chapter 32). Care depends on the client's needs and abilities.

Spinal Cord Injuries

The spinal cord is a pathway that allows communication between the brain and the rest of the body. If the spinal cord is damaged, the nerves cannot send messages between the brain and parts of the body. Partial or total paralysis may occur. **Paralysis** is the complete or partial loss of ability to move a body part or muscle group. The most common cause of spinal cord injury is motor vehicle accidents. Most spinal cord injuries are permanent.

The parts of the body that are paralyzed depend on where the spinal cord was injured. The higher up the spine the injury occurs, the greater the loss of function (Figure 31-8). Spinal cord injuries in the thoracic level (chest area) or lower may cause **paraplegia**—paralysis (*plegia*) from the waist down. Injuries in the cervical region (neck) may cause **quadriplegia**—paralysis (*plegia*) of all four (*quad*) limbs and the trunk; the person is paralyzed from the neck down. Cervical traction is often necessary (see page 541). The person in cervical traction has a special bed that keeps the spine straight at all times.

People who have had recent spinal cord injuries require rehabilitation (see Chapter 32). The rehabilitation program depends on the client's needs and remaining abilities. Paralyzed clients usually need the care listed in Box 31-6.

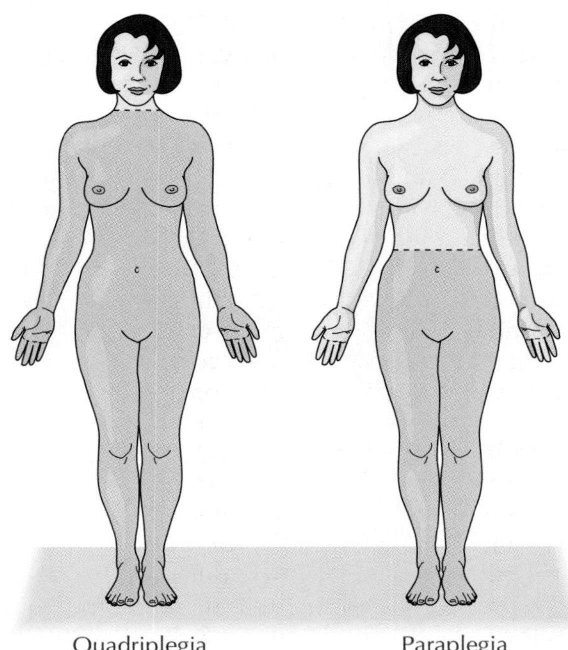

Figure 31-8 The shaded areas indicate the areas of paralysis.

Box 31-6 Care of Clients with Paralysis

- Assist with activities of daily living and home management tasks. Follow the care plan.
- Prevent falls. Follow the care plan for safety measures and the use of bed rails.
- Keep the call bell within reach (in facilities). Check the person often if he or she cannot use the call bell.
- Prevent burns. Check bathwater, heat applications, and food for the proper temperature.
- Turn and reposition the person at least every 2 hours. Follow the care plan.
- Maintain good alignment. Use supportive devices according to the care plan.
- Prevent pressure ulcers. Follow the care plan.
- Assist with transfers.
- Follow bowel and bladder training programs.
- Assist with range-of-motion and other exercises as ordered.
- Assist with food and fluids as needed. Provide self-help devices as ordered. Feed the person if necessary.
- Follow the person's rehabilitation plan.
- Give emotional support.

Musculoskeletal Disorders

Musculoskeletal disorders affect bones, joints, muscles, and the ability to move. Some disorders are caused by injury. Others result from aging or disease.

Arthritis

Arthritis means joint (*arthr*) inflammation (*itis*). It is the most common joint disease. *Inflammation* means there is swelling, redness, heat, and pain. Pain and decreased mobility occur in the affected joints. People with severe arthritis may require **arthroplasty**—surgical replacement (*plasty*) of a joint (*arthro*). Ankle, knee, hip, shoulder, wrist, finger, and toe joints can be removed and replaced with an artificial joint. The surgery relieves pain and restores joint motion.

There are many different types of arthritis. The two most common are osteoarthritis and rheumatoid arthritis.

Osteoarthritis. Osteoarthritis (OA) is the most common form of arthritis. It tends to occur in people after age 40 and becomes more common with increasing age. Approximately 80% of Canadians are affected by osteoarthritis by age 75.[7]

OA usually affects weight-bearing joints. These are the hips, knees, ankles, and spine. Joints in the fingers and thumbs can also be affected. In OA, cartilage (the material that cushions the ends of the bones) gradually breaks down. Eventually, bones may rub together. This causes pain, especially when a joint is moved. Joints are swollen, stiff, and painful.

Pain is often less severe in the morning and worsens during the day. Pain occurs with weight-bearing and joint motion. Severe pain can interfere with rest and sleep. Stiffness often occurs after the person has

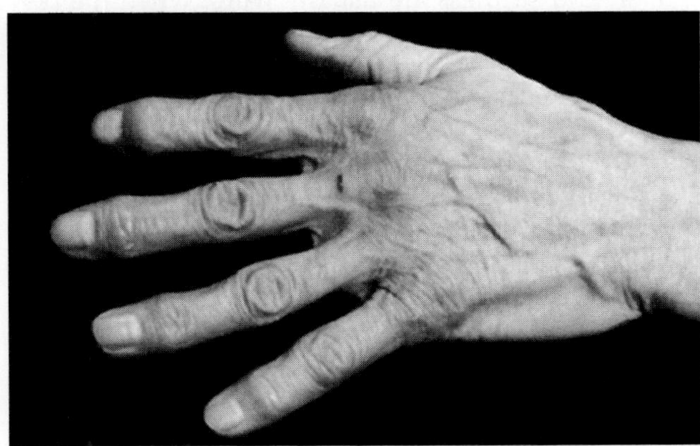

Figure 31-9 Spurs that occur in the end joints of fingers are called Heberden's nodes. Source: S.M. Lewis, M.M. Heitkemper, and S.R. Dirkson, *Medical-Surgical Nursing: Assessment and Management of Clinical Problems*, 5th ed. (St. Louis: Mosby, 2000).

not moved for a period. Cold weather and dampness can increase the symptoms.

Bones can also thicken and form growths, called spurs. Spurs called *Heberden's nodes* are common in the fingers (Figure 31-9). These growths change the shape of the bone and joint.

OA has no cure. Treatment involves relieving pain and stiffness. Physicians often order aspirin for pain. Heat or cold applications may be ordered. For obese people, weight loss is stressed. A low-fat, low-calorie diet is often ordered. When the condition is advanced, the person may need a cane or walker. Measures to prevent falls are important. Assistance with activities of daily living is given as needed. Elevated toilet seats are helpful when there is limited range of motion in the hips and knees.

Rheumatoid Arthritis. Rheumatoid arthritis (RA) is a chronic and progressive disease. It affects 1 in 100 Canadians.[8] Usually it occurs in people between the ages of 25 and 50. However, RA can also affect people of all ages, from toddlers to older adults. It is more common in women than in men. (See *Focus on Children: Arthritis* box.)

In RA, connective tissue throughout the body is affected. The immune system does not recognize the connective tissue as "normal." Therefore it attacks and destroys the connective tissue. The disease can affect connective tissue of the heart, lungs, eyes, kidneys, and skin. However, mainly the joints are affected. Smaller joints in the fingers, hands, and feet are usually affected first. Eventually larger joints are involved (wrists, elbows, and shoulders; ankles, knees, and hips). Organs then may be affected.

Joints are painful, swollen, and stiff. RA occurs on both sides of the body. For example, if the right wrist is involved, so is the left wrist. Fatigue and fever are common.

Pain and stiffness are usually worst when the person wakes in the morning but gradually decrease during the day. Eventually, the normal tissue is replaced by scar tissue. Deformities in the joints can develop (Figure 31-10).

Treatment and goals are to maintain joint motion, control pain, and prevent deformities. Rest is balanced with exercise. Adequate sleep—8 to 10 hours—is needed each night. Morning and afternoon rest periods are needed. Bed rest is needed if several joints are involved and if fever is present (see Box 31-1 on page 524).

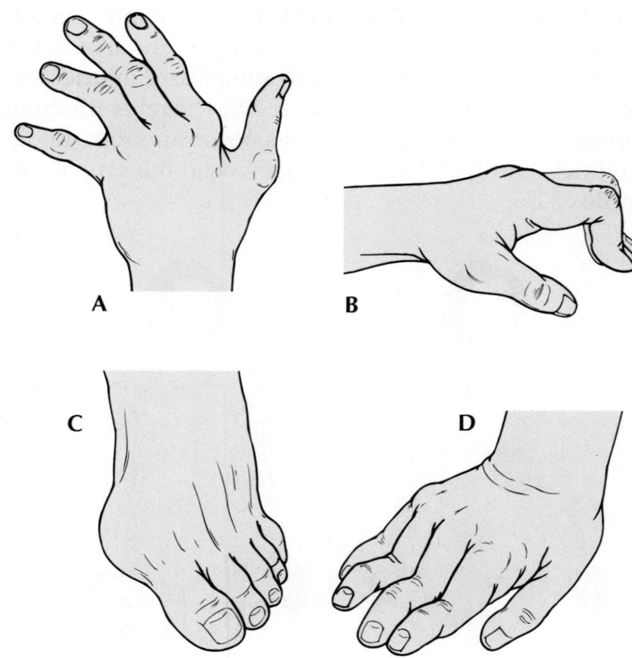

Figure 31-10 Deformities caused by rheumatoid arthritis. Source: S.M. Lewis, M.M. Heitkemper, and S.R. Dirkson, *Medical-Surgical Nursing: Assessment and Management of Clinical Problems*, 5th ed. (St. Louis: Mosby, 2000).

Range-of-motion exercises are done. Walking aids may be needed. Splints may be applied to the affected body parts. Safety measures to prevent falls are practised. The physician orders medications for pain and inflammation. Heat or cold applications may also be ordered. Many clients need joint replacement surgery.

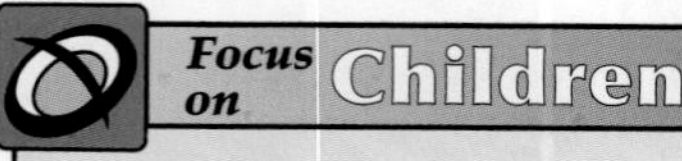

Arthritis

When RA occurs in children, it is called *juvenile rheumatoid arthritis (JRA)*. JRA can affect the child's growth and development. Eye inflammation is another complication.

Fibromyalgia

Fibromyalgia is a condition associated with aching, stiffness, and fatigue in muscles, ligaments, and tendons. The neck, shoulders, upper back, lower back, and hips are often affected. So are the legs, knees, and feet. The person has pain and stiffness in the affected parts. Fatigue and sleep disturbances are also common. Persistent fatigue makes even simple tasks difficult.

There is no cure for fibromyalgia. Heat and cold applications, massage, and regular stretching and range-of-motion exercises are helpful. Occupational therapy may be required. Medications are ordered to relieve pain and relax muscles.

Osteoporosis

Osteoporosis is a bone (*osteo*) disorder in which the bone becomes porous and brittle (*porosis*). Bones break easily. Bones of the spine, hips, and wrists are affected most often. It is common in older adults and in women after menopause. The ovaries do not produce the hormone *estrogen* after menopause. The lack of estrogen results in bone changes. Lack of dietary calcium is also a major cause of osteoporosis. Smoking, high alcohol intake, lack of exercise, prolonged bed rest, and immobility are risk factors. For bone to form properly, it must bear weight. If not, calcium is not absorbed and the bone becomes porous and brittle.

Back pain, gradual loss of height, and stooped posture occur. Fractures are a great risk if the person falls or has an accident. Sometimes bones are so brittle that the slightest activity can cause a fracture. For example, turning in bed or getting up from a chair.

Because there is no cure for osteoporosis, prevention is important. The diet must contain enough calcium and vitamins. Estrogen is often ordered for some women after menopause. Weight-bearing exercise may also prevent osteoporosis. Strength training (lifting weights), walking, jogging, dancing, and stair climbing are examples.

Some people with osteoporosis wear a back brace or corset or use walking aids. Protect the client from falls and accidents. Transfer, turn, and reposition the client gently.

FRACTURES

A **fracture** is a broken bone. Tissues around the fracture (muscles, blood vessels, nerves, and tendons) are usually injured. Fractures are open or closed (Figure 31-11). A *closed fracture* (*simple fracture*) means the bone is broken but the skin is intact. An *open fracture* (*compound fracture*) means the broken bone has come through the skin.

Fractures are caused by falls and other accidents. Fractures can also result when bones are weakened by diseases like cancer, alcoholism, and osteoporosis. Signs and symptoms of a fracture are:

- Limb looks bent or out of position
- Pain
- Swelling
- Limited movement of limb or loss of function
- Bruising and colour changes in the skin at the fracture site
- Bleeding (internal or external)

The bone has to heal. The bone ends are brought into normal position. This is called reduction. *Closed reduction* involves moving the bone back into place. The skin is not opened. *Open reduction* involves surgery. The bone is exposed and brought back into alignment.

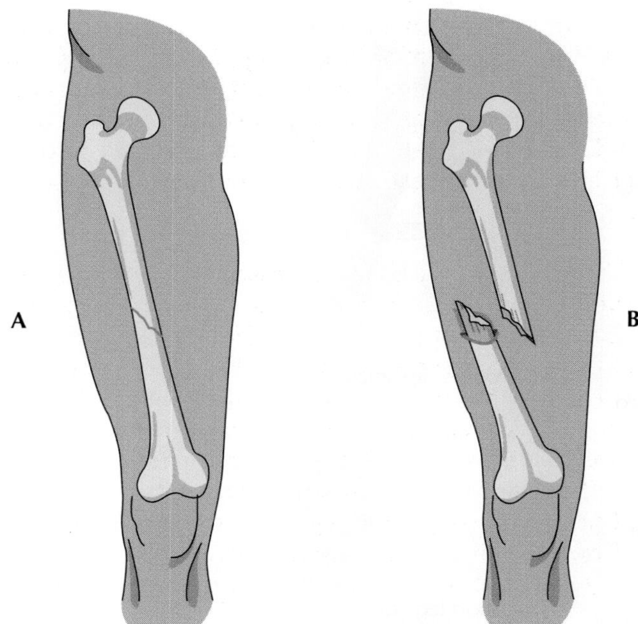

Figure 31-11 **A,** Closed fracture. **B,** Open fracture. Source: P.G. Beare and J.L. Myers, *Principles and Practice of Adult Health Nursing,* 3rd ed. (St. Louis: Mosby, 1998).

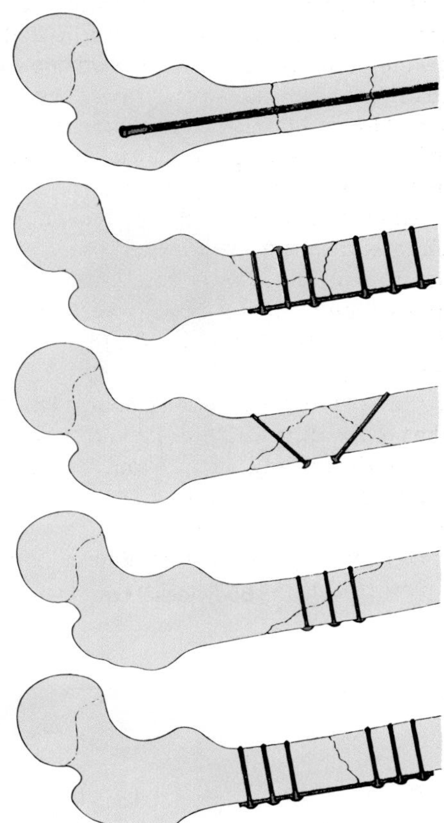

Figure 31-12 Devices used to reduce a fracture. Source: P.G. Beare and J.L. Myers, *Principles and Practice of Adult Health Nursing,* 3rd ed. (St. Louis: Mosby, 1998).

Nails, rods, pins, screws, plates, or wires are used to keep the bone in place (Figure 31-12). After reduction, the fracture is immobilized. That is, movement of the bone ends is prevented. This is done with a cast or traction. (See *Focus on Children: Fractures* box).

Cast Care. Casts are made of plaster, plastic, or fibreglass (Figure 31-13). Before casting, the injured part is covered with a stockinette. This protects the skin. Casting material comes in rolls. Moistened cast rolls are wrapped around the stockinette. Plastic and fibreglass casts dry quickly. A plaster cast dries in 24 to 48 hours. It is odourless, white, and shiny when dry. When wet, it is grey and cool and has a musty smell. Proper care of a cast is important. You may assist with care (Box 31-7).

Focus on Children

FRACTURES

Falls and accidents involving motor vehicles, bicycles, skateboards, scooters, and rollerblades are common causes of fractures in children. Fractures in infants may be a sign of child abuse.

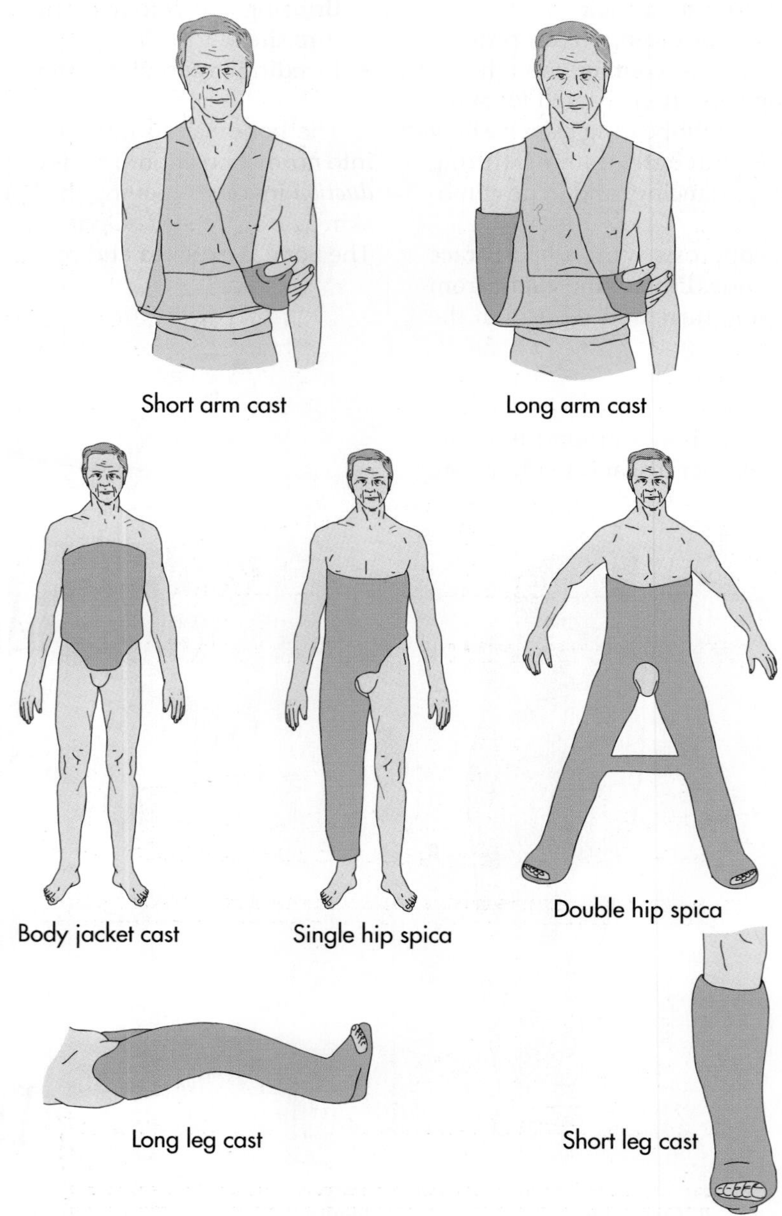

Figure 31-13 Common casts.

Box 31-7 Guidelines for Cast Care

- Do not cover the cast with blankets, plastic, or other material. A plaster cast gives off heat as it dries. Covers prevent the escape of heat. Burns can occur if the heat cannot escape.
- Turn the client as directed by the care plan. All cast surfaces are exposed to the air at one time or another. Turning promotes even drying.
- Do not place a wet cast on a hard surface because this will flatten the cast. The cast must keep its shape. Use pillows to support the entire length of the cast (Figure 31-14).
- Support a wet cast with your palms when turning and positioning the client (Figure 31-15 on page 540). Fingertips can dent the cast. The dents can cause pressure areas that can lead to skin breakdown.
- Protect the client from rough cast edges. Petalling involves covering the cast edges with tape (Figure 31-16 on page 540). If a stockinette is used, the physician pulls it up over the cast. The stockinette is secured in place with a roll of cast material.
- Keep a plaster cast dry. A wet cast loses its shape. Some casts are near the perineal area. The nurse may apply a waterproof material around the perineal area after the cast dries.
- Do not let the client insert anything into the cast. Itching under the cast causes an intense desire to scratch. Items used for scratching (pencils, coat hangers, knitting needles, back scratchers) can open the skin. An infection can develop. Items used for scratching can also wrinkle the stockinette or be lost in the cast. Both can cause pressure and lead to skin breakdown.
- Elevate a casted arm or leg on pillows. This reduces swelling.
- Have enough help when turning and repositioning the client. Plaster casts are heavy and awkward. Balance is lost easily.
- Position the client as directed by your supervisor and the care plan.
- Report these signs and symptoms immediately:
  - Pain—warns of a pressure ulcer, poor circulation, or nerve damage
  - Swelling and a tight cast, numbness, pale skin, or cyanosis—all signs of reduced blood flow to the part
  - Numbness or inability to move fingers or toes—a sign of pressure on a nerve
  - Temperature changes on the skin—cool skin means poor circulation; hot skin means inflammation
  - Chills, fever, nausea, vomiting, odour, or drainage on or under the cast —may signal an infection under the cast

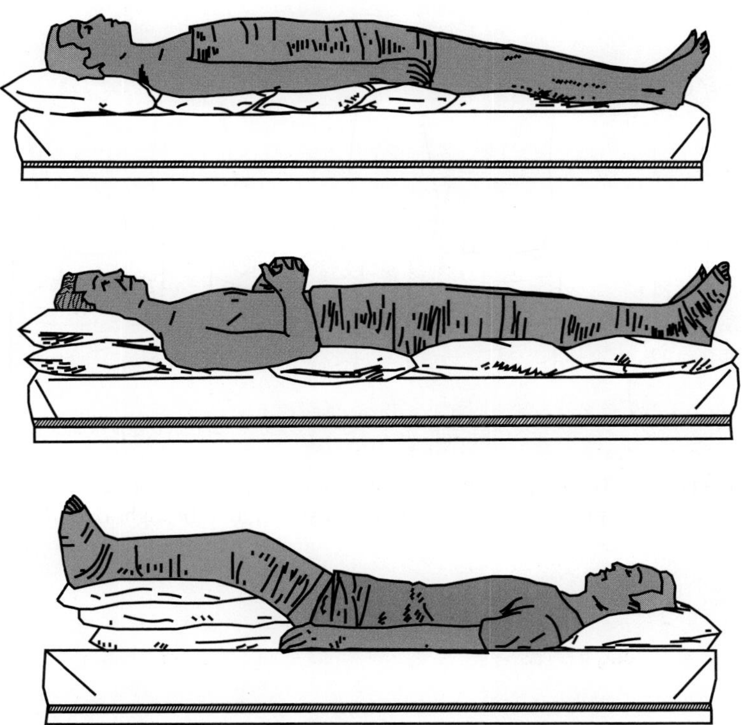

Figure 31-14 Pillows support the entire length of the wet cast. Source: G.H. Harkness and J.R. Dincher, *Medical-Surgical Nursing: Total Patient Care,* 10th ed. (St. Louis: Mosby, 1999).

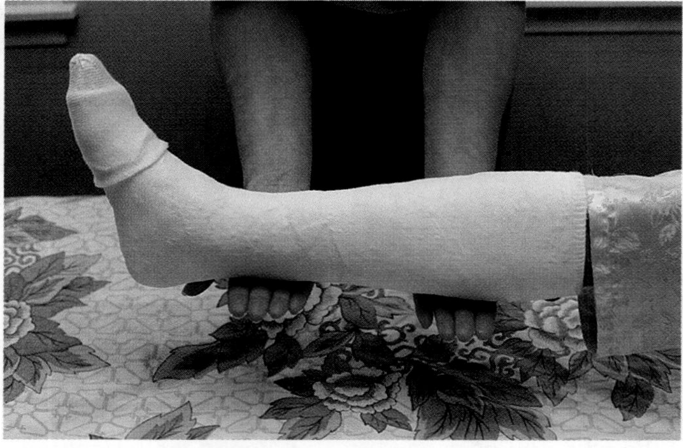

Figure 31-15 Support the cast with your palms during lifting.

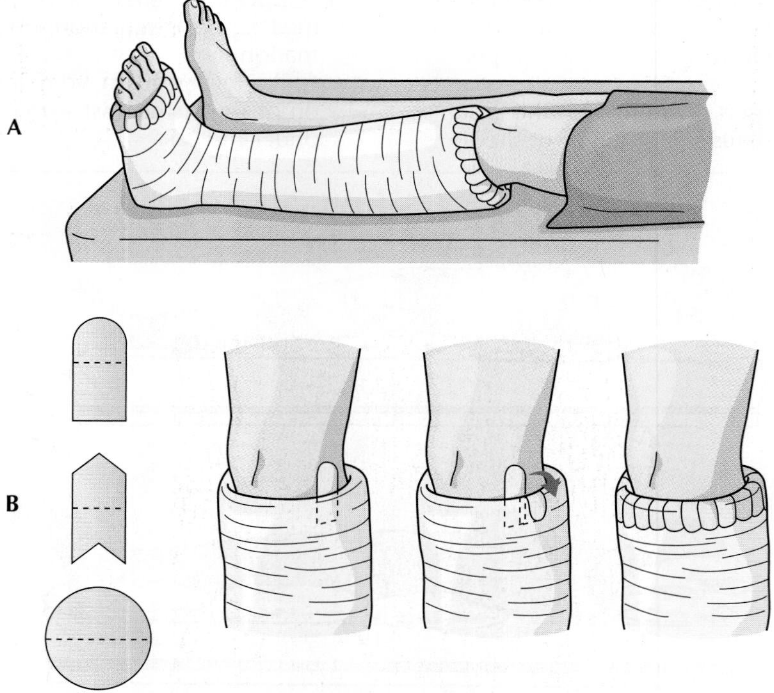

Figure 31-16 A, The edges of the cast are petalled. **B,** Pieces of tape are used to make petals. The petal is placed inside the cast and then brought over the edge.

Traction. Traction reduces and immobilizes fractures. A steady pull from two directions keeps the bone in place. Traction is also used to prevent muscle spasms, to correct or prevent deformities, and to relieve pressure on a nerve. Weights, ropes, and pulleys are used (Figure 31-17). Traction is applied to the neck, arms, legs, or pelvis.

Skin traction is applied to the skin. Tape, a boot, or a splint is used. Weights are attached to the device (see Figure 31-17). *Skeletal traction* is applied directly to the bone. Wires or pins are inserted through the bone (Figure 31-18). For *cervical traction*, tongs are applied to the skull. Weights are attached to the device.

Box 31-8 lists guidelines for caring for clients in traction.

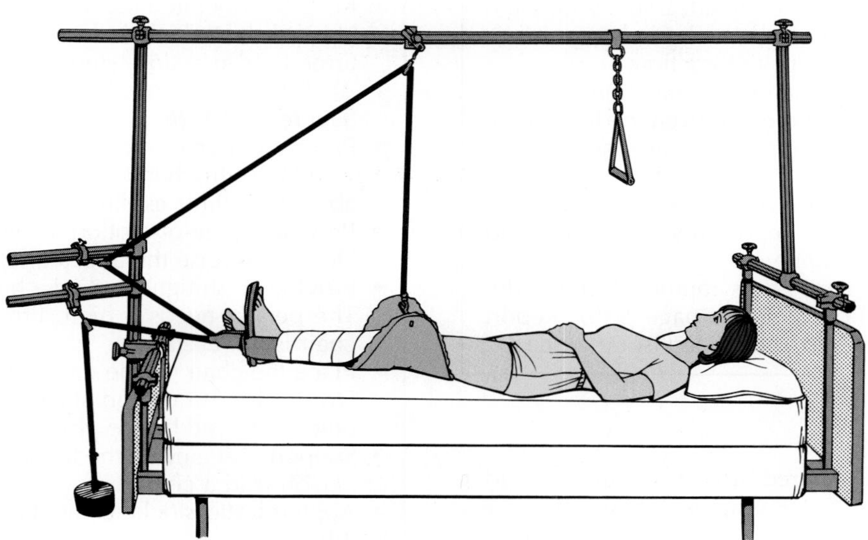

Figure 31-17 Traction setup. Note the weights, pulleys, and ropes. Source: W.J. Phipps, J.K. Sands, and J.F. Marek, *Medical-Surgical Nursing: Concepts and Clinical Practice*, 6th ed. (St. Louis: Mosby, 1999).

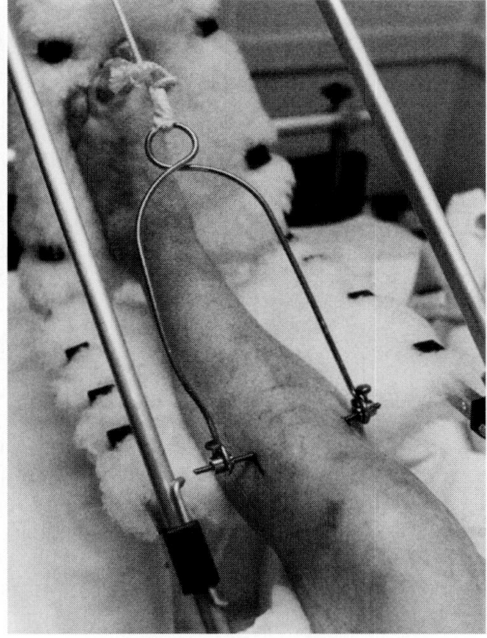

Figure 31-18 Skeletal traction is attached to the bone. Source: B.L. Christensen, E.O. Kockrow, *Adult Health Nursing*, 3rd ed. (St. Louis: Mosby, 1999).

Box 31-8 Caring for Clients in Traction

- Follow the guidelines for caring for clients confined to bed (see Box 31-1 on page 524).
- Keep the person in good alignment.
- Do not remove the traction.
- Do not touch the weights on the traction setup. You are not responsible for adding, removing, or maintaining the weights.
- Position the person as directed. Usually only the back-lying position is allowed. Slight turning is allowed with some types of traction.
- Provide the fracture pan for elimination.
- Put bottom linens on the bed from the top down. The person uses the trapeze to raise the body off the bed.
- Check pin, nail, wire, or tong sites for redness, drainage, or odours. Report any observations to your supervisor at once.
- Observe for the signs and symptoms listed under cast care (see Box 31-7 on page 539). Report these observations to your supervisor at once.

Hip Fractures. Fractured hips are common in older adults, especially in older women. They are serious because healing is slower in older people. The person is also at risk for life-threatening postoperative complications. These include pneumonia, urinary tract infections, and thrombi in the leg veins. Pressure ulcers, constipation, and confusion are other risks.

The fracture is fixed in position with a pin, nail, plate, screw, or artificial hip joint. The person needs preoperative and postoperative care (see Chapter 45). Box 31-9 describes the care required. Usually rehabilitation is needed after surgery. If home care is not possible, the person requires subacute or long-term care. Unless complications develop, the person usually returns home after successful rehabilitation. (See *Focus on Home Care: Clients Recovering from Hip Fractures* box.)

Box 31-9 Caring for Clients with Hip Fractures

- Follow the guidelines in Box 31-1 on page 524 if the person is confined to bed.
- Transfer, turn, and reposition the person as directed. Turning and positioning depend on the type of fracture and the surgery performed. Usually the person is not positioned on the operative side.
- Keep the operated leg abducted at all times. The leg is abducted when the person is supine, being turned, or in a side-lying position (Figure 31-19, *A*). Use pillows or abductor splints as directed (Figure 31-19, *B*)
- Prevent external rotation of the hip (turning outward). Use trochanter rolls, pillows, sandbags, or abductor splints as directed (see Chapter 22).
- Provide range-of-motion exercises as directed. Do not exercise the affected leg.
- Provide a straight-backed chair with armrests. The person needs a high, firm seat. A low, soft chair is not used.
- Place the chair on the unaffected side.
- Do not let the person stand on the affected leg unless allowed by the physician.
- Support and elevate the leg as directed when the person is in a chair.
- Apply elastic stockings as directed (see Chapter 28).
- Remind the person to not cross his or her legs while seated.

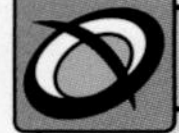

Focus on Home Care

Clients Recovering from Hip Fractures

The artificial hip joint can dislocate (move out of place) with adduction, internal rotation (turning inward), and severe hip flexion. Lying on the affected side, sitting in low seats, sitting with the legs crossed, bending from the waist, and putting on shoes and socks or stockings involve these movements. Therefore, such movements are avoided for 6 to 8 weeks after surgery.

An occupational therapist helps the client learn to do self-care activities. Self-help devices are used for dressing (see Chapter 32). The client needs a raised toilet seat for elimination and a shower chair for bathing. The client uses a pillow or abductor splint between the legs when in bed. A physical therapist helps the client learn muscle-strengthening exercises. A walker is usually needed for walking.

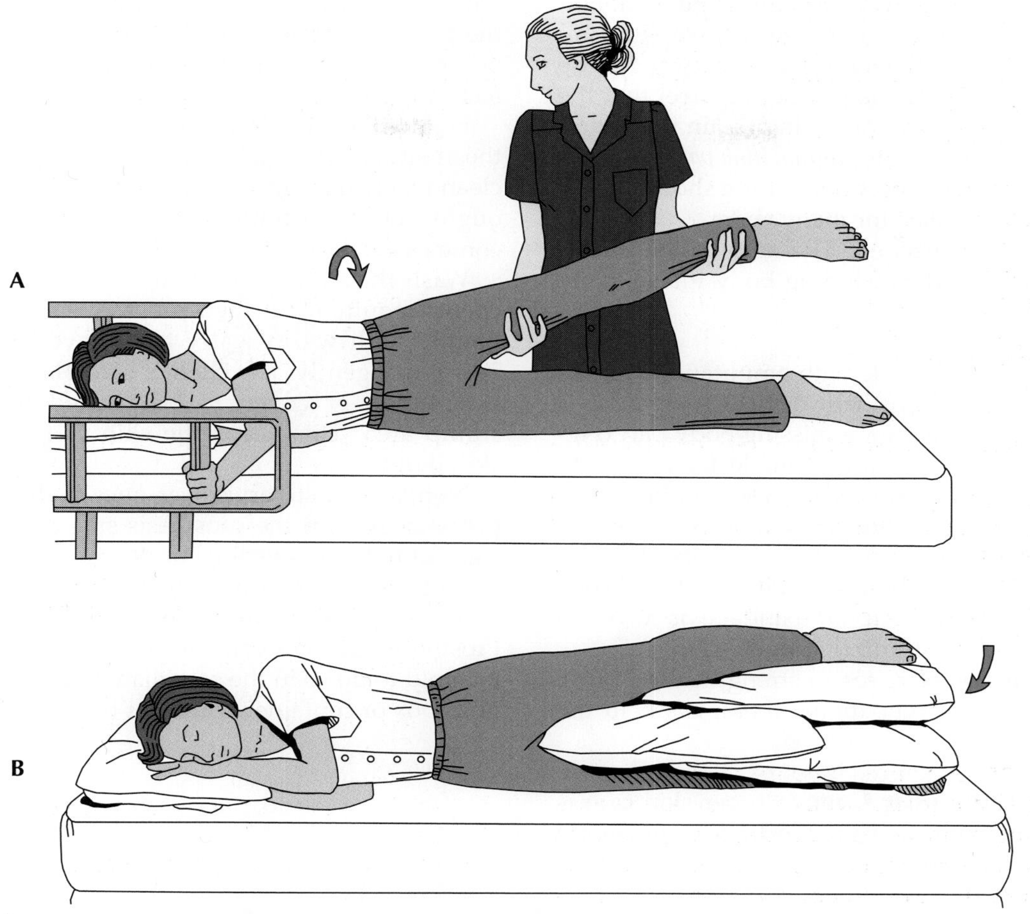

Figure 31-19 **A,** The hip is abducted when the client is turned. **B,** Pillows are used to maintain the hip in abduction. Source: W.J. Phipps, J.K. Sands, and J.F. Marek, *Medical-Surgical Nursing: Concepts and Clinical Practice*, 6th ed. (St. Louis: Mosby, 1999).

Amputation of a Limb

An **amputation** is the removal of all or part of an extremity. A *traumatic amputation* occurs by accident. *Surgical amputation* is performed when an extremity has been severely injured from a motor vehicle or other accident. Amputation may also be necessary to treat or prevent disease (such as cancer) or if gangrene has occurred. **Gangrene** is a condition in which there is tissue death. Causes include infection, frostbite, burns, injuries, and circulatory disorders. These conditions interfere with blood flow. Without good blood flow, tissues do not get enough oxygen and nutrients. Poisonous substances and waste products build up in the tissues. As a result, the tissue dies. It becomes black, cold, and shrivelled (Figure 31-20). If untreated, gangrene spreads through the body and causes death.

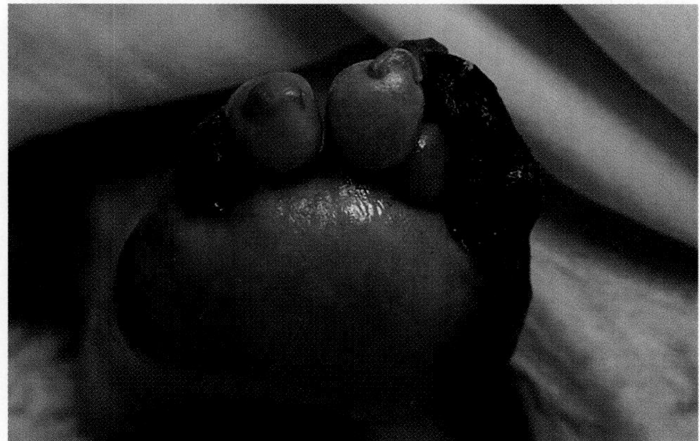

Figure 31-20 Gangrene.

All or part of an extremity may be amputated. Fingers, the hand, forearm, or entire arm may be removed. Toes, the foot, lower leg, upper leg, or entire leg may be amputated. The person may feel that the limb is still there or may complain of pain in the amputated part. This is called *phantom limb pain*. This is a normal reaction. It may occur only for a short time after surgery or it may last for many years.

Much support is needed. The amputation affects the person's whole life, including body image, daily activities, and work.

Prostheses. Most people with amputations are fitted with a prosthesis (prosthetic device). A *prosthesis* is an artificial replacement for a missing body part (Figure 31-21). A prosthesis can be made for any body part, including hands, arms, legs, eyes, and breasts.

For arm and leg prostheses, the stump (remaining limb) is conditioned so the prosthesis fits. This involves shrinking and shaping the stump into a cone shape. An elastic stocking or bandage is used to shrink and shape the stump (Figure 31-22).

The client learns exercises to strengthen the other limbs. Physical and occupational therapists help the client use the prosthesis.

Prostheses and Skin Care. Proper skin care is important for people who have prostheses. For people with leg or arm prostheses, the stump is confined in the prosthesis. The skin is not exposed to air. It may become hot and moist. Irritation, blisters, and skin infections can occur.

Follow the client's care plan. The skin at the prosthesis site requires daily skin care. Usually the skin is cleaned at the end of the day so it can dry thoroughly. Damp skin inserted into a prosthesis can become irritated.

Wash the skin with warm water and soap. Some clients require medicated soaps. Rinse the skin thoroughly with warm water to remove soap residue. Towel dry gently. The client's care plan may call for skin lotion or cream to be applied to the entire stump area. This keeps the skin soft and prevents skin damage.

Notify your supervisor at once if the client complains of pain at the prosthesis site. Also report any signs of redness, swelling, or drainage at the site.

Most prostheses are washed every day with warm, soapy water. They are rinsed well and towel dried. Prostheses are very valuable. Do not handle them unless told to do so in the care plan. Keep the prosthesis in its box or container when not in use.

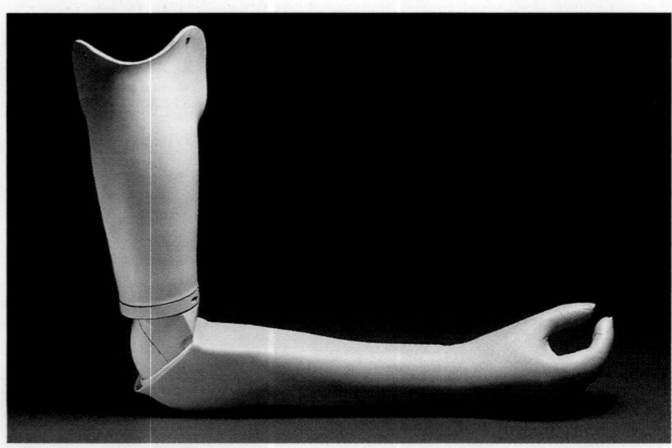

Figure 31-21 Arm prosthesis. (*Courtesy Motion Control, Subsidiary of Fillauer, Salt Lake City, UT.)*

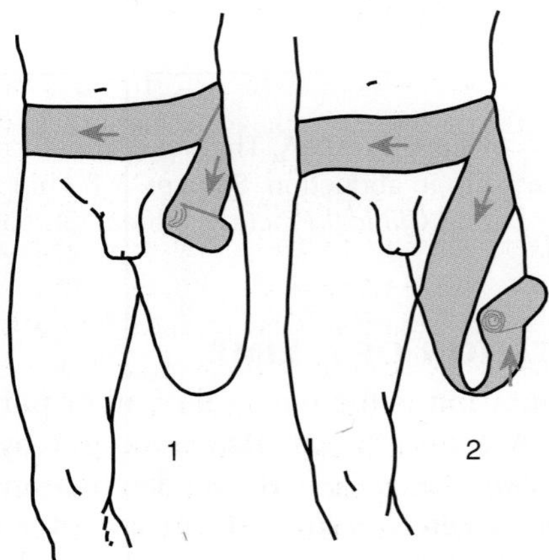

Figure 31-22 A midthigh amputation is bandaged to shrink and shape the stump. Source: W.J. Phipps, J.K. Sands, and J.F. Marek, *Medical-Surgical Nursing: Concepts and Clinical Practice*, 6th ed. (St. Louis: Mosby, 1999).

Endocrine Disorders

The endocrine system is made of glands. The endocrine glands secrete chemical messengers called *hormones*. Hormones affect other organs and glands and are essential for body function. Endocrine disorders result in hormone levels that are too high or too low. The most common endocrine disorder is diabetes.

Diabetes

Diabetes is a disorder in which the body cannot produce or use insulin properly. *Insulin* is a hormone secreted by the pancreas. It is needed for the proper use of sugar (*glucose*). Insulin helps the sugar obtained in foods to get into the cells. Without enough insulin in the body, sugar builds up in the blood. This is called *hyperglycemia*, which means high (*hyper*) sugar (*glyc*) in the blood (*emia*). When cells do not have sugar for energy, they cannot perform their functions. Left untreated, mild hypergylcemia can lead to long-term complications. Severe hyperglycemia can be life-threatening.

Over 2 million Canadians have diabetes, and one-third of them are unaware of it.[9] Diabetes can develop in children and adults. Risk factors include obesity and a family history of diabetes. The risk increases after age 40. In Canada, people of Aboriginal descent are more likely than others to have diabetes.[10]

There are three types of diabetes:

- *Type 1 diabetes*—occurs most often in children and young adults. The pancreas does not produce insulin. This leads to severe hyperglycemia. These people develop symptoms early in the disease and need treatment with daily insulin injections.
- *Type 2 diabetes*—usually develops in adulthood. This is the most common type of diabetes. The pancreas does not produce enough insulin, or the body does not effectively use the insulin that is produced. Obesity is a risk factor. The hyperglycemia is often mild, and the person may not notice symptoms. Treatment often consists of diet and exercise or oral medications. Insulin is sometimes required.
- *Gestational diabetes*—develops during pregnancy. It usually disappears after the baby is born. However, the woman is at risk for developing type 2 diabetes later in life.

A person with diabetes may experience symptoms. Remember, people with type 2 diabetes sometimes have symptoms that are so mild they do not notice them. Common signs and symptoms are:

- Increased thirst
- Frequent urination
- Constant hunger
- Unusual weight loss
- Extreme fatigue
- Dry, itchy skin
- Blurred eyesight

Diabetes must be controlled. If left untreated or poorly managed (as often happens with type 2 diabetes), the high levels of blood sugar slowly damage both the small and large blood vessels in the body. This causes many complications, including blindness, kidney disease, nerve damage, sexual dysfunction, and circulatory disorders. Circulatory disorders can lead to stroke, heart attack, and slow wound healing. Foot and leg wounds are very serious for people with diabetes. Infection and gangrene can occur. Sometimes amputation is needed.

There is no cure for diabetes, but the disease can be managed to reduce or prevent long-term complications. All people with diabetes must follow a careful diet. Overweight people need to lose weight. Exercise is included as part of the treatment plan. Regular exercise helps lower blood sugar levels, promotes weight loss, and reduces stress. Oral medications may be necessary. Regular and proper foot and nail care is extremely important. Corns, blisters, and calluses on the feet can lead to infection and amputation. Foot and nail care are provided by a professional.

Diabetes requires blood sugar monitoring. These are finger-prick blood tests that determine how much sugar is in the blood. People with type 1 diabetes test their blood sugar before each insulin dose. Those with type 2 diabetes usually monitor once daily.

People with type 1 diabetes require insulin injections, usually one to four times daily. Some people with type 2 diabetes also need insulin. Most people monitor their sugar levels and administer their insulin themselves. The exact type and dose of insulin must be taken as ordered. However, complications from insulin therapy may occur. If too much insulin is taken, hypoglycemia occurs. *Hypoglycemia* means low (*hypo*) sugar (*glyc*) in the blood (*emia*). If not corrected (by intake of sugar), it can lead to coma or death (Table 31-1 on page 546).

Table 31-1 Hyperglycemia and Hypoglycemia

	Causes	Warning signs and symptoms
Hyperglycemia (High blood sugar)	Undiagnosed diabetes Not enough insulin or diabetes medication Overeating, or eating the wrong kind of food Too little exercise Stress—physical or emotional	Tiredness or fatigue Hunger Thirst Frequent urination Leg cramps Blurred vision Dry, itchy skin Flulike achiness Headache Flushed face Rapid, weak pulse Low blood pressure Sweet breath odour Slow, deep, and laboured breathing Confusion Nausea and vomiting Convulsions Loss of consciousness
Hypoglycemia (Low blood sugar)	Too much insulin or diabetes medication Omitting or delaying a meal or snack Eating too little food Increasing exercise Vomiting	Hunger Weakness Trembling, shakiness Sweating Headache Dizziness Faintness Irritability, anxiety Confusion, disorientation Rapid pulse Low blood pressure Rapid, shallow breathing Changes in vision Cold, clammy skin Unconsciousness Convulsions

Immediately report signs and symptoms of hyperglycemia and hypoglycemia. You may prepare meals for adults and children with diabetes. Diet is a very important part of managing diabetes. Follow the client's diet carefully, and serve meals and snacks on time.

DIGESTIVE DISORDERS

The digestive system breaks down food for absorption by the body. It also eliminates solid wastes. Some digestive disorders are discussed in Chapter 30—diarrhea, constipation, flatulence, and fecal incontinence. Chapter 30 also discusses the care of clients with ostomy pouches.

DIVERTICULAR DISEASE

Many people have small pouches in their colons. The pouches bulge outward through weak spots in the colon (Figure 31-23). Each pouch is called a *diverticulum*. (*Diverticulare* means *to turn inside out.*) The condition of having these pouches is called **diverticulosis**. (*Osis* means *condition of.*)

Diverticular disease is very common in older adults. A low-fibre diet and constipation are risk factors.

When feces enter the pouches, the pouches can become inflamed and infected. This is called *diverticulitis*. (*Itis* means *inflammation.*) The person has abdominal pain and tenderness on the lower left side of the abdomen. Fever, nausea and vomiting, chills, cramping, and constipation are likely. Bloating, rectal bleeding, frequent urination, and pain while urinating can occur.

A ruptured pouch is a rare complication. Feces spill out into the abdomen. This leads to a severe, life-threatening infection. A pouch also can cause a block in the intestine (intestinal obstruction). Feces and gas cannot move past the blocked part. These problems require surgery.

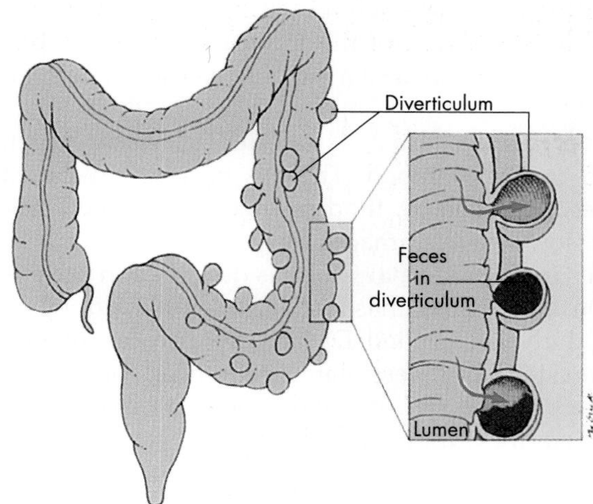

Figure 31-23 Diverticular disease.

The physician orders needed dietary changes. Sometimes antibiotics are ordered. Surgery is needed for severe disease, obstruction, and ruptured pouches. The diseased part of the bowel is removed. Sometimes a colostomy is necessary (see Chapter 30).

Vomiting

Vomiting is the act of expelling stomach contents through the mouth. It signals illness or injury. It can be life-threatening. The vomitus (material vomited) can be aspirated (inhaled into the lungs) and obstruct the airway. Vomiting large amounts of blood can lead to shock. The following measures are practised:

- Follow Standard Precautions.
- Turn the client's head well to one side. This prevents aspiration.
- Place a kidney basin or other container under the client's chin.
- Remove the vomitus from the client's immediate environment.
- Provide oral hygiene. This helps remove the taste of vomitus.
- Eliminate odours.
- Change linens or clothing as necessary.
- Observe vomitus for colour, odour, and undigested food. Vomitus that looks like coffee grounds contains digested blood. This indicates bleeding and must be reported immediately.
- Estimate the amount of vomitus. For example, is it about a cup full or a plate full? Some facilities may require you to measure and record the amount of vomitus.
- Report immediately to your supervisor that the client vomited. Also report your observations. Some facilities may require you to save the vomitus so it can be observed or sent to a laboratory.

Urinary Disorders

The kidneys, ureters, bladder, and urethra are the major urinary system structures. Disorders can occur in one or more of these structures.

Urinary Tract Infections

Urinary tract infections (UTIs) are common. Infection in one area of the urinary system can lead to infection of the entire urinary system.

Normally the urinary system is sterile. It has no microbes. Microbes can enter the system through the urethra. Catheterization, urological examinations, sexual intercourse, poor perineal hygiene, incomplete bladder emptying, and poor fluid intake are common causes. UTI is a common infection in health care settings.

Women are at high risk because microbes can easily enter the short urethra. Prostate gland secretions help protect men from UTIs. However, an enlarged prostate increases the risk of a UTI. Therefore older men are at risk.

Cystitis is inflammation (*itis*) of the bladder (*cyst*). *Pyelonephritis* is inflammation (*itis*) of the pelvis (*pyelo*) or kidney (*nephr*). Infection is the most common cause. Signs and symptoms are:

- Urinary frequency and urgency
- Oliguria—scant (*olig*) urine (*uria*)
- Dysuria—difficult or painful (*dys*) urination (*uria*)
- Pain or burning during urination
- Foul-smelling urine
- Hematuria—blood (*hemat*) in the urine (*uria*)
- Pyria—pus (*py*) in the urine (*uria*)
- Fever and chills
- Pain in the lower abdomen or back

Antibiotics are ordered. Fluids are encouraged—usually 2000 mL per day.

Renal Calculi

Renal calculi are kidney (*renal*) stones (*calculi*). White men between the ages of 20 and 40 years are at greatest risk. Prolonged bed rest, immobility, and poor fluid intake are risk factors. Stones vary in size. Signs and symptoms include:

- Severe, cramping pain in the back and side, just below the ribs
- Pain in the abdomen, thigh, and urethra
- Nausea and vomiting
- Fever and chills
- Urinary frequency and urgency
- Oliguria—scant (*olig*) urine (*uria*)
- Dysuria—difficult or painful (*dys*) urination (*uria*)
- Hematuria—blood (*hemat*) in the urine (*uria*)
- Foul-smelling urine

Treatment involves providing pain relief and encouraging fluids. The person needs to drink about 2000–3000 mL of fluid a day. Increased fluids help stones pass through the urine. All urine is strained (see Chapter 29). Surgical removal of the stone may be necessary. Some dietary changes can prevent further stones.

Renal Failure

Renal failure (kidney failure) occurs when the kidneys do not function or are severely impaired. Waste products are not removed from the blood. The body retains fluids. As fluids build up in the bloodstream, the person may become puffy and swollen in the face, hands, and feet. Hypertension and congestive heart failure can result. Renal failure can be acute or chronic.

Acute Renal Failure. Acute renal failure occurs suddenly after severely decreased blood flow to the kidneys. Causes include severe bleeding, heart attack, congestive heart failure, burns, infections, and severe allergic reactions.

Acute renal failure is usually a temporary condition. With treatment, this condition can be cured with no permanent damage to the kidneys. However, this disorder is very serious. Death can occur.

Acute renal failure occurs in phases. At first *oliguria* (scant amount of urine) occurs. Urine output is less than 400 mL in 24 hours. This phase lasts a few days to 2 weeks. Then diuresis occurs. *Diuresis* means the process (*esis*) of passing (*di*) urine (*uria*). Large amounts of urine are produced—1000 to 5000 mL per day. Kidney function improves and returns to normal during the recovery phase. This can take from one month to one year. Some people do not recover. They develop chronic renal failure.

The physician orders medications, restricted fluids, and diet therapy. The care plan will likely include:

- Measuring and recording urine output every hour; an output of less than 30 mL per hour is reported immediately
- Measuring and recording intake and output
- Restricting fluid intake
- Daily weight measurements with the same scale
- Frequent oral hygiene
- Measures to take if the client is confined to bed (see Box 31-1 on page 524)
- Measures to prevent infection

Chronic Renal Failure. In chronic renal failure the kidneys cannot meet the body's needs. Nephrons of the kidneys are destroyed over many years. Hypertension and diabetes are common causes. Infections, urinary tract obstructions, and tumours are other causes.

Signs and symptoms appear when 80 to 90% of kidney function is lost. A few of the many signs and symptoms include yellow skin; dry, itchy, or brittle skin; inflammation of the mouth; bruises and bleeding; hypertension; and a burning sensation in the legs and feet.

Every body system is affected as waste products build up in the blood. There is no cure. In the early stages, diet therapy, fluid restriction, and medications may slow kidney damage. The general care required for clients in chronic renal failure is described in Box 31-10.

Once the person has lost considerable kidney function, dialysis is needed. *Dialysis* is the process of removing wastes and excess water from the blood. Specially trained nurses perform the procedure. Some people may require kidney transplants.

Communicable Diseases

A **communicable disease** is a disease caused by microbes that spread easily. The disease can be transmitted from one person to another. Communicable diseases are spread in different ways, depending on the disease (see Chapter 18):

- *Direct contact*—with the infected person
- *Indirect contact*—with contaminated dressings, linens, or surfaces
- *Airborne transmission*—occurs when the person sneezes and coughs
- *Vehicle transmission*—occurs through blood transfusions or by ingesting contaminated food, fluids, or drugs
- *Vector transmission*—occurs via animals, fleas, ticks, mites, and mosquitoes

There are many communicable diseases. Colds, influenza, measles, mumps, and chickenpox are examples. Table 31-2 outlines common childhood communicable diseases. However, adults can also contract these diseases. This section discusses sexually transmitted diseases (STDs), hepatitis, and AIDS.

Box 31-10 Care of Clients in Chronic Renal Failure

- Limit fluids.
- Measure blood pressure in the supine, sitting, and standing positions.
- Measure weight daily with the same scale.
- Measure and record intake and output.
- Use bath oils, lotions, and creams on the skin to prevent itching. Follow the care plan.
- Provide frequent oral hygiene.
- Encourage rest.
- Prevent complications of bed rest if the person is confined to bed (see Box 31-1 on page 524).

Table 31-2 Common Communicable Childhood Diseases

Disease	Transmission	Signs and symptoms
Chickenpox (varicella)	Direct contact and airborne contact with respiratory secretions; direct contact with skin lesions	Fever, rash, and skin lesions
Measles (rubeola)	Direct or indirect contact with nasal secretions	Fever, cough, rash, inflammation of the mucous membranes of the nose, nasal discharge, bronchitis
Mumps	Direct contact with saliva droplets	Fever, headache, swollen salivary glands, earache
Pertussis (whooping cough)	Airborne or direct contact with droplets from the respiratory tract	Fever, sneezing, severe cough at night; coughs are short and rapid followed by a "whoop" or crowing sound with inhalation
Rubella (German measles)	Airborne or direct contact with secretions from the nose and pharynx	Fever, headache, loss of appetite, nasal inflammation, sore throat, cough, rash
Scarlet fever	Airborne or direct contact with nasal and pharyngeal secretions	Fever, chills, headache, vomiting, abdominal pain, red and swollen tonsils and pharynx, rash

You often cannot tell by looking at a person if he or she has a communicable disease. Sometimes even the person with the communicable disease may not know he or she has it. Therefore, you must follow Standard Precautions when working with all clients. Standard Precautions prevent the spread of communicable diseases. You may also have to follow Transmission-Based Precautions with certain clients if ordered by a physician (see Chapter 18). Follow the care plan.

HEPATITIS

Hepatitis is inflammation (*itis*) of the liver (*hepat*). It is often caused by an infection of the liver by certain viruses. When the viral infection of the liver first occurs, it is called *acute hepatitis*. Acute hepatitis may or may not cause symptoms that are recognized by the infected person. Acute hepatitis often lasts less than 1 or 2 months. Signs and symptoms of acute hepatitis include: nausea, vomiting, and pain in the abdomen. After about 2 weeks, dark urine and jaundice (a yellowish colour in the skin and whites of the eyes) develop in some, but not all, people. Some people with hepatitis have light-coloured stools, muscle pain, drowsiness, irritability, and itching. Diarrhea and general aching in the joints accompanied by redness and swelling can occur.

For mild cases of acute viral hepatitis, no medication or other treatment is available or necessary. The disease runs its course and is resolved. The primary goals for managing acute viral hepatitis are to provide good nutrition, prevent additional damage to the liver, and prevent transmission to others.

Some cases of acute hepatitis do not resolve. If hepatitis lasts longer than 6 months, it is called *chronic hepatitis*. Chronic hepatitis causes liver damage over a long period of time. The normal cells of the liver are eventually replaced with scar tissue. This condition is known as *cirrhosis*. Cirrhosis can cause complete liver failure. When the liver fails, the person needs a liver transplant. Without the transplant, the person will die.

There are three major viruses that cause hepatitis in Canada: hepatitis viruses A, B, and C. All can be passed from one person to another.

- *Hepatitis A virus*—is spread by the fecal–oral route. This means the virus is transmitted when traces of feces are ingested. Food, water, and drinking and eating vessels (cups, bowls, cutlery) can be contaminated with feces. The virus is ingested when contaminated food or water is consumed. It can also be ingested when a person eats or drinks from a contaminated vessel. Risk factors include crowded living conditions and poor sanitation and hygiene. Always wear gloves when assisting with perineal care, cleaning incontinent clients, and handling bedpans and rectal thermometers. Clients with fecal incontinence, confusion, or dementia can cause contamination. Carefully look for contaminated items and areas. Good hand washing is essential for everyone. Assist the client with hand washing if necessary. Hepatitis A does not cause chronic hepatitis. (See *Focus on Children: Hepatitis* box.)

- *Hepatitis B and C viruses*—are in an infected person's blood and certain body fluids (semen and vaginal secretions). They can be spread by having intercourse or sharing needles with an infected person. These viruses can also be spread during blood transfusions and childbirth (from the mother to the child). They can also be spread by needlestick injuries and by direct contact between open skin and infected blood or body fluids (see Chapter 18). Therefore, follow Standard Precautions when contact with blood or body fluids is likely. Transmission-Based Precautions are ordered as necessary. Hepatitis B (in 10 to 15% of the cases) and hepatitis C (in 70 to 85% of the cases) can cause chronic hepatitis.

Acquired Immunodeficiency Syndrome (AIDS)

Acquired immunodeficiency syndrome (AIDS) is a disease of the immune system caused by the *human immunodeficiency virus* (*HIV*). AIDS affects the person's ability to fight infections. People with AIDS may get infections such as pneumonia and TB. They are also at increased risk for cancers. Sometimes they experience central nervous system damage, which may cause memory loss, loss of coordination, paralysis, mental health disorders, and dementia.

A person may be infected with HIV but not have signs and symptoms of AIDS. The person is a carrier and can transmit the virus to others. There is no cure for HIV infection. However, several medications have been developed recently that slow the progress of HIV. With current treatment, infected people can remain healthy for many years.

HIV is spread from an infected person to someone else when there is an exchange of certain body fluids—blood, semen, vaginal secretions, or breastmilk. HIV is transmitted mainly by:

- Unprotected intercourse with an infected person. "Unprotected" means without a latex condom. The virus enters the bloodstream through small breaks in the mucous membranes of the rectum, vagina, penis, or mouth
- Needle-sharing among IV drug users
- HIV-infected mothers to their babies at birth or during breastfeeding

Infection can also be spread when infected body fluids come in direct contact with broken skin. Needlestick injuries can also spread HIV (see Chapter 18). HIV is not spread by saliva, tears, urine, sweat, sneezing, coughing, insects, or casual contact. Casual contact includes hugging, touching, or shaking hands with an infected person.

AIDS is the last stage of HIV infection. Without treatment, AIDS develops about 10 years after the initial HIV infection. The following are possible warning signs of HIV infection:

- Rapid weight loss
- Dry cough
- Fever or night sweats
- Fatigue
- Swollen glands in the armpits, groin, or neck
- Diarrhea that lasts for more than a week
- White spots or unusual blemishes on the tongue, in the mouth, or in the throat
- Pneumonia
- Red, brown, pink, or purplish blotches on the skin or inside the mouth, nose, or eyelids
- Memory loss, confusion, or dementia

You may care for clients who have AIDS or who are HIV carriers. You may have contact with the client's blood. Standard Precautions are necessary to protect yourself and others from the HIV virus. *These precautions apply when you are caring for all clients.* Remember, you may care for a client who has the HIV virus but

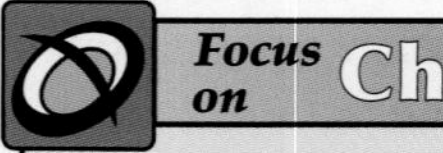

Focus on Children

Hepatitis

Hepatitis A is more common among preschool and school-aged children than among adults. This is because the virus is easily spread among children. Poor hygiene practices after defecation lead to contamination of eating and drinking vessels, toys, and other surfaces. Also, young children often put their hands, toys, and other items in their mouths.

shows no symptoms. You may also care for a client who is not yet diagnosed as having an HIV infection. As long as you strictly follow all Standard Precautions, you need not fear working with clients with HIV infection or AIDS. (See *Focus on Older Adults: HIV and AIDS* box.)

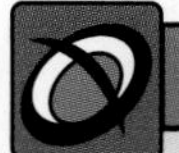

Focus on Older Adults

HIV and AIDS

AIDS is often considered a young person's disease. Also, people often think that older adults are not sexually active and not at risk for AIDS. Except for childbirth and breastfeeding, older adults get and spread the HIV virus in the same ways as younger adults. Consider every client as potentially infectious. Follow Standard Precautions with all clients.

Sexually Transmitted Diseases

Sexually transmitted diseases (STDs) are diseases that are spread by sexual contact (Table 31-3). Some people are not aware that they are infected. Others know but do not seek treatment. Embarrassment is a common reason for not seeking treatment.

STDs are usually associated with the genital area. However, other areas may be involved. These areas include the rectum, ears, mouth, nipples, throat, tongue, eyes, and nose. Most STDs are spread only by sexual contact. The use of condoms helps prevent the spread of STDs. The use of condoms is also very important for preventing the spread of HIV and AIDS. Some STDs are also spread through a break in the skin, by contact with infected body fluids (blood, semen, saliva), or by contaminated blood or needles. Standard Precautions are necessary.

Table 31-3 Sexually Transmitted Diseases

Disease	Signs and symptoms	Treatment
Genital herpes	Recurrent, painful, fluid-filled sores on or near the genitalia (Figure 31–24 on page 552) The sores may have a watery discharge Itching, burning, and tingling in the genital area Fever Swollen glands	No known cure Medications can be given to control discomfort
Venereal warts	*Males*—Warts appear on the penis, anus, or genitalia *Females*—Warts appear near the vagina, cervix, and labia	Application of special ointment that causes the warts to dry up and fall off Surgical removal may be necessary if the ointment is not effective
Gonorrhea	Burning on urination Urinary frequency and urgency Vaginal discharge (females) Urethral discharge (males)	Antibiotic medications
Syphilis	*Primary syphilis*—appears 10 to 90 days after exposure Painless chancre (a type of sore) on the penis, in the vagina, or on genitalia; the chancre may also be elsewhere on the body *Secondary syphilis*—appears about 2 months after the chancre, lasting up to one year Rash, general fatigue, loss of appetite, nausea, fever, bone and joint pain, hair loss, lesions on the lips and genitalia *Tertiary syphilis*—appears 3 to 15 years after infection Damage to the cardiovascular system and central nervous system; blindness; dementia	Antibiotic medications

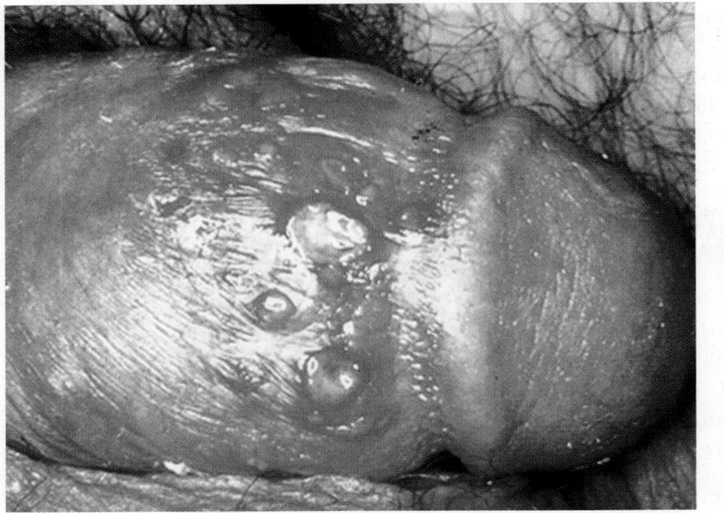

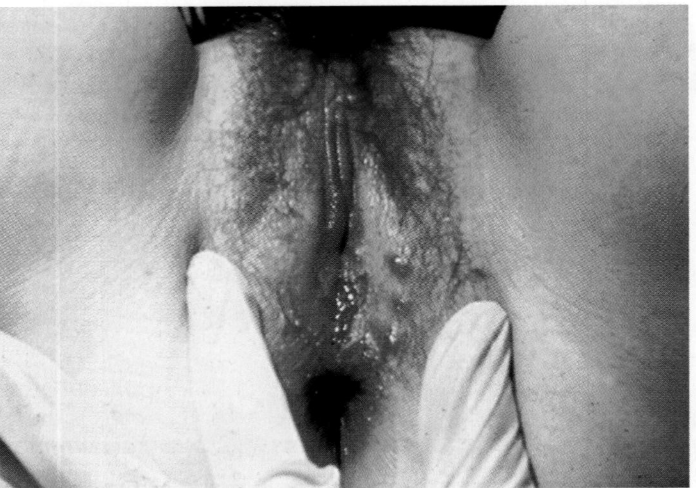

Figure 31-24 Genital herpes. **A,** Sores on the penis. **B,** Sores on the perineum. *(Courtesy USPHS, Washington, DC.)*

REVIEW

Circle T if the answer is true and F if it is false.

1. T F A sore that does not heal is a warning sign of cancer.
2. T F Stroke is a complication of hypertension.
3. T F A common treatment of hypertension is a high-sodium diet.
4. T F The pain of angina is relieved with rest and nitroglycerin.
5. T F Myocardial infarction means heart attack.
6. T F A pacemaker is a device used to treat renal failure.
7. T F People with congestive heart failure need to drink extra fluids.
8. T F Smoking is the most common cause of COPD.
9. T F The flu season in Canada is June through October.
10. T F Stroke often causes hemiplegia.
11. T F People with Parkinson's disease often have blank, expressionless faces.
12. T F People with Huntington's disease are not affected intellectually.
13. T F Canada has one of the lowest rates of MS in the world.
14. T F A person with advanced ALS cannot speak or move but can hear and understand.
15. T F People with brain or spinal cord injuries require amputations.
16. T F Arthritis usually affects bones and muscles.
17. T F Fibroymyalgia is a respiratory disorder.
18. T F People with osteoporosis have an increased risk for fractures.
19. T F When lifting a cast, support it with your palms, not your fingertips.
20. T F When caring for a client in traction, remove the weights if he or she is uncomfortable.
21. T F After a hip pinning, the operated leg is abducted at all times.
22. T F Hyperglycemia means low sugar in the blood.
23. T F Diabetes can cause circulatory disorders.
24. T F Good foot care is especially important for people with diabetes.
25. T F Vomiting can cause aspiration.
26. T F Passing a kidney stone is called cystitis.
27. T F Clients with chronic renal failure need increased fluid intake.
28. T F Hepatitis B virus is spread by the fecal–oral route.
29. T F HIV is spread by infected urine.
30. T F The HIV virus remains in the person's body for life.
31. T F STDs are usually spread by sexual contact.

Answers to these questions are on page 825.

CHAPTER

32

REHABILITATION AND RESTORATIVE CARE

OBJECTIVES

- Define the key terms listed in this chapter
- Describe the goals of rehabilitation
- Explain how rehabilitation involves the whole person
- Explain the family's role in the rehabilitation process
- Explain the role of therapy and training in rehabilitation
- Describe four rehabilitation settings
- Explain the role of the rehabilitation team in the rehabilitation process

KEY TERMS

orthosis Apparatus worn to support, align, prevent, or correct problems with the musculoskeletal system

prosthesis An artificial replacement for a missing body part

rehabilitation The process of restoring a person to the highest level of functioning possible through the use of therapy, exercise, or other methods

restorative care Care that helps a person regain health, strength, and independence

Rehabilitation is the process of restoring a person to the highest level of functioning possible through the use of therapy, exercise, or other methods. Rehabilitation may follow an acute injury or illness. Or it may be part of the treatment for a chronic illness or disability. Rehabilitation helps the person function at his or her highest level of independence.

Some people are weak. Many cannot perform activities of daily living. **Restorative care** is care that helps a person regain health, strength, and independence. Restorative care often begins during rehabilitation. It may continue longer than the rehabilitation process, or it may go on indefinitely. Restorative care may involve measures that promote:

- Self-care
- Elimination
- Positioning
- Mobility
- Communication
- Cognitive function

Many people need restorative care and rehabilitation. Often it is hard to separate restorative care and rehabilitation programs. In many facilities and agencies, they mean the same thing.

The focus of rehabilitation and restorative care is to:

- Help maintain the highest level of functioning
- Prevent unnecessary decline in function

GOALS OF REHABILITATION

Goals depend on the client's condition and circumstances. For some people, the goal is to return to work. Others want to meet self-care needs and perform activities of daily living. Most people want to reduce their reliance on others and to become more independent. The following goals are common:

- *To restore function to former levels.* A full restoration of function is the goal for most people with acute or temporary conditions. For example, a healthy person with a simple leg fracture aims for a full recovery.
- *To improve functional abilities.* A return to former levels of functioning is not possible for some people. They aim to improve their abilities to the best extent possible. For example, they may work on mobility skills or carrying out activities of daily living independently.
- *To learn new skills.* Some people need to learn new skills in order to adapt to their disability or limitations. For example, Mr. Liptak's larynx was surgically removed because of cancer. He cannot speak. His goal is to learn sign language.
- *To prevent further disability and illness.* Complications that cause further disability and illness must be prevented. For example, immobility can lead to pressure ulcers or contractures. Proper skin care, exercise and activity, good alignment, and frequent repositioning are needed.

Consider the rehabilitation goals of the following people:

- Chantal, 5, has cerebral palsy. She needs to maintain her current range of motion through specific exercises, learn how to use a wheelchair, and perform self-care.
- Mr. Cunningham, 27, is addicted to cocaine. Goals include restoring healthy physical and psychological function and preventing a relapse into addiction. He will learn how to avoid situations where drugs are present and will be encouraged to join NA (Narcotics Anonymous).
- Mr. Khan, 49, had a heart attack. His goal is to prevent another heart attack. His rehabilitation program includes exercise, nutrition counselling, and stress management techniques.
- Mr. Egri, 68, was left with hemiplegia and a severe speech impairment following a stroke. He needs to learn communication methods and restore function.

Prevention of another stroke through medication, exercise, and diet also is a goal. His family needs to learn how to help with his care.

- Mrs. Boucher, 82, fractured her hip following a fall. Her goal is to remain in her own home. She needs to restore her ability to function at former levels. She also needs to prevent another fall. (See *Focus on Older Adults: Rehabilitation* box.)

THE REHABILITATION PROCESS

Rehabilitation can be a short process. For example, a healthy person with a shoulder injury may need to do only a few simple exercises. However, rehabilitation is often a long, difficult process. Box 32-1 shows the rehabilitation process experienced by a client with a serious brain injury.

THE REHABILITATION TEAM

Rehabilitation is a team effort. Members of the team vary depending on the client's needs. They usually include the client, family members, physicians, nurses, occupational therapists, physiotherapists (physical therapists), support workers, and others. All help the client regain function and independence. The team meets often to discuss the client's progress. Changes in the rehabilitation plan are made as needed. The client and family attend the meetings when possible. Families are key members of the team.

Restorative care usually involves the client and family, nurses, and support workers. Therapists and other professionals may be consulted as needed, but the care is usually provided by nurses and support workers.

EMPHASIS ON THE WHOLE PERSON

Illness and disability affect a person's physical, emotional, social, intellectual, and spiritual health. Therefore, rehabilitation treats the whole person. It addresses all dimensions of health, not only the physical:

- *Physical health.* The client's physical condition and ability to perform activities of daily living are assessed. Complications are prevented. Range-of-motion exercises are done. The client learns or relearns self-care and mobility skills.
- *Emotional and social health.* Emotional and social health are assessed. So are work skills. Family counselling and assistance reentering the community and workplace are provided as needed.
- *Intellectual health.* Thinking, speech, memory, and organization are assessed. Measures to improve cognitive functioning are planned.
- *Spiritual health.* Counselling from spiritual advisers is provided as needed.

All aspects of rehabilitation are connected. For example, following a stroke, Mr. Silva learns how to care for himself (physical health) and how to follow instructions (intellectual health). This increases his self-esteem (emotional health). Family and friends visit often (social health), and his spiritual adviser visits every week (spiritual health).

The case study in Box 32-1 shows a rehabilitation team addressing all five dimensions of a client's health. The client's quality of life is central to care and treatment.

The rehabilitation team encourages the client to control as many aspects of his or her care as possible. Being a key member of the rehabilitation team gives the client some control.

ROLE OF THE FAMILY

Rehabilitation usually involves family members. They learn about the illness, injury, or disability. They learn how to care for their loved one. This often involves helping the person practise new skills. The family also learns new skills—for example, how to communicate with a spouse who cannot speak, how to cope with the behaviour of a mentally ill teenager, or how to dress a child with physical disabilities. Counselling is provided as needed to help people cope with changes affecting the family.

THERAPY AND TRAINING

Professionals on the rehabilitation team choose the therapy and training needed to meet goals. The client is taught how to improve a skill or how to do a task. The client practises what was learned alone, with a caregiver, or with family. You may help clients practise skills or tasks (see Chapter 12).

The client's therapy and training may involve learning how to use self-help devices. Equipment is ordered to meet the client's needs. The client is taught how to use the equipment:

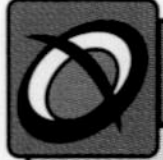

Focus on Older Adults

REHABILITATION

Rehabilitation often takes longer for older adults than for other people. Changes due to aging affect healing, mobility, vision, hearing, and other functions (see Chapter 15). Older adults often have chronic health problems that slow recovery. They are also at risk for injuries. Because older adults do not tolerate long or fast-paced programs, their rehabilitation is usually slow-paced.

Box 32-1 Case Study: Rehabilitation Following a Brain Injury

High school teacher Jeffery Butler, 34, was cycling to school when he was hit by a van. He sustained a severe blow to the head and broke several bones. After emergency care and surgery, he was placed in the intensive care unit (ICU). Because he had acquired a serious brain injury, he could not speak or recognize his family. After 10 days in the ICU, he was moved to an acute care floor, where he stayed for 2 months. Then he was transferred to the hospital's rehabilitation unit and was discharged home 3 months later. He received rehabilitation services at home and in the community for the next 6 months. During his long rehabilitation, Mr. Butler's rehabilitation team worked with him and his family (see the chart below). Regaining lost function and helping the family learn new skills were the team's main goals.

Rehabilitation team	Role
Mr. Butler and his family	• Made decisions regarding rehabilitation goals. • Involved in every aspect of care. • Learned new skills and relearned old skills.
Neurosurgeon	• Led surgical team and aspects of rehabilitation after surgery.
Orthopedic surgeon	• Led surgical team and aspects of rehabilitation after surgery.
Nurses	• Coordinated and provided care at every stage.
Specialist in rehabilitation medicine	• Led and coordinated rehabilitation.
Neuropsychologists	• Tested thinking, memory, emotions, behaviour, and personality. • Planned behaviour management treatment. • Headed adult day program.
Case manager	• Coordinated home care. • Arranged for adult day programs.
Social workers	• Provided counselling. • Headed adult day program.
Occupational therapists	• Assessed performance of activities of daily living. • Conducted home assessment prior to discharge. • Provided treatment, equipment, and devices to help attain independence.
Physiotherapists (Physical therapists)	• Evaluated strength, flexibility, and balance. • Taught mobility exercises and equipment use.
Speech-language pathologist	• Tested speech. • Taught family communication strategies.
Family physician	• Provided medical care after discharge.
Support workers	• Assisted with personal care and range-of-motion exercises. • Assisted with household management. • Assisted with eating. • Helped with physical therapy exercises.
Volunteers	• Sat with Mr. Butler when the family could not be there. • Assisted with household tasks.

- *Prostheses.* A **prosthesis** is an artificial replacement for a missing body part. Examples are prosthetic feet, knees, lower limbs, upper limbs, hands, breasts, and eyes. The goal for the prosthesis is to be like the missing body part in function and/or appearance. Artificial limbs are made from a variety of materials. Wood, aluminum, and plastics are commonly used. Most artificial limbs are powered by the person's muscles, either by muscles in the stump or by other nearby muscles. A physiotherapist works with the client to strengthen the muscles. The client learns how to use and care for the prosthesis. You might help a client get used to wearing and using a prosthesis. You might also assist the client with skin care at the prosthesis site (see Chapter 31).
- *Orthoses.* An **orthosis** is an apparatus worn to support, align, prevent, or correct problems with the musculoskeletal system. Examples are splints, foot supports, and knee and back braces (see Chapter 22). The client learns how to put on, use, and care for

the orthosis. You might help a client to put on an orthosis and practise moving or walking.

- *Eating and drinking devices*. These include glass holders, plate guards, and utensils with curved handles or cuffs (see Chapter 25).
- *Self-care devices*. These include electronic toothbrushes, combs, brushes, and sponges with long handles (Figure 32-1). There are also devices that help with dressing, cooking, writing, making phone calls, and other tasks (Figure 32-2).
- *Devices to aid mobility*. These include crutches, canes, walkers, and braces. Some clients need wheelchairs. If possible, the person learns how to transfer to and from the wheelchair using a transfer board. A transfer board is used to help the person move from one seat to another (Figure 32-3 on page 560). The person learns to transfer to and from the bed, toilet, bathtub, sofas and chairs, and cars.
- *Other equipment*. Some clients need feeding tubes (see Chapter 26) or mechanical ventilation (see Chapter 43). Some are weaned from the ventilator. Others must adapt to lifelong ventilation.

(text continues on page 560)

A

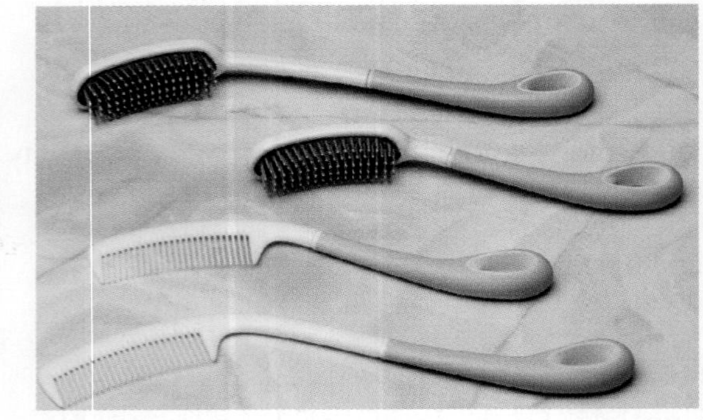

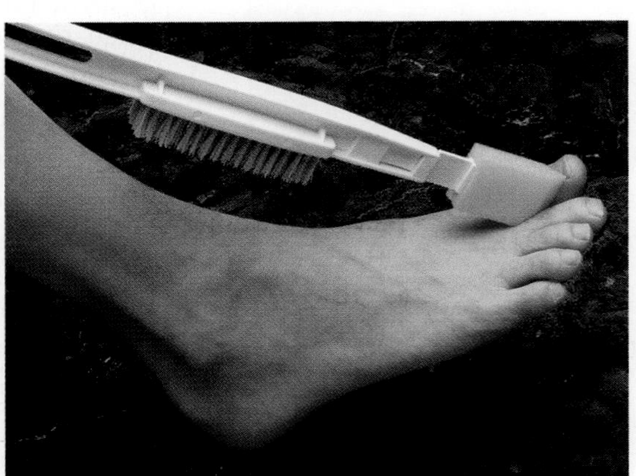

B

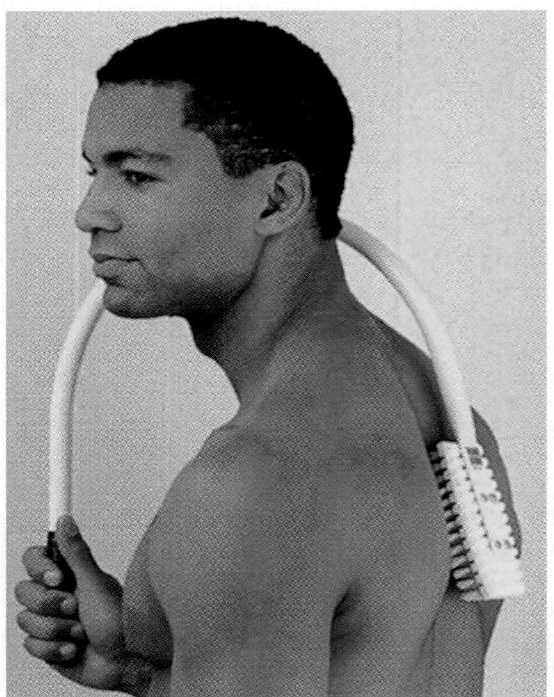

C

Figure 32-1 **A,** Long-handled combs and brushes for hair care. **B,** Long-handled brushes for bathing. **C,** Brush with a curved handle. (***A** and **B**, Courtesy Northcoast Medical, IN, Morgan Hill, CA; **C**, Courtesy Sammons Preston: An Ability One Company, Bolingbrook, IL.*)

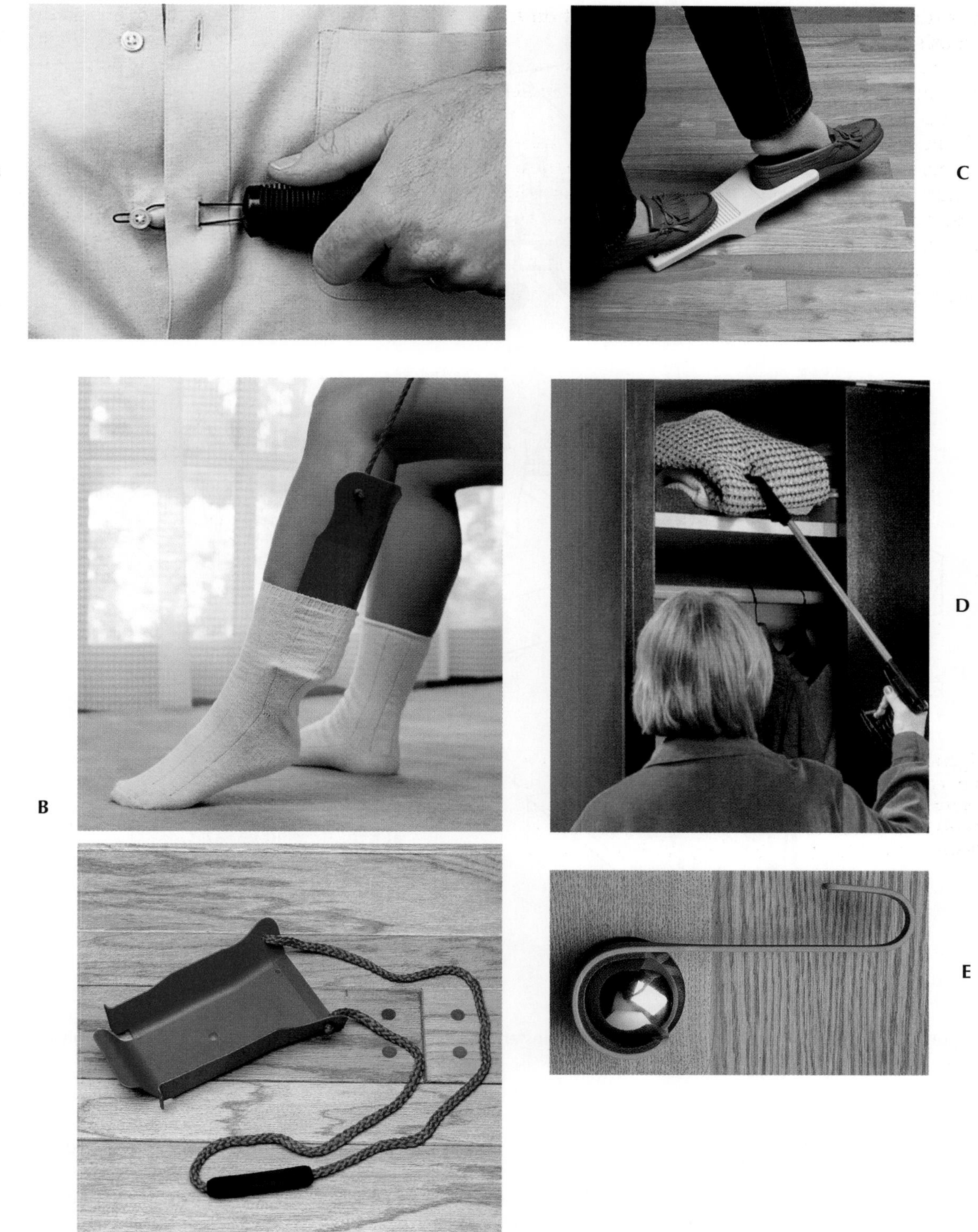

Figure 32-2 A, A button hook is used to button and zip clothing. **B,** A sock assist is used to pull on socks and stockings. **C,** A shoe remover is used to take off shoes. **D,** Reachers help to remove items from high shelves. **E,** A doorknob turner increases leverage to help turn the knob. (***A, B, C, E,*** *Courtesy Northcoast Medical Inc., Morgan Hill, CA;* ***D,*** *Courtesy AbilityOne Corporation, Germantown, WI.*)

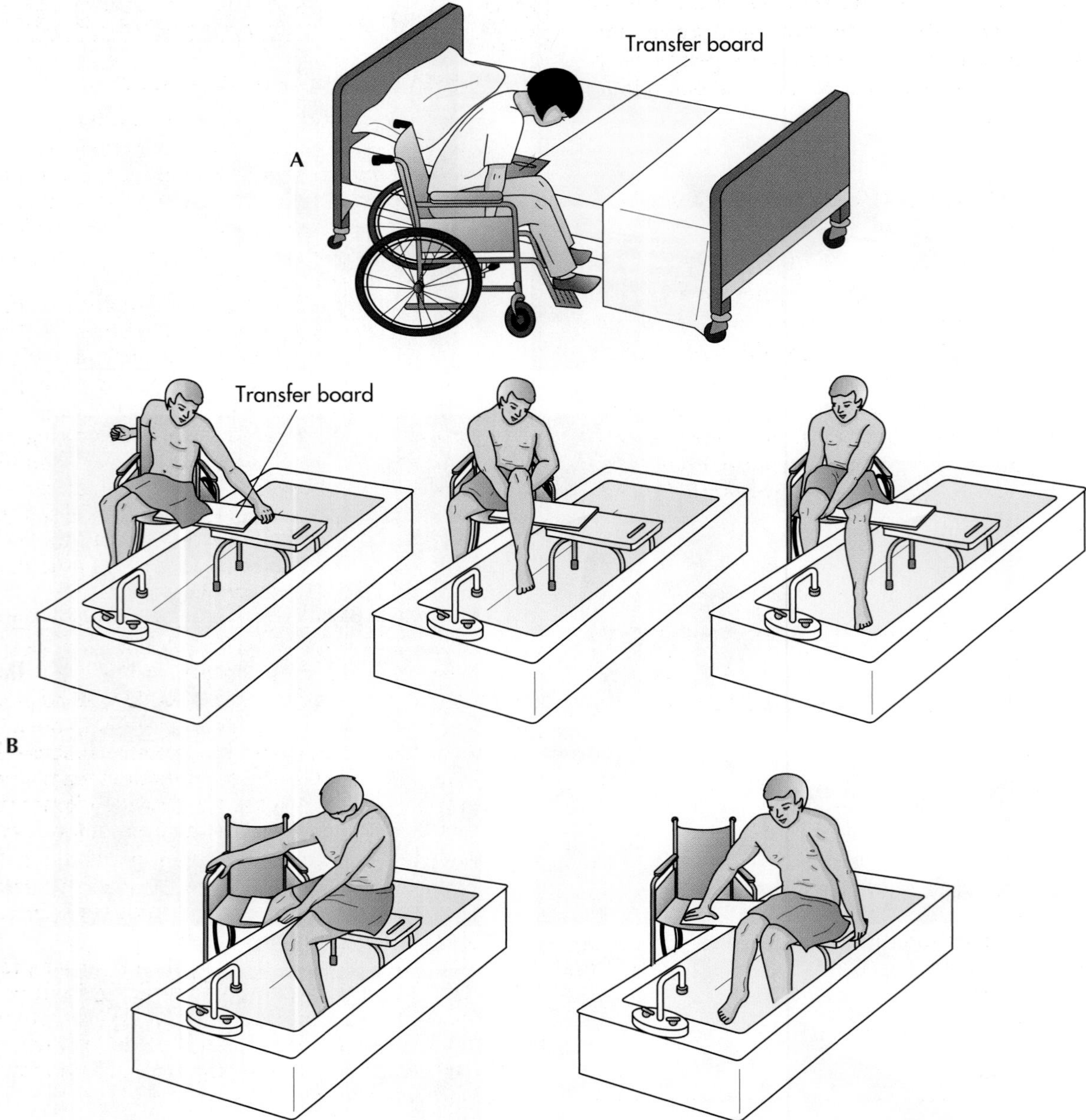

Figure 32-3 The client uses a transfer board for transferring. **A,** Transfer from a wheelchair to a bed. **B,** Transfer from a wheelchair to a bathtub.

Rehabilitation Settings

Many common health problems require rehabilitation (Box 32-2). Such services are found in most health care facilities and in the community.

- *Hospitals*. Most hospitals have rehabilitation units for inpatients and outpatients. Many programs focus on brain injury and tumours, spinal cord injury, and stroke. Some hospitals offer cardiac and respiratory rehabilitation. Some have programs for complex medical and surgical conditions such as wound care and unstable diabetes.
- *Specialized facilities*. Some health care facilities focus on specific problems. Mental illness and substance abuse/addiction are examples.
- *Long-term care facilities*. Most provide rehabilitation services similar to those found in hospitals.

- *Community care.* Home care services (see *Focus on Home Care: Home Assessment* box) and adult day programs are examples. A program for people with brain injuries may teach life skills, social behaviour, and work techniques.

Assisting with Rehabilitation and Restorative Care

Many of your clients will be undergoing some form of rehabilitation or restorative care. Some will be adjusting to overwhelming change. Rehabilitation is often slow and frustrating. Sometimes improvement is not seen for weeks or months. Some people improve quickly at first. Then the pace of improvement slows. You must be patient, supportive, and empathetic. (See *Providing Compassionate Care: Assisting with Rehabilitation* box.)

Box 32-2 Common Health Problems Requiring Rehabilitation

- Acquired brain injury
- Alcoholism
- Amputation
- Brain tumour
- Burns
- Cerebral palsy
- Chronic obstructive pulmonary disease
- Mental illness
- Myocardial infarction (heart attack)
- Parkinson's disease
- Spinal cord injury
- Spinal cord tumour
- Stroke
- Substance abuse

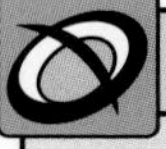

Focus on Home Care

Home Assessment

The rehabilitation team assesses a client's home (Box 32-3 on page 562). The case manager or occupational therapist discusses any safety risks and health hazards with the client and family. If necessary, changes are made to make the home more appropriate for the client.

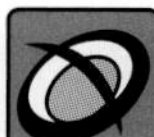

Providing Compassionate Care

Assisting with Rehabilitation

Dignity. Treat your clients with respect. Protect their right to dignity. They do not need your pity, but they do need encouragement and support. Focus on the positive. Remind them of their progress, and stress their abilities and strengths. Also provide emotional support and reassurance. Sometimes clients need someone to talk to. Be a good listener.

The process of regaining independence is often very slow. You may grow impatient with your client when repeated explanations seem to have little or no results. Never show your impatience. Imagine how the person feels. Having little control over body movements or functions is extremely frustrating. For many people, learning each new task is a reminder of the disability. Give praise when even a little progress is made. Remember that illness, disability, and fatigue can affect a person's ability to learn. People with brain injuries may have a particularly hard time learning new activities.

Independence. Independence is a key rehabilitation goal. Encourage the client to perform activities of daily living as independently as possible. Allow time for the client to complete the tasks. Do not rush the client. Be familiar with the client's self-help devices. Encourage their use whenever necessary. Practise the methods developed by the rehabilitation team when assisting the client. Practise the task the client must perform. This helps you guide and direct the client.

Preferences. Ask clients about their preferences. Allow for personal choice whenever possible. Freedom of choice helps people feel in control. Follow the client's daily routine and care plan.

Privacy. Some people feel embarrassed about practising skills (such as eating and walking) in front of others. Allow the client to practise skills in private where others cannot watch. Provide privacy for care procedures and elimination. Keep information about clients confidential.

Safety. Illness, disability, and fatigue increase the risk for accidents and injuries. Provide for safety (see Chapter 16). Never force clients to do more than they are able. Allow time for rest. Follow the care plan for safety measures needed for each client. Keep the client in good alignment. Use safe transfer methods (see Chapter 21). Perform range-of-motion exercises as directed. Turn and reposition the client as directed. Report signs and symptoms of complications. These include pressure ulcers, contractures, elimination problems, and depression. In facility settings, make sure that the call bell and overbed table are on the client's unaffected side.

Box 32-3 Home Assessment

Outdoors
- Where is parking located? What is the distance from the parking area to the door?
- Where is the mailbox?
- Where is the motor vehicle stored?
- What is the width of doors?
- Can the person turn a key?
- Can the person open and close doors?
- Are ramps needed?
- Are handrails needed?
- Are entrances lighted?
- Does the person have access to private or public transportation?
- Can the person operate a motor vehicle?
- What is the width and height of ramps and sidewalks?

Indoors
- Are there floor obstructions?
- Are there steps in the home? Where are they located?
- How is furniture arranged?
- Can the person use the furniture?
- Where are telephones located?
- Can the person raise and lower windows?
- How are floors covered (wall-to-wall carpeting, tile, hardwood floors, throw rugs)?
- Can the person use a wheelchair throughout the home?
- Where is the fuse or circuit-breaker box located?
- Can the person control the heat?
- Are walkways, doors, and halls wide enough for the person to use a wheelchair?
- Is there an elevator in an apartment or condominium building?

Kitchen
- Does the person have access to the stove, sink, cupboards, storage areas, work space, refrigerator, and other appliances?
- What is the height of the sink and countertops?
- Is there an opening under the sink for wheelchair access?
- Can the person turn faucets on and off?
- Can the person use the microwave?
- Can the person reach stove knobs?
- Are appliances arranged conveniently for the person?

Bathroom
- What is the height of the sink, toilet, shower, and tub?
- Can the person reach the faucets?
- Can the person turn the faucets on and off?
- Is there space for using a wheelchair and other mobility devices?
- Can the person get into and out of the tub or shower?
- Are there grab bars by the toilet, shower, and tub?

Bedroom
- What is the height of the person's bed?
- Can the person access the closet? Can the person reach rods and shelves?
- Can the person transfer in and out of bed safely? Is there enough space around the bed for the person to move?
- How is furniture arranged?
- Does the furniture arrangement allow for the use of a wheelchair or mobility devices?

Safety
- Is the house number clearly visible and readable during an emergency?
- Are deadbolts and locks secure? Can the person use the locks?
- Can the person see and talk to a visitor at the door without being seen?
- Are steps, porch, and front door lighted?
- Are the steps, porch, and front door protected from rain, sleet, and snow?
- Is there a nonslip doormat?
- Can the person use the telephone?
- Are emergency telephone numbers available?
- Can the person control water temperature?
- Do electrical outlets have childproof covers?
- Where are the smoke detectors? Are they working?
- Are rooms and hallways well lighted?
- Can the person control indoor and outdoor lighting?
- Can the person exit the home in an emergency?
- Is oxygen used in the home? Are safety measures for the use of oxygen in place?
- Does the person have access to the telephone, television, radio, and lights while in bed?
- Are space heaters used in the home? Are safety measures in place?
- Does the person have good judgment for cooking and stove use?
- Is there a safe play area for children?
- Can the person safely dispose of blood, body fluids, secretions, and excretions?
- Is there a pest-free method of trash storage?

Source: Adapted from S.P. Hoeman, *Rehabilitation Nursing: Process and Application,* 2nd ed. (St. Louis: Mosby, 1996).

REVIEW

Circle the BEST answer.

1. Which of the following is *not* a common goal for rehabilitation?
   A. To restore function to former levels
   B. To prepare for surgery
   C. To learn new skills
   D. To prevent further disability and illness

2. Rehabilitation is often slower for
   A. Toddlers
   B. Adolescents
   C. Middle-aged adults
   D. Older adults

3. Which member of the rehabilitation team evaluates a client's strength and balance?
   A. The physical therapist
   B. The occupational therapist
   C. The primary caregiver
   D. The nurse

4. The rehabilitation process addresses
   A. What the person cannot do
   B. Only physical health
   C. The whole person
   D. Only emotional health

5. Rehabilitation takes place
   A. Only in long-term care facilities
   B. Only in hospitals
   C. Only in specialized facilities
   D. In a variety of facility and community settings

6. Mr. Graziano needs rehabilitation after his right side is paralyzed. Personal care is
   A. Done by him to the extent possible
   B. Done by you
   C. Postponed until he can use his right side
   D. Supervised by his physician

7. Mr. Graziano is learning to use a walker. He asks to have music played. You should
   A. Tell him music is not allowed
   B. Choose some music
   C. Ask him to choose some music
   D. Ask a therapist to choose some music

8. Mr. Graziano's right side is weak. The call bell is on his right side. You move it to the left side of the bed. You have provided compassionate care to Mr. Graziano by
   A. Protecting him from abuse
   B. Providing for his safety
   C. Allowing personal choice
   D. Promoting his privacy

9. Mr. Graziano puts on his shirt using one arm. His progress is slow. You
   A. Focus his attention on learning a new task
   B. Praise him for his achievement
   C. Ask him to sit down and rest
   D. Tell him he will learn the next task more quickly

Answers to these questions are on page 826.

CHAPTER

33

MENTAL HEALTH DISORDERS

OBJECTIVES

- Define the key terms listed in this chapter
- Describe the effects of mental health disorders on everyday life
- List factors that may contribute to mental health disorders
- Describe the major mental health disorders
- Describe the stigma experienced by people with mental health disorders
- Describe the effect of mental health disorders on families
- Explain how to support clients with mental health disorders
- List the warning signals for suicide intent

KEY TERMS

affective disorders A group of mental disorders involving feelings, emotions, and moods

anxiety disorders A group of mental disorders in which anxiety is the main symptom

bipolar disorder An affective disorder in which the person experiences extremes in mood, energy, and ability to function

clinical depression Major depression

delusions False beliefs

eating disorders A group of mental disorders involving disturbances in eating behaviours and an abnormal concern with body weight and shape

emotional illness Mental illness

hallucination Seeing, hearing, or feeling something that is not real

major depression An affective disorder involving intense and prolonged feelings of sadness, hopelessness, and worthlessness; clinical depression

mental disorder Mental health disorder

mental health A state of mind in which a person copes with and adjusts to the stresses of everyday living in socially acceptable ways

mental health disorder Mental illness

mental illness A disturbance in a person's ability to cope with or adjust to stress; thinking, mood, or behaviours are affected and functioning is impaired; emotional illness; mental health disorder; psychiatric disorder

paranoia Extreme suspicion about a person or a situation

personality disorder A group of disorders involving rigid and socially unacceptable behaviours

psychosis A mental state in which perception of reality is impaired

psychiatric disorder Mental illness

psychotherapy A form of therapy in which a person explores his or her thoughts, feelings, and behaviours with a mental health specialist

schizophrenia A mental health disorder in which thinking and behaviour are disturbed

stigma A characteristic that marks a person as different or flawed

Mental health disorders can affect all aspects of a person's life: the physical, emotional, social, intellectual, and spiritual. You will support clients with physical or mental health problems. Some people have both. Sometimes physical and mental health problems are not related. Other times physical problems result from mental health problems. Or mental health problems can develop from physical problems.

You must provide your clients and their families with compassionate care. To do so, you need to understand what they are experiencing.

Mental Health and Mental Illness

Mental health is a state of mind in which a person copes with and adjusts to the stresses of everyday living in socially acceptable ways. People with optimal (complete) mental health have strong emotional, social, intellectual, and spiritual health.

Everyone feels anxiety, sadness, grief, and loneliness from time to time. People with average to good mental health can cope with life's problems and challenges. They know their own needs. They express and control their emotions appropriately. They usually form stable relationships.

Mental illness is a disturbance in a person's ability to cope with or adjust to stress. Thinking, mood, or behaviours are affected and functioning is impaired. (**Mental disorder, mental health disorder, emotional illness**, and **psychiatric disorder** also mean mental illness.) People with mental health disorders often behave differently from what is considered normal. They usually feel high levels of distress and fear. They often have trouble coping with everyday life. They may have difficulties keeping a job, staying in school, forming strong family and social relationships, and performing daily routines.

Mental illness and its symptoms range from mild to severe. The Canadian Mental Health Association (CMHA) estimates that one in five Canadian adults will experience a mental health disorder some time during their lives.[1]

The Causes of Mental Health Disorders

The causes of mental health disorders are complex. Many factors may contribute to mental health disorders, including:

- *Biological factors.* Chemical imbalances in the body can cause mental health disorders. Some disorders run in families. This suggests they can be inherited (passed from parent to child).
- *Childhood experience.* Childhood trauma or conflict, particularly when repressed, can cause mental health disorders. *Repression* means to keep unpleasant or painful thoughts from the conscious mind. For example, a woman cannot remember being sexually abused during childhood.
- *Social and cultural factors.* These include poverty, discrimination, and social isolation.
- *Stressful life events.* Family situations and workplace pressures can be stressful. Change is also stressful (see Chapter 8). Change associated with loss (such as death of a loved one or divorce) can be a source of extreme stress. This can lead to physical and mental health problems.
- *Poor physical health or disability.* People who are seriously ill, injured, or disabled are at risk for some mental health disorders.

Treating Mental Health Disorders

Until the 1960s, many people with mental health disorders lived in psychiatric facilities. Today only those who are severely ill live in facilities. Most people with mental health disorders live in the community. They are offered treatment and assistance with life skills and employment. Many people with mental health disorders live at home, in group homes, and in assisted-living facilities. Others are homeless.

The treatment of mental health disorders usually requires a team approach. The health care team may include a family physician, nurse, social worker, occupational therapist, support worker, and one or more of the following mental health specialists:

- *Psychiatrists*—physicians who specialize in mental health disorders. They can prescribe medication.
- *Psychologists and psychotherapists*—health care professionals educated to treat mental health disorders. They cannot prescribe medication.

Treatment of mental health disorders often involves **psychotherapy**. This is a form of therapy in which a person explores his or her thoughts, feelings, and behaviours with a mental health specialist. There are various forms of psychotherapy, including:

- *Psychoanalysis*—explores unconscious conflicts and underlying reasons behind the problems.
- *Behaviour therapy*—attempts to change behaviour by using various techniques. The focus is on the behaviour, not on the underlying reasons for the behaviour.
- *Group therapy*—a group of people meets regularly to discuss their problems under the guidance of a mental health specialist.
- *Family therapy*—a family meets regularly with a mental health specialist to discuss their problems.

People with mental health disorders are often helped by occupational therapy. The occupational therapist helps the person learn or relearn skills for the performance of life tasks. Social workers also provide assistance. For example, they might help a client to resolve employment problems.

Medications are ordered depending on the client's illness, signs, and symptoms. Many mental health disorders can be controlled with medication.

The care planning process is used to address the needs of clients with mental health disorders. This involves meeting the client's total needs, including physical, safety, and emotional needs.

Common Mental Health Disorders

There are many mental health disorders. They include anxiety disorders, affective (mood) disorders, schizophrenia, personality disorders, eating disorders, and substance-related disorders. Dementia is also considered a mental health disorder (see Chapter 34).

Anxiety Disorders

Anxiety disorders are a group of mental health disorders in which anxiety is the main symptom. Anxiety is a vague, uneasy feeling in response to stress. An anxious person has a sense of dread, danger, or harm. Some anxiety is normal. However, people with anxiety disorders have extreme anxiety. Their fears and worries are excessive for the situation. Normal functioning is affected.

The most common anxiety disorders are:

- *Panic disorder. Panic* is an intense and sudden feeling of fear, anxiety, terror, or dread for no obvious reason. A person with panic disorder has panic attacks. During a panic attack, the person cannot function. He or she may experience a rapid heart rate, shortness of breath, chest pain, or dizziness. Panic attacks can last for a few minutes or hours. They can occur several times a week.
- *Phobic disorder. Phobia* means fear, panic, or dread. A person with a phobic disorder has intense fear of a

particular thing or situation. Common phobias include *agoraphobia* (fear of open, crowded, public places) and *claustrophobia* (fear of enclosed places).
- *Obsessive-compulsive disorder.* An *obsession* is a persistent thought or desire. A *compulsion* is the uncontrollable urge to perform an act. The obsession is usually disturbing to the person and may be violent in nature. Usually the person tries to ignore the thought. Some people repeat an act over and over again to deal with the thought. For example, a person washes her hands over 30 times in an evening because of the fear of germs. Or a person worries that his oven is left on and must check it dozens of times before leaving the house.

Affective Disorders

Affective disorders are a group of mental health disorders that involve feelings, emotions, and moods. There are two major affective disorders.

Major Depression. **Major depression** involves intense and prolonged feelings of sadness, hopelessness, and worthlessness. It has physical and emotional effects. Sleep, eating, work, study, and other activities are affected. A person with depression may think about or attempt suicide.

Major depression may occur just once. It may be caused by a stressful event such as the death of a loved one. Divorce and job loss are other stressful events. For some people, episodes of depression occur throughout life.

Major depression occurs at any age. It is common among older adults. (See *Focus on Older Adults: Depression* box.) Learn the signs and symptoms of depression (Box 33-1).

Bipolar Disorder. *Bipolar* means two (*bi*) poles or ends (*polar*). **Bipolar disorder** involves severe extremes in mood, energy, and ability to function. A person with bipolar disorder has emotional lows (depression) and emotional highs (mania). The disorder used to be called *manic-depressive illness.* A person may be more depressed than manic, be more manic than depressed, or alternate between depression and mania.

The disorder tends to run in families. Signs and symptoms can range from mild to severe. Bipolar disorder can damage relationships and affect school or work performance. Some people with this disorder are suicidal.

Focus on Older Adults

Depression

Depression is common in older adults. They usually experience many losses—death of family and friends, loss of health, loss of body functions, and loss of independence. Loneliness and the side effects of some medications can also cause depression.

Depression in older adults is often overlooked or misdiagnosed. Sometimes the person is thought to have dementia (see Chapter 34). Therefore the depression goes untreated.

Box 33-1 Signs and Symptoms of Depression

- Depressed mood; for example, feeling sad, "blue," or hopeless
- Irritability (especially in children and adolescents)
- Reduced interest in almost all activities
- Significant weight gain or weight loss, without dieting
- Insomnia or too much sleep
- Too much or too little motor activity
- Fatigue or loss of energy
- Feelings of worthlessness or guilt
- Reduced ability to concentrate or think
- Difficulties making decisions
- Recurrent thoughts of death

Source: American Psychological Association, *Diagnostic and Statistical Manual of Mental Disorders,* 4th ed. Text Revision (Washington, DC: American Psychiatric Association, 1994).

Schizophrenia

Schizophrenia is a mental health disorder in which thinking and behaviour are disturbed. It affects about 1% of Canadians.[2] Schizophrenia affects a person's ability to function in all aspects of life, including work, school, social life, family relationships, and self-care. The word schizophrenia means split (*schizo*) mind (*phrenia*). It does not mean split personality. "Split mind" refers to the person's feelings of being "split off" from reality. The person has problems knowing what is real and what is not. The following are common with schizophrenia:

- **Psychosis**—a mental state in which perception of reality is impaired. The person cannot view or interpret reality correctly.
- **Delusions**—false beliefs. The person may believe he or she is a robot or some other person. *Delusions of grandeur* are false and exaggerated beliefs about one's importance, talent, or wealth. For example, a woman believes she is a god or the prime minister. *Delusions of persecution* are false beliefs that one is being mistreated, abused, or harassed. For example, a man believes that his neighbour wants to kill him.
- **Hallucinations**—seeing, hearing, and feeling things that are not real. For example, the person may see faces and hear voices that are not really there.

- **Paranoia**—extreme suspicion about a person or situation. For example, a person may feel he or she is being watched, followed, or controlled by someone else. A person may have delusions of persecution.

Without treatment, a person with schizophrenia has a severe mental impairment. He or she has problems relating to others. Responses are inappropriate and communication is disturbed. The person may ramble or repeat what others say. Sometimes the person's speech cannot be understood.

Some people with schizophrenia have one severe psychotic episode. Most suffer signs and symptoms throughout life but have periods of *remission*. During these times, the signs and symptoms of the disease lessen or disappear.

Some people with severe schizophrenia withdraw from others and the world. To *withdraw* means to stay away from others. They may sit for hours alone without moving, speaking, or responding.

Personality Disorders

Personality disorders are a group of disorders involving rigid and socially unacceptable behaviours. Individuals with personality disorders have problems relating to others. They may be demanding, hostile, and manipulative. Because of their behaviours, people with personality disorders cannot function well in society. Such disorders include:

- *Abusive personality*—abusive, possibly violent, behaviour toward others
- *Paranoid personality*—strong suspicion and distrust of others
- *Antisocial personality*—an inability to feel for others, poor judgment, lack of guilt and remorse, and irresponsible, often hostile, behaviour

Individuals with personality disorders do not experience normal periods. If untreated, many people with these disorders end up in trouble with the law.

Eating Disorders

Eating disorders involve disturbances in eating behaviours and an abnormal concern with body weight and shape. They occur mainly in teenage girls and young women. Eating disorders can be life-threatening. Some individuals recover. Others do not. The two most common eating disorders are anorexia nervosa and bulimia.

- *Anorexia nervosa*—occurs when a person has no appetite and has a great fear of weight gain and obesity. *Anorexia* means no (*a*) appetite (*orexia*). *Nervosa* relates to *nerves* or *emotions*. People with anorexia nervosa believe they are fat, despite being dangerously thin. They avoid food and eat only small amounts. Intense exercise and vomiting are common. Sleep problems and depression may occur. Menstruation may stop. Some people abuse laxatives and enemas to rid the body of food. Laxatives are drugs that rid the intestines of feces through defecation. Diuretic abuse also may occur. These drugs cause the kidneys to produce large amounts of urine. Extra fluid in the body is lost, causing weight loss.
- *Bulimia*—comes from the Greek words for ox (*bous*) and hunger (*limos*). Bulimia involves binge eating. That is, the person eats a large amount of food. The person then purges, or rids the body of food. Vomiting, laxatives, enemas, diuretics, fasting, and intense exercise are some methods used.

Substance-Related Disorders

Substance abuse disorder is the deliberate misuse of medications, illegal drugs, alcohol, or other substances. People with this disorder often develop relationship and work problems. They are unable to stop the substance abuse.

Abused substances affect the central nervous system. Some substances have a calming or depressing effect. Others have a stimulating effect. They all affect the mind and thinking. Many are also mood altering. After taking the substance, users may feel happy, self-confident, and relaxed. They may have an exaggerated sense of their own abilities. Or they may be emotional or aggressive. Some substances cause hallucinations.

Many people who abuse drugs, alcohol, or other substances have *substance dependence disorder*. People with this disorder show evidence of tolerance and withdrawal. *Tolerance* occurs when the person needs larger and larger amounts of the substance to produce the same effect. *Withdrawal* is a physical reaction that occurs when the person stops taking the substance. Signs and symptoms of withdrawal may include depression, agitation, abdominal cramps, nausea, diarrhea, and painful muscle spasms. The symptoms can be severe. Some people turn to criminal behaviour to support their habit. Without treatment, death is a risk. Common causes of death are overdoses, suicide, and diseases contracted from using contaminated needles.

Treatment depends on the substance being abused. Some people need *detoxification*. The detoxification process involves removing the abused substance from the body. Hospital care is usually required. Almost all treatment programs involve psychotherapy. Mental health professionals help clients to manage their problems.

Alcohol Abuse. Alcohol is abused more than any other substance. Signs and symptoms of alcohol abuse include intoxication (drunkenness), memory problems, difficulty concentrating, tremors, and loss of interest in family and friends. Liver, pancreas, and heart problems may develop. Fetal alcohol syndrome can result when a woman drinks during pregnancy (see Chapter 37). Many people with alcohol problems have poor nutrition. Many also are addicted to nicotine (cigarettes). They are at risk for lung disease and certain cancers. People with alcohol problems may be emotional, aggressive, and abusive. Their families are at risk for abuse and other problems.

Some people drink every day. Others go for days or weeks without drinking and then drink a great deal in a short period. People who are mentally ill, under stress, or lonely may turn to alcohol to help them feel better. Older adults who live alone are at risk for alcohol abuse.

The main treatment is to avoid drinking. Groups such as Alcoholics Anonymous (AA) help people stop drinking. Individual and family counselling is often needed.

The Stigma of Mental Health Disorders

A **stigma** is a characteristic that marks a person as different or flawed. People sometimes discriminate against those with mental health disorders. They may not understand mental health disorders. They may fear being with a mentally ill person. They do not know what to expect. They may believe a mentally ill person is dangerous. Or they may blame the person for his or her problems. Attitudes like these lead people to avoid and exclude people with mental health disorders. As a result, people with these disorders often feel ashamed, rejected, and isolated.

The Canadian Alliance for Mental Illness and Mental Health (CAMIMH) is an organization representing mental health professionals and individuals concerned with mental health. The main goal of the CAMIMH is to prevent stigma and discrimination against people with mental health disorders.[3] Through educational programs, the organization promotes greater understanding and acceptance of mental health disorders.

Caring for Clients and Their Families

Mental health disorders affect people in different ways. Those with mild disorders have few problems. However, severe mental illness almost always causes distress for individuals and their families. The ill person may be unable to function. His or her behaviour is often disruptive. Family members must make difficult decisions about care, treatment, and housing. They may feel anxious about an uncertain future. The stress on caregivers is significant. The financial burden of caring for a loved one may also be significant. Family members may feel guilty and blame themselves for causing the illness. They are at risk for depression.

Family members also feel the stigma of mental health disorders. Friends and acquaintances may feel uncomfortable, so they may not offer social support. One woman describes how people reacted differently to her husband's physical illness and her son's mental illness. "When my husband had cancer, neighbours and friends were very kind. The phone rang constantly with offers to help. People brought over meals and sent flowers and cards. When my son developed schizophrenia, everything was different. Nobody called. Nobody asked how we were doing. They pretended everything was fine. We felt very much alone."

Be sensitive to the feelings of your clients and their family. Examine your own attitudes about mental health and mental illness. To provide compassionate care, you must be self-aware. (See *Providing Compassionate Care: Supporting Clients with Mental Health Disorders* box on page 571. Follow the guidelines listed in Box 33-2 on page 570. Also follow the care plan.)

The Risk of Suicide

Suicide means to kill (*caedere*) oneself (*sui*). It is a common cause of death in men and women from adolescence through middle age. People with mental health disorders are at high risk for suicide. Those who attempt suicide views life as unbearable. They may believe their families and friends are better off without them.

Men commit suicide more often than women do. Men tend to use violent methods to kill themselves (hanging, firearms). Their attempts are often fatal. Women usually choose less violent methods, for example, taking an overdose of pills. With less violent methods, the person may survive.

Attempted suicide is a sign of a serious mental health problem. The person needs professional care and a suicide prevention program.

Risk factors for suicide include:

- Mental illness, especially depression, bipolar disorder, and schizophrenia
- A history of abuse
- A family history of suicide
- The suicide of a friend
- A prior suicide attempt
- A major crisis such as the loss of a relationship, family problems, loss of position in society, and work, money, or legal problems
- Pressure to succeed
- Isolation

(text continues on page 571)

Box 33-2 Guidelines for Supporting Clients with Mental Health Disorders

General Guidelines

- *Follow the care plan.* Tell your supervisor if measures are not working.
- *Provide a safe, comfortable setting.* A quiet, neat, and safe setting can calm the person.
- *Follow a consistent routine.* A routine promotes a sense of control. It can reduce uncertainty and anxiety.
- *Explain all procedures.* Understanding what will happen next reduces anxiety.
- *Be patient and supportive.* Speak calmly. Avoid speaking loudly or sharply.
- *Assist the person with medications.* As required in the care plan, remind home care clients to take medications as ordered. Assist as required (see Chapter 39).
- *Observe the person carefully.* Observe for any changes in the person's behaviour, mood, and thinking. These involve signs and symptoms of fatigue, stress, anxiety, fear, and frustration. Also observe for signs and symptoms of illness. Report and record your observations according to employer policy.

Supporting Clients with Anxiety Disorders

- *Avoid situations that are known to cause anxiety.* For example, if a person is afraid of small, closed spaces, keep him or her away from these.
- *Avoid discussing subjects that cause anxiety.* Keep the conversation on other subjects.
- *Provide comfort during periods of anxiety.* Stay with the person if he or she is extremely anxious or has a panic attack. Use touch to reassure the person, if appropriate. Report the situation to your supervisor.

Supporting Clients with Major Depression

- *Show you enjoy being with the person.* Listen to your client. Show an interest in the person's life.
- *Do not minimize the person's problems.* Do not say things like "cheer up" or "snap out of it." Such comments suggest the person is exaggerating the problem.
- *Be positive.* One positive experience may encourage further positive experiences.
- *Encourage rest.* It can refresh a person.
- *Encourage activity and social interactions.* It can improve a person's outlook and sense of well-being. However, do not tire the person.
- *Be alert for warning signals of suicide* (see Box 33-3). Report any signals to your supervisor at once.

Supporting Clients with Bipolar Disorder

- *During depression*
  - Follow the guidelines for major depression.
- *During manic periods*
  - Provide a calm environment, with few distractions.
  - Encourage periods of rest.
  - Encourage self-care; assist as required.
  - Do not argue. This could irritate the person.
  - Offer limited choices to make decisions easier.

Supporting Clients with Schizophrenia

- *Focus on one task or activity at a time.* This helps the person focus.
- *Be aware of your nonverbal communication.* Avoid body language and facial expressions that could be considered threatening.
- *Do not argue.* Never argue with the client about whether a delusion or hallucination is real. The delusion or hallucination is real to the person. Do not pretend that the delusion or hallucination is real. Rather, offer the person comfort. Show empathy. Tell your supervisor if your client is having a delusion or hallucination.
- *Use distractions.* Distract the person to avoid disturbing subjects. For example, play music or take the person for a walk.

Supporting Clients with Substance-Related Disorders

- *Report suspicions of substance abuse.* You may smell alcohol on a client's breath. Or, you may observe that a person's medication is running out more quickly than expected. Report suspected substance abuse to your supervisor at once. This information is confidential. Do not discuss the matter with anyone else.
- *Avoid confrontation.* If you think a client is abusing a substance, do not argue. Tell your supervisor immediately. Do not discuss the matter with anyone.
- *Never buy alcohol, drugs, or other substances.* Some clients may ask you to purchase alcohol, drugs, or other substances. To do so is unethical. Report any such requests to your supervisor.

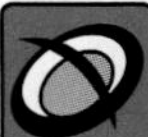

Providing Compassionate Care

SUPPORTING CLIENTS WITH MENTAL HEALTH DISORDERS

Dignity. Treat clients with mental health disorders as you would any other client. Show respect and promote dignity. Do not label them. It is not acceptable to say the person *is* a schizophrenic or drug addict. It is acceptable to say the person *has* schizophrenia or a substance dependence disorder.

Be patient and understanding. Do not patronize (talk down to) the person. Do not feel offended or hurt by the person's remarks or actions. Remember, the person may have difficulty relating to others. Help the person feel good about him or herself. Accept the person for who he or she is. Treat the person as a valued, worthy individual.

Independence. People with mental health disorders have the right to autonomy. They should be encouraged to be as independent as is safely possible.

People with mental health disorders are impaired in *some* areas. However, they are rarely impaired in *all* areas. For example, a person with schizophrenia usually has no problems with ambulation.

Preferences. Allow clients choices according to the care plan. This gives them a greater sense of control. Feelings of loss of control can cause some people with mental health disorders to withdraw. Encourage clients to express their wishes, likes, and dislikes.

Privacy. Discuss the client only with the health care team. Respect the client's and family's need for confidentiality and privacy.

Safety. Stress, fatigue, and physical illness make mental health disorders worse. They may trigger the illness. Observe the client carefully for any signs of stress or illness. Report these at once. Provide a calm, stress-free, and safe setting. The client's care plan lists activities and situations to avoid. Follow the safety guidelines in Chapter 16. For abusive situations, see Chapter 19.

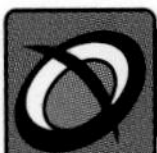

Focus on Older Adults

SUICIDE

Older adults also are at risk for suicide. They experience many losses: death of family and friends, loss of physical health, loss of cognitive (mental) abilities. Depression is common in older adults (see page 567). Some older adults choose suicide to avoid loneliness. Others are facing death because of serious illness. For them, suicide may seem better than suffering or causing hardship for their families.

- Early losses in life
- Sexual identity issues
- Feelings of deep hopelessness and helplessness
- Recent diagnosis of a life-threatening illness
- Substance abuse

See *Focus on Older Adults: Suicide* box.

The common warning signals of suicide are listed in Box 33-3. If a client talks about suicide, take the person seriously. Tell your supervisor at once. Do not leave the person alone. Encourage the person to talk. This gives your supervisor time to get help. It also shows the person that you care. Be a good listener. Do not minimize the person's concerns. Do not make comments such as:

- "You shouldn't have such thoughts."
- "Things will work out."
- "Look on the bright side."

In a home care setting, stay with the client until help arrives. Your supervisor may send a nurse, case manager, or emergency personnel to help the person.

Box 33-3 Common Warning Signals for Suicide Intent

- Signs and symptoms of depression (see Box 33-1 on page 567)
- Repeated expressions of hopelessness, helplessness, or desperation
- Expressions of interest in committing suicide
- Having a plan such as taking pills or hanging oneself at a specific place and time
- Loss of interest in friends, hobbies, or previously enjoyed activities
- Giving away prized possessions or putting personal affairs in order
- Telling final wishes to someone else
- A change in personality or mood; for example, sudden and unusually happy behaviour following a period of depression
- A change in appearance; for example, a person who is usually well groomed is untidy and unwashed
- Failure to recover from a loss or crisis
- A sudden tendency to take large risks
- Refusing to eat, drink, or take medications

Source: Health Canada, *A Report on Mental Illness in Canada*, 2002, p. 90. © Health Canada Editorial Board Mental Illnesses in Canada, Cat. No. 0-662-32817-5, www.hc-sc.gc.ca. The Canadian Mental Health Association. *Preventing Suicide*, (Toronto: National Office, 1993), http://www.cmha.ca/english/info_centre/mh_pamphlets/mh_pamphlet_12.htm.

REVIEW

Circle the BEST answer.

1. Which of the following is *false*?
   A. People with mental health disorders usually cause their own problems.
   B. Chemical imbalances in the body can cause mental health disorders.
   C. Treatment for mental health disorders might include psychotherapy and medication.
   D. Most people with mental health disorders have problems coping with daily life.

2. Mr. Mueller sees a psychologist. They explore the unconscious conflicts and underlying reasons for Mr. Mueller's problems. This kind of psychotherapy is
   A. Psychoanalysis
   B. Occupational therapy
   C. Behaviour therapy
   D. Group therapy

3. Mrs. Paré is afraid of catching a disease. She washes her hands hundreds of times a day. Mrs. Paré likely has
   A. Obsessive-compulsive disorder
   B. Panic disorder
   C. Phobic disorder
   D. Anorexia nervosa

4. Mr. Lau has bipolar disorder. This means he
   A. Is very suspicious
   B. Is hostile
   C. Has delusions
   D. Has severe mood swings

5. Mr. Duncan has an abusive personality. You know that he
   A. Has schizophrenia
   B. Has an eating disorder
   C. Has bulimia
   D. May behave violently

6. Shira, 15, has lost 30 pounds. She is terrified of becoming fat, even though she is extremely thin. She avoids food. Shira likely has
   A. Claustrophobia
   B. Anorexia nervosa
   C. Repression
   D. Bulimia nervosa

7. Mrs. Alam has major depression. Do *not*
   A. Encourage activity and social interactions
   B. Encourage periods of rest
   C. Tell her how lucky she is
   D. Show her that you care

8. You are supporting a client with bipolar disorder who is in the manic phase of the illness. Do *not*
   A. Provide a stimulating environment
   B. Encourage periods of rest
   C. Offer limited choices
   D. Encourage self-care

9. Kathy, 19, has schizophrenia. She believes she is a famous actor. This is an example of
   A. A rich fantasy life
   B. Delusions of grandeur
   C. Delusions of persecution
   D. Hallucinations

10. Kathy says giant insects are climbing the wall. She is terrified. You see nothing on the wall. You should
    A. Insist that Kathy is seeing things
    B. Pretend you also see the insects
    C. Offer Kathy comfort and report the hallucination
    D. Leave Kathy alone and call for help

11. Which of the following is *false*? People with substance dependence disorder
    A. Experience withdrawal when they stop taking the substance
    B. Are at risk of dying from infections from contaminated needles
    C. Must take the substance to feel good and avoid discomfort
    D. Have only themselves to blame

12. A client with major depression suddenly seems happy. She asks you to leave early because she is expecting friends. You should:
    A. Stay until you are scheduled to leave
    B. Leave as requested
    C. Call your supervisor to report the situation
    D. Leave as soon as the friends arrive

Answers to these questions are on page 826.

CHAPTER

34

Confusion and Dementia

OBJECTIVES

- Define the key terms listed in this chapter
- Describe confusion and delirium and their causes
- List measures that help clients who are confused
- Describe dementia and its signs and symptoms
- List different forms and causes of dementia
- Describe the common stages of dementia
- Describe the care required by a client with dementia
- List examples of challenging behaviours and possible causes
- Describe how primary caregivers may be affected by caring for family members with dementia

KEY TERMS

Alzheimer's disease (AD) A disease that gradually destroys nerve cells (neurons) in most areas of the brain; is the most common form of dementia

confusion A mental state where the person is disoriented to person, time, or place; memory and judgment are usually also impaired

delirium A state of temporary mental confusion

delusion A false belief

dementia The progressive loss of cognitive and social functions; is a symptom of changes in the brain

hallucination Seeing, hearing, or feeling something that is not real

sundowning When signs, symptoms, and behaviours of dementia increase during hours of darkness

Some changes in the brain and nervous system occur normally with aging (Box 34-1). Certain diseases also affect the brain. Some of these diseases are more common in older adults but also occur in younger people. Diseases that affect the brain can affect cognitive function. *Cognitive* relates to knowledge. Cognitive functioning involves:

- Memory
- Thinking
- Reasoning
- Ability to understand
- Judgment
- Behaviour

Loss of cognitive functioning affects all dimensions of a person's life.

CONFUSION

Confusion is a mental state where the person is disoriented to person, time, or place. Usually memory and the ability to make good judgments are impaired or lost. Behaviour changes are common. The person may be angry, restless, depressed, or irritable. Other signs and symptoms of confusion include:

- Anxiety
- Tremors
- Hallucinations (page 582)
- Delusions (page 582)
- Disorganized thinking and speech
- Attention problems
- Decline in level of consciousness

Confusion can occur suddenly and be temporary. This is called **delirium**. It is often a reaction to medications, infection, and other illness. Poor nutrition, food poisoning, and dehydration are other causes. So is emotional trauma. For example, a major life change like the death of a loved one or moving to a facility can cause delirium.

Delirium is an emergency. It often is the first or only sign of physical illness in older adults and in people with dementia. If you observe any sudden occurrence of the signs and symptoms of confusion, tell your supervisor at once. The cause must be found and treated.

Confusion is permanent when it is caused by physical changes to the structure of the brain. For example, people with dementia experience confusion. In these cases, confusion cannot be cured. Some measures improve function (Box 34-2). You must meet the client's physical and safety needs.

Box 34-1 Normal Changes in the Nervous System Associated with Aging

- Brain cells are lost
- Nerve conduction slows
- Response and reaction times are slower
- Reflexes are slower
- Vision and hearing decrease
- Taste and smell decrease
- Touch and sensitivity to pain decrease
- Reduced blood flow to the brain
- Changes in sleep patterns
- Mild word-finding problems

DEMENTIA

Dementia is a general term that describes the progressive loss of cognitive and social functions. It is not a disease, but is a symptom of changes in the brain. Usually dementia starts slowly and progresses gradually.

Box 34-2 Caring for Clients Who Are Confused

- Follow the care plan.
- Provide for safety.
- Face the person. Speak clearly and slowly.
- Call the person by name every time you are in contact with him or her.
- State your name. Show your name tag.
- Give the date and time each morning. Repeat as needed during the day or evening.
- Explain what you are going to do and why.
- Give clear, simple directions and answers to questions.
- Ask clear and simple questions. Give the person time to respond.
- Keep calendars and clocks with large numbers in the person's room and in other areas (Figure 34-1). Remind the person of holidays, birthdays, and special events.
- Have the person wear glasses and a hearing aid if needed.
- Use touch to communicate (see Chapter 12).
- Place familiar objects and pictures within the person's view.
- Provide newspapers, magazines, TV, and radio. Read to the person if appropriate.
- Discuss current events with the person.
- Maintain the day–night cycle. Open curtains, shades, and drapes during the day. Close them at night. Use a night-light at night. The person wears regular clothes during the day—not sleepwear.
- Provide a calm, relaxed, and peaceful setting. Prevent loud noises, rushing, and congested hallways and rooms.
- Follow the person's routine. Meals, bathing, exercise, TV, and other activities have a schedule. This promotes a sense of order and what to expect.
- Break tasks into small steps when helping the person.
- Do not rearrange furniture or the person's belongings.
- Encourage self-care.
- Be consistent.

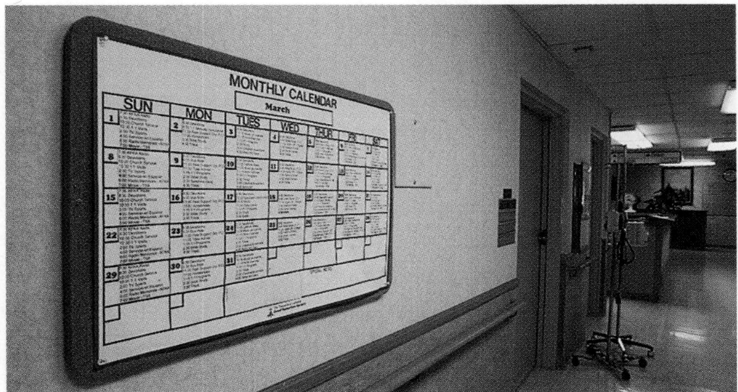

Figure 34-1 A large calendar can help clients who are confused.

Everyday skills are eventually lost. These functions are affected:

- Memory
- Thinking
- Reasoning
- Judgment
- Language
- Behaviour
- Mood
- Personality

Signs and Symptoms of Dementia

Dementia is not a normal part of aging. Most older adults do not have dementia. Only a small number of older adults are affected. Dementia can affect people in their 40s and 50s. However, dementia is more common after 65 years of age.

Early warning signs of dementia include:

- Memory loss that affects daily activities (for example, misplacing items or putting them in odd places)
- Confusion (for example, getting lost in familiar places or forgetting how to use simple, everyday items, like a calculator)
- Problems finding the right words or following conversations
- Poor judgment (for example, going outdoors in the snow without shoes)
- Problems with common tasks (for example, dressing, cooking, driving)
- Changes in mood, behaviour, or personality (for example, unfounded jealousy, suspiciousness, or poor social behaviour)
- Loss of interest in activities or hobbies (for example, a person who was once an avid gardener now lets weeds overrun the yard)

Dementia affects the ability to perform complex and simple tasks. Problems with complex tasks appear first. The person has problems driving, managing money, planning meals, and working. Over time, problems occur with simple tasks. These include bathing, dressing, eating, using the toilet, and walking. See Box 34-3 on page 576 for other signs and symptoms of dementia.

Box 34-3 Other Signs and Symptoms of Dementia

- Forgets recent events
- Forgets simple directions
- Forgets conversations
- Forgets appointments
- Forgets names (including family members)
- Forgets the names of everyday things (clock, radio, TV, and so on)
- Forgets words
- Substitutes unusual words and names for what is forgotten
- Loses train of thought
- Speaks in a native language
- Curses or swears
- Misplaces items
- Puts things in odd places
- Has problems writing cheques or balancing chequebooks
- Gives away large amounts of money
- Does not recognize or understand numbers
- Has problems following conversations
- Has problems reading
- Has problems writing
- Becomes lost in familiar settings
- Forgets where he or she is
- Wanders from home
- Does not know how to get back home
- Cannot tell or understand time
- Cannot tell or understand dates
- Cannot solve everyday problems (iron is left on, stove burners left on, food burning on the stove, and so on)
- Cannot perform everyday tasks (dressing, bathing, brushing teeth, and so on)
- Distrusts others
- Is stubborn
- Withdraws socially
- Is restless
- Becomes suspicious
- Becomes fearful
- Does not want to do things
- Sleeps more than usual

Forms and Causes of Dementia

There are many different forms and causes of dementia. Sometimes dementia is caused by conditions that are treatable. When the condition that causes the dementia is treated, the dementia is reversed (cured) or slowed. Dementias that may be reversed are those caused by:

- *Brain injury*—some brain injuries result in internal bleeding in the skull, which can cause symptoms of dementia. Surgery to correct the bleeding can correct the dementia.
- *Brain tumour*—depending on the location, size, and type of the brain tumour, delirium or dementia may result. Surgery or chemotherapy may be used to treat the tumour.
- *Alcohol*—long-term alcohol abuse can lead to dementia. If the person stops drinking, the dementia may be reversed.
- *Thyroid deficiency*—the thyroid gland produces certain hormones. An under-active thyroid can lead to dementia. It can also produce delirium. This form of dementia is reversible when the thyroid condition is corrected.

Most other forms of dementia cannot be reversed. Irreversible dementias result from changes in the brain. They have no prevention or cure. Function declines over time. Irreversible dementia eventually interferes with all daily activities and leads to death. The following are some of the most common forms of irreversible dementia:

- ***Alzheimer's disease (AD)***—the most common form of dementia. AD accounts for over 64 percent of all dementias in Canadians.[1] The disease gradually destroys nerve cells (neurons) in most areas of the brain. It results in impaired cognitive function and behaviour changes. It is progressive and irreversible. The disease is gradual in onset. It progresses over 3 to 20 years. Symptoms worsen over the years. The rate of decline varies from person to person. AD usually occurs after the age of 65 and is often diagnosed after the age of 80. However, it can also affect people in their 40s and 50s. Currently, AD has no cure. Some medications are used to slow its progress. The cause of AD is unknown. However, a family history of AD or Down syndrome are risk factors.
- *Vascular dementia* (*multi-infarct dementia*)—dementia caused by a series of small strokes. Tissues of the brain die as a result of the strokes.
- *Lewy body dementia*—progressive dementia characterized by abnormal structures in brain cells. The progression of the disease is usually more rapid than with AD.
- *Pick's disease*—a rare brain disorder that usually begins between the ages of 45 and 65. It destroys or damages brain cells in the frontal and temporal areas of the brain. Behaviour and speech are affected first, and then the general signs of dementia appear later.
- *Creutzfeldt-Jakob disease* (*CJD*)—a form of progressive dementia in which brain tissue slowly dies, causing small holes in the brain. Dementia and loss of muscle control occur.

Many health conditions can sometimes cause dementia, including the following (see Chapter 31):

- AIDS
- Huntington's disease
- Multiple sclerosis
- Parkinson's disease
- Syphilis

Delirium and depression (see Chapter 33) can easily be mistaken for dementia. They share many of the same signs and symptoms. For this reason, depression is sometimes called *pseudodementia*, meaning false (*pseudo*) dementia. However, permanent changes in the brain have not occurred with delirium and depression. They are not the same as dementia. Sometimes delirium and depression accompany dementia. A correct diagnosis by a physician is very important.

Stages of Dementia

Dementia generally has three stages. Box 34-4 describes common characteristics of each stage. These descriptions apply to Alzheimer's disease and most other forms of dementia. In the early stages, different dementias can present quite differently. However, they tend to become similar as they progress. Signs and symptoms become more severe with each stage. Eventually the person is confined to bed and becomes totally dependent on others for care. Death occurs when the brain shuts down all body systems.

Care of Clients with Dementia

Each client with dementia has unique care needs. The client's needs depend on the form of dementia, the stage of the dementia, and the care setting. Box 34-5 on pages 578–79 lists general guidelines for caring for clients with dementia. The care plan and your supervisor tell you specific instructions for each client.

Clients with Early Stage Dementia

Usually a person with dementia is cared for at home until symptoms are severe. Some people live alone in their own homes, where they receive support from family, friends, volunteers, and home care workers. Others live with family members. The primary caregiver may be the person's spouse or adult child, or it may be another family member or a friend. Other caregivers may provide relief to the primary caregiver. Respite care through adult daycare and home care provides temporary help.

(text continues on page 580)

Box 34-4 Stages of Dementia

Stage 1: Mild (Early Stage)
- Memory loss—forgetfulness; forgets recent events
- Problems finding words, finishing thoughts, following directions, and remembering names
- Poor judgment; bad decisions (including when driving)
- Confusion occurs occasionally—disoriented to person, time, and place
- Lack of spontaneity—less outgoing or interested in things
- Blames others for mistakes, forgetfulness, and other problems
- Symptoms of depression, irritability, or defensiveness
- Problems performing everyday tasks

Stage 2: Moderate (Middle Stage)
- Restlessness; increases during the evening hours
- Increasing episodes of confusion
- Sleep problems
- Memory loss increases—may not know family and friends
- Dulled senses—cannot tell the difference between hot and cold; cannot recognize dangers
- Bowel and bladder incontinence
- Needs help with activities of daily living (ADL)—bathing, feeding, and dressing self; may be afraid of bathing; may refuse to change clothes
- Loses impulse control—foul language, poor table manners, sexual aggression, rudeness
- Movement and gait problems—walks slowly, has a shuffling gait
- Communication problems—cannot follow directions; problems with reading, writing, and math; speaks in short sentences or single words; statements may not make sense
- Repeats motions and statements—moves things back and forth constantly; says the same thing over and over again
- Agitation—behaviour may be violent

Stage 3: Severe (Late Stage)
- Seizures (see Chapter 47)
- Cannot speak—may groan, grunt, or scream
- Constant state of confusion—does not recognize self, family members, or others
- Depends totally on others for all activities of daily living
- Totally incontinent of urine and feces
- Cannot swallow—choking and aspiration are risks
- Sleep problems increase
- Becomes confined to bed—cannot sit or walk
- Coma
- Death

Box 34-5 Guidelines for Caring for Clients with Dementia

Environment
- Follow established routines.
- Place picture signs on rooms, bathrooms, dining rooms, and other areas (Figure 34-2 on page 580). Follow your supervisor's directions.
- Keep personal items where the person can see them.
- Stay within the person's sight to the extent possible.
- Place memory aids (large clocks and calendars) where the person can see them.
- Keep noise levels low.
- Play music and show movies from the person's past.
- Select tasks and activities specific to the person's cognitive abilities and interests.

Communication
- Approach the person in a calm, quiet manner.
- Approach the person from the front. Do not approach from the side or back. This can startle the person.
- Call the person by name.
- Identify other people by their names. Avoid pronouns (he, she, them, and so on).
- Practise measures to promote communication (see Chapter 12).
- Use gestures and cues. Point to objects.
- Speak in a calm, gentle voice.
- Speak slowly. Use simple words and sentences.
- Let the person speak. Do not interrupt or rush the person.
- Give the person time to respond.
- Do not criticize, correct, or argue with the person.
- Present one idea, question, or instruction at a time.
- Ask simple questions having simple answers. Do not ask complex questions.
- Do not present the person with many choices.
- Provide simple explanations of all procedures and activities.
- Give consistent responses.
- Repeat information frequently. Usually, the person cannot remember new information.

Safety
- Remove harmful, sharp, and breakable objects from the area. These include knives, scissors, glass, dishes, razors, and tools.
- Provide plastic eating and drinking utensils. This helps prevent breakage and cuts.
- Place safety plugs in electrical outlets.
- Keep cords and electrical equipment out of reach.
- Remove electrical appliances from the bathroom. Examples include hair dryers, curling irons, make-up mirrors, and electric shavers.
- Store personal care items (shampoo, deodorant, lotion, and so on) in a safe place.
- Store household cleaners and medications in locked storage areas.
- Store dangerous equipment and tools in a safe place.
- Supervise the person who smokes.
- Store cigarettes, cigars, pipes, matches, and other smoking materials in a safe place.
- Practise safety measures to prevent falls, burns, choking, poisoning, and fires (see Chapter 16).
- Keep all doors to kitchens, utility rooms, and housekeeping closets locked.

Wandering
- Follow facility policy for locking doors and windows. In community settings, locks are often placed at the top and bottom of doors (Figure 34-3 on page 580). The person is not likely to look for a lock in such places.
- Keep door alarms and electronic doors turned on. The alarm goes off when the door is opened.
- Follow facility policy for fire exits. Everyone must be able to leave the building if a fire occurs.
- Make sure the person wears a facility ID bracelet or Alzheimer's Wandering Registry ID at all times.
- Exercise the person as ordered. Adequate exercise often reduces wandering.
- Involve the person in activities—folding napkins, dusting a table, sorting socks, rolling yarn, sweeping, sanding blocks of wood, or watering plants.
- Do not use restraints. Restraints require a physician's order. They tend to increase confusion and disorientation.
- Do not argue with the person who wants to leave. The person does not understand what you are saying.
- Go with the person who insists on going outside. Make sure he or she is properly dressed. Guide the person inside after a few minutes (Figure 34-4 on page 580).
- Let the person wander in enclosed areas. Many long-term care facilities have enclosed areas where clients can walk about. They provide a safe place for the person to wander.

Continued

Box 34-5 Guidelines for Caring for Clients with Dementia—cont'd

SUNDOWNING (SEE PAGE 582)
- Complete treatments and activities early in the day.
- Provide a calm, quiet setting late in the day.
- Play soft music.
- Do not restrain the person.
- Encourage exercise and activity early in the day.
- Meet nutrition needs. Hunger can increase restlessness.
- Promote elimination. The need to eliminate can increase restlessness.
- Do not try to reason with the person. Communication is impaired. He or she cannot think or speak clearly.

HALLUCINATIONS AND DELUSIONS
- Make sure the person wears eyeglasses or hearing aids as needed. Follow the care plan.
- Do not argue with the person.
- Reassure the person. Tell the person that you will protect him or her from harm.
- Distract the person with some item or activity. Taking the person for a walk may be helpful.
- Use touch to calm and reassure the person (Figure 34-5 on page 580).
- Eliminate noises that the person could misinterpret. TV, radio, stereos, furnaces, air conditioners, appliances, and other things could upset the person.
- Check lighting. Make sure there are no glares, shadows, or reflections.
- Cover or remove mirrors. The person could misinterpret his or her reflection.

SLEEP
- Follow bedtime rituals.
- Use night-lights so the person can see. They help prevent accidents and disorientation.
- Limit caffeine during the day.
- Discourage naps during the day.
- Encourage exercise during the day.
- Reduce noises.

BASIC NEEDS
- Meet food and fluid needs (see Chapter 25). Provide finger foods. Cut food and pour liquids as needed.
- Provide good skin care (see Chapters 27 and 41). Keep skin free of urine and stool.
- Promote urinary and bowel elimination (see Chapters 29 and 30).
- Provide incontinence care as needed (see Chapters 29 and 30).
- Promote exercise and activity during the day (see Chapter 22). This helps reduce wandering and sundowning behaviours. The person may also sleep better.
- Reduce intake of coffee, tea, and cola drinks. These contain caffeine. Caffeine is a stimulant. It can increase restlessness, confusion, and agitation.
- Provide a quiet, restful setting (see Chapter 20). Soft music is better than loud TV programs.
- Play soft music during care activities such as bathing and during meals.
- Promote personal hygiene (see Chapter 27). Do not force the person into a shower or tub. People with dementia are often afraid of bathing. Try bathing the person when he or she is calm. Use the person's preferred bathing method—tub bath, shower, bed bath, towel bath. Follow the care plan. Provide privacy and keep the person warm. Do not rush the person.
- Provide oral hygiene (see Chapter 27).
- Choose clothing that is comfortable and simple to put on. Front-opening garments are easy to put on. Pullover tops are harder to put on, and the person may become frightened when his or her head is inside the pullover top.
- Clothing that closes with Velcro is easy to put on and take off. Buttons, zippers, snaps, and other closures can frustrate the person.
- Offer simple clothing choices. Let the person choose between two shirts or blouses, two pants or slacks, and so on.
- Lay out clothing in the order it will be put on. Hand the person one clothing item at a time. Tell or show the person what to do. Do not rush him or her.
- Have equipment ready for any procedure. This reduces the amount of time the person is involved in care measures.
- Observe for signs and symptoms of health problems (see Chapter 31).
- Prevent infection. Assist with hand washing when necessary (see Chapter 18).

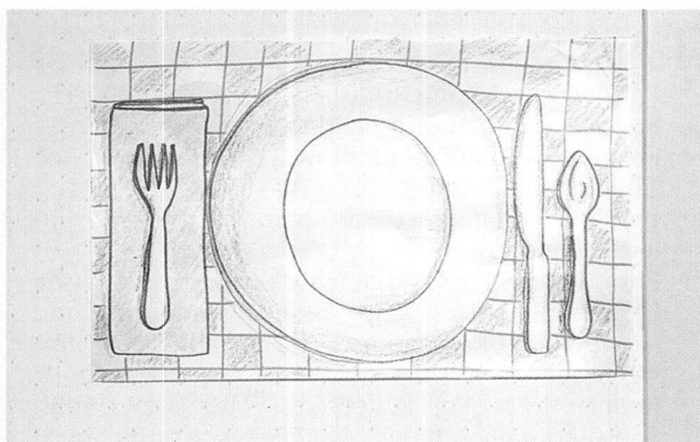

Figure 34-2 Signs provide cues to clients with dementia.

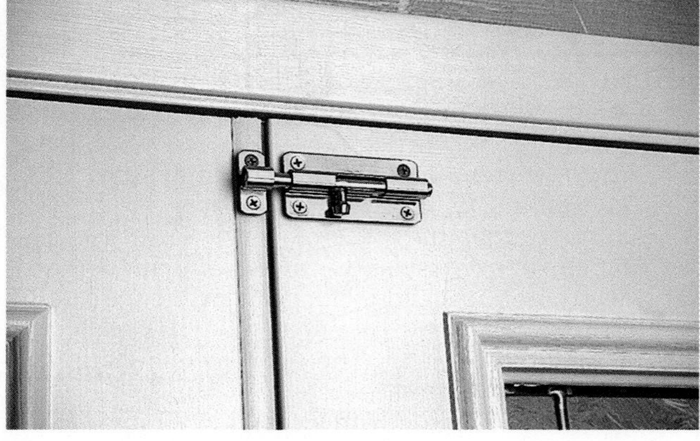

Figure 34-3 A slide lock is placed at the top of the door.

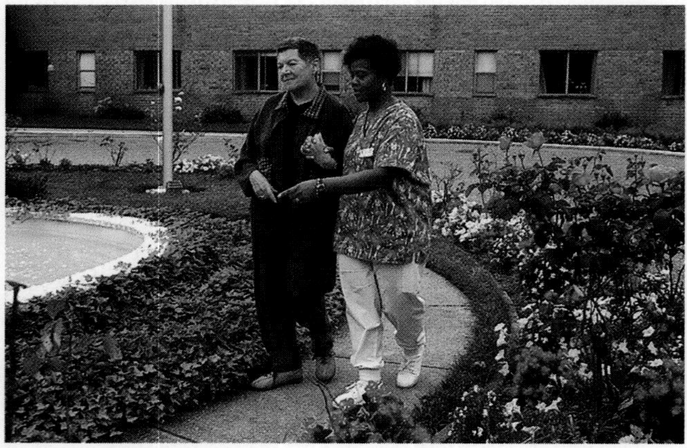

Figure 34-4 Walk outside with the client who wanders. Then guide the person back inside after a few minutes.

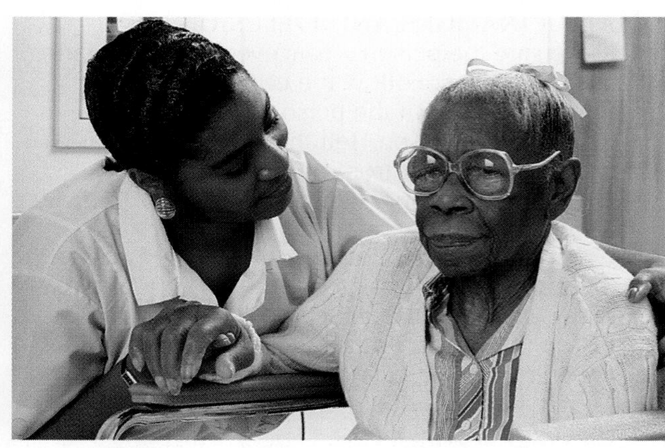

Figure 34-5 Use touch to calm the client with dementia.

People with dementia need to feel useful and to be active. Feeling useful and being active promote emotional and physical health. Adult day programs provide therapy and activities. Music programs, art programs, fitness programs, and support groups provide activity and therapy. Clients are encouraged to do what they can do and enjoy. For example, a man who was a good dancer takes part in dancing activities. A woman who likes to draw joins a painting group. The social contact may be as important as the activity itself.

In adult community settings, you often work with clients with early stage dementia. Many of these clients have some care requirements but are able to make some decisions for themselves. Your support enables these clients to remain in their homes.

These clients often need help getting organized, solving simple problems, and remembering appointments, occasions, and medications. They need support and supervision. For example, a client wants to bake cookies. You make sure that the setting is safe for the activity and that the oven is turned off when the client is finished.

You may need to help a client start an activity or task. Once the person starts, he or she may need only support and encouragement. Some people with dementia have problems completing tasks. Follow the care plan. It may specify to focus on the client's enjoyment rather than on achievement.

People with dementia need frequent cues, reminders, and restatements of facts and conversations. For example, a client wants to mail a letter but cannot remember the word for stamps or where they are kept. You help her to remember the word for stamps and then help her to find them.

Safety is a concern. A person may wander away, swallow a poisonous substance, or leave an appliance on. Provide a safe setting and supervise the client at all times. Follow the care plan. (See *Providing Compassionate Care: The Client with Dementia* box.)

Clients with Middle to Late Stage Dementia

As dementia progresses, the need for assistance increases. Usually there comes a time when family and

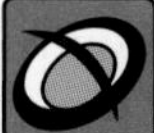

Providing Compassionate Care

The Client with Dementia

Dignity. People with dementia do not choose to be forgetful, incontinent, agitated, angry, or rude. Nor do they choose to have other behaviours, signs, and symptoms of the disease. They cannot control what is happening to them. The disease causes the behaviours. *The dementia is responsible, not the person.*

Treat all clients with dementia with dignity and respect. They have rights under human rights codes and long-term care legislation. In the advanced stages of dementia, they may not know or be able to exercise their rights. However, they are still entitled to their rights. Be patient and calm when caring for clients with dementia. Do not assume the client cannot understand you. Always explain what you are going to do.

Be careful never to make the client feel foolish about forgetting or misplacing something. Even in the later stages of dementia, people can still feel embarrassment and shame. Protect the client's dignity during care. Only those involved in the client's care should be present for care and procedures.

Independence. The client has the right to autonomy. Clients with dementia should be encouraged to be independent for as long as safely possible. Encourage clients to do what they can for themselves.

Preferences. Personal choice is important. People with early stage dementia can voice their preferences. Encourage clients with moderate stage dementia to make simple choices. For example, offer the client the choice of two sweaters. Watching or not watching TV may be a simple choice. The family or substitute decision-maker usually makes choices if the client cannot. They choose bath times, menus, clothing, activities, and other care.

A client may choose to use a special pillow or blanket. He or she may insist on wearing a particular sweater or cardigan. The item may have meaning. It may provide comfort and security. Eventually, the client may not know why the item is important or may not even recognize it. Do not remove the item. It is still important to the person.

With Alzheimer's disease and most other dementias, people continue to experience all forms of emotions well into the final stages. When a client can no longer use language, his or her emotional state can help you determine wishes, preferences, fears, likes, and dislikes.

Privacy. The client has the right to privacy and confidentiality. Provide space and privacy for the client to visit with others. Protect confidentiality. Do not share information about the client with others. Do not relate stories about the client's behaviour with others.

Safety. A safe, quiet, and calm setting promotes quality of life. Follow the safety measures in Chapter 16 and in Box 34-5 on page 578.

All people have the right to be free from restraints. Restraints require a physician's order. They are used only if it is the best way to protect the client. They are not used for the convenience of the health care team. Restraints can make confused and agitated behaviours worse. Your supervisor tells you when to use restraints.

The client must be kept free from abuse and neglect. Caring for people with dementia is often very frustrating. Some behaviours are hard to deal with. Family caregivers and health care providers can become short-tempered and angry. Protect clients with dementia from abuse. Report any signs of abuse to your supervisor at once. If you are becoming frustrated with a client, talk to your supervisor. An assignment change may be needed.

---

friends can no longer deal with the situation or meet the person's needs. Adult daycare, respite care, home care, and help from family members, friends, and volunteers are no longer enough. Long-term care is needed when at least one of the following occurs:

- Family members and friends cannot meet the person's needs
- Family members have health problems
- The person's behaviours present a danger to self or others
- The person no longer knows the caregiver

Many long-term care facilities have special care units for people with dementia. The health care team makes sure that their needs are met. Many facilities provide hospice care for people in the final stages of dementia.

When a person with dementia moves to a facility, the family or close friends usually continue to be involved in the person's care. They are an important part of the health care team. They help plan the person's care whenever possible. Some take part in facility activities. For many people with dementia, family members and close friends provide comfort and support.

Challenging Behaviours

People with dementia often display challenging behaviours. These are behaviours that may challenge the abilities of the caregivers to provide compassionate care. It is very important to know that challenging behaviours are a result of the dementia. The client is not to blame. Do not take the client's behaviours personally. Do not become upset or angry with the client. Also do not blame yourself for the client's behaviour.

Challenging behaviours can sometimes be in response to illness, infection, or physical discomfort. Report unusual or increased instances of challenging behaviours. Your supervisor and the family will try to determine the causes of the person's behaviour.

The following behaviours are common for people with dementia:

Wandering. People with dementia are not oriented to person, time, and place. They may wander away and not find their way back. Wandering may be by foot, car, bicycle, or other means. They may be with you one moment and gone the next.

Judgment is poor. They cannot tell what is safe or dangerous. Life-threatening accidents are great risks. They can walk into traffic or into a nearby lake, river, or forest. If not properly dressed, they are at risk for heat or cold exposure.

Wandering may have no cause. Or the client may be looking for something or someone—the bathroom, the bedroom, a child, a partner. Pain, side effects of medications, stress, restlessness, and anxiety are possible causes.

For people living at home or in facilities, the Alzheimer's Society of Canada provides the Alzheimer's Wandering Registry. The registry is nationwide. It serves to identify and safely return people who wander or become lost. A small fee is charged. A family member completes a form and provides a picture. These are entered into a national database. The person receives an ID card and bracelet. Anyone finding a person calls the police, who then call the family member or caregiver.

Sundowning. **Sundowning** is when signs, symptoms, and behaviours of dementia increase during hours of darkness. It occurs in the late afternoon and evening hours. As daylight ends and darkness starts, confusion and restlessness increase. So do anxiety, agitation, and other symptoms. Behaviour is worse after the sun goes down. It may continue throughout the night.

Sundowning may relate to being tired or hungry. Poor light and shadows may cause the person to see things that are not there. The person may be afraid of the dark.

Hallucinations. A **hallucination** is seeing, hearing, or feeling something that is not real. Senses are dulled. Affected people see animals, insects, or people who are not present. Some hear voices. They may feel bugs crawling or feel that they are being touched.

Sometimes the problem is made worse by impaired vision or hearing. The client needs to wear eyeglasses and hearing aids as prescribed.

Delusions. **Delusions** are false beliefs. People with dementia may believe a doll is a baby or that their spouse has been unfaithful. Some believe they are in jail, are being killed, or are being attacked. A person may believe that the caregiver is someone else. Many other false beliefs can occur. These can cause intense fear or other emotions in the person.

Catastrophic Reactions. These are extreme responses. The person reacts as if there is extreme danger, a disaster, or tragedy. The person may scream, cry, or be agitated or combative. These reactions are common from too much stimulation. Eating, hearing radio or TV noises, and being asked questions all at once can overwhelm the person.

Sometimes people have extreme reactions whenever anything out of the ordinary or unexpected happens. For example, a person may be afraid that a flickering light is a fire. He or she may scream or run away. The person may even be frightened if someone approaches too quickly or stands too close to him or her.

Agitation and Restlessness. The person may fidget, pace, hit, or yell. He or she may resist care. Common causes are pain or discomfort, anxiety, lack of sleep, and too much or too little stimulation. Hunger, thirst, and the need to eliminate may also be causes. A calm, quiet setting helps calm the person. So does meeting basic needs.

Do not overstimulate the client. Use a calm, gentle voice when talking to him or her. Do not overwhelm the client with instructions or choices. Do not rush the person or be impatient.

Aggression and Combativeness. These behaviours include hitting, pinching, grabbing, biting, or swearing. They may result from agitation and restlessness. They frighten others.

Sometimes these behaviours may be caused by pain, fatigue, too much stimulation, caregiver stress, and feeling lost or abandoned. The behaviours can occur during care measures (bathing, dressing) that upset or frighten the client. See Chapter 12 for dealing with the angry client. See Chapter 19 for workplace violence. Also follow the client's care plan.

Screaming. People with dementia have communication problems. At first, it is hard to find the right word. As dementia progresses, the person speaks in short sentences or in words. Often speech is not understandable.

Sometimes people in later stages of dementia may scream to communicate. This is common in people who are very confused and have poor communication skills. The person may scream a word or a name. Or the person just makes screaming sounds.

Possible reasons for screaming include hearing and vision problems, pain or discomfort, fear, and fatigue. Too much or not enough stimulation is another reason. A client may react to a caregiver or family member by screaming.

Sometimes these measures are helpful:

- Providing a calm, quiet setting
- Playing soft music
- Having the client wear hearing aids and eyeglasses
- Having a family member or favourite caregiver comfort and calm the client
- Using touch to calm the client

Abnormal Sexual Behaviours. Sexual behaviours are labelled abnormal because of how and when they occur. People with dementia are not oriented to person, place, or time. Sexual behaviours may involve the wrong person, the wrong place, and the wrong time. Sometimes people with dementia cannot control behaviour. Healthy people do not undress or expose themselves in front of others. They do not masturbate or engage in sexual pleasures in public. They know their sexual partners. People with dementia often mistake someone else for a sexual partner. The person kisses, hugs, or touches the other person.

Health care professionals encourage the client's sexual partner to show affection. Their normal practices are encouraged. Examples include hand holding, hugging, kissing, and touching. When a client masturbates in public, lead the client to his or her room. Provide for privacy and safety.

Sometimes behaviours are not sexual. Touching, scratching, and rubbing the genitals can signal infection, pain, or discomfort in the urinary or reproductive systems. Report when a client repeatedly touches his or her genitals. A health care professional may assess the client for health problems. Poor hygiene also may be the cause. The client may be wet or soiled from urine or stool. Clean the client quickly and thoroughly after elimination. Do not let the client stay wet or soiled.

Repetitive Behaviours. Repetitive means to repeat over and over again. People with dementia sometimes repeat the same motions over and over. For example, the person folds a napkin over and over. Or the person says the same words over and over. Or the same question is asked. Such behaviours do not hurt the client. However, they can annoy the caregivers and the family.

Harmless acts should be permitted. Music, picture books, exercise, and movies are distracting. Taking the client for a walk can help.

Meeting Basic Needs

Over time, people with dementia depend on others for all care. Safety, hygiene, grooming, dressing, and elimination needs must be met. So must nutrition and fluids, exercise, health, comfort and therapy needs. Follow the care plan (see Box 34-5 on page 578).

Safety. Clients need a safe, quiet setting. They do not recognize safety hazards and are at risk for falls. If a person with dementia falls, he or she may not understand why it is unsafe to move after the fall. You may need to let the client move about. Talk to the person in a quiet and soothing voice until someone can assist you. Never use force or hold a person down.

Clients may feel fearful even in a safe, quiet setting. They do not know what is happening. Always calmly explain what you are going to do. Be prepared to repeat information. People with dementia do not remember new information.

Hygiene, Grooming, and Dressing. People with moderate and severe dementia do not understand the need for personal hygiene and aseptic practices. They rely on the health care team to prevent the spread of infection. You assist them with hand washing:

- After urinating or having a bowel movement
- After coughing, sneezing, or blowing the nose
- Before or after handling or eating food
- Any time their hands are soiled

Good skin care is very important for people with dementia. It can help prevent skin breakdown. Skin care and other personal care threaten people with moderate and severe dementia. They may resist efforts to keep them clean and dry. They do not understand what is happening or why. They may fear harm or danger when you get too close or touch them. Therefore, they may resist care and become agitated and combative. They may shout and cry out for help. Some clients may pull away during care. Some may hit or kick. Sudden movements can cause skin tears.

If a client resists care, ask your supervisor for help. Never force care on a client. Consult with your supervisor and check the care plan before you see the client. Find out the best way to work with the person. Some measures include:

- Not rushing the person
- Using a calm, pleasant voice
- Not startling the person with sudden movements
- Giving short, simple instructions
- Diverting the person's attention
- Praising the person's attempts to cooperate or perform self-care
- Calming the person and trying again later, if necessary

During personal care, look for signs or symptoms that may cause pain (for example, skin lesions, rough pieces of clothing, or dental problems).

Elimination Needs. People with moderate and severe dementia may urinate in the wrong places. Garbage cans, planters, and heating vents are examples. Some remove incontinence products and throw them on the floor or in the toilet. Some may smear stool on themselves, furniture, and walls. Offer to assist with elimination needs frequently. Provide perineal care after bowel and bladder elimination. Ask your supervisor for help if a client resists you. Never restrict fluid intake in an effort to control elimination.

Nutrition. People with dementia may become distracted during meals. It is hard for some people to sit long enough to eat a meal. Some people with later stage dementia forget how to use eating utensils. Finger foods can be offered to clients who can no longer use utensils. Some clients have problems swallowing (see Chapter 25). Some clients have to be fed. Some resist efforts to assist them with eating. A confused person may throw or spit food. A quiet and calm dining area is often helpful. So are special mealtimes. The client may eat small amounts more often than three times per day.

Fluids. People with moderate and severe dementia are at risk for dehydration. They do not recognize thirst. Encourage them to drink. Keep water and other fluids nearby. Offer fluids whenever you are nearby.

Exercise. Inactivity and immobility are risk factors for pneumonia and pressure ulcers. Exercise is important, but people with dementia may resist it. They do not understand what is happening. They may fear harm. They may become agitated and combative or cry out for help. Do not force a client to exercise or take part in activities. Stay calm. Ask your supervisor for help if needed. Follow the care plan.

Health Problems. Many people with dementia have other health problems or injuries. However, they may not notice or recognize pain, fever, constipation, incontinence, or other signs and symptoms. Changes in usual behaviour may signal pain or discomfort. A client who normally moans and groans may become quiet and withdrawn. A client who is friendly and outgoing may become agitated and aggressive. One who is nonverbal and quiet may become restless and cry easily. Loss of appetite may also signal pain. Report any changes in a client's usual behaviour to your supervisor.

Comfort. Comfort is important. Make sure that the client is physically comfortable. A quiet environment helps. Talk in a calm voice. Massage, soothing touch, music, and aromatherapy are comforting and relaxing. Clothing should be comfortable.

Therapy and Activities. People with dementia need to feel worthwhile. As long as they are able, they need to be active. Long-term care facilities have therapy and activities. Therapists work with one client, a small group, or a large group. Therapies and activities meet the client's needs and cognitive abilities.

Secured Units

Some long-term care residents try to wander throughout the facility. This may put them at risk for injury. Some try to leave the building. These residents may be moved to a secured unit. A secured unit is an area in the facility where entrances and exits are locked. They provide a safe setting for residents to move about in. Residents cannot wander away.

Secured units are a form of environmental restraint. The facility must use the least restrictive approach. A dementia diagnosis and a physician's order are needed to place a resident on a secured unit. The health care team regularly reviews the resident's need for a secured unit. The resident's rights must always be protected.

As the dementia progresses, a secured unit is no longer needed. After a resident's condition progresses to the advanced stage, the resident cannot sit or walk and is in bed. Wandering is not a concern. The resident is transferred to another unit.

Legislation has standards of care for special care units. Staff must have special training in the care of people with dementia. The unit must have programs that promote dignity, personal freedom, and safety.

Caregiver Needs

Being a primary caregiver to a person with dementia is stressful. There are physical, emotional, social, and financial stresses. Many adult children are in the *sandwich generation.* That is, their energies are divided between their children and their parents. Both need care and attention. Caring for two families is very stressful. Many adult children have jobs as well as caregiving responsibilities.

Caregivers can suffer from anger, anxiety, and sleeplessness. Some cannot concentrate or are irritable. Depression is also common. Abuse may occur in very stressful caregiving situations.

Because they are under stress, caregivers are vulnerable to health problems. They need to take care of their own health. A healthy diet, exercise, and plenty of rest are needed. Asking for help is important. The caregiver needs to feel free to ask family and friends for help.

Caregivers need much support and encouragement. Many join support groups sponsored by hospitals, long-term facilities, and the Alzheimer's Society of Canada. The Alzheimer's Society has chapters in cities and towns across the country. Support groups offer encouragement and advice. People in similar situations share their feelings, anger, frustration, guilt, and other emotions. They also share coping and caregiving ideas.

Caregivers, family members, and friends of a person with dementia often feel helpless. No matter what is done, the person only gets worse. Much time, money, energy, and emotion are needed to care for the person. Guilty feelings are common. Family and friends know that the person does not choose to have dementia. They know that the person does not choose to have its signs, symptoms, and behaviours. Nevertheless, sometimes behaviours are frustrating, embarrassing, or threatening. Family and friends may be upset and angry that their loved one cannot show love or affection.

You play a significant role in caregiver relief. You may assist the primary caregiver or other caregivers. Or you may care for the client while the caregiver is not at home. Follow the care plan and perform your tasks competently. The caregiver should have confidence in your skill and ability so that she or he is able to relax and let go of control for a time. The care plan may ask you to encourage the caregiver to take care of his or her own needs and to leave the home for a break while you are present. You may observe signs and symptoms of caregiver stress. You may also observe signs and symptoms of depression and abuse. Report these observations immediately to your supervisor (see *Support Workers Solving Problems: Supporting Caregivers of Clients with Dementia* box).

Support Workers Solving Problems

Supporting Caregivers of Clients with Dementia

Scenario: Mrs. Munroe, 70, has AD. She has stage 2 (moderate) dementia. She lives at home with her husband, who is her primary caregiver. Leila is assigned to provide morning respite care. This is her fourth visit. Mrs. Munroe is incontinent and needs help with feeding, bathing, and dressing. She is frequently rude and aggressive. She becomes angry if someone stands too near her or tries to make her do something. Quick, sudden movements and loud noises also upset her. The care plan calls for Mr. Munroe to take a break—preferably away from the house—while Leila takes care of Mrs. Munroe's needs. Mr. Munroe is reluctant to leave. He is anxious about his wife.

Discussion: Leila's visit is for 3 hours. She knows that Mr. Munroe will not leave until he is satisfied that his wife is in competent hands. Leila starts her visit by sitting down with Mrs. Munroe at the kitchen table and talking quietly and gently. She explains that she is going to make breakfast and gives Mrs. Munroe two food choices. Leila makes breakfast, while she continues talking with Mrs. Munroe in a quiet, reassuring tone. Mr. Munroe watches anxiously from the living room. When Mrs. Munroe is settled, Leila suggests to Mr. Munroe that he go out for a coffee. He reluctantly agrees to go. When he comes back 1 hour later, Mrs. Munroe has been bathed and dressed. She is sitting quietly watching TV. Mr. Munroe feels better for having had a break. He feels confident in Leila's ability to care for his wife.

REVIEW

Circle the BEST answer.

1. Cognitive relates to the following *except*
   A. Thinking and reasoning
   B. Memory loss and personality
   C. Ability to understand
   D. Judgment and behaviour

2. A person is confused after moving to a long-term care facility. The confusion is likely to be
   A. Permanent
   B. Due to emotional stress caused by the move
   C. Due to an infection
   D. Due to brain injury

3. The following statements are about delirium. Which is *false*?
   A. It is a temporary state of confusion.
   B. It is often a reaction to medications or infection.
   C. It should be ignored so as not to embarrass the client.
   D. It is an emergency.

4. The following statements are about dementia. Which is *false*?
   A. It is a normal part of aging.
   B. It can affect people in their 40s.
   C. It is more common in people over 65 years of age.
   D. It causes loss of memory and reasoning.

5. The following statements are about AD. Which is *true*?
   A. It occurs only in older people.
   B. Diet and medications can cure the disease.
   C. AD and confusion are the same.
   D. It is the most common form of dementia.

6. Which is *not* a common sign or symptom of dementia?
   A. Memory loss, poor judgment, and behaviour changes
   B. Loss of language skills
   C. Wandering, delusions, and hallucinations
   D. Paralysis, dyspnea, and pain

7. People with early stage dementia
   A. Usually remain in their homes with support
   B. Are totally dependent on others for care
   C. Are confined to bed
   D. Are usually placed in secured units

8. Support groups do the following *except*
   A. Provide care
   B. Offer encouragement and care ideas
   C. Provide support for the family
   D. Promote the sharing of feelings and frustrations

9. Mr. Dunn has moderate dementia. He tends to wander. You should do the following *except*
   A. Make sure door alarms are turned on
   B. Make sure he wears an ID bracelet
   C. Help him with exercise as ordered
   D. Tell him what areas are safe for wandering

10. Sundowning means that
    A. The person becomes sleepy when the sun sets
    B. Behaviours become worse in the late afternoon and evening hours
    C. Behaviour improves at night
    D. The person is in the third stage of dementia

11. Safety is important for Mr. Dunn. Which is *false*?
    A. Safety plugs are placed in electrical outlets.
    B. Cleaners and medications are kept locked up.
    C. He can keep smoking materials.
    D. Sharp and breakable objects are removed from his environment.

12. You are caring for Mr. Dunn in a facility. Which is *false*?
    A. He no longer has rights.
    B. Touch can calm and reassure him.
    C. A calm, quiet setting is important.
    D. Help is needed with activities of daily living.

13. Your role with the primary caregiver does *not* include
    A. Providing support and relief
    B. Reporting signs of caregiver stress
    C. Offering advice
    D. Reporting suspicions of abuse

Answers to these questions are on page 826.

CHAPTER 35

SPEECH AND LANGUAGE DISORDERS

OBJECTIVES

- Define the key terms listed in this chapter
- Describe three types of aphasia
- Describe apraxia of speech
- Describe dysarthria
- Explain how speech and language disorders are treated
- Explain what communication aids are
- Describe the emotional effects of a language disorder
- Describe how to communicate with clients with language disorders

KEY TERMS

aphasia Partial or complete loss (*a*) of speech and language skills (*phasia*), caused by brain injury

apraxia of speech Inability (*a*) to move *(praxia)* the muscles used to speak, caused by brain injury

dysarthria Difficulty (*dys*) speaking clearly (*arthria*), caused by weakness or paralysis in the muscles used for speech

expressive aphasia Difficulty speaking or writing

expressive-receptive aphasia Difficulty speaking and understanding language

receptive aphasia Difficulty understanding language

People with speech and language disorders have problems communicating—speaking, understanding, reading, and writing. Speech and language disorders can occur at any age. There are many causes, including:

- Genetic problems or conditions present at birth
- Brain injury (may be caused by accident, infection, drug abuse, stroke, and so on)
- Disease
- Hearing loss
- Brain tumours
- Problems involving the structures used for speech

To effectively communicate with clients with speech and language disorders, use the communication methods described in Chapter 12. Also follow the measures described in this chapter.

APHASIA

Aphasia is the partial or complete loss (*a*) of speech and language skills (*phasia*) caused by brain injury. Stroke is the most common cause of aphasia. Traumas and brain tumours are other causes. Most people with dementia have aphasia (see Chapter 34). Some people with aphasia regain some or all of their language skills. In others, aphasia is permanent.

For communication to occur, a message must be sent, received, and interpreted. Some people with aphasia cannot send messages. Others cannot understand the message received. Some people can neither send nor receive messages.

There are three basic types of aphasia:

- *Receptive aphasia*—difficulty understanding language. This includes spoken and written words. People with receptive aphasia have difficulty understanding what is said or read. They cannot understand their own words. Therefore, their own speech is muddled. They may make up words or use the wrong words. For example, they may use the word "orange" when they mean "apple." They also mix up sounds within words. A person trying to say "hospital" may actually say "posital." A person trying to ask "please give me a glass of water" may actually say "ples put dat cat over tad counter." They may not be aware of their mistakes.
- *Expressive aphasia*—difficulty speaking and writing. People with expressive aphasia can understand spoken and written words. But their speech is jumbled or slurred, and difficult to understand. They think one thing but say another. For example, a person may think about food but ask for a newspaper. People with expressive aphasia cannot think of the right words or put sounds together to form words and sentences. They may leave out connecting words. For example, instead of saying "I want to go to the bathroom," a person may say "me ... uh ... room ... uh ... bathroom." Some people can only produce sounds. People with expressive aphasia are very aware of their mistakes because they can understand what they are saying. They may cry or swear for no apparent reason.
- *Expressive-receptive aphasia*—difficulty speaking and understanding language. Some people with expressive-receptive aphasia can only say "yes," "no," and make sounds such as "da da." Others have lost all speech and language skills

APRAXIA OF SPEECH

Apraxia of speech (*verbal apraxia*) is the inability (*a*) to move (*praxia*) the muscles used to speak. People with this disorder cannot control lip, jaw, or tongue movements. As a result, they cannot say the desired sounds and words. Apraxia of speech is caused by brain injury resulting from stroke, accidents, brain tumour, or infection. Some children are born with this disorder. Apraxia of speech can occur alone or with aphasia.

People with apraxia of speech are difficult to understand. Their speech is usually slow. They may use a word that sounds like the word they are trying to say. For example, a person may say "me" instead of "see." The order of sounds within words is mixed up. For example, a person may say "thootshub" instead of "toothbrush." Some people have problems putting words in the right order or finding the right words. Inconsistent speech is common. A person may say something correctly one time and incorrectly another time.

Dysarthria

Dysarthria is difficulty (*dys*) speaking clearly (*arthria*). It is caused by weakness or paralysis in the muscles used for speech. Cerebral palsy, multiple sclerosis, head injury, tumour, and infection are common causes.

People with dysarthria usually have slurred, slow, and soft speech. They speak in flat, harsh, or nasal tones. They often have problems forming words, spacing their words, and breathing while speaking. Speech errors are usually consistent and predictable. You may therefore become familiar with a client's speech.

Emotional Effects of Speech and Language Disorders

Imagine what it would be like to have a speech and language disorder. How would you feel if you could not express your thoughts and feelings? How would you feel if you could not understand what others are saying? Box 35-1 contains some comments from people who have had aphasia.

People with speech and language disorders experience many emotions. Frustration, depression, and anger are common. So are low-self esteem, shame, and guilt. Communication is important for functioning and for maintaining relationships with others. Being unable to communicate may cause the person to avoid social situations. Family and friends may avoid the person.

Speech and language disorders can be very stressful for families. Relations between all family members are affected. Sharing thoughts and feelings is often very difficult. Even everyday conversations take great effort. Financial stresses may occur. The person with a speech and language disorder may not be able to work. Routine tasks like shopping, cooking, paying bills, and doing household repairs may be impossible for the person.

Emotional reactions vary from person to person and from family to family. Observe and listen to your clients and their families. Put yourself in their place. How would you feel and want to be treated? Accept and understand displays of emotion.

Box 35-1 Comments of People Who Have Had Aphasia

"I wanted to speak, but no sounds came out of my mouth."

"I felt ... imprisoned in a tomb."

"I noticed a change in me. I was another person, someone who was unable to express the little I knew. I was ashamed."

"If you don't know words, you keep quiet ... When it's noisy, you can't talk ... People talk for us ... Anyway, when we talk, it's not the way it used to be ... you keep quiet."

"Once I had to answer the intercom. I said 'Hello? 'I heard the person speaking on the other end, but I couldn't understand him. So, to prove that it wasn't me who had the problem, I repeated 'Hello! Hello! Hello!' as if to signal the line was bad. That's how I got out of that situation."

"I feel useless ... slightly distanced from the family because I can only understand things after some time. My world has shrunk."

"I want to say something ... just before I start saying it she helps. Sometimes if she would stay back and let me finish, I would be all right."

Source: Y. Joanette, D. Lafond, and A.R. Lecours, "The Person with Aphasia," in *Living with Aphasia: Psychosocial Issues*, D. Lafond, et al., eds. (San Diego: Singular Publishing Group, 1993), pp. 19–36.

Treatment for Speech and Language Disorders

A speech therapist (also called a speech-language pathologist) helps the person with the disorder learn to communicate. The speech therapist also helps family members learn new communication techniques. Methods used depend on the disorder, its cause, and severity. Practice and exercises may help the person relearn speech and language skills. For dysarthria, the person practises muscle-strengthening exercises and learns how to breathe while speaking.

People with speech and language disorders also learn how to improve existing skills. For example, a person learns to use body language and facial expressions. Some people learn new skills such as sign language.

Those with severe speech and language problems may never regain their speech or ability to understand language. Some may be helped by the following aids:

- *Communication boards.* These are boards with pictures or words that show functions or tasks (Figure 35-1). There are pictures or words for activities of daily living, such as sleep, food, drink, medicine, and glasses. The person points to the things he or she needs. The type of communication board depends on the person's needs. For those who can read, words rather than pictures are often used. For those with quadriplegia who cannot speak, eye-gaze boards are used. The person indicates his or her needs by gazing at the picture or word on the board and either blinking or using another signal.
- *Mechanical and electronic devices.* These range in complexity and cost. Some are large computers that cannot be moved. Others are hand-held devices such as electronic talking aids (Figure 35-2). The person touches a picture displayed on the screen. The message is then spoken aloud by the device. For example, the person touches a picture of a sad face. A recorded message says "I am sad." The message may also be printed on a screen. Some devices convert words into pictures.

Communicating with Clients

To effectively communicate with clients who have speech and language disorders, you must be aware of how you communicate. Do you speak clearly? Do you mumble? Do you use gestures when you speak? You may have to change how you speak. Follow the care plan and your supervisor's instructions. Use the communication methods that are best for your client.

The effort of understanding others and making oneself understood can be exhausting. People with speech and language disorders often tire easily. Their other health problems may also cause fatigue. Be alert to signs of fatigue. These may include drooping shoulders, irritability, lack of interest, and a decline in understanding.

Some clients with speech and language disorders seem withdrawn and uninterested. Spend extra time with these clients. Social interaction can promote self-esteem and recovery. Always include them in conversations even if they cannot understand you.

Clients with speech and language disorders should be treated with respect and empathy. Remember the five priorities of support work (see *Providing Compassionate Care: Communicating with Clients with Speech and Language Disorders* box). Follow the guidelines in Box 35-2.

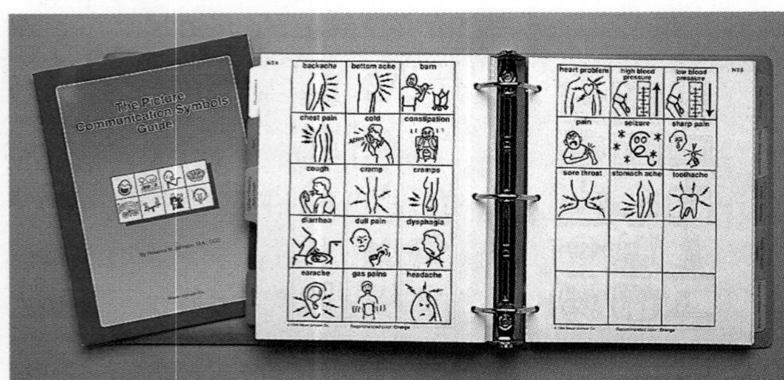

Figure 35-1 Communication board.

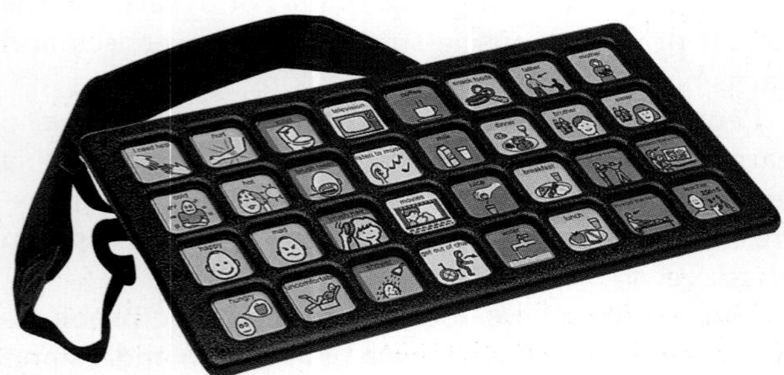

Figure 35-2 Electronic talking aid. *(Courtesy of Mayer-Johnson Co., Solana Beach, CA.)*

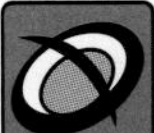

Providing **Compassionate Care**

Communicating with Clients with Speech and Language Disorders

D*ignity.* Showing respect, warmth, and compassion are important ways to promote dignity. Never talk about a client as if he or she were not present. Address questions and comments to the client, not to others who are present. Some people with language disorders are embarrassed to speak in front of others, especially strangers. Do not force a client to talk in front of others.

I*ndependence.* People with speech and language disorders must gain, regain, or maintain independence and control. Support, encouragement, and patience are important. Never show impatience, frustration, or worry when a client is having problems speaking or understanding. Do not talk down to the person. (The *Support Workers Solving Problems* box describes a support worker patiently using body language and symbols to learn a client's needs.) The care plan may list ways to encourage communication.

P*references.* Limit the number of choices to help the client express preferences. Be encouraging and supportive.

P*rivacy.* Keep information about your client confidential. Remember your role and relationship with the client at all times. Be professional in your communication. Learn to be comfortable with silence. Do not feel that you need to talk when the person is silent.

S*afety.* Take extra time to explain procedures. Do not explain all the steps at once. Explain the step just before you do it. Avoid medical terms. Speak clearly and slowly. Be alert to signs the client has not understood you.

Box 35-2 Guidelines for Communicating with Clients with Speech and Language Disorders

- **Minimize distractions**. Distractions make concentration difficult. They can also upset the person. Reduce background noise and activity. Close doors and windows. Turn off the television and radio (if the person agrees). Make sure there is nothing in your hands or on your lap.
- **Adjust the lighting**. Make sure the person can see your face clearly and that you can see the person's. Turn down lights and adjust window coverings to reduce glare. Do not position yourself between the person and a window. The person may not be able to see you in the glare.
- **Give the client your full attention.** Sit close by and face the person. Look the person in the eyes, so he or she looks directly at your face. Get the person's attention before you speak. Show that you are listening by using gestures and facial expressions. Do not do other tasks while you are talking to the person.
- **Ask the client questions to which you know the answer.** This helps you become familiar with his or her speech.
- **Determine the subject being discussed.** This helps you understand the main points. Look for nonverbal clues. Do the person's gestures, eyes, and body language tell you anything? Does the person use words or partial words that might describe an item or concept?
- **Follow the client's lead**. Change your communication method as needed. For example, Mrs. Schmidt becomes frustrated when you ask her questions. You learn that she responds better when you use gestures to act out your question. Or Mrs. Schmidt seems tired or has lost interest. Let her rest. Bring up the subject at a later time.
- **Speak slowly, clearly, and in a normal tone of voice**. Adjust your pace to suit the person's needs. Talk to adults in an adult, professional manner. Do not use slang or figures of speech. The person may not understand them.
- **Give the client time to respond.** Do not rush the person. Pause between sentences to allow the person time to think and repond. Do not answer questions addressed to the person. This includes your own questions and those asked by others.
- **Use simple words and short sentences**. Avoid long, complex sentences. Focus on key words—mostly action words and words for people, places, or things. For example, say "Let's go for lunch" instead of "It's time for me to transfer you to the dining room for lunch."
- **Be patient.** Repeat your words as needed. Rephrase your sentences if the person does not understand you.
- **Use positive statements**. These are easier to understand than negative statements. For example, say "Bend your arm" instead of "Don't straighten your arm."
- **Use appropriate questioning and paraphrasing techniques**. Ask questions that require only a short answer or a shake of the head. Paraphrase (summarize in your own words) what the person has said. Ask if you have understood correctly (see Chapter 12).
- **Provide cues as needed.** Help clients express themselves by giving them cues about a word they cannot recall. If it is an object, ask "What does it look like?" "What is it used for?" and "Where is it found?" Encourage the use of gestures and pointing. If you think you understand what the person says, test your assumption with gestures, pointing, or through the use of symbols. For example, Mrs. Lin points to her sweater. You get it for her and she puts it on. You have understood her need.
- **Try other communication methods.** Some people may write better than they speak. Follow the care plan. Use writing and communication boards as needed.

Support Workers Solving Problems

COMMUNICATING WITH A CLIENT WITH APHASIA

Scenario: Mr. Hamilton, 57, suffered a stroke several months ago. He has expressive aphasia. Marta is his support worker. Mr. Hamilton asks her a question she does not understand.

Mr. Hamilton: "Wuld ples git bassen eaten."
Marta: Could you please repeat that Mr. Hamilton?
Mr. Hamilton: (raises his voice) "Plasin get eatin puck."
Marta: "Would you like something to eat?"
Mr. Hamilton (looks puzzled and upset): "Dat stan woo."
Marta (pretends to eat): "Would you like a snack?"
Mr. Hamilton (shakes his head, but says nothing)
Marta (pretends to drink): "Something to drink?"
Mr. Hamilton (nods his head, and looks relieved)
Marta (gets a glass and cup)
Mr. Hamilton (gestures towards the cup)
Marta (gets a tea bag): "Would you like a cup of tea?
Mr. Hamilton (nods)

Discussion: Marta is not sure what Mr. Hamilton wants. The words "eaten" and "eatin" suggest that Mr. Hamilton wants something to eat. In fact, he is trying to say the word "tea." Marta does not know this, but she knows that Mr. Hamilton drinks tea. Using body language and symbols, Marta discovers what Mr. Hamilton wants. Her patience and persistence pay off. She is able to meet Mr. Hamilton's needs.

REVIEW

Circle the BEST answer.

1. People with receptive aphasia have problems with
   A. Speaking and writing
   B. Understanding language
   C. Moving the mouth, tongue, and lips
   D. Pronouncing vowels

2. People with expressive-receptive aphasia have problems with
   A. Speaking and understanding language
   B. Moving the mouth, tongue, and lips
   C. Speaking and writing
   D. Understanding language

3. Apraxia of speech is caused by
   A. Brain injury
   B. Weakness in the muscles used to speak
   C. Paralysis in the muscles used to speak
   D. Lack of coordination in the muscles used to speak

4. People with dysarthria
   A. Make unpredictable speech errors
   B. Understand what is said
   C. Can control the muscles used to speak
   D. Cannot read or write

5. People with speech and language disorders
   A. Have the same emotional reactions to their disorders
   B. Are not affected emotionally
   C. Often have problems relating to family and friends
   D. Cannot improve their communication

6. When communicating with clients who have speech and language disorders, you should *not*
   A. Speak slowly
   B. Use simple words and short sentences
   C. Leave them out of conversations
   D. Provide cues about words they cannot recall

7. You do not understand what a client has said. Do *not*
   A. Pretend that you have understood
   B. Ask the person to repeat what was said
   C. Use questioning techniques
   D. Use body language and symbols

Answers to these questions are on page 826.

CHAPTER

36

HEARING AND VISION PROBLEMS

OBJECTIVES

- Define the key terms listed in this chapter
- Describe the major ear disorders
- Describe the effects of hearing problems
- Describe aids for clients with hearing problems
- Explain how to care for clients with hearing loss
- Describe the major eye disorders
- Describe aids for clients with vision problems
- Explain how to care for clients with vision loss
- Learn the procedure described in this chapter

KEY TERMS

age-related macular degeneration (AMD; ARMD) The breakdown (degeneration) of the macula (the light-sensitive part of the retina)

Braille A writing system for the blind that uses raised dots for each letter of the alphabet

cataract A clouding of the eye's lens

diabetic retinopathy A disorder (*pathy*) caused by diabetes in which the blood vessels in the retina are damaged

dominant progressive hearing loss The impairment of nerves used to hear

glaucoma An eye disease that causes pressure within the eye and vision loss

Ménière's disease An increase of fluid in the inner ear causing pressure in the middle ear; vertigo, tinnitus, and hearing loss occur

otitis media Infection (*itis*) of the middle (*media*) ear (*ot*)

otosclerosis a condition (*osis*) in which there is hardening (*sclero*) of the ossicles in the middle ear (*oto*)

presbycusis The gradual hearing (*cusis*) loss associated with aging (*presby*)

presbyopia The gradual inability to focus (*opia*) on close objects; a condition associated with aging (*presby*)

retinal detachment The separation of the retina from its supporting tissue

tinnitus Ringing in the ear

vertigo Dizziness

The senses of sight and hearing are important for communicating, learning, moving about, and performing activities of daily living. They also help keep people safe by alerting them to danger.

Hearing and vision problems are common among all age groups. Common causes include conditions present at birth, diseases, and accidents. Some hearing and vision loss (and loss of other senses) is a natural part of aging.

You will care for many clients who have hearing and vision problems. Some people have minor problems that can be corrected with hearing aids and glasses. Others have severe losses (see *Providing Compassionate Care: Clients with Severe Hearing and Vision Loss* box).

EAR DISORDERS AND HEARING PROBLEMS

The ear is needed for hearing and balance. Hearing problems range from slight hearing impairments to complete deafness. Hearing problems may occur suddenly. However, usually they are gradual in onset. One or both ears are affected. Ear structures are shown in Figure 36-1. See page 137 for a review of the structure and function of the ear.

Common causes of hearing problems include:

- ***Otitis media***—infection (*itis*) of the middle (*media*) ear (*ot*). It is common in infants and children. The infection is acute or chronic. Chronic otitis media can damage the eardrum. It can also damage the bones of the middle ear that conduct sound to the inner ear (the *ossicles*). The eardrum and ossicles are needed for hearing. Permanent hearing loss can result from chronic otitis media.
- ***Otosclerosis***—a condition (*osis*) in which there is hardening (*sclero*) of the ossicles in the middle ear (*oto*). It is a hereditary condition that is a common cause of hearing loss in adults. The person has gradual and progressive hearing loss and **tinnitus** (ringing in the ear). Surgery can often restore some hearing.
- ***Ménière's disease***—an increase of fluid in the inner ear causing pressure in the middle ear. Usually only one ear is affected. **Vertigo** (dizziness), tinnitus, and hearing loss occur. If the person feels dizzy, he or she must lie down. Safety is important during vertigo. Severe dizziness can cause nausea and vomiting.
- ***Dominant progressive hearing loss***—the impairment of nerves used to hear. Hearing loss is progressive. Sometimes the disease starts in early childhood. However, it usually starts in early or middle adulthood.
- ***Presbycusis***—the gradual hearing (*cusis*) loss associated with aging (*presby*). It usually occurs after age 50. There is no cure. However, hearing aids and speech reading are helpful for those affected.
- *Temporary hearing loss*—The blockage of the ear canal with earwax. This is common in older adults. Hearing improves when the earwax is removed. A physician or nurse removes the wax.

(text continues on page 596)

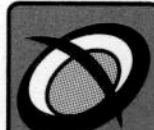

Providing Compassionate Care

Clients with Severe Hearing and Vision Loss

D*ignity.* Clients with hearing and vision loss need your patience and respect, not pity. Speak clearly in a normal tone of voice. Do not shout. Do not mumble or use slang terms. Do not talk to the client as you would to a child. Include him or her in conversations with others. Never ask another person (such as a family member) to speak for the client. When speaking of a client, always state the person's name before the disability. For example, Mrs. Kabir has hearing loss. She is not "the deaf client." If a client uses sign language and has an interpreter, speak to the client, not the interpreter.

I*ndependence.* Remember, people who are impaired in one area are not impaired in all areas. Do not make assumptions about their abilities or limitations. Clients with hearing and vision loss should do as much for themselves as possible. Tell the person what you are doing step by step. Indicate when the procedure is over. Many clients use self-care (assistive) devices to maintain independence. Make sure they have access to these needed devices.

P*references.* Follow your clients' choices and directions. Ask how you can help. Assist only if the client wants you to do so.

P*rivacy.* Respect your client's privacy. Always let the client know when you are in the room. If the person cannot hear you knock, make sure the person sees you enter the room. If the person cannot see you, clearly announce your arrival. Also tell the person if others join you in the room. Remember your role and relationship with your clients at all times. Keep information about clients confidential. Communicate in a professional manner.

S*afety.* A safe setting is critical. People with hearing loss cannot hear sounds that signal danger. People with vision loss cannot see obstacles in their path. They are at great risk for falls. Follow the safety measures in Chapter 16. Follow the care plan for safety measures specific for each client. In facilities, keep the call bell within easy reach.

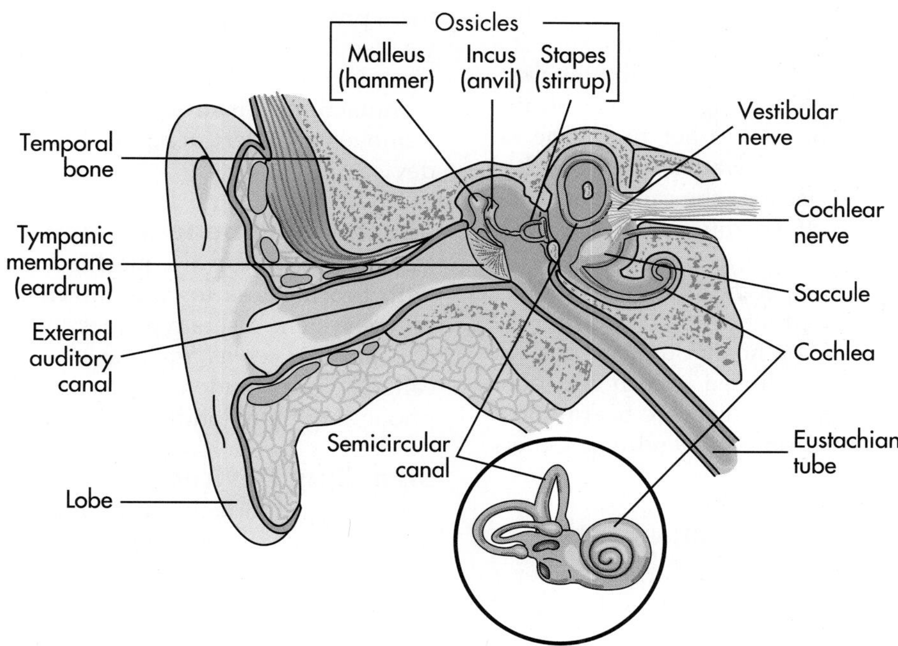

Figure 36-1 The ear.

The Effects of Hearing Problems

Signs and symptoms of hearing problems vary. They are not always obvious. A person's behaviour or attitude may change because of hearing problems. For example, a person may not respond when others talk or ask questions. He or she may become angry that others are not speaking loudly enough. Family and friends may not be aware of the hearing problems. They may become frustrated when communicating with the person. They may avoid talking with the person.

Some people deny that they have hearing problems. They may not want to believe they are different from others. Or they do not want to admit to a sign of aging. Some people refuse to get or use a hearing aid.

The obvious signs of hearing problems in adults and children include:

- Speaking too loudly
- Leaning forward to hear
- Turning and cupping the unaffected ear toward the speaker
- Responding inappropriately
- Asking for words to be repeated

Hearing problems can affect all aspects of a person's health—physical, emotional, social, intellectual, and spiritual. For example, Mrs. Lopez has hearing loss. She avoids social situations because she feels left out of conversations. She is afraid of embarrassing herself by giving the wrong response. Straining to hear a conversation makes her tired. She no longer listens to the radio or watches TV. She has stopped going to church because she cannot hear the sermon. She is by herself so much that she feels lonely and bored.

Hearing loss may cause speech problems. You hear yourself as you talk. Your pronunciation and the volume of your voice depend on how you hear yourself. Hearing loss may result in slurred speech and poor pronunciation. Some people with severe hearing loss speak in a flat tone and drop word endings. Others cannot speak at all.

Aids for People with Hearing Loss

A number of aids help people with hearing problems to communicate. These include hearing aids, special telephone systems, and signalling devices.

Hearing Aids. A *hearing aid* is a device that fits in the ear and makes sounds louder (Figure 36-2). It does not cure the hearing problem. However, it improves a person's hearing. Both background noise and speech are louder. Minimize background noise to help your client adjust to the hearing aid. Remember that the hearing aid makes speech louder—not clearer.

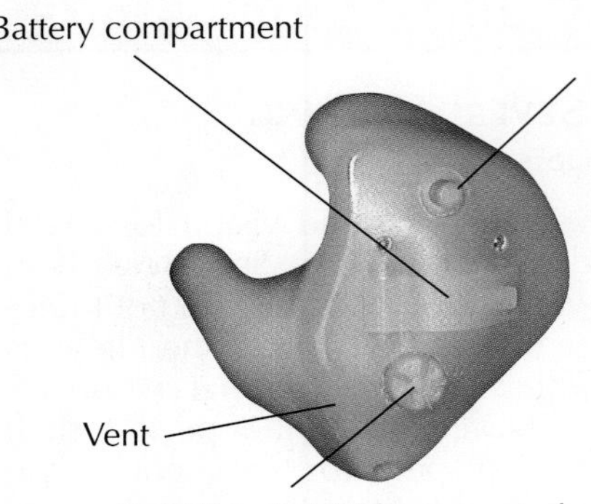

Figure 36-2 A hearing aid. *(Courtesy of Siemen Hearing Instruments Inc., Piscataway, NJ.)*

Hearing aids operate on batteries. There is an on and off switch. Sometimes hearing aids do not work properly. Often simple measures will get them to work:

- Check if the hearing aid is on.
- Check the battery position.
- Insert a new battery if needed.
- Clean the ear mould if necessary.

Hearing aids are expensive. Handle and care for them properly. Report lost or damaged hearing aids to your supervisor immediately. Check with your supervisor before washing a hearing aid. Also follow the manufacturer's instructions for proper care and use. Remove the battery at night. When not in use, turn the device off.

Special Telephone Systems. *TTYs* (once called *telephone teletypes*) are machines that allow people with hearing loss to communicate through the telephone system. Users type messages back and forth to one another. *Amplified telephone handsets* make the caller's voice louder. *Extension bells* make the telephone ring more loudly.

Signalling Devices. These attach to such items as telephones, doorbells, and smoke alarms. When the device makes a sound, a light flashes to alert the person. Some devices include a vibrating option that the person can feel.

Caring for Clients with Hearing Problems

Some people with hearing problems wear hearing aids or speech read (lip read). They watch facial expressions, gestures, and body language. Some learn sign language (Figure 36-3). Some people have *hearing* dogs. The dog alerts the person to such sounds as ringing phones, doorbells, sirens, and oncoming cars.

(text continues on page 598)

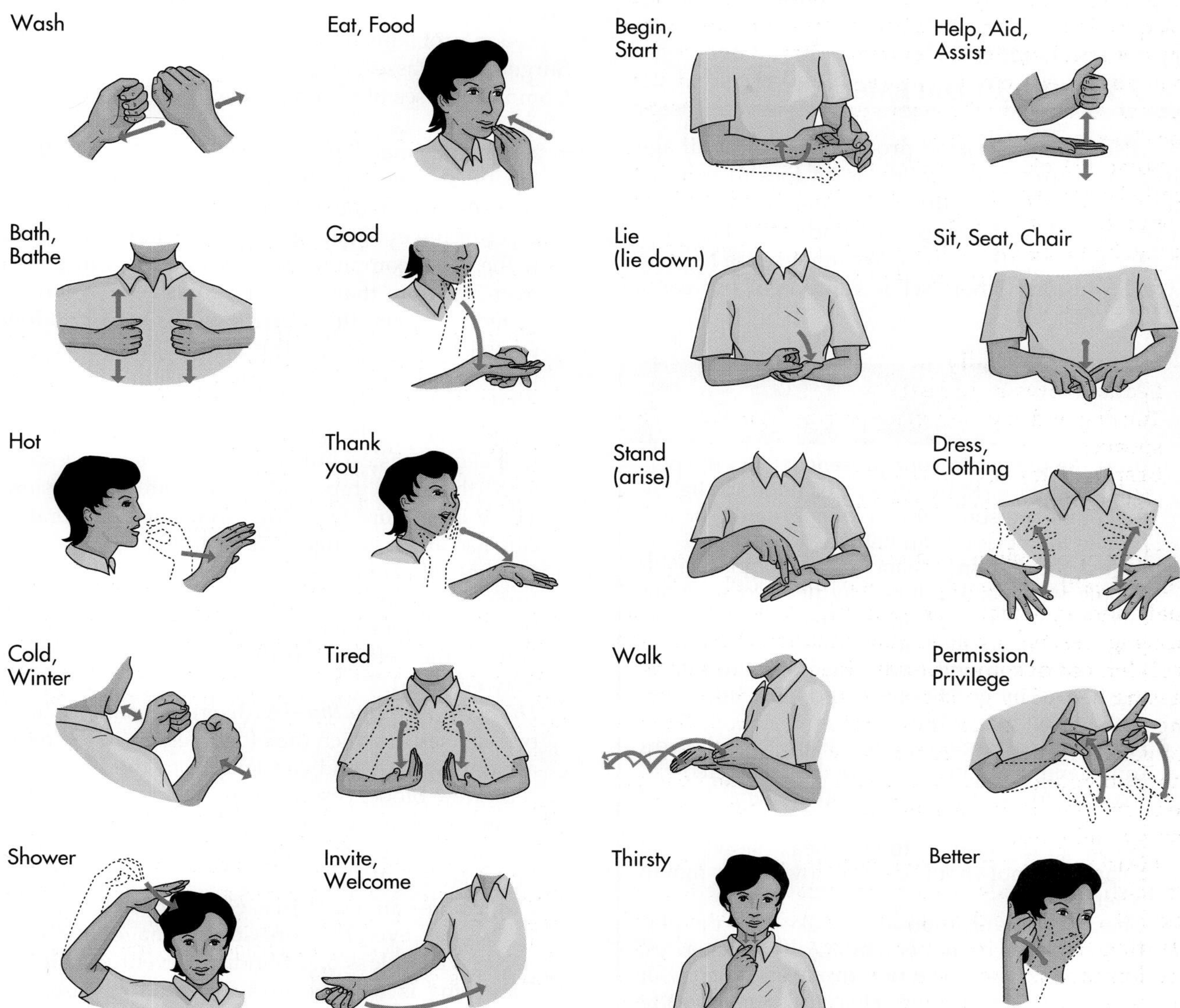

Figure 36-3 Sign language examples.

Follow the guidelines listed in Box 36-1 when caring for clients with severe hearing loss. Remember, some people with hearing loss also have speech problems. Follow the guidelines listedin Chapter 35 for communicating with clients who have speech problems.

Eye Disorders and Vision Problems

Eye disorders and vision problems occur at all ages. They range from very mild vision loss to complete blindness. Health conditions, accidents, and eye diseases are among the causes of blindness. The level of blindness varies. Some people cannot sense light and have no vision. Others sense some light but cannot see details. Still others have some vision but cannot see well. The legally blind person sees at 6 metres (20 feet) what a person with normal vision sees at 60 metres (200 feet). Eye structures are shown in Figure 36-4. See page 136 for a review of the structure and function of the eye.

Vision problems may occur suddenly or gradually. Surgery, eyeglasses, or contact lenses may be needed. Common causes of vision problems include:

- *Age-related macular degeneration (AMD; ARMD)*—the breakdown (*degeneration*) of the macula, the central part of the retina. The *retina* is the inner layer of the eye that senses light and colour. AMD is the most common cause of blindness in people over 50. More than 25% of people over 70 are affected.[1] The condition starts with slow or sudden partial loss of vision. The central vision becomes fuzzy or shadowy. Over time vision gets worse. AMD varies in severity. Some people become completely blind. Others have some sight. Many people lose central vision but still have some *peripheral* vision (the sides, top, and bottom areas of vision). There is no cure for AMD. Macular degeneration can also affect younger adults and children.
- *Retinal detachment*—the separation of the retina from its supporting tissue. The retina cannot function when detached. Permanent blindness can result. If the retina is reattached surgically, vision may be saved.
- *Diabetic retinopathy*—A disorder (*pathy*) caused by diabetes in which the blood vessels in the retina are damaged. Blood can leak from the blood vessels. New blood vessels grow over the retina. This creates scar tissue that pulls the retina away from the back of the eye. Retinal detachment and blindness may result.
- *Glaucoma*—an eye disease that causes pressure within the eye. This pressure damages the optic nerve. Vision loss and blindness eventually result. Glaucoma is usually an age-related disease. The disease is gradual or sudden in onset. Signs and symptoms include *tunnel vision* (the field of vision is reduced so the person can only see straight ahead), blurred vision, and blue-green halos around lights. Treatment involves medications and possibly surgery. The goal is to prevent further damage to the optic nerve. Damage that has already occurred cannot be reversed.
- *Cataract*—a clouding of the eye's lens. The cloudiness prevents light from entering the eye. Cataract comes from the Greek word that means *waterfall*. It is most common in older adults. Gradual blurring and dimming of vision occur. A person with a cataract is sensitive to light and glares. Vision even-

Box 36-1 Guidelines fo Caring for Clients with Hearing Loss

- **Alert the person to your presence.** Gain the person's attention. Raise an arm or hand, or lightly touch the person's arm. Do not startle or approach the person from behind.
- **Adjust the lighting.** Stand or sit in good light. People with hearing loss may need to see your face for speech reading (lip reading). Shadows and glares affect their ability to see your face.
- **Reduce background noise.** Examples are radios, televisions, air conditioners, and fans. Turn these down or off if possible.
- **Focus your attention on the client.** Face the person. Stand or sit on the side of the unaffected ear. Do not turn or walk away while talking. Do not do other tasks.
- **Speak in a normal tone.** Speak slowly and clearly. Do not shout. Do not cover your mouth when talking.
- **Check communication aids.** Make sure the person is wearing his or her hearing aids, eyeglasses, or contact lenses. The person needs to see your face for speech reading. Help the person to put them on if necessary.
- **Adjust your language.** State the topic of conversation clearly. Use simple words and short sentences. Focus on key words. Learn what works for the person. Say things in a different way if the person does not understand you.
- **Use other communication methods.** You may be unable to communicate using speech. Use nonverbal communication to send messages, including body language (see Chapter 12). Or write key words on paper.
- **Watch for signs of fatigue.** Drooping shoulders and a decline in understanding are examples. Avoid tiring the person.

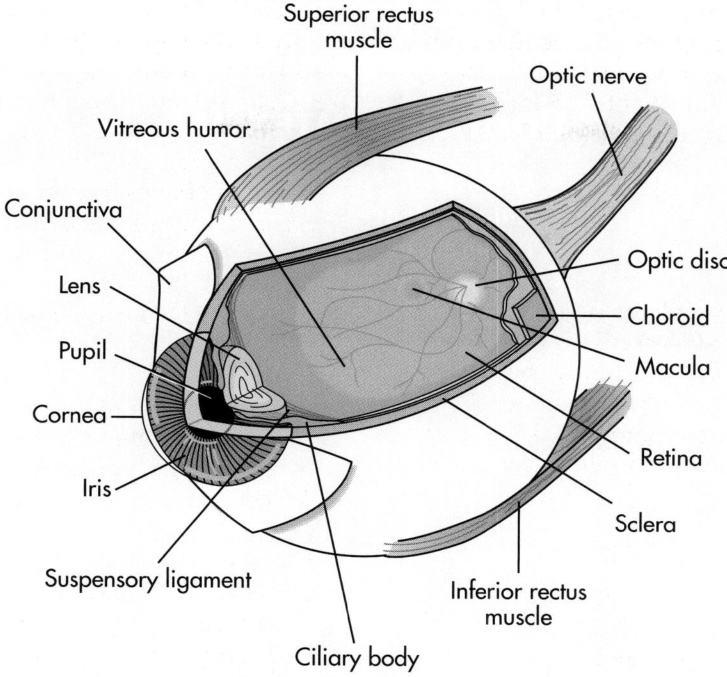

Figure 36-4 The eye.

tually is lost. A cataract can occur in one or both eyes. Surgery is the only treatment. A tiny incision is made into the eye. The cloudy lens is removed. A plastic lens is implanted into the eye. Vision returns to near normal.

- ***Presbyopia***—the gradual inability to focus (*opia*) on close objects. This condition is associated with aging (*presby*). Most people experience this normal, decline in vision, usually after age 40. Corrective and contact lenses help the problem. Good lighting is needed.

The Effects of Vision Problems

Severe vision loss affects a person's physical, emotional, social, intellectual, and spiritual health. For example, Mr. Barak, 78, has AMD. He feels the loss of his independence and self-esteem. Simple tasks such as dressing take much longer. He cannot read the newspaper. He no longer goes out alone because he is afraid of falling or getting lost. Therefore, he no longer attends his mosque.

Although the process is long and hard, many people with severe vision loss learn to lead independent lives. They learn how to move about, complete activities of daily living, and learn new reading methods.

Some people learn how to move about independently using a guide dog or white cane with a red tip. Both are recognized worldwide as signs that the person is blind. The guide dog serves as the eyes of the blind person. The dog recognizes danger and guides the person through traffic.

Aids for People with Vision Problems

A number of aids correct or help vision problems. Examples include eyeglasses and contact lenses, reading aids, communication aids, devices for entertainment, and medical devices.

Eyeglasses. Eyeglasses correct vision problems. Some people wear them for reading or seeing at a distance. Others wear them all the time while awake. People are sometimes upset when they first need glasses. However, adjustment is usually rapid. Most people know that glasses will be needed as they grow older.

Glasses are costly. Protect them from damage. When not worn, they should be kept in their case. Lenses are made of hardened glass or plastic to prevent shattering.

Glass lenses are washed with warm water and dried with soft tissue. Plastic lenses are easily scratched. Special cleaning solutions, tissues, and cloths are used to clean and dry them.

Contact Lenses. Contact lenses fit directly on the eye. There are hard and soft contacts. Many people like contacts because they cannot be seen, they do not break easily, and are worn for sports. However, contacts are easily lost. Depending on the type of lens, contacts can be worn for 12 to 24 hours or for 1 week. Contacts are usually removed for swimming and sleeping.

Contact lenses are removed and cleaned according to the manufacturer's instructions and employer policy.

(text continues on page 601)

Caring for Eyeglasses

Compassionate Care

Remember to Promote:
- **Dignity**
- **Independence**
- **Preferences**
- **Privacy**
- **Safety**

Pre-Procedure

1 Explain the procedure to the person.
2 Wash your hands.
3 Collect the following:
- Eyeglass case
- Cleaning solution or warm water
- Tissues or soft cloth

Procedure

4 Remove the person's glasses:
  a Hold the frames in front of the ear on both sides (Figure 36-5, *A*).
  b Lift the frames from the ears. Bring the glasses down away from the face (Figure 36-5, *B*).
5 Clean the lenses with cleaning solution or warm water. Dry the lenses with tissues or a soft cloth.
6 Open the eyeglass case.
7 Fold the glasses. Put them in the case. Do not touch the clean lenses.
8 Place the glass case where the person wants it. The place must be safe. Or put the glasses back on as follows:
  a Unfold the glasses.
  b Hold the frames at each side. Place them over the ears.
  c Adjust the glasses so the nosepiece rests on the nose.
  d Return the glass case to its place.
9 Wash your hands.

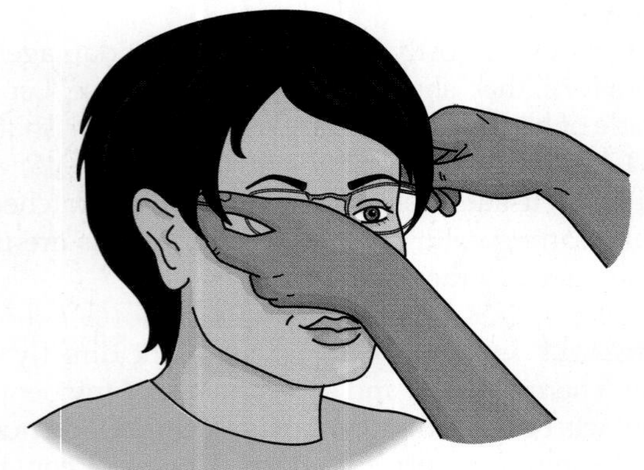

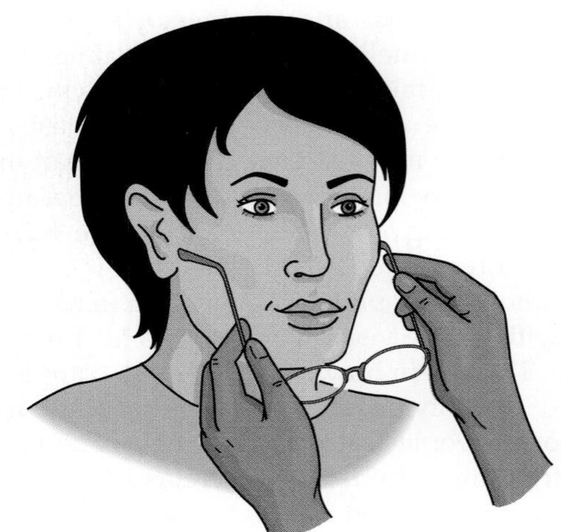

Figure 36-5 A, Remove eyeglasses by holding the frames in front of both ears. **B,** Lift the frames from the ears, and bring the glasses down away from the face.

Report any eye redness or drainage to your supervisor. Also report complaints of eye pain or blurred vision.

Aids for Reading. Many people learn to read Braille. **Braille** is a writing system for the blind that uses raised dots for each letter of the alphabet. The first 10 letters also represent numbers 0 to 9 (Figure 36-6). The person feels the arrangement of dots with his or her fingers (Figure 36-7). Many books, magazines, and newspapers are available in Braille. So are keyboards. Braille is hard to learn, especially for older adults. Some people do not learn to read Braille.

Other reading aids include books with large print, books on audiotape or compact disk, and magnifiers. Some magnifiers contain reading lamps.

Communication Aids. Examples are calendars in Braille, large-print clocks that announce the time in hours or minutes, telephones with Braille keypads and extra large numerals, and cheque and envelope writing guides.

Devices for Entertainment. Examples are playing cards and bingo cards with large letters or in Braille.

Medical Devices. Examples include pillboxes that let the person feel if the pill has been taken and "talking prescription devices" that have voice messages to describe how to take the medication.

Artificial Eyes

Removal of an eye is sometimes necessary because of injury or disease. The person is then fitted with an *ocular prosthesis,* an artificial eye made of glass or plastic that matches the other eye in colour and shape (Figure 36-8 on page 602). Some prostheses are permanent implants. Others are removable. If the prosthesis is removable, the person is taught to remove, clean, and insert it. The person performs routine prosthesis care.

You may care for clients who have artificial eyes. The eye is the client's property. Like hearing aids, eyeglasses, and other valuables, protect it from loss

a b c d e f g h i j
1 2 3 4 5 6 7 8 9 0
k l m n o p q r s t
u v w x y z Capital sign Numeral sign

Figure 36-6 Braille.

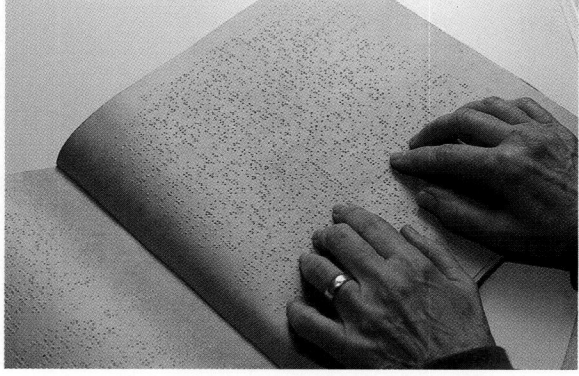

Figure 36-7 Braille is "read" with the fingers.

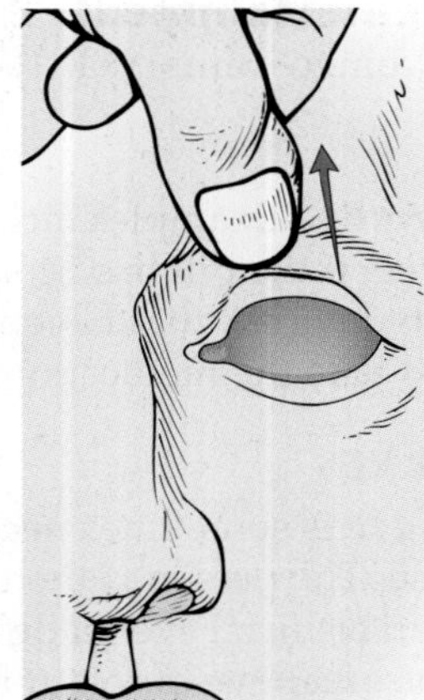
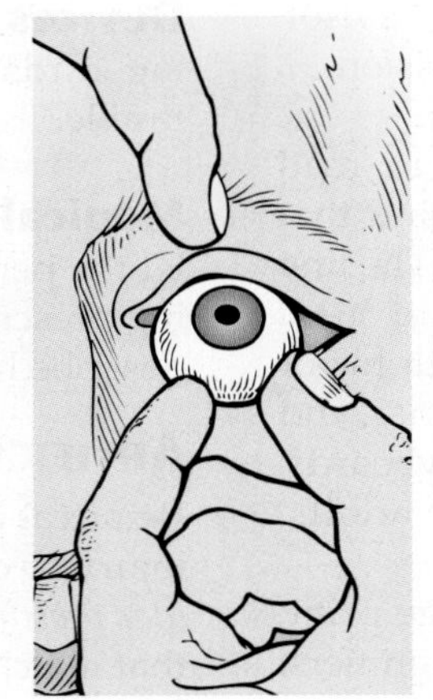
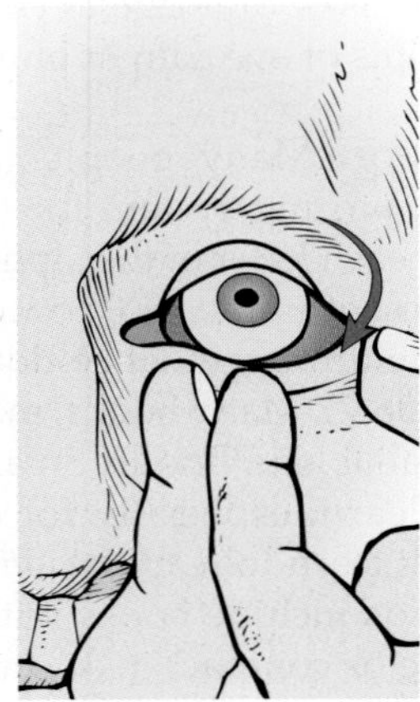

Figure 36-8 Inserting an artificial eye. Source: S.M. Lewis, M.M. Heitkemper, and S.R. Dirkson, *Medical-Surgical Nursing: Assessment and Management of Clinical Problems*, 5th ed. (St. Louis: Mosby, 2000).

and damage. Care for the eye in a safe place. Do not hold it over a sink because it can easily roll down the drain if dropped. You may assist your client in caring for the eye and the eye socket. Follow these measures if the eye is removed and will not be reinserted:

- Wash the eye with mild soap and warm water. Rinse it well.
- Line a container with a soft cloth or 4 x 4 gauze. This prevents damage.
- Fill the container with water or a saline (salt) solution.
- Place the eye in the container. Close the container.
- Label the container with the client's name (if in a facility, include the room number).
- Place the container in the drawer in the bedside stand or in another safe place as directed by the client.
- Wash the eye socket with warm water or saline. Use a washcloth or gauze square. Use a gauze square to remove excess moisture.
- Wash the eyelid with mild soap and warm water. Clean from the inner to the outer part of the eye (see Chapter 27). Dry the eyelid.

The person is blind on the side of the artificial eye. Vision in the other eye may be normal or impaired.

Caring for Clients with Vision Problems

People with vision loss often have highly developed senses of hearing, touch, smell, and taste. They are sensitive to the tone of a person's voice. When talking with clients with vision loss, pay attention to your voice. It needs to convey messages you usually show with body language. Your voice should communicate warmth and respect. Box 36-2 contains guidelines for caring for clients with vision loss.

Box 36-2 Guidelines for Caring for Clients with Vision Loss

- **Adjust the lighting.** Ask the person what type of lighting he or she prefers. Adjust blinds and shades to avoid glare (usually worse on bright, snowy days). Stand or sit in good light.
- **Alert the client to your presence.** Identify yourself when you enter a room. Give your name, title, and your reason for being there. Do not touch the person before indicating your presence. Address the person by name. Tell the person when you are leaving the room.
- **Focus your attention on the client.** Face the person. Do not turn or walk away while talking. Do not do other tasks.
- **Speak in a normal tone.** Speak slowly and clearly. Do not shout. Do not cover your mouth when talking.
- **Assist with walking.** Walk slightly ahead of the person at a normal pace (Figure 36-9). Offer your right or left arm. Tell the person which arm you are offering. The person can then take your arm. Never push, pull, or guide the person in front of you. Tell the person when approaching a curb or steps. Say if you will step up or down. Inform the person of doors, turns, furniture, and other obstructions. Give specific directions. For example, say "right behind you," "on your left," or "in front of you." Avoid phrases like "over here" or "over there."
- **Assist with eating.** Read menus to the person. Avoid table linens and china with patterns and designs. These items should be solid colours and provide contrast. For example, a white plate should be placed on a dark place mat. Explain the location of food and beverages on the tray. Use the face of a clock to describe their location (see Chapter 25). Or, guide the person's hand to each item on the tray. Cut meat, open containers, butter bread, and perform other activities as needed.
- **Provide a safe setting.** Outdoor walks and stairs must be clear of ice and snow. Tell your supervisor if they are not. Hallways and rooms must be free of clutter. Keep doors open or closed, never partially open. Otherwise the person could walk into the door. Remember that furniture and other items are arranged to meet the person's needs. Always replace items where you found them. Avoid rearranging furniture and other items. Orient the person to a new setting. Describe the layout. Identify the location and purpose of furniture or equipment. Let the person move about and touch and locate furniture if able. In facilities, keep the call bell within the person's reach.

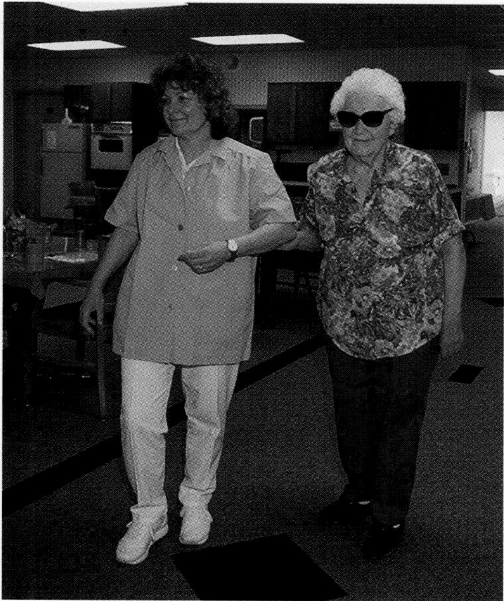

Figure 36-9 This client, who is blind, walks slightly behind the support worker and touches her arm lightly.

REVIEW

Circle the BEST answer.

1. Mr. Poulin has Ménière's disease. Which is likely *true*?
   A. He has a middle ear infection.
   B. Vertigo is a major symptom.
   C. Hearing aids will correct the problem.
   D. He has vision problems because of it.

2. Which effect of hearing problems is often not obvious to others?
   A. Loneliness and social isolation
   B. Speaking too loudly
   C. Asking to repeat things
   D. Answering questions inappropriately

3. You are talking to Mr. Poulin. You should do the following *except*
   A. Speak clearly, distinctly, and slowly
   B. Sit where there is good light
   C. Shout
   D. Sit on the side of his unaffected ear

4. Mr. Poulin's hearing aid is not working. First, you should
   A. See if it is turned on
   B. Wash the hearing aid with soap and water
   C. Have it repaired
   D. Change the batteries

5. Which is true of age-related macular degeneration?
   A. Surgery usually corrects the problem.
   B. There is no cure.
   C. Eyeglasses will improve vision.
   D. It is most common in young adults.

6. Glaucoma is
   A. An ear disorder common among children
   B. Sign language for people with hearing loss
   C. A disease that damages the optic nerve
   D. A symptom of cataracts

7. When not being worn, glasses should be
   A. Left on the bed or chair within easy reach
   B. Left out of the case on the bedside table
   C. Kept in a cleaning solution
   D. Kept in their case

8. Braille involves
   A. A white cane with a red tip for walking
   B. Raised dots arranged to represent letters of the alphabet
   C. An artificial eye
   D. Books on compact disk or audiotape

9. Mrs. Ho is blind. You should do the following *except*
   A. Offer her your arm and walk slightly ahead of her
   B. Explain procedures step by step
   C. Touch her before she knows you are present
   D. Tell her when you are leaving the room

10. Which is unsafe for Mrs. Ho?
    A. Keeping doors open or closed
    B. Informing her of steps and curbs
    C. Turning lights on
    D. Rearranging furniture

Answers to these questions are on page 826.

CHAPTER

37

Caring for Mothers, Infants, and Children

OBJECTIVES

- Define the key terms listed in this chapter
- List physical and emotional changes a new mother may experience
- Identify the signs and symptoms of postpartum complications
- Identify the signs and symptoms of illness in infants
- Describe how to hold and comfort infants
- List precautions that reduce the risk of sudden infant death syndrome (SIDS)
- Explain how to help mothers with breastfeeding and bottle-feeding
- Explain how to burp and diaper an infant
- Describe how to give cord and circumcision care
- Explain how to bathe infants
- Explain why infants are weighed
- Describe your role in providing childcare
- Learn the procedures described in this chapter

KEY TERMS

cesarean section A surgical incision into the abdominal and uterine walls; the baby is delivered through the incision

circumcision The surgical removal of foreskin from the penis

episiotomy An incision made into the perineum to increase the size of the vaginal opening for the delivery of the baby

lactation The process of producing and secreting milk from the breast

lochia Postpartum vaginal discharge

mastitis An infection of the breast

postpartum After (*post*) childbirth (*partum*)

postpartum blues Feelings of sadness or mild depression during the first 2 weeks after childbirth; baby blues

postpartum depression Major depression at any point during the first year after childbirth

postpartum psychosis The most severe form of postpartum depression; the mother may experience delusions, hallucinations, and suicidal thoughts

sudden infant death syndrome (SIDS) The sudden, unexplained death of an apparently healthy infant under 1 year of age

umbilical cord The structure that carries blood, oxygen, and nutrients from the mother to the fetus

Support workers sometimes care for new mothers, infants, and children. Usually this care is provided in a home care setting. Caring for infants or children provides a valuable service to the mother. And caring for the mother enables her to have more time and energy for her family. Respect the family's routines, schedules, and ways of doing things. Follow the care plan. Also follow the mother's standards and preferences if possible.

Caring for New Mothers

A new mother might require home care services if she:

- Experienced complications before or after the birth
- Needs help caring for her other young children at home
- Had a multiple birth (twins, triplets, or more)
- Has an infant with special needs who requires extra time and attention
- Has a physical or mental disability
- Has problems adjusting to her new responsibilities

When assisting a new mother, you usually do one or more of the following:

- Provide physical care for the mother
- Provide care for the newborn
- Help with childcare when other young children are in the home
- Help with home management tasks like meal preparation or housekeeping

Postpartum means after (*post*) childbirth (*partum*). The postpartum period starts with the birth of the baby and ends 6 weeks later. During this time, the mother adjusts physically and emotionally to the effects of childbirth.

The mother's body returns to its normal state during this time. Hormone levels change dramatically. The uterus contracts back almost to its pre-pregnant size. The body expels blood and other substances left in the uterus. This vaginal discharge is called **lochia**. (Lochia comes from the Greek word *lochos*, which means *childbirth*.) Lochia changes in colour and eventually decreases in amount. This discharge lasts for 2 to 6 weeks. Lochia increases with breastfeeding (*nursing*) and activity. It should return to normal after the mother rests. The mother wears a sanitary pad to absorb the discharge.

Because of the many changes during the postpartum period, the mother needs to rest and recover. Encourage her to rest or nap when the baby is sleeping. Encourage her to take time for herself and her partner. She also has nutritional needs (see Chapter 25).

Postpartum hemorrhage, infection of the uterine lining, and other complications are possible. Tell your supervisor immediately if you notice any of the signs or symptoms listed in Box 37-1.

Perineal Care

Some mothers have episiotomies. An **episiotomy** is an incision (*otomy*) into the perineum to increase the size of the vaginal opening for delivery of the baby. The physician or midwife performs this procedure during childbirth. The incision is sutured after the delivery.

This chapter is adapted from J. Birchenall and E. Streight, *Mosby's Textbook for the Home Care Aide* (St. Louis: Mosby, 1997). The author acknowledges the contribution of Joan Birchenall and Eileen Streight.

Box 37-1 Signs and Symptoms of Postpartum Complications

- Fever of 38° C (100.4° F) or higher
- Chills, poor appetite, fatigue, nausea, or vomiting
- Lochia that soaks a sanitary pad within 1 hour of application
- Foul-smelling lochia
- Large number of clots in the lochia
- Painful, burning, or difficult urination
- Severe abdominal or perineal pain
- Bleeding, redness, swelling, or drainage from a cesarean-section incision (see below)
- Leg pain, tenderness, or swelling
- Breast pain, tenderness, or swelling (Box 37-2)
- Feelings of depression (Box 37-3 on page 608)

Afterwards, the perineal area may be very swollen, sore, and tender. Sometimes the perineum is torn during childbirth. This also causes pain and swelling in the perineal area.

Complications can develop. These include infection and wound separation (dehiscence). Good perineal care is important. Tell your supervisor if the mother complains of pain in the perineum.

The physician may order pain-relief medications and cold packs to the perineum for the mother's comfort. Physicians may also order sitz baths for comfort and hygiene (see Chapter 42). A warm bath also may relieve perineal pain and soreness. Make sure the tub is disinfected before use. Also have clean washcloths and towels available for the mother.

Care of Abdominal Incisions

Some mothers have had cesarean sections. A **cesarean section** (c-section) is a surgical incision into the abdomen and uterine walls. The baby is delivered through the incision. A cesarean section is done when:

- The baby must be delivered quickly to save the baby's or mother's life
- The baby is too large to pass through the birth canal
- The mother has a vaginal infection that could be transmitted to the baby
- A normal vaginal delivery would be difficult for the baby or mother

The c-section incision needs to heal. See Chapter 41 for wound healing and wound care. The mother needs recovery time. In the first few weeks she may feel weak and tired. The physician may order her to avoid lifting or housework for at least the first week. You might help with housekeeping tasks and childcare. Or you might bring her the baby for feedings.

Tell your supervisor if the mother complains of pain around the incision site. Also tell your supervisor if you observe bleeding, redness, swelling, or drainage from the incision.

Breast Care

Lactation is the process of producing and secreting milk from the breasts. Lactation usually begins around the third day after childbirth. The breasts may become *engorged* (overfilled) with milk. Engorged breasts are swollen, hard, and painful. Once breastfeeding is established or the milk dries up (if the mother chooses not to breastfeed), engorgement decreases within 1 or 2 days. Cold packs applied to the breasts or warm showers promote comfort. A good nursing bra worn day and night supports the breasts and increases comfort during engorgement. Follow the care plan to promote the mother's comfort.

Sometimes mothers feel a tender lump in a breast. This usually is a symptom of a *plugged duct*. Milk drains into ducts that open onto the nipple (see Figure 13-23 on page 145). When the milk does not drain properly through the duct, the milk builds up within the breast. An untreated plugged duct can cause a breast infection. Tell your supervisor if you suspect the mother has a plugged duct. Treatment usually involves:

- Encouraging frequent nursing
- Keeping pressure off the clogged duct; make sure the clothes and bra are not too tight
- Applying warm washcloths to the affected area or having warm showers to promote drainage

Mastitis is infection (*itis*) of the breast (*mast*). It occurs when bacteria enter a milk duct through a cracked nipple. It is usually very painful. Early treatment is essential. Tell your supervisor as soon as signs or symptoms appear (see Box 37-2). Medications may be ordered. The mother also needs rest. Breastfeeding during treatment for mastitis is usually encouraged. The mother should nurse as much as possible from the affected breast, even if it is painful. This keeps the milk flowing and speeds recovery.

Box 37-2 Signs and Symptoms of Mastitis

- Pain, heat, tenderness, red streaks, or swelling in a breast
- Tender lump or hardened area in the breast
- Fever: 38° C (100.4° F) or higher
- Chills
- Fatigue
- General body aches
- Cracked nipples or cracked skin around the nipples

Postpartum Blues, Depression, and Psychosis

The postpartum period is also a time of emotional changes. Lack of sleep, more responsibilities, and her new role may affect the mother's moods. Other issues may affect the mother, including isolation, disappointment, anxiety, poor body image, or lack of support from a partner or spouse. These issues and the changes in hormone levels may contribute to **postpartum blues** (the "baby blues"), which are feelings of sadness or mild depression during the first 2 weeks after childbirth.

Common symptoms of postpartum blues include:

- Insomnia
- Mood changes
- Weepiness
- Fatigue
- Headaches
- Poor concentration
- Feelings of sadness, anger, or anxiety

Health Canada estimates that up to 80 percent of postpartum Canadian women experience postpartum blues.[1] Symptoms usually begin in the first days after birth and disappear without treatment after 1 to 2 weeks. Your encouragement and emotional support during this time may be very helpful to the mother.

About 10 to 20 percent of Canadian women suffer postpartum depression after childbirth.[2] **Postpartum depression** is major depression that begins any time within the first year after childbirth. Usually it begins within 2 weeks to 6 months after the birth. Professional care is needed as soon as possible. Postpartum depression can worsen over time.

Postpartum psychosis is a severe form of postpartum depression. It is relatively rare, affecting about 1 woman per 1000.[3] The mother with postpartum psychosis loses touch with reality. She has delusions, hallucinations, or suicidal thoughts (see Chapter 33). She could harm or neglect her child. She must not be left alone with the infant or other children. Tell your supervisor immediately if the mother shows any of the signs or symptoms listed in Box 37-3.

A mother diagnosed with postpartum depression may be ordered medications. She may need help with home management or childcare. This gives her time to rest. Your understanding and emotional support are essential.

Box 37-3 Signs and Symptoms of Postpartum Depression

- Crying
- Feelings of sadness, hopelessness, or guilt
- Difficulties sleeping
- Inability to cope with everyday problems
- Avoiding visiting with others
- Feelings of anger toward the baby
- Fatigue
- Extreme anxiety
- Delusions or hallucinations
- Thoughts of harming the baby or self

Caring for Infants

Infants are helpless and cannot protect themselves. They depend on others for their basic needs. Providing for their safety is essential (see Chapter 16). Like everyone else, infants have physical and emotional needs.

Newborns and infants change and grow quickly. Their needs change as they grow. Review the normal growth and development patterns of newborns and infants (see Chapter 14). Follow the care plan to meet the infant's needs.

Signs and Symptoms of Illness

Your observations are important for the infant's safety and well-being. Infants can become ill quickly. Signs and symptoms may be sudden. You must be very alert. If the infant has any of the signs or symptoms listed in Box 37-4, tell your supervisor immediately.

Box 37-4 Signs and Symptoms of Illness in Infants

- *Jaundice*—a yellowish colour to the skin and whites of the eyes
- Redness or drainage around the cord stump or circumcision (see pages 616 and 617)
- High temperature
- Limpness and slowness to respond
- Screaming or crying for a long time
- Flushed or pale skin
- Heavy perspiration
- Rash
- Noisy, rapid, difficult, or slow respirations
- Coughing or sneezing
- Reddened or irritated eyes
- Turning head to one side or putting a hand to one ear (signs of an ear infection)
- Not feeding
- Vomiting most of the feeding or between feedings
- Hard, formed stools
- Frequent watery, green, mucousy, or foul-smelling stools
- Signs of dehydration: fewer than 6 wet diapers a day; dark yellow urine; decreased saliva and tears; dry lips; dry, wrinkled skin; sunken eyes and top of head
- Stiff neck; head will not pull forward toward the chest

Tell your supervisor when the sign or symptom began. You may need to take an infant's or child's temperature and respirations (see Chapter 40). Axillary temperatures are taken on infants. Tympanic or axillary temperatures are taken on children younger than 5 years. Apical pulses are taken on infants and young children. Your supervisor tells you which method to use.

Holding an Infant

Most infants are comforted when held and cuddled. It helps them feel loved and secure. Use both hands to lift a newborn. Always handle the baby with gentle, smooth movements. Avoid sudden or jerking movements. These may startle or upset the baby.

A baby's neck is very weak for about the first 3 months. Always support the head and neck when lifting and holding. Also support the entire body. Do not let the arms or legs dangle. Hold the baby securely and close to your body. Figure 37-1 shows how to hold a baby.

Comforting a Crying Infant

Infants cry to communicate. They cry for many reasons, including when they are wet, hungry, hot, cold, tired, uncomfortable, in pain, overstimulated, or lonely. Respond to the baby's crying. Responding to their cries helps babies feel safe and secure. An infant cannot be spoiled with too much attention and comfort.

Some babies cry a lot and the parents have to figure out what comforts them. Ask the mother how she soothes her baby. You may have to try different things to find what works for you. Follow the guidelines in Box 37-5 on page 610. Tell your supervisor if the baby cannot be comforted.

Laying the Infant Down to Sleep

Safety precautions must be taken when laying the baby down to sleep. These are to lower the risk of **sudden infant death syndrome (SIDS)**. SIDS is the sudden, unexplained death of an apparently healthy infant under 1 year of age. It usually occurs while the infant is sleeping.

When laying the baby down to sleep, remember the following:

- *Always lay babies on their backs for sleep*. Babies who sleep on their stomachs or sides have an increased risk of SIDS. Some babies have medical conditions that require them to sleep on their stomachs. Check with your supervisor and care plan. Babies can lie on their stomachs when they are awake and being supervised.
- *Do not lay the baby on soft bedding products.* These include fluffy, plush products such as sheepskin, pillows, quilts, comforters, or soft toys. Remove these items from the crib. Soft products might cause large amounts of carbon dioxide to pool around the

A

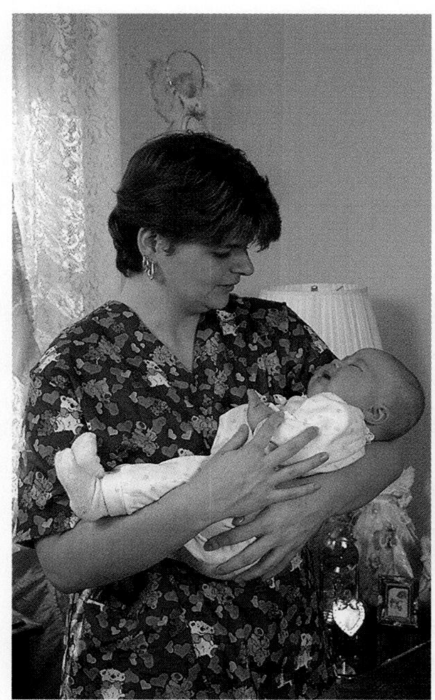

B

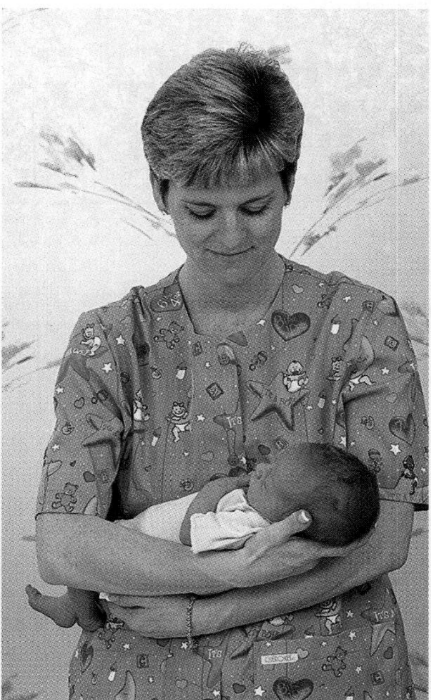

C

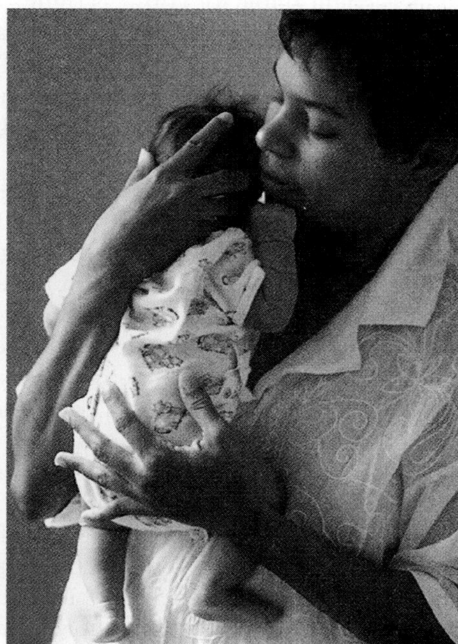

Figure 37-1 Support the head and neck with one hand and the legs and back with the other. Hold the baby close to your body. **A,** The cradle hold. **B,** The football hold. **C,** The shoulder hold.

Box 37-5 Guidelines for Soothing a Crying Infant

- Ensure all physical needs are met. Determine if the baby needs a diaper change or is hungry, hot, cold, tired, or in pain.
- Use gentle motions such as rocking, swinging, or walking back and forth with the baby.
- Hold the baby close to your chest so he or she can hear your heartbeat.
- Rub the baby's back or stomach.
- Swaddle the baby. Wrapping newborns tightly in a blanket provides warmth and security. It holds them so they cannot flail their limbs and startle themselves. Some babies like being swaddled; others dislike it. Check with the parent. To swaddle the baby, lay a blanket on a flat surface and fold a top corner down. Place the baby supine with his or her head on the folded corner. Pull the corner of the blanket near the baby's left arm across the body and tuck it under the baby's right arm. Pull the bottom corner up over the baby's body and to the chest. Bring the last free corner of the blanket over the baby's right arm and across the chest. Tuck it under the back on the baby's left side.

baby's head and cause SIDS. The soft bedding also can cover the baby's nose and mouth and cause suffocation.

- *Make sure the baby is warm but never hot.* Overheating is thought to increase the risk of SIDS. Do not overdress the baby at bedtime. If the room temperature feels comfortable for you, it is right for the baby. Use a lightweight blanket that you can add or remove depending on room temperature. To check if the baby is too hot, place your hand on the back of his or her neck. If the neck is sweaty, the baby is too warm.

Helping Mothers Breastfeed

Many mothers breastfeed their babies. Usually, mothers and babies learn how to nurse in a very short time. However, a mother and baby can have difficulties in the first few weeks. This may be a stressful time for the mother. Provide a calm, supportive, and positive atmosphere. If the mother is having problems breastfeeding, tell your supervisor. The mother may require additional support.

Breastfed newborns usually nurse every 2 to 3 hours throughout the day and night. Babies are fed on demand. In other words, they are fed when hungry, not on a schedule. When babies want to eat, they often become restless, suck on their fists, and cry.

At first, babies nurse for a short time—maybe only 5 minutes at each breast. Eventually, total nursing time may take between 20 and 30 minutes. Mothers might need help getting ready to breastfeed. Assist as needed. If you leave the room while the mother is nursing, stay within hearing distance in case she needs help. Some mothers want privacy while breastfeeding; others want you to stay. Ask the mother which she prefers. Box 37-6 describes how you can help with breastfeeding.

Box 37-6 Guidelines for Helping with Breastfeeding

- Wash your hands and remind the mother to wash her hands. Hand washing is necessary before she handles her breasts.
- Help the mother to a comfortable position. She may want to nurse sitting up in bed or in a chair. Or she may prefer the side-lying position (Figure 37-2). If the mother is recovering from a c-section or has a sore perineum she may prefer the side-lying position. Support the mother's back with pillows in whatever position she chooses.
- Change the baby's diaper if necessary. Bring the baby to the mother.
- Offer to bring the mother a glass of water or juice. Many women get thirsty while breastfeeding.
- Offer the mother a blanket to cover the baby and her breast. This promotes privacy during the feeding. For some women, using a blanket makes nursing difficult. Follow the mother's preferences.
- Help the mother burp the baby if necessary. The baby is burped after nursing at each breast.
- Change the baby's diaper after the feeding if necessary.
- Lay the baby in the crib if he or she has fallen asleep. *Remember, lay the baby on his or her back. Do not lay the baby on his or her stomach or side unless the care plan instructs you to do so.*
- Record what time the baby nursed and how long on each side. Report any problems or concerns.

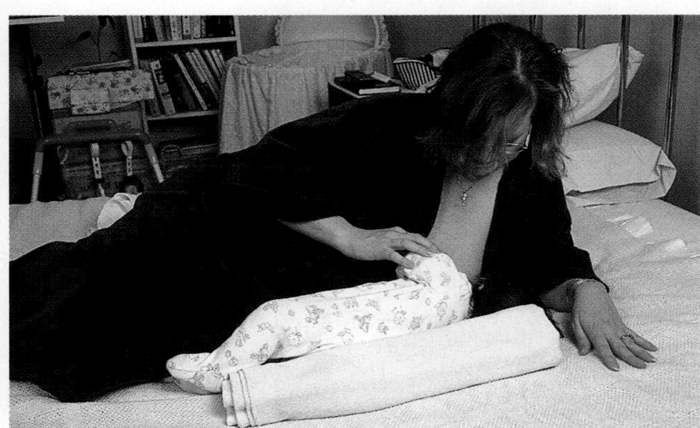

Figure 37-2 A mother breastfeeding in the side-lying position.

Helping Mothers Bottle-Feed

Formula is given to infants who are not breastfed. It provides the essential nutrients needed by the infant. Formula comes in three forms. The *ready-to-feed* form is poured directly from the can into the baby bottle (Figure 37-3). Water is added to *powdered* and *concentrated* formula. Container directions tell how much formula to use and how much water to add.

Infants must be protected from infection. Therefore, use pre-boiled, cooled tap water to mix the formula for infants under 4 months of age. Boiling the tap water for at least 2 minutes destroys microbes. Use tap water from the cold tap. Do not use hot tap water, well water, bottled water, or water that has been filtered or treated. Follow the care plan and contact your supervisor if you have any questions.

Bottles are prepared one at a time or in batches for the whole day. Extra bottles are capped (Figure 37-4) and stored in the refrigerator. These bottles should be used within 24 hours. After 24 hours, the formula must be discarded.

Cleaning the Equipment. Baby bottles, caps, and nipples must be as clean as possible. Reusable bottle-feeding equipment is carefully washed in hot, soapy water or in a dishwasher. Complete rinsing is needed to remove all soap. Some mothers use plastic nursers. They require plastic liners that are used once and then discarded.

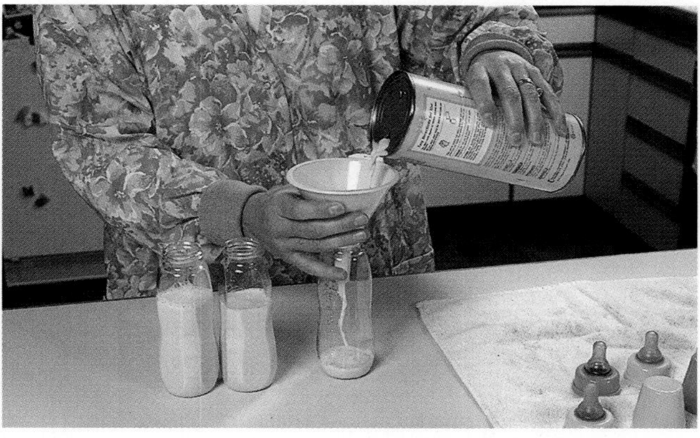

Figure 37-3 Ready-to-feed formula is poured from the can into the bottle. Use a clean funnel to prevent spilling.

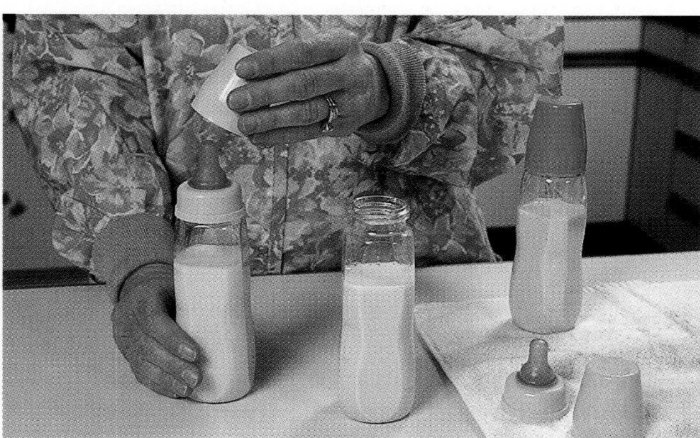

Figure 37-4 Bottles are capped for storage in the refrigerator.

Bottle-Feeding Equipment

Pre-Procedure

1 Wash your hands.

2 Collect the following:
- Bottles, nipples, and caps
- Funnel
- Can opener
- Bottle brush
- Dishwashing soap
- Other items needed to prepare formula
- Clean dishtowel

Procedure

3 Wash the bottles, nipples, caps, funnel, and can opener in hot, soapy water. Wash other items used to prepare formula.

4 Clean inside of baby bottles with the bottle brush (Figure 37-5 on page 612).

5 Squeeze hot, soapy water through the nipples (Figure 37-6 on page 612). This removes formula from them.

6 Rinse all items thoroughly in hot water.

7 Lay a clean towel on the countertop.

8 Stand the bottles upside down to drain. Place the nipples, caps, and other items on the towel. Let the items dry.

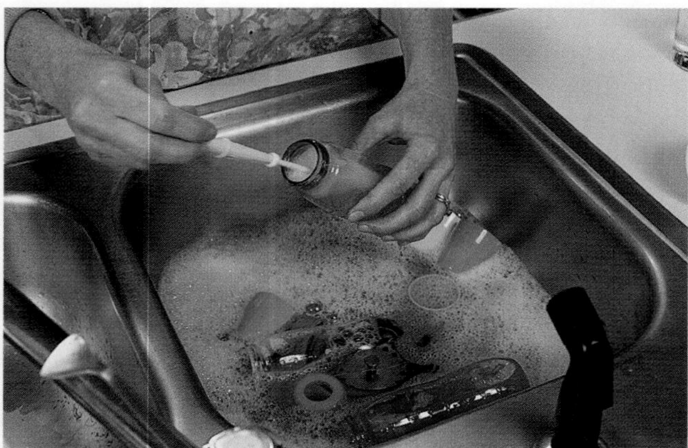

Figure 37-5 A bottle brush is used to clean the inside of the bottle.

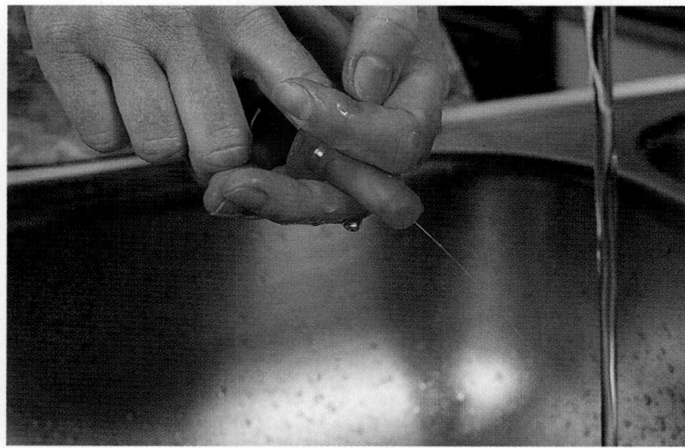

Figure 37-6 Water is squeezed through the nipples during cleaning.

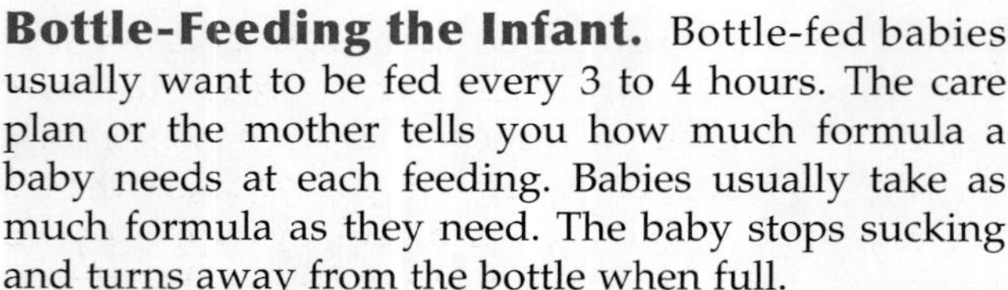

Bottle-Feeding the Infant. Bottle-fed babies usually want to be fed every 3 to 4 hours. The care plan or the mother tells you how much formula a baby needs at each feeding. Babies usually take as much formula as they need. The baby stops sucking and turns away from the bottle when full.

Babies are not given cold formula out of the refrigerator. The bottle must be warmed before the feeding. You can warm the bottle in a bowl of warm water. The formula should feel warm. Test the temperature by sprinkling a few drops on the inside of your wrist (Figure 37-7). Do not set the bottle out to warm at room temperature. This takes too long and allows the growth of microbes. Do not heat formula in microwave ovens. The formula can heat unevenly and burn the baby's mouth.

The guidelines in Box 37-7 will help you bottle-feed babies.

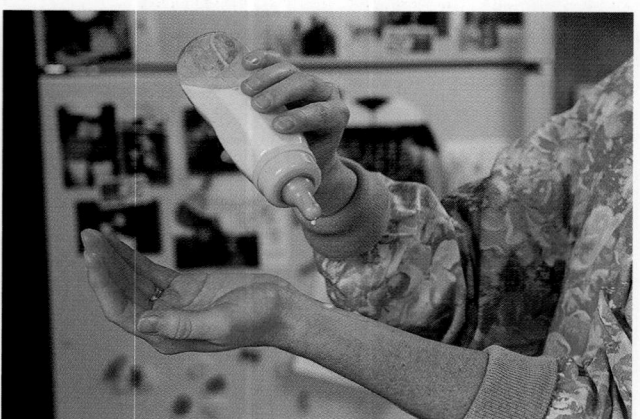

Figure 37-7 Formula should feel warm on the wrist.

Box 37-7 Guidelines for Bottle-Feeding Infants

- Place the bottle in a bowl of warm water until the formula feels warm to your wrist.
- Tilt the bottle to check the flow of formula dropping out of the nipple. Two or three drops should drip out per second. Too few drops mean the hole in the nipple is too small. Too many drops mean the hole is too large. Change the nipple if the hole is not right and test again.
- Assume a comfortable position for the feeding.
- Hold the baby close to you. Relax and snuggle the baby.
- Tilt the bottle so that the neck of the bottle and the nipple are always filled (Figure 37-8). Otherwise some air might remain in the neck or nipple. If the baby swallows air, the baby may later feel discomfort and cramping.
- Do not prop the bottle and lay the baby down for the feeding (Figure 37-9). The baby could choke.
- Burp the baby when he or she has taken about half the formula. Also burp the baby at the end of the feeding.
- Do not expect the baby to always finish all the formula. The feeding is over when the baby stops sucking and turns away from the bottle.
- Discard remaining formula.
- Wash the bottle, cap, and nipple after the feeding (see *Bottle-Feeding Equipment* on page 611).

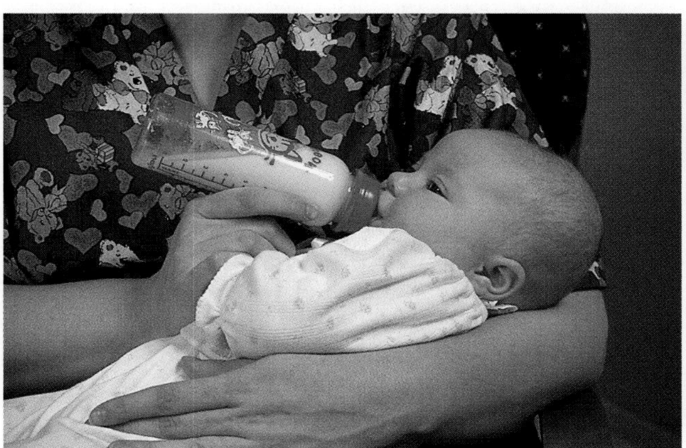

Figure 37-8 Tilt the bottle so that formula fills the bottle neck and nipple.

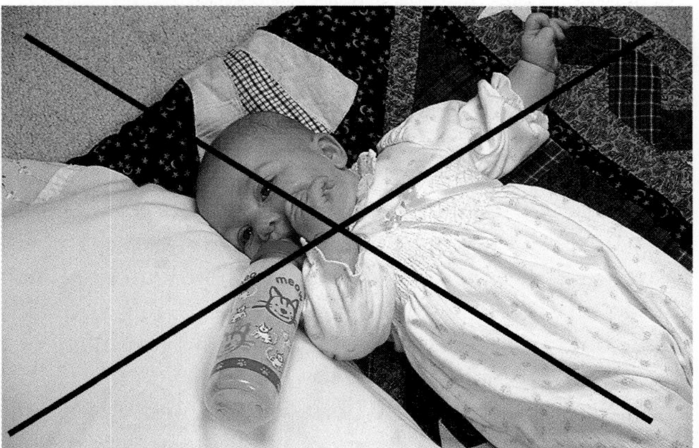

Figure 37-9 Do not prop the bottle to feed the baby.

Burping the Infant

Babies take in air when they eat. Bottle-fed babies take in more air than breastfed babies. Air in the stomach and intestines causes discomfort and cramping. This can lead to fussiness and vomiting. Burping helps to get rid of the air. Most babies burp in the middle and after the feeding.

There are two ways to position the baby for burping (Figure 37-10). One way is to hold the baby over your shoulder. First place a clean diaper or towel over your shoulder. This protects your clothing if the baby "spits up." You can also support the baby in a sitting position on your lap. If the baby is younger than 3 months, support the head and neck by cupping your hand under the baby's chin. Hold the towel or diaper in front of the baby. To burp the baby, gently pat or rub the baby's back with circular motions. Do this until the baby burps. It may take up to 2 to 5 minutes.

A

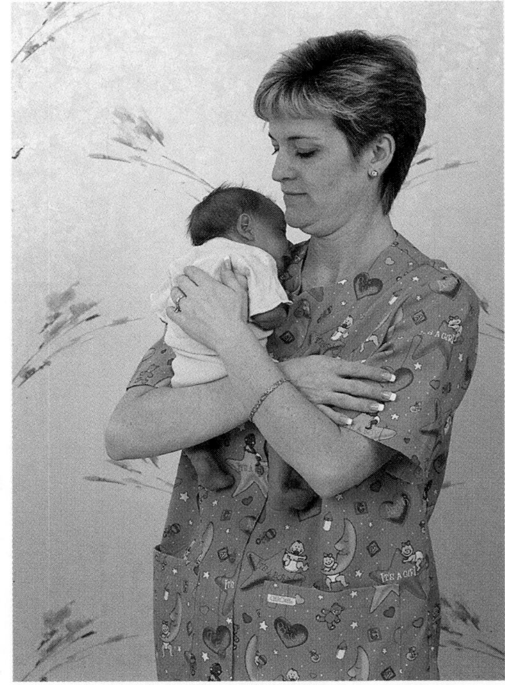

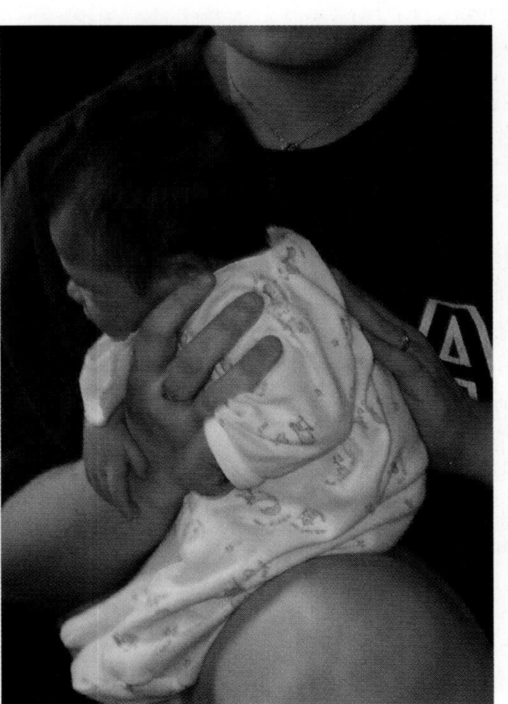

B

Figure 37-10 Burping a baby. **A,** The baby is held over the shoulder for burping. **B,** The baby is supported in the sitting position for burping.

DIAPERING

Babies urinate several times a day. Breastfed babies usually have bowel movements after feedings. Bottle-fed babies may have 3 bowel movements a day. Until they are fed solid foods, babies usually have stools that are soft and unformed. Hard, formed stools mean the baby is constipated. Watery stools mean diarrhea. Diarrhea is very serious in babies. Their water balance can be upset quickly (see Chapter 25). Tell your supervisor immediately if you suspect a baby has constipation or diarrhea.

Diapers are changed when wet or soiled. Changing the diaper after a feeding is usually necessary. The parent may have cloth or disposable diapers. Cloth diapers may be fastened with diaper pins or Velcro strips. They are covered with plastic pants to protect against leaks. When changing a soiled cloth diaper, empty the stool into the toilet, if possible. Place used diapers and plastic pants in the diaper pail until they can be laundered. They are washed in hot water with a laundry detergent made especially for baby clothes. Putting them through the wash cycle a second time without detergent helps remove all soap. Dry them thoroughly. Fold for reuse.

Disposable diapers help keep the baby dry because they absorb moisture. However, they still need to be changed whenever wet or soiled. When changing a soiled disposable diaper, empty the stool into the toilet, if possible. Place the diaper in the garbage. Do not flush disposable diapers or wipes down the toilet.

Changing diapers whenever wet helps prevent diaper rash. Moisture, stool, and urine irritate the baby's skin. If a diaper rash develops, tell your supervisor and the mother immediately. Make sure the baby is clean and dry before you apply a clean diaper. Health Canada advises that gloves are not necessary for routine diaper changes if you can avoid touching the stool or urine with your hands.[4] Check your employer's policy for the use of gloves when diapering. Always wash your hands before and after changing diapers.

To prevent falls, never turn your back on the baby when changing diapers. Gather all supplies before starting the procedure. Arrange them in an easy-to-reach place. If the baby is on a change table, keep one hand on the baby at all times.

(text continues on page 616)

Diapering a Baby

Pre-Procedure

1 Wash your hands.
2 Collect the following:
- Clean diaper
- Waterproof changing pad
- Disposable wipes, washcloth, or cotton balls
- Basin of warm water
- Baby soap
- Baby lotion or cream if necessary

Procedure

3 Place baby on the changing pad.
4 Unfasten the dirty diaper. Place diaper pins out of the baby's reach.
5 Wipe the genital area with the front of the diaper, if the diaper is dry enough (Figure 37-11). Wipe from the front to the back.
6 Fold the diaper so urine and stool are well inside. Set the diaper aside.
7 Clean the genital area from the front to back. Use a wet washcloth, disposable wipes, or cotton balls. Wash with mild soap and warm (not hot) water if there is a lot of stool or if the baby has a rash. Rinse thoroughly, and pat the area dry.
8 Give cord care (page 616) and circumcision care (page 617).
9 Apply cream or lotion to the genital area and buttocks, if in the care plan. Do not use too much. Caking can occur.
10 Raise the baby's legs. Slide a clean diaper under the buttocks.
11 For boys, fold a cloth diaper so extra thickness is in the front (Figure 37-12, *A* on page 616). For girls, fold the diaper so the extra thickness is in the back (Figure 37-12, *B* on page 616).
12 Bring the diaper between the baby's legs.
13 Make sure the diaper is snug around the hips and abdomen. It should be loose near the penis if the circumcision has not healed. The diaper should be below the cord stump.

Continued

Diapering a Baby—cont'd

Procedure—cont'd

14 Secure the diaper in place. Use the tabs on disposable diapers (Figure 37-13, *A* on page 616). Make sure the tabs stick in place. Use diaper pins or Velcro strips for cloth diapers. Pins should point away from the abdomen (Figure 37-13, *B* on page 616).

15 Apply plastic pants if cloth diapers are worn. Do not use plastic pants with disposable diapers. They already have waterproof protection.

16 Put the baby in the crib, infant seat, or other safe location.

Post-Procedure

17 Rinse the stool from the cloth diaper in the toilet. Empty stool from the disposable diaper into the toilet, if possible.

18 Store used cloth diapers in a covered pail or plastic bag. Roll the disposable diaper into a ball and secure it with its tabs. Take the disposable diaper to the garbage.

19 Clean the changing pad.

20 Wash your hands.

21 Report and record your actions and observations according to employer policy.

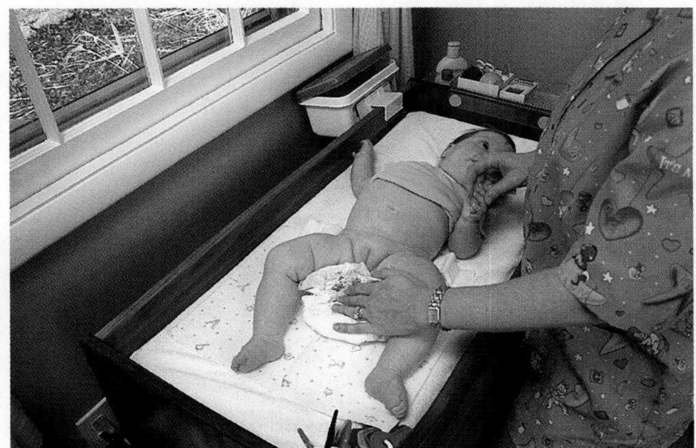

Figure 37-11 Clean the genital area with the front of the diaper.

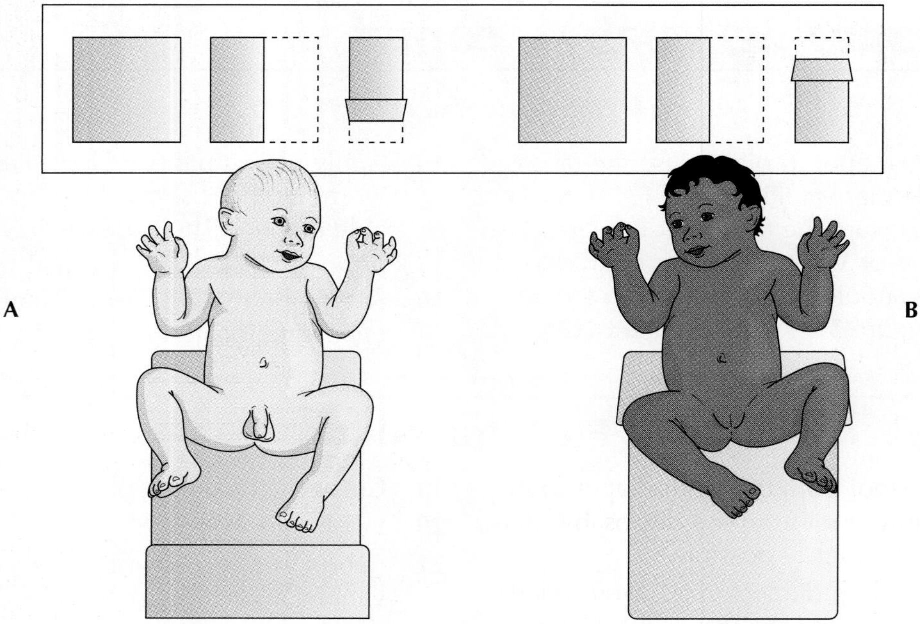

Figure 37-12 **A,** Fold a cloth diaper in front for boys. **B,** Fold the diaper in the back for girls.

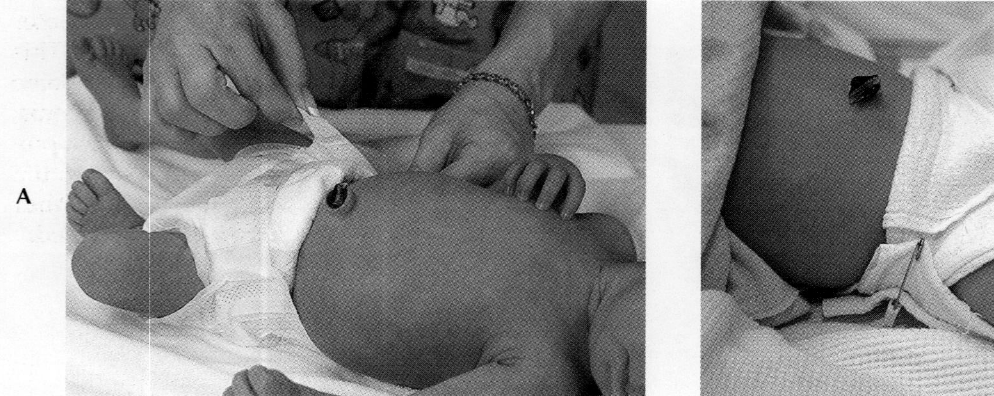

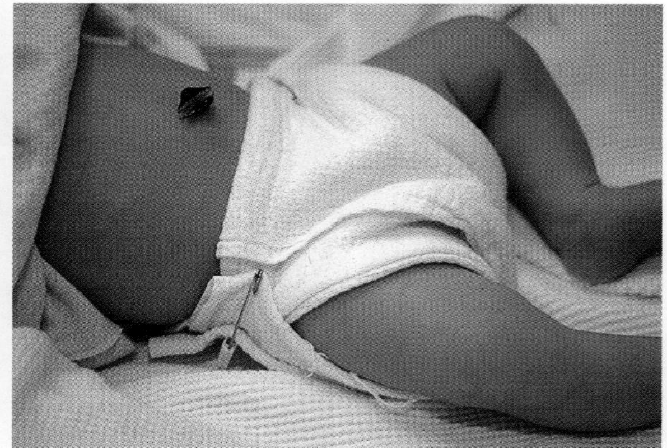

Figure 37-13 Securing a diaper. **A,** Secure disposable diaper in place with tabs. **B,** Diaper pins are sometimes used to secure cloth diapers. Point pins away from the abdomen.

Care of the Umbilical Cord

The **umbilical cord** connects the mother and the fetus (unborn baby). It carries blood, oxygen, and nutrients from the mother to the fetus (Figure 37-14). The umbilical cord is not needed after birth. Shortly after delivery, the physician or midwife clamps and cuts the cord. A stump of cord is left on the baby. The stump dries up and falls off in 7 to 10 days. Slight bleeding can occur when the cord comes off. Do not pull the cord off—even if it looks ready to fall off.

The cord stump provides an area for the growth of microbes. You need to keep it clean and dry. Cord care is done at each diaper change. Cord care is continued for 1 to 2 days after the cord comes off. The care plan and your supervisor will advise you on cord care. Cord care usually consists of the following:

- Keeping the cord dry
- Washing your hands before and after contact with the umbilical area

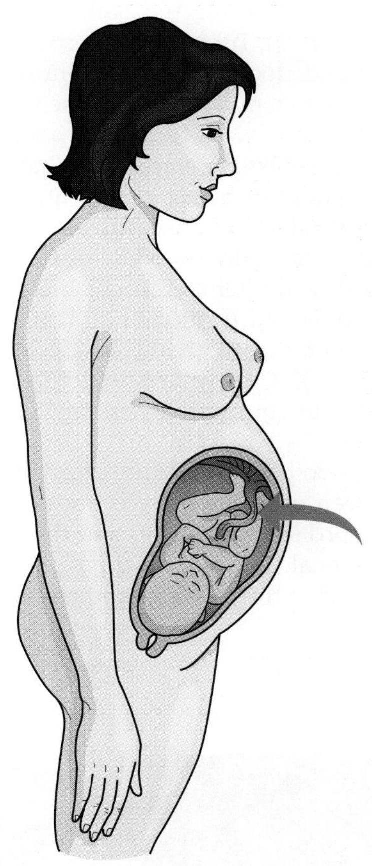

Figure 37-14 The umbilical cord connects the mother and fetus.

- Keeping the cord clean. Gently wipe around the base of the cord with a cotton ball moistened with warm water (Figure 37-15). (Alcohol swabs are not recommended.)
- Keeping the top of the diaper below the cord as in Figure 37-13. This prevents the diaper from irritating the cord. It also keeps the cord from becoming wet with urine.
- Reporting any signs of infection. These include redness, odour, or drainage from the cord.
- Giving sponge baths until the cord falls off. Then the baby can have a tub bath.

Care for a Circumcised Baby

Boys are born with foreskin on the penis. A **circumcision** is the surgical removal of foreskin. Not all boy infants are circumcised. The parents decide if they want the procedure. The procedure allows good hygiene and is thought to prevent certain cancers. Circumcision is usually done in the hospital before the baby goes home. It is a religious ceremony in the Jewish faith.

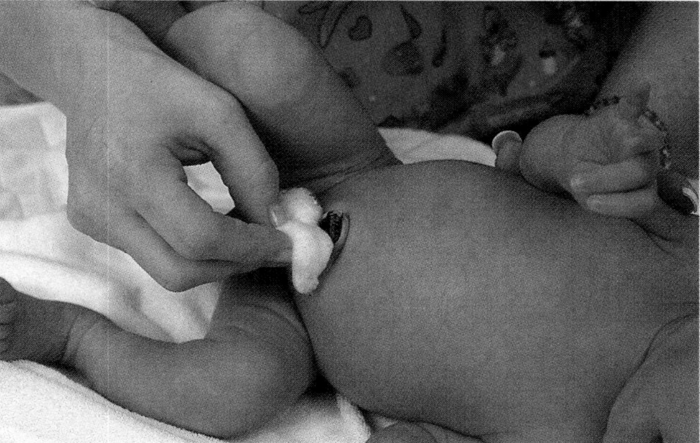

Figure 37-15 Wipe the cord stump at the base with a cotton ball moistened with warm water.

The penis will look red, swollen, and sore. However, the circumcision should not interfere with urination. Report observations of bleeding, odour, or drainage. The area should be completely healed in 10 to 14 days.

The penis should be thoroughly cleaned at each diaper change. Cleaning is especially important after the baby has a bowel movement. Use mild soap and water or commercial wipes. Apply the diaper loosely. This prevents the diaper from irritating the penis. Some physicians advise applying petroleum jelly to the penis. This protects the penis from urine and stool. It also prevents the penis from sticking to the diaper. Use a cotton swab to apply the petroleum jelly (Figure 37-16). Your supervisor will tell you if other measures are needed.

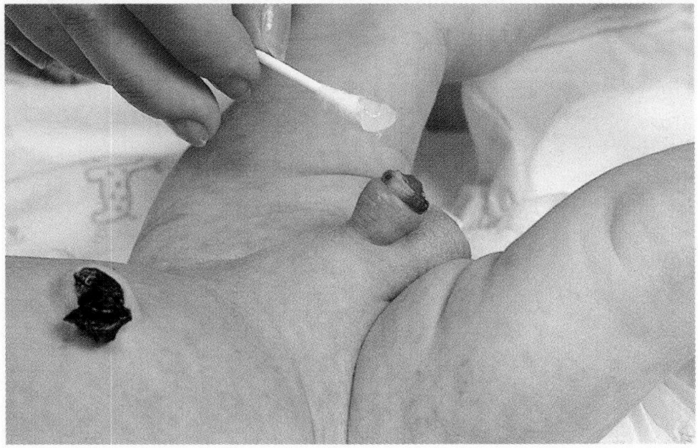

Figure 37-16 Use a cotton swab to apply petroleum jelly to the circumcised penis.

Bathing an Infant

Baths are very important for cleanliness. They also usually comfort and relax babies. They provide a wonderful time to hold, touch, and talk to babies. Bath time should be part of the baby's daily routine. Some mothers like to bathe their babies in the morning. Others prefer the evening. Follow the family's routine.

Planning is an important part of the bath. You cannot leave the baby alone if you forget something. Therefore you need to gather equipment, supplies, and the baby's clothes before you start the bath. Everything you need must be within your reach.

Safety measures are also very important:

- Never leave the baby alone on a table or in the bathtub.
- Hold the baby securely throughout the bath. Babies are very slippery when they are wet. A wet, squirming baby is hard to hold. Pay close attention to what you are doing.
- Room temperature for the bath should be 24 to 27° C (75 to 80° F). Turn up the thermostat and close windows and doors about 20 minutes before the bath. The room temperature may be uncomfortable for you. You may want to remove a sweater or roll up your sleeves before starting the bath.
- Water temperature needs special attention. Babies have delicate skin and are easily burned. Bathwater temperature should be 37.8 to 40.6° C (100 to 105° F). Bathwater temperature is measured with a bath thermometer. If one is not available, test the water temperature with the inside of your wrist (Figure 37-17). The water should feel warm and comfortable to your wrist.

There are two bath procedures for babies. Sponge baths are given until the baby is about 2 weeks old, or until the cord stump falls off and the cord site and circumcision heal. *The cord must not get wet.* The tub bath is given after the cord site and circumcision heal (Figure 37-18).

(text continues on page 621)

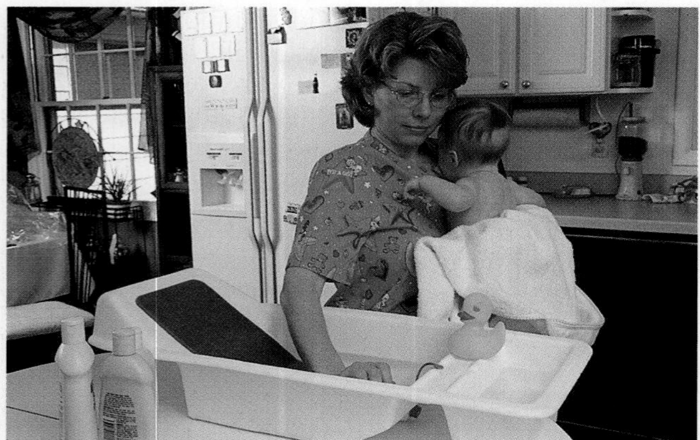

Figure 37-17 Use the inside of your wrist to test the temperature of the bathwater.

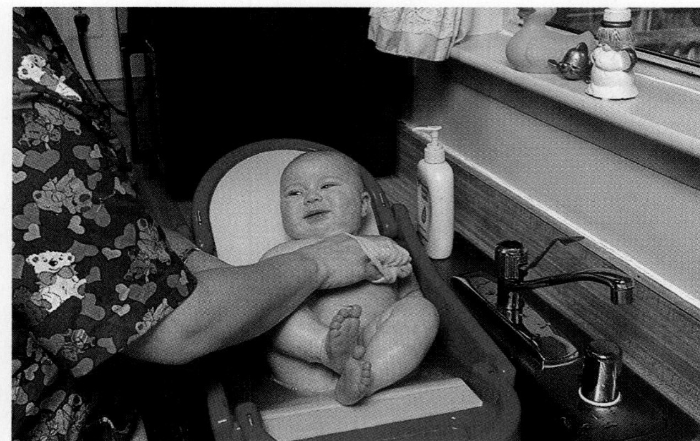

Figure 37-18 The baby is given a tub bath.

Giving a Baby a Sponge Bath

Pre-Procedure

1 Wash your hands.
2 Place the following items in your work area:
   - Bath basin
   - Bath thermometer
   - Bath towel
   - Two hand towels
   - Receiving blanket
   - Washcloth
   - Clean diaper
   - Clean baby clothing
   - Cotton balls
   - Baby soap
   - Baby shampoo
   - Baby lotion
3 Fill the bath basin with warm water. Water temperature should be 37.8 to 40.6° C (100 to 105° F). Measure water temperature with the bath thermometer or use the inside of your wrist. The water should feel warm and comfortable on your wrist.

Procedure

4 Undress the baby. Leave the undershirt and diaper on.
5 Wash the baby's eyelids (Figure 37-19 on page 620):
   a Dip a cotton ball into the water.
   b Squeeze out excess water.
   c Wash one eyelid from the inner part to the outer part.
   d Dry gently with a towel.
   e Repeat this step for the other eye with a new cotton ball.
6 Moisten the washcloth. Clean the outside of the ear and then behind the ear. Dry with the towel. Repeat this step for the other ear. Be gentle.
7 Rinse and squeeze the washcloth. Make a mitt with the washcloth (see Figure 27-8 on page 414).
8 Wash the baby's face (Figure 37-20 on page 620). Wipe around the mouth and nose, then the cheeks and forehead. *Do not use cotton swabs to clean inside the ears or nostrils.* Pat the face dry.
9 Wipe under the baby's chin and in the neck creases. Dry well.
10 Pick up the baby. Hold the baby over the bath basin using the football hold. Support the baby's head and neck with your wrist and hand.
11 Wash the baby's head (Figure 37-21 on page 620):
   a Squeeze a small amount of water from the washcloth onto the baby's head.
   b Apply a small amount of baby shampoo to the head.
   c Wash the head with circular motions.
   d Rinse the head by squeezing water from a washcloth over the baby's head. Be sure to rinse thoroughly. Avoid getting soap in the baby's eyes.
   e Use a small hand towel to dry the head.
12 Lay the baby on the table.
13 Remove the undershirt and diaper.
14 Wash the front of the body. Use a soapy washcloth. You may also apply soap to your hands and wash the baby with your hands (Figure 37-22 on page 620). Do not get the cord wet. Rinse thoroughly. Pat dry. Be sure to wash and dry all creases and folds.
15 Wash and dry baby's hands, feet, and between the fingers and toes.
16 Turn the baby to the prone position. Wash the back and buttocks using a soapy washcloth or your hands. Rinse thoroughly. Pat dry.
17 Give cord care (page 616) and circumcision care (page 617).
18 Apply baby lotion to the baby's body as directed by the care plan.
19 Put a clean diaper and clean clothes on the baby.
20 Wrap the baby in the receiving blanket. Put the baby in the crib or other safe location.

Continued

Giving a Baby a Sponge Bath—cont'd

Post-Procedure

21 Clean and return equipment and supplies to the proper place. Do this step when the baby is settled.

22 Wash your hands.

23 Report and record your actions and observations according to employer policy.

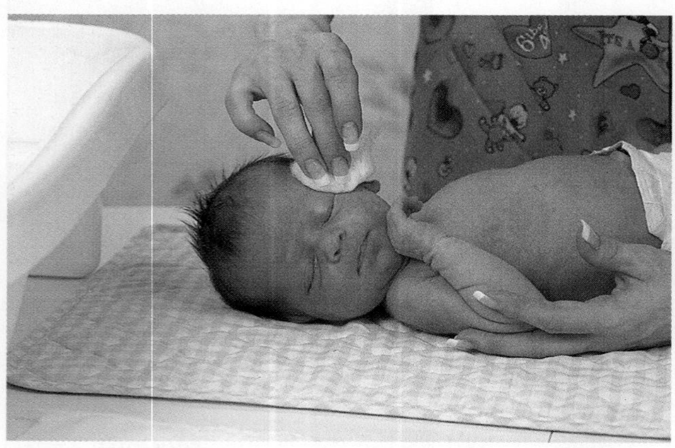

Figure 37-19 Wash the baby's eyelids with cotton balls. Clean the eyelid from the inner to the outer part. Use a fresh cotton ball for each eye.

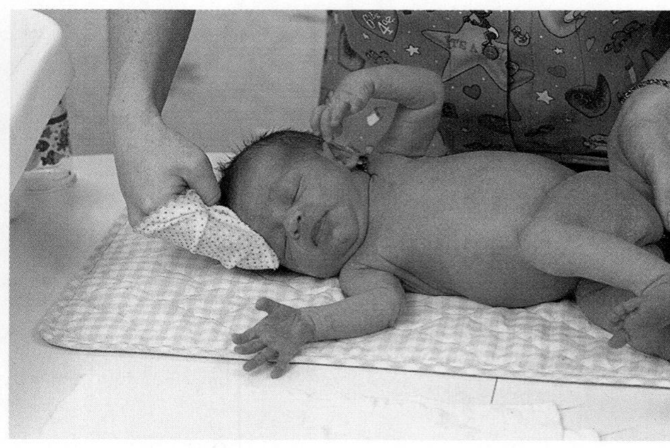

Figure 37-20 Wash the baby's face with a mitted washcloth.

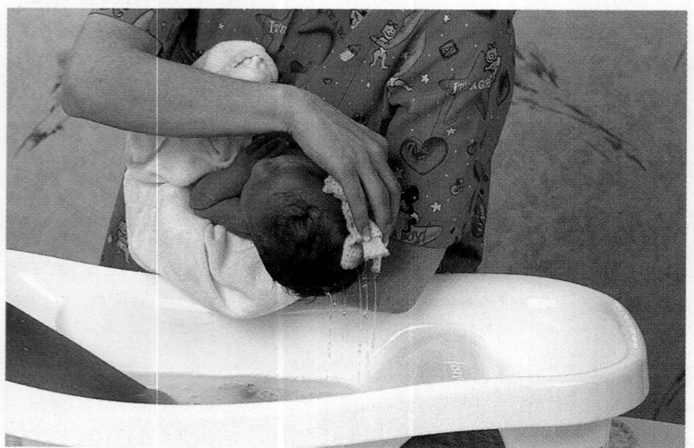

Figure 37-21 Wash the baby's head over the basin.

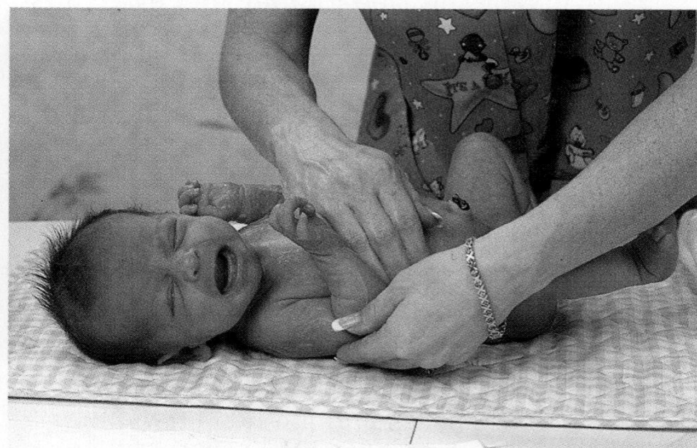

Figure 37-22 You can use your hands to wash the baby.

Giving a Baby a Tub Bath

Procedure

1. Follow steps 1 through 13 in *Giving a Baby a Sponge Bath* on page 619.
2. Hold the baby as in Figure 37-23:
   a. Place your right hand* under the baby's shoulders. Your thumb should be over the baby's right shoulder. Your fingers should be under the right arm.
   b. Use your left hand to support the baby's buttocks. Slide your left hand under the thighs. Hold the right thigh with your left hand.
3. Lower the baby into the water feet first.
4. Wash the front of the baby's body. Be sure to wash all folds and creases. Rinse thoroughly.
5. Reverse your hold. Use your left hand to hold the baby.
6. Wash the baby's back. Rinse thoroughly.
7. Reverse your hold again. Use your right hand to hold the baby.
8. Wash the genital area.
9. Lift the baby out of the water and onto a towel.
10. Wrap the baby in the towel. Also cover the baby's head.
11. Pat the baby dry. Be sure to dry all folds and creases.
12. Follow steps 18 to 23 of the *Sponge Bath* procedure.

*This procedure was written for right-handed people. Reverse the hand position if you are left-handed.

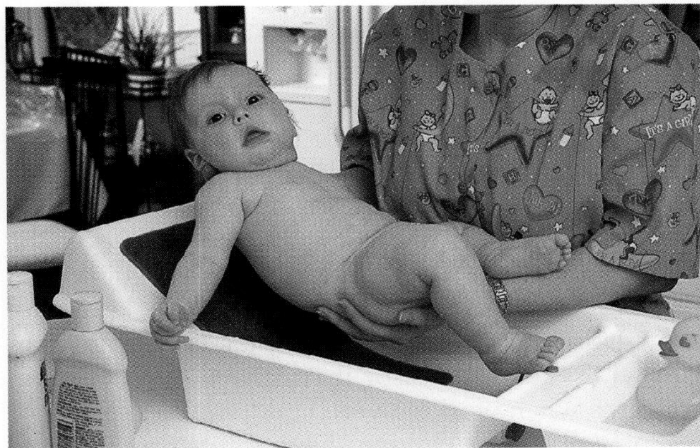

Figure 37-23 The baby is held for a tub bath.

Nail Care

The baby's fingernails and toenails should be kept short. Otherwise, the baby can scratch himself or herself and others. Nails are best cut when the baby is sleeping. That way the baby will not squirm or fuss. Use nail clippers or file nails with an emery board. If using nail clippers, clip nails straight across as for an adult (see Figure 28-7 on page 447).

Weighing Infants

Infants are weighed at birth. The birth weight is the baseline for measuring the infant's growth. Your supervisor tells you when to weigh the baby. You must meet the baby's safety needs. Protect the baby from chills. Keep the room warm and free of drafts. Also protect the baby from falling. Always keep a hand over the baby when taking the weight measurement. Remember to keep one hand on the baby if you need to look away.

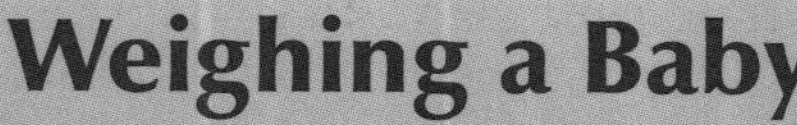

Weighing a Baby

Pre-Procedure

1 Wash your hands.
2 Collect the following:
- Baby scale
- Paper for the scale
- Items for diaper changing (see *Diapering a Baby* on page 614)

Procedure

3 Place the paper on the scale. Adjust the scale to zero (0).
4 Undress the baby and remove the diaper. Clean the genital area.
5 Lay the baby on the scale. Keep one hand over the baby to prevent falling.
6 Read the digital display (Figure 37-24) or move the pointer until the scale is balanced.
7 Diaper and dress the baby. Lay the baby in the crib.

Post-Procedure

8 Return the scale to its proper place.
9 Wash your hands.
10 Report and record the weight and your observations according to employer policy.

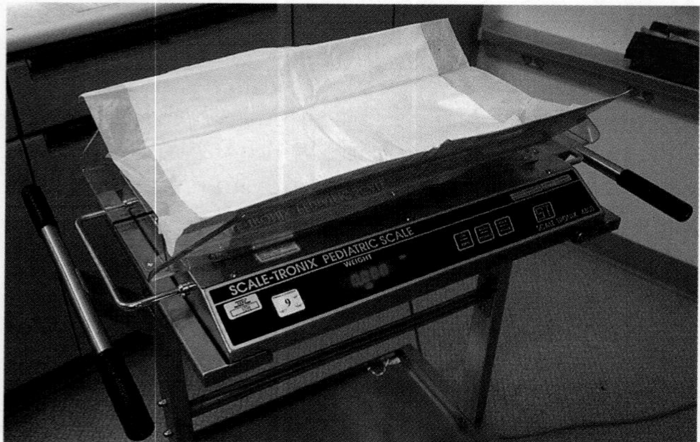

Figure 37-24 Digital infant scale.

Caring for Children

Support workers sometimes care for children. You might help parents of newborns care for other young children in the home. Or you might care for a sick or disabled child or adolescent. You might work around children if they are in a client's home. Whatever the situation, you need some understanding of children in order to work with them. Review the normal stages of growth and development in Chapter 14. Always consult with your supervisor if you have questions and concerns when working with children.

Remember that children have rights too. Promote the priorities of support work when working with children. (See *Providing Compassionate Care: Working with Children* box.)

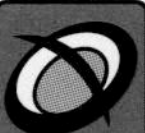

Providing Compassionate Care

WORKING WITH CHILDREN

Dignity. Children have the right to be treated with respect and in a manner that promotes their dignity. Never tease or laugh at a child. Their feelings are easily hurt. Remember to include children in conversations when appropriate. Do not talk about the child in front of him or her. Also remember to say "please" and "thank you" to children. Treat each child as an individual of worth.

Independence. Even very young children should be allowed and encouraged to do what they can for themselves.

Preferences. It is usually not difficult to find out a child's preferences. However, many times the child cannot have what he or she wants. The child's wishes may be unsafe or unhealthy. Whenever possible, offer limited choices that are equally acceptable. For example, instead of saying "What do you want for a snack?" say "Would you like a slice of apple or a piece of orange for your snack?" This way, you are able to accept the child's preference.

Privacy. Privacy is especially important to middle-school-aged children and adolescents. Unless the care plan directs otherwise, let them have privacy when using the bathroom, bathing, and using the phone. Do not pry into their affairs. Respect their belongings.

Safety. Providing for the child's safety is essential. Children are at high risk for accidental injury. Young children are curious about everything around them. Most children are very active. However, they do not usually understand danger. Provide constant supervision for babies, toddlers, and young children. When you are responsible for them, do not let them out of your sight. Review the safety measures in Chapter 16.

DISCIPLINE

When supervising or caring for children, you need to reinforce the rules of acceptable behaviour in the home. The system of rules that governs how we act is called *discipline*. Discipline is a positive way of teaching responsible behaviour. It sets limits and provides guidelines so that children can learn how to behave in an appropriate way. Discipline should be consistent. Each time a rule is broken, the consequence should be the same. For example, Noah (age 4) forgets to remove his boots and gets the floor dirty. He must get a cloth and help wipe the floor. He is not allowed to play until the mess is cleaned up. Noah knows the rules and what will happen if a rule is broken. The child feels safe knowing the caregiver's expectations.

Recognize the child's efforts when he or she tries to follow the rules of the household. Praising these efforts encourages acceptable behaviour. Being positive with children is always more effective than being negative. For example, if Noah gets the floor dirty, it is better to say "Let's clean up the mess" than "Shame on you for making that big mess." After he cleans the mess, say, "Thank you for doing such a fine job." This makes Noah feel good about his accomplishment. It also promotes the child's dignity and shows respect for the child.

Your role in disciplining the child is to:

- Know the rules of acceptable behaviour in each family situation
- Ask an appropriate family member to clarify the rules if you are unsure
- Reinforce existing rules
- Be consistent when using discipline
- Praise the child's efforts to comply with the rules

Some parents have very few rules of discipline. Or existing rules seem too harsh or too loose. Contact your supervisor for assistance. New rules may need to be set. Do not set discipline rules without the help of your supervisor.

PUNISHMENT

Punishment is a harsh response that occurs when a discipline rule is broken. Punishing a child for failing to follow the rules of the household is *not* your responsibility. If a family member asks you to do so, explain that it is not your agency's policy to carry out punishment. Ask the family member to contact your supervisor if he or she has further questions. Record this information and tell your supervisor about the situation.

YOUR ROLE

The goal is to provide a stable, secure, and safe atmosphere for the family. This is very important for sick children and for those who are experiencing stress because of an ill family member. Your responsibilities will vary in each family situation. However, the following are usually included:

- Developing positive relationships with all family members
- Maintaining the existing rules of behaviour
- Maintaining the daily routines as much as possible
- Being alert to situations that may add stress or cause harm to the family. Report these situations to your supervisor (Box 37-8 on page 624).

Follow the guidelines in Box 37-9 on page 624 when interacting with children. Check with your supervisor and the care plan for instructions for each child.

Box 37-8 Family Situations that Must Be Reported

- Violent behaviour of family member (see Chapter 19 for a description of child abuse and your responsibilities to report)
- Frequent visits by "strangers"
- Suspected drug abuse
- Excessive drinking
- Electricity, heat, or water turned off
- Severe shortage of food or clothing
- Illness of a child
- Sudden departure of caregiver
- Unexpected return of family member

Box 37-9 Guidelines for Caring for Children in the Home

COMMUNICATION

- Use active listening skills. Maintain eye contact and concentrate on what is being said.
- Watch for nonverbal communication cues from the child. These include frowning, lack of eye contact, and smiling.
- Provide nonverbal communication. Comfort the child with a hug or touch on the shoulder or arm (according to acceptable custom and culture).
- Answer questions simply, honestly, and clearly. Difficult questions about the family member's illness or death should be handled carefully. Ask your supervisor for guidance in advance.
- Offer praise for something well done.
- Give encouragement when the child attempts to improve behaviour, even when there is only slight progress.
- Use positive suggestions rather than negative words. Avoid the statements "Don't" and "No."

REST, SLEEP, PLAY, AND EXERCISE

- Follow bedtime and naptime routines. Routines and rituals are usually very important to the child. They give the child comfort. Going to sleep at the right time is also very important for most children. Otherwise, they may become overtired, overactive, or cranky.
- Supervise playtime. Encourage active exercise, if allowed.
- Avoid taking sides when disagreement occurs.
- Do not give more attention to one child and ignore others.
- Ignore tattling, if used to get attention.
- Distract the child if he or she begins to misbehave. If possible, play with the child or provide a different toy or activity.

MEALTIME

- Prepare foods that the child will eat. Follow the care plan. Check if the child has food allergies or sensitivities (see Chapter 25).
- Do not force a child to eat. When the child is full, the meal is over.
- Serve meals and snacks on time. Many children have mood swings if they do not eat on time.

REVIEW

Circle the BEST answer.

1. A mother has a red vaginal discharge the first few days after childbirth. This is
   A. Menstrual flow
   B. A postpartum complication
   C. Lochia
   D. From her episiotomy

2. A cesarean delivery involves
   A. A vaginal incision
   B. A perineal incision
   C. An abdominal incision
   D. A normal delivery through the vagina

3. A symptom of mastitis is
   A. Engorgement
   B. Thirst while breastfeeding
   C. Postpartum blues
   D. Pain in a breast

4. Zach is a newborn. Which does *not* need to be reported?
   A. Zach spits up a small amount when burped.
   B. Zach has hard, dry stools.
   C. Zach's eyes are red and irritated.
   D. Zach looks flushed and is perspiring.

5. When holding Zach, you should *not*
   A. Support his head
   B. Cuddle him
   C. Let his arms and legs dangle
   D. Swaddle him

6. The following statements are about laying infants down to sleep. Which is *false*?
   A. Lay them on their backs.
   B. Place pillows under their heads.
   C. Make sure they are not overheated.
   D. Remove soft bedding and toys from the crib.

7. A breastfed baby is burped
   A. Every 5 minutes
   B. After nursing from one breast and then again after nursing from the other
   C. After nursing from both breasts
   D. After the feeding

8. You are to warm a baby bottle. Which is *true*?
   A. The formula should feel warm on your wrist.
   B. The formula should be warmed at room temperature.
   C. The bottle is warmed for 3 minutes in the microwave.
   D. The formula is warmed on the stovetop for 5 minutes.

9. When bottle-feeding, you should
   A. Burp the baby every 5 minutes
   B. Save remaining formula for the next feeding
   C. Tilt the bottle so that formula fills the neck of the bottle and the nipple
   D. Leave the baby alone with the bottle

10. When the umbilical cord stump has not yet healed, the diaper should be
    A. Below the stump
    B. Snug over the stump
    C. Disposable
    D. Loose over the stump

11. Cord and circumcision care are given
    A. Once a day
    B. When the baby has a bowel movement
    C. Three times a day
    D. At every diaper change

12. The following statements are about bathing babies. Which is *false*?
    A. Sponge baths are given until the cord and circumcision have healed.
    B. Gather supplies before beginning the bath.
    C. Room temperature should be slightly cool.
    D. Water temperature should be between 37.8 and 40.6° C (100 to 105° F).

13. Your role when providing childcare does *not* include
    A. Maintaining the family's rules of behaviour
    B. Providing punishment when necessary
    C. Maintaining the family's daily routines
    D. Reporting situations that may add stress or cause harm to the family

Answers to these questions are on page 826.

CHAPTER

38

DEVELOPMENTAL DISABILITIES

OBJECTIVES

- Define the key terms listed in this chapter
- Identify the areas of function limited by a developmental disability
- Explain how a developmental disability affects the client and the family across the life span
- Explain when developmental disabilities occur and their causes
- Explain how various developmental disabilities affect functioning

KEY TERMS

autism A brain disorder that impairs communication, social skills, and behaviour

cerebral palsy (CP) A disorder affecting muscle control (*palsy*); is caused by an injury or abnormality in the motor region of the brain (*cerebral*)

cognitive disability Intellectual disability

congenital Present at birth

convulsion Violent and sudden contractions or tremors of muscle groups

developmental disability A disability that occurs before birth, at birth, or during childhood or adolescence; it impairs the child's development

diplegia Loss of ability to move (*plegia*) corresponding parts on both (*di*) sides of the body; both arms or both legs are affected

Down syndrome (DS) A congenital disorder caused by an extra chromosome; results in varying degrees of intellectual disability

epilepsy A condition characterized by recurrent seizures

Fetal alcohol effect (FAE) A milder form of FAS; the same symptoms may occur but to a lesser degree

Fetal alcohol syndrome (FAS) A group of physical and mental abnormalities in a child as a result of alcohol consumption by the mother during pregnancy

intellectual disability Impaired ability to learn; cognitive disability

seizure Brief disturbance in the brain's normal electrical function; affects awareness, movement, and/or sensation

spastic Uncontrolled contractions of skeletal muscles

spina bifida A congenital disorder involving improper closing of the spine before birth; *spina* means backbone and *bifida* means split in two parts

tonic-clonic seizure A seizure involving convulsions

A *disability* is any loss of physical or mental function (see Chapter 4). Many disabilities begin in adulthood. Diseases, medical conditions, and injuries can cause disabilities. Disabilities can also begin before adulthood.

A **developmental disability** is a disability that occurs before birth, at birth, or during childhood or adolescence. It impairs the child's development. It is often severe and is always permanent. Although the disability begins before adulthood, it remains for the person's entire life. Therefore, people of all ages can have developmental disabilities.

Developmental disabilities affect physical or mental function, or both. The developmental disability limits the person's ability to function in at least three of the following life activities:

- Self-care (eating, dressing, hygiene)
- Understanding and expressing speech and language
- Learning
- Mobility (getting around independently)
- Self-direction (solving problems and making choices and decisions)
- Independent living
- Economic self-sufficiency (earning enough income to support oneself financially)

Most people with developmental disabilities need lifelong assistance, support, and special services. The health care team is involved in the person's care.

Developmental Disabilities and the Family

Families of children with developmental disabilities may face many challenges. Be sensitive to the family's situation. Some families you work with may be adjusting to the news of a child's disability. They may still be working out new roles and routines for all family members. They may be under great stress. Others may have established roles and routines. Remember, every family situation is different.

Most children with disabilities live with their families at home. Being a primary caregiver for a child with disabilities can be an all-consuming task. It often takes great amounts of time, energy, and work. Many caregivers have to balance caregiving with other responsibilities, including full-time jobs and other children. The parents may not leave the child or spend time alone because they do not want to impose on family or friends to care for the child. Parents may not be able to spend as much time with their other children as they would like. Parental caregivers often worry about the stigma associated with their child's disability. They may feel that their child is considered different by society. They may encounter discrimination and other barriers. The constant stress and work of caregiving can lead to burnout (see Chapter 8). The caregiver can become physically and emotionally exhausted.

Home care and other community agencies often provide needed support and services. You will work closely with the family. You may do household tasks so that the parents can spend more time with the child and their other children. Or you may provide respite care so the parents can have a break. You also may directly assist the child according to the care plan. For example, you might help with the child's rehabilitation activities under the supervision of a physical or occupational therapist. Or you might accompany the child to and from school (Figure 38-1). Some support workers work with children in the school. Children with severe disabilities may need long-term care in special facilities.

As the child and parents grow older, caring for the adolescent or adult child is often more physically difficult. Parents may not be able to lift or move the adolescent or adult child. A parent may become ill, injured, or disabled. A parent may die. Yet the person with the developmental disability still needs care.

Some adolescents and adults with developmental disabilities live in community and residential settings. They may live in their own home. Or they may live in group homes. Others live in specially licensed long-term care facilities. Staff must receive special training to prepare them to meet the needs of residents with developmental disabilities. Often the person's family is still involved with his or her care. Remember that usually the family members have cared for the person for most of his or her life. They understand the person's condition and needs. Include family members whenever appropriate when providing care and services.

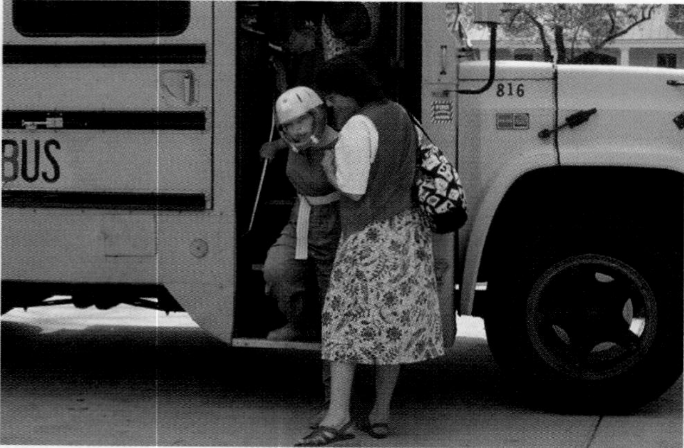

Figure 38-1 You might accompany a child with disabilities to and from school.

Types of Developmental Disabilities

There are many kinds of developmental disabilities. Generally, they are caused by conditions, illnesses, or accidents that injure the brain or body before birth, during birth, or during childhood or adolescence. These include, but are not limited to, the following:

- Intellectual disabilities
- Down syndrome
- Cerebral palsy
- Autism
- Epilepsy
- Spina bifida
- Fetal alcohol syndrome

Many children and adults have more than one condition that causes a disability. Table 38-1 lists other conditions that cause developmental disabilities.

Intellectual Disabilities

An **intellectual disability (cognitive disability)** is an impaired ability to learn. It results in below-average intelligence and limitations in the ability to function in certain areas of daily life. (*Intelligence* relates to learning, thinking, and reasoning.) The person can learn new skills, but at a slower rate than normal. A person with an intellectual disability often has difficulties with communication, self-care, and social interaction. Intellectual disability used to be called mental retardation. In Canada, the term mental retardation is no longer considered an acceptable label.

An intellectual disability can be caused by any genetic abnormality, injury, or disease that impairs development of the brain. For many people, the cause is unknown. Some common causes of intellectual disabilities are listed in Box 38-1 on page 630. People with an intellectual disability often have other disabilities as well.

Intellectual disabilities range from mild to severe. Tests that measure intelligence are called IQ tests. An average person without an intellectual disability has an IQ of about 90 to 100. People with IQ scores between 70 and 55 are considered mildly intellectually disabled. They may be slow to learn but can attend regular schools. As adults, they can function in society with some support. They can work and live in the community.

Table 38-1 Other Conditions Causing Developmental Disabilities

Acquired brain injury	Damage to brain tissue caused by disease, medical condition, accident, or violence. Some accidents and disease reduce oxygen to the brain. This destroys brain cells and can cause brain injury. For example, conditions during birth, near drownings, choking, suffocation, and stroke can cause brain injury. Certain infections or chemicals also destroy brain tissue. Meningitis, encephalitis, and mercury and lead poisoning are examples. Blows to the head that cause the brain to be battered within the skull also cause brain injury. Examples include motor vehicle accidents, falls, sport injuries, and child abuse (including shaking). Acquired brain injuries can be permanent and severe. They can result in personality changes, vision problems, speech problems, muscle control problems, and intellectual disability.
Congenital heart disease	Abnormalities in the structure or function of the heart that are present before birth. If they survive, babies and children may tire easily or experience delayed growth. Most congenital heart conditions must be corrected by surgery.
Fragile X	A genetic condition caused by changes in the X chromosome. Boys and girls can be affected, but boys are usually affected more severely. It causes intellectual disability. There is no cure.
Hydrocephalus	A condition in which fluid collects in the brain. (Hydro means water. Cephalo means head.) Left untreated, it causes the head to enlarge and increases pressure on the brain. If the child survives, intellectual disability and neurological damage may result. To treat hydrocephalus, a shunt (a long, flexible tube) is placed in the brain and connected to a body cavity, usually the abdomen or a heart chamber. The shunt is completely enclosed inside the person's body. Fluid drains from the brain through the tube into the body cavity. Shunts usually stay in place for the remainder of the person's life.
Phenylketonuria (PKU)	An inherited condition in which the body lacks an enzyme necessary to process a certain amino acid (phenylalanine). When this amino acid builds up in the blood, it injures brain tissue. Left untreated, PKU causes intellectual disability and neurological problems. PKU can be detected with a blood test in the first few days of life. With proper treatment, brain injury can be avoided. Treatment involves maintaining a strict diet throughout life.
Shaken baby syndrome	A term for the physical and cognitive impairments caused by shaking a baby or young child. Babies and young children have weak neck muscles. Shaking them causes the head to forcefully swing back and forth. As a result, the brain bangs against the skull wall. Bleeding behind the eyes and in the brain can occur. Permanent brain injury can result. So can seizures, partial or total blindness, paralysis, intellectual disability, or death. Less violent but frequent shaking of a young child can also cause long-term effects, including attention deficits and learning disabilities.

Support is not needed every day. People who have IQ scores below 55 are moderately intellectually disabled. They need daily support at home or at work. People with IQ scores below 25 are severely intellectually disabled. They need constant support in all areas.

The Canadian Association for Community Living is a national association dedicated to people with intellectual disabilities and their families. The association's goal is to ensure that people with intellectual disabilities have opportunities to live meaningful, dignified lives. The association's philosophy is that people with intellectual disabilities can and should be allowed to participate in all aspects of community living. Children should live in families and be integrated into regular schools whenever possible. They should play with others who do and do not have disabilities. Adults with intellectual disabilities have the right to control their lives to the fullest extent possible. That is, they should make choices and decisions about their care and how they live. They should have friends, work at jobs, enjoy adult activities, and contribute to their communities.

People with intellectual disabilities have sexual, emotional, and social needs and desires, just like everyone else. They have the right to privacy and to love and be loved. Remember, intellectual disabilities vary from mild to severe. Some adults with intellectual disabilities have life partners. Others marry and have children.

Most people with intellectual disabilities can control their sexual urges. A few cannot. The type and location of their sexual responses may be inappropriate.

Box 38-1 Causes of Intellectual Disability

Genetic Conditions
- Abnormal genes inherited from one or both parents—Fragile X and phenylketonuria (PKU) are genetic disorders that cause intellectual disability
- Missing or extra chromosomes—Down syndrome is a chromosome disorder that causes intellectual disability

Problems during Pregnancy
- Alcohol or drug use by the pregnant mother
- Poor nutrition
- Exposure of the pregnant mother to certain environmental hazards, such as X-rays or certain chemicals
- Illnesses of the mother, such as rubella (German measles) or syphilis
- Uncontrolled medical conditions, such as diabetes or HIV infection

Problems at Birth
- Premature birth
- Low birth weight
- Lack of oxygen to the baby's brain during birth

Problems after Birth
- Childhood diseases, such as whooping cough, chickenpox, and measles
- Infections, such as meningitis and encephalitis
- Acquired brain injury caused by accidents, disease, or abuse
- Severe malnutrition or neglect

(See Chapter 19 for how to deal with sexually aggressive clients.) Children and adults with intellectual disabilities are vulnerable to sexual abuse. Report signs of sexual abuse immediately (see Chapter 19). Children with intellectual disabilities need to learn about sexual abuse, safe sex, and other sexuality issues.

Down Syndrome

Down syndrome (DS) is a disorder caused by an extra chromosome. At fertilization, a male sex cell (sperm) unites with a female sex cell (ovum). Each sex cell has 23 chromosomes. When they unite, the cell has 46 chromosomes. With DS an extra chromosome is present. The person has 47 chromosomes. Thus DS occurs at fertilization and is a congenital condition. (**Congenital** means present at birth.)

In Canada, DS is the most common congenital chromosome disorder. There are 14 babies born with DS for every 10 000 births.[1]

DS causes varying degrees of intellectual disability—usually moderate to severe. The child also has certain physical features caused by the extra chromosome (Figure 38-2):

- Small head
- Oval-shaped eyes that slant upward
- Flat face
- Short, wide neck
- Large tongue
- Wide, flat nose
- Small ears
- Short stature
- Short, wide hands with stubby fingers
- Weak muscle tone

Many children with DS have congenital heart defects. They also tend to have vision and hearing problems. They are at risk for ear infections, respiratory infections, and thyroid gland problems. Leukemia also is a risk. After age 35, adults with DS are at risk for Alzheimer's disease.

People with DS need speech, language, physical, and occupational therapies. Most learn self-care skills. They also need health and sex education. Weight gain and constipation often are problems. They need a well-balanced diet and regular exercise.

Cerebral Palsy

Cerebral palsy (CP) is a disorder affecting muscle control (*palsy*). It is caused by an injury or abnormality in the motor region of the brain (*cerebral*). Depending on which areas of the brain have been injured, one or more of the following may occur:

- Involuntary movements
- Poor coordination and posture
- Muscle weakness
- Difficulty or inability to walk
- Difficulty or inability to speak

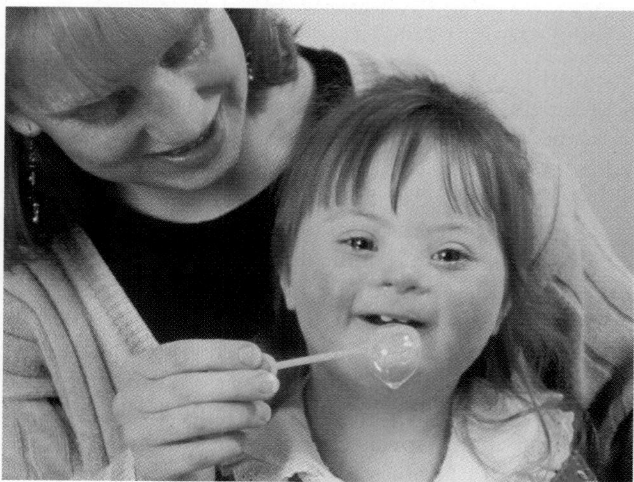

Figure 38-2 A child with Down syndrome.

CP occurs before, during, or shortly after birth. Lack of oxygen to the fetal or newborn brain is the usual cause. Infants at risk include those who:

- Are premature
- Have a low birth weight
- Do not cry in the first 5 minutes after birth
- Need mechanical ventilation
- Have bleeding in the brain
- Have heart, kidney, or spinal cord abnormalities
- Have blood problems
- Have seizures

Acquired brain injury in infancy and early childhood also can result in CP (see Table 38-1 on page 629).

Body movements and body parts are affected. These types of CP are the most common:

- *Spastic cerebral palsy*—**Spastic** means uncontrolled contractions of skeletal muscles. (*Spastic* comes from *spastikos,* meaning to draw in.) Muscles contract or shorten. They are stiff and cannot relax. One or both sides of the body may be involved. Posture, balance, and movement are affected. Movement is stiff and jerky. The person's arms may be affected. If so, he or she has problems with eating, writing, dressing, and other activities of daily living. If the person's legs are affected, he or she has problems with walking or moving. This is the most common type of CP. About half of all cases of CP are spastic CP.
- *Athetoid cerebral palsy*—The person cannot control movements. (*Athetoid* comes from *athetos,* meaning not fixed.) The person has involuntary, constant, slow weaving or writhing motions that occur in the trunk, arms, hands, legs, and feet. The person might have difficulty reaching for and grasping objects. The person might have trouble remaining upright for sitting or standing. Sometimes the tongue, face, and neck muscles are involved. As a result, the person might drool or grimace.
- *Ataxic cerebral palsy*—The person has weak muscle tone and difficulties coordinating movement. (*A* means absence of, and *taxis* means arrangement or order.) The person appears very unsteady and shaky. The person also has troubles balancing. As a result, he or she may be very unsteady when walking.

Certain terms are used to describe the body parts affected by CP (see Chapter 31):

- *Hemiplegia—Hemi* means half. *Plegia* means complete or partial loss of ability to move. The CP affects one side of the body. The right arm and leg or the left arm and leg are affected. The other side functions normally. The person may be able to walk, but might look a little awkward.
- *Diplegia—Di* means two. With **diplegia** there is loss of ability to move (*plegia*) corresponding parts on both (*di*) sides of the body. In most cases of diplegia caused by CP, both legs are affected. The person has difficulty walking, but the upper body is not affected. (In extremely rare cases, both arms are affected, but not the legs.)
- *Quadriplegia—Quad* means four. The CP affects all four limbs (both arms and both legs). The person cannot walk or use the arms. Usually the person also has difficulty moving the face and trunk. Talking and eating may be difficult. The person needs a wheelchair to get around.

Some people with CP are only mildly affected. Their movements are awkward, but they can walk independently and are not otherwise affected. They are not intellectually disabled. However, other people with CP are severely affected. They can also have many other impairments and problems. These include:

- Intellectual disability
- Learning disabilities
- Hearing impairments
- Speech impairments
- Vision impairments
- Drooling
- Bladder and bowel control problems
- Seizures
- Difficulty swallowing
- Attention deficit hyperactivity disorder (short attention span, poor concentration, and increased activity)
- Breathing problems from poor posture
- Pressure ulcers from immobility

Care depends on the severity of the CP and the needs of the person. The goal is for the person to be as independent as possible. Physical, occupational, and speech therapy can help. Some people need eyeglasses or hearing aids. Surgery and medications can help some muscle problems. You may assist with range-of-motion exercises and activities of daily living.

Autism

Autism is a brain disorder that impairs communication, social skills, and behaviour. The person has extreme difficulties relating to others. *Autos* means self; with autism, the person withdraws into the self. It may seem as if people with autism are in their own world. They often seem uninterested in others. For example, they may not notice when someone enters a room. Or they may prefer to play alone. Some avoid physical contact or become very upset when touched.

Both verbal and nonverbal communication are affected. Many people with autism do not develop speech. They often avoid eye contact or refuse to interact. Some are unable to understand the facial expressions of others.

Autism begins in early childhood—between the ages of 18 months and 3 years. In Canada, about 1 in 200 children is diagnosed with autism. It is the most common brain disorder affecting children.[2] Boys are affected more often than girls.

Autism affects each person differently. People are mildly to severely affected. The following symptoms are common:

- Develops language skills slowly, if at all
- Repeats words or phrases
- Does not start or maintain conversations
- Repeats body movements (hand flapping, finger flicking, rocking)
- Has short attention span
- Spends time alone
- Shows little reaction to pain
- Over-reacts to noise and touch
- Does not like to cuddle
- Has frequent tantrums for no apparent reason
- Forms strong attachment to a single item, idea, activity, or person
- Needs routines; does not like change
- Does not fear danger
- Does not respond to others
- Is very active or very quiet
- Displays aggressive or violent behaviour
- May injure self

There is no cure for autism. However, with therapy, the person may learn to change or control behaviours. Many therapies may be used:

- Behaviour modification—positive behaviours are rewarded and negative behaviours are corrected
- Speech and language therapy
- Music, auditory, recreation, and sensory therapies
- Occupational therapy
- Medication therapy
- Diet therapy

The person needs to develop social and work skills. Some adults with autism work and live independently. Others need support and help from family and community services. Some live in group homes or residential care facilities.

People with autism may have other disorders. Intellectual disability and epilepsy are common.

When working with children or adults with autism, remember that strict routines are usually important. The person may become very upset if his or her routine is disrupted. Follow the person's routine whenever possible. Warn the person if the routine must be changed. Children require careful supervision. Do not leave the child unattended for even a moment. The care plan provides directions for how to interact with the person.

EPILEPSY

Epilepsy is a condition characterized by recurrent seizures. (Epilepsy comes from the word *epilepsia*, meaning seizure.) Recurrent means occurring from time to time. A **seizure** is a brief disturbance in the brain's normal electrical function. Seizures affect awareness, movement and/or sensation.

Seizures that affect only one part of the brain are called *partial seizures*. Seizures that affect the whole brain are called *generalized seizures*. The area of the brain affected by the seizure temporarily loses its ability to function normally. Therefore seizures cause different reactions depending on the part of the brain affected. For example, some seizures cause the person to briefly stare and appear unresponsive. Other seizures (called **tonic-clonic seizures**) involve convulsions. A **convulsion** is violent and sudden contractions or tremors of muscle groups. The person loses consciousness and falls to the floor. All muscle groups contract and relax, causing jerking and twitching movements of the body. Urinary and bowel incontinence may occur. A tonic-clonic seizure usually lasts for 1 to 7 minutes.

A single seizure does not mean the person has epilepsy. Many factors can cause a single seizure. With epilepsy, the person has recurring seizures. The electrical system in the brain is permanently damaged, making it susceptible to seizures.

Often, the cause of a person's epilepsy is not known. Known causes of epilepsy include acquired brain injuries (see Box 38-1 on page 630), brain tumours, genetic conditions, and problems with brain development before birth.

Children and young adults are commonly affected. However, epilepsy can develop at any time during a person's life. It can occur with any problem affecting the brain. Such problems include cerebral palsy, intellectual disability, autism, Alzheimer's disease, stroke, tumours, and acquired brain injury.

There is no cure for epilepsy. A physician may order medications to prevent seizures. The medications control seizures for many people. For others, medication does not work. Some people have brain surgery to reduce the frequency of the seizures.

When controlled, epilepsy usually does not affect learning and activities of daily living. In severe cases, people may be limited in their activities. For example, a person who has frequent seizures may not be allowed to drive. This may limit job choices. Safety measures are needed for the home, workplace, transportation, and recreation.

People with epilepsy have an increased risk of death. They have higher rates of suicide and sudden, unexplained death. They also have higher rates of accidental death, especially drowning.

See Chapter 47 for emergency care of people having seizures.

Spina Bifida

Spina bifida is a congenital disorder involving improper closing of the spine before birth. (*Spina* means backbone. *Bifida* means split in two parts.) Spina bifida is a *neural tube defect (NTD)*. These are congenital conditions that involve the incomplete development of the brain, spinal cord, and protective coverings for these organs. Neural tube defects occur during the first months of pregnancy. Consuming sufficient folic acid before conception and during early pregnancy greatly reduces the risk of having a baby with neural tube defects (see Chapter 25).

Bones of the spinal column (vertebrae) protect the spinal cord. With spinal bifida, vertebrae do not close properly, leaving the spina cord unprotected. The spinal cord contains nerves that send messages to and from the brain. If the spinal cord is unprotected, nerve damage occurs. Affected body parts do not function properly and partial or complete paralysis may occur. Loss of bowel and bladder control may also result. Infection of the exposed spinal cord is a risk.

Spina bifida can occur anywhere in the spine. The lower back is the most common site. Types of spina bifida include:

- *Spina bifida occulta—Occult* means hidden. This is the mildest form of spina bifida. A slight deficiency occurs in the vertebrae closure. However, the spinal cord and the membrane that covers it (the *meninges*) remain in place. Skin usually covers the defect. In other words, the defect is hidden. The person may have a dimple or tuft of hair on the back (Figure 38-3). The spinal cord and nerves are normal. It rarely causes disability. Often there are no symptoms. Foot weakness and bowel and bladder problems can occur.
- *Spina bifida cystica—Cystica* means cyst or sac. Part of the spinal column is in a pouch or sac that protrudes from the opening in the spine. A membrane or a thin layer of skin covers the sac. It looks like a large blister. Because the pouch is easily injured, infection is a risk. There are two types of spina bifida cystica (Figure 38-4):
  - *Meningocele—Menigo* comes from *meninx*, meaning membrane. *Cele* means hernia or swelling. Meninges is the connective tissue that covers and protects the brain and spinal cord. Cerebrospinal fluid also protects the brain and spinal cord. With this type of spina bifida, a sac containing meninges and cerebrospinal fluid protrudes from the spine (see Figure 38-4, *A*, and Figure 38-5). The sac does not contain nerve tissue. The spinal cord and nerves are usually unaffected.

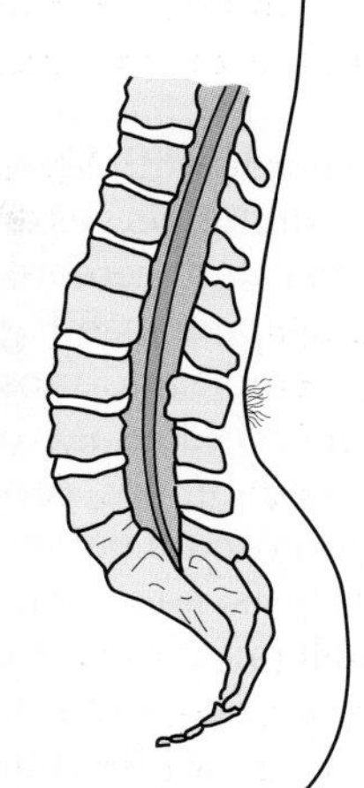

Figure 38-3 Spina bifida occulta.

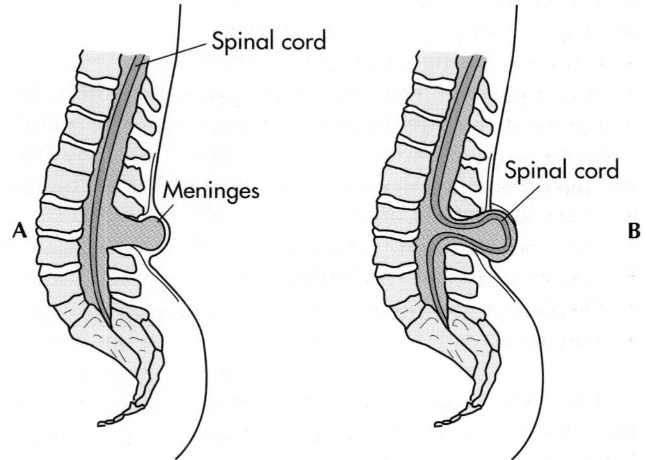

Figure 38-4 **A,** Meningocele. **B,** Myelomeningocele.

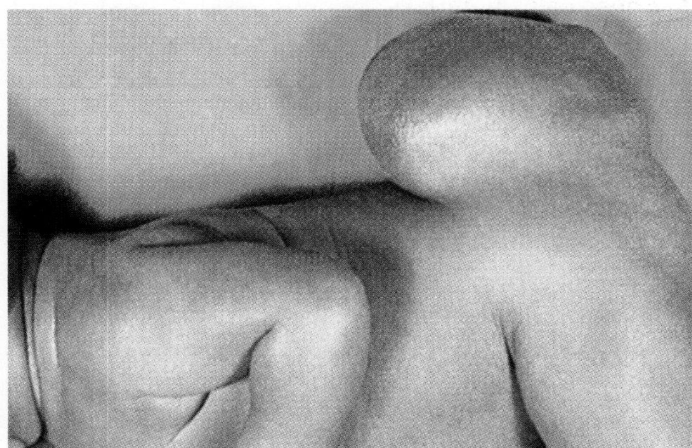

Figure 38-5 Meningocele. Surgery is performed to close the infant's back shortly after birth. Source: B.J. Zitelli and H.W. Davis, *Atlas of Pediatric Physical Diagnosis* (St. Louis: Gower Medical Publishing, 1987).

Nerve damage usually does not occur. It is corrected by surgery.
- *Myelomeningocele* (or *meningomyelocele*)—*Myelo* means spinal cord. With this type of spina bifida, a sac containing nerves, a part of the spinal cord, meninges, and cerebrospinal fluid protrudes from the spine (see Figure 38-4, *B*). This is the most common and most serious form of spina bifida. Nerve damage occurs. The spinal cord is damaged or not properly developed. Loss of function occurs below the level of damage. Leg paralysis and lack of sensation are common problems. So is lack of bowel and bladder control. The baby's back is closed with surgery, usually soon after birth. Some children and adults walk with braces or crutches. Others use wheelchairs.

People with spina bifida may have other problems or conditions. For example, some have learning problems. They may have problems with attention, language, reading, and math. They are at risk for obesity, gastrointestinal disorders, and mobility problems. Skin breakdown, depression, and social, emotional, and sexual issues are other risks. Hydrocephalus often occurs with certain types of spina bifida (see Table 38-1 on page 629).

Fetal Alcohol Syndrome

Fetal alcohol syndrome (FAS) is a group of physical and mental abnormalities in a child as a result of alcohol consumption by the mother during pregnancy. In Canada, one child is born with FAS every day.[3] It is the most common preventable developmental disability.

Physical problems include low birth weight, weak muscle tone, and poor weight gain. Heart problems, hearing loss, and abnormalities of the spine and joints may also occur. The person may have characteristic facial features, including an abnormally small head, small eye openings, thin upper lip, and a small chin.

Usually the person with FAS has an intellectual disability. The person often has many behaviour, learning, and emotional problems. These include poor attention span, hyperactivity, poor motor skills, and slow language development. Older children and adults with FAS often have memory problems, poor judgment, difficulties with daily living skills, inability to manage anger, and poor social skills. Mental health problems are common. Many adolescents with FAS drop out of school and get in trouble with the law. Many adults with FAS are unable to work or live independently. They require on-going support.

Fetal alcohol effect (FAE) is a milder form of FAS. The same symptoms may occur, but to a lesser degree. Children with FAE are not usually intellectually disabled.

Caring for Clients with Developmental Disabilities

Clients with developmental disabilities often have complicated care needs, especially if the disability is severe. You must be familiar with special equipment and self-help devices needed for each client. Follow the care plan and consult with your supervisor if you have questions. For example, Gordon, aged 10, has severe cerebral palsy. He cannot walk and has limited use of his hands. He tends to slide down in his wheelchair. Therefore he uses a postural support to help him keep in good body alignment. He must be repositioned frequently to prevent pressure ulcers. Gordon also has a hearing impairment and has hearing aids in both ears. He also uses a computer to communicate. Gordon has splints on his ankles to prevent contractures. He uses a special spoon strapped to his wrist when eating.

When working with children and adults with developmental disabilities, remember to consider the person before the disability. For example, Gordon is an intelligent, sensitive 10-year-old. He enjoys reading, going on outings, and visiting with his support worker. He also happens to have severe cerebral palsy and use a wheelchair.

People with developmental disabilities have the same rights and needs as everyone else. Each person is unique. The effects of the disability vary depending on the person. Your supervisor and the care plan tell you how to best meet each client's needs. As always, your priority when caring for these clients is to promote their dignity, independence, preferences, privacy, and safety. (See *Providing Compassionate Care: Caring for Clients with Developmental Disabilities* box.)

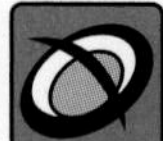

Providing Compassionate Care

Caring for Clients with Developmental Disabilities

D*ignity.* Adults and children with developmental disabilities deserve to be treated with respect and in a manner that promotes their dignity. Remember to consider the person before the disability. The words you use are an important way to show respect. For example, say "Clients with disabilities." Do not refer to them as "handicapped," "disabled," or "crippled." Also, do not say that the person is the disability. For example, it is correct to say "Mr. Joshi has autism." Do not say "Mr. Joshi is autistic." Or, say "Susan has an intellectual disability," not "Susan is retarded."

Have empathy but not pity. Remember, empathy means understanding the experiences and feelings of others. Pity means feeling sorry for others. To pity someone implies that you are superior to the person.

Also promote dignity through your actions. Extend the same courtesies and consideration that you show all clients. Be friendly. Talk with them. Be a good listener. Show interest in their lives. Children with disabilities are like all children. They need attention and love. They also need to play and have fun. Adults with disabilities are like all adults. They need support and encouragement. Treat them like adults. Shake hands when introduced. Offer to shake hands even if the person has an artificial limb, has limited function in the hand, or has to shake with the left hand. Speak directly to the person in a normal tone of voice. Address adults by their title and last name, unless they tell you otherwise.

I*ndependence.* The goal for people with disabilities is to be as independent as possible. Do not make assumptions about what the person can and cannot do. Follow the care plan. Encourage the person to use self-help devices when possible. Be patient. Do not rush the person.

P*references.* People with disabilities have the right to personal choice. Provide opportunities for the person to make choices and decisions. Ask first if the person wants help. Then ask how you can provide it. People with disabilities must consent to procedures before you start. If the person does not want you to continue, stop. Contact your supervisor. Also adapt your work to allow for the family's choices and preferences (unless told to do otherwise in the care plan).

P*rivacy.* Medical and personal information about the person is confidential. Only talk about the person with members of the health care team who need to know. Do not expose the person. Provide privacy when performing procedures. Drape the person so as not to expose the person's body. Remember that adults with disabilities have sexual needs. Many have partners or are married. Allow for privacy for sexual needs.

S*afety.* Most developmental disabilities create safety hazards for the person. Check with your supervisor and the care plan to determine how to provide for the person's safety. Practise the safety measures in Chapter 16. Also be aware of signs of abuse. Report these to your supervisor immediately. Remember, you also must report child abuse directly to a public authority (see Chapter 19).

REVIEW

Circle the BEST answer.

1. All developmental disabilities occur
   A. During adulthood
   B. From trauma
   C. During pregnancy
   D. Before birth, at birth, or during childhood or adolescence

2. These statements are about developmental disabilities. Which is *true*?
   A. Self-care, learning, and mobility are always affected.
   B. The disability is permanent.
   C. Physical and intellectual impairment always occur together.
   D. The person cannot hold a job.

3. All people with intellectual disabilities
   A. Cannot learn new skills
   B. Have IQ scores over 90
   C. Require care in a special setting
   D. Have an impaired ability to learn

4. An intellectual disability
   A. Is always severe
   B. Can occur before, during, or after birth
   C. Causes fluid to collect in the brain
   D. Affects the motor region in the brain

5. Down syndrome occurs
   A. At fertilization
   B. During the first month of pregnancy
   C. Any time before, during, or after birth
   D. From trauma

6. A person with Down syndrome always has some degree of
   A. Cerebral palsy
   B. Autism
   C. Impaired mobility
   D. Intellectual disability

7. Cerebral palsy is usually caused by
   A. An extra chromosome
   B. A high fever
   C. Lack of oxygen to the brain
   D. Infection during pregnancy

8. A person with the spastic type of cerebral palsy has problems with
   A. Learning
   B. Drooling
   C. Posture, balance, and movement
   D. Weaving motions of the trunk, arms, and legs

9. Autism begins
   A. At fertilization
   B. During pregnancy
   C. At birth
   D. In early childhood

10. A person with autism has
    A. Impaired movement
    B. Problems relating to people
    C. Diplegia
    D. A build-up of an amino acid in the blood

11. A person with epilepsy has
    A. Seizures
    B. Diplegia
    C. Weak muscle tone
    D. Low IQ

12. Which is used to control epilepsy?
    A. Physical therapy
    B. Occupational therapy
    C. Medications
    D. A shunt

13. Spina bifida involves
    A. Improper closing of the spine
    B. Seizures
    C. Abnormalities in the structure of the heart
    D. Changes in the X chromosome

14. Which is common with spina bifida?
    A. Short attention span
    B. Hearing and vision problems
    C. Seizures
    D. Bowel and bladder problems

15. Fetal alcohol syndrome is caused by
    A. Acquired brain injury
    B. Shaking an infant
    C. The mother drinking alcohol during pregnancy
    D. Abnormal chromosomes

Answers to these questions are on page 826.

CHAPTER

39

ASSISTING WITH MEDICATIONS

OBJECTIVES

- Define the key terms listed in this chapter
- Explain the difference between assisting with medications and administering medications
- Describe the different forms of medications
- Describe your role in assisting with medications
- List the five "rights" of assisting with medications
- Describe guidelines to follow when assisting with medications
- Learn the procedures described in this chapter

KEY TERMS

alternative remedies Herbal or other "natural" products that do not require a physician's prescription; not considered part of conventional medicine

medication A drug or other substance used to prevent or treat disease or illness

over-the-counter (OTC) medication A medication that can be bought without a physician's prescription

prescription (Rx) medication A medication that is prescribed by a physician and dispensed by a pharmacist

side effect An unwanted response to a medication that occurs with the intended response

Medications are drugs and other substances used to prevent or treat disease or illness. Many clients living in community settings take their medications independently. This is called *self-directed medication management*. However, some clients need assistance when taking medications. For example, some cannot reach the medicines or get them out of the container. Others have difficulties reading the labels. This chapter discusses how to assist clients with medications.

Assisting versus Administering

Assisting with medications and administering medications are two very different functions. Assist means *to help*; administer means *to give.*

Assisting with medications means helping clients self-medicate. For example, you hand them their medications. Or you open the bottles or packages for them. This is strictly a *mechanical* function, meaning that you take the place of the client's hands or feet in order for the client to obtain the medication.

Administering medications involves measuring medications or getting them into the person's body. Administering medications requires special judgment and knowledge. Patients and residents in facilities usually have medications administered to them. Some home care clients also need health care workers to administer their medications. *Administering medications is beyond your scope of practice.* Never assume this responsibility. Some provinces and territories allow support workers to administer some forms of medications under certain conditions. The function must be in your job description. You must be formally trained, supervised, and monitored.

A small mistake when assisting with or administering medications can cause serious harm. Follow employer policies and provincial/territorial laws to protect your clients, your employer, and yourself.

Types of Medications

Medications come in many forms. Table 39-1 lists some of the most common types.

Clients may take:

- ***Over-the-counter (OTC) medications***—medications that can be bought without a physician's prescription. Acetaminophen (such as Tylenol) and cough syrups are examples.
- ***Alternative remedies***—herbal or other "natural" products that do not require a physician's prescription. Alternative remedies are usually not considered part of conventional medicine. Ginseng and shark cartilage are examples.
- ***Prescription (Rx) medications***—medications that require a physician's prescription and are dispensed by a pharmacist. Antibiotics and blood pressure medications are examples.

You only assist with medications that are listed in the care plan. If a client requests your help with medications that are not in the care plan (including OTC medications and alternative remedies), notify your supervisor.

Clients might ask support workers to purchase or obtain OTC medications or alternative remedies for them. Respectfully, but firmly, refuse to do so. Inform your supervisor about the client's request.

Mixing certain medications or mixing medications with alternative remedies can cause serious harm. Therefore, clients should *never* take any medication or alternative remedy without the physician's knowledge.

Your Role

Your role in assisting with medications depends on your provincial or territorial legislation, employer

(text continues on page 640)

This chapter is adapted from J. Birchenall and E. Streight, *Mosby's Textbook for the Home Care Aide* (St. Louis: Mosby, 1997). The author acknowledges the contribution of Joan Birchenall and Eileen Streight.

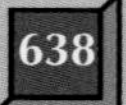

Table 39-1 Types of Medications

SOLIDS	
Capsules	Small gelatin containers that hold medications. 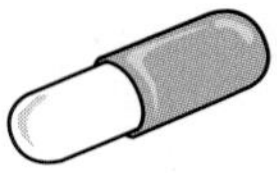
Lozenges	Flat disks containing medication in a flavoured base. Lozenges are held in the mouth, where they dissolve and slowly release medication. 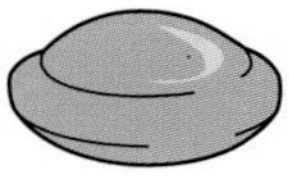
Tablets	Dry, powdered medications that have been formed into hard disks or cylinders. 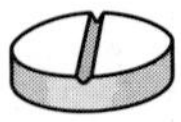
Ointments	Semisolid material containing medication. These are applied externally. 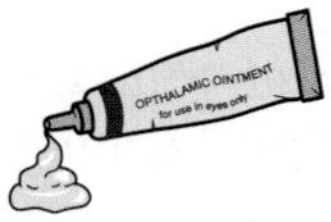
Suppositories	Solid form of medication for insertion into the rectum or vagina. Body temperature causes the suppository to melt and medication is released. 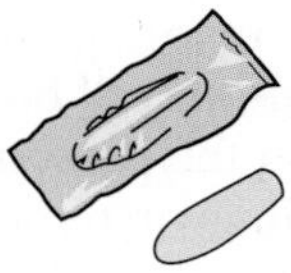
Transdermal disks or patches	Medication is on a small disk or patch that is applied to unbroken skin. The medication is absorbed through the skin over a 24-hour period. 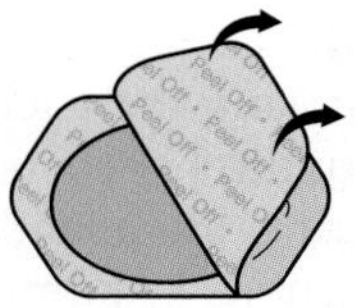
LIQUIDS	
Elixirs	Medication is dissolved in liquid containing alcohol or water and flavourings.
Suspensions	Medication is suspended in a liquid and may be labelled "Shake before using."
Syrups	Medication is dissolved in a concentrated sugar solution.

Continued

Table 39-1 Types of Medications—cont'd

Drops	Liquid form of medication in a special container that allows one drop at a time to be administered. Usual types are eye drops, ear drops, and nose drops.
Liquid for injection	Liquid form of medication that is injected using a *syringe* (a device consisting of a plastic tube filled with medication, a plunger, and an attached needle).
OTHERS	
Aerosols	Medication particles are suspended in air or gas. They are inhaled into the lungs. These are administered through a *metered dose inhaler (MDI)*. An MDI ("puffer" or "inhaler") is a small cylinder used with a special delivery system. The person uses it to inhale the medication through the mouth in specifically measured (metered) doses.

policy, and your training and education. It may involve one or more of the following:

- Reminding the client to take a medication
- Bringing medication containers to the client
- Bringing pre-poured medications, pre-filled syringes, or pill boxes to the client
- Reading the prescription label to the client
- Loosening or removing container lids or opening blister packs
- Checking the dosage against the medication label
- Providing water or other fluids as needed
- Supervising the client as he or she pours the medication into hand, measuring spoon, or cup
- Steadying the client's hand while he or she pours medications or administers eye drops, nasal sprays, etc.

You are *not* responsible for monitoring the outcome of the drug therapy. The physician, RN, or case manager is responsible for this. However, you must observe for and report any changes in the client's condition or behaviour. These changes might be caused by side effects of the medication. A **side effect** is an unwanted response to a medication that occurs with the intended response. For example, a person taking pain medication may feel pain relief, but may also experience drowsiness, nausea, and constipation. Many side effects are predictable and harmless. Other side effects can be so serious that the physician may order the medication to be stopped.

The nurse or pharmacist teaches the client about the medications he or she is taking. Clients should be able to take medications accurately. They should know the medication's desired effect, when and how to take the medication, any side effects to watch for, and foods or other medications to avoid or omit. If your client does not know this information, notify your supervisor.

Clients often store medications in a pill box (Figure 39-1). Pill boxes have compartments that organize the medications by day or by hour. They help people remember what they have taken and what medications remain to be taken each day. If the client is unable to fill the pill box, a nurse or family member may do so. This is *not* your responsibility.

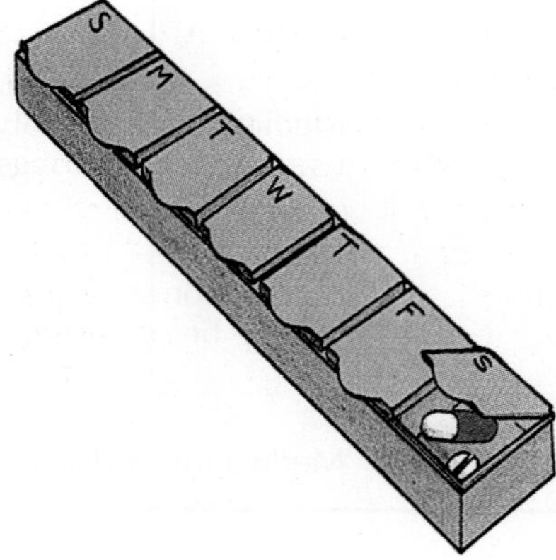

Figure 39-1 Pill boxes help clients keep track of their daily medications.

Documentation

The client's medication needs and your responsibilities are detailed in the care plan. A Medication Administration Record (MAR) also lists medication needs and serves as a record for actions taken. The exact form of the MAR varies by setting and employer. It always contains at least the following:

- The client's name
- The name, dose, and administration instructions for each medication
- A place to sign or initial after administering the medication

The MAR may also contain extra information such as the client's allergies, expected side effects, and special instructions (Figure 39-2 on page 642).

In facilities, a nurse is responsible for signing or initialling the MAR. In some facilities, an MAR is printed out daily for each client.

In community settings, an MAR is kept only when necessary to track specific medications and dosages. Clients who administer their own medications may not need an MAR. However, if an MAR is required, it is kept in the client's home. If a nurse administers the medications, the nurse signs the MAR. If the client self-medicates, the client signs the MAR. The nurse teaches the client this task. Observe as the client records after the medication was taken. Some clients may not be able to write on the MAR because of physical disability or vision problems. You may be asked to record for these clients.

Follow your employer's policies and procedures for recording. Ask your supervisor for help, if needed.

Understanding Abbreviations

Physicians, nurses, and pharmacists use many abbreviations when ordering and managing medications. The care plan and MAR should present information as clearly as possible. However, sometimes abbreviations are used in these documents. An abbreviation is a shortened form of a word or phrase. Table 39-2 on page 643 lists a few of the more common abbreviations used in health care settings (see Chapter 48).

Check with your supervisor for abbreviations used by your employer. If you are unsure about the meaning of an abbreviation, you must ask your supervisor. Never guess about the meaning of an abbreviation. Doing so can cause serious harm to the client.

Five "Rights" of Assisting with Medications

To help clients take medications accurately and safely, know and follow the five "rights" of assisting with medications: the right medication, the right person, the right dose, the right route, and the right time (Box 39-1 on page 643).

- *The right medication*. Be sure you are assisting the client to take the right medication. The name of the medication is listed on the prescription label on the medication container (Figure 39-3 on page 643). Read the label and make sure it is the same medication listed in the care plan and the MAR. Check twice.
- *The right person*. Be sure the medication is for your client. Check the prescription label on the medication container. Make sure it has the person's name on it. The label should include the person's first and last names. In some homes and facilities, two people may have the same name. Make sure you are assisting the right person. Identify the person following employer policy.
- *The right dose*. The dose is listed on the prescription label, the care plan, and the MAR. For example: "Take one tablet daily" or "Apply ointment to left elbow twice a day." The correct amount of medication must be taken. For example, Mrs. Jong removes two tablets from the container. The prescription label and her care plan say she is to take only one tablet. You must remind her to take only one tablet.

  When the medication is in a liquid form, the dose measurements may be in imperial (teaspoons or tablespoons) or in metric (millilitres) units. Be sure the client does not measure in teaspoons when the prescription calls for millilitres. Make sure the client uses measuring spoons and measuring cups—not household spoons or cups—to measure medication doses.
- *The right route*. The method in which the medication is taken is called the route. The prescription label, care plan, and MAR list the route. The routes are as follows:
  - *Oral*—taken by mouth and swallowed. Cough syrup is an example.
  - *Sublingual*—placed under the tongue. These are pills, tablets, or sprays. They are dissolved or absorbed into the body.
  - *Topical*—applied to the skin or mucous membranes. Some topical medications are contained to the area in which they are applied. Examples are ointments, eye drops, and nose drops. Others are absorbed into the bloodstream and travel throughout the body. Examples are medications applied by transdermal disks or patches. Suppositories and medicated enemas are also topical medications because they are applied to the mucous membranes (in the rectum or vagina).
  - *Inhalant*—breathed in through the mouth or nose. Medication must be in a gas or aerosol form. Examples include oxygen and medications delivered by metered dose inhalers.

(text continues on page 643)

MEDICATION ADMINISTRATION RECORD

Name	Delbert Sullivan							
Day		SUN	MON	TUE	WED	THUR	FRI	SAT
Date		7/11	7/12	7/13	7/14	7/15	7/16	7/17
Drug Name	Lasix (water pill)							
Dose	1 tablet							
Action	Increases urination							
Time	One (1) daily	8 a.m.	8 a.m.	8 a.m.	8 a.m.	8 a.m.	8 a.m.	8 a.m.
		JKS						
Special Instructions	Daily weight at 8 a.m.							
	Drink plenty of fluids.							
	Watch for and report any weight gain or swelling.							
	Do not omit or increase dosage.							
	Call doctor if unable to take medication.							
Immediately Report								
Day		SUN	MON	TUE	WED	THUR	FRI	SAT
Date		7/11	7/12	7/13	7/14	7/15	7/16	7/17
Drug Name	Ferrous Sulfate (iron pill)							
Dose	1 tablet							
Action	Replaces iron in blood.							
Time	Three (3) times daily	9 a.m.	9 a.m.	9 a.m.	9 a.m.	9 a.m.	9 a.m.	9 a.m.
		1 p.m.	1 p.m.	1 p.m.	1 p.m.	1 p.m.	1 p.m.	1 p.m.
		5 p.m.	5 p.m.	5 p.m.	5 p.m.	5 p.m.	5 p.m.	5 p.m.
		JKS						
		JKS						
		JKS						
Special Instructions	Take between meals.							
	Take with full glass of water.							
	Do not take with milk or antacids.							
	Will change color of stool to black.							
	Do not crush tablet.							
	May cause constipation.							
Immediately Report	Nausea, vomiting, and diarrhea							
	Abdominal pain							

Figure 39-2 A sample medication administration record (MAR).

Table 39-2 Common Abbreviations

Abbreviation	Meaning
bid	Twice a day
hs	Hour of sleep
npo	Nothing by mouth
po	By mouth
prn	When necessary
pr	Per rectum
qd	Every day
qh	Every (q) hour (h)
q2h, q3h, etc.	Every 2 hours, every 3 hours, and so on
qid	4 times a day
sl	Sublingual

Box 39-1 The Five "Rights" of Assisting with Medications

1. *Right medication.* Read the container label. Check against the MAR and care plan.
2. *Right person.* Read the container label. Be sure the medication is for the client. Identify the client according to employer policies.
3. *Right dose.* Be sure you know how much medication the client should be taking.
4. *Right route.* Be sure you know the correct route and form of the medication.
5. *Right time.* Bring medication to the client at correct time or remind the client to take medications.

If you have any questions or problems with any of these five "rights," notify your supervisor.

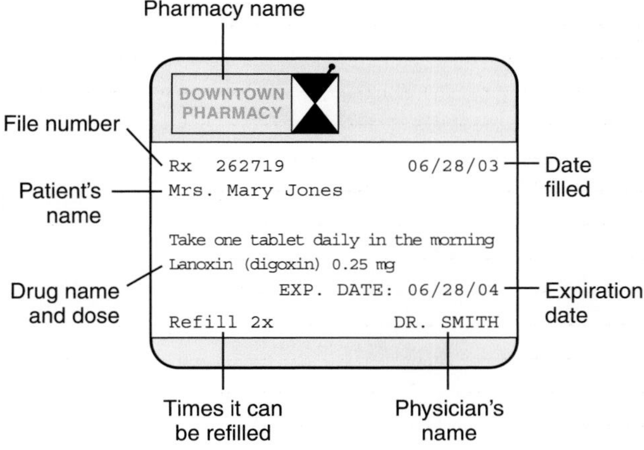

Figure 39-3 Read the prescription label before the client takes any medications.

- *Parenteral*—injected by a needle into the muscle (intramuscular), a vein (intravenous), or under the skin (subcutaneous). Insulin and IV drips are examples.

- *The right time.* To work properly, medications must be taken at the correct time. Some are taken once a day; others are taken 2, 3, or 4 times a day. The prescription label states how often the medication is to be taken. For example, Mrs. Jong's prescription label states that the medication must be taken 3 times a day. The care plan and MAR state the exact times that the client is to take the medication. For example, Mrs. Jong's care plan and MAR state she is to take her medication at 0600, 1400, and 2200.

Some medications have to be taken when the stomach is empty—that is, 1 hour before or 2 hours after eating. Other medications need to be taken at mealtime to reduce stomach upset and help with absorption. These prescription labels will say "take on empty stomach" or "take with food or milk."

Sometimes people must avoid certain foods or beverages when taking medications. Alcohol and tobacco often must be avoided. Follow the warning labels on the prescription containers. Also follow the care plan.

Sometimes people are confused about when to take their medications. A client may say, "I can never remember. Do I take two tablets at 3 o'clock, or three tablets at 2 o'clock?" Tell your supervisor if this happens. The person may need a "refresher" course on taking medications properly.

Assist the client to take all medications at the right time. If you go on an outing with the client, bring along the medications that must be taken during the outing.

Assisting with Medications

When assisting with medications, follow the guidelines in Box 39-2 on page 644. Check the care plan to see how much assistance is required.

Box 39-2 Guidelines for Assisting Clients with Medications

- Always follow employer policy.
- Review the care plan with your supervisor before assisting the person with medications. Follow the five "rights" of assisting with medications (see Box 39-1 on page 643).
- Bring the right medication containers to the person. Read the labels carefully. Compare container labels with the care plan and the MAR.
- Know the correct dose of each medication. Check the care plan and the MAR.
- Give a glass of water (or other liquid) with oral medications as ordered.
- Store medications:
  - In a special place just for the person's medications; the person's medications are stored separately from those of others
  - In a dry, cool place (not in the bathroom medicine cabinet)
  - Out of reach of children and adults with dementia
  - In the original labelled container
  - With lids tightly closed
  - According to any special storage directions; for example, "store in refrigerator"
- Do not leave medications at the bedside. Do not assume that the person will take them correctly. Remain with the person until he or she has finished taking the medications.
- Do not remove labels from medication containers.
- Never use a medication container that is unlabelled. Do not take medication from a container where the label cannot be read.
- Do not use discoloured or deteriorated medications. Check the expiry date on the labels before giving medications to the person. Notify your supervisor of expired or deteriorated medications.
- If you notice the medications are running low, tell the person or family and your supervisor.
- Check with your supervisor before discarding any unused medications.
- Listen to the person. If he or she questions something about a medication, STOP—do not assist with self-medication. Call your supervisor immediately.
- Report to your supervisor if the person:
  - Does not take medications correctly
  - Does not know why the medication is being taken, the dosage, or the time schedule
  - Refuses to take the medication, or forgets or omits a dose; the person should not take a double dose if one is omitted
  - Shows any side effects (for example, vomiting, rash, breathing difficulty, itching, or diarrhea)
  - Wants to take medications (including OTC medications or alternative remedies) that are not listed on the MAR and care plan
- Record your actions according to employer policy. When applicable, the client records on the MAR. Assist as directed.
- Report and record if a medication is not taken or is omitted. Explain why.

Assisting with Oral Medications

Compassionate Care

Remember to Promote:
- **Dignity**
- **Independence**
- **Preferences**
- **Privacy**
- **Safety**

Pre-Procedure

1. Identify the person according to employer policy.
2. Explain the procedure to the person.
3. Wash your hands.
4. Assist the person with hand washing.
5. Collect the following:
   - Oral medications
   - Standard measuring spoon, cup, or other measuring device
   - Glass of water or other cool liquid
   - Straw (optional)
6. Provide for privacy.

Procedure

7. Check label on each container (see Figure 39-3 on page 643) or on each pre-poured medication for: *right medication, right person, right dose, right route, right time*. Compare label with MAR and care plan.
8. Loosen lid(s) on container(s) if the person cannot do so. Tell the person the name of each medication (read from the label).
9. Place containers where the person can reach them. Or, hand container to the person. Let the person read the name of the medication to you. Be sure the person wears eyeglasses if needed to read.
10. Help the person to pour the correct amount of liquid or to count the correct amount of pills. Assist the person with oral medications:
    - **a** If the medication is to be swallowed:
      - **(1)** Give a sip of water to moisten mouth
      - **(2)** Support hand as necessary to pour medication
      - **(3)** Give a full glass of water or other cool liquid after the person puts medication in mouth
      - **(4)** Remind the person to lower chin while swallowing
    - **b** If the medication is to dissolve under the person's tongue:
      - **(1)** Ask the person to put the medication under the tongue
      - **(2)** Ask the person to close mouth and let the medication dissolve
      - **(3)** Remind the person not to chew or swallow the medication
      - **(4)** Do not give food or fluids while the medication is dissolving
11. Close containers.

Post-Procedure

12. Have the person record medications taken, when applicable. Or record for the person if this is a task listed in the care plan.
13. Store materials in proper locations.
14. Remove privacy measures.
15. Wash your hands.
16. Report and record your actions and observations according to employer policy.

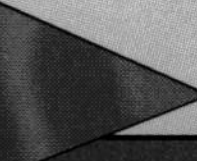

Assisting with Rectal Suppositories

Compassionate Care

Remember to Promote:
- **Dignity**
- **Independence**
- **Preferences**
- **Privacy**
- **Safety**

Pre-Procedure

1 Identify the person according to employer policy.
2 Explain the procedure to the person.
3 Wash your hands.
4 Assist the person with hand washing.
5 Collect the following:
- Suppository
- Water-soluble lubricant
- Disposable gloves
- Toilet tissue

6 Provide for privacy.

Procedure

7 Check label on the suppository for: *right medication, right person, right dose, right route, right time.* Compare label with MAR and care plan.
8 Assist the person into bed and into the Sims' position.
9 Help the person to lower or remove clothing to expose anal area.
10 Unwrap suppository.
11 Apply water-soluble lubricant to suppository. Do not use petroleum jelly because it is not water-soluble.
12 Give glove to the person to put on.
13 Hand suppository to the person to insert into rectum. Guide the person's hand if necessary. (Wear a glove.)
14 Observe as the person inserts medication and wipes anus with toilet tissue.

Post-Procedure

15 Have the person remove and discard glove into waste container.
16 Discard used materials in waste container.
17 Remind the person to remain on side for 15–20 minutes to allow suppository to melt and medication to be absorbed.
18 Assist the person with hand washing.
19 Have the person record medications taken, when applicable. Or record for the person if this is a task listed in the care plan.
20 Store materials in proper location.
21 Remove privacy measures.
22 Wash your hands.
23 Report and record your actions and observations according to employer policy.

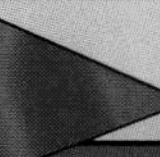

Assisting with Eye Medications or Ointments

Compassionate Care

Remember to Promote:
- **Dignity**
- **Independence**
- **Preferences**
- **Privacy**
- **Safety**

Pre-Procedure

1 Identify the person according to employer policy.
2 Explain the procedure to the person.
3 Wash your hands.
4 Assist the person with hand washing.
5 Collect the following:
- Eye medication or ointment
- Tissues or cotton balls
- Small hand mirror
- Disposable gloves (if necessary)

6 Provide for privacy.

Procedure

7 Check label on the prescription container for: *right medication* (be certain the preparation is for use in the eyes), *right person*, *right dose* (be certain the strength of the solution/ointment in the container is correct), *right route* (be certain about which eye or both eyes), *right time*. Compare label with MAR and care plan.
8 Loosen lid on container if the person cannot do so.
9 Place container within the person's reach or hand it to him or her. Be sure the person wears eyeglasses if needed.
10 Hold mirror so the person can see to administer eye medication.
11 Remove the person's eyeglasses if worn.
12 Assist the person with:
 a Eye medication:
  (1) Guide the person's hand to grasp the lower eyelid
  (2) Observe that the person looks up and releases drops into the lower lid.
  (3) Observe that the person closes eye to distribute medication
  (4) Make sure that dropper does not touch the person's eye
 b Ointment:
  (1) Guide the person's hand to grasp the lower eyelid
  (2) Observe that the person looks up and squeezes a small ribbon of ointment into the lower lid from inner corner of eye to outer corner of eye
  (3) Observe that the person closes eye to allow medication to melt and be distributed
  (4) Make sure that tip of tube does not touch eye surface

Post-Procedure

13 Reseal container.
14 Assist the person with hand washing.
15 Have the person record medications taken, if applicable. Or record for the person if this is a task listed in the care plan.
16 Store materials in proper location.
17 Remove privacy measures.
18 Wash your hands.
19 Report and record your actions and observations according to employer policy.

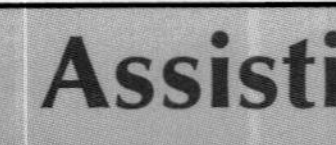

Assisting with Transdermal Disks

Compassionate Care

Remember to Promote:
- **Dignity**
- **Independence**
- **Preferences**
- **Privacy**
- **Safety**

Pre-Procedure

1 Identify the person according to employer policy.
2 Explain the procedure to the person.
3 Wash your hands.
4 Assist the person with hand washing.
5 Collect the following:
- Medicated transdermal disk
- Disposable gloves

6 Provide for privacy.

Procedure

7 Check label on the disk container for: *right medication, right person, right dose, right route, right time*. Compare label with MAR and care plan.
8 Put on gloves. Give the person a glove to put on.
9 Have the person remove and discard old disk into waste container. Wash skin that had been covered by old disk.
10 Ask the person to select new site for new disk (any area without hair). Usually the chest or upper arm site is used.
11 Observe as the person applies new disk to skin surface. Be sure that the medicated surface of the disk is not touched with ungloved fingers. (Your skin may absorb some of the drug.)

Post-Procedure

12 Discard disk wrapper and other used materials.
13 Remove gloves. Wash your hands.
14 Have the person remove the glove and discard it. Assist with hand washing.
15 Have the person record medications taken, when applicable. Or record for the person if this is a task listed in the care plan.
16 Store materials in proper location.
17 Remove privacy measures.
18 Wash your hands.
19 Report and record your actions and observations according to employer policy.

Assisting with Metered Dose Inhalers

Compassionate Care

Remember to Promote:
- **Dignity**
- **Independence**
- **Preferences**
- **Privacy**
- **Safety**

Pre-Procedure

1 Identify the person according to employer policy.
2 Explain the procedure to the person.
3 Wash your hands.
4 Help the person with hand washing.
5 Collect the following:
- Metered dose inhaler container of prescription medication
- Disposable gloves (if necessary)

6 Provide for privacy.

Procedure

7 Check label on the disk container for: *right medication, right person, right dose, right route, right time*. Compare label with MAR and care plan.
8 Hand metered dose inhaler (MDI) to the person. The person then uses it to inhale the medication (Figure 39-4).

Post-Procedure

9 Have the person record medications taken, when applicable. Or record for the person if this is a task listed in the care plan.
10 Clean inhaler according to manufacturer's instructions. Store the inhaler in proper location.
11 Remove privacy measures.
12 Wash your hands.
13 Report and record your actions and observations according to employer policy.

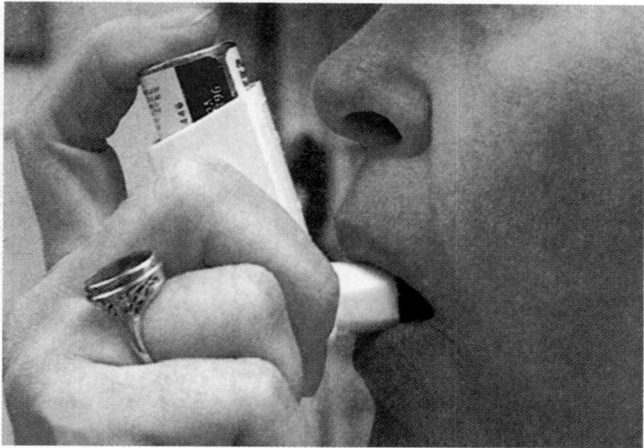

Figure 39-4 A client self-administering medication with a metered dose inhaler.

REVIEW

Circle T if the answer is true and F if it is false.

1. T F Support workers routinely administer medications.
2. T F A lozenge is a type of medication.
3. T F Over-the-counter medications require a prescription.
4. T F You can purchase OTC medications for a client.
5. T F The physician, RN, and/or case manager are responsible for monitoring the outcome of the drug therapy.
6. T F Side effects do not need to be reported.
7. T F You are responsible for filling pill boxes.
8. T F In facilities, a nurse signs or initials the MAR.
9. T F Medications can be taken at any time, as long as the correct dose is given.
10. T F When assisting with medications, you must check that the client is taking the right medication.
11. T F Medications should always be stored in the bathroom medicine cabinet.

Circle the BEST answer.

12. Mrs. Stein has sore, swollen joints in her hands. You assist with her medications. Which of the following is *not* likely to be your responsibility?
    A. Loosening and removing container lids
    B. Supporting her hand as she pours the medication
    C. Pouring the medication for her and administering it to her
    D. Closing the container for her, and putting it away
13. Which of the following is *not* one of the five "rights" of assisting with medications?
    A. The right medication
    B. The right colour
    C. The right person
    D. The right time
14. Which is *not* an accurate way to check for the right dose?
    A. Check the MAR
    B. Check the prescription label
    C. Ask the client or family member
    D. Check the care plan
15. A medication should be stored
    A. Opened, at the bedside
    B. In a warm, humid area
    C. With other family members' or residents' medications
    D. In its original labelled container
16. The following are examples of when to report to your supervisor. Which is *false*?
    A. When the client needs to use a metered dose inhaler
    B. When the client refuses to take the medication
    C. When the client vomits or has diarrhea after taking the medication
    D. When the client does not know why the medication is being taken

Answers to these questions are on page 827.

CHAPTER

40

MEASURING HEIGHT, WEIGHT, AND VITAL SIGNS

OBJECTIVES

- Define the key terms listed in this chapter
- Explain how to measure height and weight
- Explain why vital signs are measured
- List the factors affecting vital signs
- Identify the normal ranges for the temperature sites
- Know when to use each temperature site
- Identify the sites for taking a pulse
- Describe normal respirations
- Describe the factors affecting blood pressure
- Describe the practices to follow when measuring blood pressure
- Know the vital sign ranges for different age groups
- Learn the procedures described in this chapter

KEY TERMS

apical-radial pulse Taking the apical and radial pulses at the same time

blood pressure The amount of force exerted by the blood against the walls of an artery

body temperature The amount of heat in the body that is a balance between the amount of heat produced and the amount lost by the body

bradycardia A slow (*brady*) heart rate (*cardia*); the rate is less than 60 beats per minute

diastole The period of heart muscle relaxation

diastolic pressure The pressure in the arteries when the heart is at rest

dysrhythmia An irregular rhythm of the pulse; beats may be unevenly spaced or skipped

hypertension Persistent blood pressure measurements above the normal systolic (140 mm Hg) or diastolic (90 mm Hg) pressures

hypotension A condition in which the systolic blood pressure is below 90 mm Hg and the diastolic pressure is below 60 mm Hg

pulse The beat of the heart felt at an artery as a wave of blood passes through the artery

pulse deficit The difference between the apical and radial pulse rates

pulse rate The number of heartbeats or pulses felt in 1 minute

respiration The act of breathing air into (inhalation) and out of (exhalation) the lungs

sphygmomanometer The instrument used to measure blood pressure

stethoscope An instrument used to listen to the sounds produced by the heart, lungs, and other body organs

systole The period of heart muscle contraction

systolic pressure The amount of force it takes to pump blood out of the heart and into the arterial circulation

tachycardia A rapid (*tachy*) heart rate (*cardia*); the heart rate is over 100 beats per minute

vital signs Temperature, pulse, respirations, and blood pressure

The four **vital signs** of body function are temperature, pulse, respirations, and blood pressure. Vital signs reflect the function of three body processes essential for life: regulation of body temperature, breathing, and heart function. Measuring and recording vital signs provides important information for the care planning process. Measuring height and weight is also important for the care planning process.

Measuring and recording height and weight are skills you need to know for all workplace settings. Measuring and recording temperature, pulse, and respirations (TPR) are skills you need to know when working in long-term care and community settings. Measuring and recording blood pressure are additional skills that some employers may require of you. Some provinces and territories allow support workers in hospitals and other acute care settings to measure and record temperature, pulse, and respirations. Others do not. Know your employer's policies.

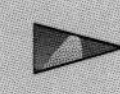

MEASURING HEIGHT AND WEIGHT

Height and weight are measured on admission to a facility. Also, some clients are weighed daily, weekly, or monthly. This is done to monitor weight gain or loss. Weigh the client at the same time of day for daily, weekly, or monthly measurements. Before breakfast is the best time. Food and fluids add weight.

The client wears only a gown or pyjamas when being weighed. Clothes add weight. Shoes or slippers also add weight and add to the height measurement. Have the client void (urinate) before being weighed. A full bladder affects the weight measurement. If a urine specimen is needed, collect it at this time.

There are balance beam, chair, and lift scales (Figure 40-1). Balance beam scales are used for clients who can stand. Chair and lift scales are used for clients who cannot stand. Follow the manufacturer's instructions and employer policy when using scales.

Mechanical and digital scales are used. Mechanical scales use a system of weights. Move the weights to zero before weighing the client. Then adjust the weights until the pointer is centred (Figure 40-2). Digital scales have LED displays that show the weight. Make sure the LED reads zero before weighing the client. (See *Focus on Children: Measuring Height and Weight* box.)

(text continues on page 657)

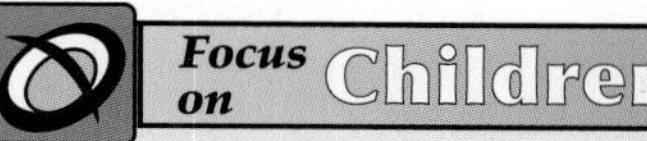

MEASURING HEIGHT AND WEIGHT

Birth weight serves as the baseline for measuring an infant's growth. Weighing infants is described in Chapter 37.

Length, not height, is measured in children younger than 2 years. The child lies on a measuring board or on a paper. Two people hold the child still. One holds the head still, and the other extends and holds the legs still. The measurement is taken from the top of the head to the heels. If using paper, mark the paper at the head and heels. Measure the distance between the two points.

A

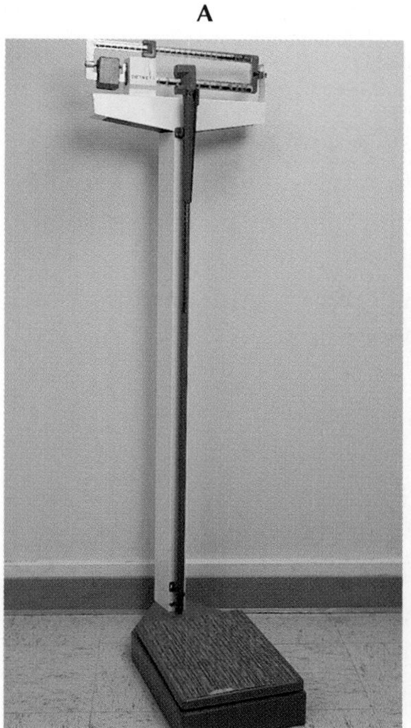

B

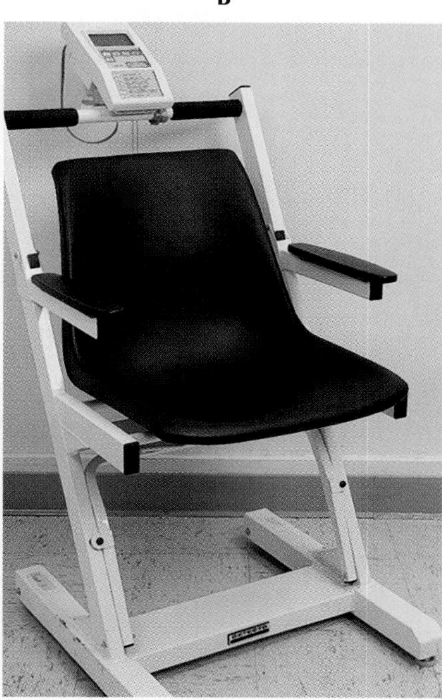

C

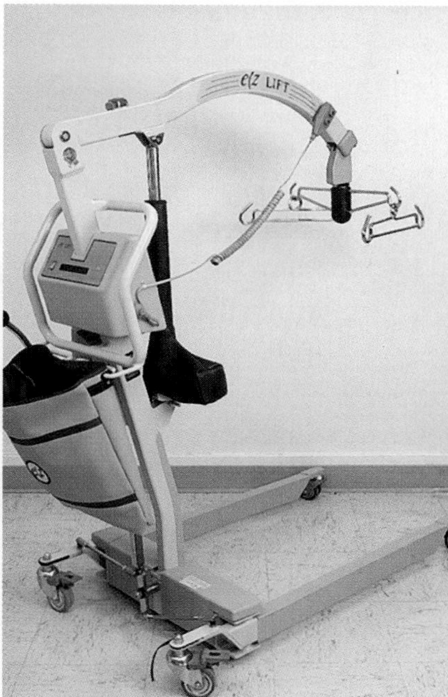

Figure 40-1 Types of scales. **A,** Balance beam scale. **B,** Chair scale. **C,** Lift scale.

A

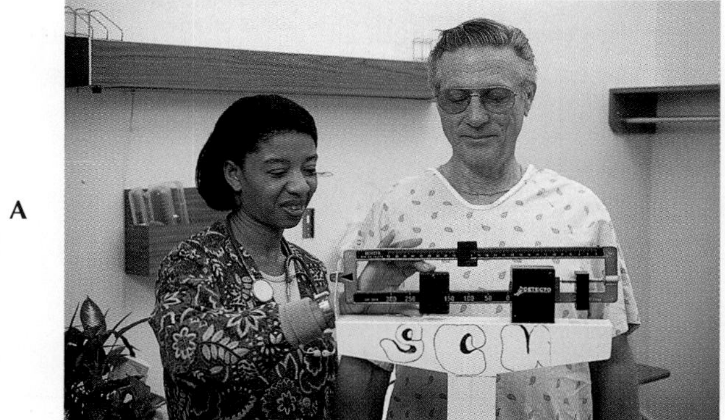

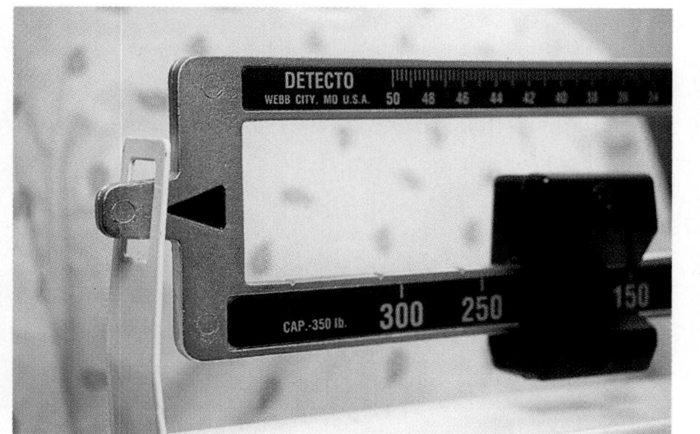

B

Figure 40-2 Using a mechanical scale. **A,** Adjust the weights. **B,** Read the weight when the balance pointer is in the middle.

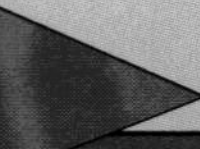

Measuring Height and Weight

Compassionate Care

Remember to Promote:

- **Dignity**
- **Independence**
- **Preferences**
- **Privacy**
- **Safety**

Pre-Procedure

1 Identify the person according to employer policy.
2 Explain the procedure to the person.
3 Ask the person to void (see Chapter 29).
4 Wash your hands.
5 Bring the scale and paper towels to the person's room.
6 Provide for privacy.

Procedure

7 *Balance beam scale (mechanical):*
  - **a** Disinfect the scale platform according to employer policy. Dry it with paper towels.
  - **b** Raise the height rod.
  - **c** Move the weights to zero (0). The pointer is in the middle.
  - **d** Have the person remove the robe and footwear. Assist as needed.
  - **e** Help the person stand on the scale platform. Arms are at the sides.
  - **f** Move the weights until the balance pointer is in the middle (see Figure 40-2 on page 653).
  - **g** Record the weight on your notepad or assignment sheet.
  - **h** Ask the person to stand very straight.
  - **i** Lower the height rod until it rests on the person's head (Figure 40-3).
  - **j** Record the height on your notepad or assignment sheet.
  - **k** Disinfect the scale platform after use according to employer policy.

8 *Chair scale (mechanical):*
  - **a** Help the person transfer from the wheelchair to the chair scale (see *Transferring the Person to a Chair or Wheelchair* on page 291).
  - **b** Place the person's feet on the foot platform.
  - **c** Move the weights until the balance pointer is in the middle.
  - **d** Record the weight on your notepad or assignment sheet.

9 *Lift scale (mechanical):*
  - **a** Attach the sling to the lift.
  - **b** Place both weights on zero.
  - **c** Level and balance the scale. Follow the manufacturer's instructions.
  - **d** Remove the sling from the scale.
  - **e** Place the person on the sling and attach it to the lift. Raise the person about 10 cm (4 inches) off the bed (see *Transferring the Person Using a Mechanical Lift* on page 300).
  - **f** Move the weights until the balance pointer is in the middle.
  - **g** Record the weight on your notepad or assignment sheet.
  - **h** Lower the person to the bed.
  - **i** Remove the sling.

10 Help the person dress if he or she will be up. Or, help the person back to bed.

Continued

Measuring Height and Weight—cont'd

Post-Procedure

11 Provide for safety and comfort.
12 Place the call bell within reach.*
13 If the person stays in bed, follow the care plan for bed rail use.*
14 Remove privacy measures.
15 Return the scale to its proper place.
16 Wash your hands.
17 Report and record the measurements and your observations according to employer policy.

*Steps marked with an asterisk may not apply in community settings.

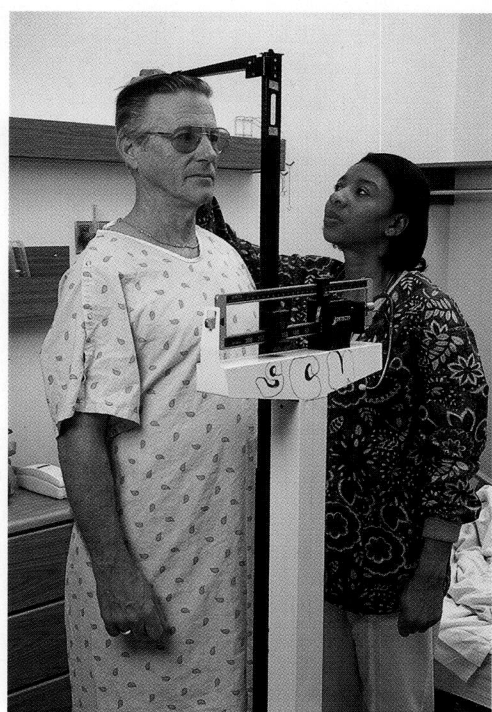

Figure 40-3 Measuring height.

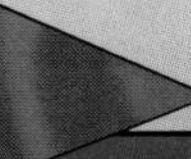

Measuring Height: The Person in Bed

Compassionate Care

Remember to Promote:
- **Dignity**
- **Independence**
- **Preferences**
- **Privacy**
- **Safety**

Pre-Procedure

1 Identify the person according to employer policy.
2 Explain the procedure to the person.
3 Wash your hands.
4 Collect a measuring tape and ruler.
5 Ask for assistance.
6 Provide for privacy.

Procedure

7 Position the person supine if this position is allowed.
8 Have your helper hold the end of the measuring tape at the person's heel.
9 Pull the measuring tape alongside the person's body until it extends past the head (Figure 40-4).
10 Place the ruler flat across the top of the person's head. It should extend from the person's head to the measuring tape. Make sure the ruler is level.
11 Record the height on your notepad or assignment sheet.
12 Help the person out of bed if appropriate.

Post-Procedure

13 Provide for safety and comfort.
14 Place the call bell within reach.*
15 If the person stays in bed, follow the care plan for bed rail use.*
16 Remove privacy measures.
17 Return equipment to its proper location.
18 Wash your hands.
19 Report and record the height and your observations according to employer policy.

*Steps marked with an asterisk may not apply in community settings.

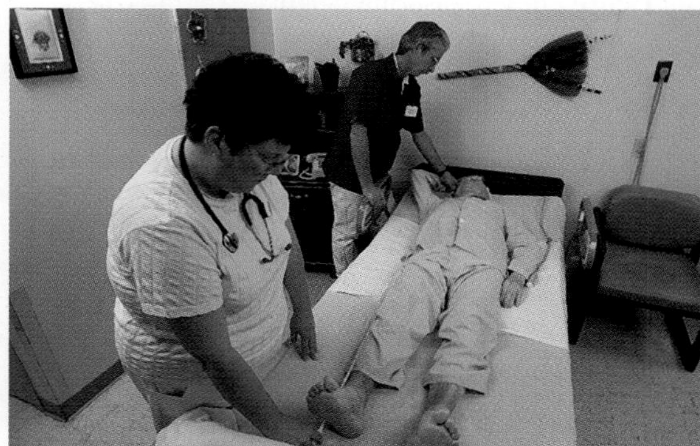

Figure 40-4 Measuring a client in bed. Extend the tape measure from the top of the client's head to the heel. Make sure the ruler is flat across the top of the client's head.

Measuring and Reporting Vital Signs

A person's vital signs vary within certain limits. Vital signs are affected by medications, pain, illness, activity, exercise, sleep, foods, fluids, and emotions such as excitement, anger, fear, and anxiety.

Vital signs are measured to detect changes in normal body function. They tell about response to treatment. They often signal life-threatening events. Vital signs are part of the assessment process. Vital signs are measured:

- During physical examinations
- When a person is admitted to a facility
- Several times a day for hospital patients and patients in subacute care units
- Before and after surgery
- Before and after complex procedures or diagnostic tests
- After certain care measures, such as ambulation
- After a fall or other injury
- When medications are taken that affect the respiratory or circulatory system
- Whenever the client complains of pain, dizziness, light-headedness, shortness of breath, rapid heart rate, or not feeling well
- As often as required by the client's condition
- As stated on the care plan (usually daily or weekly)

Vital signs show even minor changes in a person's condition. Accuracy is essential when you measure, record, and report vital signs. If unsure of your measurements, promptly ask your supervisor to take them again. Unless otherwise ordered, take vital signs with the person at rest, either lying or sitting. Immediately report:

- Any vital sign that is changed from a previous measurement
- Vital signs above the normal range
- Vital signs below the normal range

Each employer will have its own method of recording vital signs. Some use graphic flow sheets where the vital signs are graphed in red and blue ink. Others use books with pages divided into columns, where the information is to be recorded. Whatever system your employer uses, the following information must be clearly and accurately reported:

- The client's name
- The date
- The time the vital sign was measured
- The vital sign measurement

Some employers require that changed or abnormal vital signs be circled in red. The nurse or physician compares current and previous measurements.

Body Temperature

Body temperature is the amount of heat in the body. It is a balance between the amount of heat produced and the amount lost by the body. It remains within a normal, safe range when a person is healthy. Temperature normally changes slightly throughout the day and in response to different factors. It is lower in the morning and higher in the afternoon and evening. Factors affecting body temperature include age, weather, exercise, pregnancy, the menstrual cycle, emotions, and stress.

Illness also affects body temperature. Body temperature above or below the normal range signals illness or health problems.

Temperature Sites

Temperature is measured using the Centigrade or Celsius (C) and Fahrenheit (F) scales. Common sites for measuring temperature are the:

- Mouth (oral temperature)
- Ear (tympanic temperature—the tympanic membrane is in the ear)
- Underarm (axillary temperature—*axilla* means underarm)

Body temperature can also be measured in the rectum (rectal temperature). However, the rectal site is rarely used. If a rectal temperature is required, a nurse or other regulated health care provider does the procedure. Taking a rectal temperature involves inserting an instrument into a body cavity. *Therefore, support workers are not authorized to take rectal temperatures.* If you are delegated the procedure, you need to be properly trained and supervised.

Normal body temperature depends on the site. Each site has a normal range (Table 40-1 on page 658). Check with your supervisor and the care plan to determine which site to use.

Older adults have lower body temperatures than younger people. A fever for an older adult may be a normal body temperature for a younger person. Always report temperatures that are not within the client's normal range.

Table 40-1 Normal Body Temperature

Site	Average temperature	Normal range
Mouth (oral temperature)	37.0° C (98.6° F)	35.5 to 37.5° C (95.9 to 99.5° F)
Ear (tympanic temperature)	37.4° C (99.3° F)	35.8 to 38.0° C (96.4 to 100.4° F)
Underarm (axillary temperature)	36.5° C (97.8° F)	34.7 to 37.3° C (94.5 to 99.1° F)

Taking Oral Temperatures. Oral temperatures are *not* taken if the client:

- Is unconscious
- Has had surgery or an injury to the face, neck, nose, or mouth
- Has a nasogastric tube
- Is delirious, restless, confused, or disoriented
- Is paralyzed on one side of the body
- Has a sore mouth
- Has a convulsive disorder
- Is receiving oxygen therapy

Certain activities may temporarily affect oral temperatures, including:

- Eating hot or cold foods
- Drinking hot or cold fluids
- Smoking
- Chewing gum

Before taking an oral temperature, make sure the client has not done any of these activities within the previous 20 minutes.

Place the thermometer under the client's tongue (Figure 40-5). The tip of the thermometer should be at the base of the tongue. Ask the client to close his or her lips around the thermometer to hold it in place. The mouth must remain closed. Remind the client not to bite down on the thermometer or talk while it is in place.

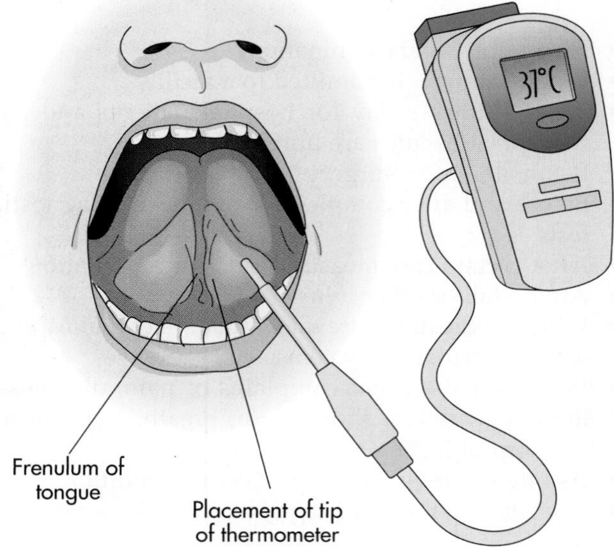

Figure 40-5 Place the thermometer at the base of the tongue.

Taking Tympanic Temperatures. If oral temperature cannot be taken, tympanic temperature is usually the next choice. Special thermometers are used for the ear (Figure 40-6).

Pull the client's ear up and back (Figure 40-7). Then gently insert the probe (the end of the thermometer that is temperature-sensitive) into the ear canal. The temperature is measured in 1 to 3 seconds. (See *Focus on Children: Taking a Tympanic Temperature* box.)

Because temperature can be measured quickly and easily, tympanic temperature is often ordered for children and clients with dementia. Tympanic temperature is not taken if there is ear drainage.

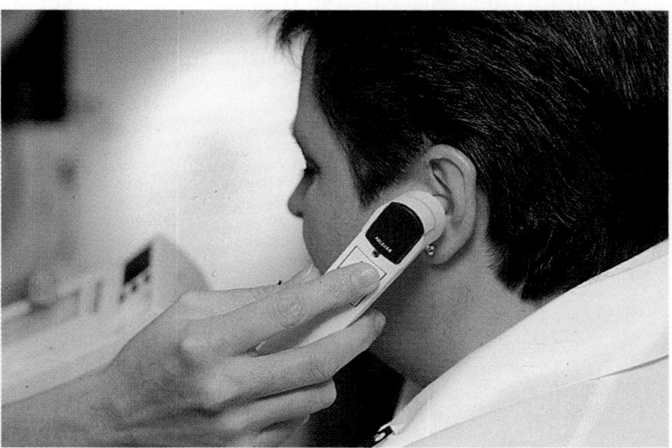

Figure 40-6 A tympanic thermometer.

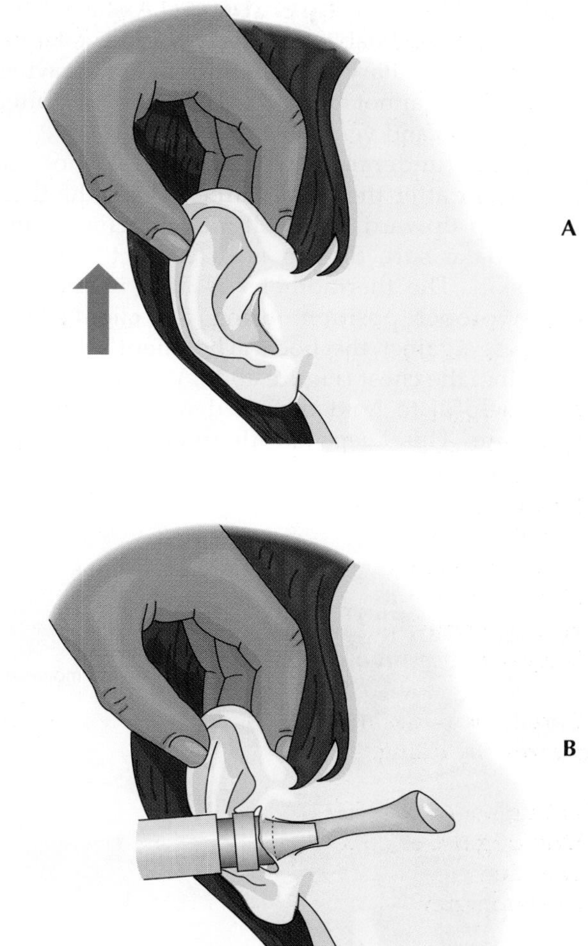

Figure 40-7 Taking an adult's tympanic temperature. **A,** Pull the ear up and back. **B,** Gently insert the probe into the ear canal.

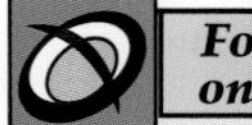

Focus on **Children**

TAKING A TYMPANIC TEMPERATURE

The shape of a child's ear canal is different from an adult's. When taking a tympanic temperature on a child, gently pull the child's ear down and forward. Then gently insert the probe.

Taking Axillary Temperatures. Axillary temperatures are less reliable than temperatures taken at the other sites. Axillary temperatures are taken when the other sites cannot be used. They also are often used for infants and very young children.

The axilla (underarm) must be dry. Do not use this site right after the client bathes. Point the thermometer tip upward and well into the client's underarm. Make sure the tip is in contact with the client's skin. The thermometer is held in place to maintain proper position. Bring the client's arm down close against the body. The client's forearm rests against the chest (Figure 40-8). With children, it may be helpful to hold the child while taking the temperature. This keeps the thermometer in place and comforts the child.

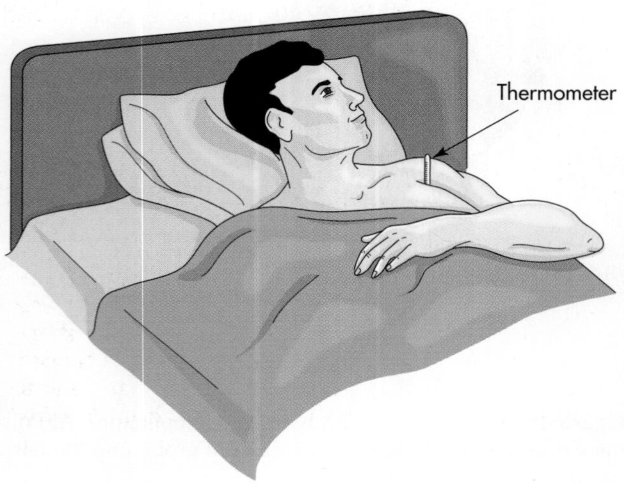

Figure 40-8 Hold the thermometer in place in the axilla by bringing the client's arm over the chest.

THERMOMETERS

A variety of thermometers are available. Most facilities and agencies use electronic thermometers. Disposable thermometers are also common. Glass thermometers are considered safety hazards and are now rarely used in any setting.

Thermometers can spread microbes. Therefore plastic covers are usually applied over the thermometer before use (Figure 40-9). A cover is used once and discarded. Thermometers must always be cleaned and stored following employer policy. Even if a plastic cover is used, clean the thermometer with warm (not hot), soapy water before and after each use. Wipe the thermometer dry. Some employers want thermometers cleaned with a disinfectant such as alcohol before and after use. Always practise medical asepsis and Standard Precautions when using thermometers.

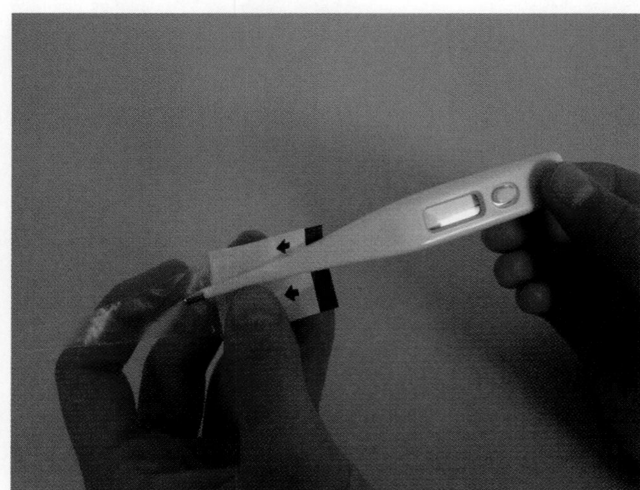

Figure 40-9 The thermometer is inserted into a disposable plastic cover; this helps prevent the spread of microbes.

Electronic Thermometers. Electronic thermometers are battery-operated. They measure temperature within 20 to 50 seconds and display a digital readout of the temperature. Some electronic thermometers consist of a hand-held unit and a probe that is inserted into the unit (Figure 40-10). The hand-held unit is kept in a battery charger when not in use.

An electronic thermometer that has a low battery charge will not record an accurate temperature. After using an electronic thermometer, replace it securely in the battery charging unit. Make sure the battery charging unit is plugged into an electrical outlet.

Electronic thermometers with probes can be used for any site. The probes may be changed depending on the site. Tympanic thermometers are electronic thermometers with probes made to fit in the ear canal (see Figure 40-6 on page 659).

A disposable plastic cover is used to cover the probe. Slide the cover onto the probe until it snaps in place. Covers are used once and then discarded. Electronic thermometers emit a tone or flashing light when the temperature reading is complete.

Other electronic thermometers are one-piece devices (Figure 40-11). They are called digital thermometers. They have a temperature-sensitive tip on one end and an on/off button on the other end. They display a digital readout of the temperature on the thermometer. Some have a memory mechanism that recalls the last temperature reading. The battery is not rechargeable, but the device shuts off after about 10 minutes. These thermometers may be used for oral or axillary temperatures. They are inserted into covers before use (see Figure 40-9). Digital thermometers are used more in home care settings than in facilities. (See *Focus on Children: Special Thermometers* box.)

(text continues on page 663)

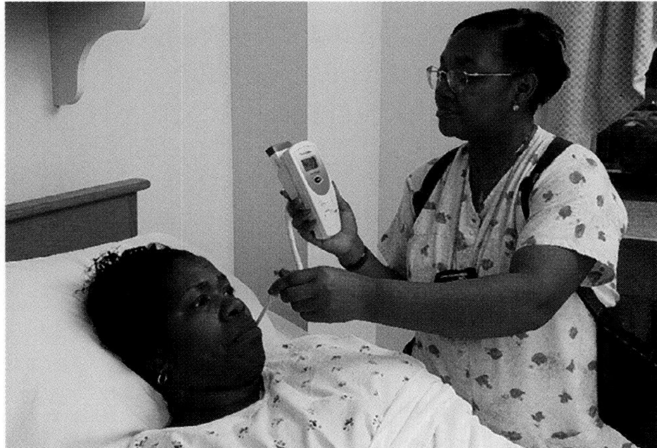

Figure 40-10 An electronic thermometer with a hand-held unit and probe.

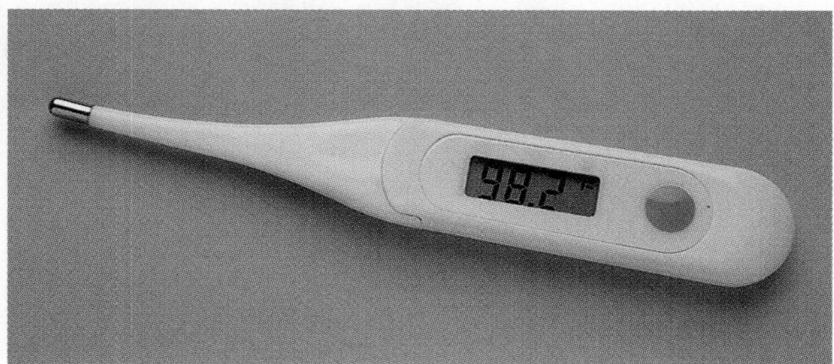

Figure 40-11 A digital thermometer.

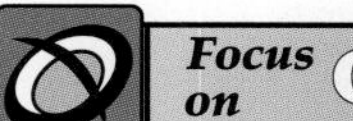

Focus on Children

SPECIAL THERMOMETERS

Pacifier thermometers are a type of electronic thermometer used for infants and toddlers. They are available in stores for home use. The pacifier thermometer has four parts: a storage cover, a nipple with a sensor, a digital display, and an on/off switch. Temperature is measured in about 5 minutes.

To use the thermometer:

- Remove it from the storage case.
- Check the pacifier for cracks or holes. These can occur if the child bites or chews on the thermometer. Do not use the thermometer if it is not intact.
- Turn it on by pressing the on/off switch.
- Place the pacifier in the child's mouth. Hold and cuddle the child.
- Read the digital display on the front of the pacifier when the thermometer beeps.
- Clean the thermometer according to employer policy. Do not use boiling water, the dishwasher, or a sterilizer to clean the thermometer.
- Wipe the thermometer dry.

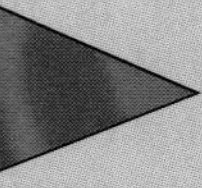

Taking a Temperature with an Electronic Thermometer

COMPASSIONATE CARE

Remember to Promote:
- **Dignity**
- **Independence**
- **Preferences**
- **Privacy**
- **Safety**

Pre-Procedure

1 Identify the person according to employer policy.
2 Explain the procedure to the person. For an oral temperature, ask the person not to eat, drink, smoke, or chew gum for at least 20 minutes beforehand.
3 Wash your hands.
4 Collect the following:
- Electronic or digital thermometer
- Probe if used. Make sure you use the correct probe for the site.
- Disposable plastic cover for thermometer or probe
- Tissues
- Towel (for axillary temperature)

5 Plug the probe into the thermometer if used.
6 Provide for privacy.

Procedure

7 Position the person for an oral, axillary, or tympanic temperature.
8 Insert the probe or thermometer tip into a disposable cover.
9 *For an oral temperature:*
   a Ask the person to open the mouth and raise the tongue.
   b Place the tip of the thermometer or probe at the base of the tongue (see Figure 40-5 on page 658).
   c Ask the person to lower the tongue and close the mouth. Remind the person not to talk or bite down on the thermometer or probe.
10 *For a tympanic temperature:*
   a Ask the person to turn his or her head so the ear is in front of you.
   b Pull up and back on the ear to straighten the ear canal (see Figure 40-7 on page 659). (With children, pull the ear down and forward.)
   c Insert the probe gently. The probe should seal the ear canal.
11 *For an axillary temperature:*
   a Help the person remove an arm from the garment. Do not expose the person.
   b Dry the axilla with the towel.
   c Place the tip of the thermometer or probe in the centre of the axilla, pointing upward. Make sure the tip of the probe is in contact with the person's skin.
   d Ask the person to place the arm over the chest to hold the thermometer or probe in place (see Figure 40-8 on page 660). Hold the arm in place if he or she cannot help.
12 Start the thermometer.
13 Keep the probe or thermometer in place until you hear a tone or see a flashing or steady light.
14 Remove the probe or thermometer.
15 Read the temperature on the display.
16 Help the person put the garment back on (for axillary temperature).
17 Record the person's name and temperature on your notepad or assignment sheet. Note the temperature site.
18 Use tissue to remove the plastic cover. Or press the eject button to remove the plastic probe cover.
19 Discard tissue and plastic cover.
20 Wash your hands.

Continued

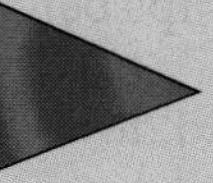

Taking a Temperature with an Electronic Thermometer—cont'd

Post-Procedure

21 Provide for safety and comfort.
22 Place the call bell within reach.*
23 Follow the care plan for bed rail use.*
24 Remove privacy measures.
25 Clean and store the equipment according to employer policy. Return electronic thermometer back to the battery charging unit.
26 Wash your hands.
27 Report and record your actions and observations according to employer policy. Include the following:
- Temperature
- Site (Write *A* for axillary, *T* for tympanic, *O* for oral)
- Abnormal temperature (report at once)

*Steps marked with an asterisk may not apply in community settings.

Dot Matrix Thermometers. Dot matrix thermometers are thin plastic strips with small chemical dots on one end (Figure 40-12). The dots change colour when heated by the body. Each dot must be heated to a certain temperature before it changes colour. These thermometers measure oral and axillary temperature. They are not for use in the ear. They must be left in place for about 3 minutes before an accurate temperature can be read. They must be discarded after one use.

Temperature-Sensitive Tape. Temperature-sensitive tape changes colour in response to body heat (Figure 40-13). The tape is applied to the forehead or abdomen. It shows if the temperature is normal or above normal. Exact body temperature is not measured. The colour change takes about 15 seconds. The tape is discarded after one use.

A

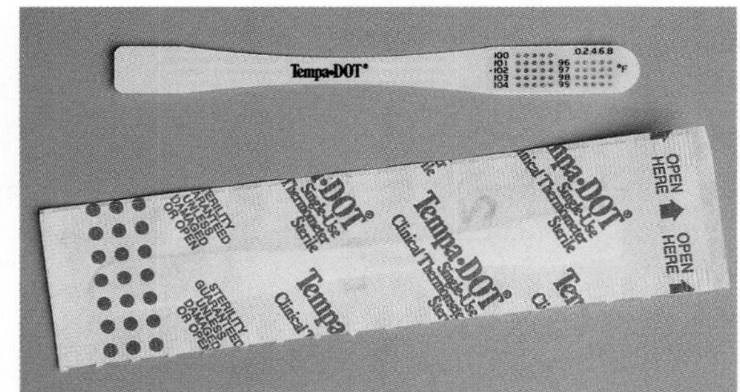

B

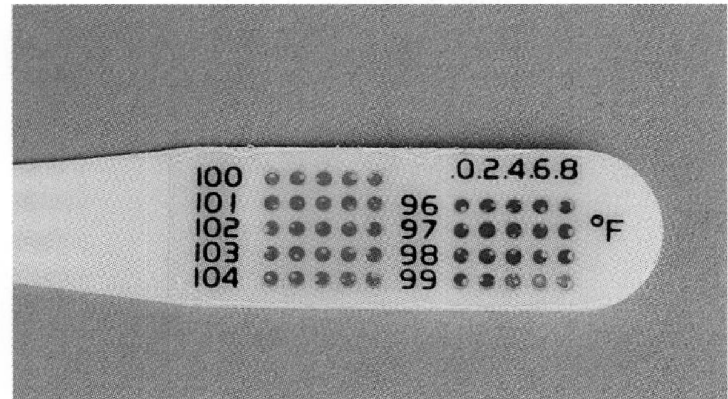

Figure 40-12 **A,** Single-use dot matrix thermometer with chemical dots. **B,** The dots change colour when the temperature is taken.

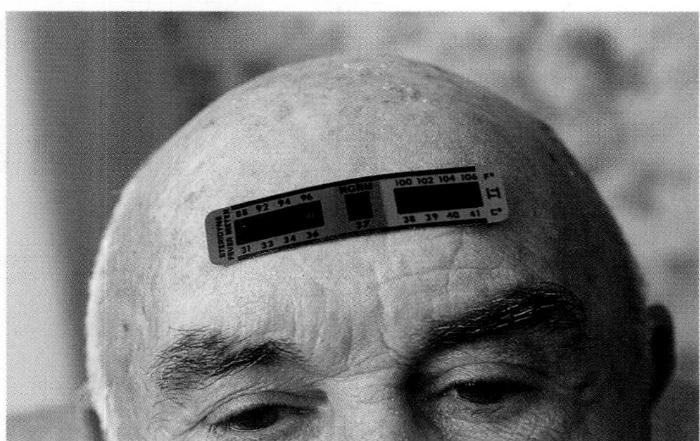

Figure 40-13 Temperature-sensitive tape.

Glass Thermometers. The glass thermometer (clinical thermometer) is a hollow glass tube filled with a liquid—usually coloured alcohol or mercury. When heated, the liquid rises in the tube to indicate the temperature.

Centigrade thermometers have long and short lines. Each long line represents 1 degree, from 34 to 42° C. Each short line represents 0.1 (one-tenth) degrees (Figure 40-14, *A*). Fahrenheit thermometers also have long and short lines. Each long line represents 1 degree, from 94 to 108° F. The short lines indicate 0.2 (two-tenths) degrees (Figure 40-14, *B*).

Glass thermometers are reusable and can be used for oral, axillary, and rectal temperatures. However, they are rarely used anymore because they have the following disadvantages:

- They can break. Broken glass is a hazard. Mercury is a hazardous substance and could cause poisoning.
- They take a long time to register—up to 10 minutes.

If you must use a glass thermometer, do the following to prevent infection, promote safety, and obtain an accurate measurement:

- Use only the client's thermometer.
- Clean before use according to employer policy.
- Check the thermometer for breaks and chips before use.
- Shake the thermometer to move the liquid down in the tube. Hold it at the stem (the part that does not touch the client). Stand away from walls, tables, or other hard surfaces. Flex and snap your wrist until the liquid is below 35° C or 95° F (Figure 40-15).
- Use plastic covers over the bulb (the part that touches the client).
- Follow the procedure for using an electronic thermometer.
- For an oral temperature, leave the thermometer in place for 2 to 3 minutes or as required by employer policy.
- For an axillary temperature, leave the thermometer in place for 5 to 10 minutes or as required by employer policy.
- Clean and store the thermometer according to employer policy.
- To read a glass thermometer:
  - Hold it at the stem. Bring it to eye level.
  - Turn it until you see both the numbers and the long and short lines.
  - Turn it back and forth slowly until you see the silver or red line.
  - Read to the nearest degree (long line).
  - Read the nearest tenth of a degree (short line)—an even number on a Fahrenheit thermometer.

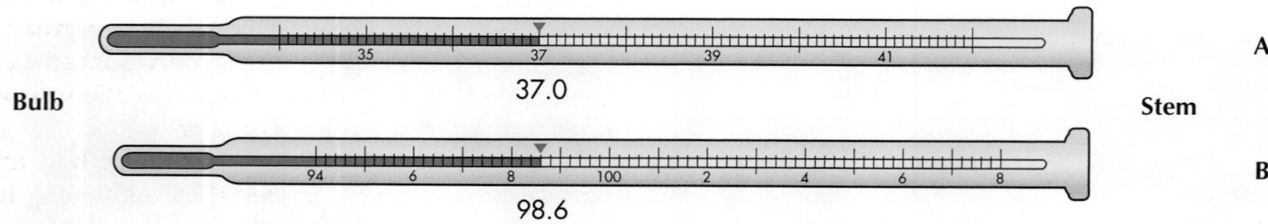

Figure 40-14 **A,** Centigrade thermometer. The temperature measurement is 37.0° C. **B,** Fahrenheit thermometer. The temperature measurement is 98.6° F.

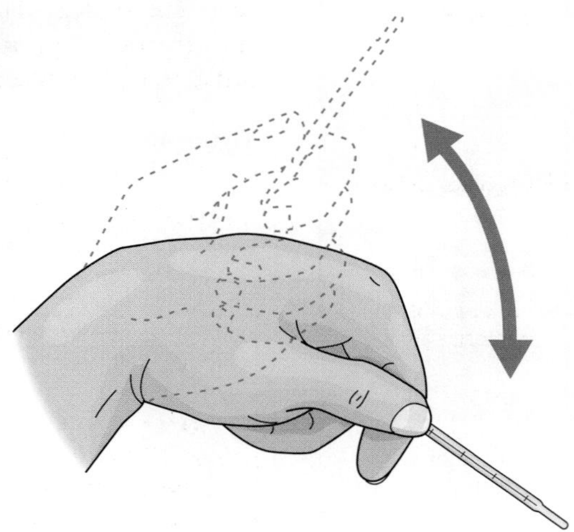

Figure 40-15 Snap your wrist to shake down the thermometer.

PULSE

The **pulse** is the beat of the heart felt at an artery as a wave of blood passes through the artery. A pulse is felt every time the heart beats. (See Chapter 13 to review the structure and function of the heart and blood vessels.)

SITES FOR TAKING A PULSE

You can feel a pulse by placing your fingertips over certain sites on the body. The temporal, carotid, brachial, femoral, popliteal, and dorsalis pedis (pedal) pulses are on both sides of the body (Figure 40-16). Pulses are easy to feel at these sites because the arteries are close to the body's surface and lie over a bone.

Support workers use the radial site to measure pulse. It is easy to reach and find. You can take a radial pulse without disturbing or exposing the client. The carotid pulse (in adults and children) and brachial pulse (in infants) are taken during cardiopulmonary resuscitation (CPR) and other emergencies (see Chapter 47).

PULSE RATE

The **pulse rate** is the number of heartbeats or pulses felt in 1 minute. The rate varies for each age group (Table 40-2). The pulse rate is affected by many factors, including:

- Elevated body temperature (caused by fever or exposure to hot environments)
- Exercise
- Pain
- Position change (pulse rate temporarily increases when a person sits or stands after lying down)
- Caffeine
- Emotions (excitement, fear, anger, anxiety)
- Medications (some increase the pulse rate; others slow down the pulse)

The adult pulse rate is between 60 and 100 beats per minute. A rate of less than 60 or more than 100 is not normal. Report abnormal rates at once:

- **Tachycardia** is a rapid (*tachy*) heart rate (*cardia*). The heart rate is over 100 beats per minute.
- **Bradycardia** is a slow (*brady*) heart rate (*cardia*). The heart rate is less than 60 beats per minute.

You need to know the client's normal pulse range. Immediately report pulse rates that are higher or lower than normal for that client.

RHYTHM AND FORCE OF THE PULSE

The rhythm of the pulse should be regular. That is, a pulse should be felt in a pattern. The same time interval should be felt between beats. An irregular pulse occurs when the beats are unevenly spaced or beats are skipped. An abnormal rhythm is called **dysrhythmia**, and must be reported at once.

Force of the pulse relates to its strength. A forceful pulse is easy to feel. It is described as strong, full, or bounding. Hard-to-feel pulses are described as weak, thready, or feeble.

Electronic blood pressure equipment (page 669) can also count pulses. The pulse rate and blood pressure are shown. However, no information is given about pulse rhythm and force. You need to feel the pulse to determine rhythm and force.

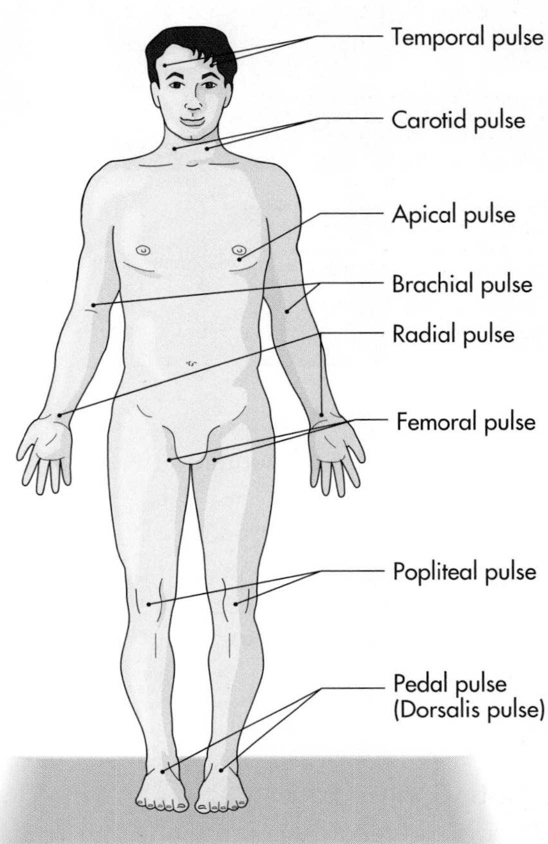

Figure 40-16 The pulse sites.

Table 40-2 Pulse Ranges for Different Ages

Age	Pulse rate (beats per minute)
Birth to 1 year	80–190
1 to 2 years	80–160
2 to 6 years	80–120
6 to 12 years	70–110
12 years and older	60–100

Taking a Radial Pulse

The radial pulse is used for routine vital signs. Place the first 2 or 3 fingers of one hand against the radial artery. The radial artery is on the thumb side of the wrist (Figure 40-17). Do not use your thumb to take a pulse. The thumb has a pulse. You could mistake the pulse in your thumb for the client's pulse.

You need a good watch or clock with a second hand. Count the pulse for 30 seconds. Then multiply the number by 2. This gives the number of beats per minute. If the pulse is irregular, count it for 1 minute.

Some employers require that all radial pulses be taken for 1 minute. Follow your employer's policy.

Report and record the following after taking a radial pulse:

- The pulse rate
- A pulse rate less than 60 or more than 100 beats per minute (report this at once)
- A pulse rate that is higher or lower than normal for the client (report this at once)
- If the pulse is regular or irregular
- The pulse force—strong, full, bounding, weak, thready, or feeble

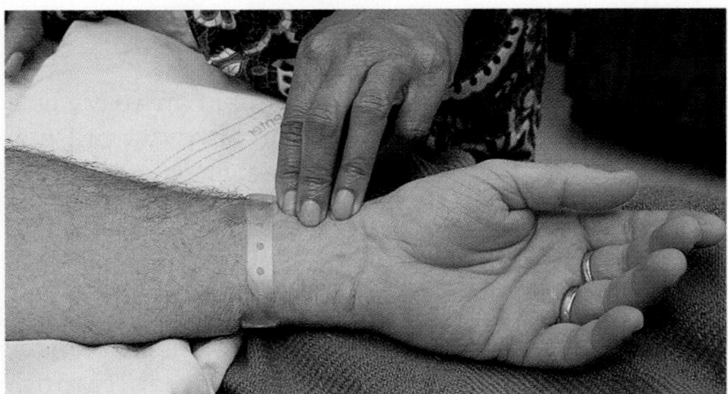

Figure 40-17 Use the middle 2 or 3 fingers to take the radial pulse.

Taking a Radial Pulse

Compassionate Care

Remember to Promote:
- **Dignity**
- **Independence**
- **Preferences**
- **Privacy**
- **Safety**

Pre-Procedure

1 Identify the person according to employer policy.
2 Explain the procedure to the person.
3 Wash your hands.
4 Provide for privacy.

Procedure

5 Have the person sit or lie down.
6 Locate the radial pulse. Use your first 2 or 3 middle fingers (see Figure 40-17).
7 Note if the pulse is strong or weak, and regular or irregular.
8 Count the pulse for 30 seconds. Multiply the number of beats by 2. Or count the pulse for 1 minute if required by employer policy.
9 Count the pulse for 1 minute if it is irregular.
10 Record the person's name and pulse on your notepad or assignment sheet. Note the strength of the pulse. Note if it was regular or irregular.

Post-Procedure

11 Provide for safety and comfort.
12 Place the call bell within reach.*
13 Remove privacy measures.
14 Wash your hands.
15 Report and record the pulse rate and your observations according to employer policy.

*Step marked with an asterisk may not apply in community settings.

The Apical-Radial Pulse

The apical pulse is on the left of the chest, slightly below the nipple. It is taken with a *stethoscope* (page 670). The apical and radial pulse rates should be equal. Sometimes heart contractions are not strong enough to create pulses in the radial artery. Then the radial pulse is less than the apical pulse. This may occur in people with heart disease.

To see if apical and radial rates are equal, two workers take the pulses at the same time (Figure 40-18). This is called an **apical-radial pulse**. The **pulse deficit** is the difference between the apical and radial pulse rates. To obtain the pulse deficit, the radial rate is subtracted from the apical rate. The apical pulse rate is never less than the radial pulse rate.

A nurse takes the apical pulse and supervises the procedure. You may be asked to take the radial pulse.

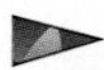

Respirations

Respiration is the act of breathing air into (inhalation) and out of (exhalation) the lungs. Oxygen enters the lungs during inhalation. Carbon dioxide leaves the lungs during exhalation. Each respiration involves one inhalation and one exhalation. The chest rises during inhalation. It falls during exhalation. (See Chapter 13 for a review of the respiratory system.)

The healthy adult has 12 to 20 respirations per minute. The respiratory rate is affected by the factors that affect temperature and pulse. Infections and heart and respiratory diseases usually increase the respiratory rate.

Respirations are normally quiet, effortless, and regular. Both sides of the chest rise and fall equally. If the chest barely moves during respiration, the breathing is called shallow. Deep breathing occurs when the chest rises and falls significantly with every breath. See Chapter 43 for abnormal respiratory patterns.

Count respirations when the client is at rest. Position the client so you can see the chest rise and fall. To a certain extent, a person can control the depth and rate of breathing. People tend to change breathing patterns when they know their respirations are being counted. Therefore the client should not know that you are counting respirations.

Respirations are counted right after taking a pulse. Keep your fingers over the pulse site. (The client assumes you are still taking the pulse.) To count respirations, watch the chest rise and fall. Count how many times the chest rises and falls in 30 seconds. Remember, each rise and fall of the chest counts as 1 respiration. Multiply the number by 2 for the number of respirations in 1 minute. If an abnormal pattern is noted, count the respirations for 1 minute.

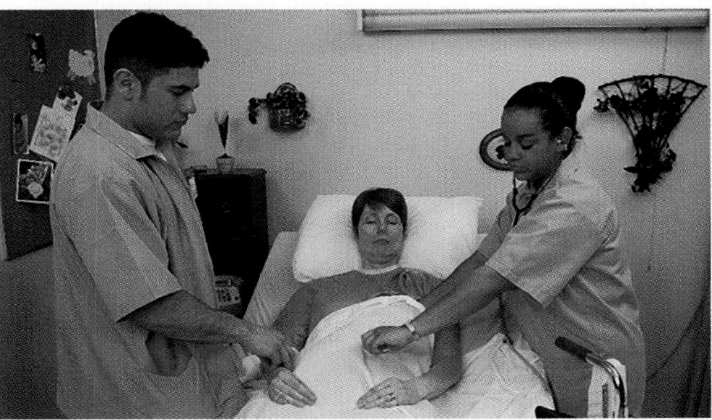

Figure 40-18 Taking an apical-radial pulse. A nurse is taking the apical pulse, and a support worker is taking the radial pulse.

Respiratory rates vary by age (Table 40-3). Infants and children have higher respiratory rates than adults. Count an infant's respiratory rate for 1 minute.

Report and record the following observations after counting respirations:

- The respiratory rate
- Equality and depth of respirations (shallow, normal, or deep)
- If the respirations were regular or irregular
- If the person has pain or difficulty breathing
- Any respiratory noises
- Any abnormal respiratory patterns (see Chapter 43)

Table 40-3 Normal Respiratory Rates by Age

Age	Respirations per minute
Newborn	30–60
Infant	30–50
Toddler	25–32
Child	20–30
Adolescent	16–19
Adult	12–20

Source: J.C. Ross-Kerr, M.J. Wood, A.G. Perry, and P.A. Potter, *Canadian Fundamentals of Nursing*, 2nd ed. (Toronto: Harcourt Canada, 2001), p. 699.

Counting Respirations

Compassionate Care

Remember to Promote:
- **Dignity**
- **Independence**
- **Preferences**
- **Privacy**
- **Safety**

Procedure

1 Continue to hold the wrist after taking the radial pulse.
2 Do not tell the person you are counting respirations.
3 Begin counting when the chest rises. Count each rise and fall of the chest as 1 respiration.
4 Note the following:
   - If respirations are regular
   - If both sides of the chest rise equally
   - The depth of the respirations
   - If the person has pain or difficulty breathing
5 Count the respirations for 30 seconds. Multiply the number by 2.
6 Count respirations for 1 minute if they are abnormal or irregular.
7 Record respiratory rate and other observations on your notepad or assignment sheet.

Post-Procedure

8 Provide for safety and comfort.
9 Place the call bell within reach.*
10 Wash your hands.
11 Report and record your actions and observations according to employer policy.

*Step marked with an asterisk may not apply in community settings.

Blood Pressure

Blood pressure is the amount of force exerted by the blood against the walls of an artery. Blood pressure is controlled by:

- The force of heart contractions
- The amount of blood pumped with each heartbeat
- How easily the blood flows through the blood vessels

The period of heart muscle contraction is called **systole**. The period of heart muscle relaxation is called **diastole**.

Both the systolic and diastolic pressures are measured. The **systolic pressure** is the higher pressure. It represents the amount of force needed to pump blood out of the heart into the arterial circulation. The **diastolic pressure** is the lower pressure. It reflects the pressure in the arteries when the heart is at rest.

Blood pressure is measured in millimetres (mm) of mercury (Hg). The systolic pressure is recorded over the diastolic pressure. The average adult has a systolic pressure of 120 mm Hg and a diastolic pressure of 80 mm Hg. This is written as 120/80 mm Hg.

Factors Affecting Blood Pressure

Blood pressure can change from minute to minute. Factors affecting blood pressure are listed in Box 40-1.

Because it varies so easily, blood pressure has normal ranges:

- *Systolic pressure*—normal range is between 100 and 140 mm Hg
- *Diastolic pressure*—normal range is between 60 and 90 mm Hg

Persistent measurements above the normal systolic and diastolic pressures are abnormal. This condition is called **hypertension** (see Chapter 31). In young and middle-aged adults, report any systolic pressure above 140 mm Hg at once. Also report if the diastolic pressure is above 90 mm Hg. Likewise, systolic pressure below 90 mm Hg and diastolic pressure below 60 mm Hg must be reported. This is called **hypotension**. Some people normally have low blood pressures. However, hypotension may signal a life-threatening problem. (See *Focus on Children: Blood Pressure* and *Focus on Older Adults: Blood Pressure* boxes.)

EQUIPMENT

A sphygmomanometer and stethoscope are used to measure blood pressure. Before using any equipment, make sure you have been properly trained. Follow manufacturer's instructions and employer's policies.

Box 40-1 Factors Affecting Blood Pressure

- *Age*—blood pressure increases with age. It is lowest in infancy and childhood and highest in adulthood.
- *Gender* (*male* or *female*)—women usually have lower blood pressures than men do. Blood pressures rise in women after menopause.
- *Blood volume*—is the amount of blood in the system. Severe bleeding lowers the blood volume. Therefore the blood pressure lowers. Giving IV fluids rapidly increases the blood volume. The blood pressure rises.
- *Stress*—includes anxiety, fear, and other emotions. Blood pressure increases as the body responds to stress.
- *Pain*—generally increases blood pressure. However, severe pain can cause shock. Blood pressure is seriously low in the state of shock (see Chapter 47).
- *Exercise*—increases blood pressure. Blood pressure should not be measured right after exercise.
- *Weight*—blood pressure is higher in overweight people. The blood pressure lowers with weight loss.
- *Ethnicity*—blood pressure tends to be higher among Canadians of South Asian, Aboriginal, and African descent.
- *Diet*—a high-sodium diet increases the amount of water in the body. The extra fluid volume increases blood pressure.
- *Medications*—medications can be given to raise or lower blood pressure. Other medications have the side effects of high or low blood pressure.
- *Position*—blood pressure is lower when a person is lying down. It is higher when a person is standing. Sudden position changes can cause sudden changes in blood pressure (orthostatic hypotension). When standing suddenly, the person may have a sudden drop in blood pressure. Dizziness and fainting can occur (see Chapter 22).
- *Smoking*—increases blood pressure. Nicotine in cigarettes causes blood vessels to narrow. The heart works harder to pump blood through narrowed vessels.
- *Alcohol*—excessive alcohol intake can raise blood pressure.

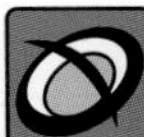

Focus on Children

BLOOD PRESSURE

As with the other vital signs, infants and children have lower blood pressures than adults do. A newborn's blood pressure is usually about 70/55 mm Hg. By 1 year of age the blood pressure increases to 90/55 mm Hg. Blood pressure continues to increase as the child grows older. Adult levels are reached between 14 and 18 years of age.

Taking an infant's or child's blood pressure is a complex task. It usually involves special equipment. Therefore, measuring blood pressure in infants and children is beyond a support worker's scope of practice. A nurse is responsible for this task.

Focus on Older Adults

BLOOD PRESSURE

Arteries narrow and lose their elasticity with aging. The heart has to work harder to pump blood through the vessels. Therefore both the systolic and diastolic pressures are higher in older adults. A blood pressure of 160/90 mm Hg is normal for many older adults. Older adults also are at risk for orthostatic hypotension (see Chapter 22).

Sphygmomanometer. A **sphygmomanometer** is an instrument used to measure blood pressure. It consists of a blood pressure cuff and a measuring device (*manometer*). There are three types of manometers:

- The *aneroid manometer*—has a round dial and a needle that points to the calibrations (Figure 40-19, *A* on page 670). These may be used in all settings.
- The *mercury manometer*—has a column of mercury within a calibrated tube (Figure 40-19, *B* on page 670). Many hospitals have wall-mounted mercury manometers in patient rooms. Remember, mercury is a hazardous substance. If a mercury manometer breaks, call for your supervisor at once. Do not touch the mercury and do not let the client touch it. If possible, move the client from the area. The facility or agency must follow special procedures for handling all hazardous materials (see Chapter 16).
- The *electronic manometer*—automatically displays the blood pressure measurement on the front of the device (Figure 40-19, *C* on page 670). The pulse rate is usually also displayed. The cuff automatically inflates and deflates on some models. Others only have automatic deflation. Electronic manometers are common in facilities. They are also available for home use.

A

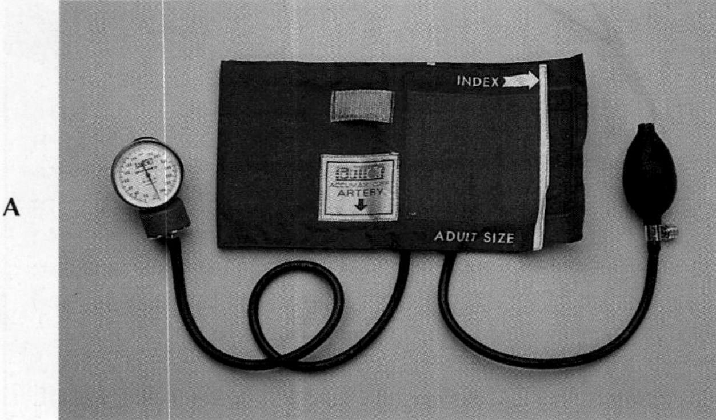

B

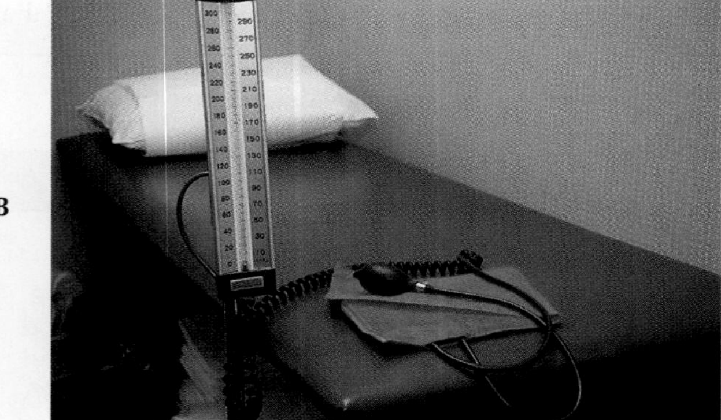

C

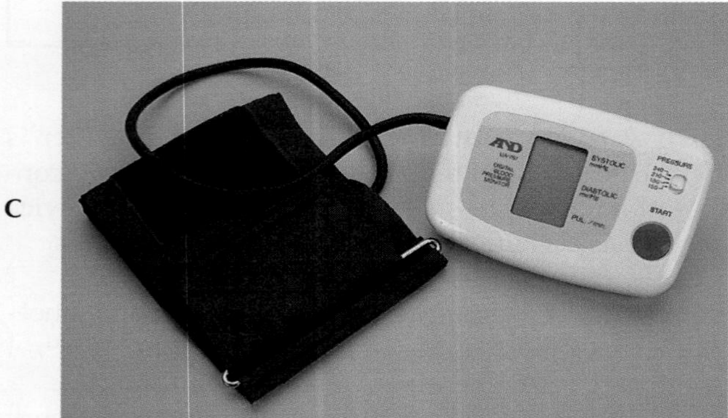

Figure 40-19 Sphygmomanometers. **A,** Aneroid manometer and cuff. **B,** Mercury manometer and cuff. **C,** Electronic manometer and cuff.

The blood pressure cuff is wrapped around the upper arm. Tubing connects the cuff to the manometer. Another tube connects the cuff to a small hand-held bulb. A valve on the bulb is turned so the cuff inflates as the bulb is squeezed. The inflated cuff causes pressure over the brachial artery. The valve is turned the other way for cuff deflation. Blood pressure is measured as the cuff is deflated.

Children and clients with very small arms may need pediatric blood pressure cuffs. Those with very large arms may need extra-large cuffs. The right size is needed for accuracy.

Stethoscope. A **stethoscope** is an instrument used to listen to the sounds produced by the heart, lungs, and other body organs (Figure 40-20). The stethoscope amplifies the sounds for easy hearing.

One of the uses of a stethoscope is to measure blood pressure. Sounds are produced as blood flows through the arteries. The stethoscope is used to listen to the sounds in the brachial artery as the cuff is deflated. Stethoscopes are not needed with electronic sphygmomanometers.

Stethoscopes are in contact with many clients and health care team members. Therefore infection control is important. The earpieces and diaphragm must be cleaned before and after use. Cleaning prevents the spread of microbes.

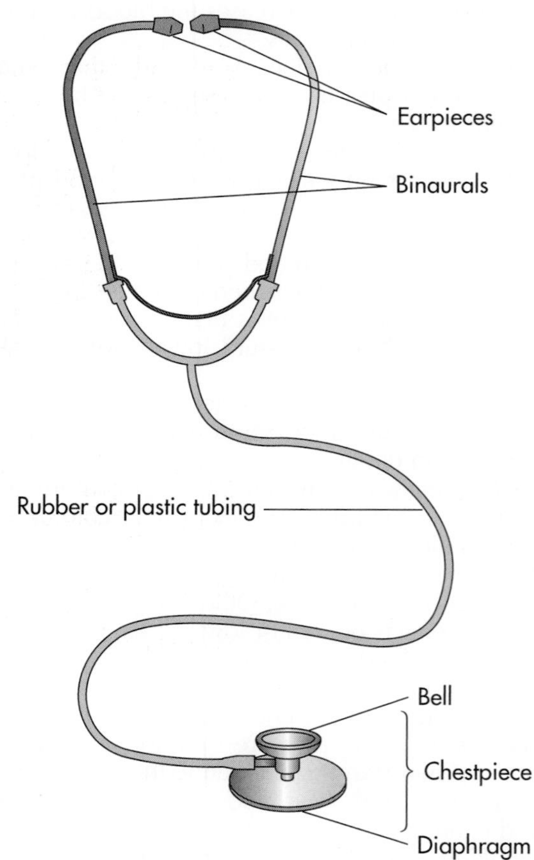

Figure 40-20 Parts of a stethoscope.

Follow these measures when using a stethoscope for taking blood pressure:

- Wipe the earpieces and diaphragm with antiseptic wipes before and after each use.
- Warm the diaphragm in your hand before touching the client with it (Figure 40-21).
- Place the earpiece tips in your ears. The bend of the tips should point forward. Earpieces should fit snugly to block out external noises. They should not cause pain or discomfort.
- Place the diaphragm over the brachial artery. Hold it in place (Figure 40-22).
- Prevent noise. Do not let anything touch the tubing. Ask the client to be silent.

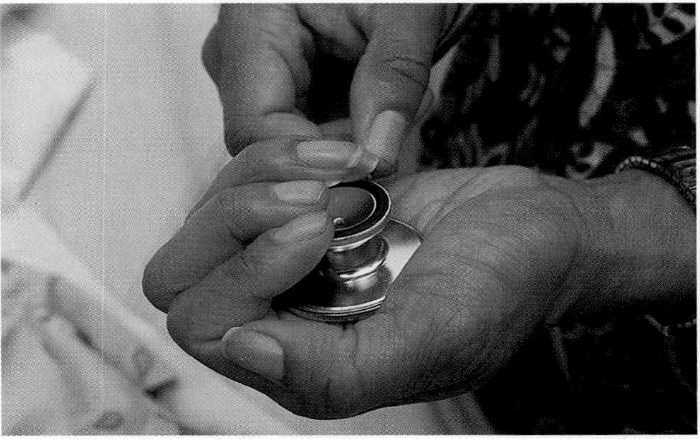

Figure 40-21 Warm the diaphragm of the stethoscope in the palm of your hand.

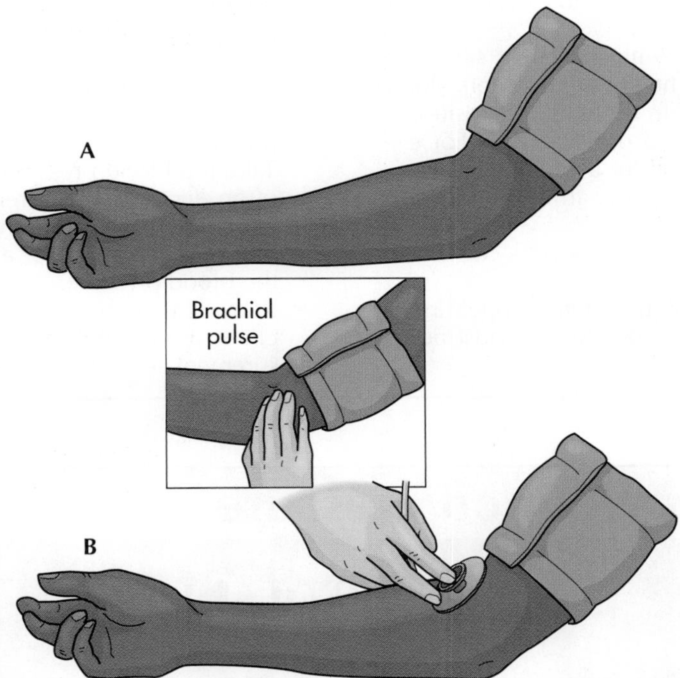

Figure 40-22 Measuring blood pressure. **A,** Apply the cuff over the brachial artery. **B,** Place the diaphragm of the stethoscope over the brachial artery.

Measuring Blood Pressure

You may be asked to measure a client's blood pressure. It is very important to be accurate when measuring blood pressure. Making an inaccurate measurement could cause the client harm. Therefore many employers do not allow support workers to measure and record blood pressure. If you are asked to measure blood pressure, make sure that:

- Your employer allows you to perform this procedure
- The procedure is in your job description
- You have received extra training
- You review the procedure with a nurse
- A nurse is available to answer questions and to supervise you

Blood pressure is normally measured in the brachial artery. Box 40-2 lists the guidelines for measuring blood pressure.

Box 40-2 Guidelines for Measuring Blood Pressure

- Do not take blood pressure on an arm with an IV infusion, a cast, or a dialysis access site. If a client had breast surgery, do not take blood pressure on that side. Avoid taking blood pressure on an injured arm.
- Let the client rest for 10 to 20 minutes before measuring blood pressure.
- Measure blood pressure with the client sitting or lying down. Sometimes the physician orders blood pressure to be measured in the standing position.
- Use the correct size blood pressure cuff. For example, use a pediatric cuff for a very small arm.
- Apply the cuff to the bare upper arm. Clothing can affect the measurement.
- Make sure the cuff is snug. Loose cuffs can cause inaccurate readings.
- Place the diaphragm of the stethoscope firmly over the artery. The entire diaphragm must be in contact with the skin.
- Make sure the room is quiet. Talking, TV, radio, and sounds from the hallway can affect an accurate measurement.
- Have the manometer clearly visible.
- Measure the systolic and diastolic pressures. Expect to hear the first blood pressure sound at the point where you last felt the radial or brachial pulse. The first sound is the systolic pressure. The point where the sound disappears is the diastolic pressure.
- Take the blood pressure again if you are not sure of an accurate measurement. Wait 30 to 60 seconds before repeating the measurement.
- Notify your supervisor at once if you cannot hear the blood pressure.
- Know the normal blood pressure ranges for the client. Immediately report any blood pressure measurement above or below the client's normal range.

Measuring Blood Pressure

Compassionate Care

Remember to Promote:

- **Dignity**
- **Independence**
- **Preferences**
- **Privacy**
- **Safety**

Pre-Procedure

1 Identify the person according to employer policy.
2 Explain the procedure to the person.
3 Wash your hands.
4 Collect the following:
   - Sphygmomanometer (blood pressure cuff)
   - Stethoscope
   - Antiseptic wipes
5 Provide for privacy.

Continued

Measuring Blood Pressure—cont'd

Procedure

6 Wipe the stethoscope earpieces and diaphragm with the wipes.

7 Have the person sit or lie down. Make sure the room is quiet and relaxing. Ask the person not to speak while you measure the blood pressure.

8 Position the person's arm level with the heart. The palm is up.

9 Stand no more than 1 metre (3 feet) away from the manometer. A mercury model must be vertical, on a flat surface, and at eye level. The aneroid type must be directly in front of you.

10 Expose the upper arm.

11 Squeeze the cuff to expel any remaining air. Close the valve on the bulb.

12 Find the brachial artery at the inner aspect of the elbow.

13 Place the arrow on the cuff over the brachial artery (see Figure 40-22, *A* on page 671). Wrap the cuff around the upper arm at least 2.5 cm (1 inch) above the elbow. It should be even and snug.

14 *Method 1:*
- **a** Place the stethoscope earpieces in your ears.
- **b** Locate the radial or brachial pulse.
- **c** Inflate the cuff until you can no longer feel the pulse. Note this point.
- **d** Inflate the cuff 30 mm Hg beyond the point where you last felt the pulse.

15 *Method 2:*
- **a** Locate the radial or brachial pulse.
- **b** Inflate the cuff until you can no longer feel the pulse. Note this point.
- **c** Inflate the cuff 30 mm Hg beyond the point where you last felt the pulse.
- **d** Deflate the cuff slowly. Note the point when you feel the pulse.
- **e** Wait 30 seconds.
- **f** Place the stethoscope earpieces in your ears.
- **g** Inflate the cuff 30 mm Hg beyond the point where you felt the pulse return.

16 Place the diaphragm over the brachial artery (see Figure 40-22, *B* on page 671). Do not place it under the cuff.

17 Deflate the cuff at an even rate of 2 to 4 mm per second. Turn the valve counterclockwise to deflate the cuff.

18 Note the point where you hear the first sound. This is the systolic reading. It should be near the point where the radial pulse disappeared.

19 Continue to deflate the cuff. Note the point where the sound disappears. This is the diastolic reading.

20 Deflate the cuff completely. Remove it from the person's arm. Remove the stethoscope.

21 Record the person's name and blood pressure on your notepad or assignment sheet.

22 Return the cuff to the case or wall holder.

Post-Procedure

23 Provide for safety and comfort.

24 Place the call bell within reach.*

25 Remove privacy measures.

26 Clean the earpieces and diaphragm with the wipes.

27 Return the equipment to its proper place.

28 Wash your hands.

29 Report and record the blood pressure and your observations according to employer policy.

*Step marked with an asterisk may not apply in community settings.

REVIEW

Circle the BEST answer.

1. The following statements are about measuring weight. Which is *false*?
   A. Before breakfast is the best time to weigh the client.
   B. Chair and lift scales are used to weigh clients who cannot stand.
   C. A digital scale should read "10" before the client is weighed.
   D. A full bladder affects weight measurement.

2. Which statement is *false*?
   A. The vital signs are temperature, pulse, respirations, and blood pressure.
   B. Vital signs detect changes in body function.
   C. Vital signs change only during illness.
   D. Sleep, exercise, medications, emotions, and noise affect vital signs.

3. Which should you report at once?
   A. An oral temperature of 37.4° C
   B. A tympanic temperature of 38.2° C
   C. An axillary temperature of 36.1° C
   D. An oral temperature of 36.6° C

4. You must take an infant's temperature. The care plan will likely tell you to take
   A. An oral temperature with a glass thermometer
   B. A rectal temperature
   C. An oral temperature with a tympanic thermometer
   D. An axillary temperature

5. Which thermometer is rarely used in health care settings?
   A. Digital
   B. Glass
   C. Electronic
   D. Dot matrix

6. Which method is usually used to take a pulse?
   A. The radial pulse
   B. The apical-radial pulse
   C. The apical pulse
   D. The brachial pulse

7. Which is reported to your supervisor at once?
   A. An adult has a pulse of 120 beats per minute.
   B. An infant has a pulse of 130 beats per minute.
   C. An adult has a pulse of 80 beats per minute.
   D. An adult has a pulse of 64 beats per minute.

8. Which statement about apical-radial pulses is *true*?
   A. The pulse can be taken by one person.
   B. The apical pulse is never less than the radial pulse.
   C. The radial pulse is never less than the apical pulse.
   D. The apical and radial pulses are always equal.

9. The following describe normal adult respirations. Which is *false*?
   A. There are between 12 and 20 per minute.
   B. They are quiet and effortless.
   C. They are regular with both sides of the chest rising and falling equally.
   D. Noises occur on inhalation.

10. Respirations are usually counted
    A. After taking the temperature
    B. After taking the pulse
    C. Before taking the pulse
    D. After taking the blood pressure

11. Which blood pressure is normal for an adult?
    A. 88/54 mm Hg
    B. 210/100 mm Hg
    C. 130/82 mm Hg
    D. 152/90 mm Hg

12. When taking a blood pressure, you should do the following *except*
    A. Take the blood pressure in the arm with an IV infusion
    B. Apply the cuff to a bare upper arm
    C. Turn off the TV and radio
    D. Locate the brachial artery

13. Which is the systolic blood pressure?
    A. The point at which the pulse is no longer felt
    B. The point where the first sound is heard
    C. The point where the last sound is heard
    D. The point 30 mm Hg above where the pulse was felt

Answers to these questions are on page 827.

CHAPTER 41

WOUND CARE

OBJECTIVES

- Define the key terms listed in this chapter
- List clients at risk for skin tears and pressure ulcers
- Describe the causes of skin tears and how to prevent them
- Describe the signs, symptoms, and causes of pressure ulcers and how to prevent them
- Identify the pressure points in the basic bed and sitting positions
- Describe the causes of leg and foot ulcers and how to prevent them
- Describe the process, types, and complications of wound healing
- Describe what to observe about wounds and wound drainage
- Explain how to secure dressings
- Explain the guidelines for applying dressings
- Explain the purpose of binders and the guidelines for applying them
- Describe how to meet the basic needs of clients with wounds
- Learn the procedure described in this chapter

KEY TERMS

abrasion A partial-thickness wound caused by the scraping away or rubbing of the skin

arterial ulcer An open wound on the lower legs and feet caused by poor arterial blood flow

bedsore Pressure ulcer, pressure sore, or decubitus ulcer

bruise Contusion

chronic wound A wound that does not heal easily

circulatory ulcer An open wound on the lower legs and feet caused by decreased blood flow through arteries or veins; vascular ulcer

clean-contaminated wound A wound occurring from the surgical entry of the urinary, reproductive, or digestive system

clean wound A wound that is not infected; microbes have not entered the wound

closed wound A wound in which tissues are injured but the skin is not broken

contaminated wound A wound with high risk of infection

contusion A closed wound caused by a blow to the body; bruise

decubitus ulcer Pressure ulcer, pressure sore, or bedsore

dehiscence The separation of wound layers

dirty wound An infected wound

edema Swelling caused by fluid collecting in tissues

evisceration The separation of the wound along with the protrusion of abdominal organs

full-thickness wound A wound in which the dermis, epidermis, and subcutaneous tissue are penetrated; muscle and bone may be involved

hematoma The collection of blood under the skin and tissues

hemorrhage The excessive loss of blood in a short period of time

incision An open wound with clean, straight edges; usually intentionally produced with a sharp instrument

infected wound A wound containing large amounts of bacteria and showing signs of infection; a dirty wound

intentional wound A wound created for therapy

laceration An open wound with torn tissues and jagged edges

open wound A wound in which the skin or mucous membrane is broken

partial-thickness wound A wound in which the dermis and epidermis of the skin are broken

penetrating wound An open wound in which the skin and underlying tissues are pierced

pressure sore Bedsore, decubitus ulcer, or pressure ulcer

pressure ulcer Any injury caused by unrelieved pressure; a decubitus ulcer, bedsore, or pressure sore

puncture wound An open wound made by a sharp object; entry of the skin and underlying tissues may be intentional or unintentional

shock The condition that results when there is not enough blood supply to organs and tissues

skin tear A break or rip in the skin; the epidermis separates from the underlying tissue

stasis ulcer An open wound on the lower legs and feet caused by poor blood return through the veins; venous ulcer

trauma An accident or violent act that injures the skin, mucous membranes, bones, or internal organs

unintentional wound A wound resulting from trauma

vascular ulcer Circulatory ulcer

venous ulcer Stasis ulcer

wound A break in the skin or mucous membrane

The skin is the body's first line of defence. It protects the body from microbes that cause infection. Giving good skin care is one of your most important tasks.

Older and disabled people are at great risk for skin breakdown. So are infants and children. Their skin is easily injured. Box 41-1 lists the common causes of skin breakdown.

A **wound** is a break in the skin or mucous membrane. It is a portal of entry for microbes. Wounds result from many causes. A surgical incision leaves a wound. Often wounds result from **trauma**—an accident or violent act that injures the skin, mucous membranes, bones, or internal organs. Falls, vehicle accidents, gun shots, stabbings, and other violent acts are causes of trauma. Pressure ulcers are wounds that occur from poor skin care and immobility. Circulatory ulcers are caused by decreased blood flow through the arteries and veins.

You must prevent skin injury and give good skin care. When injury does occur, infection is a major threat. Wound care involves preventing infection and further injury to the wound and nearby tissues.

Your role in wound care depends on your provincial or territorial laws, your job description, and the client's condition. Whatever your role, you need to know the types of wounds, how wounds heal, and how to promote wound healing.

Box 41-1 Common Causes of Skin Breakdown

- Age-related changes in the skin
- Dryness
- Fragile and weak capillaries
- General thinning of the skin
- Loss of fatty layer under the skin
- Decreased sensation to touch, heat, and cold
- Decreased mobility
- Sitting in a chair or lying in bed most or all of the day
- Chronic diseases (e.g., diabetes, high blood pressure)
- Diseases that decrease circulation
- Poor nutrition
- Poor hydration
- Incontinence
- Moisture in dark areas of the body (skinfolds, under breasts, and perineal areas)
- Pressure on bony parts (Figure 41-1 on page 678)
- Poor care of fingernails or toenails
- Friction and shearing

TYPES OF WOUNDS

Wounds are described in many ways (Box 41-2 on page 679). The following wounds are common:

- *Abrasion*—a partial-thickness wound caused by the scraping away or rubbing of the skin
- *Contusion*—a closed wound caused by a blow to the body (a **bruise**)
- *Incision*—an open wound with clean, straight edges; usually intentionally produced with a sharp instrument
- *Laceration*—an open wound with torn tissues and jagged edges
- *Penetrating wound*—an open wound in which the skin and underlying tissues are pierced
- *Puncture wound*—an open wound made by a sharp object; entry of the skin and underlying tissues may be intentional or unintentional

SKIN TEARS

A **skin tear** is a break or rip in the skin. The epidermis (top skin layer) separates from the underlying tissue (see Figure 13-4 on page 129). The hands, arms, and lower legs are common sites for skin tears. Many older adults have very thin and fragile skin. Slight pressure can cause a skin tear.

CAUSES

Skin tears are caused by friction, shearing (see Chapter 21), pulling, or direct pressure on the skin. A skin tear can occur by bumping a hand, arm, or leg on any hard surface. Beds, bed rails, chairs, wheelchair footrests, and tables are dangers. You can cause a skin tear by holding on to a client's arm or leg too tightly. Be careful when moving, repositioning, or transferring clients. Bathing, dressing, and other tasks can cause skin tears. So can pulling buttons or zippers across fragile skin.

Skin tears are painful. They are portals of entry for microbes. Tell your supervisor at once if you cause or find a skin tear.

CLIENTS AT RISK

Clients at risk for skin tears are those who:

- Require moderate to complete help in moving
- Have poor nutrition or are very thin
- Are poorly hydrated
- Have altered mental awareness; for example, clients with dementia may resist care and move quickly and without warning. These movements can cause skin tears.
- Are older

(text continues on page 679)

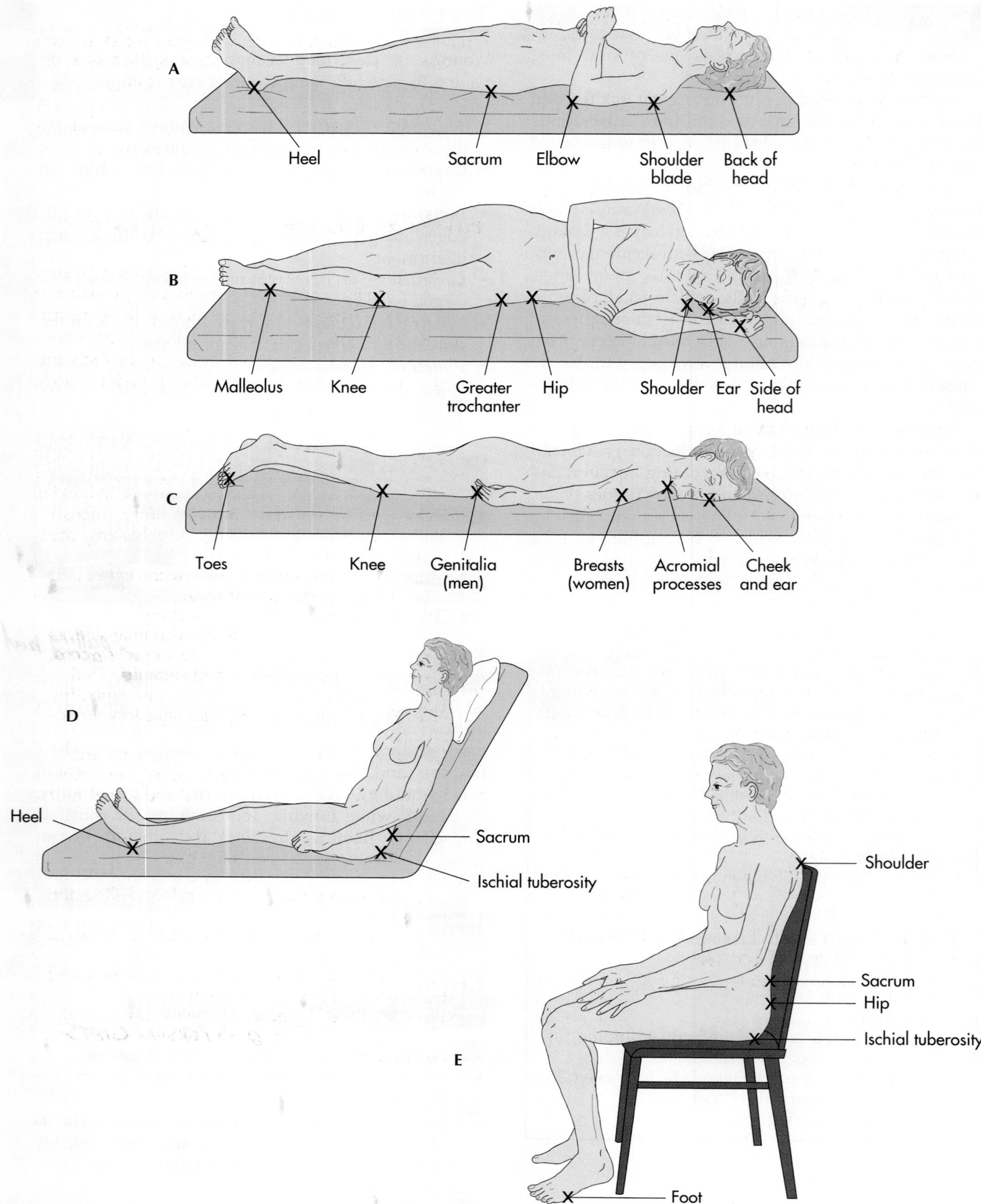

Figure 41-1 Pressure points: common pressure ulcer sites. **A,** The supine position. **B,** The lateral position. **C,** The prone position. **D,** Fowler's position. **E,** The sitting position.

Box 41-2 Types of Wounds

Intentional and Unintentional Wounds
- **Intentional wound**—is created for therapy. Surgical incisions are examples. So are venipunctures for starting IV therapy or for collecting blood specimens.
- **Unintentional wound**—results from trauma (falls, vehicle accidents, gun shots, stabbings, and other violent acts).

Open and Closed Wounds
- **Open wound**—occurs when the skin or mucous membrane is broken. Intentional and most unintentional wounds are open.
- **Closed wound**—occurs when tissues are injured but the skin is not broken (bruises, twists, and sprains).

Clean and Dirty Wounds
- **Clean wound**—is not infected. Microbes have not entered the wound. Closed wounds are usually clean. So are intentional wounds created under surgically aseptic conditions. The urinary, respiratory, and digestive systems are not entered.
- **Clean-contaminated wound**—occurs from the surgical entry of the urinary, reproductive, or digestive system. These systems are not sterile and contain normal flora.
- **Contaminated wound**—has a high risk of infection. Unintentional wounds are generally contaminated. Wound contamination also occurs from breaks in surgical asepsis and spillage of intestinal contents. Tissues may show signs of inflammation.
- **Infected wound (dirty wound)**—contains large amounts of bacteria and shows signs of infection. Examples include old wounds, surgical incisions into infected areas, and traumatic injuries that rupture the bowel.
- **Chronic wound**—does not heal easily. Pressure ulcers and circulatory ulcers are examples. Any wound that is continually exposed to friction, pressure, or moisture can become chronic.

Partial- and Full-Thickness Wounds (Describe Wound Depth)
- **Partial-thickness wound**—the dermis and epidermis of the skin are broken.
- **Full-thickness wound**—the dermis, epidermis, and subcutaneous tissue are penetrated. Muscle and bone may be involved.

Prevention and Treatment

Giving careful and safe care helps prevent skin tears and further injury. Follow the guidelines in Box 41-3.

The physician and the nurse direct skin care treatment. Dressings may be ordered. Elastic wraps protect the skin from injury. They also help the healing process (page 686). Follow the care plan and your supervisor's instructions.

Pressure Ulcers

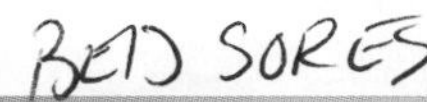

A **pressure ulcer (decubitus ulcer, bedsore, pressure sore)** is any injury caused by unrelieved pressure. It usually occurs over a bony prominence. To be prominent means to stick out. Therefore a bony prominence is an area where the bone sticks out or projects out from the flat surface of the body. The shoulder blades,

Box 41-3 Guidelines for Preventing Skin Tears

- Follow the care plan for moving, lifting, repositioning, transferring, dressing, and bathing the client.
- Keep the skin moisturized. Follow the care plan.
- Offer fluids. Follow the care plan.
- Dress and undress the client carefully.
- Dress the client in soft clothing with long sleeves and long pants. Allow for the client's preferences.
- Keep your fingernails short and smoothly filed.
- Keep the client's fingernails short and smoothly filed. Report long and rough toenails to your supervisor.
- Do not wear rings with large or raised stones.
- Follow safety guidelines when lifting and transferring the client to and from bed and wheelchair (see Chapter 21).
- Prevent friction and shearing during lifting, moving, transferring, and repositioning.
- Use a lift sheet to lift and turn the client in bed.
- Use pillows to support arms and legs. Follow the care plan.
- Be patient and calm when the client is confused or agitated or resists care.
- Pad bed rails and wheelchair arms, footrests, and leg supports. Follow the care plan.
- Provide good lighting. It helps prevent the client from bumping into furniture, walls, and equipment.

elbows, hip bones, sacrum (the bone in the lower part of the spine), knees, ankle bones, heels, and toes are bony prominences.

These bony prominences are called pressure points because they bear the weight of the body in certain positions (see Figure 41-1 on page 678). Pressure from body weight can reduce blood supply to the area. A pressure ulcer can result.

Causes

Pressure, friction, and shearing are common causes of skin breakdown and pressure ulcers. Other factors include breaks in the skin, poor circulation to an area, moisture, dry skin, and irritation by urine and stool.

Pressure occurs when the skin over a bony prominence is squeezed between hard surfaces. The bone itself is one hard surface. The other is usually the mattress or chair seat. The squeezing or pressure prevents blood flow to the skin and underlying tissues. Lack of blood flow means oxygen and nutrients cannot get to the cells. Therefore the involved skin and tissues die (Figure 41-2).

Friction scrapes the skin. The scrape is a portal of entry for microbes. The open area needs to heal. A good blood supply to the area is necessary. Infection is prevented, so healing occurs. A poor blood supply or an infection can lead to a pressure ulcer.

Shearing also exerts pressure on the skin. Shearing occurs when the skin sticks to a surface (usually the bed or chair) and deeper tissues move downward, exerting pressure on the skin (see Chapter 21). Shearing occurs when the client slides down in the bed or chair. Blood vessels and tissues are damaged. Therefore blood flow to the area is reduced. The risk of a pressure ulcer is increased.

Pressure ulcers can also occur when two bony areas are in direct contact with each other (such as when knees or ankles rub together). In obese people, pressure ulcers can develop in areas where skin is in contact with skin. Friction results when this occurs. Pressure ulcers can develop underneath the breasts, between abdominal folds, the legs, and the buttocks.

Clients at Risk

Clients at risk for pressure ulcers are those who:

- Are confined to bed or a chair
- Require moderate to complete help in moving
- Have loss of bowel or bladder control
- Have poor nutrition
- Have altered mental awareness
- Have problems sensing pain or pressure
- Have circulatory problems
- Are older
- Are obese or very thin

Signs of Pressure Ulcers

The first sign of a pressure ulcer is pale skin or a warm, reddened area. (Colour changes may be hard to notice in clients with dark skin.) The person may complain of pain, burning, itching, or tingling in the area. Some do not feel anything unusual. Box 41-4 describes pressure ulcer development. Check your client's skin every time you provide care. Immediately notify your supervisor of any signs of a pressure ulcer.

Prevention and Treatment

Pressure ulcers develop over time. The longer that pressure is exerted on the skin, the greater the risk that a pressure ulcer will develop.

Preventing pressure ulcers is much easier than trying to heal them. Good care, cleanliness, and skin care are essential. Box 41-5 on page 682 lists guidelines for preventing skin breakdown and pressure ulcers. Follow the care plan.

(text continues on page 683)

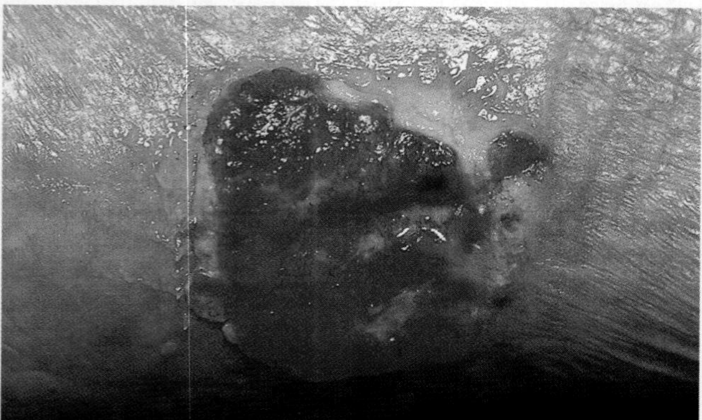

Figure 41-2 A pressure ulcer.

Box 41-4 Stages of Pressure Ulcers

Stage 1	The skin is red. The colour does not return to normal when the skin is relieved of pressure (Figure 41-3, *A*).
Stage 2	The skin cracks, blisters, or peels (Figure 41-3, *B*). There may be a shallow crater.
Stage 3	The skin is gone, and the underlying tissues are exposed (Figure 41-3, *C*). The exposed tissue is damaged. There may be drainage from the area.
Stage 4	Muscle and bone are exposed and damaged (Figure 41-3, *D*). Drainage is likely.

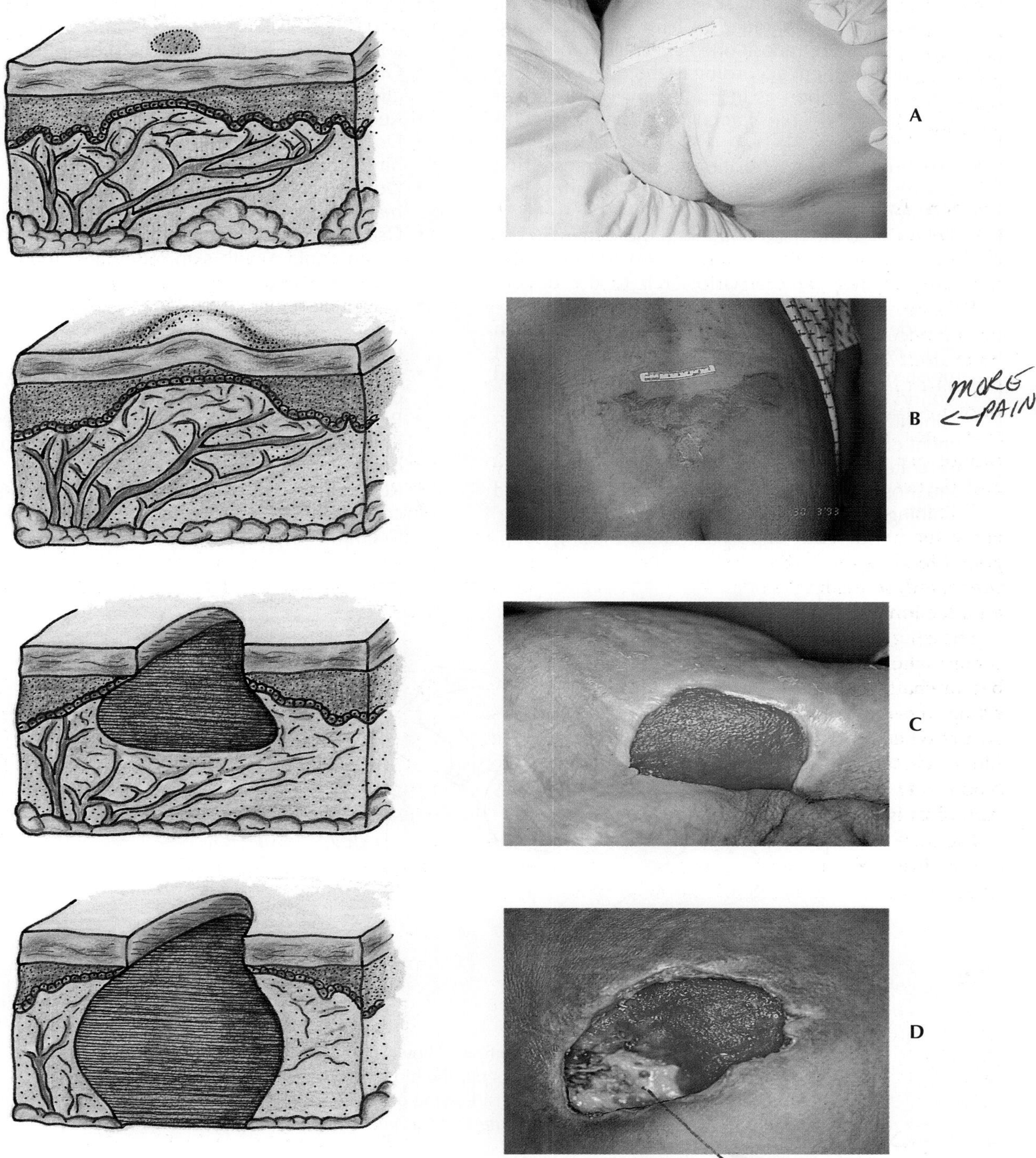

Figure 41-3 Stages of pressure ulcers. **A,** Stage 1. **B,** Stage 2. **C,** Stage 3. **D,** Stage 4. *(Courtesy Laurel Wiersema-Bryant, RN, MSN, Clinical Nurse Specialist, Barnes-Jewish Hospital, St. Louis, MO.)*

Box 41-5 Guidelines for Preventing Pressure Ulcers

- Follow the repositioning schedule in the care plan. The client is repositioned at least every 2 hours. Some clients are repositioned every 15 minutes.
- Position the client according to the care plan. Use pillows for support as instructed by your supervisor. The 30-degree lateral position is recommended (Figure 41-4).
- Use proper lifting, positioning, and transferring procedures to prevent friction and shearing (see Chapter 21).
- Do not raise the head of the bed more than 30 degrees. This prevents shearing. Follow the care plan.
- Apply a thin layer of cornstarch to the bottom sheets. This prevents friction.
- Provide good skin care. The skin must be clean and dry after bathing. The skin must be free of moisture from urine, stool, perspiration, and wound drainage.
- Minimize skin exposure to moisture. Check incontinent clients (those without bowel or bladder control) often. Also check clients who perspire heavily and those with wound drainage. Change linens and clothing as needed. Give good skin care.
- Check with your supervisor before using soap. Soap can dry and irritate the skin.
- Apply a moisturizer to dry areas—the hands, elbows, legs, ankles, and heels. Your supervisor will tell you what to use and where to apply it.
- Give a back massage when repositioning the client. Do not massage bony areas.
- Keep linens clean, dry, and wrinkle-free.
- Do not irritate the skin. Avoid scrubbing or rubbing when bathing or drying the client.
- Do not massage pressure points. *Never rub or massage reddened areas.*
- Use pillows and blankets to prevent skin from being in contact with skin. They also reduce moisture and friction.
- Keep the heels off the bed. Use pillows or other devices as directed. Place the pillows or devices under the lower legs from mid-calf to the ankles.
- Use protective devices as instructed by your supervisor and the care plan.
- Remind clients sitting in chairs to shift their positions every 15 minutes. This decreases pressure on bony points. Assist if required.
- Report any signs of skin breakdown or pressure ulcers at once. Record your observations according to employer policy.

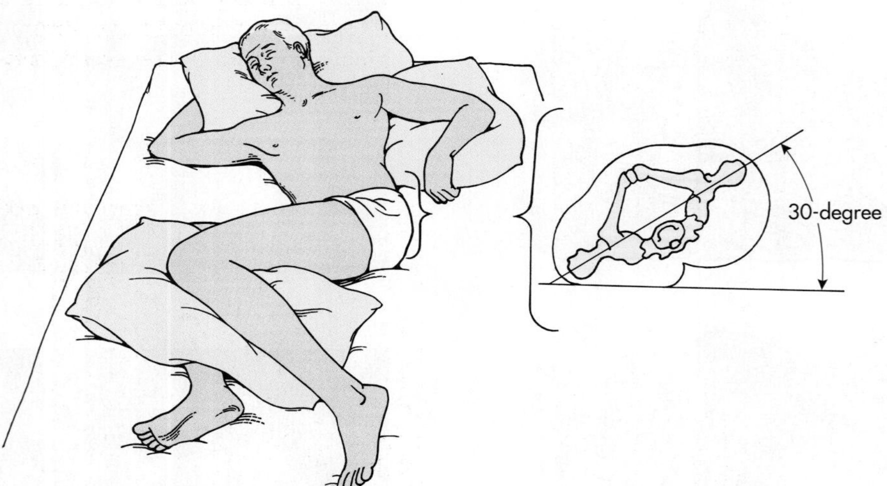

Figure 41-4 The 30-degree lateral position. Pillows are placed under the head, shoulder, and leg. This position inclines (lifts up) the hip to avoid pressure on the hip. The client does not lie on the hip as in the side-lying position. Source: R.A. Bryant et al., "Pressure Ulcer," R.A. Bryant, ed., *Acute and Chronic Wounds: Nursing Management* (St. Louis: Mosby, 1992).

Any client at risk for pressure ulcers is placed on a surface that reduces or relieves pressure. Such surfaces include foam, air, alternating air, gel, or water mattresses. The health care team decides on the best surface for the client.

A physician directs pressure ulcer treatment. Wound care products, medications, treatments, and special equipment are ordered to promote healing. Your supervisor and the care plan tell you what to do. The following protective devices are often ordered to prevent and treat pressure ulcers and other types of skin breakdown.

- *Bed cradle*—A bed cradle (Anderson frame) is a metal frame placed on the bed and over the client. Top linens are brought over the cradle to prevent pressure on the legs and feet (Figure 41-5). Top linens are tucked in at the bottom of the mattress and mitred. They are also tucked under both sides of the mattress to protect the client from air drafts and chilling. (See *Focus on Home Care: Bed Cradles* box.)

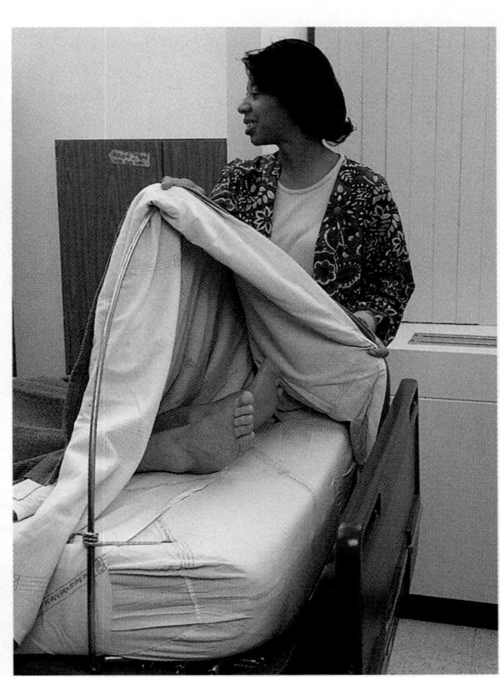

Figure 41-5 A bed cradle is placed on top of the bed. Linens are brought over the top cradle.

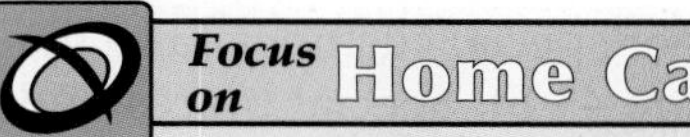

Focus on Home Care

Bed Cradles

A cardboard box is useful as a bed cradle (Figure 41-6). Your supervisor tells you how to line the box to prevent pressure on the heels.

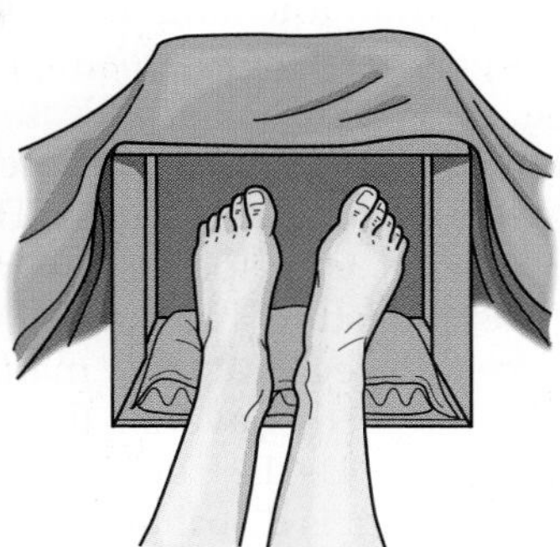

Figure 41-6 A box serves as a bed cradle. It keeps top linens off the client's feet.

- *Elbow protectors*—These devices are made of foam rubber or sheepskin. They fit the shape of the elbow (Figure 41-7). Some have straps to secure them in place. Friction is prevented between the bed and the elbow.

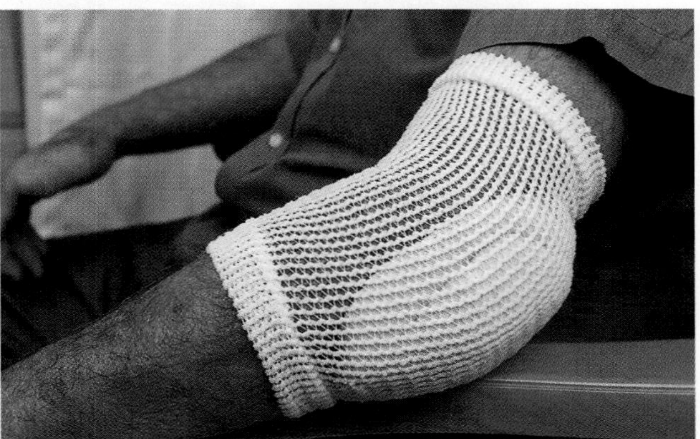

Figure 41-7 Elbow protector.

- *Heel elevators*—Pillows or special cushions raise the heels off the bed (Figure 41-8). Special braces and splints also keep pressure off the heels.
- *Flotation pads*—Flotation pads or cushions (Figure 41-9) are like water beds. They are made of a gel-like substance. The outer case is heavy plastic. They are used for chairs and wheelchairs. The pad is placed in a pillowcase or special cover. This prevents the plastic from touching the skin.
- *Eggcrate-like mattress*—This is a foam pad that looks like an egg carton (Figure 41-10). Peaks in the mattress distribute the client's weight more evenly. It is placed on top of the regular mattress. The eggcrate-like mattress is put in a special cover. The cover protects against moisture and soiling. Only a bottom sheet covers the eggcrate-like mattress.
- *Special beds*—Some beds have air flowing through the mattress (Figure 41-11). The client *floats* on the mattress. Body weight is distributed evenly. There is little pressure on bony parts. Another type of bed allows repositioning without moving the client. Depending on the bed, the client is turned to the prone or supine position or tilted various degrees. Body alignment does not change. Pressure points change as the position changes. There is little friction. Some beds constantly rotate from side to side. These beds are useful for clients with spinal cord injuries.
- *Other equipment*—Trochanter rolls and footboards are also used (see Chapter 22).

Leg and Foot Ulcers

Some diseases affect blood flow to and from the legs and feet. They can cause pain, open wounds, and edema. **Edema** is swelling caused by fluid collecting in tissues. Infection and gangrene can result from the open wound and poor circulation. *Gangrene* is a condition in which there is death of tissue (see Chapter 31).

The client needs special skin care. A physician directs the client's care. A nurse uses the care planning process to meet the client's needs. Preventing skin breakdown on the legs and feet is very important.

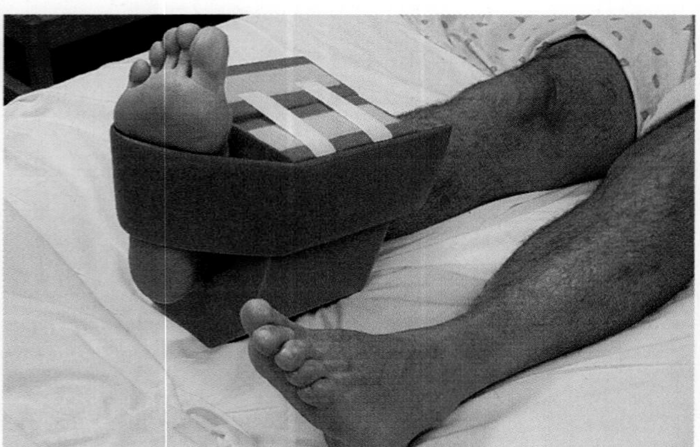

Figure 41-8 Heel elevator.

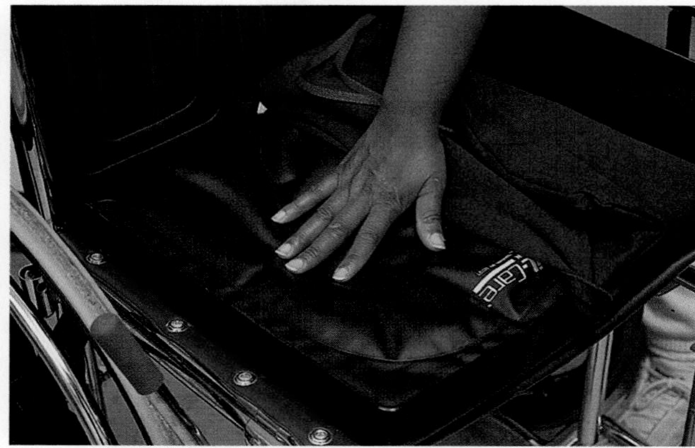

Figure 41-9 Flotation pad.

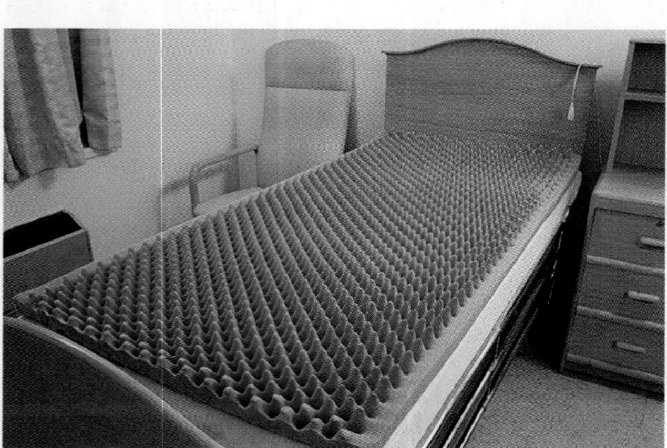

Figure 41-10 Eggcrate-like mattress on the bed.

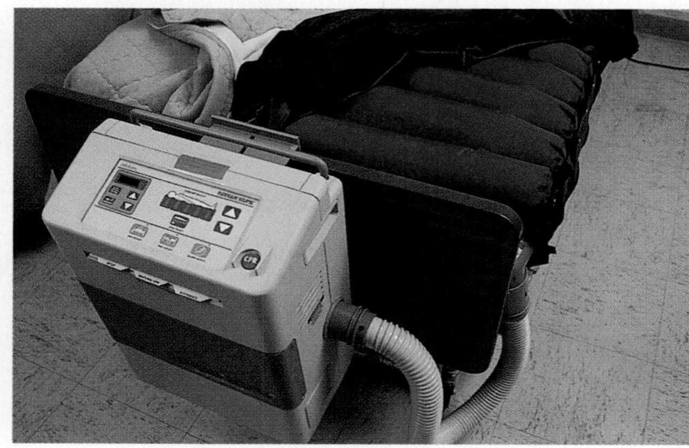

Figure 41-11 Air flotation bed.

CIRCULATORY ULCERS

Circulatory ulcers (vascular ulcers) are open wounds on the lower legs and feet caused by decreased blood flow through arteries or veins. People with diseases affecting the blood vessels are at risk for these ulcers on the legs and feet. These wounds are painful and hard to heal.

STASIS ULCERS

Stasis ulcers (venous ulcers) are open wounds on the lower legs and feet caused by poor blood return through the veins (Figure 41-12). Valves in the leg veins do not close well. Therefore the veins do not pump blood back to the heart normally. Blood and fluid collect in the legs and feet. Edema occurs in the legs and feet. Small veins in the skin can rupture. Remember, hemoglobin gives blood its red colour. When the veins rupture, hemoglobin enters the tissues. This causes the skin to turn brown. The skin also is dry, leathery, and hard. Itching is common.

The heels and inner sides of the ankles are common sites for stasis ulcers. These ulcers can occur from skin injury. Scratching is a common cause. Or the ulcers occur spontaneously. The ulcers are painful and make walking difficult. They weep fluid. Healing is slow, and infection is a great risk.

Preventing skin breakdown caused by poor circulation is very important. Stasis ulcers are hard to heal. Box 41-6 lists guidelines that help prevent stasis ulcers. They may be part of the client's care plan.

The physician may order elastic stockings or elastic bandages (see Chapter 28). They promote comfort and circulation by providing support and pressure to the veins. Professional foot care is important. The physician may also order medications or wound care products.

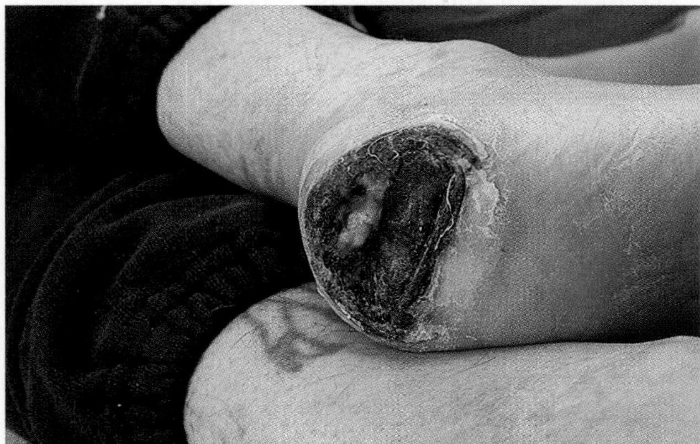

Figure 41-12 Stasis ulcer.

Box 41-6 Guidelines for Preventing Stasis Ulcers

- Apply elastic stockings or elastic wraps according to the care plan (if you are allowed to do so). See Chapter 28.
- Remind the client not to sit with legs crossed.
- Do not use elastic or rubber-band type garters to hold socks or hose in place.
- Provide good skin care daily. Clean and dry between the toes.
- Avoid injury to legs and feet.
- Keep linens clean, dry, and wrinkle-free.
- Follow the care plan for walking and exercise. They increase venous blood flow.
- Reposition the client at least every 2 hours. Follow the care plan.
- Elevate the legs according to the care plan.
- Have the client wear comfortable socks and shoes.
- Do not irritate the skin. Avoid scrubbing or rubbing when bathing or drying the client.
- Avoid massaging over the pressure point. *Never rub or massage reddened areas.*
- Keep the heels off the bed. Use pillows or other devices as instructed by your supervisor. Place the pillows or devices under the lower legs from mid-calf to the ankles.
- Use protective devices as directed by your supervisor and the care plan (page 683).
- Report signs of skin breakdown, stasis ulcers, or pressure ulcers at once.

ARTERIAL ULCERS

Arterial ulcers are open wounds on the lower legs and feet caused by poor arterial blood flow. The leg and foot may feel cold and look blue or shiny. The ulcer is often painful during rest. Pain is usually worse at night.

These ulcers are caused by diseases or injuries that decrease arterial blood flow to the legs and feet. High blood pressure and diabetes are common causes. So are narrowed arteries from aging. Smoking is another risk factor.

Arterial ulcers are found between the toes, on the tops of the toes, and on the outer sides of the ankles. The heels are common sites for people on bed rest. Arterial ulcers can also occur in pressure sites from shoes that fit poorly.

The physician directs the client's treatment. The disease causing the ulcer is treated. Medications, wound care, and a walking program are ordered. Professional foot care is important. Follow the care plan to prevent further injury. Box 41-7 on page 686 lists guidelines for preventing arterial ulcers.

Box 41-7 Guidelines for Preventing Arterial Ulcers

- Discourage the client from smoking.
- Remind clients not to sit with legs crossed.
- Avoid exposing the client to cold.
- Do not use elastic or rubber-band type garters to hold socks and hose in place.
- Make sure shoes fit well.
- Keep feet clean and dry.
- Keep pressure off heels and other bony points.
- Avoid pressure under the knees.
- Check the client's legs and feet daily. Report changes in skin colour or breaks in the skin to your supervisor.
- Avoid massaging over pressure points. *Never rub or massage reddened areas.*
- Use protective devices as directed by your supervisor and the care plan (page 683).

Wound Healing

The healing process has three phases:

- *Inflammatory phase* (3 days). Bleeding stops, and a scab forms over the wound. The scab prevents microbes from entering the wound. Blood supply to the wound increases. The blood brings nutrients and healing substances. Because blood supply increases, signs and symptoms of inflammation appear. They are redness, swelling, heat or warmth, and pain. Loss of function may occur.
- *Proliferative phase* (day 3 to day 21). Proliferate means to multiply rapidly. Tissue cells multiply to repair the wound.
- *Maturation phase* (day 21 to 1 or 2 years). The scar gains strength. The red, raised scar eventually becomes thin and pale.

Types of Wound Healing

The healing process occurs through primary intention, secondary intention, or tertiary intention. With *primary intention* (*first intention, primary closure*), the wound is closed. Sutures (stitches), staples, clips, or adhesive strips hold the wound edges together.

Secondary intention (*second intention*) is used for contaminated and infected wounds. Wounds are cleaned and dead tissue removed. Wound edges are not brought together, and the wound gapes. Healing occurs naturally. However, healing takes longer and leaves a larger scar. The threat of infection is great.

Tertiary intention (*third intention, delayed intention*) involves leaving a wound open and then closing it later. Thus tertiary intention combines secondary and primary intention. Infection and poor circulation are common reasons for tertiary intention.

Complications

Many factors affect healing and increase the risk of complications. The type of wound is one factor. Other factors include the person's age, general health, nutrition, and lifestyle.

Good circulation is important. Age, smoking, circulatory disease, and diabetes all affect circulation. Certain medications (Coumadin and heparin) prolong bleeding. Good nutrition is important. Protein is needed for tissue growth and repair.

Infection is a risk for people with immune system changes and for those taking antibiotics. Antibiotics kill pathogens. Specific antibiotics kill specific pathogens. In doing so, an environment may be created that allows other pathogens to grow and multiply.

Hemorrhage. **Hemorrhage** is excessive loss of blood in a short period of time (see Chapter 47). If bleeding is not stopped, death results. Hemorrhage may be internal or external. Internal hemorrhage cannot be seen. Bleeding occurs into tissues and body cavities. A hematoma may form. A **hematoma** is a collection of blood under the skin and tissues. The area appears swollen and has a reddish-blue colour. Shock, vomiting blood, coughing up blood, and loss of consciousness are signs of internal hemorrhage.

You can see external bleeding. Bloody drainage and dressings soaked with blood are common signs. As with internal hemorrhage, shock can occur.

Shock results when there is not enough blood supply to organs and tissues (see Chapter 47). Signs and symptoms include low or falling blood pressure, rapid and weak pulse, and rapid respirations. The skin is cold, moist, and pale. The person is restless and may complain of thirst. Confusion and loss of consciousness eventually occur.

Hemorrhage and shock are emergencies. Immediately notify your supervisor and assist as requested. Remember to practise Standard Precautions when in contact with blood. Gloves are always worn. Gowns, masks, and eye protection are necessary when blood splashes and splatters are likely.

Infection. Wound contamination can occur during or after injury. Trauma often causes contaminated wounds. Surgical wounds can be contaminated during or after surgery. An infected wound appears inflamed (reddened) and has drainage. The wound is painful and tender. The person has a fever.

Dehiscence. **Dehiscence** is the separation of the wound layers (Figure 41-13). Separation may involve the skin layer or underlying tissues. Abdominal

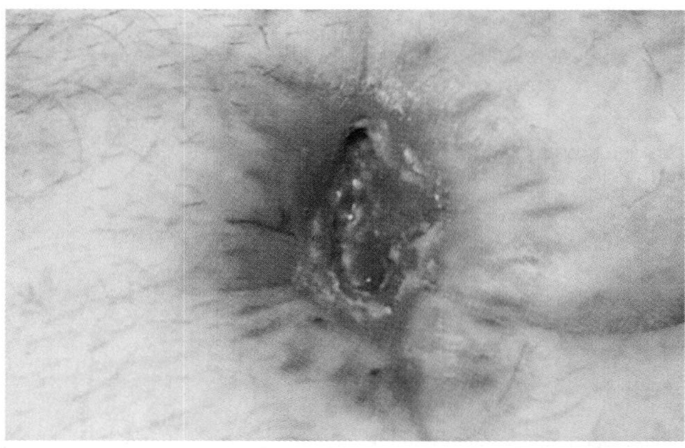

Figure 41-13 Wound dehiscence. Source: M. Morison, *A Colour Guide to the Nursing Management of Wounds* (London: Wolfe Medical Publishers, 1992).

wounds are commonly affected. Coughing, vomiting, and abdominal distention place stress on the wound. The person often describes the sensation of the wound popping open.

Evisceration. **Evisceration** is the separation of the wound along with the protrusion of abdominal organs (Figure 41-14). Causes are the same as for dehiscence.

Dehiscence and evisceration are surgical emergencies. Tell your supervisor at once if they happen. A nurse covers the wound with large sterile dressings saturated with sterile saline. The person needs emergency medical care.

Wound Appearance

During the healing process, physicians and nurses routinely observe the wound and its drainage. They observe for healing and complications. You need to make certain observations when assisting with wound care. You report your observations to your supervisor and record them according to employer policy. Box 41-8 lists questions to consider when observing wounds.

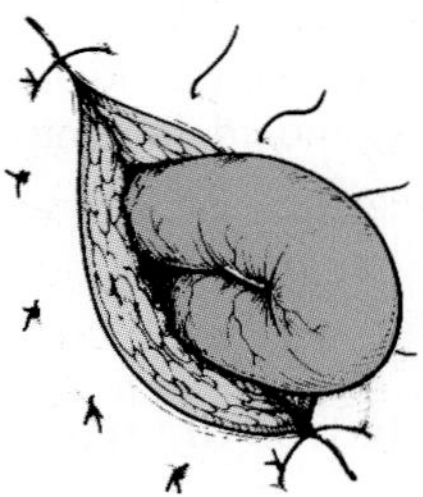

Figure 41-14 Wound evisceration. Source: *Mosby's Medical, Nursing, and Allied Health Dictionary,* 4th ed. (St. Louis: Mosby, 1994).

Box 41-8 Wound Observations

Wound Location
- Where is the wound located on the body? Is there more than one wound? (Multiple wounds may exist from surgery or trauma.)

Wound Appearance
- Is the wound red and swollen?
- Is the area around the wound warm to touch?
- Are sutures, staples, or clips intact or broken?
- Are wound edges closed or separated? Did the wound break open?

Drainage
- Is there drainage?
- What is the amount of drainage?
- Is the damage
  - Clear
  - Bloody
  - Watery and blood-tinged
  - Thick and green, yellow, or brown

Odour
- Does the wound or drainage have an odour?

Surrounding Skin
- Is surrounding skin intact?
- What is the colour of surrounding skin?
- Are surrounding tissues swollen?

Wound Drainage

During injury and the inflammatory phase of wound healing, fluid and cells escape from the tissues. The amount of drainage may be small or large, depending on wound size and location. Bleeding and infection also affect the amount and kind of drainage. Wound drainage is observed and measured.

Major types of wound drainage are as follows:

- *Serous drainage*—clear, watery fluid (Figure 41-15, *A* on page 688). The fluid in a blister is serous. Serous comes from the word *serum*, which is the clear, thin, fluid portion of blood. Serum does not contain blood cells or platelets.
- *Sanguineous drainage*—bloody drainage (Figure 41-15, *B* on page 688). Sanguineous comes from the Latin word *sanguis*, which means blood. The amount and colour of sanguineous drainage are important. Hemorrhage is suspected when large amounts are present. Bright drainage means fresh bleeding. Older bleeding is darker.
- *Serosanguineous drainage*—thin, watery drainage (*sero*) that is blood-tinged (*sanguineous*) (Figure 41-15, *C* on page 688).
- *Purulent drainage*—thick drainage that is green, yellow, or brown (Figure 41-15, *D* on page 688).

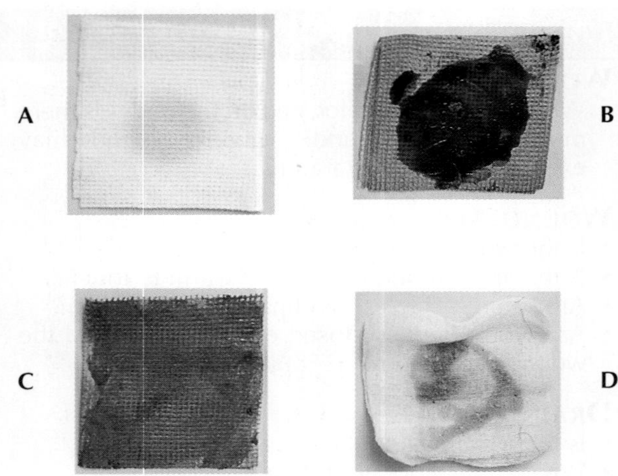

Figure 41-15 Wound drainage. **A,** Serous drainage. **B,** Sanguineous drainage. **C,** Serosanguineous drainage. **D,** Purulent drainage. Source: J.C. Ross-Kerr, M.J. Wood, A.G. Perry, and P.A. Potter, *Canadian Fundamentals of Nursing,* 2nd ed. (Toronto: Harcourt Canada, 2001).

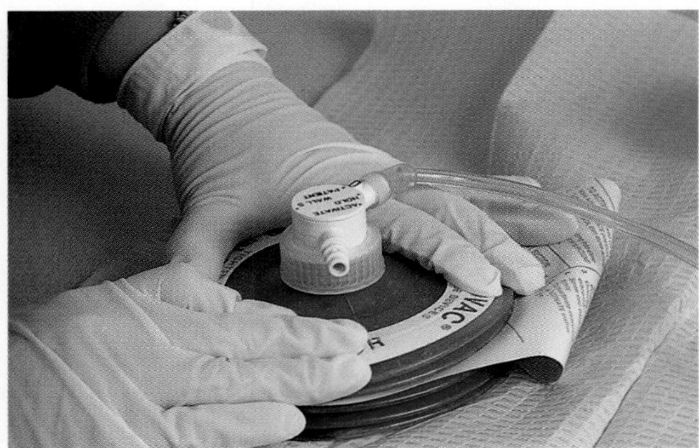

Figure 41-17 Hemovac. Drains are sutured to the wound and connected to the reservoir. Source: J.C. Ross-Kerr, M.J. Wood, A.G. Perry, and P.A. Potter, *Canadian Fundamentals of Nursing,* 2nd ed. (Toronto: Harcourt Canada, 2001).

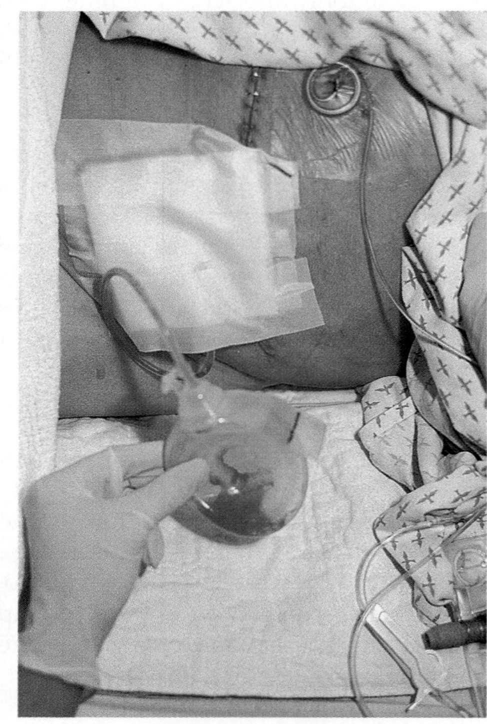

Figure 41-18 Jackson-Pratt drainage system. Source: J.C. Ross-Kerr, M.J. Wood, A.G. Perry, and P.A. Potter, *Canadian Fundamentals of Nursing,* 2nd ed. (Toronto: Harcourt Canada, 2001).

Drainage must leave the wound for healing to occur. If drainage is trapped inside the wound, underlying tissues swell. The wound may heal at the skin level, but underlying tissues do not close. Infection and other complications can occur.

When large amounts of drainage are expected, the physician inserts a drain. A Penrose drain is a rubber tube that drains onto a dressing (Figure 41-16). Because it is an open drain, it is a portal of entry for microbes.

Closed drainage systems prevent microbes from entering the wound. A drain is placed in the wound and attached to suction. The Hemovac (Figure 41-17) and Jackson-Pratt (Figure 41-18) systems are examples. Other systems used depend on the wound type, size, and location.

A nurse measures drainage in three ways:

- *Noting the number and size of dressings with drainage*—The amount and kind of drainage are described. Are dressings saturated? Is drainage on just part of the dressing? If so, which part? Is drainage through some or all layers?
- *Weighing dressings before applying them to the wound*—The weight of each dressing is noted. Dressings are weighed after removal. The dry dressing weight is

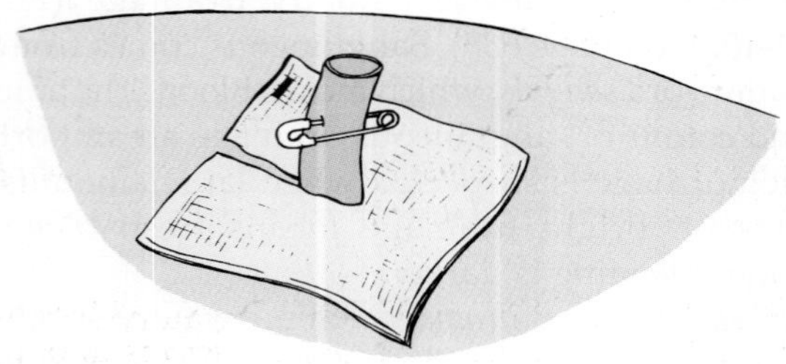

Figure 41-16 A Penrose drain. The safety pin prevents the drain from slipping into the wound. Source: J.C. Ross-Kerr, M.J. Wood, A.G. Perry, and P.A. Potter, *Canadian Fundamentals of Nursing,* 2nd ed. (Toronto: Harcourt Canada, 2001).

subtracted from the wet dressing weight. (Wet dressings weigh more.)
- *Measuring the amount of drainage in the collecting receptacle if closed drainage is used.*

DRESSINGS

Wound dressings have many functions:

- They protect wounds from injury and microbes.
- They absorb drainage.
- They remove dead tissue.
- They promote comfort.
- They cover unsightly wounds.
- They provide a moist environment for wound healing.
- When bleeding is a problem, pressure dressings help control bleeding.

The type and size of dressing used depend on many factors. These include the type of wound, its size and location, amount of drainage, and the presence or absence of infection. The dressing's function and the frequency of dressing changes are other factors. The physician and nurse choose the best type of dressing for each wound.

A dressing must always be clean and dry. A damp dressing can harbour microbes. If your client has a damp or soiled dressing, report it immediately to your supervisor.

TYPES OF DRESSINGS

Dressings are described by the material used and application method. Many products are available for dressing wounds. The following are common dressings:

- *Gauze*—comes in squares, rectangles, pads, and rolls (Figure 41-19). Gauze dressings absorb moisture.
- *Nonadherent gauze*—is a gauze dressing with a nonstick surface. It does not stick to the wound and removes easily without injuring the tissue.
- *Transparent adhesive film*—air can reach the wound but fluid and microbes cannot. The wound is kept moist. Drainage is not absorbed. The transparent film allows wound observation.

Some dressings contain special agents to promote wound healing. If you assist with the dressing change, your supervisor explains its use to you.

Dressing application methods involve dry and wet dressings:

- *Dry-to-dry dressing* (*dry dressing*)—A dry gauze dressing is placed over the wound. More dressings are placed on top of the first dressing as needed. Drainage is absorbed by the dressing and is removed with the dressing. A dry dressing can stick to the wound. The dressing is removed carefully to prevent tissue injury and discomfort.

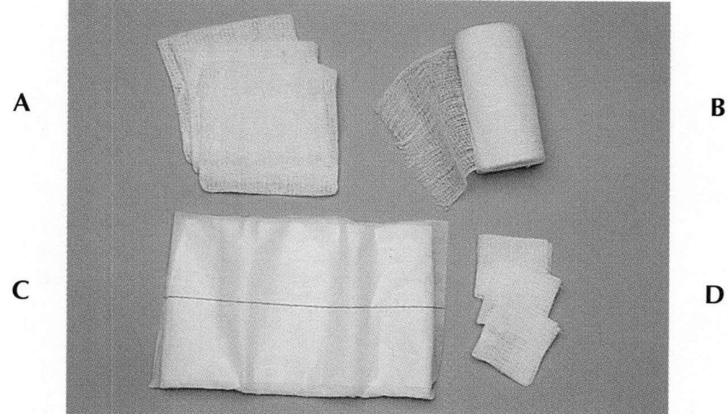

Figure 41-19 Gauze dressings. **A,** 4 × 4. **B,** Gauze roll. **C,** Abdominal pad. **D,** 2 × 2.

- *Wet-to-dry dressing*—A gauze dressing saturated with a solution is applied over the wound. More saturated dressings are applied as needed. The solution softens dead tissue in the wound. The dead tissue is absorbed by the dressing and is removed with the dressing. The dressings are removed when dry.
- *Wet-to-wet dressing*—Gauze dressings saturated with solution are placed in the wound. The dressing is kept moist.

SECURING DRESSINGS

Dressings must be secure over wounds. Microbes enter the wound and drainage can escape if the dressing is dislodged. Tape and Montgomery ties are used to secure dressings. Binders also hold dressings in place (page 692).

Tape. Adhesive, paper, plastic, and elastic tapes are common. Adhesive tape sticks well to the skin. However, adhesive remaining on the skin is hard to remove. It can irritate the skin. Sometimes skin is removed with the tape, causing an abrasion. Many people are allergic to adhesive tape. Paper and plastic tapes usually do not cause allergic reactions. Elastic tape allows movement of the body part.

Tape is applied to secure the top, middle, and bottom of the dressing (Figure 41-20 on page 690). The tape extends several centimetres beyond each side of the dressing. *The tape must not circle the entire body part. If swelling occurs, circulation to the part is impaired.*

Montgomery Ties. Montgomery ties (Figure 41-21 on page 690) are used for large dressings and when frequent dressing changes are needed. A Montgomery tie has an adhesive strip and a cloth tie. When the dressing is in place, the adhesive strips are placed on both sides of the dressing. Then the cloth ties are

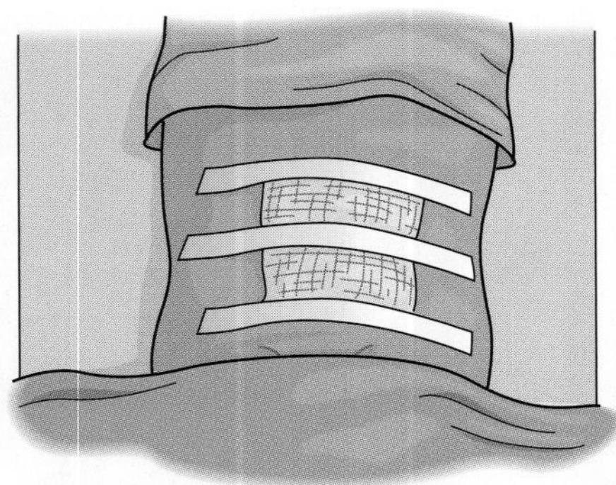

Figure 41-20 Tape is applied at the top, middle, and bottom of the dressing. Note that the tape extends several centimetres beyond both sides of the dressing.

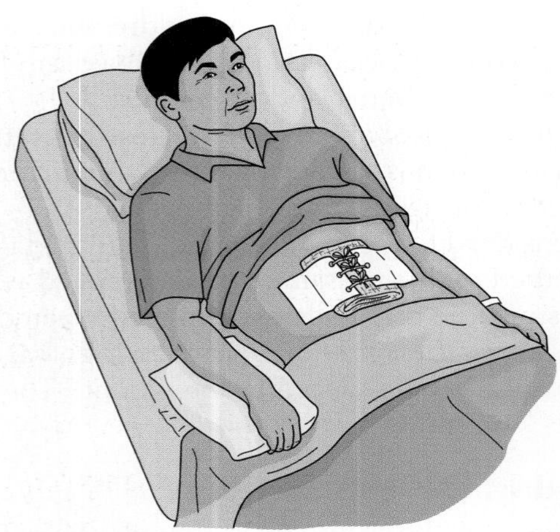

Figure 41-21 Montgomery ties.

secured over the dressing. Two or three Montgomery ties are needed on each side. The cloth ties are undone for the dressing change. The adhesive strips are not removed unless soiled.

(See *Focus on Children: Dressings* and *Focus on Older Adults: Dressings* boxes.)

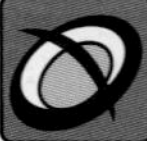

Focus on Children

Dressings

Children are often afraid of dressing changes. Tape removal is often painful for them. The wound's appearance can be frightening. It is important that the child is calm and cooperative. Otherwise the sterile field could be contaminated. A parent or caregiver holds the child so the wound can be reached with ease. Letting the child hold or play with a favourite toy is often comforting.

Focus on Older Adults

Dressings

Older adults have thin, fragile skin. Skin tears must be prevented. Extreme care is necessary when removing tape.

Applying Dressings

Your supervisor may ask you to assist with dressing changes. Some employers let support workers apply simple, dry, nonsterile dressings to simple wounds. Box 41-9 lists guidelines for applying nonsterile dressings. (See *Focus on Home Care: Changing Dressings* box.)

(text continues on page 692)

Box 41-9 Guidelines for Applying Nonsterile Dressings

- Make sure your province or territory allows you to perform the procedure.
- Make sure the procedure is in your job description.
- Apply dressings only under a nurse's direction and supervision.
- Review the procedure with the nurse.
- Allow pain medications time to take effect. The client may experience discomfort during the dressing change. The nurse gives the medication and tells you how long to wait.
- Provide for the client's fluid and elimination needs before starting the procedure.
- Collect needed equipment and supplies before you begin.
- Control your nonverbal communication. Wound odours, appearance, and drainage may be unpleasant. Do not communicate your thoughts and reactions to the client.
- Practise Standard Precautions. Wear personal protective equipment as necessary. Never touch a wound.
- Remove dressings so that the client cannot see the soiled side. The drainage and its odour may upset the client.
- Do not force the client to look at the wound. A wound can affect body image and self-esteem. The nurse helps the client deal with the wound.
- Remove tape by pulling it toward the wound.
- Remove dressings gently. The dressing may stick to the wound and surrounding skin.
- Observe the wound and report and record your observations according to employer policy (see Box 41-8 on page 687).

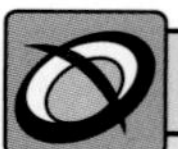

Focus on Home Care

CHANGING DRESSINGS

Your supervisor may ask you to telephone him or her after removing the old dressings. During this telephone call, you report your observations. Then your supervisor gives you instructions about how to proceed.

Follow your employer policy for disposing of dressings. Usually employers require you to:

- Place the used dressings in a plastic bag
- Fasten the bag securely
- Dispose of the bag with the household garbage

Applying a Dry Nonsterile Dressing

COMPASSIONATE CARE

Remember to Promote:

- **Dignity**
- **Independence**
- **Preferences**
- **Privacy**
- **Safety**

Pre-Procedure

1 Review the procedure with your supervisor.

2 Identify the person according to employer policy.

3 Explain the procedure to the person.

4 Allow time for pain medication to take effect.

5 Provide for the person's fluid and elimination needs.

6 Wash your hands.

7 Collect the following:
- Gloves
- Personal protective equipment as needed
- Tape or Montgomery ties as directed by the care plan
- Dressings as directed by the care plan
- Adhesive remover
- Scissors
- Leakproof plastic bag
- Bath blanket

8 Provide for privacy.

9 Arrange your work area.

10 Raise the bed to a comfortable working height. Follow the care plan for bed rail use.*

Procedure

11 Lower the bed rail near you if up.

12 Help the person to a comfortable position.

13 Cover the person with a bath blanket. Fanfold top linens to the foot of the bed.

14 Expose the affected body part.

15 Make a cuff on the plastic bag. Place it within reach.

16 Put on a gown and mask if needed.

17 Put on gloves.

18 Undo Montgomery ties or remove tape:
- a *Montgomery ties*: fold ties away from the wound.
- b *Tape*: hold the skin down and gently pull the tape toward the wound.

19 Remove adhesive from the skin. Wet a 4 × 4 gauze dressing with the adhesive remover. Clean away from the wound.

20 Remove gauze dressings. Start with the top

Continued

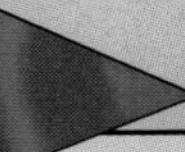

Applying a Dry Nonsterile Dressing—cont'd

Procedure—cont'd

dressing. Keep the soiled side of the dressing out of the person's sight. Place dressings in the bag. They must not touch the outside of the bag.

21 Remove the dressing directly over the wound very gently. It may stick to the wound.

22 Observe the wound and drainage (see Box 41-8 on page 687).

23 Remove gloves. Put them in the bag. Wash your hands. (If used, raise the bed rail before leaving the bedside. Lower it when you return.)

24 Put on clean gloves.

25 Open the dressings.

26 Cut the length of tape needed.

27 Apply dressings as directed by the care plan.

28 Secure the dressings in place. Use tape or Montgomery ties.

29 Remove your gloves. Put them in the bag. Wash your hands.

Post-Procedure

30 Provide for safety and comfort.

31 Cover the person and remove the bath blanket.

32 Place the call bell within reach.*

33 Return the bed to its lowest position. Follow the care plan for bed rail use.*

34 Remove privacy measures.

35 Discard supplies into the bag. Tie the bag closed. Discard the bag according to employer policy.

36 Clean your work surface following employer policy.

37 Wash your hands.

38 Report and record your actions and observations according to employer policy.

*Steps marked with an asterisk may not apply in community settings.

Binders

Binders are applied to the abdomen, chest, or perineal areas. Binders promote healing because they:

- Support wounds
- Hold dressings in place
- Reduce or prevent swelling by promoting circulation
- Promote comfort
- Prevent injury

Usually a nurse applies binders. You may provide care for clients with these binders:

- *Straight abdominal binder*—provides abdominal support and holds dressings in place (Figure 41-22). It is applied with the client supine. The top part is at the client's waist. The lower part is over the hips. The binder is secured with pins, hooks, or Velcro.
- *Breast binder*—supports the breast after breast surgery (Figure 41-23). The woman is supine when it is applied. It is pulled snugly across the chest and secured in place.
- *T binder*—secures dressings in place after rectal and perineal surgeries. The single T binder is used for women (Figure 41-24, *A*). The double T binder is for men (Figure 41-24, *B*). If perineal dressings are large, women may need double T binders. The waistbands are brought around the waist and pinned at the front. The tails are brought between the legs and up to the waistband. They are pinned in place at the waistband.

Some employers allow support workers to apply binders. You will receive training and supervision for this task. Apply a binder so there is firm, even pressure over the area. It should be snug but not affect breathing or circulation. Pins point away from the wound. Reapply the binder if it is loose, wrinkled, out of position, or if it causes discomfort. Also, change binders that are wet or soiled.

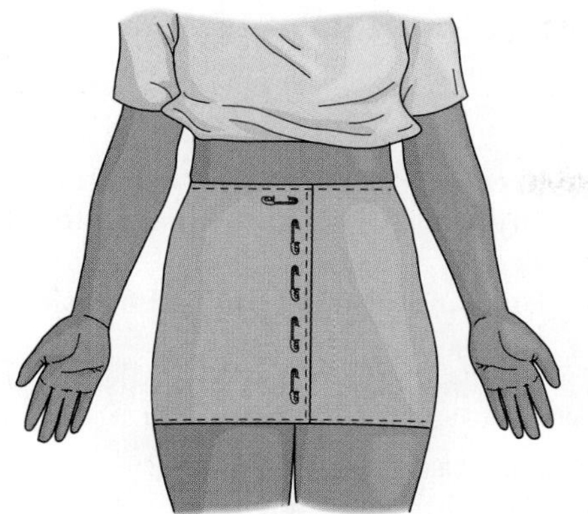

Figure 41-22 Straight abdominal binder.

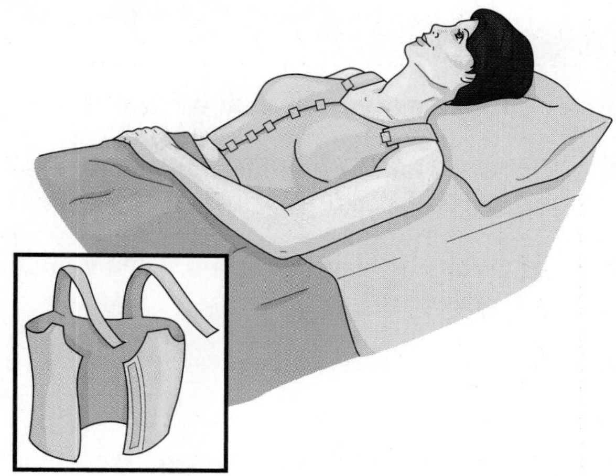

Figure 41-23 Breast binder.

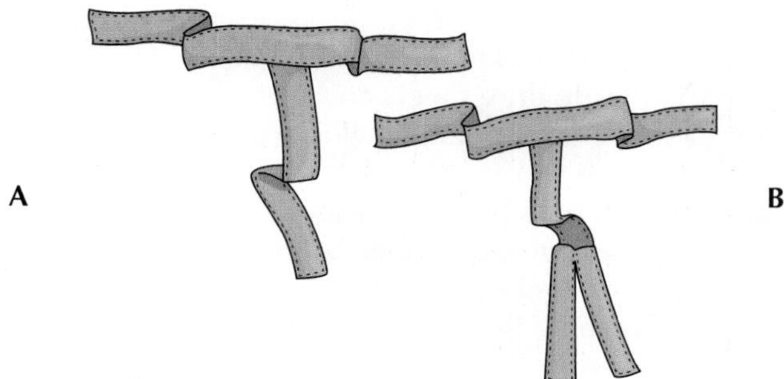

Figure 41-24 **A,** Single T binder. **B,** Double T binder.

Heat and Cold Applications

Heat and cold applications are often ordered for wound care (see Chapter 42). Physicians and nurses order them to promote healing, comfort, and to reduce tissue swelling.

Meeting Basic Needs

The wound can affect the client's basic needs. However, it is only one part of the person's care. Remember, the client has other needs as well. The client is recovering from surgery or trauma. The wound causes pain and discomfort. The wound and the pain may affect breathing and moving. Turning, repositioning, and walking may be painful. Handle the client gently. Allow pain medications to take effect before giving care.

Good nutrition is needed for healing. However, pain and discomfort can affect appetite. So can odours from wound drainage. Remove soiled dressings promptly from the room. Use room deodorizers as directed. Also keep drainage containers out of the client's sight. Tell your supervisor if the client has a taste for certain foods or beverages.

Infection is always a threat. You must practise Standard Precautions. Carefully observe the wound. Also observe for signs and symptoms of infection (see Chapter 18).

Delayed healing is a risk for clients who are older or obese or who have poor nutrition. Poor circulation and diabetes also affect healing. These conditions are risk factors for infection.

The client may have many fears. He or she may fear scarring, disfigurement, delayed healing, and infection. Fears about the wound "popping open" are common.

Victims of violence have many other concerns. Fear of future attacks, concerns about finding and convicting the attacker, and fear for family members are common. Victims of abuse often hide the true source of their injuries.

The wound may be large or small. It may be visible to others—on the face, arms, or legs—or hidden by clothing. Wound drainage may have unpleasant odours. The wound may be disfiguring. It may affect sexual performance or the person's sense of being sexually attractive. Amputation of a finger, hand, arm, toes, foot, or leg can affect the person's function, daily activities, and job. Eye injuries can affect vision. Abdominal trauma and surgery can affect eating and elimination.

Whatever the wound's location or size, function, body image, and self-esteem are often affected. Many people with serious and disfiguring wounds have increased needs for love and belonging. You must be sensitive to the client's feelings. The person may be sad and tearful or angry and hostile. Adjustments may be hard and rehabilitation necessary. Be gentle and kind, give compassionate care, and practise good communication. Other health care team members—social workers, psychiatrists, therapists, and spiritual advisers—may be involved in the client's care.

REVIEW

Circle T if the answer is true and F if it is false.

1. T F Good nutrition and hydration can help prevent skin breakdown.
2. T F White or reddened skin is a first sign of a pressure ulcer.
3. T F Pressure ulcers do not usually occur over a bony area.
4. T F Pressure ulcers can develop from failing to reposition the person often enough.
5. T F Shearing and friction can cause pressure ulcers.

Circle the BEST answer.

6. A child fell off her bike. She has a laceration on her right leg. Which is *false*?
   A. She has an open wound.
   B. She has an infected wound.
   C. She has a contaminated wound.
   D. She has an unintentional wound.
7. Mrs. Katz had rectal surgery. What type of wound does she have?
   A. A clean wound
   B. A dirty wound
   C. A clean-contaminated wound
   D. A contaminated wound
8. The skin and underlying tissues are pierced. This is
   A. A penetrating wound
   B. An incision
   C. A contusion
   D. An abrasion
9. Which can cause skin tears?
   A. Keeping your nails trimmed and smooth
   B. Dressing clients in clothing with long sleeves and pants
   C. Hurrying when lifting and transferring clients
   D. Padding wheelchair footrests
10. Which causes pressure ulcers?
    A. Repositioning the client every 2 hours
    B. Scrubbing and rubbing the skin
    C. Applying lotion to dry areas
    D. Keeping linens clean, dry, and wrinkle-free
11. Which are *not* used to treat pressure ulcers?
    A. Special beds
    B. Waterbeds and flotation pads
    C. Plastic drawsheets and waterproof pads
    D. Heel elevators and elbow protectors
12. You can help prevent stasis ulcers by
    A. Using elastic rubber-band type garters to hold socks in place
    B. Keeping the client in bed as much as possible
    C. Encouraging the client to sit with legs crossed
    D. Avoiding injury to the legs and feet when giving care
13. Which is *not* a common site for arterial ulcers?
    A. Between the toes
    B. On top of the toes
    C. On the outer side of the ankle
    D. Behind the knee
14. A wound appears red and swollen. The area around it is warm to touch. These signs occur during
    A. The inflammatory phase of wound healing
    B. The proliferative phase of wound healing
    C. Healing by primary intention
    D. Healing by secondary intention

15. A wound is healing by primary intention. While assisting with a dressing change, you note that the wound is separating. This is called
    A. Dehiscence
    B. Tertiary intention
    C. Evisceration
    D. Hematoma

16. You note a clear, watery drainage from a wound. This drainage is called
    A. Purulent drainage
    B. Serous drainage
    C. Sero-purulent drainage
    D. Serosanguineous drainage

17. A dressing does the following *except*
    A. Protect the wound from injury
    B. Absorb drainage
    C. Provide a moist environment for wound healing
    D. Support the wound and reduce swelling

18. You are securing a dressing with tape. Tape is applied
    A. Around the entire part
    B. To the top and bottom of the dressing
    C. To the top, middle, and bottom of the dressing
    D. As the client prefers

19. Mr. Heron has an abdominal binder. The binder is used to
    A. Prevent blood clots
    B. Prevent wound infection
    C. Provide support and hold dressings in place
    D. Decrease circulation and swelling

Answers to these questions are on page 827.

CHAPTER

42

Heat and Cold Applications

OBJECTIVES

- Define the key terms listed in this chapter
- Identify the purposes, effects, and complications of heat and cold applications
- List clients at risk for complications from heat and cold applications
- Describe the guidelines for application of heat and cold
- Learn the procedures described in this chapter

KEY TERMS

compress A soft pad that is moistened and applied over a body area

constrict To narrow

cyanosis Bluish skin colour

dilate To expand or open wider

pack A treatment that involves wrapping a body part with a wet or dry application

Physicians, nurses, and physical therapists order heat and cold applications to reduce tissue swelling and promote healing and comfort. Heat and cold have opposite effects on body function. Heat increases blood flow. Cold slows blood flow. Both effects can be helpful for different problems. However, there are risks associated with heat and cold applications. Severe injuries and changes in function can occur. You must thoroughly understand the purposes, effects, and complications of heat and cold applications.

Some employers allow only nurses to apply heat and cold. Others let support workers do so. Before you perform these procedures, make sure that:

- Your provincial or territorial laws and employer's policies allow you to perform the procedure
- The procedure is in your job description
- You have the necessary training
- You are familiar with the equipment
- You review the procedure with a nurse
- A nurse is available to answer questions and to supervise you

HEAT APPLICATIONS

Heat applications can be applied to almost any body part. They are often used for musculoskeletal injuries or problems (strains, low back pain, and arthritis). Heat applications are used to:

- Relieve pain
- Relax muscles
- Promote healing
- Reduce tissue swelling
- Decrease joint stiffness

When heat is applied to the skin, blood vessels in the area dilate. **Dilate** means to expand or open wider (Figure 42-1, *B*). More blood flows through the vessels. The tissues have more oxygen and nutrients for healing. Excess fluid and wastes are removed from the area faster. The skin is red and warm. Pain and swelling are reduced and muscles relax.

COMPLICATIONS

High temperatures can cause burns. Pain, excessive redness, and blisters are danger signs. Remove the application and report these signs immediately. When heat is applied too long, blood vessels **constrict** (narrow) (see Figure 42-1, C). Blood flow decreases. Tissues receive less blood. The skin becomes pale, and tissue damage occurs. Report pale skin immediately.

Some clients are at greater risk than others for burns and other complications from heat applications (Box 42-1 on page 698). Observe these clients closely. Protect your clients from injury. Follow the guidelines listed in Box 42-2 on page 698 when applying heat and cold applications.

MOIST AND DRY APPLICATIONS

A *moist heat application* means that water is in contact with the skin. Water conducts heat. Moist heat has greater and faster effects than dry heat. Heat penetrates deeper with a moist application. To prevent injury, moist heat applications have lower (cooler) temperatures than dry heat applications.

Water is not in contact with the skin with *dry heat applications*. Dry heat has advantages:

- The application stays at the desired temperature longer.
- Dry heat does not penetrate as deeply as moist heat.

(text continues on page 699)

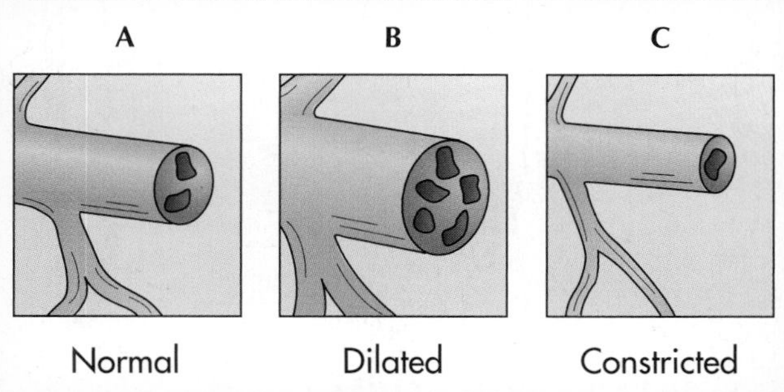

Figure 42-1 **A,** Blood vessel under normal conditions. **B,** Dilated blood vessel. **C,** Constricted blood vessel.

Box 42-1 Clients at High Risk for Complications from Heat or Cold Applications

- *People with thin, delicate, or fragile skin.* They include infants, young children, older adults, and fair-skinned people.
- *People who have decreased sensations.* Some people have difficulty sensing heat, cold, or pain. They may not realize if the application is too hot or cold and is damaging their skin. Many situations reduce a person's ability to feel pain. Loss of consciousness, scarring of the skin, and the use of some medications are examples. Diseases or conditions that affect the circulatory and nervous systems also may decrease sensations. Spinal cord injuries, stroke, and diabetes are examples. Older adults often have decreased sensations caused by changes in body function associated with aging.
- *People with dementia or confusion.* These people may not recognize pain. Or they may not be able to communicate that they are in pain. Look for changes in the person's behaviour. Behaviour changes can signal pain.
- *People with metal implants.* Metal conducts heat and cold. Deep tissues can be burned. Pacemakers and joint replacements are made of metal. Do not apply heat in the area of the implant.

Box 42-2 Guidelines for Applying Heat and Cold

- Apply only when ordered by a professional, allowed by your employer, and assigned to do so.
- Know how to use the equipment.
- Measure the temperature of moist applications before applying. Use a bath thermometer. Or follow employer policy for measuring temperature.
- Follow employer policies for safe temperature ranges. See Table 42-1 for guidelines.
- Do not apply hot applications above 41.1° C (106° F). Tissue damage can occur. A nurse applies *very hot* applications.
- Ask your supervisor what the temperature of the application should be:
  - Heat—cooler temperatures are used for clients at risk.
  - Cold—warmer temperatures are used for clients at risk.
- Know the precise site of the application. Ask your supervisor to show you the site.
- Cover dry heat or cold applications before applying them. Use a flannel or terrycloth cover, towel, or pillowcase. Follow employer policy.
- Do not leave clients at risk unattended. Observe them carefully.
- Observe the skin for signs of complications. Immediately remove the application and report the following:
  - Complaints of discomfort, pain, numbness, or burning
  - Excessive redness
  - Blisters
  - Pale, white, or grey skin
  - **Cyanosis** (bluish skin colour)
  - Shivering
- Observe for changes in the client's behaviour. These may indicate pain.
- Remind the client not to change the temperature of the application.
- Prevent chills. When moist heat is applied, the increased blood flow to the affected area may cause less blood flow to other body parts. The client may feel chilled. Cover the client with a blanket or robe. Control room drafts.
- Ask your supervisor how long to leave the application in place. Carefully watch the time. Heat and cold are applied for no longer than 20 minutes.
- Provide for privacy. Properly drape and screen the client. Expose only the body part where you will apply heat or cold.
- If it is safe to leave, place the call bell within the client's reach or remain within easy hearing distance.
- Practise Standard Precautions. Wear gloves if you or the client has non-intact skin.

Table 42-1 Heat and Cold Temperature Ranges

Temperature	Centigrade range	Fahrenheit range
Very hot	41.1 to 46.1° C	106 to 115° F
Hot	36.6 to 41.1° C	98 to 106° F
Warm	33.8 to 36.6° C	93 to 98° F
Tepid	26.6 to 33.8° C	80 to 93° F
Cool	18.3 to 26.6° C	65 to 80° F
Cold	10.0 to 18.3° C	50 to 65° F

Because water is not used, dry heat needs higher (hotter) temperatures to achieve the desired effect. Therefore, burns are still a risk. (See *Focus on Home Care: Dry Heat Applications* box.)

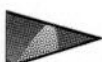

Hot Compresses

Hot compresses are moist heat applications. A **compress** is a soft pad that is moistened and applied over a body area. (Compresses can be hot or cold.) A compress is usually made of cloth. For example, a washcloth, small towel, or gauze dressing can be used as a compress.

Your supervisor tells you how long to leave the application in place. The length of time never exceeds 20 minutes. To maintain the temperature after it is applied, change the compress often. A layer of plastic wrap and/or a dry towel can be used to cover the compress and retain the heat.

Sometimes commercial compresses are ordered. These are pre-moistened and packaged in foil. Before it is unwrapped, the compress is heated under an infrared lamp as instructed by the manufacturer. After it is heated and unwrapped, a commercial compress is applied in the same manner as a regular hot compress. Commercial compresses are used once and then discarded.

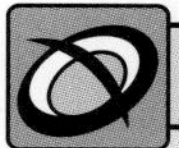

Focus on Home Care

Dry Heat Applications

Many home care clients have electric heating pads or hot-water bottles. These apply dry heat. They also create serious fire and burn risks. *Therefore, support workers are usually not permitted to apply electric heating pads or hot-water bottles.* If a client asks you to apply an electric heating pad or hot-water bottle, explain that you are not allowed to do so according to your employer's policy. Find another way to warm the client. A blanket or sweater may be helpful. Tell your supervisor about the client's request.

Applying Hot Compresses

Compassionate Care

Remember to Promote:
- **Dignity**
- **Independence**
- **Preferences**
- **Privacy**
- **Safety**

Pre-Procedure

1 Identify the person according to employer policy.
2 Explain the procedure to the person.
3 Wash your hands.
4 Collect the following:
- Basin
- Bath thermometer
- Small towel, washcloth, or gauze squares
- Plastic wrap
- Ties, tape, or rolled gauze
- Bath towel
- Waterproof pad

5 Provide for privacy.

Continued

Applying Hot Compresses—cont'd

Procedure

6 Place the waterproof pad under the body part to be treated.

7 Fill the basin ½ to ⅔ full with hot water as directed by your supervisor. Measure water temperature.

8 Place the compress in the water.

9 Wring out the compress

10 Apply the compress to the area. Note the time.

11 Ask the person if the compress feels comfortable. If the person is comfortable, cover the compress quickly with plastic wrap. Cover the plastic wrap with a bath towel (Figure 42-2). Secure the towel in place with ties, tape, or rolled gauze.

12 Place the call bell within reach. Follow the care plan for bed rail use.*

13 Check the area every 5 minutes. Check for redness and complaints of pain, discomfort, or numbness. Remove the compress if any occur and tell your supervisor immediately.

14 Change the compress if cooling occurs.

15 Remove the compress after 20 minutes or as directed by your supervisor. Pat the area dry with a towel.

Post-Procedure

16 Provide for safety and comfort.

17 Place the call bell within reach. Follow the care plan for bed rail use.*

18 Remove privacy measures.

19 Clean equipment. Discard disposable items. Wear gloves for this step.

20 Follow employer policy for soiled linen.

21 Wash your hands.

22 Report and record your actions and observations according to employer policy.

*Step marked with an asterisk may not apply in community settings.

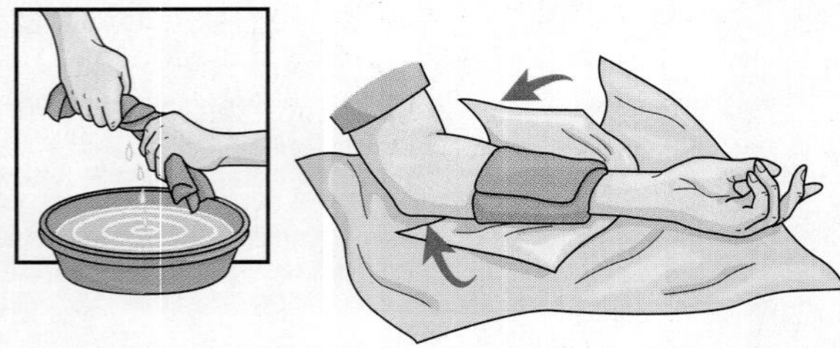

Figure 42-2 Cover a hot compress with plastic and a bath towel. These keep the compress warm.

Hot Soaks

A hot soak involves putting the body part into heated water. This promotes circulation and muscle relaxation. Hot soaks are usually used for smaller parts, such as a hand, lower arm, foot, or lower leg (Figure 42-3). A tub is used to soak larger areas (arm, leg, or torso). The soak lasts 15 to 20 minutes. Maintain the client's comfort and body alignment during the hot soak.

Remember to check the water temperature before soaking the body part. If the water is too hot, the skin can be burned as soon as it touches the water.

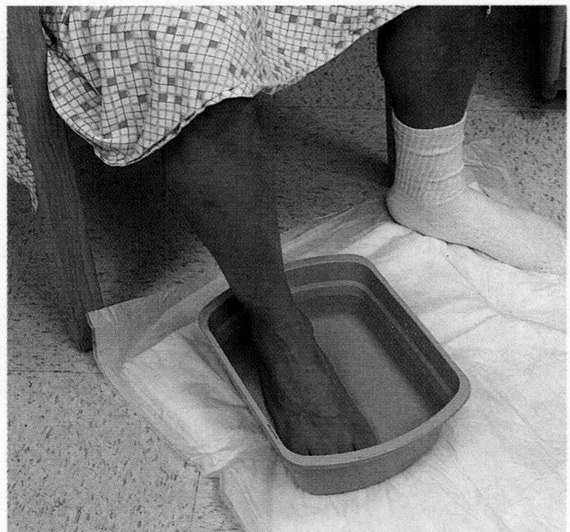

Figure 42-3 The hot soak.

The Hot Soak

Compassionate Care

Remember to Promote:
- **Dignity**
- **Independence**
- **Preferences**
- **Privacy**
- **Safety**

Pre-Procedure

1 Identify the person according to employer policy.
2 Explain the procedure to the person.
3 Wash your hands.
4 Collect the following:
- Water basin or an arm or foot bath
- Bath thermometer
- Bath blanket
- Waterproof pads

5 Provide for privacy.

Procedure

6 Position the person for treatment.
7 Place the call bell within reach.*
8 Place a waterproof pad under the area to be treated.
9 Fill the water basin ½ full with hot water as directed by your supervisor. Measure water temperature.
10 Place the body part into the water. Pad the edge of the basin with a towel. Note the time.
11 Cover the person with a bath blanket for extra warmth.
12 Check the area every 5 minutes. Check for redness and complaints of pain, discomfort, or numbness. Discontinue the soak if any of these occur. Wrap the body part in a towel and tell your supervisor at once.
13 Check water temperature every 5 minutes. Change water as necessary. Wrap the body part in a towel while changing the water.
14 Remove the body part from the water in 15 to 20 minutes. Pat dry.

Post-Procedure

15 Follow steps 16 through 22 in *Applying Hot Compresses* on page 700.

*Step marked with an asterisk may not apply in community settings.

Change the water as necessary to correct the temperature. Never add hot water while the body part is in the basin. You could burn the client. Have the client remove the body part from the basin. Assist as necessary. Then add more hot water and test the temperature.

The Sitz Bath

The sitz bath involves immersing the perineal and rectal areas in warm or hot water. (*Sitz* means *seat* in German.) The sitz bath usually lasts 20 minutes. Sitz baths are common after rectal or female pelvic surgery, after childbirth, and for hemorrhoids. They are used to:

- Clean perineal or anal wounds
- Promote healing
- Relieve pain and soreness
- Increase circulation
- Stimulate voiding

The disposable plastic sitz bath fits onto the toilet seat (Figure 42-4 on page 702). Plastic tubing runs from the bowl of the sitz bath to a water bag. A plastic clamp closes the tubing. The sitz bath is filled with water at an appropriate temperature. (Check with your supervisor to determine a safe temperature.) The water bag is filled with warmer water. As the water in the sitz bath cools, the tubing is unclamped to allow the warmer water from the bag to flow into the sitz bath.

A sitz tub is a built-in fixture with a deep seat. The client sits in a seat filled with water (Figure 42-5). The person's feet rest flat on the floor. Do not use an ordinary bathtub for a sitz bath. Immersing the legs and feet decreases the effectiveness of the procedure.

When using a sitz bath, blood flow to the perineal and rectal areas increases. Therefore less blood flows to other body parts. The client may feel chilled. Cover the client's shoulders and knees for warmth. Reduced blood flow may also make the client feel faint, dizzy, weak, or drowsy. Check the person every 5 minutes for these symptoms. Stay in the room if it is not safe to leave the person alone. Allow as much privacy as possible. If it is safe to leave, place the call bell within the person's reach or remain within easy hearing distance.

(text continues on page 704)

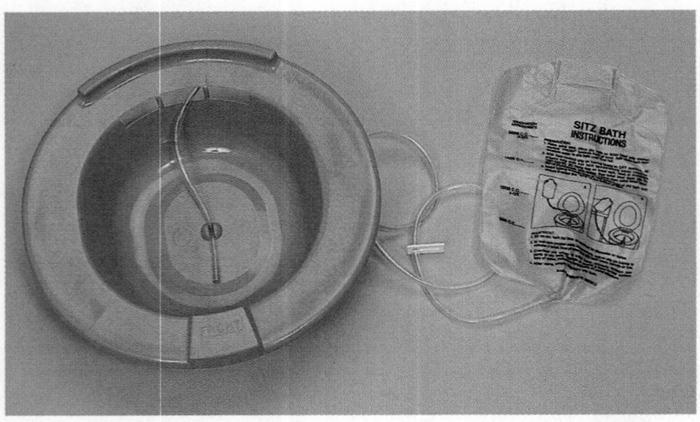

Figure 42-4 The disposable sitz bath with water bag, tubing, and clamp.

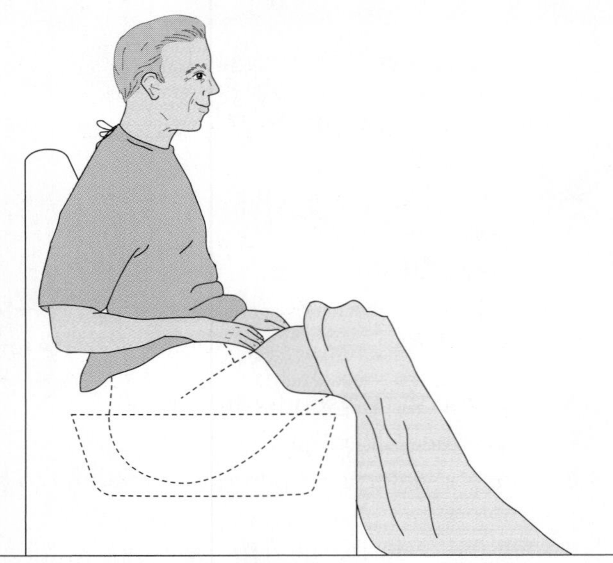

Figure 42-5 The built-in sitz tub.

Assisting the Person to Take a Sitz Bath

COMPASSIONATE CARE

Remember to Promote:
- **Dignity**
- **Independence**
- **Preferences**
- **Privacy**
- **Safety**

Pre-Procedure

1 Identify the person according to employer policy.
2 Explain the procedure to the person.
3 Wash your hands.
4 Collect the following:
   - Disposable sitz bath if used.
   - Wheelchair if the built-in sitz tub is used
   - Bath thermometer
   - Large water container
   - Two bath blankets, bath towels, and clean garments
   - Footstool if the person is short
   - Disinfectant solution
   - Utility gloves
5 Provide for privacy.

Continued

Assisting the Person to Take a Sitz Bath—cont'd

Procedure

6 Assist the person to the bathroom or commode. Encourage the person to eliminate before the procedure.

7 *If using a disposable sitz bath:*
  - a Place the disposable sitz bath on the toilet seat.
  - b Fill the sitz bath ⅔ full with water. Your supervisor tells you what water temperature to use. Measure water temperature.
  - c Close the clamp on the tubing.
  - d Fill the water bag with warmer water than that in the bowl. Your supervisor tells you what water temperature to use. Measure water temperature.
  - e Hang the bag on a towel bar or from the top of the toilet tank. The bag must be higher than the toilet seat.

8 *If using a built-in sitz tub:*
  - a Transport the person by wheelchair to the room with the sitz bath.
  - b Fill the sitz bath ⅔ full with water. Your supervisor tells you what water temperature to use. Measure water temperature.
  - c Pad the metal part of the sitz tub with towels. Pad the part in contact with the person.

9 Help the person remove or lower clothing below the waist. Or raise the person's gown above the waist.

10 Help the person sit in the sitz bath.

11 Place a bath blanket around the shoulders. Place another over the legs for warmth.

12 Provide a footstool if the edge of the sitz bath causes pressure under the knees.

13 Show the person how to open the clamp to let warmer water from the bag flow into the sitz bath (with disposable sitz baths). Assist as necessary.

14 Place the call bell within reach.*

15 Stay with a person who is weak or unsteady.

16 Check the person every 5 minutes for complaints of weakness, faintness, and drowsiness. Check for a rapid pulse. If any occur, get assistance to help the person back to bed.

17 Help the person out of the sitz bath after 20 minutes or as directed by your supervisor.

18 Assist the person with drying and dressing.

19 Assist the person back to his or her room.

Post-Procedure

20 Provide for safety and comfort.

21 Place the call bell within reach. Follow the care plan for bed rail use.*

22 Remove privacy measures.

23 Clean the sitz bath with disinfectant solution. Wear utility gloves.

24 Clean and return reusable items to their proper place. Follow employer policy for soiled linen. Wear gloves for this step.

25 Wash your hands.

26 Report and record your actions and observations according to employer policy.

*Steps marked with an asterisk may not apply in community settings.

Hot Packs

A **pack** is a treatment that involves wrapping a body part with a wet or dry application. The application can be hot or cold. There are single-use (disposable) or reusable commercial packs. Some can be used for heat or cold. The manufacturer's instructions tell you how to activate the heat or cold (Figure 42-6). For example, some hot packs are put in boiling water for a few minutes. Or they are warmed in a microwave oven. For other types, striking, kneading, or squeezing the package activates the heat. Always read warning labels and follow the manufacturer's safety instructions.

Reusable packs are cleaned after use. They are wiped with alcohol or washed with soap and water. Follow employer policy and the manufacturer's instructions.

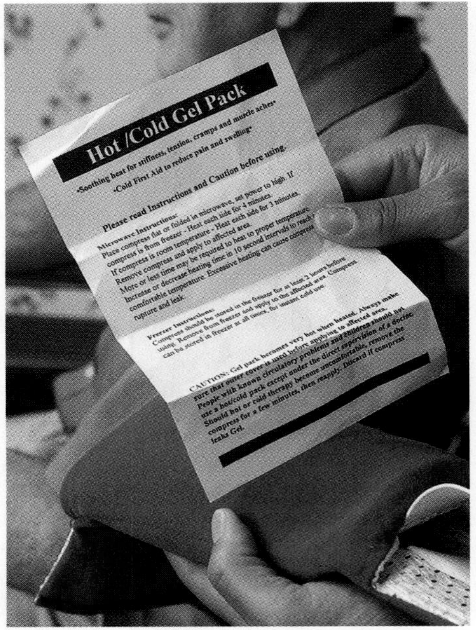

Figure 42-6 Commercial hot pack. The manufacturer's instructions explain how to activate the heat.

Applying a Hot Pack

Compassionate Care

Remember to Promote:
- Dignity
- Independence
- Preferences
- Privacy
- Safety

Pre-Procedure

1. Identify the person according to employer policy.
2. Explain the procedure to the person.
3. Wash your hands.
4. Collect the following:
   - Commercial pack
   - Towel
   - Pack cover
   - Ties, tape, or rolled gauze (if needed)
   - Waterproof pad
5. Heat the pack. Follow the manufacturer's instructions.
6. Put the pack in the cover.
7. Provide for privacy.

Continued

Applying a Hot Pack—cont'd

Procedure

8 Place the pad under the body part.
9 Apply the pack quickly. Note the time.
10 Secure the pack in place with ties, tape, or rolled gauze. Some packs are secured with Velcro straps (Figure 42-7).
11 Place the call bell within reach. Follow the care plan for bed rail use.*
12 Check the area every 5 minutes. Check for redness and complaints of pain, discomfort, or numbness. Remove the pack if any occur. Tell your supervisor at once.
13 Change the pack if cooling occurs.
14 Remove the pack after 20 minutes or as directed by your supervisor. Pat the area dry with the towel.

Post-Procedure

15 Follow steps 16 through 22 in *Applying Hot Compresses* on page 700.
16 Clean a reusable pack according to employer policy and the manufacturer's instructions.

*Step marked with an asterisk may not apply in community settings.

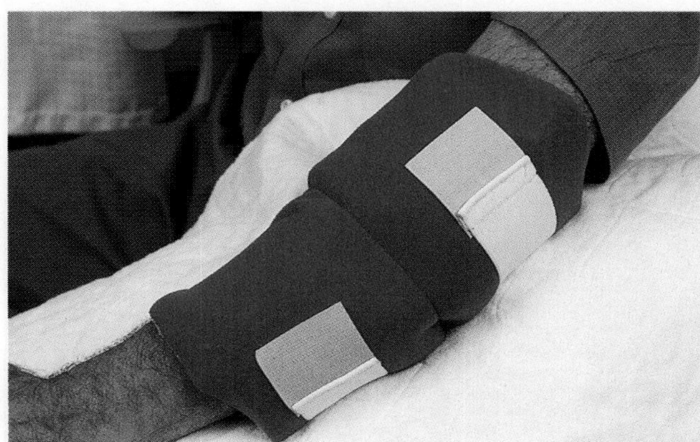

Figure 42-7 Hot pack secured with Velcro.

Cold Applications

Cold applications are often used to treat sprains, fractures, and fever. They reduce pain, prevent swelling, and decrease circulation and bleeding. Cold applications also cool the body when fever is present.

Cold has the opposite effect of heat. When cold is applied to the skin, blood vessels constrict (see Figure 42-1, *C* on page 697). Decreased blood flow results. Less oxygen and nutrients are carried to the tissues. Cold applications are useful right after injury. The decreased circulation reduces the amount of bleeding. The amount of fluid collecting in tissues is also reduced. Cold has a numbing effect on the skin. This helps reduce or relieve pain in the part.

Complications

Complications include pain, burns, blisters, and cyanosis. Burns and blisters tend to occur from intense cold. They also occur when dry cold applications are in direct contact with the skin.

When cold is applied for too long, the blood vessels dilate. Blood flow increases. This may *increase* bleeding and swelling. Often check clients who are at high risk for complications (see Box 42-1 on page 698). Prevent injuries from cold applications (see Box 42-2 on page 698).

Moist and Dry Applications

Cold applications are moist or dry.

- Dry cold—ice bag, ice collar, and ice glove
- Moist cold—cold compress
- Moist or dry—cold packs

Moist cold applications penetrate deeper than dry ones. Therefore temperatures of moist applications are not as cold as dry applications.

Ice Bags, Ice Collars, Ice Gloves, and Dry Cold Packs

Ice bags, ice collars, and ice gloves are dry cold applications. The devices are filled with crushed ice.

Commercial cold packs are reusable or single use (disposable). Single-use cold packs are discarded after use. To activate the cold, follow the manufacturer's instructions. You will need to strike, knead, or squeeze the pack. Reusable cold packs are kept in the freezer. They are cleaned after use (see *Hot Packs* on page 704).

Some devices have an outer covering. It allows direct application to the skin. If not, the device is placed in a cover. If the cover becomes moist, remove it and apply a dry one. (See *Focus on Home Care: Ice Packs* box.)

(text continues on page 708)

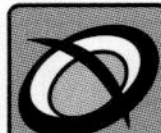

Focus on Home Care

ICE PACKS

Disposable ice packs are common in home settings. They are kept in the freezer until needed. A bag of frozen vegetables is useful as an ice pack. So are plastic bags. After filling the bag with ice, close the bag securely to prevent leaks. Then wrap the pack, bag of frozen vegetables, or plastic bag in a clean towel, dish cloth, or pillowcase. If you use a bag of frozen vegetables as an ice pack, make sure it is not later used as food. Remember, only apply an ice pack if your supervisor assigns you the task.

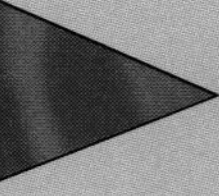

Applying an Ice Bag, Ice Collar, Ice Glove, or Dry Cold Pack

COMPASSIONATE CARE

Remember to Promote:
- **Dignity**
- **Independence**
- **Preferences**
- **Privacy**
- **Safety**

Pre-Procedure

1 Identify the person according to employer policy.
2 Explain the procedure to the person.
3 Wash your hands.
4 Collect a cold pack or the following:
- Ice bag, collar, or glove
- Crushed ice
- Flannel cover, towel, or pillowcase
- Paper towels

5 *Apply an ice bag, collar, or glove:*
   a Fill it with water. Put in the stopper. Turn the device upside down to check for leaks.
   b Empty the device.
   c Fill the device ½ to ⅔ full with crushed ice or ice chips (Figure 42-8).
   d Remove excess air. Bend, twist, or squeeze the device. Or press it against a firm surface.
   e Place the cap or stopper on securely.
   f Dry the device with the paper towels.
   g Place the device in the cover.

6 *Apply a cold pack:*
   a Squeeze, knead, or strike the disposable cold pack as directed by the manufacturer. This releases cold.
   b Place the device in the cover.

7 Provide for privacy.

Continued

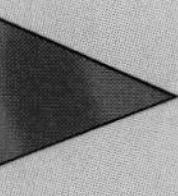

Applying an Ice Bag, Ice Collar, Ice Glove, or Dry Cold Pack—cont'd

Procedure

8 Apply the device. Secure it in place with ties, tape, or rolled gauze. Note the time.

9 Place the call bell within reach. Follow the care plan for bed rail use.*

10 Check the skin every 5 minutes. Check for blisters; pale, white, or grey skin; cyanosis; and shivering. Ask about numbness, pain, and burning. Remove the device if any occur. Tell your supervisor at once.

11 Remove the device after 20 minutes or as directed by your supervisor.

Post-Procedure

12 Follow steps 16 through 22 in *Applying Hot Compresses* on page 700.

13 Clean a reusable cold pack according to employer policy and the manufacturer's instructions.

*Step marked with an asterisk may not apply in community settings.

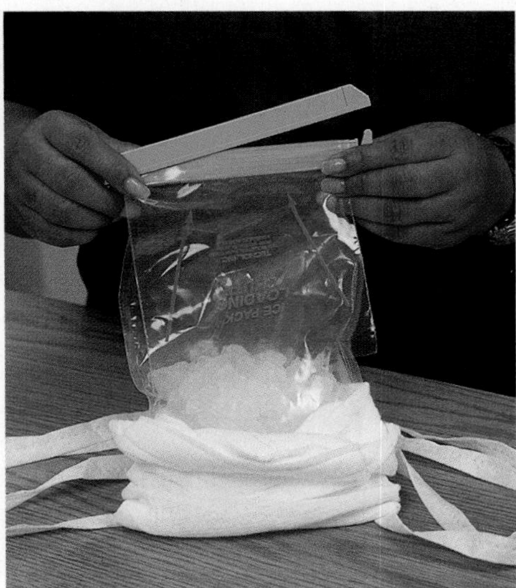

Figure 42-8 Fill the ice bag ½ to ⅔ full with ice.

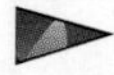

Cold Compresses

Applying a cold compress is like applying a hot compress. The cold compress is a moist application. Moist cold compresses are left in place no longer than 20 minutes.

Applying Cold Compresses

Compassionate Care

Remember to Promote:

- **Dignity**
- **Independence**
- **Preferences**
- **Privacy**
- **Safety**

Pre-Procedure

1 Identify the person according to employer policy.
2 Explain the procedure to the person.
3 Wash your hands.
4 Collect the following:
- Large basin with ice
- Small basin with cold water
- Gauze squares, washcloths, or small towels
- Waterproof pad
- Bath towel

5 Provide for privacy.

Procedure

6 Place the small basin with cold water into the large basin with ice.
7 Place the compresses into the cold water.
8 Place the pad under the body part.
9 Wring out a compress.
10 Apply the compress to the part. Note the time.
11 Place the call bell within reach. Follow the care plan for bed rail use.*
12 Check the area every 5 minutes. Check for blisters; pale, white, or grey skin; cyanosis; and shivering. Ask about numbness, pain, and burning. Remove the compress if any occur. Tell your supervisor at once.
13 Change the compress when it warms. Usually compresses are changed every 5 minutes.
14 Remove the compress after 20 minutes or as directed by your supervisor.
15 Pat the area dry.

Post-Procedure

16 Follow steps 16 through 22 in *Applying Hot Compresses* on page 700.

*Step marked with an asterisk may not apply in community settings.

REVIEW

Circle the BEST answer.

1. Heat applications have the following effects *except*
   A. Pain relief
   B. Muscle relaxation
   C. Healing
   D. Decreased blood flow

2. Which is the greatest threat from heat applications?
   A. Infection
   B. Burns
   C. Chilling
   D. Pressure ulcers

3. Who has the greatest risk of complications from a heat application?
   A. A 10-year-old boy
   B. A teenager
   C. A 40-year-old woman
   D. An older adult with diabetes

4. When checking a client with a heat application, which of the following do you *not* need to report?
   A. Warm skin
   B. Shivering
   C. Pale skin
   D. Cyanosis

5. The temperature of a hot application is usually between
   A. 26.6 and 33.8° C
   B. 33.8 and 36.6° C
   C. 36.6 and 41.1° C
   D. 41.1 and 46.1° C

6. These statements are about moist heat applications. Which is *false*?
   A. Water is in contact with the skin.
   B. Moist heat has lesser and slower effects than dry heat.
   C. Moist heat penetrates deeper than dry heat.
   D. The temperature of a moist heat application is lower than that of a dry heat application.

7. A client has a hot compress. Which is *false*?
   A. The hot compress is a moist heat application.
   B. The compress is applied no longer than 20 minutes.
   C. The area is checked every 15 minutes.
   D. A layer of plastic may cover the compress to retain heat.

8. These statements are about sitz baths. Which is *false*?
   A. The perineal and rectal areas are immersed in warm or hot water for 20 minutes.
   B. The sitz bath lasts 25 to 30 minutes.
   C. Sitz baths clean the perineum, relieve pain, increase circulation, and stimulate voiding.
   D. Weakness and fainting can occur.

9. Cold applications
   A. Reduce pain, prevent swelling, and decrease circulation
   B. Dilate blood vessels
   C. Prevent the spread of microbes
   D. Are warmed in a microwave oven

10. Which is *not* a complication of a cold application?
    A. Pain
    B. Burns and blisters
    C. Cyanosis
    D. Infection

11. Before applying an ice bag
    A. Place the bag in a freezer
    B. Measure the temperature of the bag
    C. Place the bag in a cover
    D. Ask the person to void

12. Moist cold compresses are left in place no longer than
    A. 20 minutes
    B. 30 minutes
    C. 45 minutes
    D. 60 minutes

Answers to these questions are on page 827.

CHAPTER

43

Oxygen Needs

OBJECTIVES

- Define the key terms listed in this chapter
- Describe the factors affecting oxygen needs
- Identify the signs and symptoms of hypoxia and altered respiratory function
- Describe tests used to diagnose respiratory problems
- Explain measures that promote oxygenation
- Describe devices used to administer oxygen
- Explain how to safely assist with oxygen therapy
- Describe the safety measures for suctioning
- Explain how to assist in the care of clients with artificial airways, on mechanical ventilation, and with chest tubes
- Learn the procedures described in this chapter

KEY TERMS

apnea The lack or absence (*a*) of breathing (*pnea*)

Biot's respirations Rapid and deep respirations followed by 10 to 30 seconds of apnea

bradypnea Slow (*brady*) breathing (*pnea*); respirations are fewer then 10 per minute

Cheyne-Stokes Respirations gradually increasing in rate and depth and then becoming shallow and slow; breathing may stop (*apnea*) for 10 to 20 seconds

dyspnea Difficult, laboured, or painful (*dys*) breathing (*pnea*)

hemoptysis Bloody (*hemo*) sputum (*ptysis*, meaning "to spit")

hyperventilation Respirations that are rapid (*hyper*) and deeper than normal

hypoventilation Respirations that are slow (*hypo*), shallow, and sometimes irregular

hypoxemia A deficiency (*hypo*) of oxygen (*ox*) in the blood (*emia*)

hypoxia A deficiency (*hypo*) of oxygen in the cells (*oxia*)

intubation The process of inserting an artificial airway

Kussmaul's respirations Very deep and rapid respirations; a sign of diabetic coma

mechanical ventilation The use of a machine to move air into and out of the lungs

orthopnea Breathing (*pnea*) deeply and comfortably only while sitting or standing (*ortho*)

orthopneic position Sitting up (*ortho*) and leaning over a table to breathe

oxygen concentration The amount of hemoglobin that contains oxygen (O_2)

pulse oximeter A device that measures (*meter*) oxygen (*oxi*) concentration in the arterial blood; consists of a computerized monitor and a sensor (probe)

respiratory arrest Breathing stops

respiratory depression Slow, weak respirations at a rate of fewer than 12 per minute; respirations are not deep enough to bring enough air into the lungs

sputum Mucus from the respiratory system that is expectorated (expelled) through the mouth

suction The process of withdrawing or sucking up fluid (secretions)

tachypnea Rapid (*tachy*) breathing (*pnea*); respirations are 24 or more per minute

tracheostomy A surgically-created opening (*ostomy*) through the neck into the trachea (*tracheo*)

Oxygen (O_2) is a gas. It has no taste, odour, or colour. It is a basic need required for life. Death occurs within minutes if breathing stops. Illness, surgery, and injuries affect the amount of oxygen in the blood cells.

Often you will work with clients with oxygen needs. You need to know how to give safe and effective care. Review the respiratory system in Figure 43-1 on page 712. (See Chapter 13.)

Before giving or assisting with any care described in this chapter, make sure that:

- Your province or territory allows you to perform the task
- The task is in your job description
- You have the necessary training
- You know how to use the equipment
- You review the task with a nurse
- A nurse will supervise you

FACTORS AFFECTING OXYGEN NEEDS

The respiratory and cardiovascular systems must function properly for cells to get enough oxygen. Any disease, injury, or surgery involving these systems affects the body's ability to take in oxygen and deliver it to the cells. Body systems depend on each other. Altered function of any system (for example, the nervous, musculoskeletal, or urinary system) affects oxygen needs. Major factors affecting oxygen needs are:

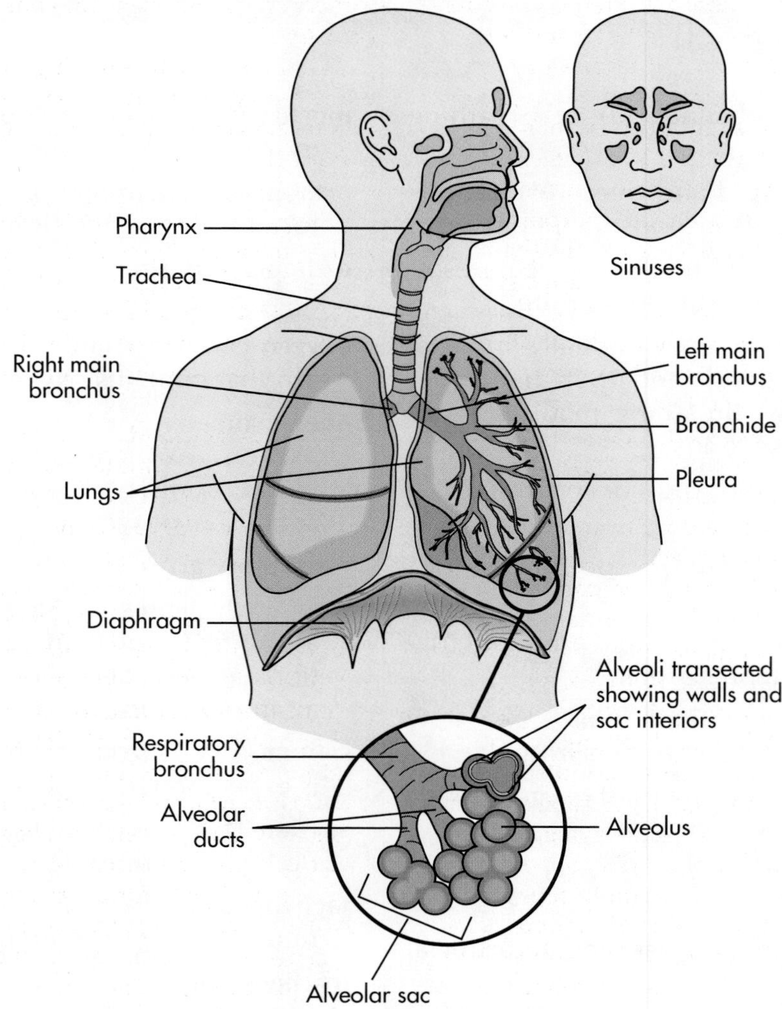

Figure 43-1 The respiratory system.

- *Respiratory system function*—Structures must be intact and functioning. The airway must be open (patent). *Alveoli* (single-celled air sacs in the lungs) must exchange O_2 and carbon dioxide (CO_2).
- *Cardiovascular system function*—Blood must flow to and from the heart. Narrowed vessels affect blood flow. Capillaries and cells must exchange O_2 and CO_2.
- *Red blood cell count*—The blood must have enough red blood cells (RBCs). RBCs contain hemoglobin, which picks up oxygen in the lungs and carries it to the cells. The bone marrow must produce enough RBCs. Poor diet, chemotherapy, and leukemia affect bone marrow function. Blood loss also reduces the number of RBCs.
- *Nervous system function*—Nervous system diseases and injuries can affect respiratory muscles. Some make breathing difficult or impossible. Brain injury affects respiratory rate, rhythm, and depth. Narcotics and depressant drugs affect the brain. They slow respirations. O_2 and CO_2 levels in the blood also affect brain function. Respirations increase when O_2 is lacking. The body tries to bring in more oxygen. Respirations also increase when CO_2 increases. The body tries to get rid of CO_2.
- *Aging*—Respiratory muscles weaken and lung tissue becomes less elastic with age. Strength for coughing decreases. Coughing removes secretions from the upper airway. If the person cannot cough, pneumonia (infection of the lungs) can develop. Older adults are at risk for respiratory complications after surgery.
- *Exercise*—O_2 needs increase with exercise. Normally, respiratory rate and depth increase to bring enough O_2 into the lungs. People with heart and respiratory diseases may have enough O_2 at rest. However, even slight activity increases O_2 needs. Their bodies may not be able to bring in O_2 and to deliver it to cells.
- *Fever*—O_2 needs increase when fever is present. Respiratory rate and depth must increase to meet the body's needs.
- *Pain*—Pain increases the need for O_2. Respirations increase to meet this need. However, chest and

abdominal injuries and surgeries often involve respiratory muscles. It hurts to breathe in and out.

- *Drugs*—Some drugs depress the respiratory centre in the brain. **Respiratory depression** involves slow, weak respirations at a rate of fewer than 12 per minute. Respirations are too shallow to bring enough O_2 into the lungs. **Respiratory arrest** occurs when breathing stops. Narcotics (morphine, Demerol, and others) can have these effects. (Narcotic comes from the Greek word *narkoun*. It means stupor or numbness.) In safe amounts, these drugs are prescribed by a physician to relieve pain. Substance abusers are at risk for respiratory depression and respiratory arrest from overdoses of drugs.
- *Smoking*—Smoking causes lung cancer and chronic obstructive pulmonary disease (COPD). It is a risk factor for coronary artery disease.
- *Allergies*—An *allergy* is a sensitivity to a substance that causes the body to react with signs and symptoms. A runny nose, wheezing, and congestion are common. Mucous membranes in the upper airway swell. With severe swelling, the airway closes. Shock and death are risks. Pollens, dust, foods, drugs, and smoke often cause allergies. People with allergies are at risk for chronic bronchitis and asthma.
- *Pollutant exposure*—A *pollutant* is a harmful chemical or substance in the air or water. Dust, fumes, toxins, asbestos, coal dust, and sawdust are some air pollutants. They damage the lungs. Pollutant exposure occurs in home, work, and community settings.
- *Nutrition*—Good nutrition is needed to produce red blood cells. The body needs iron and vitamins (vitamin B_{12}, vitamin C, and folic acid) to produce RBCs.
- *Alcohol*—Alcohol depresses the brain. Excessive amounts reduce the cough reflex and increase the risk of aspiration. Obstructed airway and pneumonia are risks from aspiration.

Altered Respiratory Function

Respiratory system function involves three processes. Respiratory function is altered if even one process is affected.

- Air moves into and out of the lungs.
- O_2 and CO_2 are exchanged at the alveoli.
- The blood transports O_2 to the cells and removes CO_2 from them.

Hypoxia

Hypoxia is a deficiency (*hypo*) of oxygen in the cells (*oxia*). They cannot function properly. Hypoxia is caused by any illness, disease, injury, or surgery affecting respiratory function. The brain is very sensitive to inadequate oxygen. Restlessness is an early sign of hypoxia. So are dizziness and disorientation. Report signs and symptoms of hypoxia immediately (Box 43-1).

Hypoxia is life threatening. All organs must receive enough oxygen to function. When hypoxia is diagnosed, oxygen is given, and the cause of the hypoxia is treated.

Abnormal Respirations

Adults normally have 12 to 20 respirations per minute. Infants and children have faster rates (see Table 40-3 on page 667). Respirations are normally quiet, effortless, and regular. Both sides of the chest rise and fall equally. The following breathing patterns are abnormal:

- ***Tachypnea***—rapid (*tachy*) breathing (*pnea*). Respirations are 24 or more per minute. Fever, exercise, pain, airway obstruction, and hypoxemia are common causes. **Hypoxemia** is a deficiency (*hypo*) of oxygen (*ox*) in the blood (*emia*).
- ***Bradypnea***—slow (*brady*) breathing (*pnea*). Respirations are fewer than 12 per minute. Drug overdoses and nervous system disorders are common causes.
- ***Apnea***—the lack or absence (*a*) of breathing (*pnea*). It occurs in cardiac arrest and respiratory arrest. Sleep apnea and periodic apnea of newborns are other types of apnea.
- ***Hypoventilation***—respirations are slow (*hypo*), shallow, and sometimes irregular. Common causes include lung disorders (such as pneumonia) that affect the alveoli. Other causes include obesity, airway obstruction, drug side effects, and nervous system and musculoskeletal disorders affecting the respiratory muscles.
- ***Hyperventilation***—respirations are rapid (*hyper*) and deeper than normal. Its many causes include asthma, emphysema, infection, fever, nervous system disorders, hypoxia, anxiety, pain, and some drugs.

Box 43-1 Signs and Symptoms of Hypoxia

- Restlessness
- Dizziness
- Disorientation
- Confusion
- Behaviour and personality changes
- Difficulty concentrating and following directions
- Apprehension
- Anxiety
- Fatigue
- Agitation
- Increased pulse rate
- Increased rate and depth of respirations
- Sitting position, often leaning forward
- Cyanosis (bluish colour to the skin, lips, mucous membranes, and nail beds)
- Dyspnea

- ***Dyspnea***—difficult, laboured, or painful (*dys*) breathing (*pnea*). Heart disease, exercise, and anxiety are common causes.
- ***Cheyne-Stokes***—respirations gradually increasing in rate and depth and then becoming shallow and slow. Breathing may stop (apnea) for 10 to 20 seconds. Drug overdose, heart failure, renal failure, and brain disorders are common causes. These respirations are common when death is near.
- ***Orthopnea***—breathing (*pnea*) deeply and comfortably only while sitting or standing (*ortho*). Common causes include emphysema, asthma, pneumonia, angina pectoris, and other heart and respiratory disorders.
- ***Biot's respirations***—rapid and deep respirations followed by 10 to 30 seconds of apnea.
- ***Kussmaul's respirations***—very deep and rapid respirations. They occur in diabetic coma.

Assisting with Assessment and Diagnostic Testing

Altered respiratory function may be an acute or chronic problem. When unable to breathe easily, a person may feel very anxious or may panic. It is also dangerous for the person. Report your observations to your supervisor promptly and accurately (Box 43-2). Quick action is necessary to meet oxygen needs. Measures are taken to correct the problem and prevent it from getting worse.

The physician orders tests to determine the cause of the problem. There are many respiratory tests available (Box 43-3). Some tests are done at hospitals or clinics. Others are done in long-term care facilities. They are done by a physician or a specially trained nurse, respiratory therapist, or laboratory technician. You may assist the client before and after a test as directed by your supervisor, the care plan, and assignment sheet.

You are likely to assist with pulse oximetry and to collect sputum specimens. Both procedures may provide the physician with information about the state of the client's respiratory system.

Pulse Oximetry.

A **pulse oximeter** is a device used to measure (*metry*) oxygen (*oxi*) concentration in arterial blood. It also measures pulse rate. **Oxygen concentration** is the amount (percent) of hemoglobin that contains oxygen. The normal range is 95 to 100%. For example, if 97% of all the hemoglobin carries O_2, tissues get enough oxygen. If only 90% of the hemoglobin contains O_2, tissues do not get enough oxygen to function. The pulse oximeter can detect low oxygen levels before any signs or symptoms appear. Measurements are used to prevent and treat hypoxia.

A pulse oximeter consists of a computerized monitor and a sensor (probe). The sensor is attached to the client's finger, toe, nose, earlobe, or forehead (Figure 43-2). Two light beams on one side of the sensor pass through the tissues. A detector on the other side measures the amount of light passing through the tissues. Using this information, the oximeter measures the O_2 concentration. The value and pulse rate are displayed on the monitor. Oximeters have alarms. The alarms sound if O_2 concentration is low, the pulse is too fast or slow, or other problems occur.

Small, hand-held oximeter units are available for home use. Usually the client's oxygen concentration is measured at the same time that vital signs are measured. Because it is portable and used for many clients, you must make sure the pulse oximeter is accurate. After applying the sensor, check the client's radial pulse and compare it with the displayed pulse. The pulse rates should be the same.

Box 43-2 Signs and Symptoms of Altered Respiratory Function

- Signs and symptoms of hypoxia (see Box 43-1 on page 713)
- Any abnormal breathing pattern
- Complaints of shortness of breath or being "winded" or "short-winded"
- Cough (note frequency and time of day)
  - Dry and hacking
  - Harsh and barking
  - Productive (produces sputum) or non-productive
- Sputum
  - Colour—clear, white, yellow, green, brown, or red
  - Odour—none or foul
  - Consistency—thick, watery, or frothy (with bubbles or foam)
  - **Hemoptysis**—bloody (*hemo*) sputum (*ptysis*, meaning "to spit"); note if the sputum is bright red, dark red, blood tinged, or streaked with blood
- Noisy respirations
  - Wheezing
  - Wet-sounding respirations
  - Crowing sounds
- Chest pain
  - Note location
  - Constant or intermittent (comes and goes)
  - Client's description (stabbing, knife-like, aching)
  - What makes it worse (movement, coughing, yawning, sneezing, sighing, deep breathing)
- Cyanosis
  - Skin
  - Mucous membranes
  - Lips
  - Nail beds
- Changes in vital signs
- Body position
  - Sitting upright
  - Leaning forward or hunched over a table

Box 43-3 Common Respiratory Tests

- *Chest X-ray (CXR)*—An X-ray is taken of the chest. It is used to evaluate changes in the lungs.
- *Lung scan*—The lungs are scanned to see what areas are not getting air or blood. The person inhales radioactive gas and is injected with a radioisotope. *Radioactive* means to give off radiation. A *radioisotope* is a substance that gives off radiation. Lung tissue getting air and blood "take up" the radioactive substances. A scanner senses areas with radioactive substances.
- *Bronchoscopy*—A scope (*scopy*) is passed into the trachea and bronchi (*broncho*). Airway structures are checked for bleeding and tumours. Tissue samples (biopsy) are taken, or mucous plugs and foreign objects are removed. After the procedure, the person is NPO and watched carefully until the gag and swallow reflexes return. They usually return in about 2 hours.
- *Thoracentesis*—The pleura (*thora*) is punctured and air or fluid is removed (*centesis*) from it. The physician inserts a needle through the chest wall into the pleural sac. Injury or disease can cause it to fill with air, blood, or fluid. This affects respiratory function. Sometimes fluid is removed for laboratory study. Sometimes anticancer medications are injected into the pleural sac. The procedure takes a few minutes. After the procedure, the person is checked often for shortness of breath, dyspnea, cough, sputum, chest pain, cyanosis, vital sign changes, and other respiratory signs and symptoms.
- *Pulmonary function tests*—Tests that measure the amount of air moving into and out of the lungs (volume) and how much air the lungs can hold (capacity). The client takes as deep a breath as possible. Using a mouthpiece, the client blows into a machine. The tests are used to evaluate people at risk for lung diseases or postoperative lung complications. They also measure the progress of lung disease and its treatment.
- *Arterial blood gases (ABGs)*—A radial or femoral artery is punctured to obtain arterial blood. Laboratory tests measure the amount of oxygen in the blood. Hemorrhage from the artery must be prevented. Pressure is applied to the artery for at least 5 minutes after the procedure. Pressure is applied longer if the person has blood clotting problems.

A good sensor site is needed. Your supervisor tells you what site to use based on the client's condition. Swollen sites are avoided. So are sites with skin breaks.

Aging and vascular disease often cause poor circulation. Sometimes blood flow to the fingers or toes is poor. Then the earlobe, nose, or forehead sites are used.

Bright light, nail polish, artificial nails, and movements affect measurements. Place a towel over the sensor to block bright light. Remove nail polish, or use another site. Do not use a finger site if the client wears artificial nails. Movements from shivering, seizures, or tremors affect finger sensors. The earlobe is a better site for these problems. Blood pressure cuffs affect blood flow. If using a finger site, do not measure blood pressure on that side.

Report and record measurements accurately. Use the abbreviation SpO_2 when recording the oxygen concentration value (S=saturation, p=pulse, O_2=oxygen). Also, report and record:

- The date and time
- What the client was doing at the time of the measurement
- Oxygen flow rate and the device used
- Reason for the measurement (routine or change in the client's condition)
- Other observations

Pulse oximetry does not lessen the need for good observations. The client's condition can change rapidly. Observe for signs and symptoms of hypoxia.

(text continues on page 717)

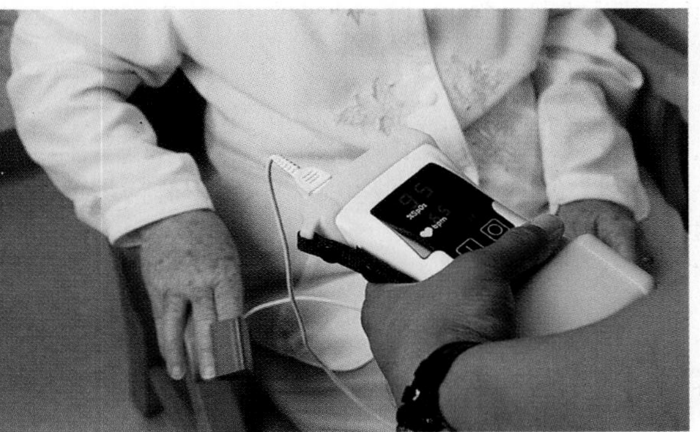

A

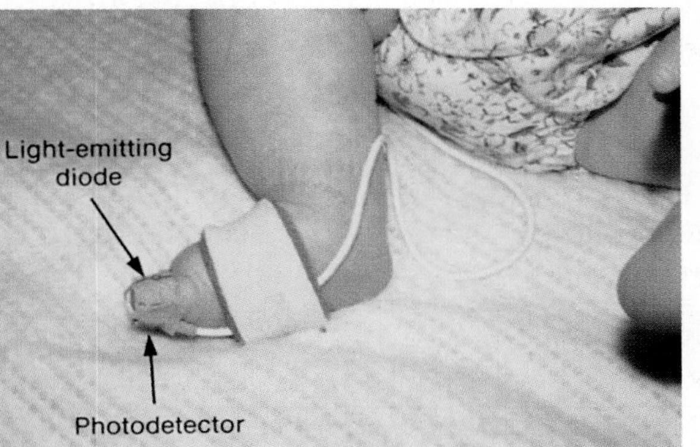

B

Figure 43-2 A, A pulse oximetry sensor is attached to a finger. **B,** The sensor is attached to an infant's toe. Source for *B:* D.L. Wong, *Whaley and Wong's Nursing Care of Infants and Children,* 6th ed. (St. Louis: Mosby, 1999).

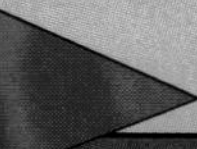

Using a Pulse Oximeter

Compassionate Care

Remember to Promote:

- **Dignity**
- **Independence**
- **Preferences**
- **Privacy**
- **Safety**

Pre-Procedure

1 Identify the person according to employer policy.
2 Review the procedure with your supervisor.
3 Find out what site to use.
4 Explain the procedure to the person.
5 Wash your hands.
6 Collect the following:
- Pulse oximeter and sensor
- Nail polish remover and cotton balls (if needed)
- SpO_2 flow sheet
- Tape (if needed)
- Towel

7 Provide for privacy.

Procedure

8 Provide for comfort.
9 Remove any nail polish if a finger or toe site is used. Use nail polish remover and a cotton ball. SAFETY NOTE: Do not use nail polish remover if the person is receiving oxygen therapy. Nail polish remover is flammable and dangerous near oxygen.
10 Dry the site with a towel.
11 Clip or tape the sensor to the site.
12 Attach the sensor cables to the oximeter.
13 Turn on the oximeter.
14 Set the high and low alarm limits for SpO_2 and pulse rate. Turn on audio and visual alarms.
15 Check the person's radial pulse with the pulse on the display. The pulses should be equal. Tell your supervisor if the pulses are not equal.
16 Read the SpO_2 and the pulse rate on the display. Note the values on the flow sheet and assignment sheet.
17 Leave the sensor in place for continuous monitoring. Otherwise, turn off the device and remove the sensor.

Post-Procedure

18 Provide for safety and comfort.
19 Place the call bell within reach.*
20 Follow the care plan for bed rail use.*
21 Remove privacy measures.
22 Return the pulse oximeter to its proper place unless monitoring is continuous.
23 Wash your hands.
24 Report and record the SpO_2, pulse rate, and other observations. Follow employer policy.

*Steps marked with an asterisk may not apply in community settings.

Collecting Sputum Specimens. Respiratory disorders cause the lungs, bronchi, and trachea to secrete mucus. Mucus from the respiratory system is called **sputum** when expectorated (expelled) through the mouth. Sputum is not saliva. Saliva (spit) is a thin, clear liquid produced by the salivary glands in the mouth.

Sputum specimens are studied for blood, microbes, and abnormal cells. The client coughs up sputum from the bronchi and trachea. This is often painful and hard to do. Specimen collection is easier in the morning when secretions are coughed up upon awakening.

The client rinses the mouth with water. Rinsing decreases saliva and removes food particles. Mouthwash is not used before the procedure. It destroys some of the microbes in the mouth.

The procedure can embarrass the client. Coughing and expectorating sounds can disturb others nearby. Also, sputum is unpleasant to look at. For these reasons, privacy is important. If possible, collect the specimen when the roommate or family members are out of the room. Cover the specimen container, and place it in a bag. Some sputum containers hide the contents. Always follow Standard Precautions when collecting a sputum specimen.

Some clients do not have the strength to cough up sputum. Coughing is made easier for them after postural drainage. Postural drainage involves draining secretions by gravity. Gravity causes fluids to flow down. The client is positioned so a lung part is higher than the airway (Figure 43-3). Positioning depends on the lung part that needs draining. The nurse or respiratory therapist does postural drainage. You may assist. Do not attempt to position the client without supervision. (See *Focus on Children: Assisting with Treatments* box.)

Report and record the following observations after collecting a sputum specimen:

- The time the specimen was collected
- The amount of sputum collected
- How easily the client raised the sputum
- The consistency of the sputum (see Box 43-2 on page 714)

(text continues on page 719)

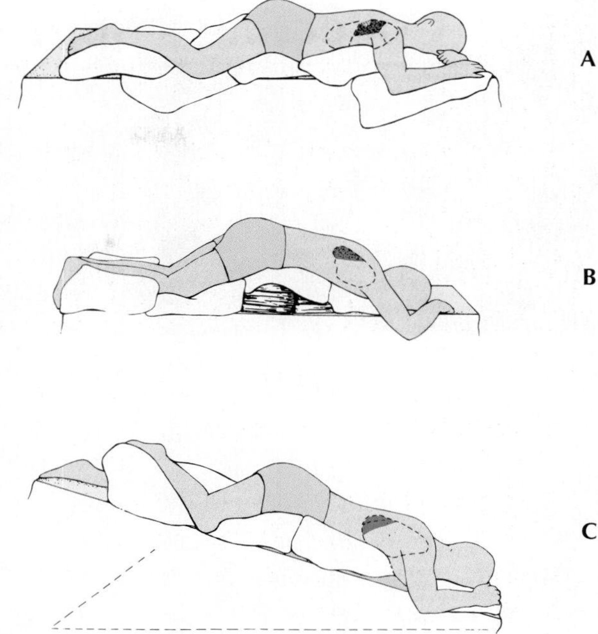

Figure 43-3 Some positions used for postural drainage. NOTE: A nurse or respiratory therapist is responsible for postural drainage. Do not place the client in these positions without supervision. **A,** Draining the right upper lobe. **B,** Draining the right middle lobe. **C,** Draining the right lower lobe. Source: P.A. Potter and A.G. Perry, *Fundamentals of Nursing: Concepts, Process, and Practice,* 5th ed. (St. Louis: Mosby, 2001).

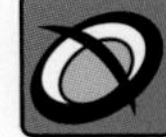

Focus on Children

Assisting with Treatments

Breathing treatments and suctioning are often needed to produce a sputum specimen in infants and small children. The nurse or respiratory therapist gives the breathing treatment. The nurse suctions the trachea for the sputum specimen. The infant or child is likely to be uncooperative during suctioning. You can assist by comforting the child. You might be asked to hold the child's head and arms still.

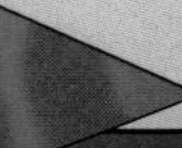

Collecting a Sputum Specimen

Compassionate Care

Remember to Promote:
- **Dignity**
- **Independence**
- **Preferences**
- **Privacy**
- **Safety**

Pre-Procedure

1 Identify the person according to employer policy.
2 Explain the procedure to the person.
3 Wash your hands.
4 Collect the following:
- Sputum specimen container and label
- Laboratory requisition
- Disposable bag
- Gloves
- Mask (if needed)
- Tissues
- Cup of water
- Kidney basin

5 Label the specimen container.
6 Provide for privacy. If able, the person uses the bathroom for the procedure.

Procedure

7 Ask the person to rinse the mouth out with clear water. If the person is in bed, offer a glass of water and let the person spit into the kidney basin.
8 Put on gloves. Put on a mask if the person has a disease that is transmitted by droplets or through the air.
9 Have the person hold the container. Only the outside is touched.
10 Ask the person to cover the mouth and nose with tissues when coughing.
11 Ask the person to take 2 or 3 deep breaths and cough up the sputum.
12 Have the person expectorate directly into the specimen container (Figure 43-4). Sputum should not touch the outside.
13 Collect 15 to 30 mL (1 to 2 tablespoons) of sputum unless told to collect more.
14 Put the lid on the container. Do not touch the inside of the lid.
15 Place the container in the bag. Attach the requisition to the bag.
16 Remove gloves. Wash your hands.

Post-Procedure

17 Provide for safety and comfort.
18 Place the call bell within reach.*
19 Remove privacy measures.
20 Wash your hands.
21 Take the bag to the appropriate area.
22 Wash your hands.
23 Report and record your actions and observations according to employer policy.

*Step marked with an asterisk may not apply in community settings.

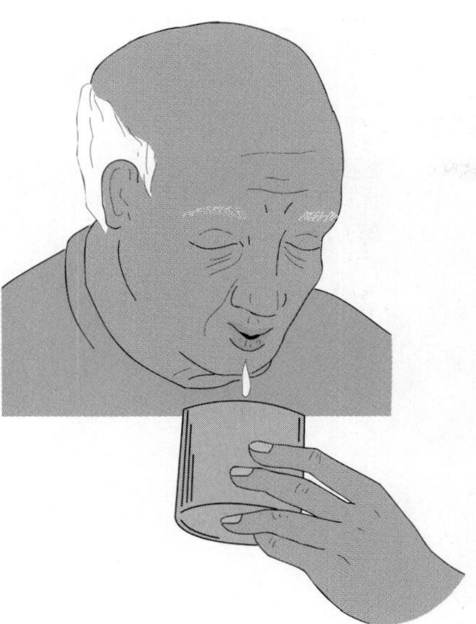

Figure 43-4 The client expectorates into the centre of the specimen container.

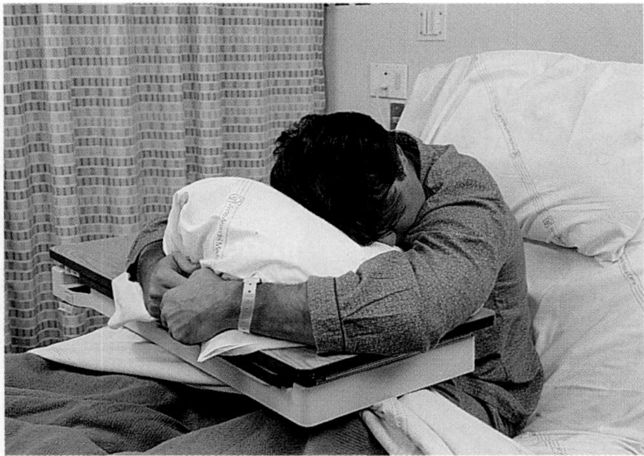

Figure 43-5 The client is in the orthopneic position. Note that a pillow is on the overbed table for the client's comfort.

PROMOTING OXYGENATION

For the body to get enough oxygen, air must move deep into the lungs. Air must reach the alveoli, where O_2 and CO_2 are exchanged. Disease and injury can prevent air from reaching the alveoli. Pain, immobility, and narcotics interfere with deep breathing and coughing up secretions. Therefore secretions collect in the airway and lungs. They interfere with air movement and lung function. Secretions also provide an environment for microbes to grow and multiply. Infection is a threat.

Oxygen needs must be met. The care plan lists measures that promote oxygenation. Often activities that involve movement and that expand the lungs are ordered. For example, taking the client for a short walk may be listed in the care plan. The following are other measures that are common in care plans.

POSITIONING

For people confined to bed, breathing is usually easier in semi-Fowler's and Fowler's position. People with difficulty breathing often prefer to sit up and lean over a table. This is called the **orthopneic position**. (*Ortho* means sitting or standing; *pnea* means breathing.) You can increase the client's comfort by placing a pillow on the table (Figure 43-5).

Frequent position changes are important. Unless the physician limits positioning, the client must not lie on one side for a long time. Otherwise, the lung cannot expand on that side. Secretions pool. Position changes are needed at least every 2 hours. Follow the care plan.

COUGHING AND DEEP BREATHING

Mucus is removed by coughing. Deep breathing moves air into most parts of the lungs. Coughing and deep breathing exercises help people with respiratory disorders. They are done after surgery and during bed rest. The exercises are painful after injury or surgery. The person may be afraid of breaking open an incision while coughing.

Coughing and deep breathing help prevent pneumonia and atelectasis. *Atelectasis* is the collapse of a portion of the lung. It occurs when mucus collects in the airway. Air cannot get to a part of the lung, and the lung collapses. Atelectasis is a risk after surgery. Bed rest, lung disease, and paralysis are other risk factors.

The frequency of coughing and deep breathing varies. Some physicians order the exercises every 1 to 2 hours while the client is awake. Others want them done 4 times a day. Your supervisor and the care plan tell you when coughing and deep breathing are done. You are told how many deep breaths and coughs the client should do. Follow the care plan.

Report and record the following observations after assisting with coughing and deep breathing:

- The number of times the client coughed and deep breathed
- How the client tolerated the procedure

(text continues on page 722)

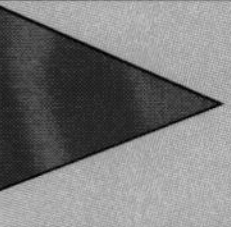

Assisting with Coughing and Deep Breathing Exercises

COMPASSIONATE CARE

Remember to Promote:
- **Dignity**
- **Independence**
- **Preferences**
- **Privacy**
- **Safety**

Pre-Procedure

1 Identify the person according to employer policy.
2 Explain the procedure to the person.
3 Wash your hands.
4 Provide for privacy.

Procedure

5 Help the person to a comfortable sitting position: dangling, semi-Fowler's, or Fowler's.
6 Have the person deep breath:
  - **a** Have the person place the hands over the rib cage (Figure 43-6).
  - **b** Ask the person to exhale. Explain that the ribs should move as far down as possible.
  - **c** Have the person take a deep breath. It should be as deep as possible. Remind the person to inhale through the nose.
  - **d** Ask the person to hold the breath for 3 seconds.
  - **e** Ask the person to exhale slowly through pursed lips (Figure 43-7). The person should exhale until the ribs move as far down as possible.
  - **f** Repeat a through e 4 more times.
7 Ask the person to cough:
  - **a** Have the person interlace the fingers over the incision (Figure 43-8, *A*). The person can also hold a pillow or folded towel over the incision (Figure 43-8, *B*).
  - **b** Have the person take in a deep breath as in step 6.
  - **c** Ask the person to cough strongly twice with the mouth open.

Post-Procedure

8 Provide for safety and comfort.
9 Place the call bell within reach.*
10 Follow the care plan for bed rail use.*
11 Remove privacy measures.
12 Wash your hands.
13 Report and record your actions and observations according to employer policy.

*Steps marked with an asterisk may not apply in community settings.

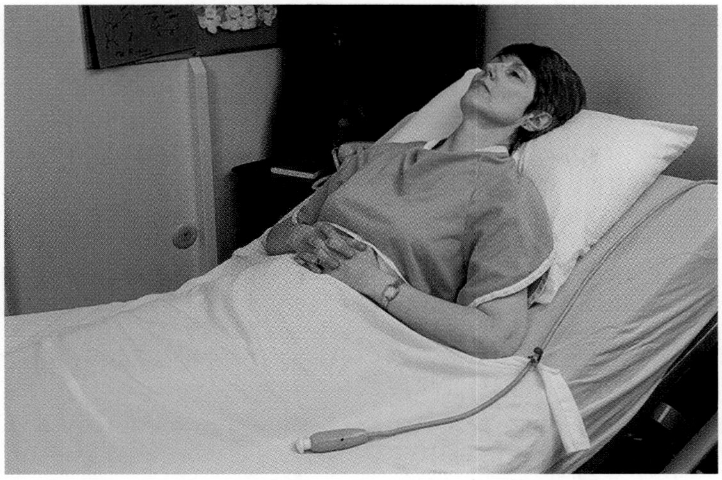

Figure 43-6 The hands are over the rib cage for deep breathing.

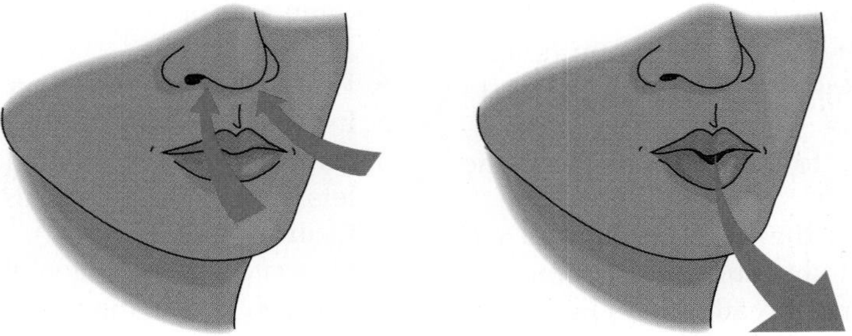

Figure 43-7 The client inhales through the nose and exhales through pursed lips during the deep-breathing exercise.

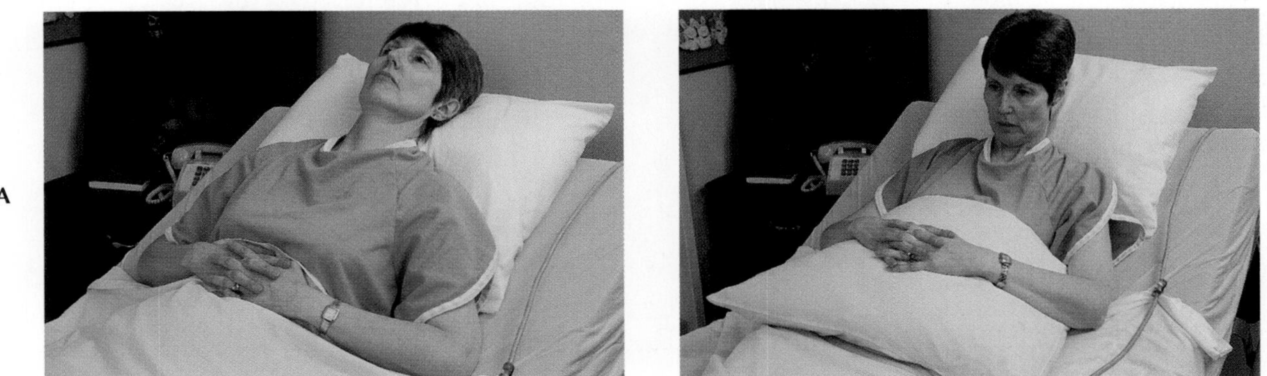

Figure 43-8 The client supports an incision for the coughing exercise. **A,** Fingers are interlaced over the incision. **B,** A pillow is held over the incision.

Incentive Spirometry

Incentive means encouragement. A *spirometer* is a machine that measures the amount (volume) of air inhaled. Balls or bars in the machine let the client see air movement when inhaling (Figure 43-9). Therefore the client is encouraged to inhale until reaching a preset volume of air. The client inhales as deeply as possible and holds that breath for a certain time, usually for at least 3 seconds. Incentive spirometry is also called *sustained maximal inspiration (SMI)*. *Sustained* means constant. *Maximal* means the most or the greatest. *Inspiration* relates to breathing in.

The goal of using a spirometer is to improve lung function and prevent respiratory complications. By taking long, slow, and deep breaths, the client moves air deep into the lungs. Secretions become loose. O_2 and CO_2 exchange occurs between the alveoli and capillaries.

The device is used as follows:

- The spirometer is placed upright.
- The client exhales normally.
- The client seals his or her lips around a mouthpiece.
- A slow, deep breath is taken until the balls rise to the desired height.
- The breath is held for 3 to 6 seconds to keep the balls floating.
- Then the client removes the mouthpiece and exhales slowly. The client may cough at this time.
- After taking some normal breaths, the client uses the device again.

Your supervisor and the care plan tell you the following:

- How often the client needs incentive spirometry
- How many breaths the client needs to take
- The desired height of the floating balls

Follow employer policy for cleaning and replacing the disposable mouthpiece.

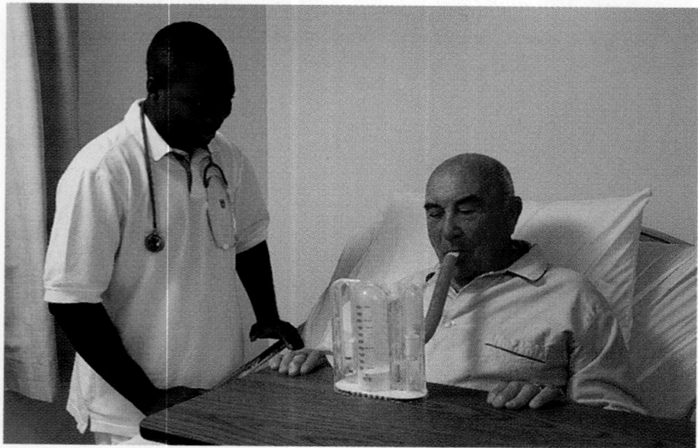

Figure 43-9 A client using a spirometer.

Assisting with Oxygen Therapy

Disease, injury, and surgery often interfere with breathing. The amount of O_2 in the blood may be less than normal (hypoxemia). If so, the physician orders oxygen therapy.

Oxygen is treated as a medication. The physician orders the amount of oxygen to give, the device to use, and when to give it. Some people need oxygen constantly. Others need it for symptom relief—chest pain or shortness of breath. Oxygen helps relieve chest pain. People with respiratory diseases may have enough oxygen while at rest but become short of breath with mild activity. Oxygen therapy helps relieve the shortness of breath.

You do not give oxygen. The nurse and respiratory therapist start and maintain oxygen therapy. You assist in providing safe care to clients receiving oxygen.

Oxygen Sources

Oxygen is supplied as follows:

- *Wall oxygen outlet*—Oxygen is delivered directly into each person's unit. Each unit is connected to a centrally located oxygen supply. Wall oxygen outlets are used in hospitals and some long-term care facilities (Figure 43-10).
- *Oxygen tank*—Oxygen is stored in a metal tank. Oxygen tanks may be placed at the bedside for

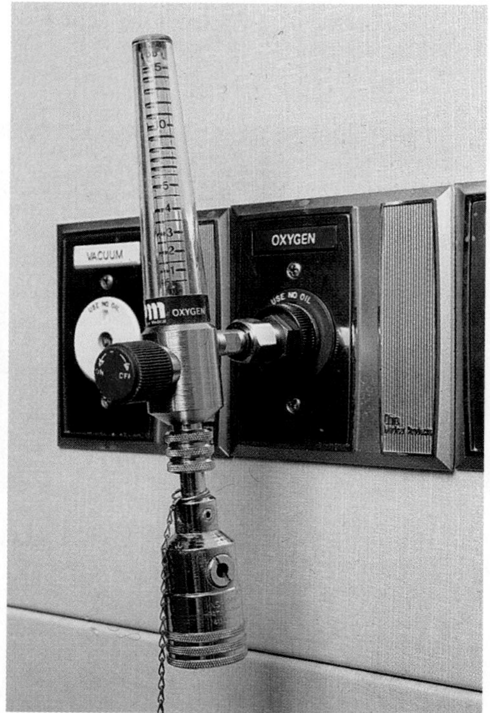

Figure 43-10 Wall oxygen outlet.

clients who are confined to bed. Some ambulatory clients need continuous oxygen as they go about their daily lives. They use portable oxygen tanks in a shoulder bag or wheeled in a cart (Figure 43-11). The gauge on the tank shows how much oxygen is left in the tank (Figure 43-12). Check the gauge often. Tell your supervisor if the oxygen in the tank is low. Oxygen tanks are used in facilities and community settings.

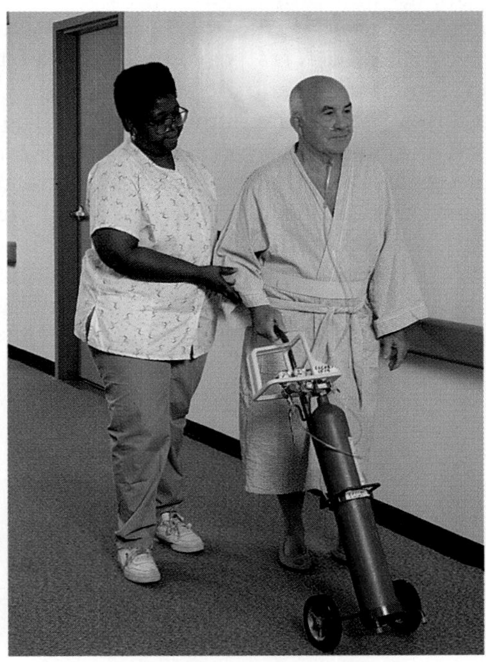

Figure 43-11 A client using a portable oxygen tank while walking.

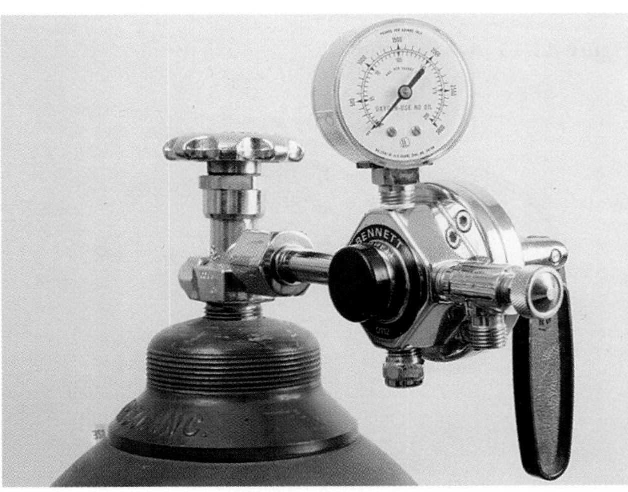

Figure 43-12 The gauge shows the amount of oxygen remaining in the tank.

- *Oxygen concentrator*—Oxygen concentrators remove oxygen from the air and store it (Figure 43-13). A power source is needed. If the concentrator is not portable, the client must stay close to the machine. Clients who use oxygen concentrators usually have portable oxygen tanks available for mobility and in case of a power failure. Oxygen concentrators are used in facilities and community settings.
- *Liquid oxygen system*—A portable unit is filled from a stationary unit (Figure 43-14 on page 724). The portable unit has enough oxygen for about 8 hours of use. A dial shows the amount of oxygen in the unit. Tell your supervisor if the unit is low. The portable unit can be worn over the shoulder. Liquid oxygen is very cold. If touched, it can freeze the skin. Follow employer procedures and the manufacturer's instructions when working with liquid oxygen. Liquid oxygen systems are used in facilities and community settings.

Oxygen and Fire Safety

Oxygen is flammable. Using oxygen puts the client at risk for burns and fire. It is very important to keep the oxygen source away from heat and open flame. Follow employer policies and the fire safety guidelines in Box 43-4 on page 724.

The physician, nurse, or respiratory therapist teaches the client and family members about oxygen safety. However, people sometimes forget or disregard safety rules. You may observe a client, visitor, or family member create a safety hazard. For example, a home care client might attempt to light a gas stove

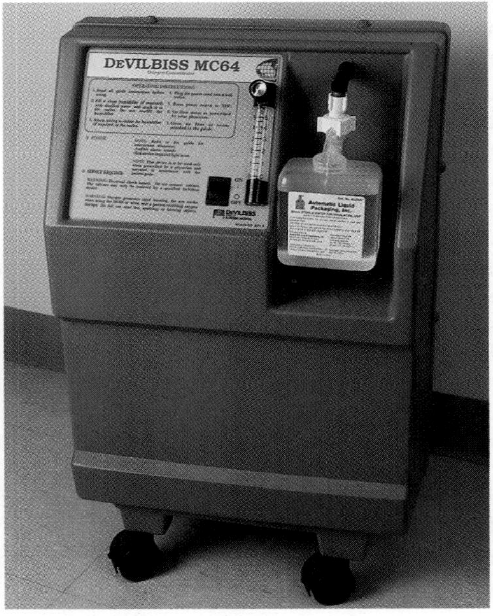

Figure 43-13 Oxygen concentrator.

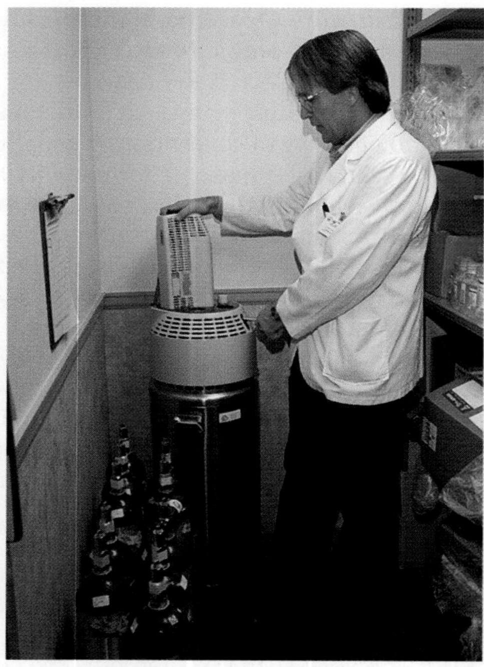

Figure 43-14 Liquid oxygen system.

while using oxygen. Or a family member might want to smoke while oxygen is running. These are very dangerous situations. Tell the person about the danger. Remind the person about safety hazards. Also call your supervisor and report the situation.

Oxygen Administration Devices

The physician orders the device used to administer oxygen. These devices are common:

- *Nasal cannula* (Figure 43-15)—plastic tubing with two prongs that project out from the tubing. The prongs are inserted into the nostrils. The prongs point downward. This prevents drying of the sinuses. An elastic headband or tubing brought behind the ears keeps the cannula in place. The client can eat and talk with a cannula in place. Nasal irritation occurs with tight prongs. Pressure on the ears and cheekbones is possible. Report signs or complaints of skin irritation or soreness.
- *Simple face mask* (Figure 43-16)—covers the nose and mouth. The mask has small holes in the sides. CO_2 escapes during exhalation. Room air enters during inhalation.

Box 43-4 Oxygen and Fire Safety Guidelines

- Place "No Smoking" signs in the room and on the room door.
- Remove smoking materials from the room (cigarettes, cigars, pipes, matches, lighters).
- Remove materials from the room that ignite easily (alcohol, nail polish remover, oils, petroleum jelly, greases).
- Keep oxygen source and tubing away from heat sources and open flames (e.g., direct sunlight, lit cigarettes, candles, lamps, stoves, heating ducts, radiators, heating pipes, space heaters, kerosene heaters).
- Turn off electrical items before unplugging them.
- Use electrical equipment that is in good repair (e.g., razor, radio, TV).
- Use only electrical equipment with three-prong plugs.
- Do not use materials that cause static electricity (wool and synthetic fabrics).
- Know the location of fire extinguishers and how to use them (see Chapter 16).
- If a fire occurs, turn off the oxygen. Then get the client to safety.
- Remind the client about oxygen safety. Report safety hazards immediately.

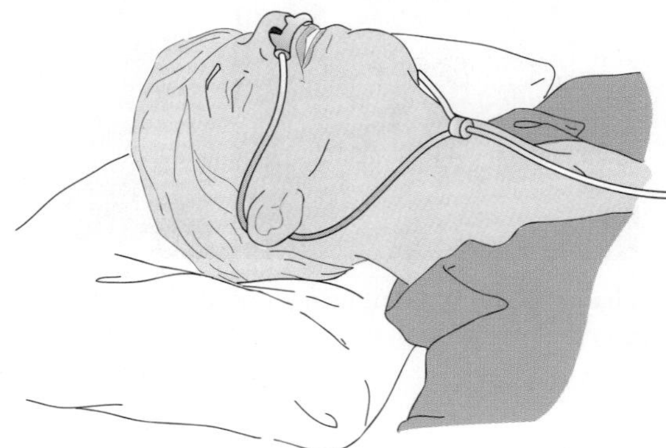

Figure 43-15 Nasal cannula.

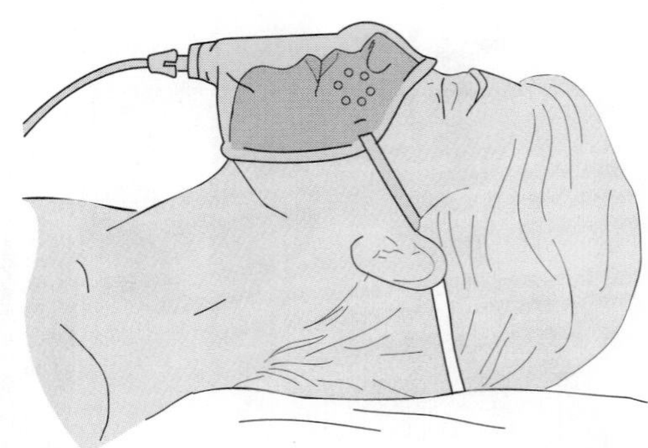

Figure 43-16 Simple face mask.

- *Partial-rebreather mask* (Figure 43-17)—a bag is added to the simple face mask. The bag is for exhaled air. When breathing in, the client inhales oxygen and some exhaled air. Some room air is also inhaled. The bag should not totally deflate during inhalation.
- *Nonrebreather mask* (Figure 43-18)—prevents exhaled air and room air from entering the bag. Exhaled air leaves through holes in the mask. Only oxygen from the bag is inhaled. The bag must not totally deflate during exhalation.
- *Venturi mask* (Figure 43-19)—allows precise amounts of oxygen to be given. Colour-coded adaptors show the amount of oxygen delivered.

Special care is needed when masks are used. Masks make talking difficult. Listen carefully to what the client is saying. Moisture can build up under masks. Keep the client's face clean and dry to help prevent irritation from the mask. Report any signs of skin irritation. Masks are removed for eating. Usually oxygen is administered by nasal cannula during meals.

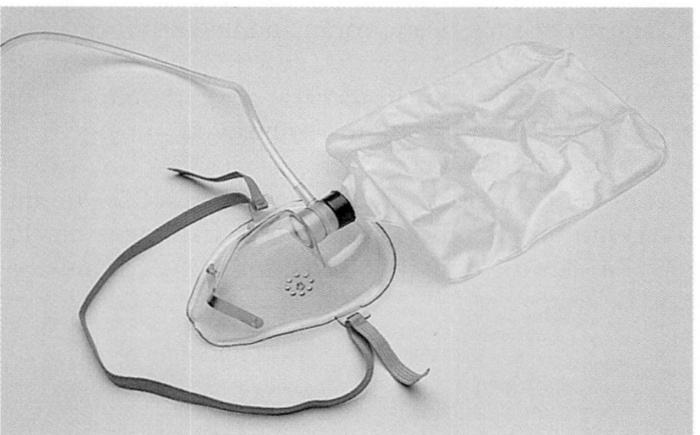

Figure 43-17 Partial-rebreather mask.

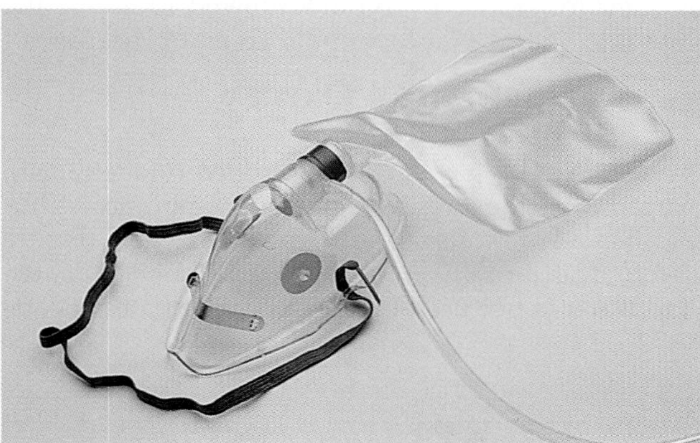

Figure 43-18 Nonrebreather mask.

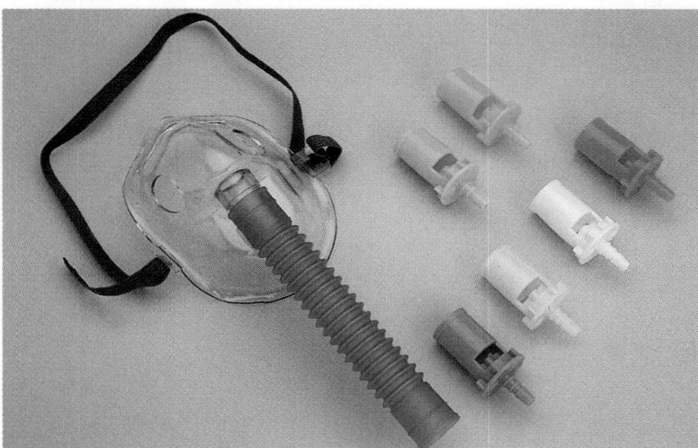

Figure 43-19 Venturi mask.

Oxygen Flow Rates

The amount of oxygen given is called the *flow rate*. This is ordered by the physician. The flow rate is measured in litres per minute (L/min). The flow rate is anywhere from 2 to 15 litres of oxygen per minute. A nurse or respiratory therapist sets the flow rate (Figure 43-20).

Your supervisor and the care plan tell you the client's flow rate. When giving care and checking clients, always check the flow rate. Tell your supervisor immediately if the flow rate is too high or too low. A nurse or respiratory therapist adjusts the flow rate. Some employers let support workers adjust oxygen flow rates. If you are allowed to adjust the flow rate, follow employer policies and procedures.

Preparing for Oxygen Administration

Oxygen is a dry gas. If not humidified (made moist), oxygen dries the airway's mucous membranes. A humidifier adds water vapour to the oxygen (Figure 43-21). The humidifier is filled with *distilled* water. (Tap water is not used because it can irritate mucous membranes and damage the equipment.) The humidifier is attached to the oxygen administration system (wall outlet, oxygen tank, oxygen concentrator). Oxygen picks up water vapour as it flows into the system. Bubbling in the humidifier means water vapour is being produced. Low flow rates (1 to 2 L/min) by nasal cannula usually do not need humidification. You may be responsible for checking the water level in the humidifier and cleaning and refilling it. Follow employer procedures and your supervisor's directions.

You do not administer oxygen, but your supervisor may ask you to set up the oxygen administration system. You are told the following:

- The client's name and room and bed number (in facilities)
- The oxygen administration device ordered
- Whether humidification was ordered

Tell your supervisor when you finish setting up the oxygen administration system. A nurse turns on the oxygen, sets the flow rate, and applies the administration device.

(text continues on page 728)

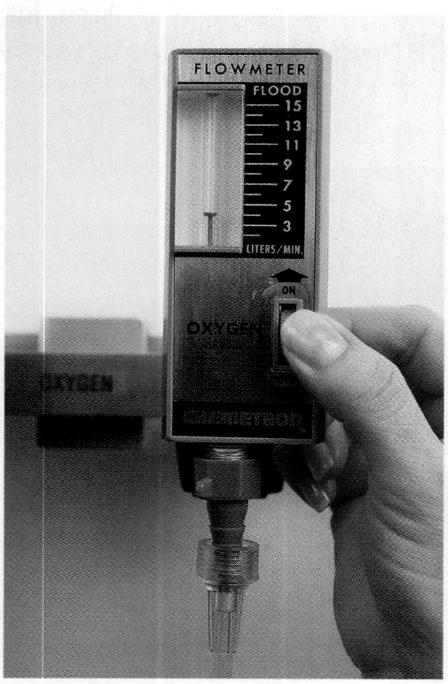

Figure 43-20 The flowmeter is used to set the oxygen flow rate.

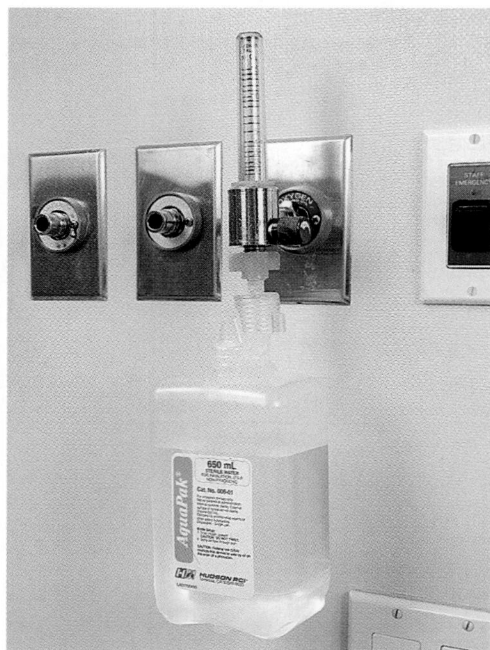

Figure 43-21 Oxygen administration system with humidifier.

Setting Up for Oxygen Administration

Compassionate Care

Remember to Promote:
- **Dignity**
- **Independence**
- **Preferences**
- **Privacy**
- **Safety**

Pre-Procedure

1. Identify the person according to employer policy.
2. Explain the procedure to the person.
3. Wash your hands.
4. Collect the following:
   - Oxygen administration device with connecting tubing
   - Flowmeter
   - Humidifier (if ordered)
   - Distilled water (if using a humidifier)

Procedure

5. Make sure the flowmeter is in the OFF position.
6. Attach the flowmeter to the wall outlet or to the tank.
7. Fill the humidifier with distilled water.
8. Attach the humidifier to the bottom of the flowmeter.
9. Attach the oxygen administration device and connecting tubing to the humidifier. *Do not set the flowmeter. Do not apply the oxygen administration device on the person.*

Post-Procedure

10. Provide for safety and comfort.
11. Place the call bell within reach.*
12. Discard packaging.
13. Make sure the cap on the distilled water bottle is secure. Store it according to employer policy.
14. Wash your hands.
15. Tell your supervisor when you are finished. A nurse will:
    - Turn on the oxygen and set the flow rate
    - Apply the oxygen administration device on the person

*Step marked with an asterisk may not apply in community settings.

Oxygen Therapy and Safety

Remember, you assist with oxygen therapy. You do not administer oxygen. However, you must give safe care to clients receiving oxygen. Follow the safety guidelines in Box 43-5. (Also follow the fire safety guidelines in Box 43-4 on page 724.)

Box 43-5 Safety Guidelines for Oxygen Therapy

- Never remove the device (cannula, mask) used to administer oxygen.
- Report to your supervisor if the client removes the device.
- Make sure the administration device is secure but not tight.
- Check for signs of irritation from the device. Check behind the ears, under the nose (cannula), and around the face (mask). Also check the cheekbones.
- Keep the face clean and dry when a mask is used.
- Never shut off oxygen flow.
- Do not adjust the flow rate unless allowed by law and your employer.
- Tell your supervisor immediately if the flow rate is too high or too low.
- Tell your supervisor immediately if the humidifier is not bubbling.
- Secure connecting tubing in place. Tape or pin it to the client's garment following employer policy.
- Make sure there are no kinks in the tubing.
- Make sure the client does not lie on any part of the tubing.
- Report signs and symptoms of hypoxia, respiratory distress, or abnormal breathing patterns to your supervisor immediately (see Boxes 43-1 on page 713 and 43-2 on page 714).
- Give oral hygiene as directed. Follow the care plan.
- Make sure the device is clean and free of mucus.
- Maintain an adequate water level in the humidifier.

Artifical Airways

Artificial airways keep the airway patent (open). They are used when:

- The airway is obstructed from disease, injury, secretions, or aspiration
- The client is semiconscious or unconscious
- The client is recovering from anesthesia
- The client needs mechanical ventilation

Intubation is the process of inserting an artificial airway. Airways are usually plastic and disposable. They come in adult, pediatric, and infant sizes. The following airways are common:

- *Oropharyngeal airway*—inserted through the mouth and into the pharynx (Figure 43-22, *A*). A nurse or respiratory therapist inserts the airway.
- *Nasopharyngeal airway*—inserted through a nostril and into the pharynx (Figure 43-22, *B*). A nurse or respiratory therapist inserts the airway.
- *Endotracheal (ET) tube*—inserted through the mouth or nose and into the trachea (Figure 43-22, *C*). A physician or RN with special training inserts it using a lighted scope. A balloon (called a *cuff*) at the end of the tube is inflated to keep the airway in place.
- *Tracheostomy tube*—inserted through a surgical incision (*ostomy*) into the trachea (*tracheo*) (Figure 43-22, *D*). Some have cuffs. The cuff is inflated to keep the tube in place. The tracheostomy is done by a physician.

You assist in caring for clients with artificial airways. The client's vital signs are checked often. The client is observed for hypoxia and other respiratory signs and symptoms. If an airway comes out or is dislodged, tell your supervisor immediately. The client needs frequent oral hygiene. Your supervisor and the care plan tell you when and how to perform oral hygiene.

Talking is hard with oropharyngeal and nasopharyngeal airways. People with endotracheal tubes cannot speak. Some tracheostomy tubes allow the person to speak. Paper and pencils, magic slates, communication boards, and hand signals are ways to communicate. Follow the care plan.

Gagging and choking sensations are common with artificial airways. Imagine something in your mouth, nose, or throat. Comfort and reassure the client. Remind the person that the airway helps breathing. Use touch to show you care.

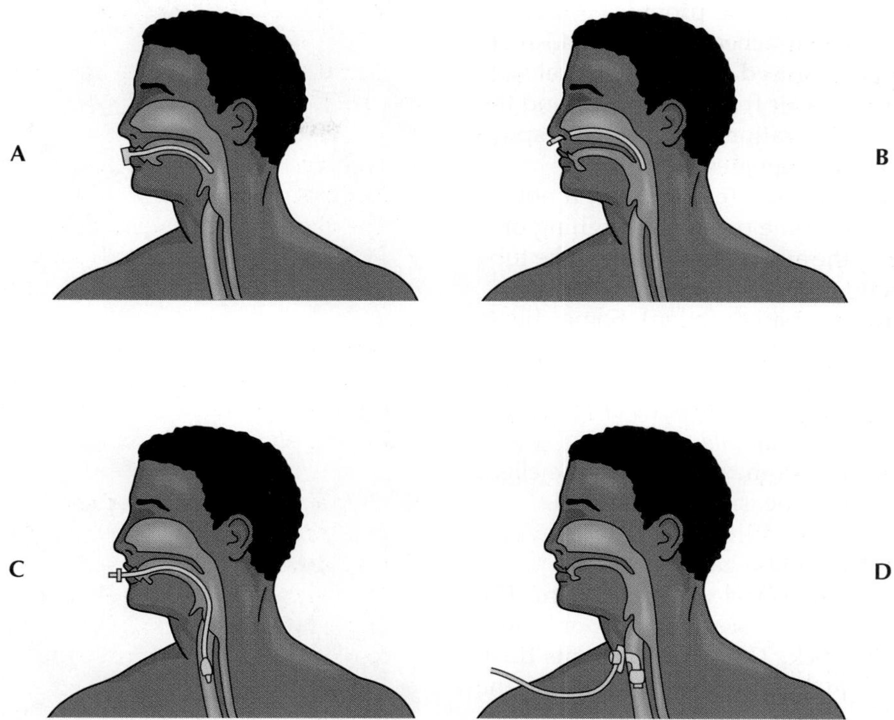

Figure 43-22 Artificial airways. **A,** Oropharyngeal airway. **B,** Nasopharyngeal airway. **C,** Endotracheal tube. **D,** Tracheostomy tube.

Tracheostomies

A **tracheostomy** is a surgically-created opening (*ostomy*) through the neck into the trachea (*tracheo*). A tracheostomy tube is usually inserted through this opening. The person breathes through the tracheostomy tube.

Tracheostomies are temporary when they are for mechanical ventilation (see page 732). They are permanent when airway structures are surgically removed. Cancer, severe airway trauma, or brain injury may require a permanent tracheostomy. (See *Focus on Children: Congenital Conditions* box.)

A tracheostomy tube is made of plastic or metal. It has three parts (Figure 43-23):

- The *obturator* has a round end. It is used to insert the outer cannula. Then it is removed. (The obturator is placed within easy reach in case the tracheostomy tube falls out and needs to be reinserted. It is taped to the wall or bedside stand.)
- The *inner cannula* is inserted and locked in place. It is removed for cleaning and mucus removal. This keeps the airway patent. Some plastic tracheostomy tubes do not have inner cannulas.
- The *outer cannula* is secured in place with ties around the neck or a Velcro collar. The outer cannula is not removed.

Focus on Children

Congenital Conditions

Some children are born with congenital conditions. (*Congenitus* is a Latin word that means born with.) Therefore congenital conditions are present at birth. Tracheostomies are needed for some congenital conditions affecting the neck and airway. Some infections cause airway structures to swell. This obstructs airflow. Foreign body aspiration also obstructs airflow. These situations can require emergency tracheostomies.

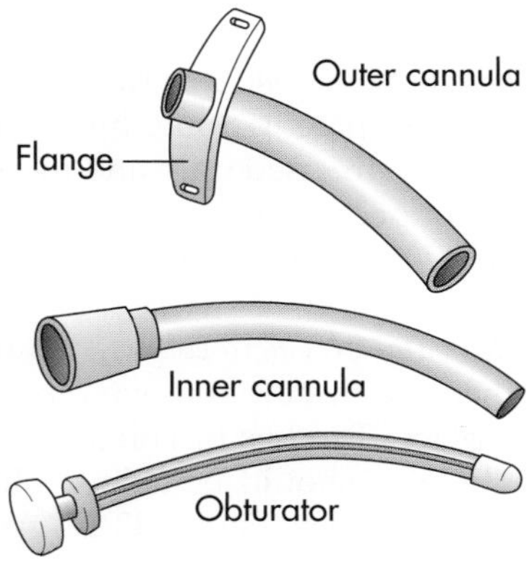

Figure 43-23 Parts of a tracheostomy tube.

The cuffed tracheostomy tube provides a seal between the cannula and the trachea (see Figure 43-22, *D* on page 729). This type is used with mechanical ventilation. The cuff prevents air from leaking around the tube. It also prevents aspiration. A nurse or respiratory therapist inflates and deflates the cuff.

The tube must not come out (extubation). If not secured properly, it could come out with coughing or if pulled on. Damage to the airway is possible if the tube is loose and moves up and down in the trachea.

The tube must remain patent (open). Some clients can cough secretions up and out of the tracheostomy. Others require suctioning. *Call your supervisor if the client shows signs and symptoms of hypoxia or respiratory distress. Also call if the outer cannula comes out.*

Nothing can enter the stoma. Otherwise the client can aspirate. These safety measures are needed:

- Dressings do not have loose gauze or lint.
- The stoma or tube is covered when outdoors. The client wears a stoma cover, scarf, or shirt or blouse that buttons at the neck. The cover prevents dust, insects, and other small particles from entering the stoma.
- The stoma is not covered with plastic, leather, or similar materials. They prevent air from entering the stoma. The client cannot breathe.
- Tub baths are taken, not showers. If showers are taken, a shower guard is worn. A hand-held nozzle is used to direct water away from the stoma.
- The client is helped with shampooing. Water must not enter the stoma.
- The stoma is covered when shaving.
- Swimming is not allowed. Water will enter the tube or stoma.
- Medical alert jewellery is worn. The client also carries a medical alert ID card.

Tracheostomy Care. Follow Standard Precautions when assisting with tracheostomy care. Such care is done every 8 to 12 hours. It is done when there are excess secretions, the ties or collar are soiled, or the dressing is soiled or moist. It involves:

- *Cleaning the inner cannula*. This removes mucus and keeps the airway patent. Some inner cannulas are disposable. They are used once and then discarded. Cleaning is not necessary.
- *Cleaning the stoma*. This prevents infection and skin breakdown.
- *Applying clean ties or Velcro collar*. This prevents infection. When the ties are removed, hold the outer cannula in place. The ties or collar must be secure but not tight. You should be able to slide a finger under the ties or collar (Figure 43-24, *A*). (See *Focus on Children: Tracheostomy Care* box.)

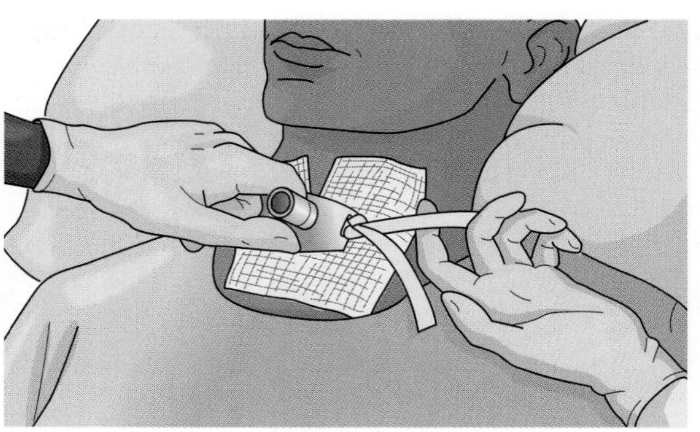
A

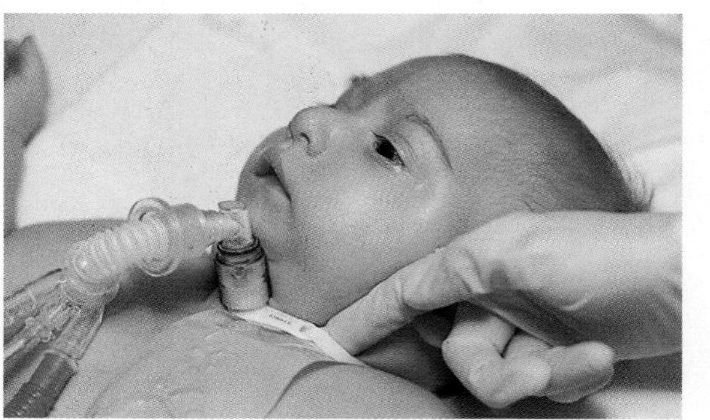
B

Figure 43-24 A, A finger is inserted under the ties. **B,** For children, only a fingertip is inserted under the ties. Source for *B*: D.L. Wong, *Whaley & Wong's Nursing Care of Infants and Children*, 6th ed. (St. Louis: Mosby, 1999).

Suctioning the Airway

Injury and illness often causes secretions to collect in the upper airway. Secretions can cause these problems:

- They obstruct air flow in and out of the airway.
- They provide an environment for microbes.
- They interfere with O_2 and CO_2 exchange.

Hypoxia can occur. Usually coughing removes secretions. Some clients cannot cough, or the cough is too weak to remove secretions. Some clients cannot

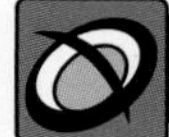
Focus on Children

Tracheostomy Care

As with adults, the ties must be secure but not tight. Only a fingertip should be able to slide under the ties (Figure 43-24, *B*). Ties are too loose if you can slide your whole finger under them.

When assisting with tracheostomy care, you must hold the child still. Position the child's head so that the neck is slightly extended.

expectorate or swallow secretions after coughing. These clients need suctioning to remove secretions.

Suction is the process of withdrawing or sucking up fluid (secretions). A tube connects to a suction source (wall outlet or suction machine) at one end and to a suction catheter at the other end. The catheter is inserted into the airway. Secretions are withdrawn through the catheter.

Suctioning Routes

The upper airway and the lower airway are suctioned. The nose, mouth, and pharynx make up the upper airway. The trachea and bronchi make up the lower airway.

- *Oropharyngeal* route—the mouth (*oro*) and pharynx (*pharyngeal*) are suctioned. A suction catheter is passed through the mouth and into the pharynx.
- *Nasopharyngeal* route—the nose (*naso*) and pharynx (*pharyngeal*) are suctioned. The suction catheter is passed through the nose and into the pharynx.
- *Lower airway* suctioning—is done through an ET (endotracheal) tube or through a tracheostomy tube.

Safety Measures

If not done correctly, suctioning can cause serious harm to the client. Suctioning removes oxygen from the airway. Therefore the client cannot breathe during suctioning. Hypoxia and life-threatening complications can arise. The respiratory, cardiovascular, and nervous systems can be affected. Cardiac arrest can occur. Infection and airway injury are possible.

The client's lungs are hyperventilated before suctioning from an ET tube or tracheostomy. *Hyperventilate* means to give extra (*hyper*) breaths (*ventilate*). An Ambu bag is used (Figure 43-25). The Ambu bag is attached to an oxygen source. Then the oxygen delivery device is removed from the ET or tracheostomy tube. The Ambu bag is attached to the ET or tracheostomy tube. To give a breath, the bag is squeezed with both hands. A nurse or respiratory therapist gives 3 to 5 breaths.

Remember, oxygen is considered a medication. You do not administer medications. Therefore you need to check if your province or territory and employer allow you to use an Ambu bag attached to an oxygen source.

Some employers limit suctioning to 10 seconds. Others allow 10 to 15 seconds for the suction cycle:

- Insert the catheter
- Apply suction
- Remove the catheter

For infants and children, suction is applied for no longer than 5 seconds.

You might be asked to assist a nurse with suctioning. You need to understand the principles and safety measures involved in safe suctioning (Box 43-6).

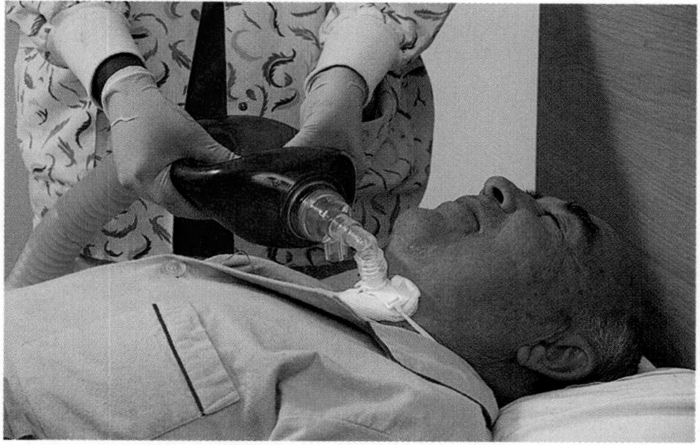

Figure 43-25 The Ambu bag. A nurse compresses it with two hands.

Box 43-6 Principles and Safety Measures for Suctioning

- Review the procedure with your supervisor (a nurse). Know what is expected of you.
- Suctioning is done as needed (*prn*). Coughing and signs and symptoms of respiratory distress signal the need for suctioning. Your supervisor tells you what signs to look for.
- Standard Precautions are followed. Secretions can contain blood and are potentially infectious.
- Sterile technique is used (see Chapter 18).
- Your supervisor tells you the size and type of catheter to collect (Figure 43-26 on page 732). Airway injury can occur if the catheter is too large.
- Needed suction equipment and supplies are kept at the bedside so that they are ready when the client needs suctioning.
- Suction is not applied while inserting the catheter. When suction is applied, air is sucked out of the airway.
- The catheter is cleared with water or saline after removal.
- The catheter is inserted smoothly. This helps prevent injury to the mucous membranes.
- The suction catheter is passed (inserted) no more than 3 times. The risk of injury increases each time the catheter is passed.
- Check the client's pulse, respirations, and pulse oximeter before, during, and after the procedure. Also observe the level of consciousness. Tell your supervisor immediately if any of the following occur:
  - A drop in pulse rate or a pulse rate less than 60 beats per minute
  - Irregular cardiac rhythms
  - A drop or rise in blood pressure
  - Respiratory distress
  - A drop in the SpO_2 (see page 715)

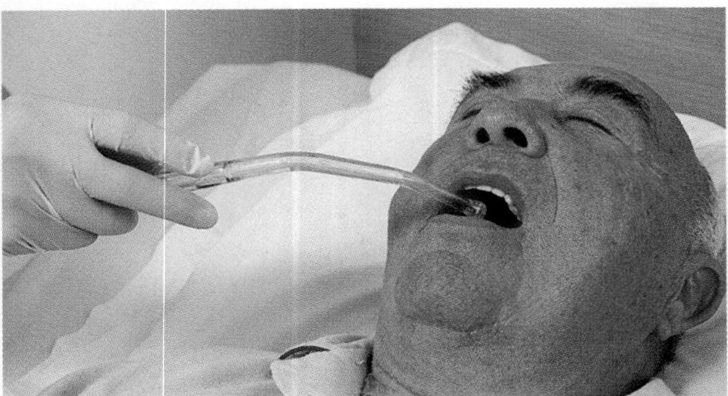

Figure 43-26 The Yankauer suction catheter is often used when there are large amounts of thick secretions.

Mechanical Ventilation

Weak muscle effort, airway obstruction, and damaged lung tissue cause hypoxia. Nervous system diseases and injuries can affect the respiratory centre in the brain. Nerve damage interferes with messages between the lungs and the brain. Drug overdose depresses the brain. With severe problems, the person cannot breathe. Or normal blood oxygen levels are not maintained. Often mechanical ventilation is needed. **Mechanical ventilation** is the use of a machine to move air into and out of the lungs (Figure 43-27). Oxygen enters the lungs and carbon dioxide leaves them.

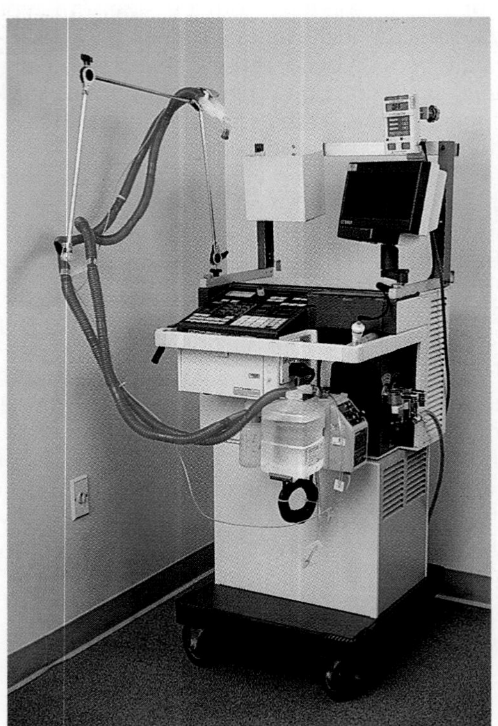

Figure 43-27 A mechanical ventilator.

Mechanical ventilation is started in hospital. Some people need it for a few hours or days. Others need it longer. An ET tube or tracheostomy tube is used.

Ventilators have alarms that sound when something is wrong. One alarm sounds when the person gets disconnected from the ventilator. Your supervisor (in this case, a nurse) shows you how to connect the ET or tracheostomy tube to the ventilator. When any alarm sounds, *first check to see if the client's tube is attached to the ventilator. If not, attach it to the ventilator. The client can die if not connected to the ventilator.* Then tell your supervisor at once about the alarm. Do not reset alarms.

People needing mechanical ventilation are very ill. Other problems and injuries are common. Some are confused, disoriented, or cannot think clearly. Many are frightened by the machine and by thoughts of dying. Some feel relieved to get enough oxygen. Many fear needing the machine for life. Mechanical ventilation can be painful for those with chest injuries or chest surgery. Tubes and hoses restrict movement. This causes more discomfort.

You may be asked to assist with the client's care. Follow the guidelines in Box 43-7.

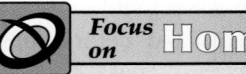

Weaning from the ventilator is often needed. That is, the client gradually needs to breathe without the ventilator. Weaning can take many weeks. A physician, respiratory therapist, and nurse plan the weaning process. (See *Focus on Home Care: Mechanical Ventilation* box.)

Focus on Home Care

Mechanical Ventilation

Home care is often arranged for clients receiving mechanical ventilation. Portable ventilators are used in home care. The RN teaches you how to care for each client. Family members are taught how to assist with the client's care. Always make sure that an RN is available by phone when you are in the client's home.

Box 43-7 Guidelines for Caring for Clients Receiving Mechanical Ventilation

- Keep the call bell within reach (in facilities).
- Make sure hoses and connecting tubing have slack. They must not pull on the artificial airway.
- Answer call bells promptly. The person depends on others for basic needs.
- Explain who you are and what you are going to do. Do this whenever you enter the room.
- Give the day, date, and time every time you give care.
- Report signs of respiratory distress or discomfort at once.
- Do not change settings on the machine or reset alarms.
- Follow the care plan for communication. The person cannot talk. Use agreed-upon hand or eye signals for "yes" and "no." All health care team members must use the same signals. Otherwise, communication does not occur. Some clients can use paper and pencils, magic slates, communication boards, and hand signals. Follow the care plan.
- Ask questions that have simple answers. It may be hard to write long responses.
- Watch what you say and do. This includes when you are near and away from the person or family. They pay close attention to your verbal and nonverbal communication. Do not say anything that could upset them.
- Comfort and reassure the person. Also talk about the weather, pleasant news events, gifts, and cards.
- Meet basic needs. Follow the care plan.
- Use touch to reassure and comfort the person.
- Tell the person when you are leaving the room and when you will return.

Chest Tubes

Air, blood, or fluid can collect in the pleural space (sac or cavity). This occurs when the chest is entered because of injury or surgery:

- *Pneumothorax* is air (*pneumo*) in the pleural space (*thorax*).
- *Hemothorax* is blood (*hemo*) in the pleural space (*thorax*).
- *Pleural effusion* is the escape and collection of fluid (*effusion*) in the pleural space (*pleural*).

Pressure occurs when air, blood, or fluid collects in the pleural sac. The pressure makes the lungs collapse. Air does not reach affected alveoli. O_2 and CO_2 are not exchanged. Respiratory distress and hypoxia may result. Sometimes there is pressure on the heart. This affects the heart's ability to pump blood and is a life-threatening situation.

Hospital care is required. A physician inserts chest tubes to remove the air, fluid, or blood (Figure 43-28). When stable, the client may need rehabilitation or subacute care.

Chest tubes attach to a drainage system (Figure 43-29). The system must be airtight. Air must not enter the pleural space. Water-seal drainage keeps the system airtight (Figure 43-30 on page 734). This is done as follows:

- A chest tube attaches to connecting tubing.
- Connecting tubing attaches to a tube in the drainage container.
- The tube in the drainage container extends under water. The water prevents air from entering the chest tube and then the pleural space.

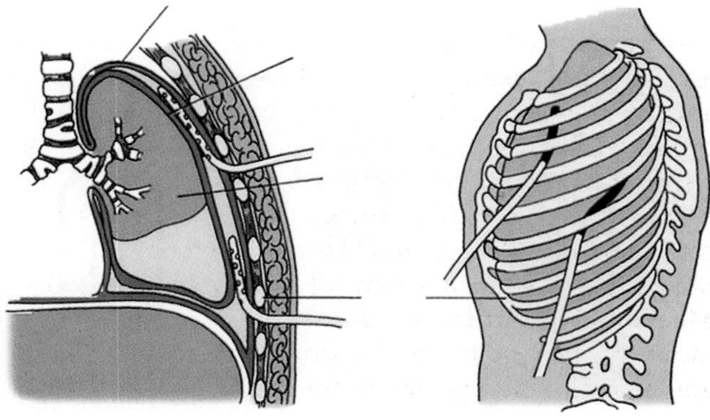

Figure 43-28 Chest tubes inserted into the pleural space. Source: M.K. Elkin, A.G. Perry, and P.A. Potter, *Nursing Interventions and Clinical Skills*, 2nd ed. (St. Louis: Mosby, 2000).

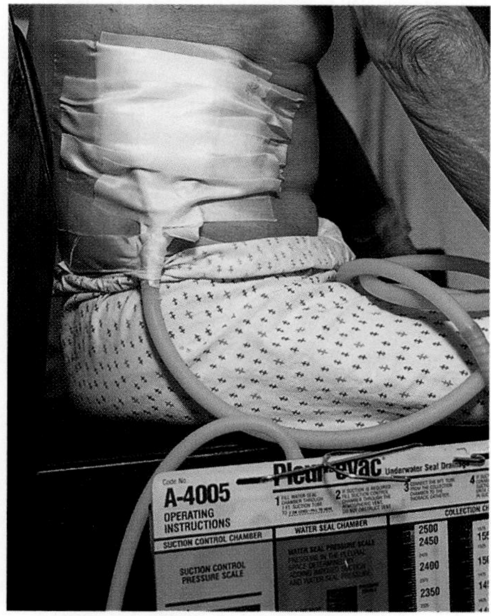

Figure 43-29 Chest tubes attached to a disposable water-seal drainage system. Source: M.K. Elkin, A.G. Perry, and P.A. Potter, *Nursing Interventions and Clinical Skills*, 2nd ed. (St. Louis: Mosby, 2000).

A 1-, 2-, or 3-bottle system can be used. Disposable systems are common (see Figure 43-29 on page 733). The bottles in Figure 43-30 show how the system works. Sometimes suction is applied to the drainage system. You might assist a nurse with the client's care. Follow the guidelines in Box 43-8.

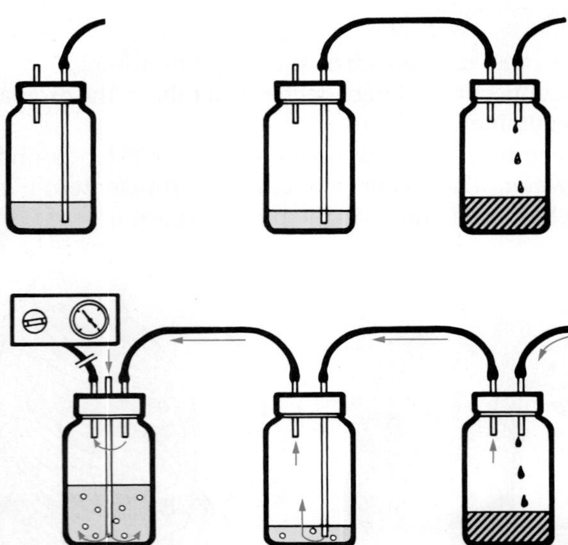

Figure 43-30 Water-seal drainage system. Source: M.K. Elkin, A.G. Perry, and P.A. Potter, *Nursing Interventions and Clinical Skills,* 2nd ed. (St. Louis: Mosby, 2000).

Box 43-8 Guidelines for Caring for Clients with Chest Tubes

- Keep the drainage system below the level of the person's chest.
- Check vital signs as directed. Report vital sign changes at once.
- Report signs and symptoms of hypoxia and respiratory distress at once. Also, report complaints of pain or difficulty breathing.
- Keep connecting tubing coiled on the bed. Allow enough slack so the chest tubes are not dislodged when the person moves. If tubing hangs in loops, drainage collects in the loop.
- Prevent tubing kinks. Kinks obstruct the chest tube. Air, blood, or fluid collects in the pleural space.
- Observe chest drainage. Report any change in chest drainage at once. This includes increases in drainage or the appearance of bright red drainage.
- Record chest drainage according to employer policy.
- Turn and position the person as directed. Be careful and gentle to prevent chest tubes from dislodging.
- Assist with coughing and deep breathing as directed.
- Assist with incentive spirometry as directed.
- Note bubbling in the drainage system. Tell your supervisor at once if bubbling increases, decreases, or stops.
- Tell your supervisor at once if any part of the system is loose or disconnected.
- Keep sterile petrolatum gauze at the bedside. It is needed if a chest tube comes out.
- Call for help at once if a chest tube comes out. Cover the insertion site with sterile petrolatum gauze. Stay with the person. Then follow the nurse's directions.

REVIEW

Circle the BEST answer.

1. Alcohol and narcotics affect oxygen needs because they
A. Depress the brain
B. Are pollutants
C. Cause allergies
D. Cause a pneumothorax

2. Hypoxia is
A. Not enough oxygen in the blood
B. The amount of hemoglobin that contains oxygen
C. Not enough oxygen in the cells
D. The lack of oxygen

3. An early sign of hypoxia is
A. Cyanosis
B. Increased pulse and respiratory rates
C. Restlessness
D. Dyspnea

4. A person can breathe deeply and comfortably only while sitting. This is called
A. Biot's respirations
B. Orthopnea
C. Bradypnea
D. Kussmaul's respirations

5. Which of the following is *not* a sign of altered respiratory function?
A. Wheezing or crowing sounds
B. Dry and hacking cough
C. Changes in vital signs
D. Joint pain

6. A client's SpO_2 is 98%. Which is *true*?
A. The pulse oximeter is wrong.
B. The client's pulse is 98 beats per minute.
C. The measurement is within normal range.
D. The client needs suctioning.

7. Which is *not* a site for a pulse oximetry sensor?
A. Toe
B. Finger
C. Ear lobe
D. Upper arm

8. The best time to collect sputum is
A. On awakening
B. After meals
C. At bedtime
D. After suctioning

9. A sputum specimen is needed. You should ask the client to
A. Use mouthwash
B. Rinse the mouth with clear water
C. Brush the teeth
D. Apply lubricant to the lips

10. You are assisting a client with coughing and deep breathing. Which is *false*?
A. The client inhales through pursed lips.
B. The client needs to be in a comfortable sitting position.
C. The client inhales deeply through the nose.
D. The client holds a pillow over an incision.

11. Which is useful for deep breathing?
A. Pulse oximeter
B. Incentive spirometry
C. Chest tubes
D. Partial-rebreather mask

12. You are assisting with oxygen therapy. You can
A. Turn the oxygen on and off
B. Start the oxygen
C. Decide what device to use
D. Keep the connecting tubing secure and free of kinks

13. A client has a tracheostomy. Which is *false*?
A. The inner cannula is removed for cleaning.
B. The obturator is inserted after the outer cannula.
C. The outer cannula must be secured in place.
D. The client must be protected from aspiration.

14. A client has a tracheostomy. He or she can do the following *except*
A. Shampoo
B. Shave
C. Shower with a hand-held nozzle
D. Swim

REVIEW

15. A client has a tracheostomy. For the client's safety, the old ties are removed after
    A. The inner cannula is removed
    B. The stoma is cleaned
    C. The dressing is removed
    D. The outer cannula is held in place

16. These statements are about suctioning. Which is *true*?
    A. Suction is applied while inserting the catheter.
    B. Suctioning is done every 2 hours.
    C. A suction cycle is no more than 10 to 15 seconds.
    D. You can perform the procedure.

17. Suctioning requires
    A. Chest tubes
    B. Sterile technique
    C. An artificial airway
    D. Mechanical ventilation

18. Which is used to hyperventilate the lungs?
    A. Incentive spirometer
    B. Pulse oximeter
    C. Ambu bag
    D. Partial-rebreather mask

19. Mr. Long requires mechanical ventilation. Which is *false*?
    A. He has an ET tube or a tracheostomy tube.
    B. His call bell must be within his reach.
    C. Touch provides comfort and reassurance.
    D. You can reset alarms on the ventilator.

20. An alarm sounds on Mr. Long's ventilator. What should you do first?
    A. Reset the alarm.
    B. Check to see if his airway is attached to the ventilator.
    C. Call your supervisor immediately.
    D. Ask him what is wrong.

21. A person has a pneumothorax. This is the collection of
    A. Fluid in the pleural space
    B. Blood in the pleural space
    C. Air in the pleural space
    D. Respiratory secretions in the pleural space

22. Chest tubes are attached to water-seal drainage. You should do the following *except*
    A. Tell your supervisor if the bubbling increases, decreases, or stops
    B. Make sure the tubing is not kinked
    C. Keep the drainage system below the client's chest
    D. Hang the tubing in loops

Answers to these questions are on page 827.

CHAPTER

44

ASSISTING WITH THE PHYSICAL EXAMINATION

OBJECTIVES

- Define the key terms listed in this chapter
- Explain what to do before, during, and after a physical examination
- Identify the equipment used during a physical examination
- Describe how to prepare a client for an examination
- Describe four examination positions and how to drape the client for each position
- Explain guidelines for assisting with a physical examination
- Learn the procedure described in this chapter

KEY TERMS

dorsal recumbent position Supine position

horizontal position Supine position

knee-chest position An examination position in which the person kneels and rests the body on the knees and chest; the head is turned to one side, the arms are above the head or flexed at the elbows, the back is straight, and the body is flexed about 90 degrees at the hips

laryngeal mirror An instrument used to examine the mouth, teeth, and throat

lithotomy position A back-lying position in which the hips are brought down to the edge of the examination table, the knees are flexed, the hips are externally rotated, and the feet are supported in stirrups

nasal speculum An instrument used to examine the inside of the nose

ophthalmoscope A lighted instrument used to examine the internal structures of the eye

otoscope A lighted instrument used to examine the external ear and the eardrum (tympanic membrane)

percussion hammer An instrument used to tap body parts to test reflexes; reflex hammer

reflex hammer Percussion hammer

Sims' position A left side-lying position; the right leg is sharply flexed so it is not on the left leg, and the left arm is positioned along the person's back

supine position A back-lying position; the legs are together; dorsal recumbent position; horizontal position

tuning fork An instrument used to test hearing

vaginal speculum An instrument used to open the vagina so that it and the cervix can be examined

Physicians and many RNs perform physical examinations (exams). They are done for many reasons. Routine health examinations are done to promote health. Pre-employment physicals are done to determine fitness for work. Physical examinations are also used to diagnose and treat disease. Some long-term care facilities require new residents to have a physical exam when they arrive. Others require residents to have physical exams at least once a year. If you work in a facility, you may be asked to assist a physician or RN with a physical exam. In the community, assisting with physical exams is unlikely to be in your job description.

YOUR RESPONSIBILITIES

Your responsibilities depend on your employer's policies and procedures. The examiner's preferences also affect what you are expected to do. You may do some or all of the following:

- Collect linens for draping the client and for the procedure
- Collect examination equipment
- Prepare the room for the examination
- Transport the client to and from the exam room
- Provide lighting
- Measure vital signs, height, and weight
- Position and drape the client
- Hand equipment and instruments to the examiner
- Stay with the client before or during the exam to provide emotional support and to prevent falls
- Label specimen containers
- Dispose of soiled linen and discard supplies
- Clean equipment
- Help the client dress or assume a comfortable position after the examination

EQUIPMENT

Instruments needed for a physical examination include, but are not limited to, the following (Figure 44-1):

- *Ophthalmoscope*—a lighted instrument used to examine the internal structures of the eye.
- *Otoscope*—a lighted instrument used to examine the external ear and the eardrum (tympanic membrane). Some scopes have parts for examining eyes and ears. They are changed into an ophthalmoscope or otoscope.
- *Percussion hammer*—used to tap body parts to test reflexes. It is also called a **reflex hammer**.

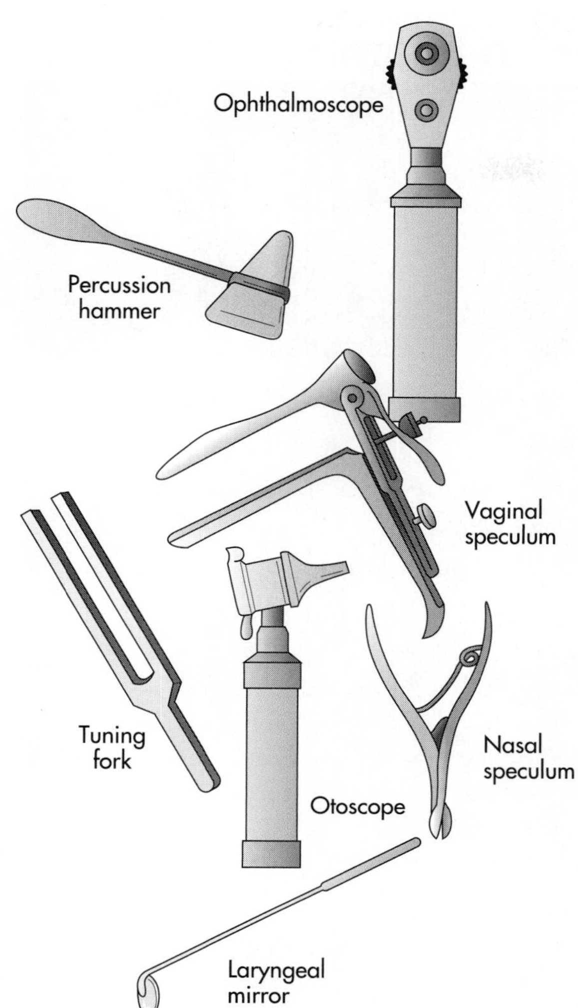

Figure 44-1 Some of the many instruments used for a physical examination.

- ***Vaginal speculum***—used to open the vagina so it and the cervix can be examined.
- ***Nasal speculum***—used to examine the inside of the nose.
- ***Tuning fork***—an instrument used to test hearing.
- ***Laryngeal mirror***—used to examine the mouth, teeth, and throat.

Many facilities have examination trays in the supply department. If not, collect the items listed in *Preparing the Person for an Examination* (page 740). Arrange them on a tray or table for the examiner.

Preparing the Client

Many people worry about having a physical examination. They may worry about possible findings. Or they are confused or fearful about what the examiner will do. Feeling discomfort and embarrassment, fearing exposure, and not knowing the procedure also may cause anxiety. You need to be sensitive to the client's feelings and concerns. The client is prepared physically and psychologically for the examination.

The client has the right to know who will do the exam, why it is done, and what to expect. The physician or nurse explains these things to the client. If a client asks you questions about an examination, tell the client you will ask your supervisor to speak to him or her.

The client has the right to personal choice. The physician or nurse must inform the client about the exam. Reasons for it are given. The client is told who will do the exam and when it will be done. The procedure is explained. The exam is done only if the client gives consent. The client may want a different examiner. Or the client may want a family member present. Some people want the exam results explained with a family member present.

The right to privacy also is protected. The person is screened and the room door closed. All clothes are removed for a complete examination. Usually a hospital gown is worn. It reduces the feeling of nakedness and the fear of exposure. The client is covered with a paper drape, bath blanket, sheet, or drawsheet. Explain that only the body part being examined is exposed. Little exposure occurs. (See *Focus on Children: Promoting Privacy* box.)

The client voids before the examination. An empty bladder lets the examiner feel the abdominal organs. A full bladder can change the normal position and shape of organs. It can also cause discomfort, especially when the abdominal organs are felt. If a urine specimen is needed, obtain it at this time. Explain how to collect the specimen (see Chapter 29). Label the container.

Warmth is a major concern during the examination. The client is protected from chilling, especially if ill, an older adult, or a child. An extra bath blanket should be nearby. Also try to prevent drafts.

The examiner may want height, weight, and vital signs measured. These are obtained before the examination starts. They are recorded on the examination form. The client is then positioned and draped for the examination. Protect the client from falls and injury. Do not leave the client unattended.

(text continues on page 741)

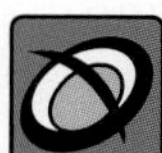
***Focus on* Children**

Promoting Privacy

Toddlers, preschool children, and school-age children are allowed to wear underpants during the examination. The underpants are lowered or removed as necessary during the procedure.

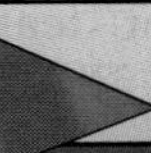

Preparing the Person for an Examination

COMPASSIONATE CARE

Remember to Promote:
- **Dignity**
- **Independence**
- **Preferences**
- **Privacy**
- **Safety**

Pre-Procedure

1 Identify the person according to employer policy.
2 Explain the procedure to the person.
3 Wash your hands.
4 Collect instruments and supplies as requested by the examiner. These may include some or all of the following:
- Flashlight
- Blood pressure cuff
- Stethoscope
- Thermometer
- Tongue depressors (blades)
- Laryngeal mirror
- Ophthalmoscope
- Otoscope
- Nasal speculum
- Percussion (reflex) hammer
- Tuning fork
- Tape measure
- Gloves
- Water-soluble lubricant
- Vaginal speculum
- Cotton-tipped applicators
- Specimen containers and labels
- Disposable bag
- Kidney basin
- Towel
- Bath blanket
- Tissues
- Drape (sheet, bath blanket, drawsheet, or disposable drape)
- Paper towels
- Cotton balls
- Waterproof bed protector
- Eye chart (Snellen chart)
- Slides
- Gown
- Alcohol wipes
- Wastebasket
- Container for soiled instruments
- Marking pencils or pens

5 Provide for privacy.

Procedure

6 Ask the person to put on the gown. Instruct him or her to remove all clothes. Assist as necessary.
7 Ask the person to void. Offer the bedpan, commode, or urinal if necessary. Provide for privacy.
8 Transport the person to the exam room.
9 Weigh and measure the person (see Chapter 40).
10 Help the person get on the examination table. Provide a footstool if necessary. (Omit this step if the exam is done in the person's room.)
11 Raise the bed to its highest level. Raise the far bed rail if used. (This step is done for an exam in the person's room.)
12 Position the person as directed.
13 Drape the person.
14 Place a bed protector under the buttocks.
15 Raise the bed rail near you if used.
16 Provide adequate lighting.
17 Press the call bell for the RN or examiner. Do not leave the person unattended.

Positioning and Draping

Sometimes a special position is needed for the exam. Some examination positions are uncomfortable and embarrassing. The examiner tells you how to position the client. Before helping the client assume and maintain the position, explain the following:

- Why the position is needed
- How to assume the position
- How the body is draped for warmth and privacy
- How long the person can expect to stay in the position

The **supine position** (also called the **dorsal recumbent** or **horizontal position**) is used to examine the abdomen, anterior chest, and breasts. The client lies flat on his or her back with the legs together. If the perineal area is to be examined, the knees are flexed and hips externally rotated (Figure 44-2, *A*). The drape is extended over the client's body, covering from the shoulders to the feet.

The **lithotomy position** (Figure 44-2, *B*) is used to examine the vagina. The client lies on her back, and her hips are brought to the edge of the examination table. The knees are flexed and the hips externally rotated. The feet are supported in stirrups. The client is draped as for perineal care (see Figure 27-26 on page 429). Some employers provide socks to cover the feet and calves. Some women cannot assume this position. In this case, the examiner tells you how to position the client.

The **knee-chest position** (Figure 44-2, *C*) is used to examine the rectum. Sometimes it is used to examine the vagina. The client kneels and rests the body on the knees and chest. The head is turned to one side. The arms are above the head or flexed at the elbows. The back is straight. The body is flexed about 90 degrees at the hips. The client wears a gown and sometimes socks. The drape is applied in a diamond shape to cover the back, buttocks, and thighs. This position is rarely used for older adults. They usually assume the side-lying position for rectal exams.

The **Sims' position** (Figure 44-2, *D*) is sometimes used to examine the rectum or vagina. The client lies on the left side. The right leg is sharply flexed so it is not on the left leg. The left arm is positioned along the client's back. The drape is applied in a diamond shape. The corner near the examiner is folded back to expose the rectum or vagina.

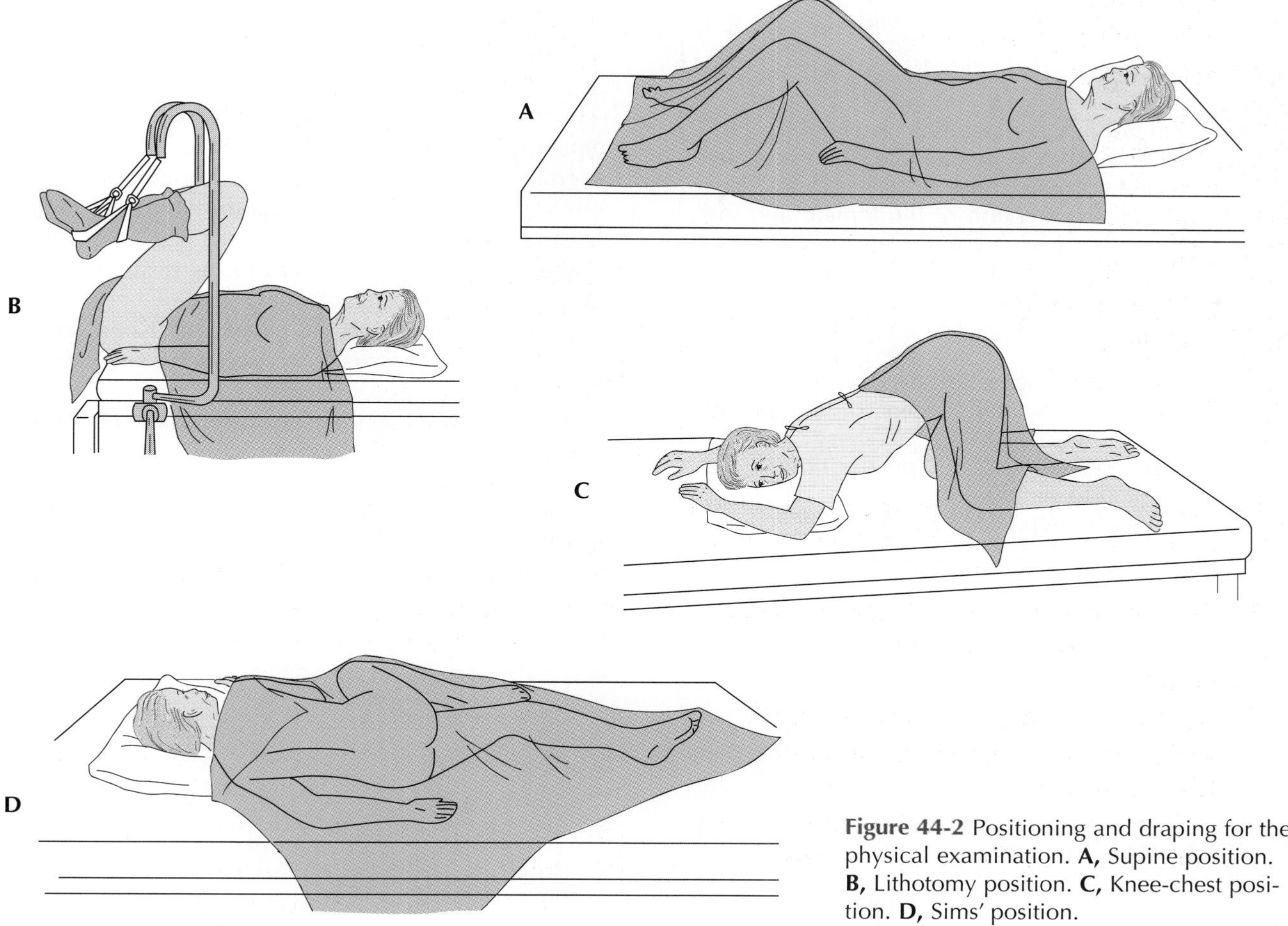

Figure 44-2 Positioning and draping for the physical examination. **A,** Supine position. **B,** Lithotomy position. **C,** Knee-chest position. **D,** Sims' position.

Assisting with the Examination

You may be asked to prepare, position, and drape the client. You may also be asked to assist the physician or RN during the exam. When assisting with an examination, follow the guidelines in Box 44-1. (See *Focus on Children: Providing Comfort during a Physical Exam* box.)

Clients with dementia may resist the examiner's efforts. The client may be agitated and physically aggressive because of confusion and fear. The client who refuses or actively resists an examination must not be restrained or forced to have the procedure. The client may react better at another time. Having a family member present may calm the client. The client's rights are always respected.

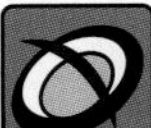

Focus on Children

Providing Comfort during a Physical Exam

The examination of an infant or child is like an adult examination. However, a parent is present. The parent may need to hold the infant or child still during some parts of the procedure if the infant or child is uncooperative. Being kept still may frighten an infant. The child may also fear separation from the parent. Some children fear being physically harmed during the examination. A calm, comforting manner helps both the child and the parent. Remember, the parent may be anxious too.

The equipment needed is like that used for the adult examination. Toys are used to assess development. Vaginal speculums are not used.

Box 44-1 Guidelines for Assisting with the Physical Examination

- Wash your hands before and after the examination.
- Provide for privacy. This is done by screening, closing doors, and draping. Expose only the body part being examined.
- Assist with positioning as directed by the examiner.
- Place instruments and equipment near the examiner.
- Stay in the room when a female is examined (unless you are a male). When a male examines a female, another female must be in the room. This is for the legal protection of the female and the male examiner. A female attendant also adds to the psychological comfort of the woman. A female examiner may want a male attendant present when she examines a male. This also is for her legal protection.
- Protect the client from falling.
- Anticipate the examiner's need for equipment and supplies.
- Place paper or paper towels on the floor if the client is asked to stand.
- Practise medical asepsis and Standard Precautions.

After the Examination

After the examination the client dresses and is taken back to the room. Assist as needed. Lubricant is used for the vaginal or rectal examination. The area is wiped or cleaned before the client dresses or returns to the room.

You also may be asked to do the following:

- Discard disposable items.
- Replace supplies for the next exam.
- Clean reusable items according to employer policy. Return them to the tray or storage place. This includes the otoscope and ophthalmoscope tips, speculum, and stethoscope.
- Remove the used drawsheet or paper from the examination table. Cover the examination table with a clean drawsheet or paper.
- Label specimens. Take them to the designated area according to employer policy.
- Clean and straighten the client's unit or examination room. Follow employer policy for soiled linens.

Remember the client's right to privacy. The results of the examination are confidential. Only members of the health care team involved in the client's care need to know the reason for the exam and its results. If the client consents, the physician tells family members. The client can share the information with others if he or she wants to. You do not tell the family or others the results of the exam.

REVIEW

Circle the BEST answer.

1. The otoscope is used to
   A. Examine the internal structures of the eye
   B. Examine the external ear and the eardrum
   C. Test reflexes
   D. Open the vagina

2. You are preparing Mrs. Janz for an exam. You should do the following *except*
   A. Have her void
   B. Ask her to undress
   C. Drape her
   D. Leave her alone while you go tell the nurse that Mrs. Janz is ready

3. Which part of Mrs. Janz's exam can you do?
   A. Test her reflexes
   B. Inspect her mouth, teeth, and throat
   C. Position and drape her
   D. Observe her perineum and rectum

4. Mrs. Janz is supine. Her hips are flexed and externally rotated. Her feet are supported in stirrups. She is in the
   A. Supine position
   B. Lithotomy position
   C. Knee-chest position
   D. Sims' position

5. You will assist with Mrs. Janz's exam. Which is *false*?
   A. Hand washing is done before and after the examination.
   B. Instruments are placed near the examiner.
   C. You leave the room when Mrs. Janz is examined.
   D. Provide for privacy by screening, closing the door, and proper draping.

6. Which statement is *true*?
   A. You can explain the reason for the exam to the client.
   B. The client must be kept safe from injury during the exam.
   C. You can tell the family the results of the exam.
   D. You explain what the examiner will do.

Answers to these questions are on page 827.

CHAPTER 45

The Patient Having Surgery

OBJECTIVES

- Define the key terms listed in this chapter
- Describe the common fears and concerns of surgical patients
- Explain how people are physically and psychologically prepared for surgery
- Describe how to prepare a room for the postoperative patient
- List the signs and symptoms to report to the nurse postoperatively
- Explain how circulation is stimulated after surgery
- Describe how to meet hygiene, nutrition, fluid, and elimination needs after surgery
- Learn the procedures described in this chapter

KEY TERMS

anesthesia The loss of feeling or sensation produced by a medication

elective surgery Surgery that is scheduled but non-urgent; delaying the surgery does not result in permanent damage, disability, or death

embolus A blood clot (thrombus) that travels through the vascular system until it lodges in a distant blood vessel

emergency surgery Surgery that must be done immediately to save a person's life or prevent disability

general anesthesia Unconsciousness and the loss of feeling or sensation produced by a medication

local anesthesia The loss of sensation in a small area, produced by a medication injected at the specific site

postoperative After surgery

preoperative Before surgery

regional anesthesia The loss of sensation or feeling in a large area of the body, produced by the injection of a medication; the person does not lose consciousness

thrombus A blood clot

urgent surgery Surgery that must be done soon to prevent further damage, disability, or disease

Surgery is done for many reasons. Common reasons include removing a diseased organ or body part, removing a tumour, or repairing injured tissue. Surgery is done also to diagnose a disease, improve appearance, and relieve symptoms. A specially trained physician called a *surgeon* performs the surgery.

Many surgeries require hospital stays. The person is admitted before the surgery and stays for a few or several days after the surgery. However, outpatient surgery (ambulatory surgery, one-day surgery, same-day surgery) is quite common. It does not require an overnight hospital stay. The person is in the hospital less than 24 hours. Many outpatient surgeries are done in clinics or surgical centres that are part of hospitals or physicians' offices.

Surgeries are elective, urgent, or emergency:

- **Elective surgery** is surgery that is scheduled but non-urgent. Delaying the surgery does not result in permanent damage, disability, or death. The surgery is scheduled anywhere from 1 day to months in advance. Often, people are placed on waiting lists for elective surgery. Hip replacement surgery is an example of elective surgery.
- **Urgent surgery** is surgery that must be done soon to prevent further damage, disability, or disease. Examples include cancer surgery and cornary artery surgery.
- **Emergency surgery** is surgery that must be done immediately to save a person's life or prevent disability. People who have been in accidents often require emergency surgery.

The person is prepared for what happens before, during, and after surgery. This involves physical and psychological preparation. Nurses and physicians prepare the patient for the surgical experience.

In hospitals you will have contact with patients before and after surgery. In long-term care facilities many residents are recovering from surgery. Many postoperative patients need home care.

Psychological Care

Illness or injury causes many fears and concerns (Box 45-1 on page 746). Surgery increases these fears. The person's deepest and worst fears are often felt. How would you feel if you needed surgery tomorrow? Would you have fears about pain or death? Who would care for your children and your home? Who would earn money while you were in the hospital? Imagine you were in an accident. You wake up hours later. You are told that your right leg was amputated during surgery.

Feelings are affected by past experiences. Some people have had surgery before. Others have not. Family and friends usually share their surgical experiences with the patient. Their experiences also can affect the patient. Most people know about tragic surgical

Box 45-1 Common Fears and Concerns of Surgical Patients

FEARS
- Disfigurement and scarring
- Disability
- Pain during surgery
- Dying during surgery
- Anesthesia and its effects
- Exposure
- Severe pain or discomfort after surgery
- Tubes, needles, and other equipment used for care
- Complications
- Prolonged recovery
- More surgery or treatments
- Separation from family and friends

CONCERNS
- Caring for children and other family members
- Pets or the house, lawn, and garden
- Monthly bills, loan payments, mortgages, or rent
- Insurance coverage for interruption of work
- Loss of control

events—surgery on the wrong person, surgery on the wrong body part, instruments left in the body, death during surgery. Some people do not talk about their fears and concerns. They may cry, be quiet and withdrawn, or constantly talk about other things. Some pace or are very cheerful.

Psychological preparation is important. You must respect the patient's fears and concerns. The health care team must show the patient warmth, sensitivity, and caring.

PATIENT INFORMATION

The physician explains the need for surgery to the patient and family. They are told about the surgical procedure, risks, and possible complications. Options other than surgery are explained. Risks from not having surgery are also explained. Information is given about who will do the surgery, when it is scheduled, and how long it will take. The person and family may have questions about the surgery and what to expect. Questions and misunderstandings are cleared up. Instructions about care also are given. All information before surgery is given by the physician or nurse. It is beyond the scope of your job to give this information.

After surgery the physician tells the patient and the family about the results. The physician decides what and when to tell them. Often the health care team knows the results before the patient does. Patients and families are usually anxious to know the results. They may ask you, nurses, and other health care workers. They may ask if reports are back from the laboratory or what the reports say. Knowing what the person was told is very important. You do not tell of any diagnosis. If the patient asks you questions about the surgery or test results, explain that you cannot give this information and that you will get your supervisor to help him or her. Your supervisor tells you what and when the patient and family were told. This is confidential information. Do not repeat it to anyone.

YOUR ROLE

You can assist in the psychological care of the surgical patient. Do the following if you are involved in preoperative and postoperative care:

- Listen to the patient who voices fears or concerns about surgery.
- Refer any questions about the surgery or its results to the nurse.
- Explain to the patient procedures you will perform and why they are being done.
- Communicate effectively. Use verbal and nonverbal communication (see Chapter 12).
- Report to your supervisor verbal and nonverbal signs of patient fear or anxiety.
- Report to your supervisor a patient's request to see a spiritual adviser.

THE PREOPERATIVE PERIOD

The **preoperative** (before surgery) period may be many days or just a few minutes. If time permits, the patient is prepared psychologically and physically for the effects of anesthesia and surgery. Good preoperative preparation prevents complications after surgery.

PREOPERATIVE TEACHING

A nurse does the preoperative teaching. The nurse explains to the patient what to expect before and after surgery. Teaching includes explaining the following:

- *Preoperative activities*—These include tests and their purpose, skin preparation, personal care, and the purpose and effects of medications.
- *Deep-breathing, coughing, and leg exercises*—These are done after the surgery. They are taught and practised before the surgery.

- *The recovery room*—This is where the patient wakes up (Figure 45-1). Care in the recovery room is explained.
- *Food and fluids*—The patient cannot eat or drink and has an IV infusion after surgery. The physician orders food and oral fluids when the patient's condition is stable.
- *Turning and repositioning*—The patient usually is turned and repositioned every 2 hours after surgery. The patient is taught what to expect.
- *Early ambulation*—Usually the patient walks as soon as possible after surgery.
- *Pain*—The patient is told about the type and amount of pain to expect and about medications for pain relief.
- *Needed treatments and equipment*—The patient may need a urinary catheter, NG tube, oxygen, wound suction, a cast, or traction. The patient is told about these.
- *Position restrictions*—The patient is told if a certain position is required after surgery. For example, after hip replacement surgery, the hip is abducted.

(See *Focus on Children: Preparing for Surgery* box.)

Special Tests

Before surgery the physician orders tests to evaluate the patient's circulatory, respiratory, and urinary systems. These tests include a chest X-ray, a complete blood count (CBC), and urinalysis. An electrocardiogram (ECG or EKG) detects any cardiac (heart) problems. If blood loss is expected, the patient's blood is tested to determine blood type. This is called *type and crossmatch.* Other tests depend on the patient's condition and the surgery. The patient is prepared for the tests as needed. The results must be on the chart by the time of surgery.

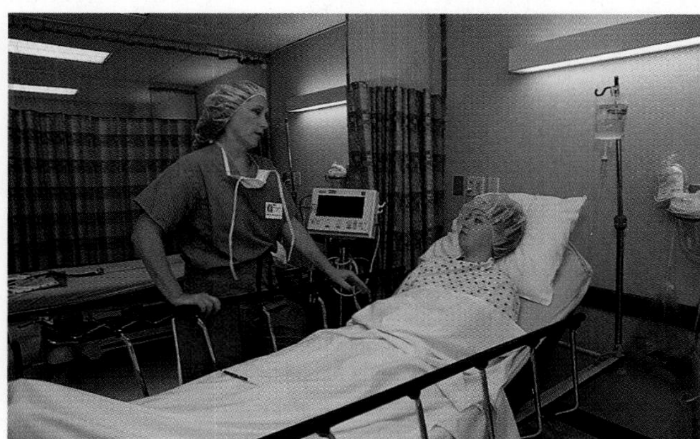

Figure 45-1 Recovery room.

Nutrition and Fluids

A light meal is usually allowed. Then the patient is NPO (not allowed to eat or drink by mouth) for 6 to 8 hours before the surgery. These measures reduce the risk of vomiting and aspiration during anesthesia and after surgery. An NPO sign is placed in the patient's room. Remember, the water pitcher and glass are removed when the patient is NPO.

Elimination

Abdominal surgeries usually require a preoperative enema. Cleansing enemas are common before intestinal surgeries. They are ordered in order to clear the colon of feces. This is done so that feces do not spill into the abdominal cavity when the intestine is opened.

Enemas are also given when straining or a bowel movement could cause postoperative problems. Such problems include pain, severe bleeding (hemorrhage), or stress on the operative area. The physician orders what enema to give and when. Usually a nurse administers the enema.

Some surgeries require catheters. For pelvic and abdominal surgeries, the bladder must be empty. A full bladder is easily injured during surgery. Catheters also allow accurate output measurements during and after surgery.

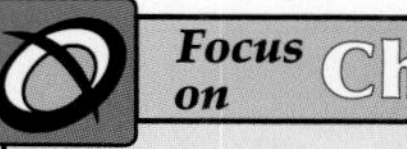

Focus on Children

Preparing for Surgery

The child and parents are prepared for the surgery. Often play is used to help the child understand what will happen. For example, anatomical dolls are used to show the site of surgery. A tour of the operating and recovery rooms also is common. The child and parents are introduced to the members of the health care team who will care for the child.

Personal Care

Personal care before surgery usually involves the following:

- Giving a complete bed bath, shower, or tub bath. A special soap or cleanser may be ordered. A shampoo is included. The bath and shampoo reduce the number of microbes on the body at the time of surgery.
- Removing make-up and nail polish. The skin, lips, and nail beds are observed for colour and circulation during and after surgery.
- Braiding long hair. All hairpins, clips, combs, and similar items are removed. So are wigs and hairpieces. Some hospitals have both men and women wear surgical caps. A cap keeps hair out of the face and the operative area.
- Giving oral hygiene to promote comfort. Being NPO causes thirst and a dry mouth. The patient must not swallow any water during oral hygiene. (See *Focus on Children: Preoperative Oral Hygiene* box.)
- Removing dentures. They are removed before preoperative medications are given. They are cleaned and kept moist in a denture cup. They are kept in a safe place. Some people do not like being seen without their dentures. Let them wear their dentures as long as possible. This promotes the person's sense of dignity and esteem.

> ***Focus on* Children**
>
> **Preoperative Oral Hygiene**
>
> Check for loose teeth when giving oral hygiene. Report any loose teeth to the nurse. The nurse notes the observation on the preoperative checklist and informs the OR staff. A loose tooth can fall out during anesthesia. The child can aspirate the tooth.

Valuables

Valuables are removed for safekeeping. These include dentures, glasses, contact lenses, hearing aids, and jewellery. Artificial eyes and limbs also are removed. These items are easily lost or broken during surgery. Transfers to the operating room (OR), recovery room, and back to the patient's room also present safety risks. A note is made on the patient's chart about the valuables removed and where they are kept. The patient may want to wear a wedding band or religious medal. The item is secured in place with gauze or tape according to hospital policy.

Skin Preparation

The skin and hair shafts contain microbes that could enter the body through the surgical incision. A serious infection could result. The skin cannot be sterilized. However, a *skin prep* can reduce the number of microbes.

Hospital policy and the surgeon's preferences determine the area to be prepared for a specific surgery (Figure 45-2). The incision site and a large area around the site are *prepped.*

The skin prep is done right before the surgery. It is done in the patient's room or in the OR. Hair is removed by applying a depilatory (cream hair remover) or shaving.

Disposable prep kits are used for shaving. A kit has a razor, a sponge filled with soap, a basin, and a drape and towel (Figure 45-3 on page 750). The skin is lathered with soap. Then the skin is shaved in the direction of hair growth (Figure 45-4 on page 750). Any skin break is a possible infection site. If you do a skin prep, be very careful not to cut, scratch, or nick the skin. Report and record any nicks, cuts, and scratches. Follow Standard Precautions.

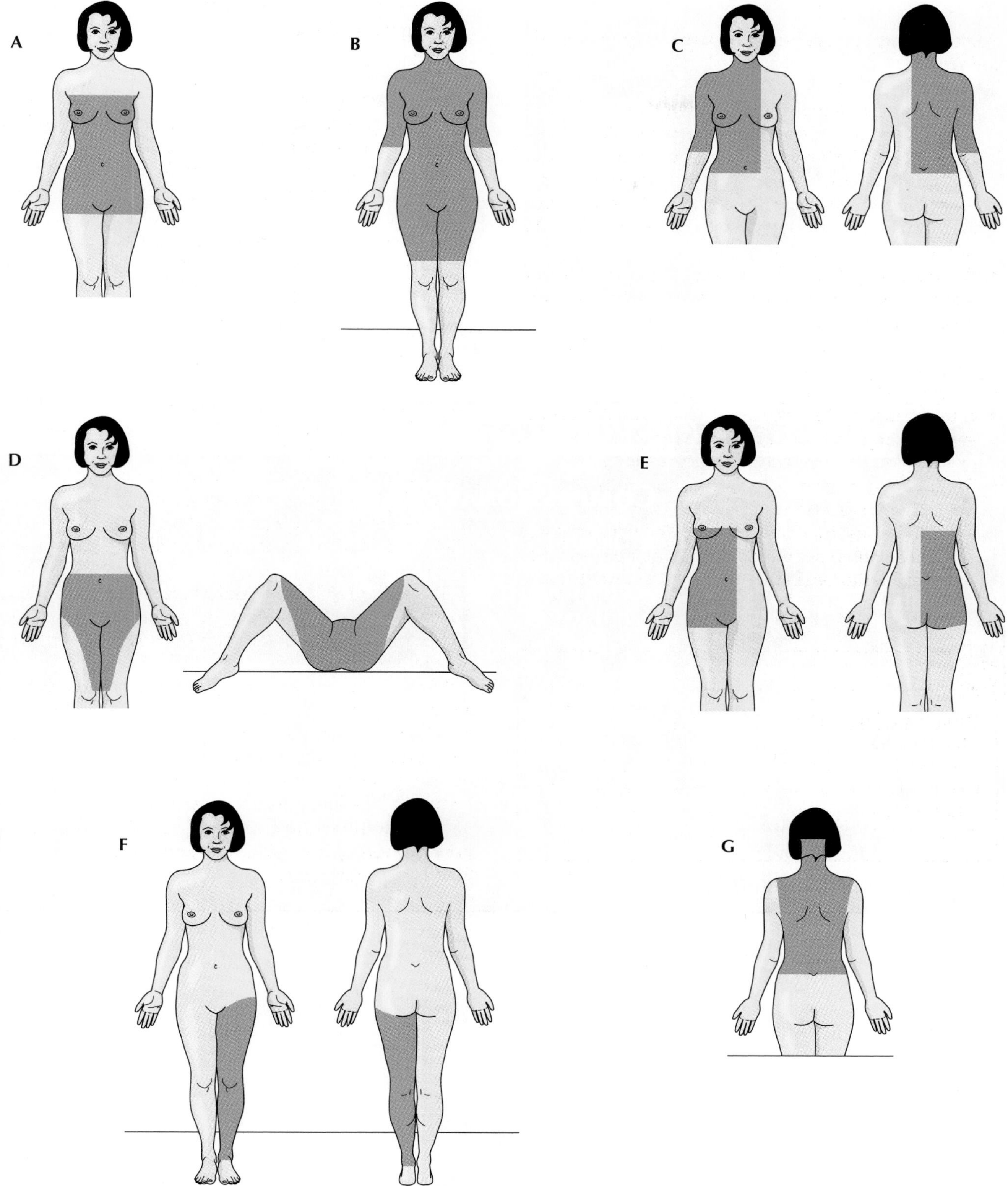

Figure 45-2 Common skin preparation sites. The shaded areas are those shaved preoperatively. **A,** Abdominal surgery. **B,** Open-heart surgery. **C,** Breast surgery. **D,** Vaginal, rectal, and perineal surgery. **E,** Kidney surgery. **F,** Knee surgery. **G,** Cervical spine surgery.

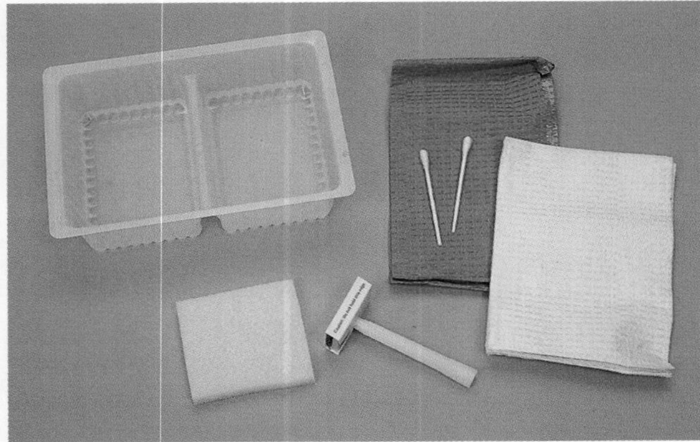

Figure 45-3 Skin prep kit.

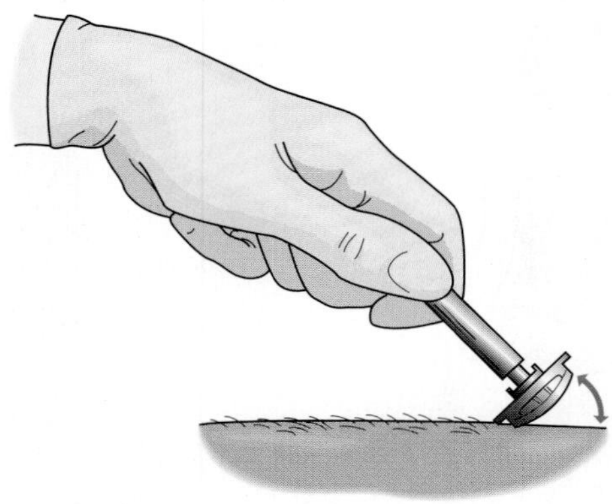

Figure 45-4 Hold the skin taut. Shave in the direction of hair growth.

The Surgical Skin Prep

Compassionate Care

Remember to Promote:
- **Dignity**
- **Independence**
- **Preferences**
- **Privacy**
- **Safety**

Pre-Procedure

1 Identify the person according to employer policy.
2 Explain the procedure to the person.
3 Wash your hands.
4 Collect the following:
   - Disposable skin prep kit
   - Bath blanket
   - Warm water
   - Gloves
   - Waterproof pad
   - Bath towel
5 Provide for privacy.

Continued

The Surgical Skin Prep—cont'd

Procedure

6 Make sure you have good lighting. There should be no glares or shadows.
7 Raise the bed to a comfortable working height. Follow the care plan for bed rail use. Lower the bed rail near you if up.
8 Cover the person with a bath blanket. Fan-fold top linens to the foot of the bed.
9 Place the waterproof pad under the area you will shave.
10 Open the skin prep kit.
11 Position the person for the skin prep. Drape him or her with the disposable drape.
12 Add warm water to the basin. Check water temperature. Put on gloves.
13 Apply soap to the skin with the sponge. Work up a good lather.
14 Hold the skin taut. Shave in the direction of hair growth (see Figure 45-4).
15 Shave outward from the centre, using short strokes.
16 Rinse the razor often.
17 Check to see that the entire area is free of hair. Also check for cuts, scratches, or nicks.
18 Rinse the skin thoroughly. Pat dry.
19 Remove the drape and waterproof pad. Remove gloves. Wash your hands.
20 Return top linens. Remove the bath blanket.

Post-Procedure

21 Provide for safety and comfort.
22 Return the bed to its lowest position.
23 Follow the care plan for bed rail use.
24 Place the call bell within reach.
25 Remove privacy measures.
26 Return equipment to its proper place.
27 Discard supplies and soiled linen following employer policy.
28 Wash your hands.
29 Report and record your actions and observations according to employer policy.

The Preoperative Checklist

A preoperative checklist (Figure 45-5 on page 752) is placed on the front of the patient's chart. The RN makes sure the checklist in completed. The patient is ready for surgery when the list is complete. The nurse may ask you to do some things on the list. Promptly report when you complete each task. Also report any observations. Except for the bed rails, the entire checklist is completed before preoperative medications are given.

Preoperative Medication

About 45 minutes to 1 hour before surgery, the preoperative medications are given by a physician or nurse. One medication helps the patient relax and feel drowsy. The other dries up respiratory secretions to prevent aspiration. Drowsiness, lightheadedness, thirst, and dry mouth are normal and expected.

After the medications are given, measures are taken to prevent falls. Bed rails are raised, and the patient is not allowed out of bed. Therefore the patient voids before the medications are given. After the medications are given, the bedpan or urinal is used for voiding.

(text continues on page 753)

CREDIT · VALLEY
THE CREDIT VALLEY HOSPITAL

PRE-OPERATIVE CHECKLIST

Date: ______________

Procedure: ______________________________

____

Allergies: ______________________________

____

Allergy Band: ❑ Yes ❑ No

Infectious Disease Risk: ❑ Yes ❑ No ❑ Unknown

	YES	NO	N/A	OR
Addressograph Plate				
Identification Bracelet				
Consent				
Blood Consent				
History & Physical				
Surgical Consultation				
Pre Anaesthetic Questionnaire				
Pre-op Teaching				
Old Chart to OR				
Dentures Removed				
Capped/Loose Teeth - Braces				
Contact Lenses Removed				
Hearing Aid Removed				
Prostheses Removed				
Jewellery Removed/Taped				
Nail Polish Removed				

Operative Side ❑ Bil. ❑ RT ❑ LT ❑ N/A

Last Voided Time __________

NPO Since __________

Vital Signs:

Temp _______ Pulse _______ Respirations _______

BP _______ Weight _______kg

PHYSICAL AND EMOTIONAL ASSESSMENT

❑ Oriented ❑ Confused

❑ Semi-Conscious ❑ Anxious

❑ Unconscious ❑ Language Barrier

Language Spoken at Home______________

IMPLANTS

AV FISTULA	❑ (R) ARM	❑ (L) ARM
TOTAL HIP	❑ (R)	❑ (L)
TOTAL KNEE	❑ (R)	❑ (L)
PACEMAKER	❑ YES	❑ NO

LAB RESULTS/REPORTS

❑ Hemoglobin
❑ Urinalysis
❑ Sickle Cell
❑ Electrolytes
❑ Glucose
❑ PT / PTT
❑ Group & Reserve/OB Mom
❑ Cross Match ____ Units
❑ Autologous ____ Units
❑ X-ray (Chest or other)
❑ ECG

OTHER PERTINENT LAB TESTS AND/OR RELATED INFORMATION:

SPECIAL INFORMATION

Date: ______________________

Pre-Op Nurse Signature: ______________________

Date: ______________________

OR Nurse Signature: ______________________

5322 D HR (01/22/2002) PRE-OPERATIVE CHECKLIST

Figure 45-5 Preoperative checklist.

The bed is kept in the lowest position or raised to the highest position following hospital policy. Move furniture out of the way to make room for the stretcher. Also clean off the overbed table and the bedside stand. This prevents damage to equipment and valuables. Raise the bed to the highest position for transferring the patient from the bed to a stretcher.

Transport to the Operating Room

A nurse or an OR attendant brings a stretcher to the room. The patient is transferred onto the stretcher and covered with a bath blanket. Assist with the transfer as required. The blanket provides warmth and prevents exposure. Falling is prevented. Safety straps are secured and the side rails raised. A small pillow is sometimes placed under the patient's head for comfort.

Identification checks are made. Then the patient's chart is given to the OR staff member.

The nurse responsible for preoperative care may go with the patient to the OR entrance. Often the family also is allowed to go this far. (See *Focus on Children: Preoperative Medications* box.)

Anesthesia

Anesthesia is the loss of feeling or sensation produced by a medication. Anesthetics are given by specially trained physicians called *anesthetists*. There are three types of anesthesia:

- **General anesthesia** produces unconsciousness and the loss of feeling or sensation. A medication is given intravenously or a gas is inhaled.
- **Regional anesthesia** produces loss of sensation or feeling in a large area of the body. The person does not lose consciousness. A medication is injected into a body part.
- **Local anesthesia** produces loss of sensation in a small area. A medication is injected at the specific site.

The Postoperative Period

After surgery (**postoperative**) the patient is taken to the recovery room (RR). This is often called the postanesthesia room (PAR) or postanesthesia care unit (PACU). The recovery room is near the OR. There the patient recovers from the anesthetic. This can take 1 to 2 hours. The patient is watched very closely. Vital signs are taken and observations are made often. The patient leaves the recovery room when:

- Vital signs are stable
- The patient has good respiratory function
- The patient can respond and call for help when it is needed

The physician gives the transfer order when appropriate.

Preparing the Patient's Room

The room must be ready for the patient's return from the recovery room. A surgical bed is made (see Chapter 24). Equipment and supplies needed for the patient's care are brought to the room. The nurse tells you if special measures and equipment are needed. The room is prepared after the patient is taken to the OR. Preparations include:

- Making a surgical bed
- Placing equipment and supplies in the room:
  - Thermometer
  - Stethoscope
  - Sphygmomanometer
  - Kidney basin
  - Tissues
  - Waterproof bed protector
  - Vital signs flow sheet
  - I&O record
  - IV pole
  - Other items as directed by the nurse
- Raising the bed to its highest position
- Lowering bed rails
- Moving furniture out of the way for the stretcher

Return from the Recovery Room

The recovery room nurse calls the nursing unit when the patient is ready for transfer. The patient is transported by the recovery room nurses. A nurse meets the patient on the nursing unit, and the patient is transferred from the stretcher to bed. Assist as needed in the transfer. Also help position the patient.

Have an extra blanket ready for the patient. Patients often feel cold after surgery.

Vital signs are taken by a nurse. Vital signs are usually measured:

- Every 15 minutes the first hour
- Every 30 minutes for 1 to 2 hours
- Every hour for 4 hours
- Then every 4 hours

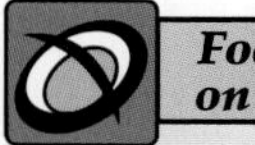

Focus on Children

Preoperative Medications

Some hospitals allow a parent to be with the child while anesthesia is given. The parent stays in the OR until the child is asleep.

The nurse also observes the patient. The nurse checks dressings for bleeding. Catheters, IV infusions, and other tube placement and function are checked. Bed rails are raised, and the call bell is placed within the patient's reach. Necessary care and treatments are given. Then the family can see the patient.

Observations

The patient requires careful monitoring during the postoperative period. After the patient is stable, you may be asked to check the patient. The nurse tells you how often to check the patient. This is an important function. Always be alert for the signs and symptoms listed in Box 45-2. Report them to the nurse immediately.

Box 45-2 Postoperative Observations

- Choking
- A drop or rise in blood pressure
- Bright red blood from the incision, drainage tubes, or suction tubes
- A pulse rate of more than 100 or less than 60 beats per minute
- A weak or irregular pulse
- A rise or drop in body temperature
- Hypoxia (see Chapter 43)
- The need for upper-airway suctioning, signalled by any of the following:
  - Tachypnea (rapid breathing)
  - Dyspnea (difficult, laboured, or painful breathing)
  - Moist-sounding respirations
  - Gurgling or gasping
  - Restlessness
  - Cyanosis (bluish colouring to the skin, lips, and nails)
- Shallow, slow breathing
- Weak cough
- Complaints of thirst
- Cold, moist, clammy, or pale skin
- Increased drainage on or under dressings or on bed linens (including drawsheets, bottom sheets, and pillowcases)
- Complaints of pain or nausea
- Vomiting
- Confusion or disorientation
- Other measurements and observations as directed by a nurse:
  - The amount, character, and time of the first voiding after surgery
  - Intake and output
  - IV flow rate
  - The appearance of drainage from a urinary catheter, NG tube, or wound suction
  - Any other observation that can mean a change in the patient's condition

Positioning

Proper positioning promotes comfort and prevents complications. The type of surgery affects positioning. Position restrictions may be ordered. The patient is usually positioned for easy and comfortable breathing. Also, stress on the incision is prevented. When the patient is supine, the head of the bed is usually raised slightly. The patient's head may be turned to the side. These positions prevent aspiration if vomiting occurs.

Repositioning every 1 to 2 hours helps prevent respiratory and circulatory complications. It may be painful for the patient to be turned. Provide support, and turn the patient with smooth, gentle motions. Pillows and other positioning devices are often used (see Chapters 21 and 22).

The nurse tells you when to reposition the patient and the positions allowed. Usually you assist the nurse. Sometimes you turn and reposition the patient yourself. This occurs when the patient's condition is stable and care is simple. (See *Focus on Older Adults: Postoperative Positioning* box.)

Coughing and Deep Breathing

Respiratory complications must be prevented. There are two major complications. One is *pneumonia*—an inflammation and infection in the lung. The other is *atelectasis*—the collapse of a portion of the lung. Coughing and deep-breathing exercises and incentive spirometry help prevent these complications (see Chapter 43). They are done every 1 to 2 hours when the patient is awake. (See *Focus on Older Adults: Respiratory Complications after Surgery* box.)

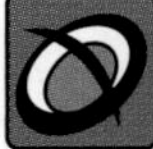

Focus on Older Adults

Postoperative Positioning

Many older adults have stiff and painful joints. Sore muscles, bones, and joints occur from positioning on the operating room table. Remember to turn and reposition older adults slowly and gently.

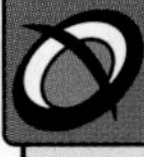

Focus on Older Adults

Respiratory Complications after Surgery

The changes associated with aging increase the older adult's risk for respiratory complications. Respiratory muscles are weaker. Lung tissue is less elastic. The person has less strength for coughing. Coughing, deep breathing, and incentive spirometry are very important.

Stimulating Circulation

After surgery, circulation must be stimulated. This is especially true for blood flow in the legs. If blood flow is sluggish, blood clots may form. A blood clot (**thrombus**) can form in the deep leg veins (Figure 45-6, *A*). Part of the thrombus can break loose and travel through the bloodstream. It then becomes an embolus. An **embolus** is a blood clot that travels through the vascular system until it lodges in a distant vessel (Figure 45-6, *B*). An embolus from a vein can eventually lodge in the lungs (pulmonary embolus). A pulmonary embolus can cause severe respiratory problems and death.

Leg Exercises. Leg exercises increase venous blood flow. Therefore they help prevent thrombi. Leg exercises are easy to do. You assist if the patient is weak. If the patient had leg surgery, a physician's order is needed for the exercises. Your supervisor tells you when to do the exercises. They are done with the patient supine, at least every 1 or 2 hours while the patient is awake. The following exercises are done 5 times (see Chapter 22):

- Ask the person to make circles with the toes. This rotates the ankles.
- Have the person dorsiflex and plantar flex the feet.
- Have the person flex and extend one knee and then the other (Figure 45-7).
- Ask the person to raise and lower one leg off the bed (Figure 45-8). Repeat this exercise with the other leg.

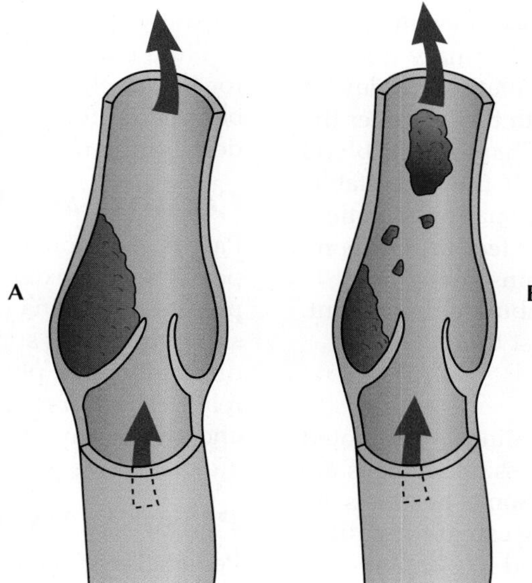

Figure 45-6 A, A thrombus (blood clot) is attached to the wall of a vein. The arrows show the direction of blood flow. **B,** Part of the thrombus broke off and has become an embolus. The embolus will travel in the bloodstream until it lodges in a distant vessel.

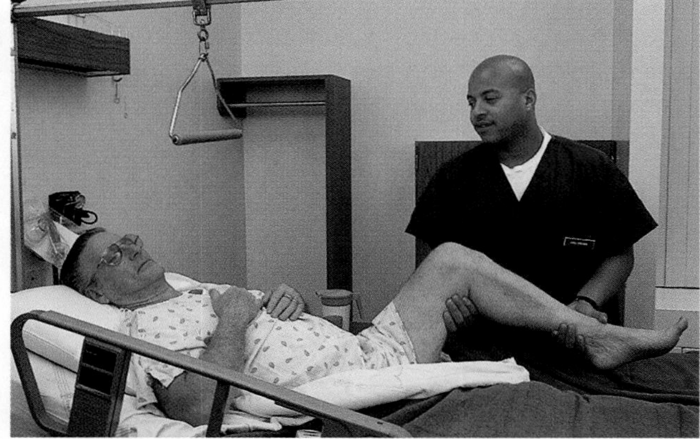

Figure 45-7 Flex and then extend the knee during postoperative leg exercises.

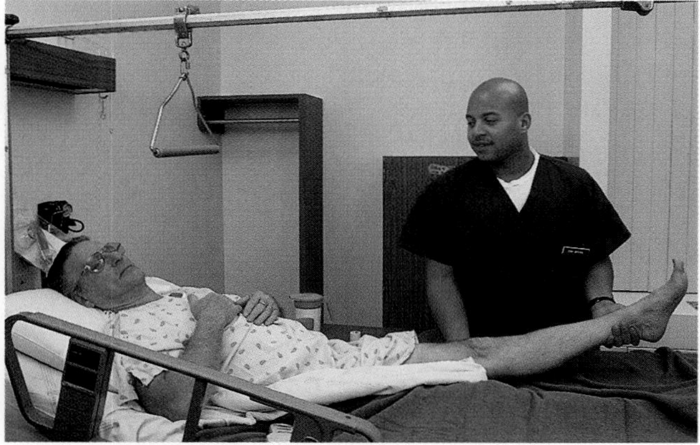

Figure 45-8 Assist the patient with raising and lowering the leg.

Elastic Stockings and Bandages. Elastic stockings and bandages help prevent thrombi. The elastic exerts pressure on the veins, promoting venous blood flow to the heart. Elastic stockings or bandages are often ordered for postoperative patients and for those with heart disease and circulatory disorders.

Both elastic stockings and bandages could harm the patient if applied improperly. Therefore, most hospitals allow only nurses to apply them to acute-care patients. If you are assigned this task, make sure it is in your scope of practice and employer policy allows you to do it. Also make sure you have been properly trained and have close supervision. Application of elastic stockings and bandages is discussed in Chapter 28.

Early Ambulation

Early ambulation prevents postoperative circulatory complications such as thrombi. It also prevents pneumonia, atelectasis, constipation, and urinary tract infections. The patient usually ambulates the day of surgery. The patient first sits up with the legs over the edge of the bed (dangling) (see Chapter 21). Blood pressure and pulse are measured. If they are stable, the patient is assisted out of bed. Usually the patient does not walk very far—just a few feet in the room. Distance increases as the patient gains strength.

The nurse tells you when to ambulate the patient. Usually you assist the nurse the first time.

Wound Healing

The incision needs protection. Healing is promoted and infection prevented. Sterile dressing changes are done by the physician or nurse. Some hospitals let support workers do simple dressing care if the patient is stable. Wound healing is discussed in Chapter 41.

Nutrition and Fluids

The patient has an IV infusion on return from the OR. Continued IV therapy depends on the type of surgery and the patient's condition. Anesthesia can cause nausea and vomiting. The patient's diet progresses from NPO to clear liquids, to full liquids, to a light diet, to a regular diet. The diet is ordered by the physician. Frequent oral hygiene is important when the patient is NPO.

Some patients have nasogastric (NG) tubes (see Chapter 26). Often the NG tube is attached to suction to keep the stomach empty. The patient is NPO and receives IV therapy.

Elimination

Anesthesia, the surgery, and being NPO affect normal bowel and urinary elimination. Medications for pain relief can cause constipation. The measures to promote elimination are practised as directed by the nurse (see Chapters 29 and 30).

Intake and output are measured postoperatively. The patient must urinate within 8 hours after surgery. Report the time and amount of the patient's first voiding. If the patient does not void within 8 hours, a catheterization is usually ordered. Some patients have catheters after surgery. See Chapter 29 for care of the person with a catheter.

Fluid intake and return to a regular diet are needed for bowel elimination. Suppositories or enemas may be ordered for constipation. Rectal tubes may be ordered for flatulence (see Chapter 30).

Comfort and Rest

Pain is common after surgery. The degree of pain depends on the extent of surgery, incision site, and the presence of drainage tubes, casts, or other devices. Positioning during surgery can cause muscle strains and discomfort. The physician orders medications for pain relief. The nurse tells you how to promote comfort and rest. Many of the guidelines listed in Chapter 20 are part of the person's care plan.

Personal Hygiene

Personal hygiene is important for the patient's physical and mental well-being. Wound drainage and skin prep solutions can irritate the skin and cause discomfort. NPO causes a dry mouth and breath odours. Moist, clammy skin from blood pressure changes or elevated body temperatures also cause discomfort. Frequent oral hygiene, hair care, and a complete bed bath the day after surgery help refresh and renew the patient physically and psychologically. The gown is changed whenever it becomes wet or soiled (see Chapter 27).

REVIEW

Circle T if the answer is true and F if it is false.

1. T F Hair is kept out of the face for surgery by using pins, clips, or combs.
2. T F Nail polish is removed before surgery.
3. T F Women can wear make-up to surgery.
4. T F Pyjamas are worn to the operating room.
5. T F Contact lenses are removed before surgery.
6. T F A surgical bed is made for the patient's return from the recovery room.
7. T F A drop in a patient's blood pressure is reported to the nurse immediately.
8. T F The patient ambulates the first time the day after surgery.
9. T F Intake and output are measured after surgery.
10. T F A surgical patient should void within 8 hours after surgery.

Circle the BEST answer.

11. Which is *true* of elective surgery?
    A. The surgery is done immediately.
    B. The need for surgery is sudden and unexpected.
    C. Surgery is scheduled for a later date.
    D. General anesthesia is always used.
12. You can assist in Mr. Long's psychological preparation by explaining
    A. The reason for the surgery
    B. The procedures you are doing
    C. The risks and possible complications of surgery
    D. What to expect during the preoperative and postoperative periods
13. Preoperatively, Mr. Long is
    A. NPO
    B. Allowed only water
    C. Given a regular breakfast
    D. Given a tube feeding
14. Cleansing enemas are ordered for Mr. Long preoperatively. The enemas are given
    A. To clean the colon of feces
    B. To prevent bleeding
    C. To relieve flatus
    D. To prevent pain
15. Mr. Long's skin prep is done preoperatively to
    A. Completely bathe the body
    B. Sterilize the skin
    C. Reduce the number of microbes on the skin
    D. Destroy nonpathogens and pathogens
16. When shaving the skin before surgery
    A. Shave in the direction opposite of hair growth
    B. Shave toward the centre of the specific area
    C. Be careful not to cut, scratch, or nick the skin
    D. Use an electric razor
17. Mr. Long's preoperative medication was given. He
    A. Must remain in bed
    B. Is allowed to walk within his room
    C. Can use the commode to void
    D. Is allowed only sips of water
18. General anesthesia
    A. Is injected into a body part
    B. Produces unconsciousness and the loss of feeling or sensation
    C. Is a specially educated physician
    D. Produces loss of sensation or feeling in a body part
19. Mr. Long must cough and deep breathe after surgery to prevent
    A. Bleeding
    B. A pulmonary embolus
    C. Respiratory complications
    D. Pain and discomfort

REVIEW

20. **Leg exercises are ordered for Mr. Long. Which is *false*?**
    A. **Leg exercises stimulate circulation.**
    B. **Leg exercises prevent thrombi.**
    C. **Leg exercises are done 5 times every 1 or 2 hours.**
    D. **Leg exercises are done only for leg surgery.**

21. **Postoperatively, Mr. Long's position is changed**
    A. **Every 2 hours**
    B. **Every 3 hours**
    C. **Every 4 hours**
    D. **Every shift**

Answers to these questions are on page 828.

CHAPTER

46

Caring for a Client Who Is Dying

OBJECTIVES

- Define the key terms listed in this chapter
- Explain how culture, religion, and age influence attitudes toward death
- Describe the five stages of grief
- Explain how to help meet a dying person's needs
- Describe the needs of the family of a dying person
- Describe palliative care
- Explain the importance of an advance directive
- Identify the signs of approaching death and the signs of death
- Describe how to assist in giving postmortem care
- Learn the procedure described in this chapter

KEY TERMS

advance directive A legal document in which a person states his or her wishes about future health care, treatment, and personal care; the document is put into effect when the person is unable to make or express these wishes; living will

anticipatory grief The sense of loss and sorrow experienced before an expected loss happens

grief The process of moving from deep sorrow caused by loss toward healing and recovery

living will Advance directive

palliative care Services for people (and their families) living with or dying from a progressive, life-threatening illness; these services aim to relieve suffering and improve comfort, not cure the illness

postmortem care Care of the body after (*post*) death (*mortem*)

rigor mortis The stiffness or rigidity (*rigor*) of skeletal muscles that occurs after death (*mortis*)

People who are dying are cared for in facilities or at home. The health care team sees death often. Some members of the team may be unsure of their feelings about death. They may be uncomfortable with dying people and the subject of death. Dying people may represent helplessness and the failure to cure. Dying people may also remind them of their own eventual death or the death of loved ones.

You will help meet the physical, social, emotional, intellectual, and spiritual needs of clients who are dying. Your feelings and beliefs about death and dying affect the care you give. You need to understand both the dying process and your own attitudes toward death and dying. This will help you provide compassionate care. Before reading on, reflect on the following:

- What has been your experience with death?
- What are your feelings and beliefs about death and dying?
- How have your experiences and culture shaped your beliefs?

LIFE-THREATENING ILLNESS

Many life-threatening illnesses have no cure. Some injuries are so serious that the body cannot function. In these cases, recovery is not expected. The illness or injury ends in death.

Health care professionals cannot predict the exact time of death. A person may have days, months, weeks, or years to live. People expected to live for a short time have lived for many years. Others expected to live longer have died much sooner. Hope and the will to live can influence dying and living. Some people die sooner than expected when they lose the will to live.

ATTITUDES TOWARD DEATH

Personality, culture, religion, age, and experience influence attitudes toward death. Many people fear death. Others do not believe they will die. Some look forward to and accept death. A person's attitude toward death often changes with age and experience.

Until the beginning of the last century, many Canadians died at home. Families cared for loved ones who were dying. Death was a natural part of life. Today most Canadians die in facilities. Many people have never seen a dying person or a dead body. Therefore, death is frightening to them.

CULTURE AND RELIGION

Practices and attitudes about death differ among cultures. Attitudes toward death are closely related to religion (see *Respecting Diversity: Death and Dying Rituals* box). Some believe that life after death is free of suffering and hardship. They may also believe in reunion with loved ones. Many believe sins and misdeeds are punished in the afterlife. Others believe there is no afterlife.

Religious beliefs exist about the body's form after death. Some people believe that the body keeps its physical form. Others believe that only the spirit or soul is present in the afterlife. *Reincarnation* is the belief that the spirit or soul is reborn in another human body or in another life form.

Many people strengthen their religious beliefs when dying. Religion often provides comfort to the dying person and the family.

Respecting Diversity

Death and Dying Rituals

Hinduism	The dying person may lie on the floor. A priest ties a thread around the neck or wrist. This should not be removed. A priest pours water in the person's mouth. The family washes the body before cremation.
Sikhism	The deceased needs the five Ks: *Kesh*, uncut hair; *Kangra*, wooden comb; *Kara*, wrist band; *Kirpan*, sword; *Kach*, shorts.
Buddhism	A priest is called before death. Last rites and chanting are done at the bedside. Burial or cremation is acceptable.
Shinto	Jewellery is removed; the body is washed and dressed in a white kimono and straw shoes.
Islam	The dying confess their sins. The body is washed and wrapped in white cloth; the head is turned toward the right shoulder; the body faces east, toward Mecca.
Judaism	The body is washed by burial society, and someone remains with the body (Orthodox and Conservative Jews). Whenever possible, burial is to take place within 24 hours after death.
Christianity	Rituals vary greatly among groups. Many give last rites or communion. Many prefer burial to cremation.

Note: Remember, individuals may not follow every belief and practice of their culture and religion. Each person is unique. Do not judge the person by your own standards.

Source: J.C. Ross-Kerr, M.J. Wood, P.A. Potter, and A.G. Perry, *Canadian Fundamentals of Nursing*, 2nd ed. (Toronto: Mosby, 2001), p. 600.

Age

People's attitudes and responses to dying are highly individual. However, age and stage of life influence many people's feelings and reactions.

Infants and toddlers have no concept of death. Between the ages of 3 and 5 years, children are curious and have ideas about death. They know when family members or pets die. They notice dead birds and insects. They may think that death is temporary. Misleading answers to questions about death can cause fear and confusion. For example, children who are told "He is sleeping" may be afraid to go to sleep. Children between ages 5 and 7 know that death is final, though they may not think it will happen to them.

Adults usually have more fears about death than children. They may fear pain and suffering, dying alone, separation from loved ones, and loss of dignity. They may worry about the care and support of those left behind. Some people have regrets about missed opportunities, failed relationships, or unfulfilled hopes and dreams. Some feel that their life did not have meaning. Others feel that their life has made a difference.

Older adults usually have fewer fears. They expect to die. Many have experienced the deaths of friends and loved ones. Some feel they have lived a full and complete life. Others have regrets. Some welcome death as freedom from pain, suffering, and disability. Like younger adults, older adults often fear dying alone.

Although age and stage of life influence a person's response to dying, you cannot predict how an individual will respond.

The Stages of Grief

Grief is the process of moving from deep sorrow caused by loss toward healing and recovery. Both the person who is dying and his or her loved ones experience a range of emotions when faced with loss. Many people experience **anticipatory grief**. This is the sense of loss and sorrow experienced before an expected loss happens.

Dr. Elisabeth Kübler-Ross identified five stages of grief that a dying person experiences. They are denial, anger, bargaining, depression, and acceptance.

- *Denial.* During the first stage, the person refuses to believe that he or she is dying. "No, not me" is a common response. The person does not accept that the condition will end in death. He or she cannot deal with problems or decisions about the illness or injury. This stage can last for a few hours, days, or much longer. Some people may still be in denial when they die.
- *Anger.* During this stage, the person thinks "Why me?" He or she feels anger and, sometimes, rage. The person may envy and resent those with life and health. Family, friends, and the health care team are often targets of anger. The person may blame him or herself. Or the person may blame others and find fault with those who are loved and needed the most. If a client is angry with you, remember that anger is a normal stage of grief. Do not take the anger personally. Control any urge to argue with the person.
- *Bargaining.* After anger passes, the person enters the third stage. The person now says "Yes, me, but …" Often the person bargains with God for more time. Promises are made in exchange for more time.

The person may want to see a child marry, see a grandchild, have one more summer, or live for some other event. You may not see this stage. Bargaining usually is private and on a spiritual level.
- *Depression.* During the fourth stage, the person thinks "Yes, me" and is very sad. He or she mourns things that have been lost and for the future loss of life. The person may cry or say little. Some people may talk about loved ones and things that will be left behind.
- *Acceptance.* This is the final stage. The person is at peace and has said what needs to be said. He or she has completed unfinished business. The person accepts death. This stage may last for many months or years. Reaching acceptance does not mean that death is near.

People who are dying do not always go through all five stages. A person may never get beyond a certain stage. Some accept death without experiencing the other stages. Some move back and forth between stages. For example, a client may reach the depression stage, move back to bargaining, and then move forward to acceptance. Some people stay in one stage until death.

The family also experiences the five stages of grief. Often family members do not go through the stages at the same time as the person who is dying. For example, a woman may still be angry at her husband's diagnosis when her husband has reached the acceptance stage. Family members may experience all or some of the stages and may move back and forth among them.

Members of the health care team also experience the stages of grief. Caring for a dying person is a moving and emotional experience. Supporting a grieving family can be very difficult. You will grieve the loss of clients you have cared for. It is important that you examine your feelings about loss and grief. Do not turn away from these feelings. Develop your own support system, including your supervisor and co-workers (Box 46-1).

Box 46-1 Case Study: Support Worker Grief

Indira works in a long-term care facility. She relates this experience about her grief following the death of a resident:

"I cared for Mrs. Giovanni on and off for 5 years. We always talked while I gave care, and I got to know her quite well. She told me about her early life in Italy before she came to Canada. She showed me photographs of her family.

"I was with her the day before she died. She wanted me to stay with her. I didn't realize the end was so near. When I heard the next day that she had died, I was really upset. I had not been this sad when other residents died. I felt sad for several weeks afterwards.

"I shared my feelings with the RN on my unit and a co-worker. It helped to talk about it. Gradually, I accepted that my feelings were a natural reaction to loss and death. Looking back, I'm glad I got to know Mrs. Giovanni so well and made time for her the day before she died."

Palliative Care

Palliative care refers to the services offered to people (and their families) living with or dying from a progressive, life-threatening illness. The goals of palliative care are to relieve pain and suffering, improve comfort, and promote dignity. Palliative care does not attempt to cure illness. Nor does it attempt to prolong life when a person is near death. Rather, palliative care focuses on meeting the physical, social, emotional, intellectual, and spiritual needs of the person and family. This allows the person to maintain a meaningful life and have a dignified death.

Palliative care can be provided in a person's home or in a facility setting. Palliative care in the home is usually offered through home care agencies.

Some cities and towns have community hospice organizations. These are usually non-profit organizations run by volunteers. The organizations may work closely with home care programs.

Separate facilities called hospices also provide palliative care. Many hospices provide care in houses that once were private homes. They are often located in quiet neighbourhoods in park-like settings. The goal is to provide a comfortable, peaceful setting. Some hospices provide palliative care to specific client groups, such as those with AIDS or cancer.

The most common facility setting is the palliative care unit within a hospital. Many long-term care facilities also provide palliative care.

Many people work together as a team to provide palliative care. Team members vary depending on the situation. The team often includes physicians, nurses, case managers, social workers, psychologists, spiritual advisers, support workers, and volunteers. The person and family members are also key members of the team. Some people choose to have a close friend on the team. Family members and close friends provide much emotional and physical care. Even in facility settings, families and close friends are encouraged to help with the person's care. The person is an active participant in his or her own care.

Caring for a Person Who is Dying

Dying people have emotional, social, spiritual, intellectual, and physical needs. The health care team helps to meet those needs. Every effort is made to promote physical and emotional comfort. The person has the right to die in peace and dignity. See Box 46-2 and *Providing Compassionate Care: The Dying Person* box.

(text continues on page 764)

Box 46-2 The Dying Person's Bill of Rights

- I have the right to be treated as a living human being until I die.
- I have the right to maintain a sense of hopefulness, however changing its focus may be.
- I have the right to be cared for by those who can maintain a sense of hopefulness, however changing this might be.
- I have the right to express my feelings and emotions about my approaching death, in my own way.
- I have the right to participate in decisions concerning my care.
- I have the right to expect continuing medical and nursing attention even though "cure" goals must be changed to "comfort" goals.
- I have the right not to die alone.
- I have the right to be free of pain.
- I have the right to have my questions answered honestly.
- I have the right not to be deceived.
- I have the right to have help from and for my family in accepting my death.
- I have the right to die in peace and dignity.
- I have the right to retain my individuality and not to be judged for my decisions, which may be contrary to the beliefs of others.
- I have the right to discuss and enlarge my religious and/or spiritual experiences, regardless of what they may mean to others.
- I have the right to expect that the sanctity of the human body will be respected after death.
- I have the right to be cared for by caring, sensitive, knowledgeable people who will attempt to understand my needs and will be able to gain some satisfaction in helping me face my death.

Source: A.J. Barbus, *American Journal of Nursing* 75 (1) (1975), 99.

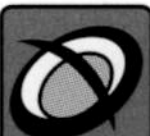

Providing Compassionate Care

THE DYING PERSON

D*ignity.* Treat the client who is dying with respect, dignity, warmth, and empathy. Be sensitive to the person's wishes. Listen when the person wants to talk. Respect the person's need for quiet and silence. Do not avoid the person if you feel uncomfortable or sad. Imagine how the person feels.

Whether a person is dying at home or in a facility, the environment should be comfortable and pleasant, quiet, well lit, and well ventilated. Try to keep equipment and supplies out of view. Some people find equipment like suction machines and drainage containers upsetting to look at. Keep expressions of concern (such as flowers and cards) in view. Many people find these comforting.

Be sensitive to the person's needs. Provide comfort through care and touch, if culturally appropriate.

Respect the person's religious views and practices. Do not impose your views on the person. Treat religious items and other personal possessions with care and respect.

I*ndependence.* Let the person do things without help, if able. Offer assistance before helping. Encourage the person. The person has the right to autonomy.

P*references.* The person has the right to make choices about his or her care, treatment, and environment. Respect these choices. Ask before providing care. Respect a person's decision to refuse treatment and not prolong life. In all health care settings, the client and family should be free to arrange the room as they wish. The room should reflect the client's choices. This shows respect and helps the person feel cared for.

P*rivacy.* The dying person has the right to privacy. Remember, do not expose the person during care. The person has the right not to have his or her body seen by others. Follow proper screening and privacy procedures. Provide privacy during prayer and spiritual moments. The person and family have the right to visit in private. In facilities, privacy may need to be arranged. A roommate may have to leave while the family visits. Some people may ask to see a spiritual adviser. The person also has the right to confidentiality. Protect this right before and after death. Share information about diagnosis, health, and treatment only with those involved with the person's care. Keep the person's final moments and cause of death, as well as statements and reactions of the family, confidential.

S*afety.* People who are dying are at high risk for falls, choking, and other accidents. Know the safety measures required for the client. The dying person has the right to be free from abuse, mistreatment, and neglect. Family members or health care team members may abuse or mistreat the person. The person has the right to be free of restraints (see Chapter 17). They are used only if ordered by a physician. Follow the safety measures in Chapter 16.

Emotional, Social, Intellectual, and Spiritual Needs

People who are dying need accurate information to make informed decisions. They may want to talk about their fears, worries, and anxieties. Some may want family and friends present. Some want to be alone. Others may want someone from the health care team to stay with them. Often a person needs to talk at night when things are quiet and there are few distractions. Sometimes, a person's fears and anxieties are worse at night. The following are ways you can meet a client's needs:

- *Listening.* The person may need to share worries and concerns with you. Let the person talk. Just being there and listening are helpful. You do not need to talk. Do not worry about saying the wrong thing or finding comforting words. Nothing need be said. Being there for the person is what counts. Sometimes the person does not want to talk but needs you nearby. If the person requests medical information, spiritual guidance, or counselling, immediately tell your supervisor. Remember, it is not your role to give clients information about their medical condition.
- *Touch.* Touch shows caring and support when words cannot. Touch, along with silence, is a powerful and compassionate way to communicate.
- *Respect.* The person may share thoughts about his or her religious or spiritual beliefs. Respect the person's beliefs.

Physical Needs

Dying may take a few minutes, hours, days, or weeks. Body processes slow down. The person becomes weak. Changes occur in levels of consciousness. The health care team encourages the person to do as much as possible independently. As the person weakens, more help is provided with personal care. The person may need to depend on others for all basic needs and activities of daily living.

- *Pain relief and comfort.* Some people have severe pain. Health care professionals administer medications to relieve pain. The care plan may call for other measures such as back massages and relaxation techniques. Skin care, personal hygiene, and good alignment promote comfort. Follow the care plan.
- *Comfort and positioning.* Frequent position changes and supportive devices also promote comfort. You may need help to turn the person slowly and gently. Semi-Fowler's position (Fowler's position with the knees slightly bent) is usually best for breathing problems.
- *Vision and eye care.* At the end of life, vision blurs and gradually fails. The person may find a darkened room frightening. The room should be well lit (if the person wishes). However, bright lights and glares should be avoided. Since the person's vision may be failing, explain what you are doing. Secretions may collect in the corners of the person's eyes. Ease the person's discomfort by providing eye care. Follow the care plan. It may call for a protective ointment and moist pads to be applied to the person's eyes.
- *Hearing.* Hearing is one of the last functions lost. Many people hear until the moment of death. Even unconscious people may hear. Always assume that the person can hear. Speak in a normal voice. Provide explanations and reassurance about care. Offer words of comfort. Avoid topics that could upset the person.
- *Speech.* The person may have difficulty speaking. It may be hard to understand the person. Some people cannot speak. Anticipate the person's needs. Ask "yes" or "no" questions. Avoid asking questions needing long answers. Do not tire the person with questions. However, do talk to the person.
- *Mouth care.* The person's mouth may feel dry, uncomfortable, or sore. Swallowing may be difficult and uncomfortable. Oral hygiene promotes comfort. Routine mouth care is given if the person can eat and drink. Frequent oral care is given as death nears and when the person has difficulty taking oral fluids. Oral hygiene is needed if mucus collects in the mouth and the person cannot swallow. Offer ice chips or small sips of fluids if the person has a dry mouth. Apply moisturizer to relieve dry, chapped lips. Follow the care plan.
- *Nostril care.* The person's nostrils may become crusted and irritated. Nasal secretions, an oxygen cannula, or a nasogastric tube are common causes. Carefully clean the nose. Apply lubricant as directed by the care plan.
- *Skin care.* Circulation to the arms and legs slows as death approaches. The hands and feet may feel especially cool. The skin colour may change and appear pale or mottled (blotchy). Although the person's skin may feel cool, the person is not usually aware of feeling cold. The upper parts of the body may sweat as circulation to the peripheral parts fails. The body temperature may rise. Only light bed coverings are needed. Blankets may make the person too warm and cause restlessness. Skin care, bathing, and frequent changes of linens and garments help keep the person comfortable. Measures must be taken to prevent pressure ulcers.
- *Elimination.* The person may have urinary or fecal incontinence. Follow the care plan for the use of incontinence products or bed protectors. Keep the person dry and clean. Give perineal care as needed. Constipation and urinary retention are common. The care plan may call for the use of enemas and

catheter care. This care may be delegated to you. Remember to follow Standard Precautions.

Comforting the Family

This is a stressful time for family members. They may be very tired, sad, and tearful. Watching a loved one die is very painful. So is dealing with the eventual loss of that person. If the family tells you they want to see a spiritual adviser, let your supervisor know immediately.

It may be very hard to find comforting words. Show your feelings by being respectful, empathetic, and supportive. You may need to listen to a family member who wants to talk. Do not feel the need to talk. Use touch to show your concern. In a home care setting, you can show your support in many ways. You might help by doing household management tasks while the family cares for the person who is dying. Or you might provide respite care to give the family a break. Follow the care plan.

In facilities, family members are usually allowed to stay as long as they wish. Sometimes they spend the night. The health care team helps make them as comfortable as possible.

No matter what the setting, you need to respect the family's right to privacy. At the same time, you cannot neglect care because the family is present. Most facilities let family members give care. You can suggest they take a break for a beverage or a meal.

Legal Issues

Much attention is given to the right to die. Many people do not want machines or other measures keeping them alive. Consent is needed for any treatment. All provinces and territories have legislation about the need for consent (see Chapter 10). Most clients give or withhold consent and make their own decisions about care. Some are unable to do so due to confusion, dementia, or other impairments. A substitute decision maker often makes decisions for these clients.

Advance Directive

An **advance directive (living will)** is a legal document in which a person states his or her wishes about future health care, treatment, and personal care. Health care includes all medical treatment: diagnostic, therapeutic, preventative, and palliative. Personal care includes shelter, hygiene, nutrition, clothing, and safety.

An advance directive is used when the person can no longer make or express his or her wishes. Advance directives allow people to control their future health care. Without an advance directive, family members sometimes have to make difficult decisions on behalf of a loved one. This can result in family conflict.

Every province and territory has legislation about advance directives. Most advance directives have a dual function. They allow a person to:

- Appoint a representative (proxy) to make medical care and treatment and/or personal care decisions
- Give written instructions about medical care and treatment and/or personal care

People often use advance directives to forbid certain types of treatment and care when there is no hope of recovery. For example, some people do not want life-sustaining measures to keep them alive. Life-sustaining measures are those that support or maintain life. Tube feedings, ventilators, and CPR (cardiopulmonary resuscitation) are examples. These measures and other machines keep a person alive when death is likely. An advance directive may instruct physicians

- Not to start measures that prolong dying
- To remove measures that prolong dying

Advance directives are known by different names and have different powers, depending on provincial or territorial legislation. For example, in Alberta advance directives are called *Personal Directives.* In Manitoba they are called *Health Care Directives.* And in Ontario they are called *Powers of Attorney for Personal Care.*

Most people appoint a family member or friend to be their representative or proxy. In some cases, someone else is named, such as a lawyer. The advance directive *only* comes into effect when a client can no longer make decisions about his or her own health care and personal care. When this happens, the proxy steps in to make decisions on behalf of the client. This person has been given the legal right to make decisions for the client.

In most provinces and territories, residents name a proxy to make decisions about personal care as well as medical care and treatment. However, in some parts of the country, a proxy can be used only for decisions about medical care and treatment.

Not all clients name a proxy. When no proxy is named, family members usually have the legal authority to make decisions on behalf of the client. Some provinces, however, require a court application before any decision can be made on behalf of an incapable person.

"Do Not Resuscitate" Orders

When death is sudden and unexpected, every effort is made to save the person's life. An emergency response system is activated. CPR is started (see Chapter 47). In facilities, nurses, physicians, and emergency staff rush to the person's bedside. In the community, ambulances and paramedics rush to the scene. They bring emergency and life-saving equipment with them. CPR and other life-support measures are continued until the person is resuscitated or until a physician declares the person dead.

Physicians often write "do not resuscitate" (DNR) or "no code" orders for patients who are not expected to recover. This means that the person will not be resuscitated. The person is allowed to die in peace and with dignity. The orders are written after consulting with the client and/or family. The family and/or the proxy in consultation with the physician make the decision if the client is not mentally able. Some people prepare an advance directive that contains DNR orders.

You may not agree with care and resuscitation decisions. However, you must follow the client's (or proxy's) wishes and physician's orders. These may be against your personal, religious, and cultural values. If you are not comfortable with care and resuscitation decisions, discuss the matter with your supervisor.

Signs of Death

There are signs that death is near. These signs may occur rapidly or slowly:

- Movement, muscle tone, and sensation are lost. This usually begins in the feet and legs. It eventually spreads to other parts. When a person's mouth muscles relax, the jaw drops. The mouth may stay open. The person's face often looks peaceful.
- Peristalsis and other digestive functions slow. Abdominal distention, fecal/urinary incontinence, fecal impaction, nausea, and vomiting are common. The person usually refuses to eat or drink.
- Body temperature rises. The person feels cool or cold, looks pale, and perspires heavily.
- Circulation fails. The pulse is fast, weak, and irregular. Blood pressure begins to fall. Skin may have a mottled appearance.
- The respiratory system fails. *Cheyne-Stokes* respirations are common. These are respirations that gradually increase in rate and depth, and then become shallow, slow, and stop for a few seconds. Mucus collects in the airway. This causes a wet, gurgling sound as the person breathes, known as the *death rattle*.
- Pain decreases as the person loses consciousness. Some people are conscious until the moment of death.

The signs of death include no pulse, respirations, or blood pressure. The pupils are fixed and dilated. A physician determines that death has occurred and pronounces the person dead. In some parts of the country, RNs are able to pronounce death in the home when the death is expected (see *Focus on Home Care: When Death Occurs* box).

Care of the Body after Death

Care of the body after (*post*) death (*mortem*) is called **postmortem care**. Postmortem care begins after the person is pronounced dead and when there is no autopsy required. (An *autopsy* is an examination of the body to determine the cause of death.) You may be asked to assist with postmortem care. During this process, you may have contact with blood or body fluids. Follow Standard Precautions.

Postmortem care is done to maintain the body's appearance. It helps prevent discolouration and skin damage. Remember, the right to privacy and the right to be treated with dignity and respect apply after death.

Within 2 to 3 hours after death, rigor mortis develops. **Rigor mortis** is the stiffness or rigidity (*rigor*) of skeletal muscles that occurs after death (*mortis*).

Postmortem care involves positioning the body in normal alignment before rigor mortis sets in. The family may want to see the body before it is taken to the morgue or funeral home. The body should be placed in a natural position for this viewing.

In some cases, the body is prepared only for viewing. Postmortem care is completed later at the funeral home. If the person dies at home, the funeral home usually does postmortem care.

Postmortem care may involve repositioning the body. This may be necessary to bathe soiled areas and to put the body in good alignment. Movement of the body can cause sounds from the body as air is expelled. Do not be frightened by these sounds. They are normal and expected.

You will not have full responsibility for postmortem care, but you may assist in the procedure.

Focus on Home Care

When Death Occurs

Some people die at home. You may be present at the time of death. Know your employer's policies and procedures. Call your supervisor and follow his or her directions. Be supportive of the family.

Assisting with Postmortem Care

Pre-Procedure

1 Wash your hands.
2 Collect the following:
- Postmortem kit (shroud or body bag, ID tags, gauze squares, and safety pins)
- Bed protectors
- Washbasin
- Bath towels and washcloths
- Tape
- Dressings
- Gloves
- Cotton balls
- Gown or clean garments

3 Provide for privacy.
4 Raise the bed to a comfortable working height. Make sure it is flat. *

Procedure

5 Put on gloves.
6 Position the body supine. Straighten the arms and legs. Place a pillow under the head and shoulders (Figure 46-1 on page 768).
7 Close the eyes. Gently pull the eyelids over the eyes. Apply moist cotton balls gently over the eyelids if the eyes will not stay closed.
8 Insert dentures if it is employer policy. If not, put them in a labelled denture container.
9 Close the mouth. If necessary, place a rolled towel under the chin to keep the mouth closed.
10 Follow employer policy about jewellery. Remove all jewellery, except for wedding rings if this is employer policy. List the jewellery that you removed. Place the jewellery and the list in a valuables envelope.
11 Place a cotton ball over the ring. Tape it in place.
12 Follow employer policy and instructions for drainage containers, tubes, and catheters.
13 Bathe soiled areas with plain water. Dry thoroughly.
14 Place a bed protector under the buttocks.
15 Remove soiled dressings and replace with clean ones.
16 Put a clean gown, pyjamas, nightgown, or clothes on the body, as instructed. Position the body as in step 6.
17 Brush and comb the hair if necessary.
18 Cover the body to the shoulders with a sheet if the family will view the body.
19 Put the person's belongings in a bag labelled with the person's name.*
20 Remove supplies, equipment, and linens. Straighten the room. Provide soft lighting.*
21 Remove gloves. Wash your hands.
22 If the family views the body, leave the room. Return after the family leaves.
23 Wash your hands. Put on gloves.
24 Fill out the ID tags. Tie one to an ankle or to the right big toe.*
25 Place the body in the body bag or cover it with a sheet.* Or apply the shroud (Figure 46-2 on page 769):
  a Bring the top down over the head.
  b Fold the bottom up over the feet.
  c Fold the sides over the body.
  d Pin or tape the shroud in place.
26 Attach the second ID tag to the shroud, sheet, or body bag.*
27 Leave the denture cup with the body.
28 Provide for privacy.
29 Remove gloves. Wash your hands.

Continued

Assisting with Postmortem Care—cont'd

Post-Procedure

30 Strip the bed after the body has been removed. Wear gloves.*

31 Remove gloves. Wash your hands.

32 Report the following to your supervisor:

- The time the body was taken by the funeral director
- What was done with jewellery, personal items, etc.
- What was done with dentures

*Steps marked with an asterisk may not apply in community settings.

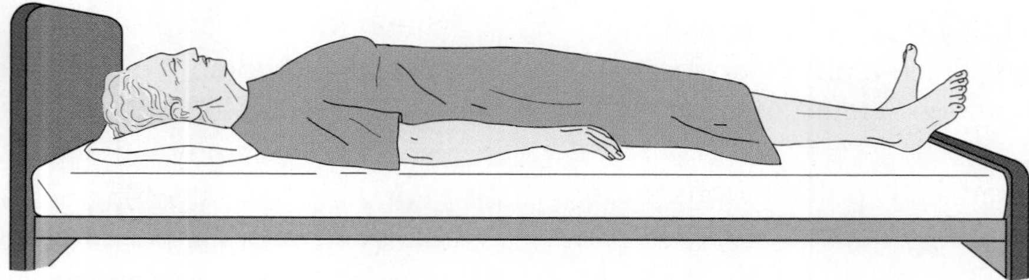

Figure 46-1 The body is in the supine position. Arms are straight at the sides. A pillow is under the head and shoulders.

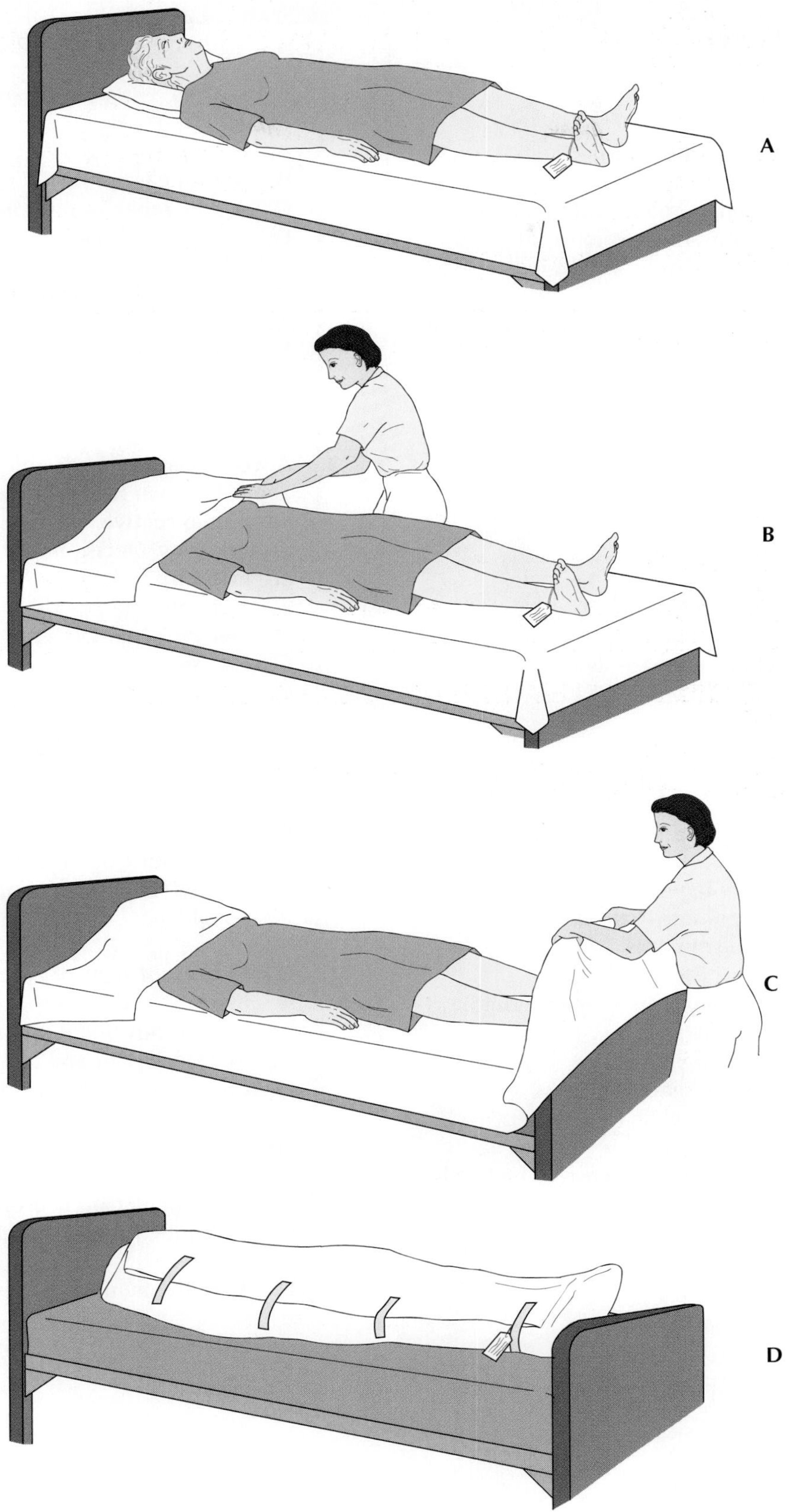

Figure 46-2 Applying a shroud. **A,** Place the body on the shroud. **B,** Bring the top of the shroud down over the head. **C,** Fold the bottom up over the feet. **D,** Fold the sides over the body. Tape or pin the sides together. Attach the ID tag.

REVIEW

Circle the BEST answer.

1. Reincarnation is the belief that
   A. There is no afterlife
   B. The spirit or soul is reborn into another human body or another form of life
   C. The body keeps its physical form in the afterlife
   D. Only the spirit or soul is present in the afterlife

2. Adults of all ages often fear
   A. Dying alone
   B. Reincarnation
   C. The five stages of grief
   D. Advance directives

3. People in the stage of denial
   A. Are angry
   B. Make "deals" with God
   C. Are sad or quiet
   D. Refuse to believe they are dying

4. Palliative care is
   A. Treatment that prolongs life
   B. Physical therapy for people with severe back pain
   C. Massage therapy and relaxation techniques to relieve pain
   D. Services for people with a progressive and life-threatening illness that relieve or reduce uncomfortable symptoms

5. When caring for a dying person, you should
   A. Listen and use touch
   B. Do most of the talking
   C. Keep the room darkened
   D. Speak in a loud voice

6. As death approaches, the last sense to be lost is
   A. Sight
   B. Taste
   C. Smell
   D. Hearing

7. Care of the dying person includes the following *except*
   A. Eye care
   B. Mouth care
   C. Active range-of-motion exercises
   D. Position changes

8. The dying person is positioned in
   A. The supine position
   B. Fowler's position
   C. Good body alignment
   D. The dorsal recumbent position

9. A woman is no longer able to make decisions about her own health care. Through an advance directive, she has appointed her sister as her proxy. Decisions about her health care are made by
   A. Her son
   B. Her physician
   C. Her sister
   D. Her lawyer

10. A "do not resuscitate" order has been written for a client. This means
    A. CPR will not be done
    B. The person has a living will
    C. Life-prolonging measures will be carried out
    D. The person will be kept alive as long as possible

11. Which are *not* signs of approaching death?
    A. Increased body temperature and rapid pulse
    B. Loss of movement and muscle tone
    C. Increased pain and blood pressure
    D. Cheyne-Stokes respirations

12. Postmortem care is done
    A. After rigor mortis sets in
    B. After the person is pronounced dead
    C. When the funeral director arrives for the body
    D. After the family has viewed the body

Answers to these questions are on page 828.

CHAPTER

47

BASIC EMERGENCY CARE

OBJECTIVES

- Define the key terms listed in this chapter
- Describe the signs, symptoms, and emergency care for cardiac arrest and obstructed airway
- Describe the signs, symptoms, and emergency care for hemorrhage
- Describe the signs, symptoms, and emergency care for shock
- Describe different types of seizures and how to care for a person during a seizure
- Describe the causes, types, and emergency care for burns
- Identify common causes of and emergency care for fainting
- Describe the signs of and emergency care for stroke
- Learn the procedures described in this chapter

KEY TERMS

anaphylaxis A life-threatening sensitivity to an antigen

cardiac arrest The heart and breathing stop suddenly and without warning

cardiopulmonary resuscitation (CPR) Emergency procedure used to restore breathing and circulation after cardiac arrest

convulsion Violent and sudden contractions or tremors of muscles

fainting The sudden loss of consciousness from an inadequate blood supply to the brain

first aid Emergency care given to an ill or injured person before medical help arrives

foreign body airway obstruction (FBAO) The blockage of the airway by an object, causing the person to choke

hemorrhage Excessive loss of blood in a short time

respiratory arrest Breathing stops

seizure Brief disturbances in the brain's normal electrical function; affects awareness, movement, and/or sensation

shock A condition that results when organs and tissues do not get enough blood

tonic-clonic seizure A type of generalized seizure where the person has convulsions

Emergencies can occur anywhere. Sometimes you can save a life if you know what to do. Most support workers are required to take a first aid course and a basic life support course. These courses prepare you to give care when emergencies occur. Once you are in the workforce, it is important to keep your skills up-to-date. You will need to keep your certification current by taking additional courses every year or so.

The basic life support procedures in this chapter are given as information. They do not replace certification training. You need to take a basic life support course for people who assist in health care settings.

EMERGENCY CARE

First aid is the emergency care given to an ill or injured person before medical help arrives. Its goals are to:

- Prevent death
- Prevent injuries from becoming worse

In an emergency, the Emergency Medical Service (EMS) system should be activated. Emergency personnel (paramedics, emergency medical technicians) rush to the scene. They know how to treat, stabilize, and transport people with life-threatening problems. Their ambulances have emergency equipment, supplies, and medications. Emergency personnel communicate with physicians in hospital emergency rooms. The physicians tell them what to do. To activate the EMS system, dial 911. Or, in areas without 911 service call the local police or fire department or telephone operator. Be prepared. Have these numbers readily available before an emergency.

In facilities, a nurse decides when to activate the EMS system. The nurse tells you how to help. If the person stops breathing or is having a cardiac arrest, the nurse may start cardiopulmonary resuscitation (CPR) (page 774). Some facilities allow support workers to start CPR. Others do not. Know your employer's policy about CPR.

In community settings, you decide when to activate the EMS system. Home care agencies have guidelines about when to activate the EMS system and when to call your supervisor. Some home care agencies do not allow support workers to start CPR. Know your employer's policies.

Sometimes death is expected, especially for people receiving palliative care. Sometimes people who are very ill and expect to die have "do not resuscitate" (DNR) orders. This means that the person wishes not to be resuscitated (see Chapter 46). Make sure you know if a client has DNR orders. This information is in the care plan. Also check with your supervisor.

Each emergency is different. However, the guidelines in Box 47-1 apply to any emergency.

Box 47-1 Guidelines for Providing Emergency Care

- Know your limits. Do not do more than you are able. Do not perform an unfamiliar procedure. Do what you can under the circumstances.
- Stay calm. This helps the person feel more secure.
- Practise Standard Precautions to the extent possible. During emergencies, contact with blood, body fluids, secretions, and excretions is likely. Be prepared for emergencies. For home care visits, always have two pairs of gloves and a barrier device (for mouth-to-mouth rescue breathing) in your bag. In facilities, know where to find emergency supplies.
- Check the scene for safety. The situation that caused the injury may also be hazardous to you. Proceed with caution.
- Determine responsiveness (consciousness). Tap the person's shoulder and ask loudly in each ear, "Are you okay?" Tap infants on the feet to check for responsiveness.
- Check for breathing, a pulse, and bleeding.
- Keep the person lying down or as you found him or her. Moving the person could make an injury worse.
- Activate the EMS system or tell someone else to do so. An operator will send emergency vehicles and personnel to the scene. *If you make the call, do not hang up until the operator has hung up.* Give the operator the following information:
  - Your location—street address and city or town, cross streets or roads, and landmarks
  - Telephone number you are calling from
  - What happened (for example, heart attack, accident, fire)—police, fire equipment, and ambulances may be needed
  - How many people need help
  - Condition of the person, obvious injuries, and life-threatening situations
- Perform necessary emergency measures.
- Do not remove the person's clothing unless you have to. If you must remove clothing, tear or cut garments along the seams.
- Keep the person warm. Cover the person with a blanket, coat, or sweater.
- Reassure the responsive person. Explain what is happening and that help is on the way.
- Do not give the person food or fluids.
- Keep bystanders away. They invade privacy and tend to stare, give advice, and comment about the person's condition. They may increase the person's anxiety.

Basic Life Support

When the heart and breathing stop, the person is clinically dead. Blood and oxygen are not circulated through the body. Brain injury and other organ damage occur within minutes. Basic life support (BLS) procedures support breathing and circulation. These life-saving measures require speed, skill, and efficiency.

The basic life support discussion and procedures that follow assume that the person does not have injuries from trauma. If injuries are present, special measures are needed to position the person and open the airway. Such measures are learned when you take a basic life support certification course.

Cardiac Arrest

The heart and breathing can stop suddenly and without warning. This is a state of **cardiac arrest**. A person who has a cardiac arrest suddenly collapses. Common causes include heart disease, drowning, electric shock, airway obstruction (choking), and drug overdose. A blow to the chest can also cause cardiac arrest.

Immediately after cardiac arrest, the person's heart usually has abnormal heart rhythms. The heart cannot pump blood. Oxygen is not circulated through the body. Unless breathing and circulation are restored (with CPR), permanent brain injury and other organ damage occur within minutes. A regular heartbeat also must be restored. This is done with a defibrillator (see page 789). If the heartbeat is not restored, the person will die.

Respiratory Arrest

Respiratory arrest occurs when breathing stops. Heart action continues for several minutes. If breathing is not restored, cardiac arrest occurs. Causes of respiratory arrest include:

- Drowning
- Stroke
- Foreign body airway obstruction (FBAO)—choking on an object (see page 784)
- Drug overdose
- Electric shock (including lightning strikes)
- Smoke inhalation
- Suffocation
- Heart attack
- Coma
- Injuries from motor vehicle accidents or other trauma

Chain of Survival

The Heart and Stroke Foundation of Canada's basic life support courses teach the *Chain of Survival*. The actions in the chain are taken for heart attack, cardiac arrest, stroke, and FBAO (choking). They also apply to other life-threatening problems. They are done as soon as possible. Any delay reduces the person's chance of surviving.

Chain of Survival first aid actions include:

- *Early recognition*—This means that you must realize that a person is having a medical emergency. You must recognize the warning signs of heart attack, cardiac arrest, stroke (see Chapter 31), and choking (see page 784).
- *Early access to the emergency response system*—This means activating the EMS system. It is essential to get help as quickly as possible. The Heart and Stroke Foundation of Canada teaches to "phone first." You must phone the emergency number before you do anything else. This ensures emergency personnel are on the way while you help the person. Remember, the emergency number is 911 in most Canadian cities and towns. Confirm the EMS number in your community. Facilities have codes that are called for life-threatening emergencies.
- *Early CPR*—See below.
- *Early defibrillation*—See page 789.
- *Early advanced care*—This is given by EMS staff, physicians, and nurses. They give medications and perform other life-saving measures.

Cardiopulmonary Resuscitation (CPR)

Cardiopulmonary resuscitation (CPR) is an emergency procedure used to restore breathing and circulation during cardiac arrest. It must be started at once when a person is in cardiac arrest. It provides oxygen to the brain and heart until defibrillation or advanced emergency care is given.

There are three major signs of cardiac arrest:

- No response
- No breathing or visible signs of circulation—coughing or movement
- No pulse

The person's skin is cool, pale, and clammy. The person is not coughing or moving.

CPR has three basic parts (the ABCs of CPR):

- **A**irway
- **B**reathing
- **C**irculation

Airway. The respiratory passages (airway) must be open to restore breathing. The airway often is obstructed (blocked) during cardiac arrest. The person's tongue falls toward the back of the throat and blocks the airway. The *head-tilt/chin-lift manoeuvre* opens the airway (Figure 47-1):

- Position the person supine on a hard, flat surface.
- Kneel or stand at the person's side.
- Place the palm of one hand on the forehead.
- Tilt the head back by pushing down on the forehead with your palm.
- Place the fingers of the other hand under the bony part of the chin.
- Gently lift the chin up as you tilt the head backward with your other hand.

The head-tilt/chin-lift manoeuvre is used only if you do not suspect a head, neck, or spinal injury. If head, neck, or spinal injury is likely, use the *jaw-thrust manoeuvre* (Figure 47-2). This method opens the airway without moving the neck:

- Place one hand on each side of the person's head. Rest your elbows on the surface on which the person is lying.
- Grasp the lower jaw (the back corners below the ears). Lift upward and outward with both hands.
- Ensure that the person's head is not tilted backward or turned from side to side.

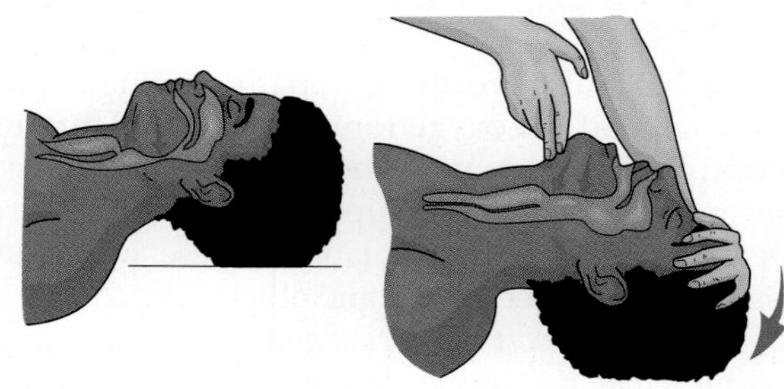

Figure 47-1 The head-tilt/chin-lift manoeuvre opens the airway. Place one hand on the person's forehead. Apply pressure to tilt the head back. Lift the chin with the fingers of your other hand.

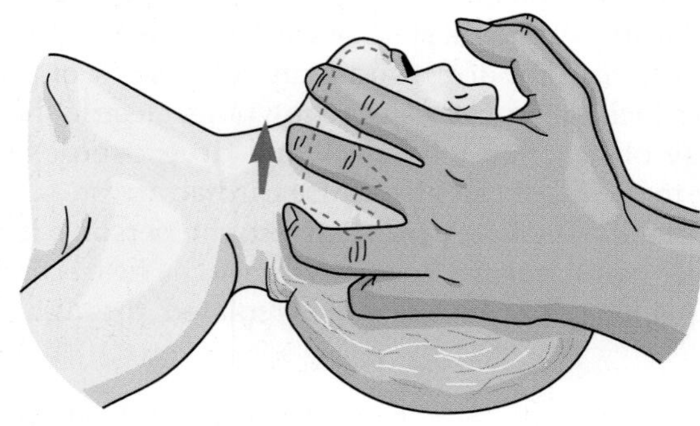

Figure 47-2 Jaw-thrust without head tilt. Grasp the lower jaw on both sides of the head. Lift the jaw upward and outward.

When the airway is open, check for vomitus, loose dentures, or other objects. These can obstruct the airway during rescue breathing. Remove dentures and wipe vomitus away with your index and middle fingers. Wear gloves or cover your fingers with a cloth. Although you must not waste time, try to protect the dentures from loss or damage.

Breathing. Air is not inhaled when breathing stops. The person must get oxygen. Otherwise, permanent brain injury and organ damage occur. Breathing is done for the person. This is called *rescue breathing*.

Before you start rescue breathing, check for normal breathing (Figure 47-3). It should take no more than 10 seconds to do the following:

- Maintain an open airway.
- Place your ear over the person's mouth and nose.
- Observe the person's chest.
- *Look* to see if the person's chest rises and falls.
- *Listen* for the escape of air.
- *Feel* for the flow of air on your cheek.

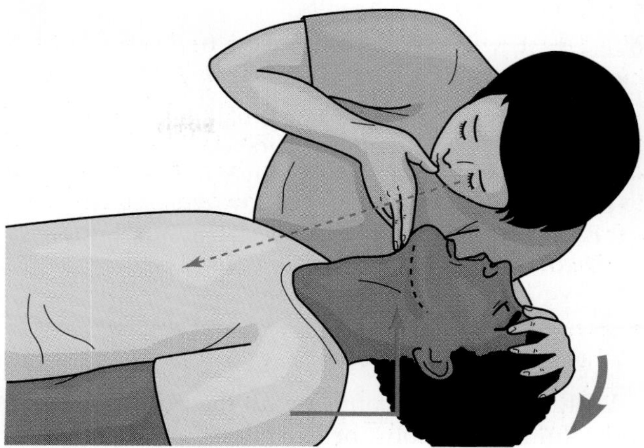

Figure 47-3 Determining breathing. *Look* to see if the chest rises and falls. *Listen* for the escape of air. *Feel* for the flow of air on your cheek.

Gasping or weak attempts to breathe are not normal. If you are unsure if breathing is normal, proceed with rescue breathing.

Rescue breathing involves inflating the person's lungs. There are several types of rescue breathing, depending on the situation. *Mouth-to-mouth* rescue breathing (Figure 47-4) involves placing your mouth over the person's mouth. (See *Focus on Children: Rescue Breathing* box on page 776.) To give mouth-to-mouth rescue breathing:

- Keep the airway open.
- Pinch the person's nostrils shut. Use your thumb and index finger. Place your hand on the forehead. Pinching the nostrils prevents air from escaping through the nose.
- Take a deep breath.
- Place your mouth tightly over the person's mouth.
- Blow air into the person's mouth slowly. Be sure the person's chest rises each time. This means the lungs are filling with air.
- Remove your mouth from the person's mouth. You should hear the escape of air when the person exhales.
- Then take another deep breath and give another slow rescue breath.
- Give 1 rescue breath about every 5 seconds. Each rescue breath should last about 2 seconds. Giving rescue breaths too quickly causes the air to enter and fill the stomach (gastric distension), which may cause the person to vomit.

A

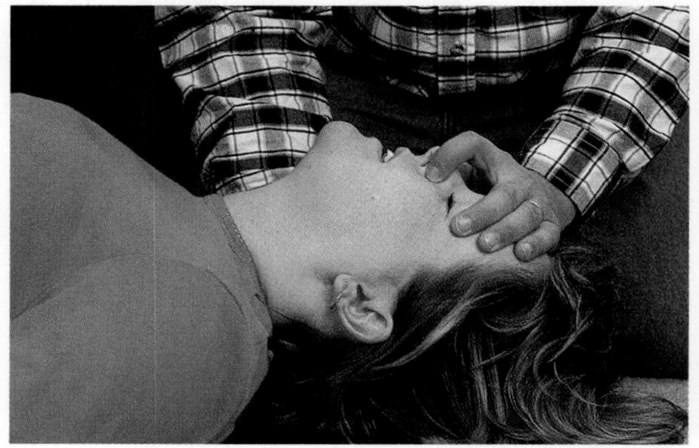

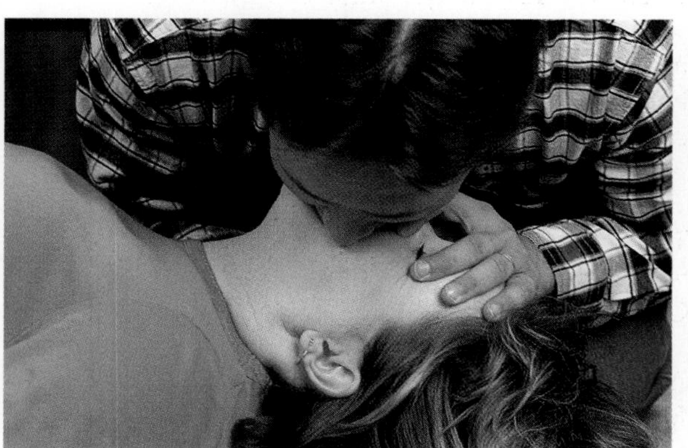

B

Figure 47-4 Mouth-to-mouth rescue breathing. **A,** Open the person's airway. Pinch the nostrils shut. **B,** Seal the person's mouth with your mouth.

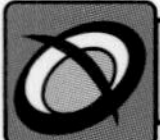

Focus on Children

RESCUE BREATHING

The mouth position for rescue breathing is the same for children as for adults. However, for infants, cover the *mouth and nose* tightly with your mouth. For children and infants:

- Each rescue breath should last about 1 to 1½ seconds
- Give 1 breath every 3 seconds

With this method, contact with the person's blood, body fluids, secretions, or excretions is likely. Therefore, *mouth-to-barrier device* rescue breathing is used whenever possible. A barrier device is placed over the person's mouth and nose. It prevents contact with the person's mouth, blood, body fluids, secretions, and excretions (Figure 47-5). The seal must be tight.

The Ambu bag (see Chapter 43) is another barrier device. It can be used to provide oxygen during rescue breathing.

Mouth-to-mouth rescue breathing is not always possible. *Mouth-to-nose* rescue breathing is used when:

- You cannot ventilate through the person's mouth
- You cannot open the mouth
- You cannot make a tight seal for mouth-to-mouth breathing
- The mouth is severely injured
- Rescuing a drowning victim.

The mouth is closed for mouth-to-nose rescue breathing. The head-tilt/chin-lift manoeuvre opens the airway. Pressure is placed on the chin to close the mouth. To give a breath, place your mouth over the person's nose and blow air into the nose (Figure 47-6). After giving a rescue breath, remove your mouth from the person's nose.

Some people breathe through openings (*stomas*) in their necks (Figure 47-7). They need *mouth-to-stoma* rescue breathing during cardiac or respiratory arrest. Seal your mouth around the stoma and blow air into the stoma (Figure 47-8). Before giving mouth-to-mouth or mouth-to-nose rescue breathing, always check to see if the person has a stoma. Other rescue breathing methods are not effective if the person has a stoma.

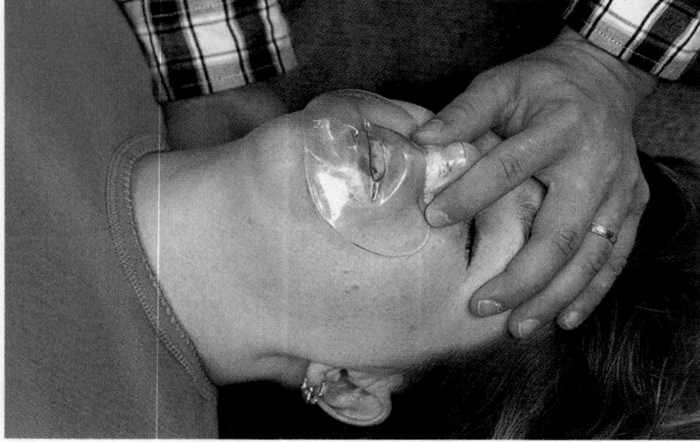

Figure 47-5 Barrier device.

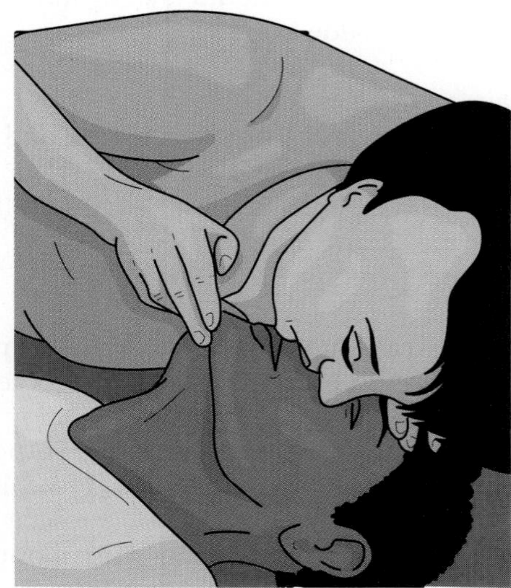

Figure 47-6 Mouth-to-nose rescue breathing.

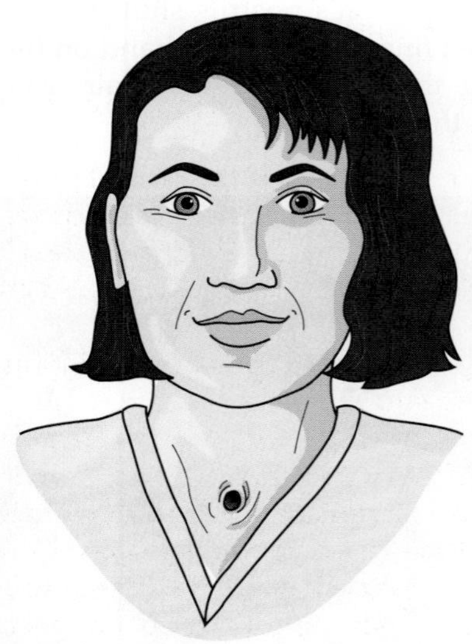

Figure 47-7 A stoma in the neck. The person breathes in and out of the stoma.

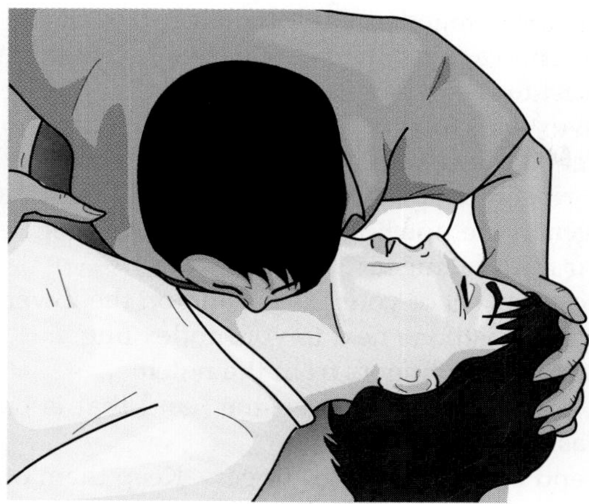

Figure 47-8 Mouth-to-stoma rescue breathing.

When CPR is started, 2 rescue breaths are given at first. Always check to make sure the chest rises and falls with each breath. Then breaths are given at a rate of about 1 every 5 seconds. During CPR, 2 breaths are given after every 15 chest compressions (see below).

Circulation. The brain and other organs must receive blood. Otherwise, permanent damage results. In cardiac arrest the heart has stopped beating. Therefore blood must be pumped through the body in some other way. Chest compressions force blood through the circulatory system. A *chest compression* is pressure applied to the breastbone (sternum).

Before starting chest compressions, check for signs of circulation:

- Look for normal breathing, coughing, or movement in response to rescue breathing.
- Check for a pulse.

If a pulse or signs of circulation are present, do not proceed with chest compressions.

To check for a pulse, use the carotid pulse for adults and children. Use the brachial pulse for infants. Take no longer than 10 seconds to perform the check.

To find the carotid pulse in adults and children:

- Maintain the head-tilt position with your hand on the person's forehead.
- Place 2 or 3 fingers of your other hand on the person's trachea (windpipe).
- Slide your fingertips down off the trachea to the groove of the side of the neck nearest to you (Figure 47-9). Press the neck gently with your fingers to feel the pulse. Do not use your thumb to check the pulse.

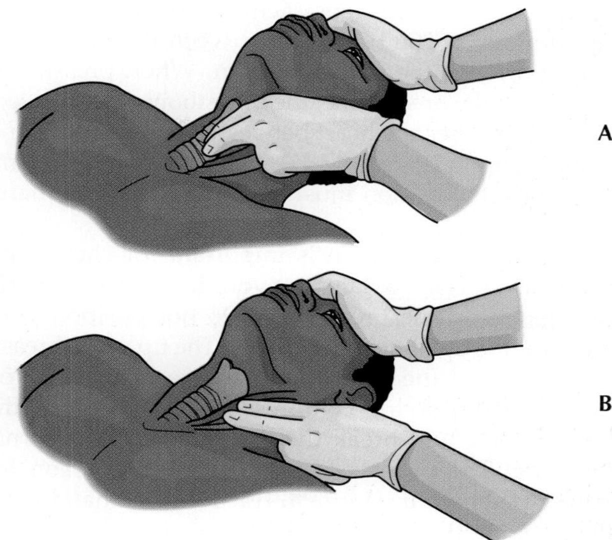

Figure 47-9 Locating the carotid pulse. **A,** Place 2 or 3 fingers on the trachea. **B,** Move your fingers down into the groove of the neck where the carotid pulse is located. Do not use your thumb to check the pulse.

To find the brachial pulse in infants:

- Maintain the head-tilt position with your hand on the infant's forehead.
- Place your thumb on the outside of the infant's arm, just above the elbow.
- Place your middle and index fingers on the inside of the arm between the elbow and the shoulder (Figure 47-10). Press gently to feel the pulse.

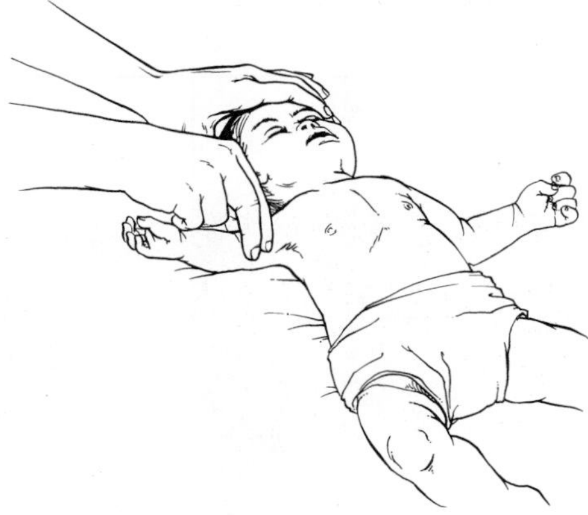

Figure 47-10 Locating the brachial pulse for an infant. Place your thumb on the outside of the infant's arm. Place your middle and index fingers on the inside of the arm between the elbow and shoulder. Press gently. Source: Reproduced with permission. Basic Life Support for Healthcare Providers, 1997–1999.

If you do not find signs of circulation, provide chest compressions. The heart lies between the breastbone (sternum) and the spinal column. When pressure is applied to the breastbone, the breastbone is depressed. This compresses the heart between the breastbone and spinal column (Figure 47-11). For effective chest compressions, the person must be supine and on a hard, flat surface.

Proper hand position is important for chest compressions. It is important that your hands are properly positioned on the breastbone. Do not position your hands at the tip of the breastbone. (The tip of the breastbone is called the *zyphoid process*. See Figure 13-5 on page 130.) Applying compressions at the tip of the breastbone could break the bone and cause internal bleeding. The process of locating hand position for adults is shown in Figure 47-12. To locate hand positions for adults:

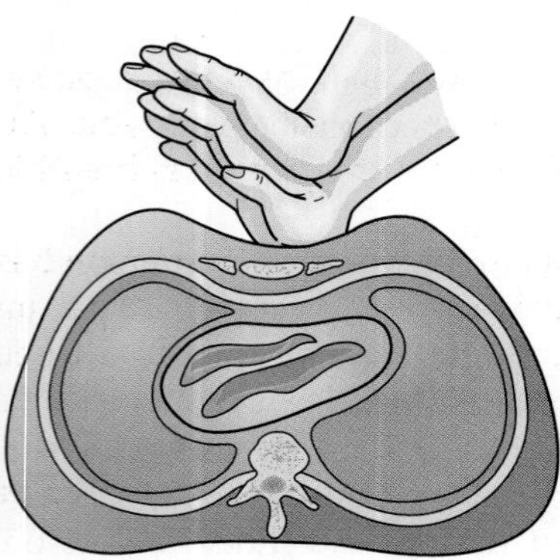

Figure 47-11 The heart lies between the breastbone and spinal column. The heart is compressed when pressure is applied to the breastbone.

- Use 2 or 3 fingers to find the lower part of the person's rib cage on the side near you. Use the hand closest to the person's feet.
- Move your fingers up along the rib cage to the notch at the centre of the chest. The notch is where the ribs and breastbone meet. Place your middle finger in the notch. Place your index finger beside your middle finger.
- Place the heel of your other hand on the lower half of the breastbone next to your index finger.
- Remove your fingers from the notch.
- Place your other hand on the hand that is on the breastbone.
- Extend or interlace your fingers. Keep them off the chest (see Figure 47-11).

You must be positioned properly for chest compressions. Keep your arms straight and lock your elbows. Your shoulders are directly over your hands (Figure 47-13). Push straight down to depress the breastbone about 4 to 5 cm (1½ to 2 inches). Then release pressure without removing your hands from the chest. Give compressions in a regular rhythm at a rate of 100 compressions per minute.

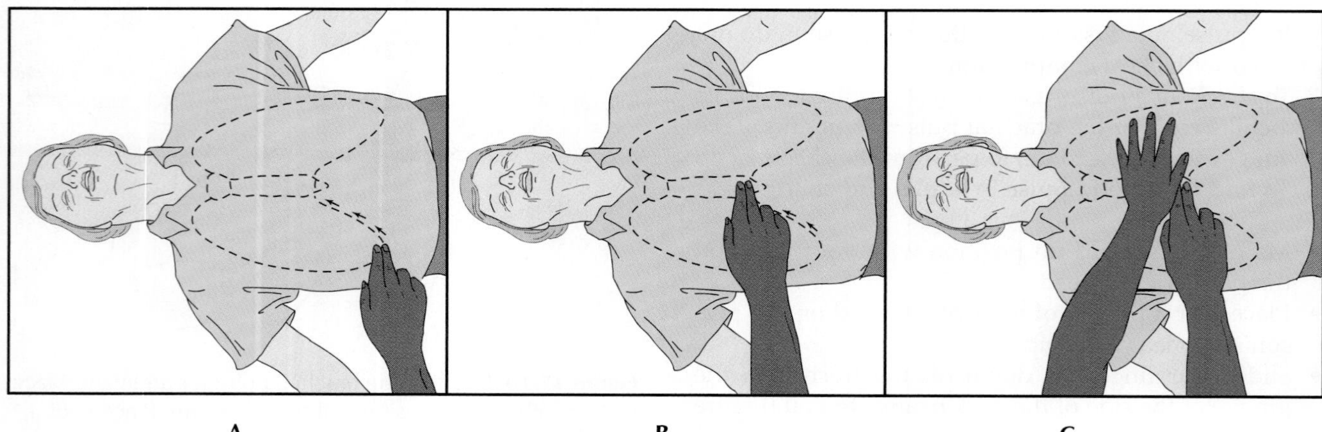

A B C

Figure 47-12 Proper hand position for adult CPR. **A,** Find the rib cage. **B,** Move your fingers along the rib cage to the notch. **C,** Place the heel of your other hand next to your index finger.

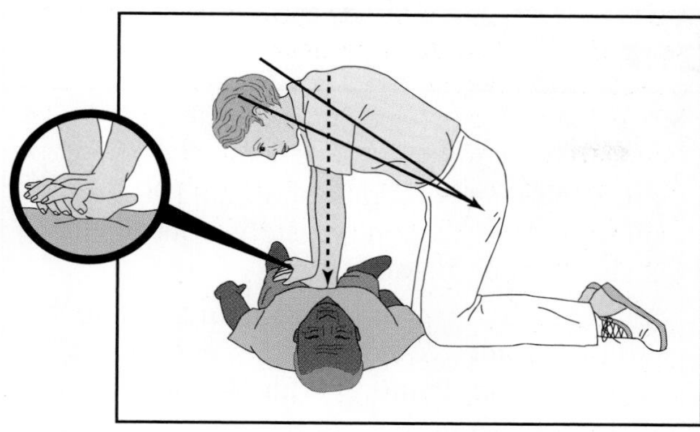

Figure 47-13 To give chest compressions, keep your arms straight and shoulders over your hands.

 Performing CPR on Adults

CPR is done for cardiac arrest. You must determine if cardiac arrest or fainting has occurred. *CPR is done when the person does not respond, is not breathing, and has no pulse.* Basic life support involves the following sequence:

1. See if the person is responding. Tap or gently shake the person, call the person by name, and shout "Are you okay?" If there is no response, the person is unconscious.
2. *Activate the EMS system at once if the person does not respond.* Long-term care facilities and hospitals have an emergency response system. If a person has a cardiac or respiratory arrest in a hospital or long-term care facility, the facility's emergency response system is activated. In community settings, dial 911 (see Box 47-1 on page 773).
3. Get the automated external defibrillator (AED) if one is available (see page 789).
4. Open the airway using the head-tilt/chin-lift manoeuvre. Or if you suspect a head, neck, or spinal injury, use the jaw thrust manoeuvre (see Figure 47-2 on page 774).
5. Check for breathing. *Look* at the person's chest to see if it rises and falls. *Listen* for the escape of air during expiration. *Feel* for the flow of air. To feel for air, place your cheek near the person's nose.
6. Give 2 slow rescue breaths if the person is not breathing. The chest rises when air enters the lungs. If the chest rises with the first breath, give the second breath. If the chest does not rise with the first breath, change the tilt of the head and the lift of the chin. Give the second breath. If the chest still does not rise, the person may have an obstructed airway (see page 784).
7. Check for circulation. Check for a pulse using the carotid artery on the side near you. At the same time, look to see if the person is breathing, coughing, or moving.
8. Start chest compressions if the person has no pulse. Give compressions at a rate of 100 per minute.
9. Give 15 compressions followed by 2 rescue breaths. Do this for 1 minute (4 sets of 15 compressions and 2 rescue breaths). Then check for circulation. Continue CPR if there are no signs of circulation.

Cardiopulmonary resuscitation is done alone or with another person. *Never practise CPR on another person.* Serious damage can be done. Mannequins are used to learn CPR.

(text continues on page 781)

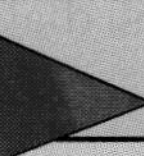

Adult CPR—One Rescuer

Procedure

1 Check the scene for safety. Use a barrier device and gloves.
2 Determine unresponsiveness.
3 Activate the EMS system or the facility's emergency response system. Or have someone else do so.
4 Position the person supine. Logroll the person so there is no twisting of the spine. The person must be on a hard, flat surface. Place the person's arms alongside the body.
5 Open the airway. Use the head-tilt/chin-lift manoeuvre.
6 Check for breathing. (Look, listen, and feel for breathing.)
7 Give 2 slow rescue breaths if the person is not breathing or not breathing adequately. Each breath should take 2 seconds. If the chest rises with the first breath, give the second breath. Let the person's lungs deflate between breaths. If the chest does not rise with the first breath, change the tilt of the head and the lift of the chin. Give the second breath.
8 Check for a carotid pulse and for visible signs of circulation (breathing, coughing, and moving). This should take 5 to 10 seconds. Use your other hand to keep the airway open with the head-tilt/chin-lift manoeuvre.
9 Give 15 chest compressions if there is no pulse or visible signs of circulation. Compress the chest at a rate of about 100 per minute. After 15 compressions, follow with 2 slow rescue breaths.
  a Establish a rhythm, and count out loud. (Try: "1 and, 2 and, 3 and, 4 and, 5 and, 6 and, 7 and, 8 and, 9 and, 10 and, 11 and, 12 and, 13 and, 14 and, 15.")
  b Open the airway, and give 2 slow rescue breaths.
  c Repeat this step until 4 sets of 15 compressions and 2 breaths are given.
10 Check for carotid pulse. Also check for visible signs of circulation (breathing, coughing, and moving).
11 Continue CPR if the person has no signs of circulation. Begin with chest compressions.
12 Continue the set of 15 compressions and 2 breaths. Check for circulation every few minutes.
13 Do the following if the person has signs of circulation:
  a Check for breathing.
  b Position the person in the recovery position (page 788) if the person is breathing.
  c Monitor breathing and circulation.
14 Do the following if the person has signs of circulation but breathing is absent:
  a Give 1 rescue breath every 5 seconds.
  b Monitor circulation.

Adult CPR—Two Rescuers

Procedure

1 Check the scene for safety. Use barrier devices and gloves.
2 Determine unresponsiveness.
3 One rescuer activates the EMS system or the facility's emergency response system.
4 Position the person supine. Logroll the person so there is no twisting of the spine. The person must be on a hard, flat surface. Place the person's arms alongside the body.
5 Open the airway using the head-tilt/chin-lift manoeuvre.
6 Check for breathing. (Look, listen, and feel for breathing.)
7 Give 2 slow rescue breaths if the person is not breathing or if breathing is inadequate. If the chest rises with the first breath, give the second breath. Let the person's lungs deflate between breaths. If the chest does not rise after the first breath, change the tilt of the head and the lift of the chin. Give the second breath.
8 Check for a carotid pulse and for visible signs of circulation (breathing, coughing, and moving).
9 Perform two-person CPR (Figure 47-14) if there are no signs of circulation.
   a Rescuer #2 gives chest compressions at a rate of 100 per minute. Count out loud in a rhythm. (Try: "1 and, 2 and, 3 and, 4 and, 5 and, 6 and, 7 and, 8 and, 9 and, 10 and, 11 and, 12 and, 13 and, 14 and, 15.")
   b Rescuer #1 gives 2 slow rescue breaths after every 15 compressions. While rescuer #1 gives the rescue breaths, rescuer #2 stops the compressions. Rescuer #2 continues chest compressions after the rescue breaths.
10 After 4 sets of 15 compressions and 2 rescue breaths, rescuer #1 checks for circulation—carotid pulse, breathing, coughing, and moving.
11 Continue with 15 compressions and 2 slow rescue breaths if the person has no signs of circulation. Start with chest compressions.

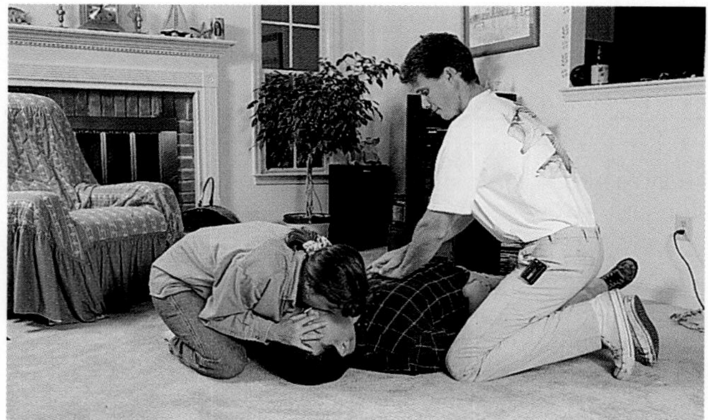

Figure 47-14 Two people performing CPR.

Performing CPR on Infants and Children

Cardiac arrest caused by heart disease is rare in children. More common causes involve diseases and injuries that lead to respiratory arrest or circulatory failure. Sudden infant death syndrome (SIDS), respiratory diseases, airway obstruction, drowning, infection, and nervous system diseases are the most common causes of cardiac arrest in children under 1 year of age. Injuries are the most common cause in children older than 1 year. They include motor vehicle injuries, sports injuries, bicycle injuries, drowning, and burns.

Basic life support for infants and young children (1 to 8 years) also involves activating the EMS system and determining unresponsiveness, breathing, and pulse. However, there are some important differences from the adult procedures:

- Injuries are a likely cause of respiratory or cardiac arrest. Head, neck, and spinal cord injuries are possible. Therefore do not move or shake the child to determine responsiveness. Check unresponsiveness by tapping or shouting to get a response.
- If there are no injuries and if the child is small, carry the child to the telephone. This makes calling the EMS system easier.
- Move the child from a dangerous location. Also move the child if you cannot perform CPR where the child is lying.
- If you must move the child, make sure the head does not roll, twist, or tilt. Hold the head and body straight without twisting. Use the logrolling procedure to turn the child.
- Use the head-tilt/chin-lift manoeuvre for infants and children. Do not hyperextend the head as in the adult. Rather, tilt the head to a normal (neutral) or *sniffing* position (Figure 47-15).
- If neck injury is suspected, use the jaw thrust manoeuvre (see Figure 47-2 on page 774).
- In children under 1 year of age, use the brachial pulse to determine pulselessness (see page 777).
- Keep the airway open throughout CPR. *Use only one hand to give chest compressions on a child. Use only 2 or 3 fingers to give chest compressions on an infant.* Keep the other hand on the forehead to maintain head tilt. Steps 8a and 9a of *CPR for Infants and Children (8 Years of Age and Under)* describe how to locate proper hand position for chest compressions.
- For children, use both hands for the head-tilt/chin-lift manoeuvre when giving breaths.
- Compress the chest at a rate of 100 per minute.
- *Give 5 chest compressions followed by 1 slow rescue breath.*
- *Repeat 20 sets of 5 compressions followed by 1 rescue breath. Twenty sets will take slightly longer than 1 minute to complete.*

See Table 47-1 for the Heart and Stroke Foundation of Canada's summary of the basic life support requirements for adults, children, and infants.

(text continues on page 784)

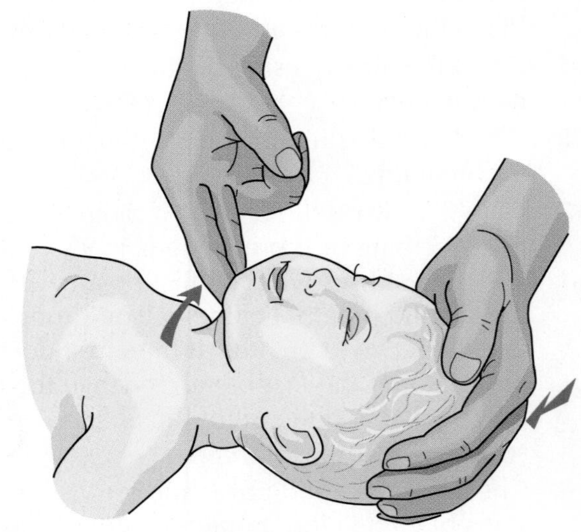

Figure 47-15 The head-tilt/chin-lift manoeuvre is used for infants. The infant's head is not tilted as far back as that of the adult. The infant's head is in a neutral or "sniffing" position.

Table 47-1 Heart and Stroke Foundation of Canada's Basic Life Support Summary

	Adult	Child	Infant
RESCUE BREATHING			
Volume	Breathe slowly until the chest visibly rises—about 2 seconds per breath	Breathe slowly until the chest visibly rises—about 1 to 1½ seconds per breath	Breathe slowly until the chest visibly rises—about 1 to 1½ seconds per breath
Rate	1 breath every 5 seconds	1 breath every 3 seconds	1 breath every 3 seconds
COMPRESSIONS			
Hand Position	Place both hands on the lower half of the breastbone	Place one hand on the lower half of the breastbone	Place two fingers on the lower half of the breastbone (one finger-width below the nipple line)
Depth	4 to 5 cm (1½ to 2 inches)	2.5 to 4 cm (1 to 1½ inches)	1 to 2.5 cm (½ to 1 inch)
Rate	About 100 per minute	About 100 per minute	About 100 per minute
CPR			
Ratio (1 and 2 rescuers)	15 compressions : 2 rescue breaths	5 compressions : 1 rescue breath	5 compressions : 1 rescue breath
Sets per minute	4	About 20	About 20

Source: Heart and Stroke Foundation of Canada, 2003.

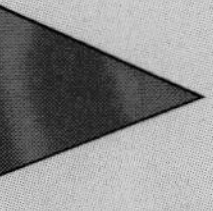

CPR for Infants and Children (8 Years of Age and Under)

Procedure

1 Check the scene for safety. Use a barrier device and gloves.

2 Determine unresponsiveness.

3 Activate the EMS system or the facility's emergency response system. Or have someone else do so.

4 Open the airway. Use the head-tilt/chin-lift manoeuvre.

5 Check for breathing. (Look, listen, and feel for breathing.)

6 Give 2 slow rescue breaths if the infant or child is not breathing or is not breathing adequately. Each rescue breath should take 1 to 1½ seconds. If the chest rises with the first breath, give the second breath. Let the lungs deflate between breaths. If the chest does not rise with the first breath, change the tilt of the head and the lift of the chin. Give the second breath.

7 Check for a brachial pulse (infants) or a carotid pulse (children) and for visible signs of circulation (breathing, coughing, and moving). Use your other hand to keep the airway open. Proceed with chest compressions if there is no pulse or signs of circulation.

8 Give chest compressions to an *infant*:

a Locate hand position (Figure 47-16 on page 784):

(1) Maintain head-tilt position with one hand. Imagine there is a line between the infant's nipples.

(2) Place your index finger on one nipple, then slide it along the imaginary line to the breastbone. (Use your hand closest to the infant's feet.)

(3) Place your middle and ring fingers next to your index finger on the breastbone.

(4) Lift your index finger off the chest. Your middle and ring fingers are now in the correct position.

b Press straight down on the breastbone to a depth of 1 to 2.5 cm (½ to 1 inch). Maintain the head-tilt with one hand while compressing the chest with the other hand.

c Do 5 chest compressions. Count out loud in a rhythm. (Try: "1, 2, 3, 4, 5.") Compress the chest at a rate of 100 compressions per minute. Release pressure after each compression. Do not remove your fingers from the chest.

9 Give chest compressions to a *child* (use the adult method if the child is large or older than age 8):

a Locate hand position (Figure 47-17 on page 784):

(1) Run your middle finger up along the rib cage to the notch at the centre of the chest.

(2) Mark the notch with your middle finger.

(3) Place your index finger next to your middle finger.

(4) Place the heel of the same hand next to where the index finger was located.

b Push straight down to a depth of 2.5 to 4 cm (1 to 1½ inches). Maintain the head-tilt with one hand while compressing with the heel of your other hand. Keep your fingers off the chest.

c Do 5 chest compressions. Count out loud in a rhythm. (Try: "1 and 2 and 3 and 4 and 5.") Compress the chest at a rate of 100 compressions per minute.

10 Give 1 breath after every fifth compression.

11 Complete 20 sets of 5 compressions and 1 breath (which will take slightly longer than 1 minute).

12 Check for a brachial pulse (infants) or a carotid pulse (children) and visible signs of circulation (breathing, coughing, moving).

13 If the infant or child has no visible signs of circulation or pulse, continue with sets of 5 compressions and 1 breath, beginning with chest compressions.

14 Reassess every few minutes thereafter until help arrives or signs of circulation resume.

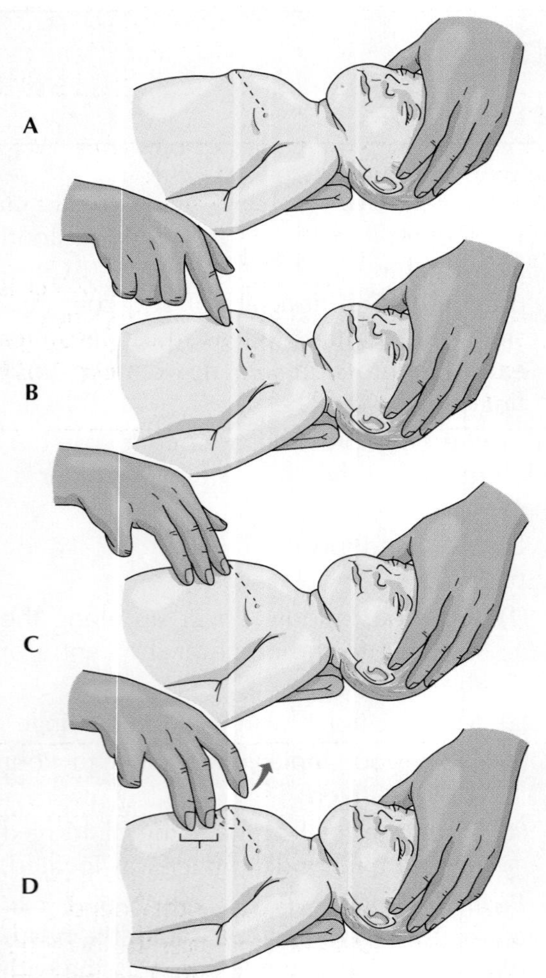

Figure 47-16 Locating hand position for infant chest compressions. **A,** Imagine a line between the nipples. **B,** Place your index finger on one nipple, then slide it along the imaginary line to the breastbone. **C,** Place your middle and ring fingers next to your index finger on the breastbone. **D,** Lift your index finger off the chest, and give compressions using your middle and ring fingers.

Foreign Body Airway Obstruction (FBAO) in Adults and Children

A **foreign body airway obstruction (FBAO)** is the blockage of the airway by an object. The person chokes. Air cannot pass through the air passages to the lungs. The body does not get oxygen. FBAO can lead to cardiac arrest and death.

The most common cause of airway obstruction in adults is improperly chewed food. Laughing and talking while eating also are common causes. Older adults are at risk for airway obstruction. Weakness, poorly fitting dentures, dysphagia (difficulty swallowing), and chronic illness are common causes in older adults. Infants and young children also have a high risk of choking because they can easily put small objects in their mouths. Many foods such as hot dogs and popcorn can easily cause FBAO in children (see Chapter 16).

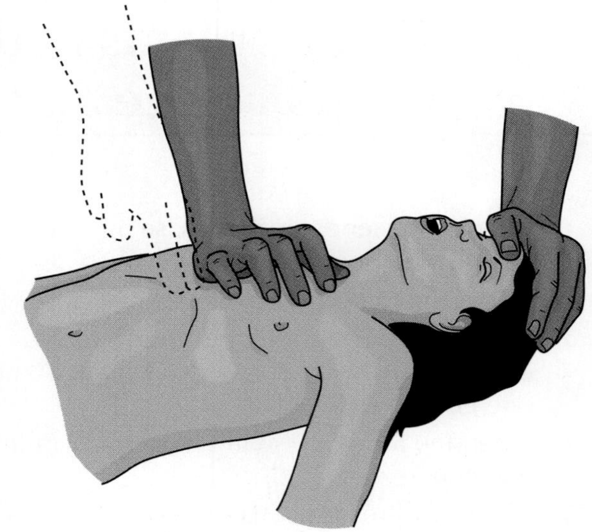

Figure 47-17 Use the heel of one hand for CPR on a child. Place the heel over the lower end of the breastbone as for an adult.

Airway obstruction can also occur in unconscious people. Common causes are aspiration of vomitus and the tongue falling back into the airway. These can occur during cardiac arrest.

Foreign bodies can cause partial or complete airway obstruction. With *partial obstruction,* the person can move some air into and out of the lungs. The person is responsive. Usually the person can speak. Often forceful coughing can remove the object. If the person can speak and cough, do not interfere. Stay close by.

With *complete airway obstruction,* the person clutches at the throat (Figure 47-18). The person cannot breathe, speak, or cough. The person is pale and cyanotic (has a bluish colour). Air does not move into and out of the lungs. The responsive person is very frightened. If the obstruction is not removed, the person will become unresponsive and eventually die. FBAO is an emergency. Activate the EMS system at once.

The *Heimlich manoeuvre* is used to relieve an obstructed airway caused by a foreign body. It involves abdominal thrusts. The manoeuvre is performed with the responsive person standing or sitting. It can be used on responsive adults and children.

The Heimlich manoeuvre is not effective with extremely obese people or pregnant women. Chests thrusts are used for them (Box 47-2). The Heimlich manoeuvre is also not given when a choking person becomes unresponsive. Instead of abdominal thrusts, proceed with chest compressions as with CPR (see page 777).

(text continues on page 786)

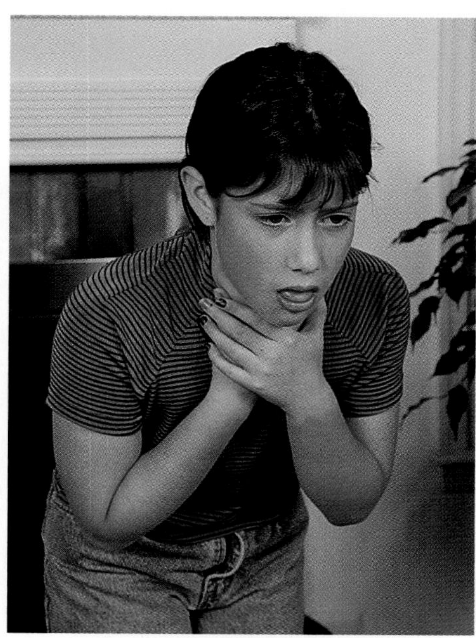

Figure 47-18 A choking person will usually clutch the throat.

Box 47-2 FBAO: Chest Thrusts for Obese or Pregnant People

1. Stand behind the person.
2. Place your arms under the person's arms. Wrap your arms around the person's chest.
3. Make a fist. Place the thumb side of the fist on the middle of the breastbone (sternum).
4. Grasp the fist with your other hand.
5. Give backward chest thrusts until the object is expelled or the person becomes unresponsive. If the person becomes unresponsive, follow the steps in *FBAO—The Unresponsive Adult, Child, or Infant* on page 788.

FBAO—The Responsive Adult or Child

Procedure

1 Ask, "Are you choking?"

2 If the person can speak, breathe, or cough, do not interfere.

3 Perform the Heimlich manoeuvre (abdominal thrusts) if the person cannot cough, breathe, or speak (Figure 47-19 on page 786):

- **a** Stand behind the person.
- **b** Wrap your arms around the person's waist.
- **c** Make a fist with one hand.
- **d** Place the thumb side of your fist against the person's abdomen. Your fist must be in the middle of the abdomen, slightly above the navel but well below the end of the breastbone (sternum).
- **e** Grasp your fist with your other hand.
- **f** Press your fist and hand into the person's abdomen with a quick, upward and inward thrust (like a "J").

4 Repeat thrusts until the object is expelled or the person becomes unresponsive. Each thrust should be a separate movement.

5 If the person becomes unresponsive, lower him or her to the floor.

6 Position the person supine.

7 Follow the procedure for *FBAO—The Unresponsive Adult, Child, or Infant* on page 788.

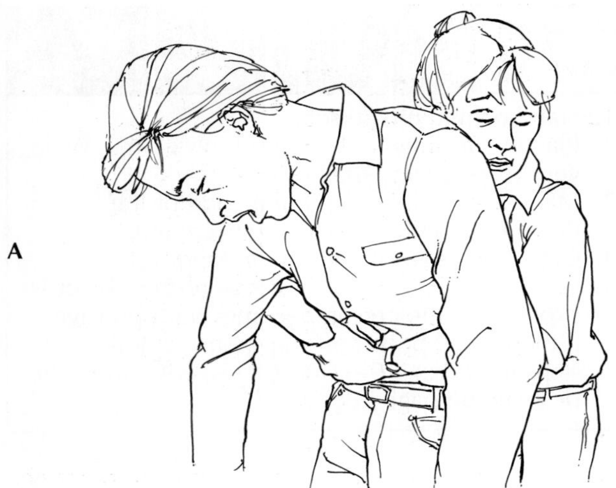

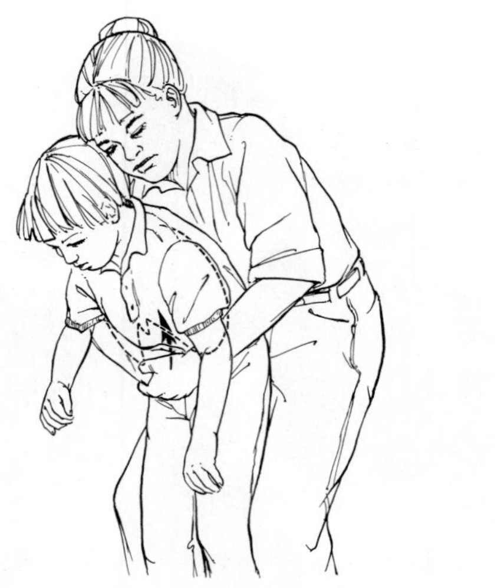

Figure 47-19 A, Abdominal thrusts on a responsive adult. **B,** Abdominal thrusts on a responsive child. Reproduced with permission. Basic Life Support for Healthcare Providers, 1997–1999. © 2003, Copyright American Heart Association.

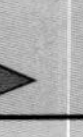

FBAO in Infants

Responsive infants with airway obstruction require back blows and chest thrusts, not the Heimlich manoeuvre. If the infant becomes unresponsive, follow the procedure in *FBAO—The Unresponsive Adult, Child, or Infant.*

The following procedure should be given only if you witnessed or strongly suspect that the infant has an FBAO. Infections or allergic reactions can also cause airway obstruction. Do *not* waste time by trying to clear this type of obstruction. The infant may drool or have a fever, a barking cough, or noisy breathing. Activate the EMS system at once.

FBAO—The Responsive Infant

Procedure

1. Determine if the infant has an airway obstruction. Observe for sudden onset of difficulty breathing, coughing or gagging, high-pitched noise, weak cry, or grey-blue colour to the lips.
2. Give back blows:
   a. Hold the infant face down over your forearm. Support your arm on your thigh. The infant's head should be lower than the trunk. Hold the infant's jaw to support the head (Figure 47-20).
   b. Give up to 5 back blows with the heel of one hand. Give the blows between the infant's shoulder blades in the middle of the back (see Figure 47-20).
3. Turn the infant. Support the infant's head, neck, jaw, and chest with one hand. Support the back with your other hand.
4. Place the infant over your thigh. The baby's head is lower than the trunk.
5. Give chest thrusts:
   a. Locate hand position as for chest compressions—near the lower half of the breastbone, approximately one finger's width below the mid-nipple line (Figure 47-21).
   b. Give up to 5 quick, downward chest thrusts, at a rate of about 1 per second.
6. Repeat back blows and chest thrusts until the object is expelled or the infant becomes unresponsive.
7. If the infant becomes unresponsive, follow the procedure in *FBAO—The Unresponsive Adult, Child, or Infant* on page 788.

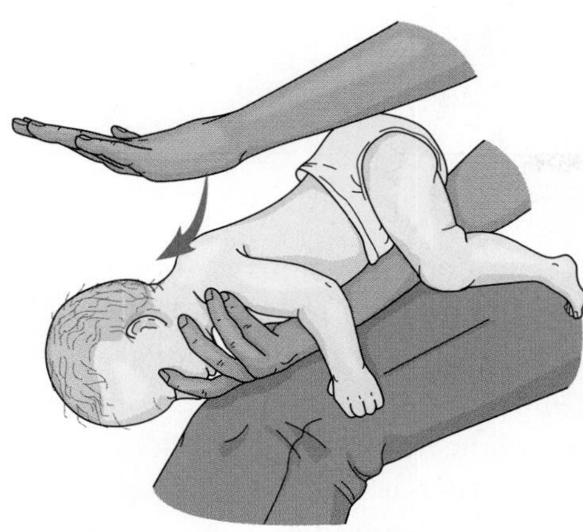

Figure 47-20 Back blows. Hold the infant face down and support with one hand. Support your arm on your thigh. Give back blows with the heel of one hand. Give the blows between the infant's shoulder blades.

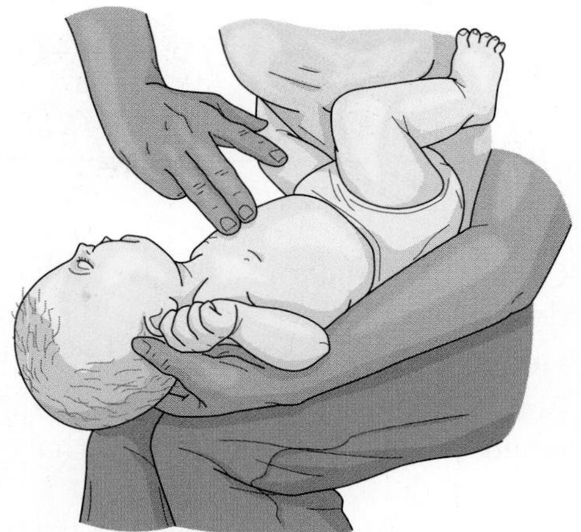

Figure 47-21 Chest thrusts. Position the infant on your thigh. Hand position for chest thrusts in the infant is the same as for chest compressions.

The Unresponsive Adult, Child, or Infant

You may find an unresponsive adult, child, or infant. If you did not see the person lose consciousness, you cannot know the cause. You cannot assume the person is choking. Therefore you need to establish unresponsiveness. Remember, always activate the EMS system (or have someone else do so) before doing anything else.

Open the airway and check for breathing. Start rescue breathing if necessary. If you cannot ventilate the person (the chest does not rise and fall with rescue breaths), the person may have an airway obstruction. Start chest compressions right away. These may dislodge the object. Look in the mouth for a foreign object after the cycle of chest compressions.

If you saw the person become unresponsive because of an airway obstruction, do the following:

- Open the airway
- Look in the mouth for the object
- Remove the object if it is visible

If you cannot see and remove the object, continue with attempting rescue breaths and giving chest compressions. Look in the mouth again after the cycle of chest compressions.

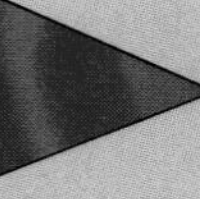

FBAO—The Unresponsive Adult, Child, or Infant

Procedure

1 Check the scene for safety. Use a barrier device and gloves.
2 Determine unresponsiveness.
3 Activate the EMS system or the facility's emergency response system. Or have someone else do so.
4 Open the airway. Use the head-tilt/chin-lift manoeuvre.
5 If the person was responsive and obstructed and became unresponsive, look in the mouth for an object. Remove the object if it is visible.
6 Check for breathing. (Look, listen, and feel for breathing.)
7 Give 2 slow rescue breaths if the person is not breathing (*adult:* 2 seconds per rescue breath; *child and infant:* 1 to 1½ seconds per rescue breath). If the chest rises with the first breath, give the second breath. If the chest does not rise with the first breath, change the tilt of the head and the lift of the chin. Give the second breath.
8 Give chest compressions if rescue breaths do not go in (that is, the chest does not rise):
   a *Adult:* 15 chest compressions.
   b *Child or infant:* 5 chest compressions. Maintain the head-tilt while giving chest compressions.
9 Look in the mouth. Open the mouth by lifting the jaw. Look at the back of the throat. If you see an object, use a finger to move it to the front of the mouth and then remove it.
10 Open the airway with the head-tilt/chin-lift manoeuvre.
11 Give 2 slow rescue breaths. If the chest rises with the first breath, give the second breath. If the chest does not rise with the first breath, change the tilt of the head and the lift of the chin. Give the second breath. If the chest still does not rise, continue with chest compressions.
12 Repeat steps 8 through 11 (chest compressions, looking in the mouth, and rescue breathing) until rescue breathing is effective or emergency help arrives.

Recovery Position

The recovery position is a side-lying position (Figure 47-22). It is used when the person is breathing and has a pulse but is unresponsive. The position helps keep the airway open. Because the side-lying position allows fluids to drain from the mouth, it helps prevent aspiration of mucus and vomitus. It also prevents the tongue from falling toward the back of the throat.

Logroll the person into the recovery position. Keep the head, neck, and spine straight. Then keep the person in good alignment. Position the person's hand to support the head. *Do not use this position if the person might have neck injuries or other trauma.* Check the person's breathing and circulation often. Activate the EMS system if you have not already done so.

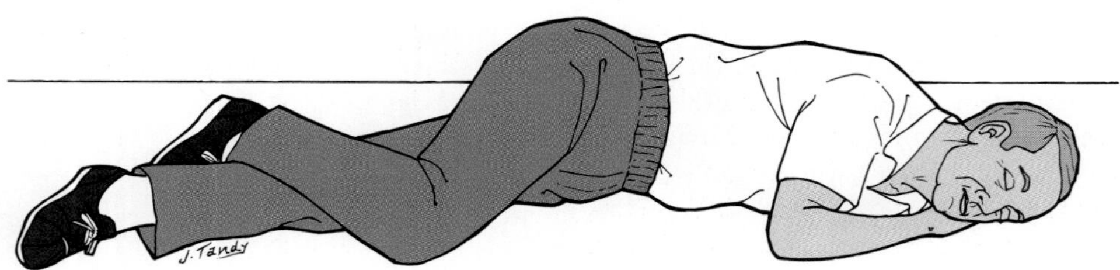

Figure 47-22 Recovery position.

Self-Administered Heimlich Manoeuvre

You yourself may choke. You can perform the Heimlich manoeuvre to relive the obstructed airway. To do so:

- Make a fist with one hand.
- Place the thumb side of the fist above your navel and below the lower end of the breastbone.
- Grasp your fist with your other hand.
- Press inward and upward quickly.
- Press the upper abdomen against a hard surface if the thrust did not relieve the obstruction. Use the back of a chair, a table, or a railing.
- Use as many thrusts as needed.

Automated External Defibrillators (AEDs)

Early defibrillation is the fourth link in the Heart and Stroke Foundation of Canada's *Chain of Survival*. An abnormal heart rhythm, called *ventricular fibrillation* (VF, V-fib), causes cardiac arrest. Rather than beating in a regular rhythm, the heart muscle shakes and quivers like a bowl of jelly. No blood is pumped out of the heart. Therefore the heart, brain, and other organs do not receive blood and oxygen.

VF must be stopped and a regular heart rhythm restored. If not, the person dies. A device called a *defibrillator* is used to stop the VF. It delivers a shock to the heart. The shock stops the VF. This allows the return of a regular heart rhythm. Defibrillation done as soon as possible after the onset of VF increases the person's chance of survival.

Automated external defibrillators (AEDs) are computerized devices. Hospitals, long-term care facilities, and other health care agencies have them. Many businesses and institutions that deal with the public also have them, including some airports, health clubs, malls, office buildings, restaurants, and schools. Most basic life support courses now teach health care providers and members of the general public how to use them. Remember, the goal is early defibrillation.

Hemorrhage

Life and body functions require an adequate blood supply. Blood must circulate through the body. If a blood vessel is torn or cut, bleeding occurs. The larger the blood vessel, the greater the bleeding and blood loss. **Hemorrhage** is excessive loss of blood in a short time. If the bleeding is not stopped, the person will die.

Hemorrhage may be internal or external. You cannot see internal hemorrhage. Bleeding occurs inside the body into the tissues and body cavities. Pain, shock, vomiting blood, coughing up blood, and loss of responsiveness signal internal hemorrhage. There is little you can do for internal bleeding. Activate the EMS system. Then keep the person warm, flat, and quiet until help arrives. Do not give fluids.

External bleeding is usually seen. However, it may be hidden by clothing. Hemorrhage may be from an injured artery or vein. Bleeding from an artery is bright red and occurs in spurts. There is a steady flow of blood from a vein. To control external bleeding:

- Follow the guidelines in Box 47-1 on page 773. This includes activating the EMS system.
- Have the person lie down.
- Do not remove any objects that have pierced or stabbed the skin.
- Practise Standard Precautions. Wear gloves if possible. If the person is able, have the person place his or her bare hand over the wound while you put on gloves and get the dressing.
- Place a sterile dressing directly over the wound. Use any clean material (handkerchief, towel, cloth, or sanitary napkin) if there is no sterile dressing.
- Apply pressure with your hand directly over the bleeding site (Figure 47-23). Do not release the pressure until the bleeding stops. If blood seeps through the dressing, put additional dressings over the first dressing.
- If direct pressure does not control bleeding, apply pressure over the artery above the bleeding site (Figure 47-24 on page 790). Use your first three fingers. For example, if bleeding is from the lower arm, apply pressure over the brachial artery. The brachial artery supplies blood to the lower arm. Continue to apply pressure to the wound with your other hand.
- Bind the wound when the bleeding stops. Tape or tie the dressing in place. You can tie the dressing with items such as clothing, a scarf, or a belt. If the dressing is around a limb, check the fingers and toes frequently for good circulation. If they are bluish or cold, the dressing may be too tight.

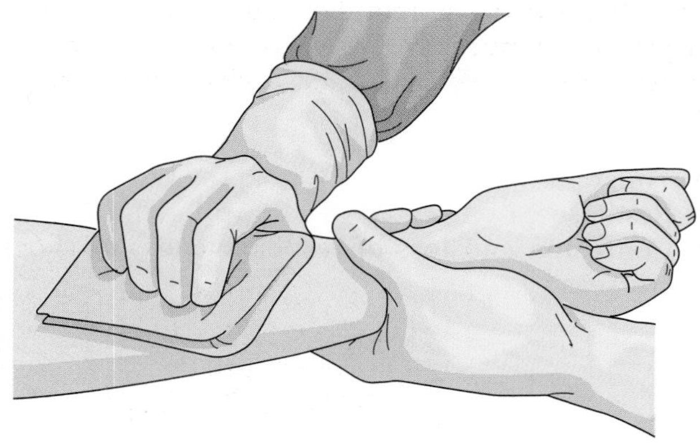

Figure 47-23 Apply direct pressure to the wound to stop bleeding. Place your hand over the wound.

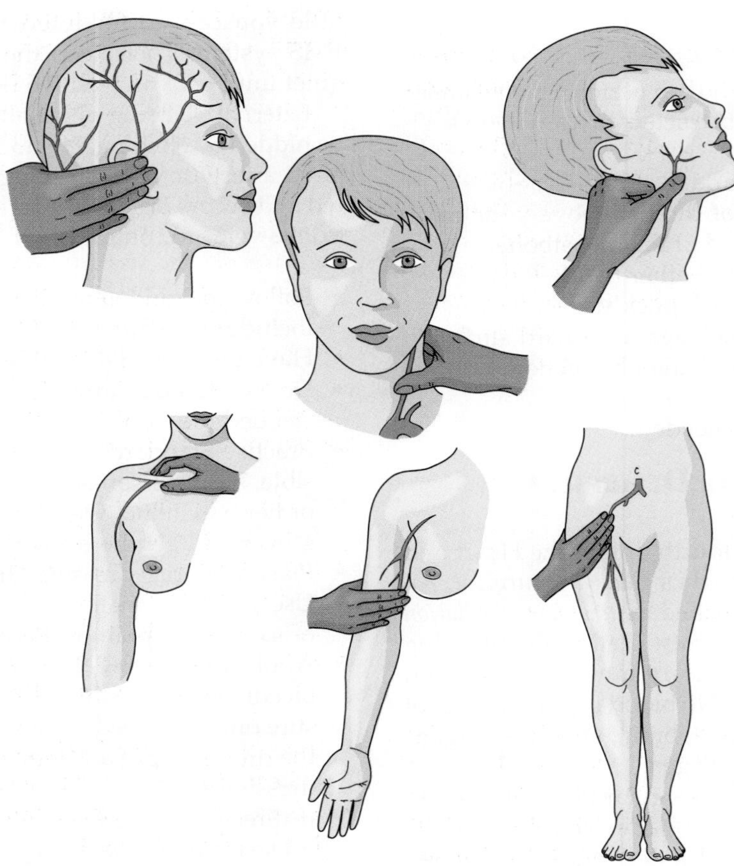

Figure 47-24 Pressure points to control bleeding.

SHOCK

Shock results when organs and tissues do not get enough blood. Blood loss, heart attack (myocardial infarction), burns, and severe infection can cause shock. Signs and symptoms include:

- Low or falling blood pressure
- Rapid and weak pulse
- Rapid respirations
- Cold, moist, and pale skin
- Thirst
- Restlessness
- Confusion and loss of responsiveness as shock worsens

Shock is possible in any person who is acutely ill or injured. Do the following to prevent or to treat shock:

- Follow the guidelines in Box 47-1 on page 773. This includes activating the EMS system and following Standard Precautions.
- Keep the person lying down.
- Maintain an open airway.
- Control hemorrhage.
- Keep the person warm. Place blankets over and under the person if possible.
- Reassure the person.

ANAPHYLACTIC SHOCK

Some people are allergic or sensitive to various substances such as foods, insects, chemicals, and medications. Many people are allergic to penicillin. An antigen is a substance the body reacts to. The body fights or attacks the antigen by releasing chemicals. The reaction may be a local area of redness, swelling, or itching. Or the reaction can involve the entire body.

Anaphylaxis is life-threatening sensitivity to an antigen. It comes from the Greek words that mean without (*ana*) protection (*phylaxis*). In severe cases, anaphylactic shock can occur within seconds. Signs and symptoms include:

- Sweating
- Shortness of breath
- Low blood pressure
- Irregular pulse
- Respiratory congestion
- Swelling of the larynx (laryngeal edema)
- Hoarseness
- Dyspnea

Anaphylactic shock is an emergency. The EMS system must be activated. The person needs special medications to reverse the allergic reaction. Until emergency help arrives, keep the person lying down. Also keep the airway open. CPR is necessary if cardiac arrest occurs.

SEIZURES

Seizures are brief disturbances in the brain's normal electrical function. They affect awareness, movement, and/or sensation. Causes include brain injury during birth or from trauma, high fever, brain tumours, poisoning, seizure disorders, and central nervous system infections. Lack of blood flow to the brain also can cause seizures.

The major types of seizures are *partial seizures* and *generalized seizures*. Only a part of the brain is involved with a partial seizure. A body part may jerk. Or the person has hearing or vision problems or stomach discomfort. The person does not lose consciousness.

With generalized seizures, the whole brain is involved. The **tonic-clonic seizure** is a type of generalized seizure where the person has convulsions. A **convulsion** is the violent and sudden contraction or tremor of muscles. A tonic-clonic seizure occurs in two phases. First, the person becomes unresponsive. If standing or sitting, the person falls to the floor. The body is rigid because all muscles contract at once. Next, muscle groups contract and relax. This causes jerking and twitching movements. Urinary and fecal incontinence may occur. After the seizure, the person usually falls into a deep sleep. The person may have confusion and headache on awakening.

The *absence seizure* is another type of generalized seizure. With absence seizures, the person becomes briefly unresponsive, usually for only a few seconds. The person's speech or activity stops, and the person stares. After the seizure, the person resumes normal speech and activity. Absence seizures are more common in children than in the other age groups. They usually disappear by adolescence. No first aid is necessary.

You cannot stop a seizure. However, you can protect the person from injury during a seizure. The following measures are performed for a tonic-clonic seizure:

- Follow the guidelines in Box 47-1 on page 773. This includes activating the EMS system.
- Do not leave the person alone.
- If the person is not in bed, lower the person to the floor. This protects the person from falling.
- Place a folded blanket, towel, cushion, pillow, or other soft item under the person's head (Figure 47-25).
- Turn the person onto his or her side. (The left side is best.) Make sure the head is turned to the side.
- Loosen jewellery and clothing (ties, scarves, or collars) around the neck.
- Move furniture, equipment, and sharp objects away from the person. The person may strike these objects during the uncontrolled body movements.
- Do not restrain body movements during the seizure.
- Do not put your fingers between the person's teeth. The person can bite down on your fingers during the seizure.
- Do not insert any object into the person's mouth. It is not necessary and could cause the person to choke.

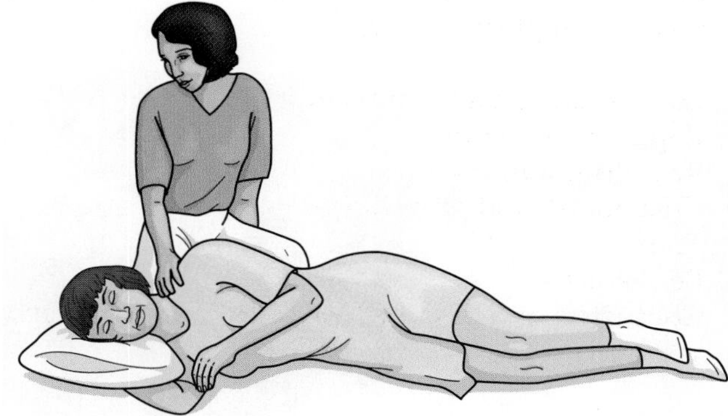

Figure 47-25 Place a pillow or other soft item under the person's head during a seizure.

BURNS

Burns can severely disfigure and disable a person (Figure 47-26). They can also cause death. Most burn injuries occur in the home. Infants and children are at risk. So are older adults. Burns are caused by:

- Dry heat—fire, stoves, space heaters
- Moist heat—hot liquids, steam
- Chemicals—oven cleaner, drain cleaner, rust remover, and so on
- Electricity—Faulty electrical equipment, live wires, or lightning (Figure 47-27)
- Radiation—sunlight

Some burns are minor; others are severe. Burns are more severe and require emergency help when:

- They are located on the head, face, neck, hands, feet, or genitals
- They are spread over a large area of the body
- The burned person is under 2 or over 50 years of age or has a pre-existing medical condition (such as diabetes or hypertension)

The size and depth of the burn also affect its severity. Remember, the skin has two layers: the dermis and epidermis.

- *First-degree burns*—are the least severe. Only the top layer of skin (the dermis) is affected. The skin is red or discoloured, and mild swelling and a moderate amount of pain are present. Depending on the situation, these burns may not require medical attention. Having mild sunburn and briefly touching a heat source may cause first-degree burns.
- *Second-degree burns*—involve the dermis and part of the epidermis. The skin is red or mottled and blistering. These burns are very painful because nerve endings are exposed. These burns are also known as *partial-thickness burns*. Severe sunburn and burns caused by hot liquids are examples. They are serious and require emergency medical attention.
- *Third-degree burns*—are very deep, affecting the dermis and the entire epidermis. These burns are the most severe and require emergency medical attention. Fat, muscle, and bone may be injured or destroyed. The skin may look black, white, or charred. The burn often covers a large surface area (see Figure 47-27). The person may feel excruciating pain or, if the nerve endings have been destroyed, no pain at all. These burns are also known as *full-thickness burns*. Burns caused by fire or electric shock are usually third-degree burns.

For minor first-degree burns that are limited to a small area, do the following:

- Immediately cool the injury to reduce pain, swelling, blistering, and tissue damage. Immerse the burn in a sink of cool water, run cool water over it, or cover it with a clean, wet, cool cloth.

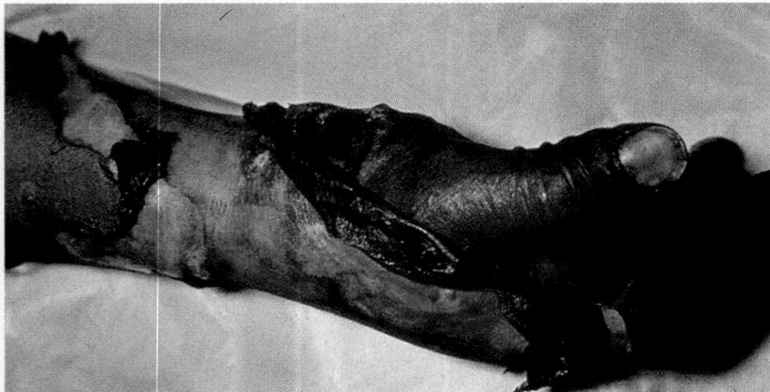

Figure 47-26 Full-thickness (third-degree) burn. Source: D.D. Ignatavicius and M.L. Workman, *Medical-Surgical Nursing: Critical Thinking and Collaborative Care*, 4th ed. (Philadelphia: Saunders, 2002).

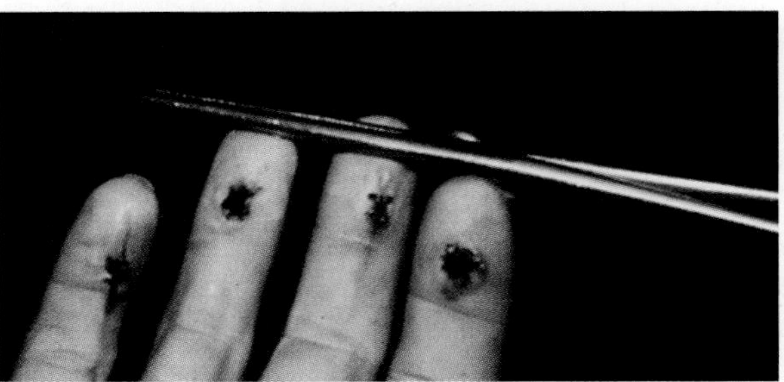

A

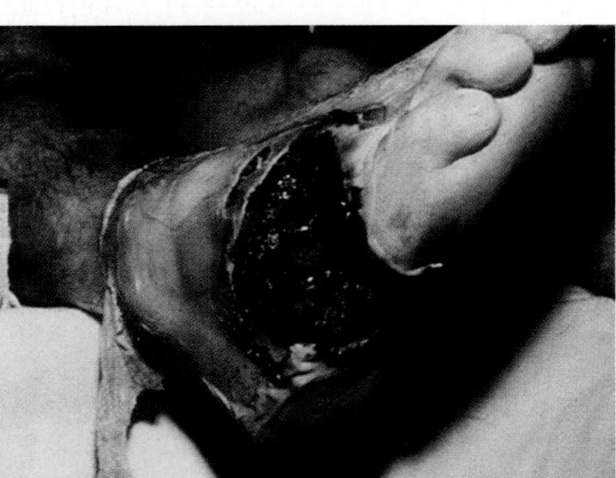

B

Figure 47-27 An electrical burn. **A,** The electrical current enters through the hand. **B,** The electrical current exits through the foot. Source: M. Sanders, *Mosby's Paramedic Textbook* (St. Louis: Mosby, 1994).

- Once pain is reduced, gently pat the skin dry and cover it with dry, lint-free, clean cloth or gauze. Secure the dressing with tape, being careful not to touch the burn with the tape.
- Do not apply oil, butter, salve, or ointments on a burn.
- Report the burn to your supervisor. Seek medical attention if necessary.

Emergency care of second- and third-degree burns includes the following:

- Follow the guidelines in Box 47-1 on page 773. This includes activating the EMS system and following Standard Precautions.
- For chemical burns, carefully and quickly brush off any loose chemical powder with a cloth. Flush the area with large amounts of cool water (such as in a shower) for 15 to 20 minutes. Carefully remove contaminated clothing while flushing the area.
- For electrical burns, secure your safety first. Do not touch the person if he or she is in contact with an electrical source. Have the power source turned off or remove the electrical source first. Use an object that does not conduct electricity (rope or wood) to remove the electrical source. Do not apply water onto the burn. Water may increase the risk of shock.
- For heat source burns, stop the burning process. Protect yourself from the source of the burn. Extinguish flames with water, or roll the person in a blanket, coat, sheet, or towel.
- Remove hot clothing that is not sticking to the skin. Do not pull at clothing that sticks to the burn. Remove jewellery and tight clothing or belts before the injury swells.
- Provide rescue breathing and CPR as needed.
- Cool the burned skin with cool water, not ice. Do not use cold water on large, third-degree burns. Do not immerse in ice water. Cover the burn with a clean, cool, moist compress. (Use towels, sheets, or any other clean cloth.) Reapply the cool compress for up to 20 minutes (for burns on the hands, feet, or face) or up to 1 hour (for second-degree burns). Pat dry.
- Loosely cover the burn wounds with a clean, dry covering. Thick, sterile gauze is preferable, but you can use towels, sheets, or any other clean cloth. Tape the covering in place, being careful not to touch the burn with the tape.
- Do not put oil, butter, salve, or ointments on the burn.
- Do not break the blisters.
- Cover the person with a blanket or coat to prevent heat loss.
- Watch for signs of shock. Stay with the person until help arrives.

POISONING

Many household products can cause poisoning (see Chapter 16). Children and people with confusion or dementia are at risk. In community settings, the phone number for the local poison control centre should always be posted near the telephone or carried in your bag. Signs of poisoning include empty pill bottles or hazardous products lying out. Or the person suddenly collapses, vomits, or has difficulty breathing. If you suspect poisoning:

- Follow the guidelines in Box 47-1 on page 773. This includes activating the EMS system. The EMS system operator will give you instructions.
- Gather any empty pill bottles or other evidence of poisoning to determine what has been ingested and how much.

FAINTING

Fainting is the sudden loss of consciousness from an inadequate blood supply to the brain. Hunger, fatigue, and pain are common causes. Some people faint at the sight of blood or injury. Standing in one position for a long time or being in a warm, crowded room are other causes. Dizziness, perspiration, and blackness before the eyes are warning signals. The person looks pale. The pulse is weak. Respirations are shallow if the person loses consciousness. Emergency care for fainting includes the following:

- Have the person sit or lie down before fainting occurs.
- If sitting, have the person bend forward and place the head between the knees (Figure 47-28 on page 794).
- If the person is lying down, elevate his or her legs.
- Loosen tight clothing (belts, ties, scarves, collars, and so on).
- Keep the person lying down if fainting has occurred. Elevate the legs.
- Do not let the person get up until symptoms have subsided for about 5 minutes.
- Help the person to a sitting position after recovery from fainting. Observe for symptoms of fainting.
- Notify your supervisor.

STROKE

Stroke (cerebrovascular accident) is described in Chapter 31. A stroke occurs when the brain is suddenly deprived of its blood supply. Usually only part of the brain is affected. A stroke may be caused by a

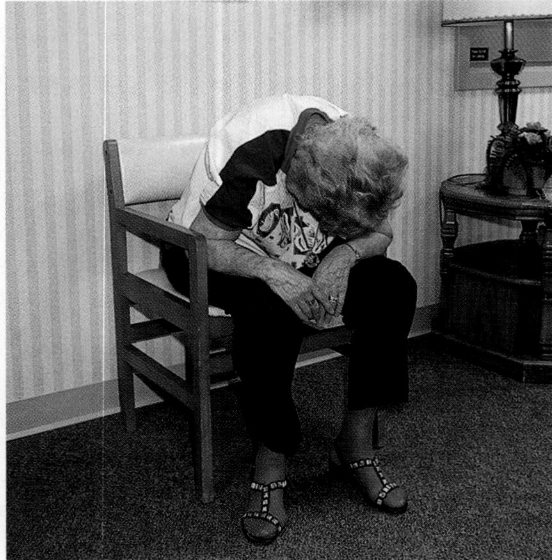

Figure 47-28 Have the person bend forward and place the head between the knees to prevent fainting.

thrombus, an embolus, or cerebral hemorrhage if a blood vessel ruptures.

Signs of stroke vary. They depend on the size and location of brain injury. Loss of consciousness or semiconsciousness, rapid pulse, laboured respirations, elevated blood pressure, vomiting, and hemiplegia are signs of stroke. The person may have slurred speech or aphasia (the inability to speak). Seizures may occur.

Emergency care includes the following:

- Follow the guidelines in Box 47-1 on page 773. This includes activating the EMS system. The EMS system operator will give you instructions.
- Place the person in the recovery position on the unaffected side (see Figure 47-22 on page 788). The affected side is limp, and the cheek appears puffy.
- Elevate the head without flexing the neck.
- Loosen tight clothing (belts, ties, scarves, collars, and so on).
- Keep the person quiet and warm.
- Reassure the person.
- Provide rescue breathing and CPR if necessary.
- Provide emergency care for seizures if necessary.

Compassionate Care

Compassionate care must be provided during emergencies. (See *Providing Compassionate Care: Emergencies* box.)

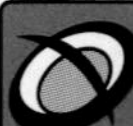

Providing Compassionate Care

Emergencies

Dignity. The person must be treated with dignity and respect at all times. The person may feel very frightened. Reassure the person whenever you can. A touch or kind word may be comforting. Stay with the person during the emergency. Tell the person that help is on the way.

Protect personal possessions from loss and damage. Dentures and eyeglasses often are lost or broken in emergencies. Watches and other jewellery are easily lost. Clothing may be torn or cut. You must be very careful to protect the person's property. In public places, personal items are given to family members, police, or EMS personnel.

Independence. Depending on the injury and situation, the person may be able to help in the care. For example, the person may be able to hold a cold compress in place. If the person is willing, allow him or her to participate in care. If you have time and the person is responsive, explain what you are doing. Remember, however, in many emergency situations, your priority is to provide care as quickly as possible.

Preferences. Protect the right to personal choice. It is often hard to give choices in emergencies. They are given when possible. Hospital care may be required. The person has the right to choose which hospital to be taken to.

Privacy. Protect the right to privacy and confidentiality. Do not expose the person unnecessarily. You may be in a place where you cannot close doors, shades, and curtains. The person may be in a lounge, dining area, or public place. Do what you can to protect privacy.

Onlookers are major threats to privacy and confidentiality. When giving emergency care, your main concern is the person's illness or injuries. You cannot give care and manage onlookers at the same time. Ask someone to deal with onlookers. If someone else is giving care, keep onlookers away from the person.

People are naturally curious. They want to know what happened, the extent of injuries or illness, and if the person will be okay. You must not discuss the situation. Information about the person's care, treatment, and condition is confidential.

Safety. Provide a safe setting. Physical and psychological safety are important. The person must be protected from further injury. For example, a person is protected from falls after a stroke. The person having a seizure is protected from head injuries. The person needs to feel safe and secure. Reassurance, explanations about care, and a calm approach are important. They help the person feel safe and secure.

REVIEW

Circle the BEST answer.

1. The goals of first aid are to
A. Call for help and keep the person warm
B. Prevent death and prevent injuries from becoming worse
C. Stay calm and wait for others to perform emergency measures
D. Reassure the person and bystanders

2. When giving first aid you should
A. Be aware of your limits
B. Move the person
C. Give the person fluids
D. Call for help after doing all you can

3. Cardiac arrest is
A. The same as stroke
B. The sudden stopping of heart action and breathing
C. The sudden loss of consciousness
D. The condition that results when organs and tissues do not get enough blood

4. Which is *not* a sign of cardiac arrest?
A. No pulse
B. No breathing
C. Clutching the throat
D. No response

5. When giving mouth-to-mouth rescue breathing to an adult, you should do the following *except*
A. Pinch the person's nostrils shut
B. Place your mouth tightly over the person's mouth
C. Blow air into the person's mouth as you exhale
D. Cover the person's nose and mouth

6. When giving CPR to an adult, the chest is compressed
A. 1 to 2.5 cm (½ to 1 inch) with the index and middle fingers
B. 2.5 to 4 cm (1 to 1½ inches) with the heel of one hand
C. 4 to 5 cm (1½ to 2 inches) with two hands
D. 5 to 6 cm (2 to 2½ inches) with one hand in the middle of the breastbone

7. When giving CPR to an infant, the chest is compressed
A. 1 to 2.5 cm (½ to 1 inch) with the index and middle fingers
B. 2.5 to 4 cm (1 to 1½ inches) with the heel of one hand
C. 4 to 5 cm (1½ to 2 inches) with two hands
D. 5 to 6 cm (2 to 2½ inches) with one hand in the middle of the breastbone

8. Which does *not* determine adequate breathing?
A. Looking to see if the chest rises and falls
B. Counting respirations for 30 seconds
C. Listening for the escape of air
D. Feeling for the flow of air

9. Which is used to feel for a pulse during CPR on an adult or child?
A. The apical pulse
B. The brachial pulse
C. The carotid pulse
D. The dorsalis pedis pulse

10. How many rescue breaths are given at the beginning of CPR?
A. 1
B. 2
C. 3
D. 4

11. You are performing adult CPR alone. Which is *false*?
A. Give 2 breaths after every 15 compressions.
B. Check for a pulse after every 4 sets of 15 compressions and 2 breaths.
C. Give 1 breath after every 5 compressions.
D. Count out loud.

12. CPR is being given on an adult by two rescuers. Two rescue breaths are given
A. After every fifth compression
B. After every fifteenth compression
C. After every compression
D. Only when positions are changed

13. If complete airway obstruction occurs, the person usually will
A. Clutch at the throat
B. Be able to speak, cough, and breathe
C. Be calm
D. Have a seizure

REVIEW

14. The Heimlich manoeuvre (abdominal thrusts) is used to relieve an obstructed airway in responsive adults and children. Which statement is *false*?
    A. The person can be standing or sitting.
    B. The rescuer stands behind the person; the rescuer wraps his or her arms around the person's waist.
    C. The thrusts are given inward and upward on the breastbone.
    D. The hands are positioned above the navel and well below the breastbone.

15. An infant has an obstructed airway. Which statement is *false*?
    A. Chest thrusts and back blows are given on an unresponsive infant.
    B. Activate the EMS system at once.
    C. Chest thrusts and back blows are given on a responsive infant.
    D. Chest compressions, mouth check, and rescue breathing are done on an unresponsive infant.

16. A person has a partially obstructed airway and can cough and talk. Abdominal thrusts should be given.
    A. True
    B. False

17. Arterial bleeding is suspected. Arterial bleeding
    A. Cannot be seen
    B. Occurs in spurts
    C. Is dark red
    D. Oozes from the wound

18. A person is hemorrhaging from the left forearm. The *first* action should be to
    A. Lower the body part
    B. Apply pressure to the brachial artery
    C. Apply direct pressure to the wound
    D. Cover the person

19. These statements relate to tonic-clonic seizures. Which statement is *false*?
    A. There is a contraction of all muscles at once.
    B. Incontinence may occur.
    C. The seizure usually lasts for a few seconds.
    D. There is loss of consciousness during the seizure.

20. The signs of shock are
    A. Rising blood pressure, rapid pulse, and slow respirations
    B. Rapid pulse, rapid respirations, and warm skin
    C. Falling blood pressure, slow pulse and respirations, thirst, restlessness, and warm, flushed skin
    D. Falling blood pressure, rapid pulse and respirations, and cool skin

21. A person is in shock. You should
    A. Open the airway
    B. Remove the person's clothing
    C. Keep the person lying down
    D. Elevate the person's head

22. A person is about to faint. Which statement is *false*?
    A. Take the person outside for some fresh air.
    B. Have the person sit or lie down.
    C. Loosen tight clothing.
    D. Elevate the legs if the person is lying down.

23. A person is having a stroke. Emergency care includes all of the following *except*
    A. Positioning the person on the unaffected side
    B. Giving the person sips of water
    C. Loosening tight clothing
    D. Keeping the person quiet and warm

24. A second-degree burn
    A. Is the least severe type of burn
    B. Affects only the dermis
    C. Causes blistering
    D. Is not painful

25. For second- and third-degree burns, cover the burn with
    A. A clean, cool, moist cloth or dressing
    B. Butter, oil, or salve
    C. Ice water
    D. Nothing

26. Which is *not* an example of compassionate care in emergency situations?
    A. Providing privacy
    B. Protecting personal items from loss or breakage
    C. Protecting the person from further injury
    D. Telling concerned onlookers what happened

Answers to these questions are on page 828.

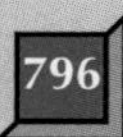

CHAPTER

48

MEDICAL TERMINOLOGY

OBJECTIVES

- Define the key terms listed in this chapter
- Identify three word elements used in medical terms
- Learn the meanings of common Greek and Latin prefixes, roots, and suffixes
- Combine word elements into medical terms
- Learn the meanings of common medical terms
- Identify the four abdominal regions
- Define the directional terms that describe the positions of the body in relation to other body parts
- Identify and define some of the abbreviations used in health care

KEY TERMS

abbreviation A shortened form of a word or phrase

anterior Located at or toward the front of the body or body part; ventral

combining vowel A vowel added between two roots or a root and a suffix to make pronunciation easier

distal The part farthest from the centre or from the point of attachment

dorsal Located at or toward the back of the body or body part; posterior

lateral Relating to or located at the side of the body or body part

medial Relating to or located at or near the middle or midline of the body or body part

posterior Dorsal

prefix A word element placed at the beginning of a word to change the meaning of the word

proximal The part nearest to the centre or to the point of origin

root A word element containing the basic meaning of the word

suffix A word element placed at the end of a root to change the meaning of the word

ventral Anterior

word element A part of a word

Many people find medical language mysterious and secretive—the private code of physicians and nurses. Yet people use medical terms every day. Examples are *flu*, *diarrhea*, *cancer*, *appendectomy*, *cardiac*, and *pneumonia*. Health and medicine get a lot of attention in the media. Because of so much news coverage, many medical terms are commonly understood.

Knowing medical terminology is important in your work. As you gain more knowledge and experience, you will understand and use medical terms often and with ease. Learning medical terms for illnesses, diseases, and common things like bruises, baldness, and a "runny nose" can be fun and educational. This chapter introduces medical terminology and the common abbreviations used in health care.

WORD ELEMENTS

Like all words, medical terms are made up of parts or **word elements**. These elements are combined in various ways to form medical terms. A term is translated by separating the word into its elements. Important word elements are prefixes, roots, and suffixes.

PREFIXES

A **prefix** is a word element placed at the beginning of a word. A prefix changes the meaning of the word. The prefix *olig* (scant, small amount) is placed before the word *uria* (urine) to make *oliguria*. It means a scant amount of urine. Prefixes are always combined with other word elements. They are never used alone. Most prefixes are Greek or Latin. You need to learn the following prefixes to begin understanding medical terminology:

Prefix	Meaning
a-, an-	without, not, lack of
ab-	away from
ad-	to, toward, near
ante-	before, forward, in front of
anti-	against
auto-	self
bi-	double, two, twice
brady-	slow
circum-	around
contra-	against, opposite
de-	down, from
dia-	across, through, apart
dis-	apart, free from
dys-	bad, difficult, abnormal
ecto-	outer, outside
en-	in, into, within
endo-	inner, inside
epi-	over, on, upon
eryth-	red
eu-	normal, good, well, healthy
ex-	out, out of, from, away from
hemi-	half
hyper-	excessive, too much, high
hypo-	under, decreased, less than normal
in-	in, into, within, not
infra-	within
inter-	between
intro-	into, within
leuk-	white
macro-	large
mal-	bad, illness, disease
meg-	large
micro-	small
mono-	one, single
neo-	new
non-	not
olig-	small, scant
para-	beside, beyond, after
per-	by, through
peri-	around
poly-	many, much
post-	after, behind
pre-	before, in front of, prior to
pro-	before, in front of
re-	again, backward
retro-	backward, behind
semi-	half
sub-	under, beneath
super-	above, over, excess
supra-	above, over
tachy-	fast, rapid
trans-	across
uni-	one

Roots

The **root** contains the basic meaning of the word. It is combined with another root, with prefixes, and with suffixes in various combinations to form a medical term. Roots are mainly from Greek and Latin.

A vowel is added when two roots are combined or when a suffix is added to a root. The vowel is called a **combining vowel** and is usually an *o*. An *i* is sometimes used. An *i* is used when there is no vowel between the two combined roots or between the root and the suffix. A combining vowel makes pronunciation easier.

The most common roots and their combining vowels are listed here:

Root (combining vowel)	Meaning
abdomin (o)	abdomen
aden (o)	gland
adren (o)	adrenal gland
angi (o)	vessel
arterio	artery
arthr (o)	joint
broncho	bronchus, bronchi
card, cardi (o)	heart
cephal (o)	head
chole, chol(o)	bile
chondr (o)	cartilage
colo	colon, large intestine
cost (o)	rib
crani (o)	skull
cyan (o)	blue
cyst (o)	bladder, cyst
cyt (o)	cell
dent (o)	tooth
derma	skin
duoden (o)	duodenum
encephal (o)	brain
enter (o)	intestines
fibr (o)	fibre, fibrous
gastr (o)	stomach
gloss (o)	tongue
gluc (o)	sweetness, glucose
glyc (o)	sugar
gyn, gyne, gyneco	woman
hem, hema, hemo, hemat (o)	blood
hepat (o)	liver
hydr (o)	water
hyster (o)	uterus
ile (o), ili (o)	ileum
laparo	abdomen, loin, or flank
laryng (o)	larynx
lith (o)	stone
mamm (o)	breast, mammary gland

Root (combining vowel)	Meaning
mast (o)	mammary gland, breast
meno	menstruation
my (o)	muscle
myel (o)	spinal cord, bone marrow
necro	death
nephr (o)	kidney
neur (o)	nerve
ocul (o)	eye
oophor (o)	ovary
ophthalm (o)	eye
orth (o)	straight, normal, correct
oste (o)	bone
ot (o)	ear
ped (o)	child, foot
pharyng (o)	pharynx
phleb (o)	vein
pnea	breathing, respiration
pneum (o)	lung, air, gas
proct (o)	rectum
psych (o)	mind
pulmo	lung
py (o)	pus
rect (o)	rectum
rhin (o)	nose
salping (o)	eustachian tube, uterine tube
splen (o)	spleen
sten (o)	narrow, constriction
stern (o)	sternum
stomat (o)	mouth
therm (o)	heat
thoraco	chest
thromb (o)	clot, thrombus
thyr (o)	thyroid
toxic (o)	poison, poisonous
toxo	poison
trache (o)	trachea
urethr (o)	urethra
urin (o)	urine
uro	urine, urinary tract, urination
uter (o)	uterus
vas (o)	blood vessel, vas deferens
ven (o)	vein
vertebr (o)	spine, vertebrae

SUFFIXES

A **suffix** is placed at the end of a root to change the meaning of the word. Suffixes are not used alone. Like prefixes and roots, they are from Greek and Latin. When translating medical terms, begin with the suffix. For example, *nephritis* means inflammation of the kidney. It is formed by combining *nephro* (kidney) and *itis* (inflammation).

You need to learn the suffixes listed below:

Suffix	Meaning
-algia	pain
-asis	condition, usually abnormal
-cele	hernia, herniation, pouching
-centesis	puncture and aspiration of
-cyte	cell
-ectasis	dilation, stretching
-ectomy	excision, removal of
-emia	blood condition
-genesis	development, production, creation
-genic	producing, causing
-gram	record
-graph	a diagram, a recording instrument
-graphy	making a recording
-iasis	condition of
-ism	a condition
-itis	inflammation
-logy	the study of
-lysis	destruction of, decomposition
-megaly	enlargement
-meter	measuring instrument
-metry	measurement
-oma	tumour
-osis	condition
-pathy	disease
-penia	lack, deficiency
-phasia	speaking
-phobia	an exaggerated fear
-plasty	surgical repair or reshaping
-plegia	paralysis
-ptosis	falling, sagging, dropping, down
-rrhage, -rrhagia	excessive flow
-rrhaphy	stitching, suturing
-rrhea	profuse flow, discharge
-scope	examination instrument
-scopy	examination using a scope
-stasis	maintenance, maintaining a constant level
-stomy, -ostomy	creation of an opening
-tomy, -otomy	incision, cutting into
-uria	condition of the urine

Combining Word Elements

Medical terms are formed by combining word elements. A root can be combined with prefixes, roots, or suffixes. The prefix *dys* (difficult) can be combined with the root *pnea* (breathing). This forms the term *dyspnea,* meaning difficulty in breathing.

Roots can be combined with suffixes. The root *mast* (breast) combined with the suffix *ectomy* (excision or removal) forms the term *mastectomy.* It means the removal of a breast.

Combining a prefix, root, and suffix is another way to form medical terms. *Endocarditis* consists of the prefix *endo* (inner), the root *card* (heart), and the suffix *itis* (inflammation). *Endocarditis* means inflammation of the inner part of the heart.

There are more complex combinations of prefixes, roots, and suffixes:

- Two prefixes, a root, and a suffix
- A prefix, two roots, and a suffix
- Two roots and a suffix

The important things to remember are that prefixes always come before roots and suffixes always come after roots. You can practise forming medical terms by combining the word elements listed in this chapter.

Abdominal Regions

The abdomen is divided into regions (Figure 48-1) in order to help describe the location of body structures, pain, or discomfort. The regions are:

- Right upper quadrant (RUQ)
- Left upper quadrant (LUQ)
- Right lower quadrant (RLQ)
- Left lower quadrant (LLQ)

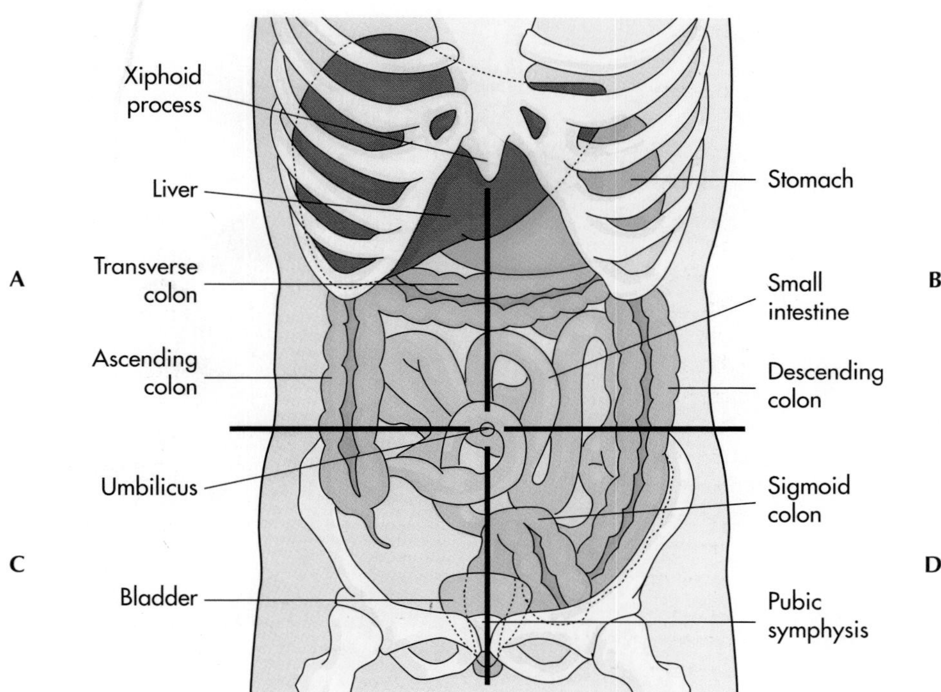

Figure 48-1 The four regions of the abdomen. **A,** Right upper quadrant. **B,** Left upper quadrant. **C,** Right lower quadrant. **D,** Left lower quadrant.

Directional Terms

Certain terms describe the position of one body part in relation to another. These terms give the direction of the body part when a person is standing and facing forward. The following directional terms come from some of the prefixes listed in this chapter:

- ***Anterior (ventral)***—located at or toward the front of the body or body part
- ***Distal***—the part farthest from the centre or from the point of attachment
- ***Lateral***—relating to or located at the side of the body or body part
- ***Medial***—relating to or located at or near the middle or midline of the body or body part
- ***Posterior (dorsal)***—located at or toward the back of the body or body part
- ***Proximal***—the part nearest to the centre or to the point of origin

Abbreviations

Abbreviations are shortened forms of words or phrases. They save time and space in written communication. Each employer has a list of accepted abbreviations. Obtain the list when you are hired, and use only the abbreviations accepted by the employer. If you are unsure an abbreviation is acceptable, write the term out in full to communicate accurately.

Common abbreviations are listed on the inside of the back cover for easy reference.

REVIEW

Fill in the blanks.

1 Word elements used in medical terminology are
   a ______________________________
   b ______________________________
   c ______________________________

2 A ______ is placed at the beginning of a word to change the meaning of the word.

3 A ______ is placed at the end of a word to change the meaning of the word.

4 The four regions of the abdomen are
   a ______________________________
   b ______________________________
   c ______________________________
   d ______________________________

Match the item in column A with the item in column B.

Column A		Column B	
5	Distal	a	The part nearest to the centre or point of origin
6	Proximal	b	Relating to or located at the side of the body or body part
7	Anterior (ventral)	c	Located at or toward the front part of the body or body part
8	Medial	d	The part farthest from the centre or point of attachment
9	Posterior (dorsal)	e	Located at or toward the back of the body or body part
10	Lateral	f	Relating to or located at or near the middle or the midline of the body or body part

Write the definition of the following prefixes.

11 a- ______________________________
12 dys- ______________________________
13 bi- ______________________________
14 ab- ______________________________
15 trans- ______________________________
16 post- ______________________________
17 olig- ______________________________
18 hyper- ______________________________
19 per- ______________________________
20 hemi- ______________________________
21 hypo- ______________________________
22 ad- ______________________________

Write the definition of the following suffixes.

23 -algia ______________________________
24 -itis ______________________________
25 -ostomy ______________________________
26 -ectomy ______________________________
27 -emia ______________________________
28 -osis ______________________________
29 -rrhage ______________________________
30 -penia ______________________________
31 -pathy ______________________________
32 -otomy ______________________________
33 -rrhea ______________________________
34 -plasty ______________________________

Write the definition of the following roots.

35 cranio ______________________________
36 cardio ______________________________
37 mammo ______________________________
38 veno ______________________________
39 urino ______________________________
40 pnea ______________________________
41 cyano ______________________________
42 arterio ______________________________
43 colo ______________________________
44 arthro ______________________________
45 litho ______________________________
46 gastro ______________________________
47 encephalo______________________________
48 gluco ______________________________
49 hemo ______________________________
50 hystero ______________________________
51 hepato ______________________________
52 myo ______________________________
53 nephro ______________________________

REVIEW

54 phlebo ________
55 oculo ________
56 osteo ________
57 neuro ________
58 pneumo ________
59 toxico ________
60 psycho ________
61 thoraco ________

Match the item in column A with the item in column B.

Column A	Column B
62 Intravenous	a Inflammation of a joint
63 Apnea	b Blood in the urine
64 Hemiplegia	c Excessive flow of blood
65 Thoracotomy	d Paralysis on one side
66 Arthritis	e Surgical removal of the uterus
67 Bronchitis	f No breathing
68 Anuria	g Inflammation of the bronchi
69 Hematuria	h Incision into the chest
70 Hysterectomy	i No urine
71 Hemorrhage	j Within a vein

Write the abbreviation for the following terms.

72 Bathroom privileges ________
73 As desired ________
74 Complains of ________
75 Twice a day ________
76 Hour of sleep ________
77 Intake and output ________
78 Nothing by mouth ________
79 When necessary ________
80 Postoperative ________
81 Every ________
82 Wheelchair ________
83 At once, immediately ________

Answers to these questions are on page 828.

CHAPTER

49

YOUR JOB SEARCH

OBJECTIVES

- Learn the key terms listed in this chapter
- List three tools you need to organize yourself for your job search
- Explain the difference between a chronological résumé and a functional résumé
- List three sources of advertised positions
- Identify methods for finding out about unadvertised positions
- List five details that are important in a letter of application
- Explain why you should take time completing application forms
- List what interviewers are trying to determine during an interview
- Explain why the interview is a key element in the job search
- Explain why it is important to practise and plan before an interview
- Describe three ways to make a good impression at an interview
- Explain why it is important to write a thank-you note following an interview

KEY TERMS

chronological résumé A résumé that highlights employment history, starting with the most current employment and working in reverse chronological order (backward) through earlier jobs

cover letter Letter of application

functional résumé A résumé that highlights skills or functions and briefly lists positions held

letter of application A letter that is included with a résumé; can be solicited or unsolicited; cover letter

reference A person who can speak to a potential employer about your skills, abilities, and personal qualities

résumé A concise one- to two-page summary of experience, education, work-related skills, and personal qualities

solicited letter of application A letter of application that responds to an advertised position

unsolicited letter of application A letter of application that enquires about potential openings

Finding a job takes discipline, focus, and hard work. For many people, the process is stressful because the end result is uncertain. However, with good preparation and a sound plan, the job search can be exciting and rewarding. It gives you the opportunity to learn about yourself and to meet new people.

Getting Organized

Your job search will be more successful if you get organized before you start. Choose a place in your home where you will work. Then make sure you have the following tools in your workspace:

- *A computer and printer*—There are many benefits to having a computer. A computer enables you to store letters and résumés; it also can give you Internet and e-mail access. Many employers today post job openings on the Internet and correspond by e-mail. Letters and résumés prepared on the computer look more professional than hand-written letters. If you do not own a computer, you need access to one. Most public libraries have computers available to the public. You can obtain an e-mail account whether or not your have your own computer.
- *A telephone with an answering machine*—Prospective employers need to be able to reach you. The message on your answering machine should sound professional.
- *Office supplies*—Make sure that you have a supply of good-quality paper, notebooks, envelopes, file folders, a stapler, paper clips, Post-It notes, pens, pencils, and stamps.
- *Resources*—Many excellent books and websites can help in your job search. Look for books and websites that show you how to prepare a résumé and cover letter. Your college library or local public library should have extensive resources on the job search. Box 49-1 contains a list of useful resources.

Setting Priorities and Goals

Before writing your résumé, think about your priorities and goals. Decide the following:

- What type of support work do you want to pursue?
- Would you prefer to work in a facility or a community setting?
- Do you want full-time or part-time work?

As discussed in Chapter 3, there are many different kinds of support work settings. If you have experience in health care, you probably know the setting you prefer. If you are inexperienced, your course may have helped you make the decision. If you are still undecided, you may want to apply for work in a variety of settings.

Preparing Your Résumé

A **résumé** is a concise one- to two-page summary of your experience, education, work-related skills, and personal qualities. It is the first step to a job interview. A résumé introduces you to possible employers. It must look and sound professional. Employers use résumés to decide which job applicants to interview. Even small errors like typos and spelling mistakes influence the employer's decision.

As you prepare your résumé, keep the needs of the prospective employer in mind. It is best to prepare your résumé before you begin your job search. This

Box 49-1 Useful Resources for Your Job Search

Resource	Description
What Color Is Your Parachute?	Well-known guide on job hunting
www.jobhuntersbible.com	Website for *What Color Is Your Parachute?*
jobfutures.ca/en/home.shtml	Website address for Job Futures, a Canadian site that provides information on the world of work, including an overview of the labour market
www.careerbookstore.ca	Website with a comprehensive catalogue of books on all aspects of the job search
www.resumeedge.com	Free sample résumés and cover letters
accent-resume-writing.com/tips/	Tips on résumé writing
www.job-interview.net	Sample interview questions
www.workopolis.com	Comprehensive website on all aspects of the job search. It posts positions in health care on the website. You can post your résumé on the Workopolis website for employers to view.

gives you time to do it properly without rushing. Consider what most employers look for in support workers (see Chapter 1). However, each job is unique. Revise your résumé to fit the needs of each employer and setting. Keep a copy of the résumé on a disk in a safe place so you can change or update it at any time.

Elements of a Résumé

All résumés include information on the following:

- *Experience*—Employers want to know what you have done that qualifies you for the position. Experience does not have to be paid work. It can include volunteer work, field placements, special projects, and recreational activities. Stress your skills and accomplishments rather than your duties and responsibilities.
- *Education*—Employers want to know if you have the educational qualifications for the position. Your résumé should include the exact name of your certificate, the name of your educational institution, and the year you graduated. Also include additional training and any awards or honours you received.

The following elements are optional:

- *Objective*—An objective on a résumé states your career goal and briefly lists relevant skills, abilities, and personal qualities. It appears at the top of the first page of your résumé, underneath your name.
- *Profile*—A career profile summarizes your qualifications, highlighting particular skills and experience in one brief paragraph. It usually appears at the top of the first page of your résumé, underneath your name. Most people include either an objective or a profile, but rarely both.
- *Interests*—Most career consultants advise against including a separate section on interests because it takes up valuable space. Instead, they suggest incorporating accomplishments in sports or hobbies into other sections of the résumé. Only include information on sports or hobbies if it is relevant to the job. For example, mention your skills in curling only if you can use it to show you are an experienced team player.

Getting Started on Your Résumé

Think of a résumé as an advertisement for those experiences, skills, and qualities that an employer might be seeking. Start by making a list of the skills and qualities an employer would want in a support worker. Then make a list of your own skills and qualities. Also list the experiences that helped you to develop those qualities.

If you cannot identify your skills and qualities, start by thinking about your experiences. Ask yourself what you learned from each experience. How have your experiences influenced you?

Organizing Your Résumé

There are two basic résumé styles: the chronological résumé and the functional résumé.

Chronological Résumé. A **chronological résumé** highlights employment history, starting with the most current employment and working in reverse chronological order (backward) through earlier jobs (Figure 49-1 on page 808). Because of its emphasis on work history, it is best for those who have:

- A steady history of employment in their chosen field
- At least two years' employment with one employer
- Few gaps between jobs

Sean Tootoosis

16 Uptown Street, Apt. 4, Edmonton, AB T9Q 2P1, (403) 765-4321, stootoosis@elsewhere.net

PROFILE

- Experienced support worker has cared for clients with diverse needs
- Skilled at motivating clients to regain their independence
- Dedicated to creating a caring, compassionate environment
- Discreet, hard-working, and loyal

EXPERIENCE

Support Worker, Hummingbird Agency, Edmonton, AB, August 1999–Present
- Provide personal care and support to diverse client population
- Skilled at caring for clients with quadriplegia and severe physical disabilities
- Selected to assist in training new staff and writing procedures for manual
- Praised for my calm, composed, empathetic manner with clients
- Demonstrated ability to work independently under minimal supervision

Support Worker, Primrose Group Home, Edmonton, AB, June 1996–July 1999
- Assisted developmentally disabled adolescents with activities of daily living
- Developed good listening and other interpersonal skills
- Demonstrated flexibility in meeting multiple needs and finishing tasks on time
- Commended by supervisor for initiative and problem-solving skills
- Served as leader of four-person team to redesign the home's living space

Lamantia Brickworks and Patios, Edmonton, AB, March 1990–May 1995
- Demonstrated leadership skills while supervising team of four bricklayers.

EDUCATION AND TRAINING

- Certificate in Personal Support Work, Western Canadian College, Edmonton, AB, 1996
- St. John's Ambulance First Aid and CPR Level C, Certification, Edmonton, AB, yearly 1996–2003

OTHER

- Spoken languages: English and Cree

Figure 49-1 Chronological résumé.

Functional Résumé. A **functional résumé** highlights skills or functions and briefly lists positions held (Figure 49-2). Because it emphasizes skills and abilities rather than specific jobs, a functional résumé is best for those who have:

- Little work experience in their chosen field
- Long periods in which they were not in the workforce
- Frequent job changes

A functional résumé should include an outline of your employment history with dates. A résumé that excludes this information might suggest that you have something to hide.

(text continues on page 810)

KAYLEE SAUVÉ

105 Pine Avenue, Hamilton, ON L4W 5Y3, (905) 725-9589, ksauve@link.com

OBJECTIVE

To provide support to clients in their homes and to deliver compassionate personal care.

SKILLS AND ABILITIES

- Listening skills: composed, respectful, and empathetic
- Speaking skills: won public speaking award in secondary school
- Language skills: speak English and French fluently
- Organizational skills: ability to complete work while meeting multiple demands
- Leadership skills: strong ability to motivate others; captain of winning basketball team
- Meal preparation skills: experienced; sound knowledge of food safety and nutrition
- Mature and responsible: childcare worker for two families for six years
- Flexible: able to work in a variety of settings and adapt to different situations
- Self-reliant: confident working under minimal supervision
- Physically strong: unloaded trucks and lifted boxes at local food bank

EDUCATION

- Certificate in Personal Support Work, Ontario Institute for Applied Health Sciences, Hamilton, ON, 2003
- St. John's Ambulance First Aid and CPR Level C, Certification, Hamilton, ON, 2003
- Food Safety course, River College, Toronto, ON, 2002

EXPERIENCE

Sunset Nursing Home, Field Placement, Hamilton, ON, February 2002–April 2002
- Prepared and delivered meals for 35 residents

Ricky's Restaurant, Waitress, Hamilton, ON, Summers, May 1998–August 2002
- Greeted customers, served meals, prepared salads

Children's Caregiver, Hamilton, ON, Part-time, 1995–2001
- Cared for children ages 4 months through 9 years

Volunteer, Daily Food Bank, Hamilton, ON, January 1998–March 2001
- Unloaded trucks, stocked shelves, helped customers

Figure 49-2 Functional résumé.

Writing Your Résumé

You will probably need to write several drafts of your résumé before you are satisfied. As you write your drafts, ask yourself these questions:

- *Is the information relevant?* You have limited space to make an impression. Mention only those experiences that say something about how you would perform on the job.
- *Have I been completely honest?* Make the most of your strengths. However, do not misrepresent yourself. It is unethical to lie. Do not change your qualifications, job titles, and dates of employment. Do not exaggerate if you are lacking experience. Remember that some employers prefer to hire inexperienced workers, who may be more motivated and flexible than those with experience.
- *Have I expressed myself clearly?* Be concise and avoid using long words. Revise your work to make sure it is clear. Avoid writing paragraphs. Use bulleted points instead. Sentences should be short and direct. Start them with action words and avoid the use of the word "I." Remember, your résumé should be only one or two pages.
- *Is my résumé consistent?* Set up the page, headings, and sentences consistently. Use bullets, bolding, italics, and underlining the same way throughout the document. Use the same grammatical form for each point.
- *Is my résumé correct?* Read over the final document several times slowly and carefully. Some people have problems proofreading their own work because they read what they think they have written rather than what is actually on the page. Read your document backwards. Starting at the end of the résumé, read each sentence backwards. You are more likely to catch typos and spelling mistakes when you read this way. Do not depend on computer spell-checks to find errors. Ask at least two reliable people to proofread your résumé.

Formatting and Printing

To make a good impression, your résumé must look neat and professional:

- Choose a simple, professional-looking font (typeface) such as Times New Roman or Ariel.
- Do not use more than one font.
- Keep the use of graphic devices, such as bolding, to a minimum.
- Do not crowd too much type onto the page.

Most computer programs have preset résumé designs that you can use to format your résumé. Many books and websites present a variety of designs that you can use. Some websites offer to format your résumé so that it can be posted on the web. You can also have your résumé formatted by a professional. Look in the Yellow Pages under "Résumé Service" to find a résumé centre near you. Your college may also provide this service through the career centre.

Print your résumé on good-quality white or ivory bond paper that is 8½" × 11". If your résumé is two pages, staple the pages together.

Finding and Following Leads

The main sources for advertised positions are local newspapers, the Internet, and college career services.

- *Employment advertisements.* Check your local newspaper daily for advertisements. If your community has a weekly newspaper, check that as well.
- *The Internet.* Many health care facilities post job openings on their websites. To search the Internet, try using the headings "Health Care," "Home Health Care," "Home Care," "Home Health Services," "Community Health Care," "Retirement Homes," "Nursing Homes," and "Nursing Services." Also try "Not-For-Profit Jobs/Careers." General job search websites such as Workopolis (see Box 49-1 on page 807) also post health care positions.
- *College career services.* Some colleges offer a career service to students and members of the community. Employers post job openings on bulletin boards at the college or on the college website.

Some positions are not advertised. To find out about unadvertised positions, try the following:

- *Contact people you know.* Friends, acquaintances, and professional contacts may help you to find work and advance your career. Make a list of people you know in the health care field, including course instructors and employers you worked for in your program placement. Ask these people if any positions are available at their workplace. They may be aware of jobs posted on bulletin boards, or jobs that may become available.
- *Check with your district home care program.* The websites of your health district's home care program or community care access centre may list agencies used to deliver home care in the community. They may also list long-term care agencies.
- *Look in the Yellow Pages.* Look under the headings "Home Health Care," "Home Care," "Home Health Services," "Community Health Care," "Retirement Homes," "Nurses and Nurses Registries," "Nursing Homes," and "Nursing Services."
- *Check your local library.* Libraries often have lists of health care facilities and agencies.

- *Attend job fairs.* Job fairs are often held at community colleges or elsewhere in the community. The fairs are advertised in the local newspapers, on local cable channels, or at your college.
- *Check with your Canada Employment Centre.* These centres often have information about local area employers. They may also have information about specific job openings.

SELECTING REFERENCES

A **reference** is a person who can speak to a potential employer about your skills, abilities, and personal qualities. Choose the people you want as references early in the job search. Do not use family members or friends as references. Previous employers are usually the best people to use as references. Other possibilities are people in positions of authority such as teachers and camp directors. Here are some basic tips about references:

- *Ask for the reference*—Do not use someone as a reference without asking. Explain the type of work you are looking for. Do not assume the person will speak positively about you. Ask the person what he or she would say are your strengths and weaknesses. Be reasonably certain the person will speak positively about you before listing him or her as a reference.
- *Make sure contact information is correct*—Make sure you provide accurate phone numbers or e-mail addresses to give prospective employers.
- *Keep your references informed*—Let your references know when you are going for a job interview so that they can prepare for a phone call. They are more likely to give you a good reference if they are prepared.
- *Follow up*—Keep your references informed about your job search. If you got the job, thank them for their help. If you did not get the job, let them know.

PREPARING A LETTER OF APPLICATION

A **letter of application**, also called a **cover letter**, is a letter included with a résumé. There are two kinds of letters of application:

- A **solicited letter of application** responds to an advertised position (Figure 49-3 on page 812)
- An **unsolicited letter of application** inquires about potential job openings (Figure 49-4 on page 813)

A letter of application should not simply summarize the information in your résumé. It should focus on what you can *offer* by demonstrating how your skills and experiences are relevant to the job you are seeking. A good letter of application is persuasive, professional, and personalized. It should be addressed to a prospective employer by name. It should also be written specifically for the position you are seeking.

(text continues on page 814)

ADVERTISEMENT

Ferndale Lodge has two positions available for support workers. Reporting to the Director of Nursing Services, the successful candidates will provide personal care to residents. They must have excellent communications, problem-solving, and organizational skills. They must be able to cope with the demands of personal care services while remaining calm and courteous with clients and their families. They must be available to work days, evenings, nights, and weekends. Experience preferred, but not required.

Reply in confidence to Derek Sykes, Human Resources Director, Ferndale Lodge, Box 101, Littletown, BC, V6X 2Z1.

453 Lower Town Road
Littletown, BC
V6N 4N3

September 5, 2003

Mr. Derek Sykes
Human Resources Director
Ferndale Lodge
Box 101
Littletown, BC
V6X 2Z1

Dear Mr. Sykes:

I am writing to apply for one of the support worker positions that were advertised in the September 4th issue of *The Star Daily*.

You specified that Ferndale Lodge is seeking qualified support workers with excellent communications, problem-solving, and organizational skills. I attended the support worker program at Central Vancouver College, where I developed strong organizational skills and finished in the top third of the class. Before enrolling in the support worker program, I worked as a full-time cashier while raising three children. In my position as a cashier for *Fresh Food,* I interacted with the public and treated all customers with respect, tact, and courtesy. I was promoted to the customer service desk, where I learned how to solve customers' problems efficiently and diplomatically.

I am a mature, hard-working person who enjoys working with people. I am also assertive, persuasive, and adaptable to new situations. Because I am highly motivated to begin a new career in support work, I would be a productive and enthusiastic employee. I am available to work all the times that you listed in your advertisement, including weekends.

Enclosed you will find a résumé that details my skills and experience. At your convenience, I would like to meet to discuss how I can contribute to Ferndale Lodge.

Sincerely,

Belinda Lau

Belinda Lau
(604) 345-6789
bflau@internet.ca

Enclosure

Figure 49-3 A sample advertisement and a solicited letter of application.

Letter	Annotation
105 Pine Avenue Hamilton, ON L4W 5Y3	Include return address
October 15, 2003	Include today's date
Ms. Katherine Ferrero Director of Personnel Mapleview Health Care Agency 1572 Maple Road Hamilton, ON L9P 8B2	Identify the name and title of contact, and address of prospective employer
Dear Ms. Ferrero:	Include a greeting
I read in *The Sun Daily* on October 14th that Mapleview Health Care Agency is expanding its home care services. I am writing to ask you to consider me if you need support workers.	Identify the position
The article in *The Sun Daily* indicated that Mapleview Health Care Agency offers a wide range of services to people in their homes, including personal care, meal preparation, and housekeeping. While completing a support worker course at Ontario Institute for Applied Health Sciences, I acquired skills in all those areas. For my six-week field placement, I worked in the kitchen at Sunset Nursing Home, where I prepared and delivered meal trays. In this position, I learned how to balance multiple demands by delivering hot meals on time and meeting the different dietary needs of residents.	Indicate your knowledge of the facility or agency Indicate your qualifications Link your skills to the job requirements; explain what you have learned from experience
I am a mature, responsible person who works well independently and as part of a team. Because I enjoy helping people, I know you would find me a competent and enthusiastic support worker.	Highlight personal qualities and other skills relevant to the job
Please find enclosed my résumé, which outlines my skills and experience in detail. I hope to have the opportunity to meet you to discuss how I can contribute to Mapleview Health Care Agency. Next week I will call you to discuss the possibility of an interview.	Indicate that your résumé is enclosed Ask for an interview
Sincerely, *Kaylee Sauvé* Kaylee Sauvé (905) 725-9589 ksauve@link.com	Include a signature block
Enclosure	

Figure 49-4 Unsolicited letter of application.

Determining the Employer's Needs

If the letter is solicited, study the advertisement to decide what the employer is looking for. Describe your experiences and skills that match what the employer wants. Think about some of the skills and qualities that are not listed in the advertisement. Even if you are new to support work, your course should have provided you with information about those qualities.

If you write an unsolicited letter, find out as much as you can about the employer first. As mentioned, many agencies and facilities have websites that contain information about their health care goals and practices. For example, a facility's website might emphasize respect, compassion, and innovation. In your letter, you could indicate experiences in which you have demonstrated some of these qualities.

Organizing a Letter of Application

Use standard letter format to organize your letter. The sample letter in Figure 49-4 on page 813 shows different parts of a standard letter.

Front Matter

- *Return address.* Put your mailing address at the top left-hand corner of the page.
- *Today's date.* Include today's date on the left-hand side of the letter beneath your return address.
- *Name, title, and address of prospective employer.* Include a contact person's name, title, and address flush with the left-hand margin. Ensure that this information is correct. You may have to call the facility or agency to check. If you are unable to find out the person's name, you may have to exclude this information.
- *Greeting.* Greet the person you are writing to in a professional manner. If you do not know the name, write "Dear Sir or Madam."

Body

- *Paragraph one.* Identify the job, indicate how it came to your attention, and explain your purpose for writing. For unsolicited letters, use this opening paragraph to ask about potential opportunities.
- *Paragraph two.* Explain how your qualifications, experience, and skills relate to the position you are seeking.
- *Paragraph three.* Describe personal qualities or additional skills that make you a suitable candidate.

Closing

- *Paragraph four.* Use your concluding paragraph to ask for an interview. If the letter is unsolicited, say that you will contact the reader at a future date. Refer the reader to the enclosed résumé.
- *Signature block.* End the letter in a professional manner by writing "Sincerely" or "Yours Truly." Type your name at the end of the letter. Sign in ink above the typed name. Add your phone number and e-mail address (if you have one) following your name. Type "Enclosure" at the bottom of the page to indicate that your résumé is enclosed.

Writing Your Letter

You will probably have to write several drafts to produce a convincing letter. First concentrate on getting down your main points. As you revise, ask yourself the following questions:

- *Have I emphasized relevant skills and qualities?* Mention experiences that demonstrate the skills, qualities, and attitudes necessary to support work. For example, if you have worked as a sales clerk, emphasize your positive interactions with clients.
- *Have I emphasized accomplishments and skills?* Rather than simply listing duties, explain what your experience has taught you. You might say "Working as a sales clerk taught me how to interact with the public in a warm, courteous, and respectful manner."
- *Have I used an appropriate tone?* Your letter should be written in a respectful, capable, and professional tone. Be persuasive without being boastful. Minimize the use of the word "I" to sound more modest. If you lack experience, avoid an apologetic tone.
- *Is my letter concise?* Your letter should not be more than one page. If it is longer, eliminate some of the detail.
- *Does my letter sound and look professional?* Proofread your letter carefully and have at least two reliable people do the same. Prepare it on a computer. Use standard business letter format and print it on high-quality paper. Double-check that your contact information is correct. You want to be completely sure that a prospective employer can reach you.

Delivering Your Letter

Hand-deliver your letter of application and résumé whenever possible to make sure they arrive on time. Another alternative method of delivery is to courier the information to a prospective employer. Follow up with a telephone call to the appropriate person to check that the information arrived. If you respond to an advertisement, deliver your letter and résumé as soon as possible. Sometimes the earliest applicants get more attention simply because their applications arrived first.

Many employers request that letters and résumés be submitted by e-mail. Because technologies vary, your résumé could lose its formatting. Or a prospective employer may have difficulty opening it. If you send your letter and résumé by e-mail, deliver a hard copy as well. (If the employer asks the applicant not to submit a hard copy, you need to abide by this request.)

Completing a Job Application Form

For some positions, you are expected to complete a job application form. Employers use applications to find out specific information. Some also use forms to make sure applicants have acceptable reading and writing skills. It is a good idea to attach your résumé to the job application form, even if one is not required.

Most application forms ask for information about the following:

- Your legal eligibility to work in Canada
- Your education
- Your work-related skills
- Your employment history
- Names and phone numbers of employers
- Reasons for leaving previous jobs
- The names and phone numbers of three references

Remember that the completed application form says something about you. It should be professional looking, with no spelling and grammar mistakes and no blank spaces. Do a thorough job with the form. If possible, take two copies of the form home with you. Use one as a rough copy and the other as your final copy. Ask someone reliable to read the final copy. If you make an error on the final copy, use eraser fluid to make the correction.

Application forms often require detailed information such as the reason for leaving a job. You must answer every question truthfully. If you have been fired, or if you have an inconsistent work history, consider attaching a note of explanation.

Some employers require you to submit an on-line application form. Be just as careful with an on-line application as you would with a hard copy. Ask someone reliable to read it over before you send it.

The Interview

You will not be hired as a support worker unless someone first interviews you and decides you are the right person for the job. During the interview, a prospective employer is trying to determine the following:

- Do you have the educational qualifications for the job?
- Do you have the skills necessary to do the job, or can you learn those skills?
- Will clients and co-workers respond well to you?
- Will you be a reliable, responsible, and motivated employee?

The interview is a key factor in any job search. From the interview, prospective employers decide if you have essential personal qualities like compassion, respect, and enthusiasm. They can also judge if you are a good listener, if you speak clearly, and if you are at ease with others.

Interviewers may ask questions to find out the following:

- Can you handle the stress of working with seriously ill people?
- Can you deal with interpersonal conflict?
- Would you respond calmly and responsibly to an emergency?
- Are you capable of being firm and assertive with clients?
- Are you flexible enough to adapt to a variety of situations?
- Can you handle multiple demands and conflicts?
- Can you work under minimal supervision?
- Do you have initiative?
- Are you an effective team player?
- Can you handle routine problems on your own?
- Are you discreet?
- Do you respect individual differences?
- Are you a quick learner?
- Are you effective at managing your time?

Many interviewers ask situational questions. These are questions that are designed to find out what you would do in a certain situation. You may be asked a question about an imaginary situation. Or you may be asked to describe what you did in a particular situation.

Always prepare for an interview. When you are nervous, it can be difficult to think and speak clearly. If you have thought about possible questions and answers, you are more likely to be at ease. To prepare for an interview, think about the following:

- *The position.* Make sure you understand the nature of the position. Learn about the employer's services, clients, and philosophy. This may require research. Check information that is available to the general public such as websites and brochures. Talk to friends, instructors, and acquaintances who know the agency or facility. Review the skills and qualities that are essential to support work.
- *Your qualities, skills, and experience.* Develop a clear understanding of yourself: your values, skills, qualities, interests, goals, strengths, and weaknesses. Write these down, along with specific experiences that illustrate each.
- *The interviewer.* Put yourself in the interviewer's place. Review your cover letter and résumé. Why do you think you were selected for an interview? What concerns might the reviewer have about you? For example, if you are young and inexperienced, the interviewer may be concerned about your maturity level. If you have never remained in a job for more than a

year, the interviewer may be concerned about your commitment. Be prepared to address these concerns.

PRACTISING

Practice will give you confidence. When practising, focus on listening skills, relaxation techniques, and responses to questions you think might be asked.

Developing Listening Skills. The ability to listen is an important interviewing skill. If you fail to listen, you will not make a good impression. Since listening is essential in support work, an employer is unlikely to hire a poor listener as a support worker. Be a good listener during the interview by avoiding the following:

- Failing to concentrate on what the interviewer is saying
- Failing to ask for clarification if the question is unclear
- Talking too much
- Responding to questions too quickly without thinking first about the answer

Practising Relaxation Techniques. You will probably listen more attentively if you feel relaxed in the interview. Deep breathing exercises and other relaxation techniques can help you relax (see Chapter 8).

Practising Your Responses. Most interviewers ask similar questions. See Box 49-2 for a list of commonly asked questions. Practise your responses to these questions in front of a mirror or with a friend.

Box 49-2 Common Interview Questions

- Tell me a little about yourself.
- What are your strengths?
- What are your weaknesses?
- Tell me about your last job.
- What did you like best/least about your last job?
- Why did you leave your last job?
- Why do you want to be a support worker?
- What do you think are the three most important qualities in a support worker?
- What do you think you can bring to support work?
- What do you think is the biggest challenge in support work?
- What do you like best/least about support work?
- Describe a situation in which you have met several demands.
- Describe a typical day in your last job.
- How did you manage your time in your last job?
- What did you learn from your last job?
- Give me an example of how you have worked as part of a team.
- Tell me about a time you showed initiative on the job.
- Tell me about a problem you had in your last job. How did you handle it?
- Tell me about a conflict you had with a client or co-worker. How did you handle it?
- What would your former supervisor tell me about your strengths and weaknesses?
- I'm going to give you a made-up situation. How would you handle it?

PLANNING

Plan ahead so that things go smoothly on the interview day.

- Decide what you are going to wear and make sure that the clothing is cleaned and pressed. Get a haircut if you need one.
- If the route is unfamiliar, do a practise run so you will not get lost on the interview day. Leave yourself at least half an hour to spare in case of traffic hold-ups on the way to the interview.
- Prepare a portfolio with a fresh copy of your résumé, notepaper, and a pen that works. Include a list of references with contact information. It is a good idea to include a list of questions to ask during the interview.

MAKING A GOOD IMPRESSION

In an interview, first impressions are crucial. Poor impressions can be difficult to change, no matter how well your interview goes. From the moment you meet a prospective employer, you need to present a calm and professional image. This applies even when you stop by to pick up an application form. Pay attention to your grooming, your clothing, and your conduct.

Grooming

- Make sure your hair is freshly washed, neat, and away from your face.
- Brush and floss your teeth. If you are a heavy coffee drinker or a smoker, bring breath mints with you (but do not have them in your mouth during the interview).
- Be careful not to wear too much make-up.
- Keep jewellery to a minimum. Avoid large bracelets, rings, and earrings.
- Remove body ornaments such as nose rings and eyebrow studs; cover tattoos.
- Do not use perfume.
- Make sure your nails are trimmed. If you wear nail polish, use a neutral colour.
- If possible, wash your hands before you shake hands with the interviewer, especially if your palms perspire when you are nervous.

Clothing

- Men should wear a business suit, or jacket and separate pants, with a tie. Women should wear a business suit, dress, jacket and skirt, or jacket and tailored pants. Do not wear jeans, T-shirts, or shorts.

Avoid tight clothing. Your outfit should be coordinated and should fit properly. It should also be in good repair.
- Women should make sure that hosiery is in good repair. Carry an extra pair of stockings in your purse.
- Shoes should be in good repair and freshly polished. Avoid casual shoes such as running shoes or sandals and shoes with very high heels.

Conduct

- Arrive in the lobby 5 to 10 minutes before the interview.
- Do not bring anyone with you. If someone has driven you, ask the person to wait outside.
- Do not chew gum, smoke, or eat as you wait for the interviewer.
- Do not ask to use the phone or talk on a cell phone.
- Do not talk with the receptionist, unless he or she starts the conversation.
- If you feel nervous, take deep breaths to calm yourself.

Interview Tips

Being adequately prepared should help you feel relaxed during the interview. If you feel calm, you are more able to focus on details that may help you get the job. Some of these are discussed below.

Use a Firm Handshake. When you meet the interviewer, shake hands and smile. Use a firm handshake. A limp, clammy handshake makes a poor impression. Make sure your hands are dry. If your palms are perspiring, wipe them on a tissue as you wait in the lobby.

Do Not Use the Interviewer's First Name. The exception is if you are asked to do so. However, do call the interviewer by name.

Project a Confident Image. Stand and sit straight, breathe deeply to relax, and avoid nervous habits such as picking at your fingernails or fiddling with your hair. Be aware of gestures and body language that might be perceived negatively such as crossed arms. Look the interviewer in the eye, and keep your hands folded in your lap.

Listen Carefully. If you listen carefully, you should be able to answer questions concisely and directly. Do not be afraid to ask the interviewer to repeat a question.

Take Your Time. Many people speak quickly when they are nervous. Slow down, take a deep breath, and think about the question before you answer. A question answered too quickly may sound rehearsed.

Answer Questions Honestly. You must be honest in your answers. If you do not understand a question or you are unsure of an answer, say so. Do not try to hide aspects of your past that you think may disqualify you from the job. Instead, explain how you have learned from past mistakes. For example, if you were fired from your last position, explain the reason and give examples of how you have corrected the behaviour.

Speak Positively about Your Previous Job. Do not demean, ridicule, appear upset with, or speak critically about your previous employer, regardless of the circumstances. To do otherwise may suggest a negative attitude.

Use Experiences to Support Opinions. When you are asked your opinion, support your answer with examples from your experience. For instance, after saying "I think it's important for support workers to know their scope of practice," describe a situation that illustrates this point. If you are inexperienced, use an example from your course of study.

Ask the Right Questions. Most interviewers conclude by asking if you have any questions. The questions you prepared in advance may have been answered during the interview. Rather than trying to think up new questions, it is acceptable to say something like "No, I don't have any questions. You have addressed all the questions that I had during our discussion." If you do have a question, make sure that it is appropriate. Do not ask questions about the salary, benefits, hours, and vacation times. You can ask about these if you are offered the position.

Concluding the Interview. At the end of the interview, thank the interviewer for his or her time. Show confidence and enthusiasm by saying something like "I am really interested in working for your facility, and I am sure I could be a productive member of your staff." Whatever you say, it is important to be genuine.

Follow-Up

Send a brief thank-you note after an interview. Write the note as soon as possible, no later than the day following the interview. The thank-you note will indicate that you are enthusiastic and courteous. It might set you apart from other candidates.

The note can be hand-written or prepared on a computer. If you write the note by hand, use a plain white note card. Write at least one draft before you write the final copy. Ask someone else to read the note before you send it. Mail the note rather than send it by e-mail. It shows the employer you are prepared to make an effort.

Express your thanks for the interview and reinforce your interest in the position. Sign your name on the card. Figure 49-5 on page 818 contains a sample note.

(text continues on page 819)

October 03, 2003

Dear Ms. Frye,

Thank you for the interview on Wednesday morning. I appreciated the opportunity to meet you and to discuss your needs for the support worker position at Greenacres.

As I mentioned at the end of the interview, I am very interested in the position. I am sure that my recent experience in home care would enable me to make an immediate contribution to your care team.

Once again, thank you for your time and interest. I look forward to hearing from you.

All the best,

Sumi Ramarashan
(604) 432-7376

Figure 49-5 Sample thank-you note.

The Employment Offer

You may be offered the position at the end of the interview or within a few days following the interview. Or you may wait weeks before hearing anything. Instead of waiting by the phone, continue to explore other opportunities.

Even if you are not offered a job, the interview experience will have been worthwhile if you can learn from it. Review the interview process by asking yourself the questions in Box 49-3.

If you are not offered the job, contact the employer to see if you can learn why. Ask if you can talk to the person who interviewed you, either in person or on the phone. Most employers are willing to help people who are genuinely interested in improving their skills.

Box 49-3 Learning from the Interview Experience

- Was I prepared enough? Did I practise my listening skills, relaxation techniques, and responses to potential questions?
- Did I arrive for the interview in plenty of time?
- Did I pay enough attention to my grooming, my clothing, and my conduct?
- Did I project a calm, professional, positive image?
- Did I listen attentively?
- Did I speak clearly and calmly?
- Did I answer all questions honestly?
- Did I use my experiences to support my opinions?
- Did I relate my skills and experience to the requirements of the job?
- Did I show enthusiasm for the job?
- Did I express interest in the job at the end of the interview?
- Did I send a thank-you note after the interview?

Accepting an Offer

Before you accept an offer of employment, find out as much as you can about the terms of your employment. Find out if the offer is conditional and if the job begins with a trial period.

Terms of Employment. At the time of the job offer, make sure that you clarify your wages, your hours of work, requirements, and expectations. If, for example, a car is required for the position, find out the employer's policy on car mileage and repairs. Many employers publish procedure manuals that should address your questions.

If the job is a contract position, find out the length of the contract, the terms of the contract, and what is and is not included in the contract prior to accepting.

If you are hired directly by a client or a client's family, you must clarify the terms of your employment. The client may be required to pay benefits such as unemployment insurance and Canada Pension. He or she may also be required to submit your taxes directly to the government. Before you accept employment directly with a client, read Revenue Canada's booklet *Employee or Self-Employed* (Catalogue Number: RC4110(E) 1219). This booklet is available at your local Canada Customs and Revenue Agency Office.

Conditional Offer. In the health care field an offer of employment is often conditional, meaning that you must meet certain conditions or requirements before you are hired. These usually include a health report signed by your family physician that verifies that you are in good health and a police record check that shows that you do not have a criminal record. You are responsible for providing all documents that are required. Some employers may also require that you have certain equipment necessary to perform the job. For example, in community settings a cell phone may be required.

Probation. Most employers hire new staff for a probationary (trial) period that lasts 3 to 6 months. During this time, both you and the employer can decide if you are the right fit for the job. Within this period, the employer can end your employment at any time and you can leave without giving the usual two-week notice.

Benefits. Find out what you can about an employer's benefits package. Many employers publish booklets that explain their benefit plan. Benefits do not usually begin until the end of the probationary period. If you work part-time you may not be eligible for benefits. Be especially careful to find out about benefits if you are working directly for a client in his or her home.

REVIEW

Circle T if the answer is true and F if it is false.

1. T F It is best to prepare your résumé before you begin your job search.
2. T F A résumé is revised for each position applied for.
3. T F Every résumé should include an objective and a career profile.
4. T F A chronological résumé is best for those with a steady work history in their chosen field.
5. T F A functional résumé should not include employment history.
6. T F Résumés should make extensive use of graphics.
7. T F It is best to ask your references what they plan to say about you.
8. T F A letter of application should summarize the information from your résumé.
9. T F A solicited letter of application inquires about potential job openings.
10. T F A letter of application should list duties held in previous positions.
11. T F Most employers overlook small mistakes on letters, résumés, and applications.
12. T F It is acceptable to wear jeans to an interview, as long as they are clean.
13. T F It is unacceptable to bring a friend to an interview, even if she or he stays in the lobby.
14. T F The ability to listen is one of the most important interviewing skills.
15. T F It is a good idea to bring a prepared list of questions to an interview.
16. T F It is usually not necessary to practise answering questions before an interview.
17. T F Assume you can address the interviewer by his or her first name.
18. T F It is best not to ask about salary, benefits, and holidays during an interview.
19. T F Never admit in an interview that you have been fired from a previous position.
20. T F If an offer is conditional, it is usually firm.

Answers to these questions are on page 829.

ANSWERS TO REVIEW QUESTIONS

Chapter 1
The Role of the Support Worker

1. C
2. C
3. B
4. D
5. A
6. D
7. B
8. C
9. A
10. A
11. B
12. A

Chapter 2
The Canadian Health Care System

1. A
2. C
3. B
4. C
5. A
6. D
7. B
8. A
9. C
10. B
11. C

Chapter 3
Workplace Settings

1. C
2. A
3. D
4. B
5. C
6. B
7. D
8. A
9. D

Chapter 4
Health, Wellness, Illness, and Disability

1. C
2. B
3. C
4. D
5. A
6. C
7. A
8. D
9. B
10. C

Chapter 5
Working with Others: Teamwork, Supervision, and Delegation

1. A
2. C
3. D
4. B
5. B
6. D
7. B
8. D
9. A
10. A

Chapter 6
Working with Clients and Their Families

1. B
2. A
3. D
4. B
5. A
6. C
7. B
8. C
9. A
10. A
11. B

Chapter 7
Client Care: Planning, Processes, Reporting, and Recording

1. A
2. D
3. A
4. B
5. B
6. A
7. B
8. A
9. C
10. C
11. D

Chapter 8
Managing Stress, Time, and Problems

1. B
2. A
3. B
4. D
5. B
6. C
7. D
8. B
9. A
10. C
11. A

Chapter 9
Ethics

1. F
2. F
3. T
4. T
5. F
6. D
7. C
8. B
9. A
10. D

Chapter 10
Legislation: The Client's Rights and Your Rights

1. B
2. C
3. A
4. C
5. D
6. A
7. D
8. A
9. D
10. C
11. A
12. C

Chapter 11
Caring about Culture

1. F
2. T
3. T
4. F
5. T
6. F
7. F
8. B
9. C
10. A
11. B

Chapter 12
Interpersonal Communication

1. A
2. B
3. D
4. C
5. A
6. D
7. A
8. D
9. B
10. D
11. B
12. A

Chapter 13
Body Structure and Function

1. A
2. B
3. C
4. C
5. A
6. B
7. C
8. D
9. D
10. B
11. A
12. B
13. B
14. C
15. A
16. B

Chapter 14
Growth and Development

1. B
2. C
3. D
4. B
5. A
6. A
7. C
8. C
9. C
10. A
11. B
12. C
13. A
14. D
15. C

Chapter 15
Caring for Older Adults

1. C
2. A

3. C
4. A
5. B
6. C
7. D
8. C
9. C
10. A
11. B
12. A

Chapter 16
Safety
1. T
2. T
3. F
4. F
5. T
6. T
7. F
8. T
9. F
10. T
11. F
12. F
13. F
14. T
15. C
16. C
17. B
18. D
19. C
20. D
21. D
22. B
23. B
24. C
25. C
26. A
27. B
28. C
29. D
30. D
31. C
32. C

Chapter 17
Restraint Alternatives and Safe Restraint Use
1. F
2. F
3. T
4. T
5. T
6. T
7. F
8. T
9. T
10. F
11. D
12. A
13. C
14. C
15. A
16. D
17. B
18. C

Chapter 18
Preventing Infection
1. F
2. T
3. F
4. T
5. F
6. T
7. F
8. F
9. F
10. T
11. F
12. T
13. F
14. T
15. F
16. T
17. T
18. F
19. F
20. F
21. T
22. T
23. B
24. D
25. C
26. A
27. D
28. A

Chapter 19
Abuse
1. D
2. B
3. C
4. C
5. C
6. B
7. A
8. A
9. C
10. D
11. A
12. B

Chapter 20
The Client's Environment: Promoting Well-Being, Comfort, and Rest

1. T
2. T
3. T
4. F
5. F
6. C
7. C
8. C
9. A
10. B
11. C
12. D

Chapter 21
Body Mechanics: Moving, Positioning, and Transferring the Client

1. F
2. T
3. F
4. T
5. F
6. T
7. T
8. F
9. T
10. T
11. F
12. T
13. F
14. T
15. T
16. F
17. T
18. F
19. T
20. F
21. B
22. C
23. B
24. C
25. B
26. A
27. A
28. D

Chapter 22
Exercise and Activity

1. A
2. B
3. C
4. B
5. B
6. C
7. A
8. B
9. C
10. B
11. F
12. F
13. T
14. F
15. T

Chapter 23
Home Management

1. C
2. C
3. C
4. A
5. C
6. D
7. A
8. B
9. D
10. A

Chapter 24
Beds and Bedmaking

1. C
2. B
3. D
4. B
5. A
6. A
7. C
8. B
9. D
10. C

Chapter 25
Basic Nutrition and Fluids

1. B
2. A
3. D
4. A
5. C
6. D
7. C
8. A
9. A
10. D
11. B
12. B
13. C
14. C

Chapter 26
Enteral Nutrition and IV Therapy

1. B
2. D
3. A
4. C
5. A
6. D
7. B
8. C
9. C

Chapter 27
Personal Hygiene

1. T
2. T
3. F
4. F
5. F
6. F
7. F
8. T
9. F
10. F
11. F
12. T
13. T
14. T
15. T
16. D
17. B
18. B
19. C
20. C
21. D

Chapter 28
Grooming and Dressing

1. D
2. C
3. A
4. D
5. C
6. B
7. D
8. B
9. D
10. A
11. A
12. F
13. F
14. T
15. T

Chapter 29
Urinary Elimination

1. B
2. D
3. A
4. B
5. B
6. A
7. D
8. C
9. D
10. B
11. A
12. B
13. D

Chapter 30
Bowel Elimination

1. A
2. B
3. D
4. A
5. C
6. D
7. B
8. C
9. B
10. D
11. D
12. A

Chapter 31
Common Diseases and Conditions

1. T
2. T
3. F
4. T
5. T
6. F
7. F
8. T
9. F
10. T
11. T
12. F
13. F
14. T
15. F
16. F
17. F
18. T
19. T
20. F
21. T
22. F

23. T
24. T
25. T
26. F
27. F
28. F
29. F
30. T
31. T

Chapter 32
Rehabilitation and Restorative Care

1. B
2. D
3. A
4. C
5. D
6. A
7. C
8. B
9. B

Chapter 33
Mental Health Disorders

1. A
2. A
3. A
4. D
5. D
6. B
7. C
8. A
9. B
10. C
11. D
12. C

Chapter 34
Confusion and Dementia

1. B
2. B
3. C
4. A
5. D
6. D
7. A
8. A
9. D
10. B
11. C
12. A
13. C

Chapter 35
Speech and Language Disorders

1. B
2. A
3. A
4. B
5. C
6. C
7. A

Chapter 36
Hearing and Vision Problems

1. B
2. A
3. C
4. A
5. B
6. C
7. D
8. B
9. C
10. D

Chapter 37
Caring for Mothers, Infants, and Children

1. C
2. C
3. D
4. A
5. C
6. B
7. B
8. A
9. C
10. A
11. D
12. C
13. B

Chapter 38
Developmental Disabilities

1. D
2. B
3. D
4. B
5. A
6. D
7. C
8. C
9. D
10. B
11. A
12. C
13. A

14. D
15. C

Chapter 39
Assisting with Medications

1. F
2. T
3. F
4. F
5. T
6. F
7. F
8. T
9. F
10. T
11. F
12. C
13. B
14. C
15. D
16. A

Chapter 40
Measuring Height, Weight, and Vital Signs

1. C
2. C
3. B
4. D
5. B
6. A
7. A
8. B
9. D
10. B
11. C
12. A
13. B

Chapter 41
Wound Care

1. T
2. T
3. F
4. T
5. T
6. B
7. C
8. A
9. C
10. B
11. C
12. D
13. D
14. A
15. A
16. B
17. D
18. C
19. C

Chapter 42
Heat and Cold Applications

1. D
2. B
3. D
4. A
5. C
6. B
7. C
8. B
9. A
10. D
11. C
12. A

Chapter 43
Oxygen Needs

1. A
2. C
3. C
4. B
5. D
6. C
7. D
8. A
9. B
10. A
11. B
12. D
13. B
14. D
15. D
16. C
17. B
18. C
19. D
20. B
21. C
22. D

Chapter 44
Assisting with the Physical Examination

1. B
2. D
3. C
4. B
5. C
6. B

Chapter 45
The Patient Having Surgery

1. F
2. T
3. F
4. F
5. T
6. T
7. T
8. F
9. T
10. T
11. C
12. B
13. A
14. A
15. C
16. C
17. A
18. B
19. C
20. D
21. A

Chapter 46
Caring for the Person Who Is Dying

1. B
2. A
3. D
4. D
5. A
6. D
7. C
8. C
9. C
10. A
11. C
12. B

Chapter 47
Basic Emergency Care

1. B
2. A
3. B
4. C
5. D
6. C
7. A
8. B
9. C
10. B
11. C
12. B
13. A
14. C
15. A
16. B
17. B
18. C
19. C
20. D
21. C
22. A
23. B
24. C
25. A
26. D

Chapter 48
Medical Terminology

1. A Prefix
   B Root
   C Suffix
2. Prefix
3. Suffix
4. A Right upper quadrant
   B Left upper quadrant
   C Right lower quadrant
   D Left lower quadrant
5. D
6. A
7. C
8. F
9. E
10. B
11. Without or not
12. Bad, difficult, abnormal
13. Double, two, twice
14. Away from
15. Across, over
16. After, behind
17. Scant, small
18. Excessive, too much
19. By, through
20. Half
21. Decreased, less than normal
22. Toward
23. Pain
24. Inflammation
25. Creation of an opening
26. Removal of, excision
27. Blood condition
28. Condition
29. Excessive flow

30. Lack, deficiency
31. Disease
32. Incision, cutting into
33. Profuse flow, discharge
34. Surgical repair or reshaping
35. Skull
36. Heart
37. Breast
38. Vein
39. Urine
40. Breathing, respiration
41. Blue
42. Artery
43. Colon, large intestine
44. Joint
45. Stone
46. Stomach
47. Brain
48. Glucose, sweetness
49. Blood
50. Uterus
51. Liver
52. Muscle
53. Kidney
54. Vein
55. Eye
56. Bone
57. Nerve
58. Lung
59. Poison
60. Mind
61. Chest
62. J
63. F
64. D
65. H
66. A
67. G
68. I
69. B
70. E
71. C
72. BRP
73. Ad lib
74. C/o
75. Bid
76. HS (hs)
77. I&O
78. NPO (npo)
79. prn
80. postop (post op)
81. q
82. w/c
83. stat

Chapter 49
Your Job Search

1. T
2. T
3. F
4. T
5. F
6. F
7. T
8. F
9. F
10. F
11. F
12. F
13. T
14. T
15. T
16. F
17. F
18. T
19. F
20. F

GLOSSARY

abbreviation A shortened form of a word or phrase

abduction Moving a body part away from the midline of the body

abrasion A partial-thickness wound caused by the scraping away or rubbing of the skin

abuse Physical or mental harm caused by someone in a position of trust—such as a family member, partner, or caregiver

accountable Being responsible for the outcome; involves answering questions and explaining actions

acetone A compound that appears in the urine from the rapid breakdown of fat for energy; ketone body

acquired brain injury Damage to brain tissue caused by disease, medical condition, accident, or violence

acquired immunodeficiency syndrome (AIDS) Immune system disease caused by the human immunodeficiency virus (HIV)

act Another term for a specific law

active listening Paying close attention to a person's verbal and nonverbal communication

activities of daily living (ADL) Self-care activities people perform daily to remain independent and to function in society

acute care Health care that is provided for a relatively short time (usually days to weeks) and is intended to diagnose and treat an immediate health issue

acute illness An illness that appears suddenly and lasts a short time, usually less than three months; symptoms can be severe

acute pain Sudden pain due to injury, disease, trauma, or surgery; it generally lasts less than 6 months

adduction Moving a body part toward the midline of the body

admission Official entry of a person into a hospital or other health care facility

adolescence A time of rapid growth and psychological and social maturity

adult daycare Community day program

advance directive A legal document in which a person states his or her wishes about future health care, treatment, and personal care; the document is put into effect when the person is unable to make or express these wishes; living will

affective disorders A group of mental disorders involving feelings, emotions, and moods

afternoon care Routine care given in a facility after lunch and the evening meal

ageism Bias and discrimination against older adults

age-related macular degeneration (AMD; ARMD) The breakdown (degeneration) of the macula (the light-sensitive part of the retina)

allergy Sensitivity to a substance that causes the body to react with signs and symptoms

alopecia Hair loss

alternative remedies Herbal or other "natural" products that do not require a physician's prescription; not considered part of conventional medicine

Alzheimer's disease (AD) A disease that gradually destroys nerve cells (neurons) in most areas of the brain; is the most common form of dementia

AM care Routine care given in a facility before breakfast; early morning care

ambulation The act of walking

amputation The removal of all or part of an extremity

amyotrophic lateral sclerosis (ALS) A neurological disorder that results in loss of all muscle control but does not affect intelligence; Lou Gehrig's disease

anal incontinence Fecal incontinence

anaphylaxis A life-threatening sensitivity to an antigen

anesthesia The loss of feeling or sensation produced by a medication

angina pectoris Chest (*pectoris*) pain (*angina*) due to coronary artery disease

anterior Located at or toward the front of the body or body part; ventral

anticipatory grief The sense of loss and sorrow experienced before an expected loss happens

anxiety A vague, uneasy feeling, including a sense of impending danger or harm

anxiety disorders A group of mental disorders in which anxiety is the main symptom

aphasia Partial or complete loss (*a*) of speech and language skills (*phasia*), caused by brain injury

apical-radial pulse Taking the apical and radial pulses at the same time

apnea The lack or absence (*a*) of breathing (*pnea*)

apraxia of speech Inability (*a*) to move (*praxia*) the muscles used to speak, caused by brain injury

arrhythmia Abnormal (*a*) heart rhythm (*rhythmia*)

arterial ulcer An open wound on the lower legs and feet caused by poor arterial blood flow

artery A blood vessel that carries blood away from the heart

arthritis Joint (*arthr*) inflammation (*itis*)

arthroplasty Surgical replacement (*plasty*) of a joint (*arthro*)

asepsis The state of being free of pathogens; clean

aseptic technique Medical asepsis

aspiration Inhaling fluid or an object into the lungs

assault Intentionally attempting or threatening to touch a person's body without the person's consent

assertiveness A style of communication in which thoughts and feelings are expressed positively and directly without offending others

assessment Collecting information about the client; a step in the care planning process

assigning Giving responsibility for providing care

assisted-living facility A residential facility where residents live in their own apartments and are provided support services; supportive housing facility

assistive personnel A broad term applied to staff who assist nurses and other health care professionals in giving care

asthma Respiratory disease characterized by narrowed air passages; episodes of difficulty breathing (asthma attacks) occur

atrophy A decrease in size or a wasting away of tissue

authority The legal right to do something

autism A brain disorder that impairs communication, social skills, and behaviour

autonomy Having free choice involving decisions that affect one's life; self-determination

base of support The area on which an object rests

battery The touching of a person's body without the person's consent

bedsore Pressure ulcer, pressure sore, or decubitus ulcer

beneficence Doing or promoting good

benign Noncancerous

biohazardous waste Items that may be harmful to others because they are contaminated with blood, body fluids, secretions, or excretions; bio means life and hazardous means dangerous or harmful

Biot's respirations Rapid and deep respirations followed by 10 to 30 seconds of apnea

bipolar disorder An affective disorder in which the person experiences extremes in mood, energy, and ability to function

blood pressure The amount of force exerted by the blood against the walls of an artery

body alignment The way in which body parts (head, trunk, arms, and legs) are positioned in relation to one another; posture

body language Posture, appearance, facial expressions, body movements, eye contact, and gestures that send messages to others

body mechanics The movement of the body in an efficient and careful way

body temperature The amount of heat in the body that is a balance between the amount of heat produced and the amount lost by the body

brace An apparatus worn to support or align weak body parts or to prevent and correct problems with the muscoskeletal system; othosis

bradycardia A slow (*brady*) heart rate (*cardia*); the rate is less than 60 beats per minute

bradypnea Slow (*brady*) breathing (*pnea*); respirations are fewer then 10 per minute

Braille A writing system for the blind that uses raised dots for each letter of the alphabet

bruise Contusion

burnout A state of physical, emotional, and mental exhaustion

call bell A safety device for hospital patients and long-term care residents that enables them to call for assistance

calorie The amount of energy produced as the body burns food

Canada Health Act (1984) Federal legislation that clarifies the types of health care services that are insured; it also outlines five principles that must be met for provinces and territories to qualify for federal health money

cancer A group of diseases characterized by out of control cell division and growth

capillary A tiny blood vessel; food, oxygen, and other substances pass from the capillaries to the cells

cardiac arrest The heart and breathing stop suddenly and without warning

cardiopulmonary resuscitation (CPR) Emergency procedure used to restore breathing and circulation after cardiac arrest

care plan A document that details the care and services the client should receive

care planning process The method used by nurses and case managers to plan and deliver care

case manager A health care professional who assesses, monitors, and evaluates a client's needs in a community care setting; also coordinates team services

cataract A clouding of the eye's lens

catheter A tube used to drain or inject fluid through a body opening

catheterization The process of inserting a catheter

cell The basic functional unit of body structure

cerebral palsy (CP) A disorder affecting muscle control (*palsy*); is caused by an injury or abnormality in the motor region of the brain (*cerebral*)

cerebral vascular accident (CVA) Stroke

cesarean section A surgical incision into the abdominal and uterine walls; the baby is delivered through the incision

chart Document that details a person's condition or illness and responses to care; record

charting Recording

chemical restraints Medications used to control behaviour or movement; they are not otherwise required for a person's medical condition

Cheyne-Stokes Respirations gradually increasing in rate and depth and then becoming shallow and slow; breathing may stop (*apnea*) for 10 to 20 seconds

chronic illness An on-going illness, slow or gradual in onset, that usually grows worse over time and cannot be cured

chronic obstructive pulmonary disease (COPD) A chronic lung disorder that obstructs (blocks) the airways; refers to chronic bronchitis and emphysema

chronic pain Pain that lasts longer than 6 months; it may be constant or occur off and on

chronic wound A wound that does not heal easily

chronological résumé A résumé that highlights employment history, starting with the most current employment and working in reverse chronological order (backward) through earlier jobs

circulatory ulcer An open wound on the lower legs and feet caused by decreased blood flow through arteries or veins; vascular ulcer

circumcision The surgical removal of foreskin from the penis

civil law Laws that deal with the relationships between people

clean technique Medical asepsis

clean wound A wound that is not infected; microbes have not entered the wound

clean-contaminated wound A wound occurring from the surgical entry of the urinary, reproductive, or digestive system

client A person receiving care or support services in a community setting; a general term for all people receiving health care or support services: hospital patients, facility residents, and clients in the community

clinical depression Major depression

closed questions Questions that focus on specific information

closed wound A wound in which tissues are injured but the skin is not broken

cognitive disability Intellectual disability

colostomy An artificial opening (*stomy*) between the colon (*colo*) and abdominal wall

combining vowel A vowel added between two roots or a root and a suffix to make pronunciation easier

communicable disease A disease caused by microbes that spread easily

community day program A daytime community-based program for people with physical and/or mental health problems or older adults who need assistance; adult daycare

community-based services The health care and support services provided outside of a facility setting and in a community setting

compassion Caring about another person's misfortune and suffering

competence Performing your job well

compress A soft pad that is moistened and applied over a body area

condom catheter A sheath that slides over the penis; tubing connects the catheter and drainage bag

confidentiality Respecting and guarding personal and private information about another person

conflict A clash between opposing interests and ideas

confusion A mental state where the person is disoriented to person, time, or place; memory and judgment are usually also impaired

congenital Present at birth

congestive heart failure (CHF) Condition occurring when the heart cannot pump blood normally; causes a build-up (congestion) of fluid in the tissues

consent Agreeing to medical treatment, health care, or personal care services

constipation A condition in which bowel movements are less frequent than usual; the stool is hard, dry, and difficult to pass

constrict To narrow

contagious disease Communicable disease

contaminated wound A wound with high risk of infection

contamination The process of being exposed to pathogens

contracture The lack of joint mobility caused by abnormal shortening of a muscle

contusion A closed wound caused by a blow to the body; bruise

convalescent care Subacute care

convulsion Violent and sudden contractions or tremors of muscles

coronary artery disease (CAD) A condition in which the coronary arteries are narrowed or blocked

cover letter Letter of application

crime A violation of a criminal law

criminal law Laws concerned with offences against the public and against society in general

cross-contamination The spread of pathogens from one source to another

culture The characteristics of a group of people—the language, values, beliefs, habits, ways of life, rules of behaviour, and traditions—that are passed from one person to the next and from one generation to the next

cyanosis Bluish skin colour

Daily Value (DV) How a serving fits into the daily diet; expressed as a percentage based on recommended daily intake

dandruff Excessive amount of dry, white flakes on the scalp

deconditioning The loss of muscle strength from inactivity

decubitus ulcer Pressure ulcer, pressure sore, or bedsore

defamation Injuring the name and reputation of a person by making false statements to a third person

defecation The process of excreting feces from the rectum through the anus; a bowel movement

defence mechanism An unconscious reaction that blocks unpleasant or threatening feelings

dehiscence The separation of wound layers

dehydration The excessive loss of water from tissues

delegation A process by which an RN authorizes another health care provider to perform certain tasks; transfer of function

delirium A state of temporary mental confusion

delusion A false belief

dementia The progressive loss of cognitive and social functions; is a symptom of changes in the brain

dependence The state of relying on others for support; being unable to manage without help

development Changes in a person's psychological and social functioning

developmental disability A disability that occurs before birth, at birth, or during childhood or adolescence; it impairs the child's development

developmental task An activity that must be mastered during a stage of development

diabetes A disorder in which the body cannot produce or use insulin properly; causes sugar (glucose) to build up in the blood

diabetic retinopathy A disorder (*pathy*) caused by diabetes in which the blood vessels in the retina are damaged

diarrhea The frequent passage of liquid stools

diastole The period of heart muscle relaxation

diastolic pressure The pressure in the arteries when the heart is at rest

digestion The process of physically and chemically breaking down food so that it can be absorbed for use by the cells

dignity The state of feeling worthy, valued, and respected

dilate To expand or open wider

diplegia Loss of ability to move (*plegia*) corresponding parts on both (*di*) sides of the body; both arms or both legs are affected

dirty wound An infected wound

disability The loss of physical or mental function

discharge Official departure of a client from a hospital or other health care facility

discretion Good judgment

discrimination Behaviour that treats people unfairly based on their group membership

disease prevention Strategies that prevent the occurrence of disease or injury

disinfection The process of destroying pathogens

distal The part farthest from the centre or from the point of attachment

diverticulosis The condition (*osis*) of having small pouches in the colon that bulge outward (*diverticulum*)

dominant progressive hearing loss The impairment of nerves used to hear

dorsal Located at or toward the back of the body or body part; posterior

dorsal recumbent position Supine position

dorsiflexion Bending the toes and foot up at the ankle

Down syndrome (DS) A congenital disorder caused by an extra chromosome; results in varying degrees of intellectual disability

drawsheet A small sheet placed over the middle of the bottom sheet; it helps keep the mattress and bottom linens clean and dry; can be used to turn and move the client in bed; the cotton drawsheet

dysarthria Difficulty (*dys*) speaking clearly (*arthria*), caused by weakness or paralysis in the muscles used for speech

dysphagia Difficulty (*dys*) swallowing (*phagia*)

dyspnea Difficult, laboured, or painful (*dys*) breathing (*pnea*)

dysrhythmia An irregular rhythm of the pulse; beats may be unevenly spaced or skipped

dysuria Painful or difficult (*dys*) urination (*uria*)

early morning care AM care

eating disorders A group of mental disorders involving disturbances in eating behaviours and an abnormal concern with body weight and shape

edema Swelling caused by fluid collecting in tissues

ejaculation The release of semen

elective surgery Surgery that is scheduled but non-urgent; delaying the surgery does not result in permanent damage, disability, or death

embolus A blood clot (thrombus) that travels through the vascular system until it lodges in a distant blood vessel

emergency surgery Surgery that must be done immediately to save a person's life or prevent disability

emotional abuse Words or actions that inflict mental harm; psychological abuse

emotional health Well-being in the emotional dimension achieved when people feel good about themselves

emotional illness Mental illness

empathetic listening Being attentive to a person's feelings

empathy Being open to and trying to understand the experiences and feelings of others

enema The introduction of fluid into the rectum and lower colon

enteral nutrition Giving nutrients through the gastrointestinal tract (*enteral*)

environmental restraints Barriers, furniture, or devices that prevent free movement

epilepsy A condition characterized by recurrent seizures

episiotomy An incision made into the perineum to increase the size of the vaginal opening for the delivery of the baby

ethics The moral principles or values that guide us when deciding what is right and what is wrong, what is good and what is bad

ethnicity Refers to groups of people who share a common history, language, geography, national origin, religion, and identity

evaluation Assessing and measuring; a step in the care planning process

evening care HS care or PM care

evisceration The separation of the wound along with the protrusion of abdominal organs

expressive aphasia Difficulty speaking or writing

expressive-receptive aphasia Difficulty speaking and understanding language

extension Straightening a body part

external rotation Turning the joint outward

fainting The sudden loss of consciousness from an inadequate blood supply to the brain

false imprisonment Unlawful restraint or restrictions of a person's freedom of movement

family A biological, legal, or social network of people who provide support for one another

family conference A meeting attended by the health care team and family members to discuss a client's care

fecal impaction The prolonged retention and accumulation of feces in the rectum

fecal incontinence The inability to control the passage of feces and gas through the anus; anal incontinence

feces The semisolid mass of waste products in the colon

fetal alcohol effect (FAE) A milder form of FAS; the same symptoms may occur but to a lesser degree

fetal alcohol syndrome (FAS) A group of physical and mental abnormalities in a child as a result of alcohol consumption by the mother during pregnancy

fibromyaliga A condition associated with aching, stiffness, and fatigue in muscles, ligaments, and tendons

financial abuse The misuse of a person's money or property

first aid Emergency care given to an ill or injured person before medical help arrives

flatulence The excessive formation of gas in the stomach and intestines

flatus Gas or air from the stomach or intestines passed through the anus

flexion Bending a body part

flow rate The number of drops per minute (gtt/min)

focusing Limiting the conversation to a certain topic

Foley catheter A retention or indwelling catheter

foodborne illness An illness caused by improperly cooked or stored food

footdrop The foot falls down at the ankle (permanent plantar flexion)

foreign body airway obstruction (FBAO) The blockage of the airway by an object, causing the person to choke

Fowler's position A semi-sitting position in bed; the head of the bed is elevated 45 to 60 degrees or the person is propped up with a backrest or pillows

fracture A broken bone

friction The rubbing of one surface against another

full-thickness wound A wound in which the dermis, epidermis, and subcutaneous tissue are penetrated; muscle and bone may be involved

functional incontinence The loss of urine that occurs when the person has bladder control but cannot use the toilet in time

functional résumé A résumé that highlights skills or functions and briefly lists positions held

gait belt A transfer belt used when helping a client to walk

gangrene A condition in which there is tissue death

gastrostomy tube A tube inserted through an opening (*stomy*) into the stomach (*gastro*)

gavage Tube feeding

general anesthesia Unconsciousness and the loss of feeling or sensation produced by a medication

geriatrics The branch of medicine that provides care for older adults

gerontology The study of the aging process

glaucoma An eye disease that causes pressure within the eye and vision loss

glucosuria Sugar (*glucos*) in the urine (*uria*); glycosuria

glycosuria Glucosuria

grief The process of moving from deep sorrow caused by loss toward healing and recovery

group home A residential facility in which a small number of people with physical and/or mental disabilities live together and are provided with supervision and/or care and support services

growth The physical changes that can be measured and that occur in a steady, orderly manner

hallucination Seeing, hearing, or feeling something that is not real

harassment Troubling, tormenting, offending, or worrying a person by one's behaviour or comments

hazardous material Any substance that presents a physical hazard or a health hazard in the workplace

health The state of well-being in all dimensions of one's life

health care ethics The philosophical study of what is morally right and wrong when providing health care services

health promotion Strategies that improve or maintain health and independence

heart attack Myocardial infarction

hematoma The collection of blood under the skin and tissues

hematuria Blood (*hemat*) in the urine (*uria*)

hemiplegia Paralysis (*plegia*) of one side (*hemi*) of the body; the right arm and leg or left arm and leg could be affected

hemoglobin The substance in red blood cells that carries oxygen and gives blood its colour

hemoptysis Bloody (*hemo*) sputum (*ptysis*, meaning "to spit")

hemorrhage The excessive loss of blood in a short period of time

hepatitis Inflammation (*itis*) of the liver (*hepat*) caused by a viral infection

hirsutism Excessive body hair in women and children

holism A concept that considers the whole person; the whole person has physical, social, emotional, intellectual, and spiritual dimensions

home care Health care and support services provided to people in their places of residence

home management The cleaning and organizing of a home

horizontal position Supine position

hormone A chemical substance secreted by specialized glands into the bloodstream

hospice A facility that provides care for people who are dying

HS care Routine care given in a facility in the evening at bedtime (HS means hour of sleep); evening care or PM care

Huntington's disease An inherited neurological disorder; causes uncontrolled movements, emotional disturbances, and cognitive losses

hyperextension Excessive straightening of a body part

hypertension Persistent blood pressure measurements above the normal systolic (140 mm Hg) or diastolic (90 mm Hg) pressures

hyperventilation Respirations that are rapid (*hyper*) and deeper than normal

hypotension A condition in which the systolic blood pressure is below 90 mm Hg and the diastolic pressure is below 60 mm Hg

hypoventilation Respirations that are slow (*hypo*), shallow, and sometimes irregular

hypoxemia A deficiency (*hypo*) of oxygen (*ox*) in the blood (*emia*)

hypoxia A deficiency (*hypo*) of oxygen in the cells (*oxia*)

ileostomy An artificial opening (*stomy*) between the ileum (small intestine; *ileo*) and the abdominal wall

illness The loss of physical or mental health

immunity Protection against a certain disease or infection; the person will not get or be affected by the disease

implementation Carrying out or performing; a step in the care planning process

incident report A report submitted whenever an accident, error, or unexpected problem arises in the workplace; occurrence report

incision An open wound with clean, straight edges; usually intentionally produced with a sharp instrument

independence The state of not depending on others for control or authority

indwelling catheter A catheter that is left in place in the bladder so urine drains constantly into a drainage bag; Foley or retention catheter

infected wound A wound containing large amounts of bacteria and showing signs of infection; a dirty wound

infection A disease state resulting from the invasion and growth of microbes in the body

infection control Policies and procedures used to prevent the spread of infection within health care settings

influenza Respiratory tract infection; the "flu"

informed consent Consent based on accurate and complete information

inpatient A patient who is assigned a bed and is admitted to stay in a facility overnight or longer

insomnia A chronic condition in which the person cannot go to sleep or stay asleep throughout the night

intake The amount of fluids taken in by the body

intellectual disability Impaired ability to learn; cognitive disability

intellectual health Well-being in the intellectual dimension achieved through an active, creative mind

intentional wound A wound created for therapy

interdependence The state of depending on one another

internal rotation Turning the joint inward

interpersonal communication The exchange of information between two people, usually face to face

intervention An action or measure taken by the health care team to help the client meet a goal in the care plan

intravenous (IV) therapy Fluids given through a needle or catheter inserted into a vein; IV, IV therapy, and IV infusion

intubation The process of inserting an artificial airway

invasion of privacy Violating a person's right not to have his or her name, photograph, private affairs, health information, or any personal information exposed or made public without consent

isolation precautions Guidelines for preventing the spread of pathogens; includes Standard Precautions and Transmission-Based Precautions

jejunostomy tube A tube inserted into the intestines through an opening (*stomy*) into the middle part of the small intestine (*jejunum*)

justice Treating people in a fair and equal manner

ketone body Acetone

knee-chest position An examination position in which the person kneels and rests the body on the knees and chest; the head is turned to one side, the arms are above the head or flexed at the elbows, the back is straight, and the body is flexed about 90 degrees at the hips

Kussmaul's respirations Very deep and rapid respirations; a sign of diabetic coma

laceration An open wound with torn tissues and jagged edges

lactation The process of producing and secreting milk from the breast

laryngeal mirror An instrument used to examine the mouth, teeth, and throat

lateral Relating to or located at the side of the body or body part

lateral position A side-lying position

laundry symbols Symbols on garment tags that indicate care for that garment

legislation A body of laws that govern the behaviour of a country's residents

letter of application A letter that is included with a résumé; can be solicited or unsolicited; cover letter

liable Legally responsible

libel Making false statements in print, writing, or through pictures or drawings

licensed practical nurse (LPN) Registered practical nurse

lithotomy position A back-lying position in which the hips are brought down to the edge of the examination table, the knees are flexed, the hips are externally rotated, and the feet are supported in stirrups

living will Advance directive

local anesthesia The loss of sensation in a small area, produced by a medication injected at the specific site

lochia Postpartum vaginal discharge

logrolling Turning the person as a unit, in alignment, with one motion

long-term care Medical, nursing, and/or support services provided over the course of months or years to people who cannot care for themselves

long-term care facility A facility that provides accommodations, 24-hour nursing care, and support services to people who cannot care for themselves at home but do not need hospital care

major depression An affective disorder involving intense and prolonged feelings of sadness, hopelessness, and worthlessness; clinical depression

malignant Cancerous

mastitis An infection of the breast

mechanical ventilation The use of a machine to move air into and out of the lungs

medial Relating to or located at or near the middle or midline of the body or body part

medical asepsis Practices that reduce the number of microbes and prevent their spread; clean technique or aseptic technique

medical diagnosis The identification of a disease or condition by a physician

medicare Canada's national health care insurance system; publicly funds all the cost of medically necessary health services

medication A drug or other substance used to prevent or treat disease or illness

melena A black, tarry stool

menarche The time when menstruation first begins

Ménière's disease An increase of fluid in the inner ear causing pressure in the middle ear; vertigo, tinnitus, and hearing loss occur

menopause The time when menstruation stops

menstruation The process in which the lining of the uterus breaks up and is discharged from the body through the vagina

mental health A state of mind in which a person copes with and adjusts to the stresses of everyday living in socially acceptable ways

mental health disorder Mental illness

mental health services Services for people with mental disorders or emotional and behavioural problems

mental illness A disturbance in a person's ability to cope with or adjust to stress; thinking, mood, or behaviours are affected and functioning is impaired; emotional illness; mental health disorder; psychiatric disorder

metabolism The burning of food for heat and energy by the cells

metastasis The spread of cancer to other parts of the body

microbe Microorganism

microorganism A form of life (*organism*) that is so small (*micro*) it can be seen only with a microscope; a microbe

micturition Urination

middle-old People between 75 and 84 years of age

morning care Routine care given in a facility after breakfast; hygiene measures are more thorough at this time

multidisciplinary team A team of health care providers from a variety of backgrounds and specialties who work together to meet the client's needs

multiple sclerosis (MS) Progressive neurological disease in which nerve impulses are not sent to and from the brain in a normal manner

multi-resistant organism (MRO) A strain of bacteria that is very difficult to treat with common antibiotics; examples are MRSA and VRE

myocardial infarction (MI) Death (infarction) of heart tissue (*myocardium*) caused by lack of oxygen to the heart; heart attack

nasal speculum An instrument used to examine the inside of the nose

nasogastric (NG) tube A tube inserted through the nose (*naso*) into the stomach (*gastro*)

nasointestinal tube A tube inserted through the nose (*naso*) into the small intestine (*intestinal*)

need That which is necessary or desirable for maintaining life and psychosocial well-being

neglect The failure to meet the basic needs (physical or emotional) of a dependent person

negligence Failing to act in a careful or competent manner and thereby harming a person or damaging property

nocturia Frequent urination (*uria*) at night (*noct*)

nonmaleficence Seeking to do no harm

nonpathogen A microbe that does not usually cause infection

nonverbal communication Messages sent without words

nosocomial infection An infection acquired after admission to a health care facility

nursing diagnosis A statement describing a health problem that is treated by nursing measures

nutrient A substance that is ingested, digested, absorbed, and used by the body

nutrition The many processes involved in the ingestion, digestion, absorption, and use of foods and fluids by the body

objective data Information that is observed; signs

observation The act of noticing a truth or fact

occurrence report Incident report

OH&S (occupational health and safety) legislation Laws designed to protect employees from injuries and accidents in the workplace; these laws outline the rights and responsibilities of employers, supervisors, and workers

old-old People older than 85 years

oliguria Scant amount (*olig*) of urine (*uria*); usually less than 500 mL in 24 hours

open wound A wound in which the skin or mucous membrane is broken

open-ended questions Questions that invite a person to share thoughts, feelings, or ideas

ophthalmoscope A lighted instrument used to examine the internal structures of the eye

oral hygiene Measures performed to keep the mouth and teeth clean; mouth care

organ Groups of tissues that work together to perform special functions

orthopnea Breathing (*pnea*) deeply and comfortably only while sitting or standing (*ortho*)

orthopneic position Sitting up (*ortho*) and leaning over a table to breathe

orthosis Apparatus worn to support, align, prevent, or correct problems with the musculoskeletal system

orthostatic hypotension A drop in (*hypo*) blood pressure when the person stands (*ortho* and *static*); postural hypotension

osteoporosis A bone disorder (*osteo*) in which the bone becomes porous and brittle (*poros*)

ostomy The surgical creation of an artificial opening

otitis media Infection (*itis*) of the middle (*media*) ear (*ot*)

otosclerosis A condition (*osis*) in which there is hardening (*sclero*) of the ossicles in the middle ear (*oto*)

otoscope A lighted instrument used to examine the external ear and the eardrum (tympanic membrane)

outpatient A patient who does not stay overnight in a facility

output The amount of fluid lost by the body

overflow incontinence The leaking of urine when the bladder is too full

over-the-counter (OTC) medication A medication that can be bought without a physician's prescription

oxygen concentration The amount of hemoglobin that contains oxygen (O_2)

pack A treatment that involves wrapping a body part with a wet or dry application

palliative care Services for people (and their families) living with or dying from a progressive and life-threatening illness; these services aim to relieve suffering and improve comfort, not cure the illness

paralysis Complete or partial loss of ability to move a limb or muscle group

paranoia Extreme suspicion about a person or a situation

paraphrasing Restating someone's message in your own words

paraplegia Paralysis (*plegia*) from the waist down

Parkinson's disease Neurological disorder in which cells in certain parts of the brain are gradually destroyed; causes tremors, muscle stiffness, slow movement, and poor balance

partial-thickness wound A wound in which the dermis and epidermis of the skin are broken

pathogen A microbe that can cause an infection

patient A person receiving care in a hospital setting

pediculosis (lice) Infestation with lice

pediculosis capitis Infestation of the scalp (*capitis*) with lice

pediculosis corporis Infestation of the body (*corporis*) with lice

pediculosis pubis Infestation of the pubic (*pubis*) hair with lice

penetrating wound An open wound in which the skin and underlying tissues are pierced

percussion hammer An instrument used to tap body parts to test reflexes; reflex hammer

percutaneous endoscopic gastrostomy (PEG) tube A tube inserted into the stomach (*gastro*) through a stab or puncture wound (*stomy*) made through (*per*) the skin (*cutaneous*); a lighted instrument (*scope*) allows the physician to see inside the body cavity or organ (*endo*)

pericare Perineal care

perineal care Cleansing the genital and anal areas

peristalsis Involuntary muscle contractions in the digestive system that move food through the alimentary canal

personal protective equipment (PPE) Special clothing and equipment that act as a barrier between microbes and your hands, eyes, nose, mouth, and clothes; includes gloves, gowns, masks, and eye protection

personal space The area immediately around one's body

personality disorder A group of disorders involving rigid and socially unacceptable behaviours

phantom pain Pain felt in a body part that is no longer there

physical abuse Force or violence that causes pain, injury, and sometimes death

physical health Well-being in the physical dimension achieved when the body is strong, fit, and free of disease

physical restraints Garments or devices used to restrict movement of the whole body or parts of the body

planning Establishing priorities and goals and developing measures or actions to help the client meet the goals; a step in the care planning process

plantar flexion The foot (*plantar*) is bent (*flexion*)

plaque A thin film that sticks to the teeth; it contains saliva, microbes, and other substances

plastic drawsheet A drawsheet placed between the bottom sheet and the cotton drawsheet to keep the mattress and bottom linens clean and dry

PM care HS care or evening care

pneumonia Infection of the lung tissue

podiatrist A professional who provides foot care

polyuria The production of abnormally large amounts (*poly*) of urine (*uria*)

posterior Dorsal

postmortem care Care of the body after (*post*) death (*mortem*)

postoperative After surgery

postpartum After (*post*) childbirth (*partum*)

postpartum blues Feelings of sadness or mild depression during the first 2 weeks after childbirth; baby blues

postpartum depression Major depression at any point during the first year after childbirth

postpartum psychosis The most severe form of postpartum depression; the mother may experience delusions, hallucinations, and suicidal thoughts

postural hypotension Orthostatic hypotension

posture Body alignment

prefix A word element placed at the beginning of a word to change the meaning of the word

prejudice An attitude that judges a person based on his or her membership in a group

preoperative Before surgery

presbycusis The gradual hearing (*cusis*) loss associated with aging (*presby*)

presbyopia The gradual inability to focus (*opia*) on close objects; a condition associated with aging (*presby*)

prescription (Rx) medication A medication that is prescribed by a physician and dispensed by a pharmacist

pressure sore Bedsore, decubitus ulcer, or pressure ulcer

pressure ulcer Any injury caused by unrelieved pressure; a decubitus ulcer, bedsore, or pressure sore

primary caregiver A person—usually a family member or close friend—who assumes the responsibilities of caring for an ill or disabled person in the home

professionalism An approach to work that demonstrates respect for others, commitment, competence, and appropriate behaviour

prognosis The expected course of recovery based on the usual outcome of the illness

pronation Turning downward

prone position A front-lying position on the abdomen, with the head turned to one side

prosthesis An artificial replacement for a missing body part

proximal The part nearest to the centre or to the point of origin

psychiatric disorder Mental illness

psychological abuse Emotional abuse

psychosis A mental state in which perception of reality is impaired

psychosocial health Well-being in the social, emotional, intellectual, and spiritual dimensions of one's life

psychotherapy A form of therapy in which a person explores his or her thoughts, feelings, and behaviours with a mental health specialist

puberty The period when the reproductive organs begin to function and secondary sex characteristics appear

pulse The beat of the heart felt at an artery as a wave of blood passes through the artery

pulse deficit The difference between the apical and radial pulse rates

pulse oximeter A device that measures (*meter*) oxygen (*oxi*) concentration in the arterial blood; consists of a computerized monitor and a sensor (*probe*)

pulse rate The number of heartbeats or pulses felt in 1 minute

puncture wound An open wound made by a sharp object; entry of the skin and underlying tissues may be intentional or unintentional

quadriplegia Paralysis (*plegia*) of all four (*quad*) limbs and the trunk; paralysis from the neck down

race Refers to groups of people who share similar features, such as skin colour, hair colour and texture, facial characteristics, and bone structure

radiating pain Pain felt at the site of tissue damage and in nearby areas

range of motion (ROM) The movement of a joint to the extent possible without causing pain

receptive aphasia Difficulty understanding language

record Chart

recording The process of documenting care provided and observations made; charting

reference A person who can speak to a potential employer about your skills, abilities, and personal qualities

reflex An involuntary movement in response to a stimulus

reflex hammer Percussion hammer

reflex incontinence The loss of urine at predictable intervals

regional anesthesia The loss of sensation or feeling in a large area of the body, produced by the injection of a medication; the person does not lose consciousness

registered nurse (RN) A health care professional licensed and regulated by the province or territory to maintain overall responsibility for the planning and provision of client care

registered practical nurse (RPN) A health care professional licensed and regulated by the province or territory to carry out basic nursing techniques and client care; licensed practical nurse

regulation Detailed rules that implement the requirements of a legislative act

regurgitation The backward flow of food from the stomach into the mouth

rehabilitation The process of restoring a person to the highest level of functioning possible through the use of therapy, exercise, or other methods

rehabilitation services Therapies and educational programs designed to restore or improve the person's independence and functional abilities

relationship The connection between two or more people, shaped by the roles, feelings, and interactions of those involved

renal calculi Kidney (*renal*) stones (*calculi*)

reservoir The environment in which microbes live and grow; host

resident A person living in a residential facility

residential facility A facility that provides living accommodations and services; includes assisted-living facilities and retirement residences

respect Showing acceptance and regard for another person

respiration The act of breathing air into (inhalation) and out of (exhalation) the lungs

respiratory arrest Breathing stops

respiratory depression Slow, weak respirations at a rate of fewer than 12 per minute; respirations are not deep enough to bring enough air into the lungs

respite care Temporary care of a person with a serious illness or disability that gives the person's caregivers a break from their duties

restorative care Care that helps a person regain health, strength, and independence

restraint Any device, garment, barrier, furniture, or medication that limits or restricts freedom of movement or access to one's body

résumé A concise one- to two-page summary of experience, education, work-related skills, and personal qualities

retention catheter A Foley or indwelling catheter

retinal detachment The separation of the retina from its supporting tissue

retirement residence A facility that provides accommodation and supervision for older adults

reverse Trendelenburg's position The opposite of Trendelenburg's position; the head of the bed is raised and the foot of the bed is lowered

right Something to which a person is justly entitled

rigor mortis The stiffness or rigidity (*rigor*) of skeletal muscles that occurs after death (*mortis*)

root A word element containing the basic meaning of the word

rotation Turning the joint

Routine Practices Standard Precautions

schizophrenia A mental health disorder in which thinking and behaviour are disturbed

scope of practice The legal limits of your role

seizure Brief disturbance in the brain's normal electrical function; affects awareness, movement, and/or sensation

self-actualization Experiencing one's potential

self-awareness Understanding one's own feelings, moods, attitudes, preferences, biases, and limitations

self-determination Autonomy

self-esteem Thinking well of yourself and being well thought of by others

semi-Fowler's position The head of the bed is raised 45 degrees and the knee portion is raised 15 degrees; or the head of the bed is raised 30 degrees and the knee position is not raised

sexual abuse Unwanted sexual activity

sexual harassment Any conduct, comment, gesture, threat, or suggestion that is sexual in nature; a form of sexual abuse

sexually transmitted disease (STD) A disease that is spread by sexual contact

sharp Equipment or item that may pierce the skin; includes needles, razor blades, and broken glass

shearing The process in which skin sticks to a surface and muscles slide in the direction the body is moving

shock A condition that results when organs and tissues do not get enough blood

side effect An unwanted response to a medication that occurs with the intended response

signs Objective data

Sims' position A left side-lying position; the right leg is sharply flexed so it is not on the left leg, and the left arm is positioned along the person's back.

skin tear A break or rip in the skin; the epidermis separates from the underlying tissue

slander Making false statements orally

social health Well-being in the social dimension achieved when people have stable and satisfying relationships

social support system An informal group of people who help each other or others

solicited letter of application A letter of application that responds to an advertised position

spastic Uncontrolled contractions of skeletal muscles

sphygmomanometer The instrument used to measure blood pressure

spina bifida A congenital disorder involving improper closing of the spine before birth; spina means backbone and bifida means split in two parts

spiritual health Well-being in the spiritual dimension achieved through the belief in a purpose greater than the self

sputum Mucus from the respiratory system that is expectorated (expelled) through the mouth

Standard Precautions Guidelines to prevent the spread of infection from blood, body fluids, secretions, excretions, nonintact skin, and mucous membranes; Routine Practices

stasis ulcer An open wound on the lower legs and feet caused by poor blood return through the veins; venous ulcer

stereotype An overly simple or exaggerated view of a group of people

sterile Free of all microbes—pathogens and nonpathogens

sterile field A work area free of all microbes—pathogens and nonpathogens

sterile technique Surgical asepsis

sterilization The process of destroying all microbes

stethoscope An instrument used to listen to the sounds produced by the heart, lungs, and other body organs

stigma A characteristic that marks a person as different or flawed

stoma An artificial opening

stool Excreted feces

straight catheter A catheter that drains the bladder and is removed

stress The emotional, behavioural, or physical response to an event or situation

stress incontinence The leaking of urine during exercise and certain movements

stressor An event or situation that causes stress

stroke Sudden loss of brain function; cerebral vascular accident (CVA)

subacute care Care provided to people who are recovering from surgery, injury, or serious illness; convalescent care

subjective data Information reported by a client that cannot be directly observed by others; symptoms

substitute decision maker A person authorized to give or withhold consent on an incapable person's behalf

suction The process of withdrawing or sucking up fluid (secretions)

sudden infant death syndrome (SIDS) The sudden, unexplained death of an apparently healthy infant under 1 year of age

suffix A word element placed at the end of a root to change the meaning of the word

suffocation Occurs when breathing stops due to lack of oxygen

sundowning When signs, symptoms, and behaviours of dementia increase during hours of darkness

supination Turning upward

supine position A back-lying position; the legs are together; dorsal recumbent position; horizontal position

support worker A worker who provides personal care and support services

supportive housing facility Assisted-living facility

suppository A cone-shaped, solid medication that is inserted into a body opening; it melts at body temperature

suprapubic catheter A catheter that is surgically inserted into the bladder through the abdomen

surgical asepsis Practices that keep equipment and supplies free of all microbes; sterile technique

symptoms Subjective data

syncope A brief loss of consciousness; fainting

system Organs that work together to perform special functions

systole The period of heart muscle contraction

systolic pressure The amount of force it takes to pump blood out of the heart and into the arterial circulation

tachycardia A rapid (*tachy*) heart rate (*cardia*); the heart rate is over 100 beats per minute

tachypnea Rapid (*tachy*) breathing (*pnea*); respirations are 24 or more per minute

tartar Hardened plaque on teeth

task A function, procedure, or activity that you assist with or perform for the client

thrombus A blood clot

tinnitus Ringing in the ear

tissue A group of cells with similar functions

tonic-clonic seizure A type of generalized seizure where the person has convulsions

tort A wrongful act committed by an individual against another person or the person's property

tracheostomy A surgically created opening (*ostomy*) through the neck into the trachea (*tracheo*)

transfer Moving a client from one room or unit to another

transfer belt A belt used to hold onto a person during a transfer or when walking with the person

transfer of function Delegation

Transmission-Based Precautions Guidelines to contain pathogens within a certain area, usually the client's room

trauma An accident or violent act that injures the skin, mucous membranes, bones, or internal organs

Trendelenburg's position The head of the bed is lowered and the foot of the bed is raised

tuberculosis (TB) A bacterial infection, usually affecting the lungs

tumour An abnormal lump or mass caused by cells growing out of control; tumours are benign or malignant

tuning fork An instrument used to test hearing

umbilical cord The structure that carries blood, oxygen, and nutrients from the mother to the fetus

unintentional wound A wound resulting from trauma

unsolicited letter of application A letter of application that enquires about potential openings

ureterostomy An artificial opening (*stomy*) between the ureter (*uretero*) and the abdomen

urge incontinence The loss of urine in response to a sudden, urgent need to void

urgent surgery Surgery that must be done soon to prevent further damage, disability, or disease

urinary frequency Voiding at frequent intervals

urinary incontinence The loss of bladder control

urinary urgency The inability to control the loss of urine from the bladder; the need to void immediately

urination The process of emptying urine from the bladder; micturition or voiding

vaginal speculum An instrument used to open the vagina so that it and the cervix can be examined

vascular ulcer Circulatory ulcer

vein A blood vessel that carries blood back to the heart

venous ulcer Stasis ulcer

ventral Anterior

verbal communication Messages sent through the spoken word

verbal report A spoken account of care provided and observations made

vertigo Dizziness

vital signs Temperature, pulse, respirations, and blood pressure

voiding Urination

wellness The achievement of the best health possible in all dimensions of one's life

word element A part of a word

Workplace Hazardous Materials Information System (WHMIS) A national system that provides safety information about hazardous materials; includes labelling, material safety data sheets (MSDSs), and employee education

workplace violence Any physical assault or threatening behaviour that occurs in a work setting

wound A break in the skin or mucous membrane

young-old People between 60 and 74 years of age

REFERENCES

Chapter 8

1. M.E. Douglas, and D.N. Douglas, *Manage Your Time, Your Work, Yourself*, updated ed. (New York: American Management Association, 1993), pp. 16–17.

Chapter 11

1. R.E. Davidhizar and J.N. Giger, *Canadian Transcultural Nursing: Assessment and Intervention* (St. Louis: Mosby, 1998), p. 29.
2. S. Sorrentino, *Mosby's Textbook for Nursing Assistants*, 5th ed. (St. Louis: Mosby, 1998), p. 98.
3. Ibid.
4. P.A. Potter, A. Perry, J.C. Ross-Kerr, and M.J. Wood, *Canadian Fundamentals of Nursing*, 2nd ed. (Toronto: Harcourt Canada, 2001), p. 119.
5. Davidhizar and Giger, *Canadian Transcultural Nursing*, p. 51.
6. Ibid., p. 31.
7. Ibid.
8. Ibid.
9. Ibid., p. 30
10. Sorrentino, *Mosby's Textbook for Nursing Assistants*, 5th ed., p. 101.
11. Ibid.
12. Ibid.
13. Potter, Perry, Ross-Kerr, and Wood, *Canadian Fundamentals of Nursing*, 2nd ed., p. 126.
14. Davidhizar and Giger, *Canadian Transcultural Nursing*, p. 28.
15. Sorrentino, *Mosby's Textbook for Nursing Assistants*, 5th ed., p. 102.
16. Davidhizar and Giger, *Canadian Transcultural Nursing*, p. 115.

Chapter 16

1. *For the Safety of Canadian Children and Youth: From Injury Data to Preventive Measures* (Ottawa: Health Canada, 1997), p. 14.
2. *Statistical Report on the Health of Canadians* (Ottawa: Health Canada, 1997), p. 243.
3. *For the Safety of Canadian Children and Youth*, p. 136.
4. "Falls in Nursing Homes: National Center for Injury Prevention and Control," CDC http://www.cdc.gov/ncipc/factsheets/nursing.htm. Accessed 2001.
5. *For the Safety of Canadian Children and Youth*, p. 158.
6. M. Lesperance, *Kids for Keeps: Preventing Injuries to Children* (Cochrone, AB: Kids for Keeps, 1995), p. 47.

Chapter 17

1. C. Cohen, R.R. Neufeld , J. Dunbar, and B. Breuer, "Old Problem, Different Approach: Alternatives to Physical Restraints before and after a Clinical Intervention Program," *Journal of Gerontological Nursing* (1996), 23–29.
2. Ontario Hospital Association, *Minimizing the Use of Restraints in Ontario Hospitals*, Report of the Restraints Task Force (Toronto: Ontario Hospital Association, 2001), p. 47.

Chapter 19

1. Statistics Canada, *Family Violence in Canada: A Statistical Profile* (2000), p. 11. http://www.statcan.ca:80/English/freepub/83-224-XIE/0000085-224-XIE.pdf
2. N. Trocme and D. Wolfe, *Child Maltreatment in Canada: Canadian Incidence Study of Reported Child Abuse and Neglect* (Ottawa: Health Canada, The National Clearinghouse on Family Violence, 2001), p. 29. http://www.hc-sc.gc.ca/hpb/lcdc/publicat/cissr-ecirc/pdf/cmic-e.pdf

3. Statistics Canada, *Family Violence in Canada: A Statistical Profile*, p. 11.

4. P.L. McDonald, J.P. Hornick, G.B. Robertson, and J.E. Wallace, *Elder Abuse and Neglect in Canada* (Toronto: Butterworths, 1991), p. 29.

Chapter 31

1. National Cancer Institute of Canada, *Canadian Cancer Statistics*, 2002.

2. Heart and Stroke Foundation of Canada website: http://www.heartandstroke.ca. Accessed February 2003.

3. Ontario Lung Association website: http://www.on.lung.ca/ola/aboutus.html. Accessed February 2003.

4. Heart and Stroke Foundation of Canada website: http://www.heartandstroke.ca. Accessed February 2003.

5. Multiple Sclerosis Society of Canada website: http://www.mssociety.ca/en/information/default.htm. Accessed February 2003.

6. ALS Society of Canada website: http://www.als.ca. Accessed February 2003.

7. Laboratory Centre for Disease Control website: http://www.hc-sc.gc.ca/hpb/lcdc/publicat/cdic/cdic173/cd173b_e.html. Accessed February 2003.

8. Arthritis Society website: http://www.arthritis.ca/types%20of%20arthritis/ra/default.asp?s=1. Accessed February 2003.

9. Canadian Diabetes Association website: http://www.diabetes.ca/Section_About/prevalence.asp. Accessed February 2003.

10. Ibid.

Chapter 33

1. Canadian Mental Health Association, "Mental Health and Mental Illness in Canada: Facts and Figures," http://www.cmha.ca/mhw2002/facts_fig.htm. Accessed January 27, 2003.

2. Health Canada, *A Report on Mental Illness in Canada*, cat. no. 0-662-32817-5 (2002), p. 49.

3. Ibid., p. 21.

Chapter 34

1. Alzheimer's Society of Canada website: http://www.alzheimer.ca/english/disease/stats-people.htm. Accessed April 7, 2003.

Chapter 36

1. "AMD Awareness: About Age-Related Macular Degeneration (AMD)," The Canadian National Institute for the Blind (CNIB), http://www.cnib.ca/amd/edu/amd_info.htm. Accessed April 30, 2003.

Chapter 37

1. Health Canada, *Family-Centred Maternity and Newborn Care: National Guidelines* (Ottawa: Minister of Public Works and Government Services 2000), p. 6.19.

2. Ibid., p. 6.20.

3. Ibid., p. 6.21.

4. Health Canada, "Routine Practices and Additional Precautions for Preventing the Transmission of Infection in Health Care," *Canadian Communicable Disease Report* (July 1999), p. 78.

Chapter 38

1. Health Canada, *Congenital Anomalies in Canada: A Perinatal Health Report* (2002), p. 2.

2. Geneva Centre for Autism website: http://www.autism.net. Accessed March 2003.

3. Health Canada website: http://www.hcsc.gc.ca/english/media/releases/2000/2000_75ebk1.htm. Accessed March 2003.

INDEX

C

F

I

J

K

L

M

N

O

Q

R

T

U